Length of Stay
by Operation
United States, 1997

LOS

Length of Stay

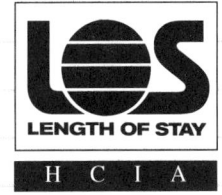
LENGTH OF STAY

HCIA

Statistics reported in the 1997 edition are drawn from individual patient discharge records for the time period October 1, 1995, through September 30, 1996. This volume is one of the books in the *Length of Stay by Diagnosis and Operation* series:

Length of Stay by Diagnosis and Operation, United States
ISSN 0895-9824

Length of Stay by Diagnosis and Operation, Northeastern Region
ISSN 0895-9838

Length of Stay by Diagnosis and Operation, North Central Region
ISSN 0895-9846

Length of Stay by Diagnosis and Operation, Southern Region
ISSN 0895-9854

Length of Stay by Diagnosis and Operation, Western Region
ISSN 0895-9862

Pediatric Length of Stay by Diagnosis and Operation, United States
ISSN 0891-1223

Geriatric Length of Stay by Diagnosis and Operation, United States
ISSN 0891-2173

HCIA Inc.
300 East Lombard Street
Baltimore, Maryland 21202
(800) 568-3282

Length of Stay by Diagnosis and Operation, United States, 1997

© 1997 by HCIA Inc.
All rights reserved. Published 1997
Printed and bound in the United States of America

HCIA Guarantee
Books may be returned for a full refund within 10 business days of receipt only if they are returned in good condition. Books damaged by the customer will not be accepted for return. Books damaged in shipping must be returned to HCIA within 5 business days for replacement. Should you need to return a book, please contact HCIA Customer Service at (800) 568-3282 for return authorization. Diskettes and magnetic tapes are not returnable.

Price: $295

ISSN 0895-9824
ISBN 1-57372-068-2

CONTENTS

INTRODUCTION

The *Length of Stay* Series

The *Length of Stay by Diagnosis and Operation* series incorporates length of stay and demographic data on patients treated in nonfederal, short-term, general hospitals in the United States during federal fiscal year 1996. This book is one volume in a set of seven books; the complete set is the latest in a series of publications on length of stay that is compiled from HCIA's all-payor projected inpatient database, which contains 12 million discharges and represents one-third of the all-payor universe.

The *Length of Stay by Diagnosis and Operation* series is designed to be user-friendly. The front section of each book includes information on practical application of the data, a description of the data source, and a step-by-step guide to using the tables. The LOS tables themselves include data organized by ICD-9-CM code for the most frequently occurring diagnoses and procedures—covering 90 percent of all inpatient admissions. All remaining codes are represented at the three-digit level (as diagnosis groups). The tables examine average, median, and percentile length of stay for patients in five age groups, with single and multiple diagnoses or procedures, and according to whether the patient's stay included an operation. The appendices include counts of U.S. hospitals by bed size, region, census division, setting (rural or urban), and teaching intensity; a list of the states included in each LOS comparative region; and a table showing operative status of every procedure code included in the book. The glossary defines all of the terms used in the tables. An alphabetical index of diagnoses and procedures grouped according to classification categories has been included to assist users who do not know the ICD-9-CM code for a particular diagnosis.

HCIA's *Length of Stay* series includes *Length of Stay by Diagnosis and Operation, Psychiatric Length of Stay,* and *Length of Stay by DRG and Payment Source.* Each book in the series is updated annually. These three versions are available in editions for the United States and for Northeastern, North Central, Southern, and Western regions. *Pediatric Length of Stay* (19 years old and younger) and *Geriatric Length of Stay* (65 years and older) are also available in the *Length of Stay by Diagnosis and Operation* series for the United States. For every series, data files (electronic media) are available for all of the editions listed above.

About HCIA

HCIA is a leading health care information content company that develops and markets clinical and financial decision support systems used by hospitals, integrated delivery systems, managed care organizations, employers, and pharmaceutical manufacturers. The Company's databases and products are used to benchmark clinical performance and outcomes, profile best practices, and manage the cost and delivery of health care.

HCIA maintains the industry's largest health care database, containing more than 325 million patient discharge records. Each year, HCIA collects data from more than 6,500 hospitals and 35,000 alternate care facilities including nursing homes, retirement facilities, medical rehabilitation facilities, and other providers. HCIA also maintains exclusive rights to unique classification methodologies, including the International Classification of Clinical Services (ICCS). These methodologies allow for standardization of patient-level data across settings and longitudinally over time.

Serving a client base of more than 7,000 customers, HCIA provides decision support systems to more than 1,500 hospitals, as well as 18 of the largest U.S. health insurance companies, 16 of the largest U.S. managed care organizations, and 21 of the largest pharmaceutical manufacturers. These systems are utilized by the following major health care constituencies in different ways:

Providers, such as hospitals, physician groups, and integrated delivery systems, use HCIA's decision support systems to measure and analyze the cost and quality of medical interventions. The Company's entry-level systems provide users with competitor-specific information such as market share by product line, local market utilization rates compared with regional and national norms, and customer-specific analyses of product line and physician-level resource consumption. All systems incorporate benchmarks for specific medical resource consumption, and are designed to help providers understand the best practice for a medical intervention.

Buyers, such as managed care organizations, indemnity insurers, and employers, use the information and analyses of medical resource usage and outcomes derived from HCIA's decision support systems. This information helps them select and monitor the performance of network providers, channel specific types of patients toward the most clinically effective providers, negotiate fair prices and appropriate utilization criteria, and identify superior and efficient hospitals and physicians. It also allows them to manage the overall health status of a covered population.

Suppliers, such as pharmaceutical, biotechnology, and medical supply and device companies, use HCIA's decision support systems in market analysis, product positioning, and pharmacoeconomic analysis. Pharmacoeconomic analysis provides suppliers with information needed to measure the specific benefit/cost and outcome of an individual product against those of competing products, alternative therapies, or in the case of a new drug or product, the industry standard therapy.

Using proprietary technologies, HCIA transforms raw health care data into decision support systems that provide value-added information. All of HCIA's systems and products rely on three principal components—the core competencies: DataBridge™, SoleSource®, and Databases —as the basis for creating health care information. HCIA's products and systems can be broadly classified as follows:

Decision Support Systems: HCIA offers a wide range of specialized and customized health care information systems, including SoleSource® and CHAMP™. These systems assist health care providers, payors, consultants, and suppliers in analyzing different performance measures within the industry, allowing them to:

- profile best practices;

- analyze market share;

- assess competitive position;

- evaluate disease management strategies;

- measure clinical outcomes and costs; and

- measure patient health status and satisfaction.

Syndicated Products: These products include publications and standardized databases, ranging from database directories (e.g., health care industry professionals, nursing homes, and managed care organizations) to more complex data analyses (e.g., cost and outcome summaries for each U.S. hospital). Available in a variety of formats, Syndicated Products fall into four general categories: Market Analysis Studies, Industry Publications, Health Care Directories, and Reference Guides.

Patient-Based Assessments: HCIA offers state-of-the-art patient profiling and information management systems, as well as consultation services for the development of customized assessment tools, reports, and programs. Through the development of data capture technology, HCIA is able to provide diverse health care applications, ranging from health education and promotion to hospital quality, patient satisfaction and health status, and detailed disease-specific outcomes. HCIA's Response product line has pioneered the use of point-of-service, patient-centered data collection and analysis systems for health care providers, managed health care, and pharmaceutical industries.

Headquartered in Baltimore, Maryland, HCIA Inc. (NASDAQ:HCIA) has offices throughout the United States and in Europe.

DESCRIPTION OF THE PROJECTED INPATIENT DATABASE

The data appearing in the *Length of Stay* series were derived from HCIA's Projected Inpatient Database (PIDB), the largest all-payor inpatient database available in the marketplace. The PIDB supports publications, products, and custom studies, the results of which are applicable to all short-term, general, nonfederal (STGNF) hospitals in the United States. This exclusive database combines data from both public and proprietary state data as well as individual and group hospital contracts and contains 12 million all-payor discharges for fiscal year 1996, representing one-third of all discharges from all U.S. STGNF hospitals. Updated quarterly, the PIDB is used to create the *Length of Stay* series, the *National Inpatient Profile*, the *National Link Study*, and other HCIA products.

Data Projection and Methodology

The PIDB was created as an external, stable, consolidated database to enable users to make accurate projections about the entire universe of U.S. short-term, general, nonfederal (STGNF) hospitals. First, data from all sources are standardized to create an aggregated patient record database. Each discharge record is then assigned a weight (or projection factor) to indicate the number of discharges it represents. In this way, the data are projected to represent the universe of all inpatient episodes.

To create the projection factors, accurate external sources that describe the target universe of hospitals must be available. HCIA uses two sources: the National Hospital Discharge Survey (NHDS) and the Medicare Provider Analysis and Review File (MedPAR). NHDS is a survey produced and published by the National Center for Health Statistics (NCHS) that has itself been projected to represent the entire universe of nonfederal, general (medical or surgical) or children's general, short stay hospitals in the United States. MedPAR is produced by the Health Care Financing Administration (HCFA) and contains 100 percent of all Medicare inpatient discharges. When the projection factors are summed over all discharges, they match this universe and are known as a *weighted sum*. Similarly, a count of the number of discharges in a particular patient subgroup would equal the estimated number of such patients in the STGNF universe, not just those in the database. Also, when the weights are properly applied, a mean length of stay (LOS), for example, represents the mean LOS for all such patients in the STGNF universe, rather than just those in the database. This measure is a *weighted mean*. The projection process takes into account the age and sex of the patient; the HCIA-assigned bed service of the inpatient episode; and the census region, bed size, and teaching status of the hospital.

The universe of inpatients discharged from all short-term, general, nonfederal U.S. hospitals is defined using the HCFA's MedPAR and the NHDS. These hospital characteristics are defined according to the American Hospital Association criteria:

Short-Term: The average length of stay for all patients at the facility is less than 30 days, or more than 50 percent of all patients are admitted to units in which the average length of stay is less than 30 days.

General: The primary function of the institution is to provide patient services, diagnostic and therapeutic, for a variety of medical conditions.

Nonfederal: The facility is controlled by a state, county, city, city-county, hospital district or authority, or church.

U.S. hospitals include those in the 50 states and the District of Columbia. Data from long-term specialty institutions, *e.g.,* long-term psychiatric or rehabilitation facilities, are excluded. For the average length of stay data, several exclusions are applied to eliminate discharge records that do not represent a typical short-term inpatient stay. These exclusions include: admission from other short-term hospital; discharge to other short-term hospital; discharge against medical advice; and death.

Data Quality

The PIDB is the cleanest consolidated source of data available. All data are run through a set of standard edit screens to ensure their quality. Examples of discrepancies detected by the audit include records with invalid diagnosis or procedure codes, invalid or unrecorded principal diagnosis, sex- or age-specific diagnosis or procedure inconsistencies, and incalculable age or length of stay. All records from hospitals with more than 5 percent of discharges failing any screen are deleted from the database.

Validation

The projection methodology ensures that the PIDB will be representative of the inpatient universe defined by NHDS and MedPAR. By comparing PIDB data with NHDS and MedPAR, the validity of the PIDB has been demonstrated on the ICD-9-CM diagnosis and procedure level, as well as on the DRG level.

To perform such a comparison between PIDB data and NHDS and MedPAR data, the weighted discharges in the PIDB were grouped within ICD-9-CM diagnosis and procedure chapters, as were the discharges in NHDS and MedPAR. PIDB patients under the age of 65 were compared to NHDS patients for the same age range, and PIDB patients aged 65 and older were compared to MedPAR patients for the same age range. The findings show that the chapter distributions of the PIDB were highly representative of NHDS and MedPAR.

Concordance between DRG-specific Medicare estimates from the PIDB and the actual Medicare counts in MedPAR is illustrated in the figure below. The correlation between the PIDB and MedPAR count is 99.9 percent. Because the PIDB projection methodology incorporates payor data, the validity of the PIDB applies not only to the Medicare population, but across all payors.

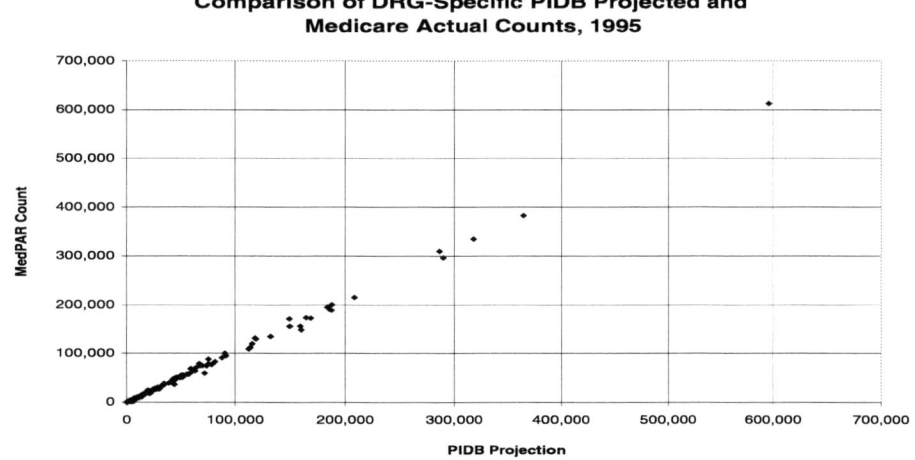

Comparison of DRG-Specific PIDB Projected and Medicare Actual Counts, 1995

BENEFITS AND APPLICATIONS

HCIA's *Length of Stay* series is an invaluable supplement and reference for health care professionals who want to measure inpatient utilization across a variety of settings. Users of the hospital stay data found in this series can compare regional and national norms to an individual institution or a special population. Specifically, the *Length of Stay* series allows the user to:

- project extended stay reviews;

- identify candidates for utilization review;

- establish baselines (benchmarking);

- develop forecasts;

- pre-authorize procedures; and

- review network providers, both prospectively and retrospectively.

Patient severity, managed care market presence, and varying practice patterns all have significant impact on actual LOS statistics. As technological advances and financial pressures reduce inpatient days and increase outpatient volumes, only the most severely ill patients are left in the hospitals. Consequently, health care professionals must have detailed measurement criteria to make truly accurate, patient-focused assessments of appropriate lengths of stay. Using the *Length of Stay* series, professionals can tailor LOS analyses to a particular patient age group, or compare the norms for patients with single or multiple diagnoses. Users may also study regional variations, as well as specialized groups including pediatric, geriatric, and psychiatric patient populations. HCIA's LOS data can help pinpoint whether patients are being cared for efficiently, targeting areas that may need further clinical analysis.

The recent proliferation of new laws regulating utilization management procedures—in part, by requiring the disclosure of criteria used—is also fueling the demand for high quality data. To comply with these new legal stipulations and to track fluctuating LOS trends, utilization managers must have reliable, industry-accepted criteria sets. Because HCIA updates the *Length of Stay* series annually with millions of new patient records, it provides extremely useful trend information—including significant developments from one year to the next and over even longer periods of time. Compiled from HCIA's exclusive Projected Inpatient Database (PIDB), the largest all-payor inpatient database available in the marketplace, this series is the most comprehensive, current source for length of stay data available.

HOW TO USE THE TABLES

The data in each volume are organized numerically by the *International Classification of Diseases, 9th Revision, Clinical Modification (ICD-9-CM)*. Each Diagnosis volume contains every three-digit diagnosis code (including both summary and valid detail codes) and the 1,200 four- and five-digit codes highest in projected volume. Each Operation volume contains every three-digit procedure code (including both summary codes and valid detail codes) and the 850 four-digit codes highest in projected volume. If a patient's ICD-9-CM code is not known, refer to the index, which provides an alphabetical listing of the descriptive titles for all codes included in the book.

Data are categorized by number of observed patients, average length of stay, variance, and distribution percentiles. In addition, two subtotals and a grand total are included. All data elements except the number of observed patients are calculated using the projection methodology described on page vii.

Specific length of stay norms can be obtained by taking the following steps:

Step 1: Find the desired ICD-9-CM code in the tables in one of the *Length of Stay* volumes; the code precedes the title of each table.

The Observed Patients column represents the number of observed patients in the stratified group. Patients with stays longer than 99 days (>99) are not included. This data element does not use the projection factor. Many of the numbers in this column have increased this year due to a larger available data sample.

Step 2: Find the appropriate portion of the table for review:

- Single or Multiple Diagnoses

- Not Operated or Operated (for Diagnosis groups only)

- Patient's Age (on day of admission)

For each diagnosis code, patients are stratified by single or multiple diagnoses, operated or not operated status, and age. For diagnosis codes V30-V39, which pertain exclusively to newborns, age is replaced by birth weight in grams. Newborns with unrecorded birth weights with secondary diagnosis codes in the 764.01-764.99 and 765.01-765.19 ranges have been assigned to the appropriate birth weight category on the basis of the fifth digit of these codes. Data for patients whose birth weights cannot be determined by using this method are included only in the Subtotal and Total rows of the table. For each procedure code, patients are stratified by single or multiple diagnoses and age.

Patients are classified in the multiple diagnoses category if they had at least one valid secondary diagnosis in addition to the principal one. The following codes are not considered valid secondary diagnoses for purposes of this classification:

1. Manifestation codes (conditions that evolved from underlying diseases [etiology] and are in italics in *ICD-9-CM, Volume 1*)

2. Codes V27.0-V27.9 (outcome of delivery)

3. E Codes (external causes of injury and poisoning)

In the diagnosis tables, operated patients are those who had at least one procedure that is classified by the Health Care Financing Administration (HCFA) as an operating room procedure. HCFA physician panels classify every ICD-9-CM procedure code according to whether the procedure would in most hospitals be performed in the operating room. This classification system differs slightly from that used in Length of Stay publications published before 1995, in which patients were categorized as "operated" if any of their procedures were labeled as Uniform Hospital Discharge Data Set (UHDDS) Class 1. Appendix C contains a list of procedure codes included in this series and their HCFA-defined operative status.

Step 3: Find the 50th percentile of stay for similar patients at the point where the 50th percentile column of the table intersects the horizontal line containing the pertinent patient variables.

You may also wish to observe the average length of stay. The average length of stay is calculated from the admission and discharge dates by counting the day of admission as the first day; the day of discharge is not included. The average is figured by adding the lengths of stay for each patient and then dividing by the total number of patients. Patients discharged on the day of admission are counted as staying one day. Patients with stays over 99 days (>99) are excluded from this calculation.

For further information, the other percentile columns may be studied (e.g., if a patient's stay was approved for extension beyond the 50th percentile, an extended stay review may be based on the 75th, 90th, 95th, or 99th percentile).

A length of stay percentile for a stratified group of patients is determined by arranging the individual patient stays from low to high. Counting up from the lowest stay to the point where one-half of the patients have been counted yields the value of the 50th percentile. Counting one-tenth of the total patients gives the 10th percentile, and so on. The 10th, 25th, 50th, 75th, 90th, 95th, and 99th percentiles of stay are displayed in days. If, for example, the 10th percentile for a group of patients is four, then 10 percent of the patients stayed four days or fewer. The 50th percentile is the median. Any percentile with a value of 100 days or more is listed as >99. Patients who were hospitalized more than 99 days (>99) are not included in the total patients, average stay, and variance categories. The percentiles, however, do include these patients.

Step 4: Consult the total patient sample and variance to consider the homogeneity of the data, i.e., to what extent length of stay averages are clustered or spread out within a particular patient group.

The subtotal ("Total") represents the total patients in each of the two patient groups. The grand total represents the total number of patients in the specified diagnosis or procedure category.

The variance is a measure of the spread of the data (from the lowest to the highest value) around the average. The smallest variance is zero, indicating that all lengths of stay are equal. In tables in which there is a large variance and the patient group size is relatively small, the average stay may appear high. This sometimes occurs when one or two patients with long hospitalizations fall into the group.

FEATURES OF A DIAGNOSIS TABLE

ICD-9-CM diagnosis code and title ⎯⎯⎯⎯⎯⎯

Diagnosis group(s) previously used.

008.8: VIRAL ENTERITIS NOS. Formerly included in diagnosis group(s) 001.

Type of Patients	Observed Patients	Avg. Stay	Vari-ance	Percentiles						
				10th	25th	50th	75th	90th	95th	99th
1. SINGLE DX										
A. Not Operated										
0–19 Years	1346	1.9	2	1	1	2	2	3	4	5
20–34	416	1.7	<1	1	1	2	2	3	3	5
35–49	213	2.3	3	1	1	2	3	3	5	10
50–64	89	2.0	3	1	1	1	3	3	4	12
65+	55	2.8	3	1	2	2	3	6	6	9
B. Operated										
0–19 Years	24	2.5	1	1	2	2	3	4	5	6
20–34	21	2.6	<1	1	2	3	3	3	3	4
35–49	6	4.2	2	2	4	5	5	5	5	6
50–64	1	2.0	0	2	2	2	2	2	2	2
65+	0									
2. MULTIPLE DX										
A. Not Operated										
0–19 Years	5020	2.3	5	1	1	2	3	4	5	8
20–34	1625	2.2	3	1	1	2	3	4	5	7
35–49	1453	2.7	3	1	1	2	3	5	6	9
50–64	1301	2.9	3	1	2	2	4	5	6	9
65+	2964	3.6	7	1	2	3	4	7	9	13
B. Operated										
0–19 Years	35	4.3	9	2	2	4	4	8	9	13
20–34	32	3.8	9	1	2	3	4	8	12	12
35–49	23	5.7	20	1	3	4	8	11	20	20
50–64	10	8.0	50	3	4	6	7	25	25	28
65+	27	14.0	92	4	7	10	18	30	31	43
SUBTOTALS:										
1. SINGLE DX										
A. Not Operated	2119	1.9	2	1	1	2	2	3	4	7
B. Operated	52	2.9	1	1	2	3	3	5	5	6
2. MULTIPLE DX										
A. Not Operated	12363	2.7	5	1	1	2	3	5	6	10
B. Operated	127	6.7	46	2	3	4	8	15	20	31
1. SINGLE DX	2171	2.0	2	1	1	2	2	3	4	7
2. MULTIPLE DX	12490	2.7	6	1	1	2	3	5	7	10
A. NOT OPERATED	14482	2.6	5	1	1	2	3	5	6	9
B. OPERATED	179	5.2	31	2	2	3	5	10	15	30
TOTAL										
0–19 Years	6425	2.3	4	1	1	2	3	4	5	8
20–34	2094	2.1	3	1	1	2	3	4	4	7
35–49	1695	2.7	4	1	1	2	3	5	6	10
50–64	1401	2.8	4	1	2	2	3	5	6	9
65+	3046	3.7	8	1	2	3	5	7	9	15
GRAND TOTAL	14661	2.6	5	1	1	2	3	5	6	10

Length of stay (in days) by percentile

Patients are stratified by single or multiple diagnoses, operated or not operated status, and age.

Total number of patients

Observed Patients reflects the actual number of patient discharges. Length of stay figures are derived from data projected to represent the inpatient universe. See "Description of the Projected Inpatient Database" for further explanation.

A measure of the spread of the data around the average

Average length of stay, in days, calculated from the admission and discharge dates

FEATURES OF AN OPERATION TABLE

ICD-9-CM procedure code and title ⎯⎯⎯

Operation group(s) previously used.

01.1: SKULL/BRAIN DX PROCEDURE. Formerly included in operation group(s) 501, 512.

Patients are stratified by single or multiple diagnoses and age.

Type of Patients	Observed Patients	Avg. Stay	Vari-ance	Percentiles						
				10th	25th	50th	75th	90th	95th	99th
1. SINGLE DX										
0–19 Years	78	4.4	20	1	1	3	6	11	11	28
20–34	62	2.6	8	1	1	1	3	5	7	14
35–49	82	4.1	21	1	1	4	4	7	10	18
50–64	92	3.5	17	1	1	2	4	7	9	26
65+	68	5.6	32	1	1	2	10	15	15	17
2. MULTIPLE DX										
0–19 Years	425	15.6	236	2	4	11	21	38	56	71
20–34	347	14.1	238	1	3	7	19	42	49	71
35–49	429	11.0	137	1	3	6	15	29	35	>99
50–64	471	8.5	77	1	3	5	9	21	31	37
65+	665	10.8	120	1	3	7	14	25	33	48
TOTAL SINGLE DX	**382**	**4.1**	**21**	1	1	2	5	10	15	18
MULTIPLE DX	**2337**	**11.7**	**159**	1	3	7	16	29	40	62
TOTAL										
0–19 Years	503	14.1	222	1	3	9	21	34	56	71
20–34	409	12.6	223	1	2	7	17	39	49	67
35–49	511	9.6	121	1	2	6	14	27	31	77
50–64	563	7.7	71	1	2	5	9	18	28	37
65+	733	10.4	115	1	3	7	14	25	30	48
GRAND TOTAL	**2719**	**10.7**	**147**	1	2	7	14	28	37	59

Length of stay (in days) by percentile

Total number of patients ⎯⎯⎯

Observed Patients reflects the actual number of patient discharges. Length of stay figures are derived from data projected to represent the inpatient universe. See "Description of the Projected Inpatient Database" for further explanation.

A measure of the spread of the data around the average

Average length of stay, in days, calculated from the admission and discharge dates

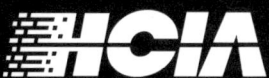
The Comparative Performance of U.S. Hospitals: The Sourcebook

The Sourcebook features comprehensive information on the performance of the U.S. hospital industry for the latest five-year period. Included in the book are 52 key measures of hospital performance, with median and quartile values presented for more than 160 hospital comparison groups. Published with Deloitte & Touche every fall. $399*

The DRG Handbook: Comparative Clinical and Financial Standards

The Handbook focuses on key clinical and financial measures for the 50 highest volume Diagnosis-Related Groups (DRGs). For each DRG, *The Handbook* identifies the top 20 hospitals (based on volume of cases) and provides average charge and length of stay information for more than 90 hospital comparison groups. Includes all-payor data. Published with Ernst & Young every winter. $399*

The Guide to the Nursing Home Industry

The Guide presents aggregate financial operating performance data for more than 10,000 nursing homes. It provides an overview of each state's Medicaid and certificate of need programs, with median values presented for 19 key financial and operating indicators. Published with Arthur Andersen every summer. $249*

Profiles of U.S. Hospitals

This publication presents more than 30 key measures of financial, clinical, and operating performance for every U.S. hospital. Decile rankings for financial indicators such as profitability, leverage, and liquidity are also included. In addition, *Profiles of U.S. Hospitals* lists the number of cases, average charge, and average length of stay for each of the hospital's top five DRGs. Published every fall. $299*

Length of Stay Publications

Organized by individual ICD-9-CM codes or by DRGs, and broken down by diagnosis, operation, and payment source, *LOS* publications serve as a comprehensive guide to one of the most important issues in hospital care. The publications contain detailed patient and clinical data, including breakouts by age groups, single versus multiple diagnoses, and operated versus non-operated populations. Published every summer. Please call for prices.*

The Guide to the Managed Care Industry

A comprehensive listing of the nation's HMOs and PPOs, *The Guide* features enrollment information, names of key industry contacts, and an analysis of major industry trends. Published every fall. $245*

* Also available on magnetic tape and diskette. Please call for prices.

(continued on other side)

HCIA Inc.
300 East Lombard Street
Baltimore, MD 21202

3 WAYS TO ORDER

❶ Call (800) 324-1746

❷ Fax Your Order to (410) 865-4321

❸ Return the Attached Order Cards

Essential Information for the Health Care Industry

Item	Qty.	Price	Total
❏ The Comparative Performance of U.S. Hospitals: The Sourcebook		$ 399	
❏ The DRG Handbook: Comparative Clinical and Financial Standards		399	
❏ The Guide to the Nursing Home Industry		249	
❏ Profiles of U.S. Hospitals		299	
❏ Length of Stay Publications		*call*	
❏ The Guide to the Managed Care Industry		245	
❏ 50 Top Outpatient Procedures: Benchmarks, Standards & Trends		245	
❏ The APG Handbook		295	
❏ Market Profiles for Medicare Risk Contracting: A Provider Perspective		310	

Subtotal _____

(AL, CA, CT, FL, GA, IL, KY, MA, MD, MI, NC, OH, RI, SC, TN, TX, UT, WA) Sales Tax _____

Shipping and Handling ___$7.95___

❏ Enclosed is a check made payable to HCIA Inc. for $_____   **Total** _____

❏ Please bill my: ❏ VISA ❏ MasterCard ❏ American Express

   Account #_____ Expiration Date_____

   Purchase Order #_____ Signature *(required)*_____

Name and Title_____

Company_____

Address_____

(cannot be delivered to a P.O. box)

City_____ State_____ Zip_____

Telephone_____ Fax_____

Target Selected Markets — With HCIA's Specialized Directories

Item	Qty.	Price	Total
❏ The Directory of Nursing Homes		$ 249	
❏ The Directory of Retirement Facilities		249	
❏ The Directory of Health Care Professionals		299	

Subtotal _____

(AL, CA, CT, FL, GA, IL, KY, MA, MD, MI, NC, OH, RI, SC, TN, TX, UT, WA) Sales Tax _____

Shipping and Handling ___$7.95___

                                  Total _____

❏ Enclosed is a check made payable to HCIA Inc. for $_____

❏ Please bill my: ❏ VISA ❏ MasterCard ❏ American Express

   Account #_____ Expiration Date_____

   Purchase Order #_____ Signature *(required)*_____

Name and Title_____

Company_____

Address_____

(cannot be delivered to a P.O. box)

City_____ State_____ Zip_____

Telephone_____ Fax_____

HCIA Inc.
300 East Lombard Street
Baltimore, MD 21202

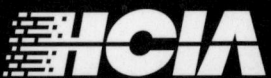

**Your Complete Resource
For Health Care Information**

# 3 WAYS TO ORDER

❶ Call (800) 324-1746

❷ Fax Your Order to (410) 865-4321

❸ Return the Attached Order Cards

The APG Handbook
The APG Handbook is the complete guide to both the implementation and use of an APG system. Beginning with a detailed overview of the history and implementation requirements of APGs, *The Handbook* provides detailed information on APG Initial Classification Variable, Significant Surgical Procedures, and Medical and Ancillary APGs. $295*

Market Profiles for Medicare Risk Contracting: A Provider Perspective
Market Profiles presents charge, reimbursement, and utilization figures on the county level. Use it to investigate regional markets prior to negotiating a risk contract. Available in regional editions. $310*

50 Top Outpatient Procedures: Benchmarks, Standards & Trends
50 Top Outpatient Procedures provides a broad range of information on 50 of the most significant outpatient procedures. Reflective of the heavy growth in outpatient services, it is an excellent tool for analyzing ongoing shifts in use rates, charges, and reimbursement — by setting, patient demographics, or region. For each studied procedure, detailed information is broken down across hospital-based outpatient, physician office, ambulatory surgery center, and inpatient settings. $245*

HCIA DIRECTORIES

The Directory of Nursing Homes
This publication lists more than 16,000 licensed nursing homes across the U.S., alphabetically arranged by state and city. *The Directory* features addresses, contact names, service offerings, and ownership/management information. Published every winter. $249*

The Directory of Retirement Facilities
Profiles of more than 18,000 assisted living, congregate care, independent living, and continuing care facilities in the U.S. are featured. Conveniently catalogued by state and city, facilities are listed with addresses, contact names, number of residents, average monthly fees, social/recreational service offerings, ownership, and affiliation. Published every fall. $249*

The Directory of Health Care Professionals
The Directory is a comprehensive source of contact names arranged by hospital, system headquarters, and primary job function. More than 175,000 hospital professionals and 7,000 hospitals are listed in an easy-to-use format. Published every fall. $299*

* Also available on magnetic tape and diskette. Please call for prices.

Prices are subject to change without notice.

**NO POSTAGE
NECESSARY
IF MAILED
IN THE
UNITED STATES**

BUSINESS REPLY MAIL

FIRST CLASS MAIL   PERMIT NO. 302   BALTIMORE, MD

POSTAGE WILL BE PAID BY ADDRESSEE

ATTN PUBLICATION SALES
HCIA INC
300 EAST LOMBARD ST
BALTIMORE MD 21298-6213

**NO POSTAGE
NECESSARY
IF MAILED
IN THE
UNITED STATES**

BUSINESS REPLY MAIL

FIRST CLASS MAIL   PERMIT NO. 302   BALTIMORE, MD

POSTAGE WILL BE PAID BY ADDRESSEE

ATTN PUBLICATION SALES
HCIA INC
300 EAST LOMBARD ST
BALTIMORE MD 21298-6213

HCIA GUARANTEE

Books may be returned for a full refund if they are returned in good condition within 10 business days of receipt. Books damaged in shipping should be returned to HCIA within 5 business days for replacement. If you need to return a book, please contact HCIA Customer Service at (800) 568-3282 for return authorization. Diskettes and magnetic tapes are not returnable.

LENGTH OF STAY TABLES
OPERATION CODES

United States, October 1995–September 1996 Data, by Operation

Summary of All Patients in Operation Codes

Type of Patients	Observed Patients*	Avg. Stay	Vari-ance	Percentiles 10th	25th	50th	75th	90th	95th	99th
1. SINGLE DX										
0–19 Years	342200	2.1	4	1	1	2	2	3	4	9
20–34	395751	1.9	3	1	1	2	2	3	4	7
35–49	144301	2.5	6	1	1	2	3	5	6	12
50–64	70509	2.9	8	1	1	2	4	6	7	12
65+	54039	3.5	12	1	1	3	4	7	8	16
2. MULTIPLE DX										
0–19 Years	661765	4.8	68	1	1	2	4	10	17	51
20–34	811467	3.4	20	1	2	2	4	6	10	23
35–49	717758	4.9	36	1	2	3	6	10	14	31
50–64	747634	6.0	46	1	2	4	7	12	17	35
65+	1582034	7.1	50	2	3	5	9	14	20	37
TOTAL SINGLE DX	1006800	2.2	5	1	1	2	2	4	5	10
MULTIPLE DX	4520658	5.5	46	1	2	3	6	11	16	35
TOTAL										
0–19 Years	1003965	3.8	47	1	1	2	3	7	12	40
20–34	1207218	2.9	15	1	1	2	3	5	8	20
35–49	862059	4.4	31	1	2	3	5	9	13	29
50–64	818143	5.7	43	1	2	4	7	11	16	33
65+	1636073	7.0	49	2	3	5	9	14	19	36
GRAND TOTAL	5527458	4.8	39	1	2	3	6	10	15	32

*Observed Patients reflects the actual number of patient discharges. Length of stay figures are derived from data projected to represent the inpatient universe. See "Description of the Projected Inpatient Database" (p. viii) for further explanation.

Length of Stay by Diagnosis and Operation, United States, 1997

United States, October 1995–September 1996 Data, by Operation

01.0: CRANIAL PUNCTURE. Formerly included in operation group(s) 501.

Type of Patients	Observed Patients	Avg. Stay	Variance	10th	25th	50th	75th	90th	95th	99th
1. SINGLE DX										
0–19 Years	36	2.7	7	1	1	2	3	7	10	11
20–34	6	3.2	3	2	2	3	5	5	7	7
35–49	6	4.3	18	1	1	2	7	10	10	10
50–64	6	5.0	7	1	2	7	7	7	7	7
65+	2	1.6	<1	1	1	1	3	3	3	3
2. MULTIPLE DX										
0–19 Years	517	5.7	30	1	2	4	8	13	17	27
20–34	76	6.3	32	2	3	4	6	15	19	24
35–49	59	7.6	84	2	3	4	7	16	29	35
50–64	64	10.6	84	2	4	8	15	23	23	46
65+	111	9.3	42	2	2	11	15	15	18	21
TOTAL SINGLE DX	56	3.2	8	1	1	2	4	7	10	11
MULTIPLE DX	827	6.8	41	1	2	4	9	15	18	33
TOTAL										
0–19 Years	553	5.5	29	1	2	4	8	13	17	27
20–34	82	6.1	31	2	3	4	6	15	19	24
35–49	65	7.2	78	1	2	4	7	16	29	35
50–64	70	9.8	78	2	4	7	14	23	23	46
65+	113	9.2	42	2	2	10	15	15	18	21
GRAND TOTAL	883	6.6	40	1	2	4	9	15	18	29

01.09: CRANIAL PUNCTURE NEC. Formerly included in operation group(s) 501.

Type of Patients	Observed Patients	Avg. Stay	Variance	10th	25th	50th	75th	90th	95th	99th
1. SINGLE DX										
0–19 Years	15	2.7	6	1	1	1	4	7	7	10
20–34	2	3.1	6	1	1	5	5	5	5	5
35–49	3	4.8	20	1	1	7	10	10	10	10
50–64	6	5.0	7	1	2	7	7	7	7	7
65+	1	1.0	0	1	1	1	1	1	1	1
2. MULTIPLE DX										
0–19 Years	103	8.2	56	2	4	5	13	18	24	>99
20–34	25	8.5	53	1	3	6	16	21	23	24
35–49	24	10.3	124	1	4	7	12	29	29	65
50–64	30	12.5	109	2	3	7	23	23	36	41
65+	55	9.6	44	2	2	14	15	15	18	21
TOTAL SINGLE DX	27	3.7	10	1	1	2	7	10	10	10
MULTIPLE DX	237	9.2	60	2	3	6	15	18	23	40
TOTAL										
0–19 Years	118	7.7	53	2	4	4	10	18	24	40
20–34	27	8.3	52	1	3	5	16	19	23	24
35–49	27	8.8	102	1	2	6	10	23	29	65
50–64	36	10.6	94	1	3	7	18	23	23	41
65+	56	9.5	44	1	2	14	15	15	18	21
GRAND TOTAL	264	8.7	58	1	3	6	15	18	23	40

01.02: VENTRICULOPUNCT VIA CATH. Formerly included in operation group(s) 501.

Type of Patients	Observed Patients	Avg. Stay	Variance	10th	25th	50th	75th	90th	95th	99th
1. SINGLE DX										
0–19 Years	21	2.7	7	1	1	2	3	3	11	11
20–34	4	3.3	3	2	2	3	3	7	7	7
35–49	2	2.0	0	2	2	2	2	2	2	2
50–64	0									
65+	0									
2. MULTIPLE DX										
0–19 Years	413	4.9	20	1	2	3	7	10	14	21
20–34	49	5.6	27	2	3	4	5	15	15	23
35–49	32	6.6	67	2	2	4	6	16	35	35
50–64	31	9.0	61	2	6	8	11	17	17	46
65+	49	6.6	30	2	3	4	9	12	14	33
TOTAL SINGLE DX	27	2.8	6	1	1	2	3	3	11	11
MULTIPLE DX	574	5.4	27	1	2	4	7	11	15	24
TOTAL										
0–19 Years	434	4.8	20	1	2	3	7	10	14	21
20–34	53	5.5	26	2	3	4	5	15	15	23
35–49	34	6.5	66	2	3	4	6	16	35	35
50–64	31	9.0	61	2	6	8	11	17	17	46
65+	49	6.6	30	2	3	4	9	12	14	33
GRAND TOTAL	601	5.3	26	1	2	4	7	11	15	24

01.1: DXTIC PX ON SKULL/BRAIN. Formerly included in operation group(s) 501, 512.

Type of Patients	Observed Patients	Avg. Stay	Variance	10th	25th	50th	75th	90th	95th	99th
1. SINGLE DX										
0–19 Years	74	2.3	6	1	1	1	2	6	8	14
20–34	60	3.3	24	1	1	1	3	12	15	24
35–49	95	3.1	13	1	1	1	4	7	11	12
50–64	83	2.5	8	1	1	1	3	7	7	16
65+	77	3.3	6	1	1	2	5	5	7	14
2. MULTIPLE DX										
0–19 Years	496	14.0	260	2	4	10	17	31	49	>99
20–34	403	13.4	139	2	4	10	24	27	33	47
35–49	543	8.3	121	1	1	4	11	23	27	57
50–64	567	10.5	109	1	3	7	15	21	28	55
65+	887	9.4	118	1	2	6	13	20	30	53
TOTAL SINGLE DX	389	2.8	11	1	1	1	3	7	8	16
MULTIPLE DX	2896	10.8	154	1	2	7	15	25	32	70
TOTAL										
0–19 Years	570	12.2	239	1	3	7	15	31	39	98
20–34	463	12.1	135	1	2	9	20	25	32	47
35–49	638	7.5	108	1	1	3	10	21	25	57
50–64	650	8.8	99	1	1	6	12	21	27	54
65+	964	8.9	112	1	2	5	12	20	27	53
GRAND TOTAL	3285	9.7	142	1	1	6	13	25	31	61

Percentiles columns span 10th, 25th, 50th, 75th, 90th, 95th, 99th.

Length of Stay by Diagnosis and Operation, United States, 1997

United States, October 1995–September 1996 Data, by Operation

01.13: CLSD (PERC) BRAIN BX. Formerly included in operation group(s) 501.

Type of Patients	Observed Patients	Avg. Stay	Variance	10th	25th	50th	75th	90th	95th	99th
1. SINGLE DX										
0–19 Years	39	1.7	4	1	1	1	1	3	4	14
20–34	39	1.6	4	1	1	1	1	3	3	11
35–49	67	2.6	9	1	1	1	3	6	11	11
50–64	70	2.2	5	1	1	1	2	7	7	9
65+	59	3.2	5	1	1	2	5	5	7	14
2. MULTIPLE DX										
0–19 Years	61	6.1	50	1	1	4	6	14	25	32
20–34	186	7.7	103	1	1	4	11	21	30	43
35–49	303	4.6	55	1	1	1	6	13	18	33
50–64	365	6.8	51	1	1	5	9	14	20	37
65+	581	7.1	75	1	1	4	11	16	20	49
TOTAL SINGLE DX	274	2.2	6	1	1	1	2	5	7	11
MULTIPLE DX	1496	6.5	68	1	1	3	9	15	21	43
TOTAL										
0–19 Years	100	3.5	28	1	1	1	4	8	14	32
20–34	225	6.2	86	1	1	2	8	14	25	42
35–49	370	4.2	47	1	1	1	5	11	15	33
50–64	435	5.4	42	1	1	4	9	13	17	37
65+	640	6.7	69	1	1	4	10	16	19	49
GRAND TOTAL	1770	5.6	58	1	1	2	7	14	18	38

01.18: DXTIC PX BRAIN/CEREB NEC. Formerly included in operation group(s) 512.

Type of Patients	Observed Patients	Avg. Stay	Variance	10th	25th	50th	75th	90th	95th	99th
1. SINGLE DX										
0–19 Years	18	4.1	15	1	1	3	7	8	8	16
20–34	8	12.0	61	2	3	12	16	24	24	24
35–49	3	5.5	5	3	3	7	7	7	7	7
50–64	2	2.0	2	1	1	3	3	3	3	3
65+	1	1.0	0	1	1	1	1	1	1	1
2. MULTIPLE DX										
0–19 Years	364	15.2	285	2	5	10	18	31	52	>99
20–34	169	17.9	115	5	9	17	25	29	36	47
35–49	86	22.0	307	4	10	21	25	48	57	88
50–64	60	24.9	398	6	10	17	33	56	65	97
65+	52	12.6	151	2	5	7	18	27	40	51
TOTAL SINGLE DX	32	6.6	40	1	2	4	8	16	24	24
MULTIPLE DX	731	16.6	248	3	6	13	25	32	47	98
TOTAL										
0–19 Years	382	14.9	281	2	4	10	18	31	51	>99
20–34	177	17.7	114	5	9	16	25	29	36	47
35–49	89	21.2	305	4	9	20	25	45	57	88
50–64	62	24.4	400	6	10	17	32	56	65	97
65+	53	12.5	151	2	3	7	18	27	40	51
GRAND TOTAL	763	16.3	244	2	6	12	24	32	47	98

01.14: OPEN BIOPSY OF BRAIN. Formerly included in operation group(s) 501.

Type of Patients	Observed Patients	Avg. Stay	Variance	10th	25th	50th	75th	90th	95th	99th
1. SINGLE DX										
0–19 Years	16	4.0	7	1	2	3	6	8	8	8
20–34	10	3.9	2	1	3	4	5	5	6	6
35–49	19	5.0	30	2	2	5	5	6	12	41
50–64	9	9.0	39	2	2	7	16	16	16	16
65+	13	4.7	10	1	2	5	6	8	12	12
2. MULTIPLE DX										
0–19 Years	63	12.6	183	2	4	7	17	35	52	>99
20–34	41	9.7	48	2	5	8	14	20	20	36
35–49	126	11.2	72	4	8	10	16	25	25	50
50–64	121	14.1	55	4	8	13	21	23	23	31
65+	216	14.6	164	2	5	11	19	32	53	53
TOTAL SINGLE DX	67	5.0	20	2	2	4	6	8	16	16
MULTIPLE DX	567	13.1	114	2	5	10	20	25	35	53
TOTAL										
0–19 Years	79	11.2	164	2	3	6	13	31	47	>99
20–34	51	8.8	45	2	4	6	9	20	20	22
35–49	145	10.5	71	2	4	8	16	25	25	44
50–64	130	13.9	55	4	8	13	21	21	22	31
65+	229	14.3	163	2	5	11	19	30	53	53
GRAND TOTAL	634	12.5	111	2	4	10	19	25	34	53

01.2: CRANIOTOMY & CRANIECTOMY. Formerly included in operation group(s) 502.

Type of Patients	Observed Patients	Avg. Stay	Variance	10th	25th	50th	75th	90th	95th	99th
1. SINGLE DX										
0–19 Years	317	4.1	7	2	3	4	4	6	9	14
20–34	91	4.6	14	3	3	3	5	9	11	19
35–49	122	4.3	12	2	3	3	5	8	11	18
50–64	88	4.5	23	2	2	4	4	7	11	35
65+	51	5.6	33	2	2	4	5	11	21	26
2. MULTIPLE DX										
0–19 Years	616	13.4	351	2	3	5	12	63	64	64
20–34	399	9.9	105	2	4	7	13	19	26	59
35–49	500	10.6	85	3	4	9	14	19	27	48
50–64	500	12.0	135	3	4	8	14	27	38	50
65+	813	10.6	91	3	5	8	13	20	27	55
TOTAL SINGLE DX	669	4.4	13	2	3	4	4	7	10	21
MULTIPLE DX	2828	11.5	172	3	4	7	13	24	39	64
TOTAL										
0–19 Years	933	10.1	250	2	3	4	8	24	63	64
20–34	490	8.4	85	2	3	5	11	17	24	45
35–49	622	9.2	75	3	4	6	13	17	27	42
50–64	588	9.8	115	3	4	5	12	26	33	49
65+	864	10.4	90	3	5	8	12	20	27	54
GRAND TOTAL	3497	9.7	142	2	3	5	11	20	31	64

United States, October 1995–September 1996 Data, by Operation

01.24: OTHER CRANIOTOMY. Formerly included in operation group(s) 502.

Type of Patients	Observed Patients	Avg. Stay	Variance	10th	25th	50th	75th	90th	95th	99th
1. SINGLE DX										
0–19 Years	229	4.1	9	2	3	4	4	6	9	20
20–34	68	4.3	10	3	3	4	5	8	11	13
35–49	98	5.1	15	2	3	3	6	9	12	18
50–64	63	4.6	29	2	3	4	4	7	15	35
65+	41	6.1	38	2	2	4	6	21	21	26
2. MULTIPLE DX										
0–19 Years	458	13.9	357	3	4	6	12	64	64	64
20–34	304	10.9	111	3	4	8	14	20	26	60
35–49	345	12.1	98	3	5	10	16	22	29	64
50–64	349	12.3	124	3	4	8	15	27	34	50
65+	664	11.0	94	3	5	8	13	23	28	56
TOTAL SINGLE DX	499	4.5	15	2	3	4	5	7	11	23
MULTIPLE DX	2120	12.1	174	3	4	8	14	26	38	64
TOTAL										
0–19 Years	687	10.5	258	2	3	4	8	27	64	64
20–34	372	8.8	88	3	3	6	11	17	24	54
35–49	443	10.8	90	3	4	9	16	20	27	48
50–64	412	10.1	109	2	4	8	12	26	33	49
65+	705	10.8	92	3	5	8	13	22	27	56
GRAND TOTAL	2619	10.3	146	3	4	6	12	21	31	64

01.3: INC BRAIN/CEREB MENINGES. Formerly included in operation group(s) 501.

Type of Patients	Observed Patients	Avg. Stay	Variance	10th	25th	50th	75th	90th	95th	99th
1. SINGLE DX										
0–19 Years	84	4.6	9	1	3	4	5	9	9	15
20–34	53	4.8	22	2	2	4	6	8	10	29
35–49	88	4.5	9	1	3	4	6	8	10	15
50–64	83	3.9	6	3	3	3	4	7	7	10
65+	187	5.7	11	3	4	5	7	8	11	17
2. MULTIPLE DX										
0–19 Years	453	13.7	173	3	4	10	17	27	40	73
20–34	323	13.6	143	4	5	10	18	29	39	68
35–49	589	14.8	139	4	6	12	21	26	36	86
50–64	867	13.8	222	2	4	8	18	31	54	62
65+	2985	12.3	110	4	6	9	15	23	35	55
TOTAL SINGLE DX	495	4.9	11	2	3	4	6	8	9	16
MULTIPLE DX	5217	13.0	142	4	5	9	16	26	37	62
TOTAL										
0–19 Years	537	12.4	160	2	4	9	17	26	39	66
20–34	376	12.3	134	3	5	8	16	27	36	65
35–49	677	13.6	135	4	5	11	19	26	32	70
50–64	950	12.4	203	2	4	7	15	30	53	62
65+	3172	11.7	105	4	5	8	15	22	33	55
GRAND TOTAL	5712	12.1	134	3	5	8	15	25	35	62

01.25: OTHER CRANIECTOMY. Formerly included in operation group(s) 502.

Type of Patients	Observed Patients	Avg. Stay	Variance	10th	25th	50th	75th	90th	95th	99th
1. SINGLE DX										
0–19 Years	84	3.9	4	3	3	3	4	6	8	9
20–34	18	7.0	46	1	2	4	11	18	19	21
35–49	18	3.2	6	2	2	2	4	5	8	13
50–64	18	4.2	7	3	4	4	4	4	5	19
65+	9	2.8	2	1	2	3	4	4	4	5
2. MULTIPLE DX										
0–19 Years	134	12.4	364	2	3	4	8	63	63	63
20–34	77	7.0	88	2	2	4	7	16	27	45
35–49	102	6.2	24	3	4	4	6	13	14	33
50–64	101	12.8	202	2	4	7	17	44	44	45
65+	114	9.8	92	4	5	7	11	17	25	64
TOTAL SINGLE DX	147	4.1	8	2	3	4	4	6	9	19
MULTIPLE DX	528	10.1	195	2	3	5	10	21	44	63
TOTAL										
0–19 Years	218	9.2	243	2	3	4	6	21	63	63
20–34	95	7.0	82	2	3	4	7	18	21	45
35–49	120	5.7	22	2	3	4	6	12	13	27
50–64	119	9.8	151	2	4	4	10	24	44	45
65+	123	9.4	89	3	5	6	10	16	23	54
GRAND TOTAL	675	8.5	152	3	3	4	7	18	40	63

01.31: INC CEREBRAL MENINGES. Formerly included in operation group(s) 501.

Type of Patients	Observed Patients	Avg. Stay	Variance	10th	25th	50th	75th	90th	95th	99th
1. SINGLE DX										
0–19 Years	31	5.0	13	1	2	4	8	9	9	15
20–34	29	4.2	19	2	2	4	5	7	8	24
35–49	52	4.2	11	1	2	3	5	8	15	15
50–64	66	3.7	3	3	3	3	4	6	7	9
65+	154	5.8	11	3	4	6	7	8	10	16
2. MULTIPLE DX										
0–19 Years	246	13.9	187	3	5	11	17	27	39	96
20–34	160	15.0	181	4	6	12	18	38	50	74
35–49	315	12.5	117	4	5	11	15	24	33	>99
50–64	519	13.9	250	2	4	7	17	32	62	62
65+	2309	11.8	116	4	5	8	14	23	36	55
TOTAL SINGLE DX	332	4.9	10	2	3	4	6	8	9	15
MULTIPLE DX	3549	12.5	144	3	5	9	15	26	37	62
TOTAL										
0–19 Years	277	12.9	175	2	4	10	17	26	39	95
20–34	189	12.9	167	2	4	10	15	31	47	74
35–49	367	11.5	111	3	4	9	15	22	31	86
50–64	585	11.6	213	3	3	6	13	30	62	62
65+	2463	11.2	108	3	5	8	14	22	34	55
GRAND TOTAL	3881	11.5	134	3	5	8	14	24	36	62

Length of Stay by Diagnosis and Operation, United States, 1997

United States, October 1995–September 1996 Data, by Operation

01.39: OTHER BRAIN INCISION. Formerly included in operation group(s) 501.

Type of Patients	Observed Patients	Avg. Stay	Variance	10th	25th	50th	75th	90th	95th	99th
1. SINGLE DX										
0–19 Years	51	4.1	5	2	3	4	5	6	6	13
20–34	21	5.9	28	1	3	5	6	9	11	29
35–49	33	4.9	15	3	3	4	6	8	10	10
50–64	16	6.7	44	3	3	5	8	10	10	34
65+	33	4.9	9	2	4	4	5	8	12	17
2. MULTIPLE DX										
0–19 Years	180	14.2	169	3	4	12	21	29	40	64
20–34	154	13.0	117	4	5	8	18	26	29	65
35–49	262	17.5	153	4	8	15	26	26	38	70
50–64	347	13.7	189	2	6	9	18	30	45	68
65+	674	13.7	91	5	7	12	16	23	31	51
TOTAL SINGLE DX	154	4.9	13	2	3	4	6	8	10	17
MULTIPLE DX	1617	14.3	137	4	6	11	19	26	36	63
TOTAL										
0–19 Years	231	12.4	154	2	4	8	17	27	40	64
20–34	175	12.2	112	2	5	8	18	26	29	56
35–49	295	16.5	152	4	6	14	26	26	37	66
50–64	363	13.5	186	2	5	9	18	30	45	68
65+	707	13.2	91	4	6	11	16	23	31	51
GRAND TOTAL	1771	13.6	134	4	6	10	18	26	35	63

01.42: GLOBUS PALLIDUS OPS. Formerly included in operation group(s) 501.

Type of Patients	Observed Patients	Avg. Stay	Variance	10th	25th	50th	75th	90th	95th	99th
1. SINGLE DX										
0–19 Years	0									
20–34	0									
35–49	20	3.0	1	2	2	3	4	4	4	6
50–64	86	2.2	1	1	1	2	3	4	4	5
65+	85	2.2	1	1	1	2	3	3	4	6
2. MULTIPLE DX										
0–19 Years	0									
20–34	3	7.4	37	2	2	3	14	14	14	14
35–49	16	4.0	10	2	3	3	3	10	12	13
50–64	92	3.0	6	1	2	3	4	5	6	16
65+	125	3.8	9	1	2	3	5	9	9	13
TOTAL SINGLE DX	191	2.3	1	1	1	2	3	4	4	5
MULTIPLE DX	236	3.6	9	1	2	3	4	9	10	14
TOTAL										
0–19 Years	0									
20–34	3	7.4	37	2	2	3	14	14	14	14
35–49	36	3.5	6	2	2	3	4	5	10	13
50–64	178	2.6	3	1	1	3	3	5	5	12
65+	210	3.1	6	1	2	3	5	7	9	10
GRAND TOTAL	427	3.0	6	1	2	3	3	6	9	13

01.4: THALAMUS/GLOBUS PALL OPS. Formerly included in operation group(s) 501.

Type of Patients	Observed Patients	Avg. Stay	Variance	10th	25th	50th	75th	90th	95th	99th
1. SINGLE DX										
0–19 Years	0									
20–34	2	2.1	1	1	1	3	3	3	3	3
35–49	26	2.8	1	1	2	3	4	4	4	6
50–64	95	2.1	1	1	1	2	3	3	3	5
65+	94	2.2	1	1	1	2	3	3	4	6
2. MULTIPLE DX										
0–19 Years	0									
20–34	9	2.8	14	1	1	1	3	3	14	14
35–49	29	3.6	8	1	2	3	3	7	12	13
50–64	114	2.7	4	1	2	2	3	6	6	14
65+	152	4.0	43	1	2	3	5	9	9	14
TOTAL SINGLE DX	217	2.2	1	1	1	2	3	4	4	6
MULTIPLE DX	304	3.4	23	1	2	2	4	7	9	14
TOTAL										
0–19 Years	0									
20–34	11	2.7	13	1	1	1	3	3	14	14
35–49	55	3.2	5	1	2	3	3	4	10	13
50–64	209	2.5	3	1	2	2	3	4	5	12
65+	246	3.2	26	1	2	2	3	7	9	10
GRAND TOTAL	521	2.9	14	1	2	2	3	5	8	13

01.5: EXC/DESTR BRAIN/MENINGES. Formerly included in operation group(s) 501.

Type of Patients	Observed Patients	Avg. Stay	Variance	10th	25th	50th	75th	90th	95th	99th
1. SINGLE DX										
0–19 Years	456	5.5	17	3	3	4	7	10	12	20
20–34	290	5.0	5	3	3	5	6	8	9	12
35–49	426	4.8	5	3	4	4	6	7	9	14
50–64	351	5.8	11	2	3	5	8	10	11	15
65+	166	6.0	9	3	3	6	8	9	9	17
2. MULTIPLE DX										
0–19 Years	1184	11.1	139	3	4	7	13	24	35	>99
20–34	831	9.2	68	3	4	6	10	25	25	38
35–49	1665	7.5	42	3	4	5	9	14	20	36
50–64	2220	8.2	55	3	4	6	10	15	20	41
65+	2342	10.9	108	3	5	8	13	22	29	55
TOTAL SINGLE DX	1689	5.4	10	3	3	5	7	9	10	17
MULTIPLE DX	8242	9.4	84	3	4	7	11	19	27	53
TOTAL										
0–19 Years	1640	9.4	109	3	4	6	11	21	31	>99
20–34	1121	8.2	56	3	4	6	9	19	25	36
35–49	2091	6.9	35	3	4	6	8	13	17	34
50–64	2571	7.9	49	3	4	6	10	14	19	41
65+	2508	10.4	101	3	5	8	13	20	29	51
GRAND TOTAL	9931	8.6	72	3	4	6	10	17	25	48

Length of Stay by Diagnosis and Operation, United States, 1997

United States, October 1995–September 1996 Data, by Operation

01.51: EXC CEREB MENINGEAL LES. Formerly included in operation group(s) 501.

Type of Patients	Observed Patients	Avg. Stay	Vari-ance	Percentiles						
				10th	25th	50th	75th	90th	95th	99th
1. SINGLE DX										
0–19 Years	17	3.5	3	1	2	3	5	6	6	8
20–34	33	5.0	7	2	3	5	6	9	11	11
35–49	116	4.6	4	3	4	4	5	7	8	12
50–64	108	4.0	3	2	3	4	5	6	8	11
65+	53	6.4	5	3	4	8	8	8	8	10
2. MULTIPLE DX										
0–19 Years	41	8.5	140	2	3	5	9	16	31	41
20–34	67	7.0	24	3	4	7	8	9	19	31
35–49	332	6.8	34	2	3	5	8	13	22	32
50–64	464	8.6	59	3	4	6	10	15	25	41
65+	597	10.3	63	3	5	8	14	19	24	43
TOTAL SINGLE DX	**327**	**4.7**	**5**	**3**	**3**	**4**	**5**	**8**	**8**	**11**
MULTIPLE DX	**1501**	**8.6**	**55**	**3**	**4**	**6**	**10**	**16**	**23**	**41**
TOTAL										
0–19 Years	58	6.7	97	1	3	5	7	13	21	41
20–34	100	6.6	21	3	4	6	8	9	11	26
35–49	448	6.2	27	2	3	5	7	12	15	30
50–64	572	7.7	51	3	4	6	10	13	23	41
65+	650	9.9	59	3	5	8	13	18	24	43
GRAND TOTAL	**1828**	**7.8**	**48**	**3**	**4**	**6**	**9**	**15**	**22**	**39**

01.59: EXC/DESTR BRAIN LES NEC. Formerly included in operation group(s) 501.

Type of Patients	Observed Patients	Avg. Stay	Vari-ance	Percentiles						
				10th	25th	50th	75th	90th	95th	99th
1. SINGLE DX										
0–19 Years	411	5.6	17	3	3	4	7	10	12	23
20–34	218	4.9	5	3	3	5	6	7	9	12
35–49	270	4.8	6	3	4	5	6	7	9	15
50–64	230	6.6	13	3	4	6	9	11	11	19
65+	111	5.9	11	3	3	6	8	9	9	23
2. MULTIPLE DX										
0–19 Years	1053	11.0	139	3	4	7	13	24	35	>99
20–34	691	9.5	74	3	4	6	11	25	25	38
35–49	1248	7.6	44	3	4	6	9	14	19	36
50–64	1676	8.1	51	3	5	6	10	14	19	40
65+	1673	10.8	120	3	5	7	13	22	29	55
TOTAL SINGLE DX	**1240**	**5.5**	**12**	**3**	**3**	**5**	**7**	**9**	**11**	**19**
MULTIPLE DX	**6341**	**9.4**	**89**	**3**	**4**	**7**	**11**	**19**	**27**	**55**
TOTAL										
0–19 Years	1464	9.4	109	3	4	6	10	21	31	>99
20–34	909	8.4	61	3	4	6	9	21	25	36
35–49	1518	7.0	37	3	4	5	9	13	17	34
50–64	1906	7.9	47	3	4	6	10	14	18	40
65+	1784	10.4	112	3	4	7	12	21	29	55
GRAND TOTAL	**7581**	**8.7**	**77**	**3**	**4**	**6**	**10**	**17**	**25**	**50**

01.53: BRAIN LOBECTOMY. Formerly included in operation group(s) 501.

Type of Patients	Observed Patients	Avg. Stay	Vari-ance	Percentiles						
				10th	25th	50th	75th	90th	95th	99th
1. SINGLE DX										
0–19 Years	27	5.6	19	3	3	4	7	12	14	20
20–34	39	5.9	8	3	4	5	7	9	9	17
35–49	40	6.2	10	3	4	5	8	9	11	22
50–64	13	5.4	4	3	5	6	6	7	9	14
65+	2	6.7	33	3	3	3	12	12	12	12
2. MULTIPLE DX										
0–19 Years	54	13.9	187	4	5	10	23	42	61	>99
20–34	67	8.9	51	3	4	5	13	19	21	32
35–49	84	8.5	60	4	4	6	11	17	23	50
50–64	78	9.8	145	3	5	7	12	16	21	93
65+	70	15.5	62	5	11	14	19	26	26	36
TOTAL SINGLE DX	**121**	**5.8**	**10**	**3**	**4**	**5**	**7**	**9**	**11**	**20**
MULTIPLE DX	**353**	**11.5**	**102**	**4**	**4**	**9**	**15**	**26**	**26**	**82**
TOTAL										
0–19 Years	81	11.0	143	3	4	6	14	24	45	>99
20–34	106	7.8	38	3	4	5	9	18	20	32
35–49	124	7.7	44	4	4	5	9	15	18	50
50–64	91	8.5	106	3	5	6	9	15	19	54
65+	72	15.4	62	5	11	14	19	26	26	36
GRAND TOTAL	**474**	**9.9**	**83**	**3**	**4**	**7**	**13**	**22**	**26**	**61**

01.6: EXCISION OF SKULL LESION. Formerly included in operation group(s) 501.

Type of Patients	Observed Patients	Avg. Stay	Vari-ance	Percentiles						
				10th	25th	50th	75th	90th	95th	99th
1. SINGLE DX										
0–19 Years	75	2.2	6	1	1	1	2	4	7	13
20–34	25	2.6	2	1	1	2	3	5	5	7
35–49	32	2.6	5	1	2	2	2	4	5	11
50–64	10	2.2	2	1	1	2	2	5	6	6
65+	5	2.2	2	1	1	1	4	4	4	4
2. MULTIPLE DX										
0–19 Years	57	5.0	22	1	1	3	8	10	15	19
20–34	23	7.3	20	2	4	7	9	12	12	32
35–49	39	6.5	104	1	1	3	7	11	38	48
50–64	59	7.4	77	1	1	4	13	22	23	39
65+	43	3.4	16	2	2	2	3	7	12	14
TOTAL SINGLE DX	**147**	**2.4**	**5**	**1**	**1**	**2**	**2**	**4**	**7**	**13**
MULTIPLE DX	**221**	**5.7**	**46**	**1**	**1**	**3**	**7**	**13**	**16**	**39**
TOTAL										
0–19 Years	132	3.1	13	1	1	1	4	8	12	19
20–34	48	5.6	19	1	2	5	7	12	12	12
35–49	71	3.7	33	1	1	2	4	6	11	42
50–64	69	6.7	70	1	2	2	9	16	23	39
65+	48	3.2	15	1	2	2	3	6	11	14
GRAND TOTAL	**368**	**4.0**	**29**	**1**	**1**	**2**	**4**	**9**	**13**	**28**

Length of Stay by Diagnosis and Operation, United States, 1997

United States, October 1995–September 1996 Data, by Operation

02.0: CRANIOPLASTY. Formerly included in operation group(s) 503.

Type of Patients	Observed Patients	Avg. Stay	Vari-ance	10th	25th	50th	75th	90th	95th	99th
1. SINGLE DX										
0–19 Years	844	3.2	2	2	2	3	4	5	5	7
20–34	112	2.8	5	1	2	3	6	6	8	12
35–49	56	2.3	3	1	1	2	3	4	5	8
50–64	28	2.8	4	1	2	2	3	4	8	8
65+	12	3.4	2	2	2	4	4	4	6	6
2. MULTIPLE DX										
0–19 Years	1190	5.2	37	2	3	4	5	9	13	28
20–34	464	6.2	48	2	3	4	8	14	20	36
35–49	341	7.1	94	1	2	4	8	15	21	67
50–64	162	6.7	88	1	2	4	8	15	28	47
65+	115	7.3	42	2	3	6	11	11	18	36
TOTAL SINGLE DX	1052	3.1	3	1	2	3	4	5	5	9
MULTIPLE DX	2272	5.9	51	2	2	4	6	11	17	36
TOTAL										
0–19 Years	2034	4.3	23	2	2	3	5	7	11	23
20–34	576	5.3	39	1	2	3	7	11	17	32
35–49	397	6.5	85	1	2	3	7	14	20	63
50–64	190	5.9	74	1	2	3	8	15	28	47
65+	127	7.0	40	2	3	5	11	11	18	36
GRAND TOTAL	3324	4.9	36	2	2	3	5	10	13	29

02.02: ELEVATION SKULL FX FRAG. Formerly included in operation group(s) 503.

Type of Patients	Observed Patients	Avg. Stay	Vari-ance	10th	25th	50th	75th	90th	95th	99th
1. SINGLE DX										
0–19 Years	206	3.4	3	1	2	3	5	5	6	6
20–34	65	4.0	8	1	2	3	6	8	9	13
35–49	20	2.4	4	1	1	2	3	4	6	15
50–64	4	4.5	36	1	1	1	3	14	14	14
65+	0									
2. MULTIPLE DX										
0–19 Years	391	6.6	47	2	3	4	7	14	23	33
20–34	281	7.8	58	1	3	5	10	16	23	41
35–49	182	10.5	158	2	4	6	13	21	31	67
50–64	48	11.0	163	2	3	8	11	28	33	79
65+	34	10.2	32	5	7	11	11	13	23	36
TOTAL SINGLE DX	295	3.5	4	1	2	3	5	5	6	12
MULTIPLE DX	936	7.9	75	2	3	5	10	17	23	46
TOTAL										
0–19 Years	597	5.4	33	2	2	4	5	11	16	29
20–34	346	7.1	51	1	3	5	10	14	23	36
35–49	202	9.5	147	2	3	5	12	20	29	67
50–64	52	10.8	160	2	3	8	11	28	33	79
65+	34	10.2	32	5	7	11	11	13	23	36
GRAND TOTAL	1231	6.7	60	2	3	5	8	13	21	42

02.01: OPENING CRANIAL SUTURE. Formerly included in operation group(s) 503.

Type of Patients	Observed Patients	Avg. Stay	Vari-ance	10th	25th	50th	75th	90th	95th	99th
1. SINGLE DX										
0–19 Years	321	2.9	<1	2	2	3	4	4	4	5
20–34	0									
35–49	1	4.0	0	4	4	4	4	4	4	4
50–64	0									
65+	0									
2. MULTIPLE DX										
0–19 Years	223	3.7	3	2	3	3	4	6	7	11
20–34	1	37.0	0	37	37	37	37	37	37	37
35–49	1	2.0	0	2	2	2	2	2	2	2
50–64	1	9.0	0	9	9	9	9	9	9	9
65+	2	8.2	1	7	7	9	9	9	9	9
TOTAL SINGLE DX	322	2.9	<1	2	2	3	4	4	4	5
MULTIPLE DX	228	3.8	5	2	3	3	4	6	9	11
TOTAL										
0–19 Years	544	3.3	2	2	2	3	4	5	6	10
20–34	1	37.0	0	37	37	37	37	37	37	37
35–49	2	2.9	2	2	2	2	4	4	4	4
50–64	1	9.0	0	9	9	9	9	9	9	9
65+	2	8.2	1	7	7	9	9	9	9	9
GRAND TOTAL	550	3.3	3	2	2	3	4	5	6	11

02.06: CRANIAL OSTEOPLASTY NEC. Formerly included in operation group(s) 503.

Type of Patients	Observed Patients	Avg. Stay	Vari-ance	10th	25th	50th	75th	90th	95th	99th
1. SINGLE DX										
0–19 Years	240	3.1	2	2	2	3	4	5	5	8
20–34	32	2.1	<1	2	2	2	2	3	3	7
35–49	23	2.4	2	1	1	2	4	4	5	5
50–64	20	2.7	2	2	2	3	4	4	8	8
65+	8	3.8	1	2	3	4	4	6	6	6
2. MULTIPLE DX										
0–19 Years	396	4.2	9	2	3	4	5	7	8	12
20–34	128	4.0	29	1	1	2	4	9	16	24
35–49	115	3.8	15	1	2	2	4	8	10	17
50–64	81	4.0	26	1	2	2	5	14	15	28
65+	53	6.4	54	2	4	4	7	11	19	36
TOTAL SINGLE DX	323	2.9	2	2	2	2	4	5	5	8
MULTIPLE DX	773	4.2	19	1	2	3	5	7	11	24
TOTAL										
0–19 Years	636	3.7	7	2	2	3	5	6	7	11
20–34	160	3.3	20	2	2	2	3	7	12	20
35–49	138	3.6	14	1	2	2	4	8	10	14
50–64	101	3.6	19	1	1	2	3	8	15	28
65+	61	6.1	47	2	2	4	7	11	19	36
GRAND TOTAL	1096	3.8	13	1	2	3	4	6	9	17

Length of Stay by Diagnosis and Operation, United States, 1997

United States, October 1995–September 1996 Data, by Operation

02.1: CEREBRAL MENINGES REPAIR. Formerly included in operation group(s) 505.

Type of Patients	Observed Patients	Avg. Stay	Vari-ance	Percentiles						
				10th	25th	50th	75th	90th	95th	99th
1. SINGLE DX										
0–19 Years	68	3.7	6	1	2	3	4	7	8	10
20–34	19	5.1	2	3	3	6	6	6	8	7
35–49	28	4.2	4	3	3	3	6	8	8	9
50–64	13	5.5	2	3	5	6	6	7	8	8
65+	6	5.7	6	3	4	4	8	8	9	9
2. MULTIPLE DX										
0–19 Years	196	9.6	109	3	4	7	10	21	25	72
20–34	75	7.5	35	2	4	6	9	15	20	23
35–49	123	7.9	53	3	4	6	9	15	18	38
50–64	110	8.2	63	2	4	6	8	21	32	32
65+	62	14.4	202	3	5	9	17	37	45	75
TOTAL SINGLE DX	134	4.4	4	2	3	4	6	6	8	9
MULTIPLE DX	566	9.2	92	3	4	7	10	20	25	52
TOTAL										
0–19 Years	264	7.8	84	2	3	5	8	15	21	63
20–34	94	6.1	17	3	3	6	6	10	15	22
35–49	151	7.1	44	3	3	5	8	13	17	38
50–64	123	7.9	58	2	3	6	7	19	31	32
65+	68	13.9	194	3	5	9	16	31	45	75
GRAND TOTAL	700	7.7	70	2	3	6	8	15	22	45

02.12: REP CEREBRAL MENING NEC. Formerly included in operation group(s) 505.

Type of Patients	Observed Patients	Avg. Stay	Vari-ance	Percentiles						
				10th	25th	50th	75th	90th	95th	99th
1. SINGLE DX										
0–19 Years	63	3.7	7	1	2	3	4	8	8	19
20–34	18	5.1	2	3	3	6	6	6	6	7
35–49	28	4.2	4	3	3	3	6	8	8	9
50–64	13	5.5	2	3	5	6	6	7	8	8
65+	6	5.7	6	3	4	4	8	8	9	9
2. MULTIPLE DX										
0–19 Years	181	9.9	118	3	4	7	10	21	26	72
20–34	69	7.4	36	2	3	6	9	15	20	23
35–49	116	7.7	49	3	4	6	9	13	18	38
50–64	104	7.6	58	2	3	6	7	15	32	32
65+	60	12.3	144	3	5	9	16	22	31	75
TOTAL SINGLE DX	128	4.5	5	2	3	4	6	6	8	9
MULTIPLE DX	530	8.9	87	2	4	7	9	19	25	52
TOTAL										
0–19 Years	244	8.0	93	2	3	6	8	17	23	72
20–34	87	6.0	16	3	3	6	6	9	15	23
35–49	144	6.8	41	3	3	5	8	13	16	38
50–64	117	7.4	52	2	3	6	7	14	32	32
65+	66	11.9	137	3	5	8	16	22	31	75
GRAND TOTAL	658	7.5	66	2	3	6	8	15	21	39

02.2: VENTRICULOSTOMY. Formerly included in operation group(s) 504.

Type of Patients	Observed Patients	Avg. Stay	Vari-ance	Percentiles						
				10th	25th	50th	75th	90th	95th	99th
1. SINGLE DX										
0–19 Years	91	3.1	15	1	1	2	3	6	9	25
20–34	22	7.6	29	1	3	7	13	13	13	20
35–49	19	3.5	12	1	1	2	5	6	6	21
50–64	11	4.9	37	1	1	1	7	16	16	16
65+	12	5.6	40	1	1	1	7	19	19	19
2. MULTIPLE DX										
0–19 Years	466	14.4	337	1	3	8	17	40	69	>99
20–34	180	16.5	233	2	6	12	22	35	45	95
35–49	284	17.4	269	2	4	11	27	46	53	65
50–64	312	21.4	230	3	7	18	37	37	39	59
65+	305	17.5	207	4	7	12	23	42	42	52
TOTAL SINGLE DX	155	4.2	23	1	1	2	5	13	14	20
MULTIPLE DX	1547	17.4	274	2	5	12	26	39	48	94
TOTAL										
0–19 Years	557	12.6	302	1	2	7	16	34	60	>99
20–34	202	14.8	207	2	5	12	19	33	39	73
35–49	303	16.8	266	2	3	10	26	46	53	65
50–64	323	21.1	231	3	7	18	37	37	38	55
65+	317	17.0	206	3	6	11	22	42	42	52
GRAND TOTAL	1702	16.2	265	2	4	11	22	37	46	89

02.3: EXTRACRANIAL VENT SHUNT. Formerly included in operation group(s) 504.

Type of Patients	Observed Patients	Avg. Stay	Vari-ance	Percentiles						
				10th	25th	50th	75th	90th	95th	99th
1. SINGLE DX										
0–19 Years	479	2.7	5	1	1	2	3	5	6	14
20–34	52	3.1	7	1	2	2	4	5	7	18
35–49	48	3.5	5	1	2	3	4	5	6	13
50–64	53	3.3	7	2	2	2	3	7	10	13
65+	132	5.0	7	2	3	5	7	7	8	14
2. MULTIPLE DX										
0–19 Years	1428	10.2	201	2	2	5	13	28	45	>99
20–34	250	10.6	150	2	3	6	13	30	43	53
35–49	323	10.8	159	2	3	7	12	23	41	64
50–64	425	12.1	183	2	4	6	16	41	44	47
65+	1181	8.7	79	2	3	6	10	21	26	43
TOTAL SINGLE DX	764	3.3	7	1	2	3	4	7	7	14
MULTIPLE DX	3607	10.0	154	2	3	5	12	24	39	91
TOTAL										
0–19 Years	1907	8.4	164	1	2	4	9	22	39	>99
20–34	302	9.3	134	2	3	5	10	25	39	53
35–49	371	9.9	146	2	3	5	11	21	35	64
50–64	478	11.3	173	2	3	5	14	35	44	47
65+	1313	8.2	72	2	3	6	9	20	24	40
GRAND TOTAL	4371	8.8	134	2	3	5	10	22	34	82

Length of Stay by Diagnosis and Operation, United States, 1997

United States, October 1995–September 1996 Data, by Operation

02.34: VENT SHUNT TO ABD CAVITY. Formerly included in operation group(s) 504.

Type of Patients	Observed Patients	Avg. Stay	Vari-ance	10th	25th	50th	75th	90th	95th	99th
1. SINGLE DX										
0–19 Years	458	2.5	4	1	1	2	3	4	5	9
20–34	49	3.0	7	1	1	2	3	5	7	18
35–49	43	3.6	5	1	2	3	5	5	6	13
50–64	51	3.3	6	2	2	3	3	5	10	13
65+	128	5.1	7	2	3	5	7	7	8	14
2. MULTIPLE DX										
0–19 Years	1256	9.8	204	1	2	4	11	28	48	>99
20–34	212	10.4	159	1	3	5	13	33	47	63
35–49	268	9.8	152	2	3	6	11	19	40	64
50–64	378	11.7	177	2	3	5	15	41	44	47
65+	1085	8.4	75	2	3	5	10	20	24	40
TOTAL SINGLE DX	729	3.2	6	1	2	3	4	7	7	12
MULTIPLE DX	3199	9.5	151	2	3	5	11	24	40	91
TOTAL										
0–19 Years	1714	7.9	161	1	2	3	8	23	39	>99
20–34	261	9.0	139	2	3	4	10	20	43	53
35–49	311	9.0	137	2	3	5	11	18	35	60
50–64	429	10.8	166	2	3	5	12	33	44	47
65+	1213	8.0	67	2	3	5	8	19	24	36
GRAND TOTAL	3928	8.3	129	2	2	4	9	21	33	82

02.4: VENT SHUNT REV/RMVL. Formerly included in operation group(s) 505.

Type of Patients	Observed Patients	Avg. Stay	Vari-ance	10th	25th	50th	75th	90th	95th	99th
1. SINGLE DX										
0–19 Years	768	2.8	9	1	1	2	3	5	8	16
20–34	82	2.7	4	1	2	2	3	4	6	13
35–49	22	3.3	9	1	1	2	5	9	8	11
50–64	10	1.9	11	2	2	1	5	9	8	24
65+	17	3.3	3	1	2	3	5	6	6	6
2. MULTIPLE DX										
0–19 Years	4040	5.9	78	1	2	3	6	14	22	46
20–34	570	6.2	61	1	2	3	8	14	23	36
35–49	315	8.7	107	1	3	5	10	28	35	49
50–64	191	8.9	115	2	3	7	10	21	26	57
65+	355	9.0	115	2	3	6	10	20	33	48
TOTAL SINGLE DX	899	2.8	9	1	2	2	3	5	8	16
MULTIPLE DX	5471	6.3	82	1	2	3	7	15	23	46
TOTAL										
0–19 Years	4808	5.4	69	1	2	2	5	13	20	42
20–34	652	5.8	56	1	2	3	7	14	18	36
35–49	337	8.4	103	1	2	5	9	24	35	49
50–64	201	7.9	106	1	3	5	9	19	24	57
65+	372	8.8	112	1	2	6	10	18	33	48
GRAND TOTAL	6370	5.9	73	1	2	3	6	14	22	43

02.42: REPL VENTRICULAR SHUNT. Formerly included in operation group(s) 505.

Type of Patients	Observed Patients	Avg. Stay	Vari-ance	10th	25th	50th	75th	90th	95th	99th
1. SINGLE DX										
0–19 Years	726	2.6	7	1	1	2	3	4	6	11
20–34	74	2.7	4	1	1	2	3	4	6	13
35–49	22	3.3	9	1	2	2	5	5	9	11
50–64	7	4.8	43	2	2	2	3	8	24	24
65+	15	3.2	3	1	2	3	4	6	6	6
2. MULTIPLE DX										
0–19 Years	3606	4.7	57	1	2	2	4	11	18	39
20–34	496	5.5	48	1	3	3	7	12	18	33
35–49	257	6.1	63	1	3	5	6	12	17	44
50–64	155	8.1	92	2	3	5	9	19	26	57
65+	295	8.1	110	2	3	5	9	15	26	48
TOTAL SINGLE DX	844	2.7	7	1	1	2	3	4	6	12
MULTIPLE DX	4809	5.1	60	1	2	3	5	11	18	40
TOTAL										
0–19 Years	4332	4.4	49	1	2	2	4	9	16	39
20–34	570	5.2	44	1	2	3	6	11	17	32
35–49	279	5.9	60	2	2	4	5	12	16	44
50–64	162	8.0	90	1	3	5	9	19	24	57
65+	310	7.9	106	2	3	5	9	14	24	48
GRAND TOTAL	5653	4.8	53	1	2	2	5	10	17	39

02.43: RMVL VENTRICULAR SHUNT. Formerly included in operation group(s) 505.

Type of Patients	Observed Patients	Avg. Stay	Vari-ance	10th	25th	50th	75th	90th	95th	99th
1. SINGLE DX										
0–19 Years	41	5.9	29	1	1	4	9	16	16	23
20–34	7	2.1	<1	1	2	2	3	3	3	3
35–49	0									
50–64	3	1.3	3	2	2	1	1	1	1	12
65+	2	4.4	5	2	2	6	6	6	6	6
2. MULTIPLE DX										
0–19 Years	423	14.4	146	5	8	12	16	26	36	69
20–34	72	13.4	146	4	5	10	17	27	39	>99
35–49	57	15.3	162	2	6	10	35	35	35	51
50–64	36	13.2	226	4	5	10	14	24	26	86
65+	59	12.7	121	4	5	10	15	31	36	37
TOTAL SINGLE DX	53	4.3	24	1	1	1	7	13	16	16
MULTIPLE DX	647	14.3	148	4	8	11	17	28	35	69
TOTAL										
0–19 Years	464	13.7	142	3	8	11	16	24	33	62
20–34	79	12.6	144	2	5	10	17	26	38	>99
35–49	57	15.3	162	2	6	10	35	35	35	51
50–64	39	7.5	155	1	1	4	10	16	26	86
65+	61	12.6	120	3	5	10	15	30	36	37
GRAND TOTAL	700	13.4	145	2	6	10	16	26	35	69

Length of Stay by Diagnosis and Operation, United States, 1997

United States, October 1995–September 1996 Data, by Operation

02.9: SKULL & BRAIN OPS NEC. Formerly included in operation group(s) 505.

Type of Patients	Observed Patients	Avg. Stay	Variance	Percentiles						
				10th	25th	50th	75th	90th	95th	99th
1. SINGLE DX										
0–19 Years	132	6.7	71	2	2	4	8	14	20	51
20–34	194	5.2	14	1	3	4	6	10	13	18
35–49	162	6.0	19	2	2	6	7	11	14	20
50–64	40	4.6	12	1	2	4	5	10	13	13
65+	18	3.4	7	1	1	3	6	7	9	9
2. MULTIPLE DX										
0–19 Years	296	8.7	67	2	4	6	11	15	20	48
20–34	413	8.2	102	2	3	5	9	18	24	45
35–49	401	9.9	61	3	4	7	14	19	26	40
50–64	196	8.0	50	2	3	6	10	16	21	40
65+	255	10.5	87	2	5	8	14	21	30	>99
TOTAL SINGLE DX	546	5.8	33	2	2	4	7	11	15	24
MULTIPLE DX	1561	9.1	77	2	4	7	11	18	25	48
TOTAL										
0–19 Years	428	8.1	69	2	3	6	11	15	20	51
20–34	607	7.4	79	2	3	5	8	15	21	41
35–49	563	8.7	51	2	4	7	11	16	24	34
50–64	236	7.5	45	2	3	6	9	13	20	32
65+	273	10.1	86	2	4	7	13	20	30	>99
GRAND TOTAL	2107	8.2	68	2	3	6	11	16	22	47

02.96: INSERT SPHENOID ELECTROD. Formerly included in operation group(s) 505.

Type of Patients	Observed Patients	Avg. Stay	Variance	Percentiles						
				10th	25th	50th	75th	90th	95th	99th
1. SINGLE DX										
0–19 Years	52	5.8	22	2	3	4	7	10	19	21
20–34	110	5.8	10	3	4	5	7	10	12	18
35–49	96	6.1	7	3	4	6	7	8	10	16
50–64	20	5.3	5	2	4	5	7	9	9	10
65+	2	4.0	0	4	4	4	4	4	4	4
2. MULTIPLE DX										
0–19 Years	90	7.8	160	2	3	5	7	11	21	80
20–34	130	6.4	10	3	4	6	7	10	12	17
35–49	150	7.0	20	3	4	6	8	13	16	24
50–64	38	6.6	14	3	5	5	9	11	14	21
65+	7	5.8	3	4	5	6	7	8	8	8
TOTAL SINGLE DX	280	5.9	11	3	4	5	7	9	11	19
MULTIPLE DX	415	7.0	54	3	4	6	8	11	15	38
TOTAL										
0–19 Years	142	7.1	112	2	3	5	7	10	20	80
20–34	240	6.1	10	3	4	5	7	10	12	18
35–49	246	6.6	14	3	4	6	7	10	15	23
50–64	58	6.2	11	3	4	5	8	10	12	21
65+	9	5.6	3	4	4	6	7	8	8	8
GRAND TOTAL	695	6.5	36	3	4	6	7	10	14	23

02.94: INSERT/REPL SKULL TONGS. Formerly included in operation group(s) 505.

Type of Patients	Observed Patients	Avg. Stay	Variance	Percentiles						
				10th	25th	50th	75th	90th	95th	99th
1. SINGLE DX										
0–19 Years	30	4.1	5	1	3	4	6	7	7	10
20–34	51	2.9	4	1	1	2	4	4	6	13
35–49	36	2.7	4	1	2	2	3	6	8	11
50–64	11	5.0	21	1	1	4	7	13	13	13
65+	10	3.7	8	1	1	3	5	9	9	9
2. MULTIPLE DX										
0–19 Years	111	8.3	40	3	6	6	11	15	15	31
20–34	222	8.0	138	1	2	4	8	20	26	82
35–49	195	10.9	76	3	4	8	16	19	27	48
50–64	131	8.3	61	2	3	6	10	17	20	40
65+	221	10.5	95	3	5	8	12	27	33	>99
TOTAL SINGLE DX	138	3.3	6	1	2	2	4	7	8	13
MULTIPLE DX	880	9.3	86	2	4	6	11	18	27	50
TOTAL										
0–19 Years	141	7.8	37	2	4	6	11	13	15	26
20–34	273	7.0	116	1	2	4	7	15	22	49
35–49	231	9.3	73	2	3	6	14	19	26	43
50–64	142	7.9	57	2	3	6	10	16	20	40
65+	231	10.3	93	2	5	8	12	27	31	>99
GRAND TOTAL	1018	8.4	79	2	3	6	11	16	24	48

03.0: SPINAL CANAL EXPLORATION. Formerly included in operation group(s) 506.

Type of Patients	Observed Patients	Avg. Stay	Variance	Percentiles						
				10th	25th	50th	75th	90th	95th	99th
1. SINGLE DX										
0–19 Years	127	4.0	7	2	3	3	5	7	9	13
20–34	445	2.4	5	1	1	2	3	5	6	10
35–49	1384	2.2	2	1	1	2	3	4	5	8
50–64	1404	2.4	3	1	2	2	3	4	5	8
65+	1079	2.9	3	1	2	3	4	5	6	8
2. MULTIPLE DX										
0–19 Years	428	11.3	223	2	3	5	10	44	50	50
20–34	764	5.0	33	1	2	3	6	11	15	25
35–49	3105	4.0	18	1	2	3	5	7	11	23
50–64	5476	4.2	17	1	3	3	5	8	11	22
65+	11242	5.5	36	2	3	4	6	10	14	30
TOTAL SINGLE DX	4439	2.5	3	1	1	2	3	4	5	9
MULTIPLE DX	21015	5.0	34	1	2	4	6	9	13	30
TOTAL										
0–19 Years	555	9.8	188	2	3	5	8	27	50	50
20–34	1209	3.9	24	1	1	3	4	8	13	23
35–49	4489	3.4	13	1	2	3	4	6	9	19
50–64	6880	3.7	14	1	2	3	4	7	10	20
65+	12321	5.2	34	2	2	4	6	9	14	30
GRAND TOTAL	25454	4.5	29	1	2	3	5	8	12	26

Length of Stay by Diagnosis and Operation, United States, 1997

United States, October 1995–September 1996 Data, by Operation

03.1: INTRASPIN NERVE ROOT DIV. Formerly included in operation group(s) 507.

Type of Patients	Observed Patients	Avg. Stay	Vari-ance	10th	25th	50th	75th	90th	95th	99th
1. SINGLE DX										
0–19 Years	75	6.7	22	3	5	6	7	9	9	31
20–34	7	5.5	14	1	1	7	7	7	14	14
35–49	11	2.4	2	1	1	2	3	4	5	5
50–64	5	2.2	1	1	1	2	3	4	4	4
65+	0									
2. MULTIPLE DX										
0–19 Years	137	7.9	40	5	5	6	7	10	20	46
20–34	10	3.9	3	2	2	4	4	7	7	8
35–49	17	4.0	6	2	2	4	4	9	9	10
50–64	19	8.9	42	1	4	9	13	13	13	38
65+	20	7.2	32	1	3	6	8	19	19	25
TOTAL SINGLE DX	98	6.1	21	3	4	6	7	9	9	31
MULTIPLE DX	203	7.4	37	3	5	6	7	12	20	38
TOTAL										
0–19 Years	212	7.5	35	4	5	6	7	10	20	37
20–34	17	4.3	7	1	1	4	7	7	7	14
35–49	28	3.4	5	1	2	3	4	6	9	10
50–64	24	7.4	41	1	3	8	13	13	13	38
65+	20	7.2	32	1	3	6	8	19	19	25
GRAND TOTAL	301	7.0	32	3	4	6	7	10	19	31

03.2: CHORDOTOMY. Formerly included in operation group(s) 507.

Type of Patients	Observed Patients	Avg. Stay	Vari-ance	10th	25th	50th	75th	90th	95th	99th
1. SINGLE DX										
0–19 Years	6	2.6	<1	2	2	2	3	4	4	4
20–34	0									
35–49	2	6.4	2	3	7	7	7	7	7	7
50–64	1	5.0	0	5	5	5	5	5	5	5
65+	0									
2. MULTIPLE DX										
0–19 Years	48	5.5	7	3	4	5	6	10	11	13
20–34	7	10.8	106	3	3	6	21	29	29	29
35–49	18	11.1	300	4	4	4	8	19	44	80
50–64	11	6.2	24	2	2	3	6	13	21	21
65+	11	6.3	26	3	3	3	9	14	19	19
TOTAL SINGLE DX	9	4.0	4	2	2	3	7	7	7	7
MULTIPLE DX	95	7.2	81	2	3	5	7	13	19	44
TOTAL										
0–19 Years	54	5.0	7	2	3	5	6	10	11	13
20–34	7	10.8	106	3	3	6	21	29	29	29
35–49	20	10.2	247	4	4	6	8	19	44	80
50–64	12	6.2	23	3	3	6	6	13	15	21
65+	11	6.3	26	3	3	3	9	14	19	19
GRAND TOTAL	104	6.9	73	2	3	5	7	12	19	44

03.02: REOPEN LAMINECTOMY SITE. Formerly included in operation group(s) 506.

Type of Patients	Observed Patients	Avg. Stay	Vari-ance	10th	25th	50th	75th	90th	95th	99th
1. SINGLE DX										
0–19 Years	0									
20–34	32	1.7	1	1	1	1	2	3	3	8
35–49	62	2.3	3	1	1	1	4	5	5	6
50–64	34	1.8	2	1	1	1	2	4	4	7
65+	15	2.4	2	1	2	2	3	4	6	6
2. MULTIPLE DX										
0–19 Years	13	10.4	104	3	4	7	11	34	34	34
20–34	62	5.5	12	1	4	5	6	10	14	16
35–49	215	4.8	17	1	3	4	5	9	12	24
50–64	208	4.6	14	1	2	3	5	10	12	19
65+	241	8.0	37	2	4	6	13	14	14	21
TOTAL SINGLE DX	143	2.1	2	1	1	1	3	4	5	7
MULTIPLE DX	739	5.8	25	2	3	4	7	13	14	22
TOTAL										
0–19 Years	13	10.4	104	3	4	7	11	34	34	34
20–34	94	3.6	10	1	1	3	5	7	10	15
35–49	277	4.1	14	1	2	3	5	9	11	23
50–64	242	4.2	13	1	2	3	5	9	11	19
65+	256	7.7	36	2	4	6	12	14	14	21
GRAND TOTAL	882	5.0	22	1	2	4	6	12	14	21

03.09: SPINAL CANAL EXPLOR NEC. Formerly included in operation group(s) 506.

Type of Patients	Observed Patients	Avg. Stay	Vari-ance	10th	25th	50th	75th	90th	95th	99th
1. SINGLE DX										
0–19 Years	123	4.0	7	2	3	3	5	7	9	13
20–34	411	2.4	5	1	1	2	3	5	6	10
35–49	1321	2.2	2	1	1	2	3	4	5	8
50–64	1370	2.4	3	1	2	2	3	4	5	8
65+	1064	2.9	3	1	2	3	4	5	6	8
2. MULTIPLE DX										
0–19 Years	398	7.3	81	2	3	5	7	16	21	67
20–34	685	4.8	34	1	2	3	6	9	15	25
35–49	2873	3.9	17	1	2	3	5	7	11	23
50–64	5258	4.1	17	1	2	3	5	8	11	22
65+	10996	5.4	36	2	3	4	6	11	14	30
TOTAL SINGLE DX	4289	2.5	3	1	1	2	3	4	5	9
MULTIPLE DX	20210	4.9	30	1	2	4	6	9	13	27
TOTAL										
0–19 Years	521	6.5	66	2	3	5	7	13	18	40
20–34	1096	3.9	24	1	1	2	4	7	12	23
35–49	4194	3.3	13	1	2	3	4	6	9	18
50–64	6628	3.7	14	1	2	4	6	7	9	20
65+	12060	5.2	33	2	3	4	6	9	13	30
GRAND TOTAL	24499	4.4	25	1	2	3	5	8	11	24

Length of Stay by Diagnosis and Operation, United States, 1997

United States, October 1995–September 1996 Data, by Operation

03.3: DXTIC PX ON SPINAL CANAL. Formerly included in operation group(s) 507, 512.

Type of Patients	Observed Patients	Avg. Stay	Vari-ance	10th	25th	50th	75th	90th	95th	99th
1. SINGLE DX										
0–19 Years	11391	3.0	6	1	2	3	3	5	7	11
20–34	1537	3.2	5	1	2	3	4	6	7	12
35–49	937	3.1	6	1	2	2	4	6	7	11
50–64	271	3.9	9	1	2	4	5	8	8	14
65+	122	4.7	18	1	2	3	6	9	11	19
2. MULTIPLE DX										
0–19 Years	36725	5.1	40	2	2	3	6	10	14	36
20–34	6283	5.4	32	1	2	3	7	10	15	28
35–49	7566	6.5	44	2	3	4	8	13	19	34
50–64	4675	7.2	44	2	3	5	9	15	19	32
65+	8282	9.0	69	2	4	7	11	17	24	44
TOTAL SINGLE DX	14258	3.0	6	1	2	3	3	5	7	11
MULTIPLE DX	63531	5.9	45	2	2	4	7	12	16	35
TOTAL										
0–19 Years	48116	4.6	32	2	2	3	5	9	12	30
20–34	7820	4.9	27	1	2	3	6	10	13	26
35–49	8503	6.0	40	1	2	4	7	12	17	32
50–64	4946	7.0	42	2	3	5	9	15	18	32
65+	8404	9.0	68	2	4	7	11	17	24	44
GRAND TOTAL	77789	5.4	38	2	2	3	6	11	15	32

03.31: SPINAL TAP. Formerly included in operation group(s) 512.

Type of Patients	Observed Patients	Avg. Stay	Vari-ance	10th	25th	50th	75th	90th	95th	99th
1. SINGLE DX										
0–19 Years	11388	3.0	6	1	2	3	3	5	7	11
20–34	1534	3.2	5	1	2	3	4	6	7	12
35–49	930	3.1	6	1	2	2	4	5	7	11
50–64	265	3.9	9	1	2	4	5	8	8	14
65+	120	4.7	18	1	2	3	6	9	11	19
2. MULTIPLE DX										
0–19 Years	36689	5.1	39	2	2	3	6	10	14	35
20–34	6257	5.4	31	1	2	3	7	10	15	28
35–49	7507	6.4	43	2	3	4	7	13	19	34
50–64	4609	7.2	44	2	3	5	9	15	19	32
65+	8176	9.0	68	2	4	7	11	17	24	44
TOTAL SINGLE DX	14237	3.0	6	1	2	3	3	5	7	11
MULTIPLE DX	63238	5.9	45	2	2	4	7	12	16	35
TOTAL										
0–19 Years	48077	4.6	32	2	2	3	5	9	12	29
20–34	7791	4.9	26	1	2	3	6	10	13	26
35–49	8437	6.0	40	1	2	4	7	12	17	32
50–64	4874	7.0	42	2	3	5	9	15	18	32
65+	8296	8.9	68	2	4	7	11	17	24	44
GRAND TOTAL	77475	5.3	38	2	2	3	6	11	15	32

03.4: EXC SPINAL CORD LESION. Formerly included in operation group(s) 507.

Type of Patients	Observed Patients	Avg. Stay	Vari-ance	10th	25th	50th	75th	90th	95th	99th
1. SINGLE DX										
0–19 Years	93	4.9	7	2	3	4	6	7	11	15
20–34	82	4.0	10	1	2	3	4	9	9	18
35–49	133	5.3	14	2	3	3	5	8	10	18
50–64	97	3.0	5	1	1	3	4	6	6	9
65+	52	3.8	6	2	2	3	4	6	9	15
2. MULTIPLE DX										
0–19 Years	306	7.3	51	2	4	5	8	14	19	46
20–34	164	7.5	58	3	4	5	8	15	17	39
35–49	375	6.7	45	2	3	5	7	12	18	41
50–64	480	7.6	69	2	3	5	9	15	22	55
65+	609	8.0	46	2	3	6	11	16	23	32
TOTAL SINGLE DX	457	4.2	9	1	2	4	5	7	9	18
MULTIPLE DX	1934	7.5	53	2	3	5	9	15	21	41
TOTAL										
0–19 Years	399	6.7	41	2	3	5	7	13	15	46
20–34	246	6.2	44	2	3	4	7	11	16	29
35–49	508	6.5	40	2	3	5	7	11	18	32
50–64	577	6.7	60	1	3	5	8	13	21	55
65+	661	7.6	44	2	3	5	10	16	22	32
GRAND TOTAL	2391	6.8	46	2	3	5	8	14	19	35

03.5: SPINAL CORD PLASTIC OPS. Formerly included in operation group(s) 507.

Type of Patients	Observed Patients	Avg. Stay	Vari-ance	10th	25th	50th	75th	90th	95th	99th
1. SINGLE DX										
0–19 Years	144	4.7	7	2	3	4	5	8	9	14
20–34	51	4.5	4	2	4	4	6	7	8	11
35–49	71	6.0	19	3	4	5	7	10	11	16
50–64	27	9.4	367	5	5	3	6	9	77	77
65+	9	5.5	3	5	5	5	5	6	11	11
2. MULTIPLE DX										
0–19 Years	793	10.3	127	3	4	6	12	27	38	51
20–34	239	8.2	58	2	4	5	9	17	20	41
35–49	282	9.1	94	2	4	7	11	17	25	69
50–64	208	7.4	46	1	3	6	11	15	17	26
65+	211	10.5	68	3	5	7	17	23	23	29
TOTAL SINGLE DX	302	5.3	35	2	3	4	6	9	11	16
MULTIPLE DX	1733	9.5	96	2	4	6	11	21	32	51
TOTAL										
0–19 Years	937	9.5	115	3	4	5	10	23	38	51
20–34	290	7.7	53	2	4	5	9	17	18	39
35–49	353	8.4	79	2	4	6	10	16	21	64
50–64	235	7.6	73	2	3	5	11	15	17	43
65+	220	10.3	66	3	5	7	15	22	23	29
GRAND TOTAL	2035	8.9	90	2	4	6	10	19	28	48

Length of Stay by Diagnosis and Operation, United States, 1997

United States, October 1995–September 1996 Data, by Operation

03.53: VERTEBRAL FX REPAIR. Formerly included in operation group(s) 507.

Type of Patients	Observed Patients	Avg. Stay	Vari-ance	10th	25th	50th	75th	90th	95th	99th
1. SINGLE DX										
0–19 Years	16	6.8	26	2	2	5	14	14	15	15
20–34	34	4.1	6	1	2	4	5	6	7	8
35–49	19	6.4	45	3	4	5	6	9	16	11
50–64	6	28.8	>999	2	4	5	77	77	77	77
65+	2	5.5	1	3	6	6	6	6	6	6
2. MULTIPLE DX										
0–19 Years	79	10.3	119	3	5	7	10	18	39	48
20–34	162	9.4	71	3	5	7	12	17	23	41
35–49	133	13.0	156	4	7	9	15	24	38	69
50–64	74	7.6	67	1	3	6	10	15	18	40
65+	101	12.9	85	1	5	11	21	23	23	38
TOTAL SINGLE DX	77	7.1	138	2	3	5	6	11	14	77
MULTIPLE DX	549	10.6	96	3	5	8	14	21	25	48
TOTAL										
0–19 Years	95	9.7	104	2	5	7	10	17	30	48
20–34	196	8.9	67	2	5	6	11	17	22	41
35–49	152	12.2	146	4	6	8	14	23	38	69
50–64	80	8.5	129	1	3	6	10	15	19	77
65+	103	12.8	84	1	5	11	21	23	23	38
GRAND TOTAL	626	10.3	101	2	5	7	13	21	25	61

03.59: SPINAL STRUCT REPAIR NEC. Formerly included in operation group(s) 507.

Type of Patients	Observed Patients	Avg. Stay	Vari-ance	10th	25th	50th	75th	90th	95th	99th
1. SINGLE DX										
0–19 Years	98	3.9	2	2	3	4	5	5	6	7
20–34	10	5.0	1	4	4	4	6	6	6	7
35–49	40	6.0	14	2	3	5	8	11	16	16
50–64	13	4.9	8	2	3	4	9	9	9	10
65+	5	5.0	<1	5	5	5	5	5	5	9
2. MULTIPLE DX										
0–19 Years	435	5.3	20	2	3	4	6	7	11	30
20–34	65	5.9	22	2	3	5	6	12	15	27
35–49	116	5.9	20	2	2	5	7	11	15	25
50–64	104	7.4	27	2	3	6	11	14	16	21
65+	94	7.5	34	3	5	6	9	13	18	28
TOTAL SINGLE DX	166	4.6	5	2	3	4	5	6	9	16
MULTIPLE DX	814	5.8	23	2	3	5	6	11	14	29
TOTAL										
0–19 Years	533	5.1	18	2	3	4	5	7	10	30
20–34	75	5.7	18	2	4	5	6	10	14	25
35–49	156	5.9	19	2	3	5	7	11	15	25
50–64	117	7.2	26	2	3	6	11	14	16	20
65+	99	7.2	31	3	5	5	8	12	18	28
GRAND TOTAL	980	5.6	21	2	3	4	6	10	13	27

03.6: SPINAL CORD ADHESIOLYSIS. Formerly included in operation group(s) 507.

Type of Patients	Observed Patients	Avg. Stay	Vari-ance	10th	25th	50th	75th	90th	95th	99th
1. SINGLE DX										
0–19 Years	10	3.3	2	2	2	3	4	4	7	7
20–34	13	2.1	2	1	1	2	2	3	5	5
35–49	16	2.2	<1	1	2	2	2	3	3	8
50–64	10	2.5	2	1	1	2	4	5	6	6
65+	2	1.4	<1	1	1	1	2	2	2	2
2. MULTIPLE DX										
0–19 Years	26	6.4	35	3	3	5	7	9	21	32
20–34	18	4.1	6	1	2	5	7	7	9	9
35–49	67	4.2	32	2	2	3	4	6	11	39
50–64	49	4.7	16	1	2	4	6	11	15	17
65+	40	6.5	10	2	3	8	8	8	10	14
TOTAL SINGLE DX	51	2.4	2	1	2	2	3	4	5	7
MULTIPLE DX	200	5.2	21	2	2	4	8	8	11	26
TOTAL										
0–19 Years	36	5.3	26	2	3	4	5	9	11	32
20–34	31	3.2	5	2	2	3	4	7	7	9
35–49	83	3.7	25	2	2	3	3	5	9	39
50–64	59	4.3	14	1	2	3	6	8	12	17
65+	42	6.4	10	2	3	8	8	8	10	14
GRAND TOTAL	251	4.7	18	2	2	3	7	8	10	21

03.7: SPINAL THECAL SHUNT. Formerly included in operation group(s) 507.

Type of Patients	Observed Patients	Avg. Stay	Vari-ance	10th	25th	50th	75th	90th	95th	99th
1. SINGLE DX										
0–19 Years	13	4.7	1	3	5	5	5	5	5	5
20–34	30	3.0	7	1	1	2	4	7	7	13
35–49	16	5.7	8	2	3	7	7	7	9	15
50–64	8	4.3	11	1	1	6	6	10	10	10
65+	7	2.4	1	1	2	3	3	4	4	4
2. MULTIPLE DX										
0–19 Years	84	5.6	52	1	2	3	6	16	20	68
20–34	77	5.7	11	2	3	7	7	9	9	15
35–49	90	6.1	27	2	2	4	8	10	18	25
50–64	47	12.3	88	3	3	7	23	23	23	42
65+	77	10.3	97	2	4	6	14	26	34	34
TOTAL SINGLE DX	74	4.5	4	1	3	5	5	7	7	12
MULTIPLE DX	375	7.6	56	2	3	6	8	20	23	34
TOTAL										
0–19 Years	97	5.2	31	1	2	5	5	9	20	28
20–34	107	5.3	11	2	3	6	7	7	9	15
35–49	106	6.0	23	2	3	6	7	10	18	25
50–64	55	11.8	86	2	3	6	23	23	23	23
65+	84	10.0	95	1	3	6	14	22	34	34
GRAND TOTAL	449	6.9	47	2	3	5	7	15	23	34

Length of Stay by Diagnosis and Operation, United States, 1997

United States, October 1995–September 1996 Data, by Operation

03.71: SUBARACH-PERITON SHUNT. Formerly included in operation group(s) 507.

Type of Patients	Observed Patients	Avg. Stay	Vari-ance	10th	25th	50th	75th	90th	95th	99th
1. SINGLE DX										
0–19 Years	7	4.8	<1	5	5	5	5	5	5	5
20–34	21	2.7	9	1	1	1	3	7	11	13
35–49	13	4.2	13	1	2	3	4	9	12	15
50–64	5	4.2	13	1	1	6	6	10	10	15
65+	6	2.2	<1	1	1	2	3	3	3	3
2. MULTIPLE DX										
0–19 Years	38	3.8	29	1	2	2	4	9	18	>99
20–34	49	5.9	11	2	4	7	7	9	11	14
35–49	38	5.7	43	2	2	2	9	18	18	34
50–64	28	14.3	89	3	3	23	23	23	23	23
65+	48	11.1	127	1	2	6	16	34	34	34
TOTAL SINGLE DX	52	4.4	4	1	3	5	5	5	6	12
MULTIPLE DX	201	7.7	65	1	2	5	7	23	23	34
TOTAL										
0–19 Years	45	4.3	14	1	2	5	5	5	8	21
20–34	70	5.4	12	1	2	7	7	7	7	14
35–49	51	5.4	36	1	2	3	8	14	18	34
50–64	33	13.6	90	2	3	16	23	23	23	23
65+	54	10.4	123	1	2	6	15	29	34	34
GRAND TOTAL	253	6.8	50	1	2	5	7	21	23	34

03.9: SPINAL CORD OPS NEC. Formerly included in operation group(s) 507, 512.

Type of Patients	Observed Patients	Avg. Stay	Vari-ance	10th	25th	50th	75th	90th	95th	99th
1. SINGLE DX										
0–19 Years	136	2.1	3	1	1	2	2	4	4	13
20–34	863	2.1	5	1	1	2	2	4	5	9
35–49	747	2.8	4	1	1	2	2	5	7	10
50–64	336	3.1	5	1	1	2	4	6	7	12
65+	219	3.3	7	1	1	3	4	6	9	12
2. MULTIPLE DX										
0–19 Years	327	4.7	28	1	1	3	6	9	17	32
20–34	1281	3.9	16	1	2	3	4	8	11	22
35–49	2392	4.8	21	1	2	3	4	9	14	23
50–64	2050	5.4	19	2	3	4	7	10	13	24
65+	4598	6.7	28	2	3	5	9	13	16	26
TOTAL SINGLE DX	2301	2.6	5	1	1	2	3	5	6	10
MULTIPLE DX	10648	5.5	24	1	2	4	7	11	15	24
TOTAL										
0–19 Years	463	3.8	21	1	1	2	4	7	13	31
20–34	2144	3.2	12	1	1	3	4	6	9	19
35–49	3139	4.3	18	1	2	3	5	8	12	20
50–64	2386	5.1	18	2	2	4	6	10	13	21
65+	4817	6.5	28	2	3	5	9	13	16	26
GRAND TOTAL	12949	4.9	21	1	2	4	6	10	14	23

03.8: DESTR INJECT-SPINE CANAL. Formerly included in operation group(s) 507.

Type of Patients	Observed Patients	Avg. Stay	Vari-ance	10th	25th	50th	75th	90th	95th	99th
1. SINGLE DX										
0–19 Years	18	5.3	2	4	5	5	6	7	7	10
20–34	0									
35–49	0									
50–64	2	4.0	4	1	1	5	5	5	5	5
65+	0									
2. MULTIPLE DX										
0–19 Years	735	4.9	24	2	2	3	5	10	15	26
20–34	29	7.8	42	3	3	6	11	15	27	27
35–49	27	11.2	61	2	5	9	18	24	24	27
50–64	15	18.0	124	5	8	17	22	34	34	45
65+	36	7.7	43	2	3	6	10	18	19	36
TOTAL SINGLE DX	20	5.2	2	4	5	5	6	7	7	10
MULTIPLE DX	842	5.4	30	2	2	3	6	11	17	29
TOTAL										
0–19 Years	753	5.0	24	2	2	3	5	10	15	26
20–34	29	7.8	42	3	3	6	11	15	27	27
35–49	27	11.2	61	2	5	9	18	24	24	27
50–64	17	16.9	129	2	7	17	22	34	34	45
65+	36	7.7	43	2	3	6	10	18	19	36
GRAND TOTAL	862	5.4	29	2	2	3	6	11	17	29

03.90: INSERT SPINAL CANAL CATH. Formerly included in operation group(s) 512.

Type of Patients	Observed Patients	Avg. Stay	Vari-ance	10th	25th	50th	75th	90th	95th	99th
1. SINGLE DX										
0–19 Years	73	2.1	4	1	1	2	2	4	4	13
20–34	426	1.6	<1	1	1	1	2	3	3	5
35–49	175	2.6	6	1	2	2	3	5	8	10
50–64	48	3.8	4	1	2	4	5	6	7	9
65+	45	3.3	8	1	2	3	4	4	6	20
2. MULTIPLE DX										
0–19 Years	97	5.1	32	1	1	3	7	13	17	32
20–34	403	4.3	25	1	2	3	4	10	15	22
35–49	646	5.0	17	2	2	4	6	9	11	25
50–64	531	5.6	22	2	3	4	7	12	14	25
65+	917	8.0	42	2	3	6	12	15	18	31
TOTAL SINGLE DX	767	2.0	3	1	1	2	2	4	5	10
MULTIPLE DX	2594	5.9	30	2	2	4	8	13	17	27
TOTAL										
0–19 Years	170	3.5	19	1	1	2	4	7	13	17
20–34	829	2.8	13	1	1	2	2	5	9	22
35–49	821	4.6	16	2	2	4	6	8	10	23
50–64	579	5.5	21	2	3	4	7	12	14	24
65+	962	7.8	41	2	3	6	12	15	18	31
GRAND TOTAL	3361	4.8	25	1	2	3	6	11	15	25

Length of Stay by Diagnosis and Operation, United States, 1997

United States, October 1995–September 1996 Data, by Operation

03.91: INJECT ANES-SPINAL CANAL. Formerly included in operation group(s) 512.

Type of Patients	Observed Patients	Avg. Stay	Variance	Percentiles						
				10th	25th	50th	75th	90th	95th	99th
1. SINGLE DX										
0–19 Years	34	2.0	2	1	1	2	2	4	4	8
20–34	169	2.5	5	1	1	2	3	5	8	9
35–49	139	3.3	4	1	2	3	5	5	7	9
50–64	77	3.6	3	2	2	4	5	5	6	8
65+	50	4.9	9	2	3	5	6	10	11	11
2. MULTIPLE DX										
0–19 Years	42	3.2	20	1	1	2	2	8	18	18
20–34	238	3.6	10	1	1	2	5	8	10	16
35–49	455	6.0	33	2	2	4	8	14	18	20
50–64	451	6.2	19	2	3	6	7	11	15	20
65+	1223	6.9	28	2	3	5	8	12	17	29
TOTAL SINGLE DX	469	3.0	5	1	1	2	4	5	8	11
MULTIPLE DX	2409	6.0	26	2	3	5	8	12	16	23
TOTAL										
0–19 Years	76	2.8	14	1	1	2	2	4	13	18
20–34	407	3.1	8	1	1	4	4	7	8	15
35–49	594	5.4	28	2	2	4	6	14	18	18
50–64	528	5.7	17	2	3	5	6	10	15	19
65+	1273	6.8	28	2	3	5	8	12	16	29
GRAND TOTAL	2878	5.4	23	1	2	4	7	11	15	21

03.92: INJECT SPINAL CANAL NEC. Formerly included in operation group(s) 512.

Type of Patients	Observed Patients	Avg. Stay	Variance	Percentiles						
				10th	25th	50th	75th	90th	95th	99th
1. SINGLE DX										
0–19 Years	9	2.3	3	1	1	2	3	4	4	8
20–34	117	4.0	25	1	2	3	5	6	10	35
35–49	253	2.9	4	1	1	2	4	5	6	10
50–64	131	2.9	6	1	1	2	4	5	8	12
65+	97	3.2	7	1	1	3	4	7	8	12
2. MULTIPLE DX										
0–19 Years	101	4.8	19	1	3	4	6	6	8	42
20–34	207	3.8	13	2	2	3	4	7	9	25
35–49	644	5.0	24	1	2	4	6	10	15	25
50–64	735	5.4	16	2	3	5	6	10	13	24
65+	2192	6.4	21	2	3	5	8	12	14	22
TOTAL SINGLE DX	607	3.1	8	1	1	2	4	6	7	12
MULTIPLE DX	3879	5.6	20	2	3	4	7	11	14	23
TOTAL										
0–19 Years	110	4.5	18	1	2	4	6	6	8	42
20–34	324	3.9	17	1	2	3	4	7	9	27
35–49	897	4.3	18	1	2	3	5	6	11	19
50–64	866	5.0	15	2	3	5	6	9	12	22
65+	2289	6.2	20	2	3	5	8	12	14	21
GRAND TOTAL	4486	5.2	19	1	2	4	7	10	13	22

03.93: INSERT SPINAL NEUROSTIM. Formerly included in operation group(s) 507.

Type of Patients	Observed Patients	Avg. Stay	Variance	Percentiles						
				10th	25th	50th	75th	90th	95th	99th
1. SINGLE DX										
0–19 Years	1	5.0	0	5	5	5	5	5	5	5
20–34	49	2.4	4	1	1	2	3	5	6	11
35–49	98	1.9	2	1	1	1	3	4	4	7
50–64	50	2.5	4	1	1	2	4	6	6	9
65+	21	1.7	<1	1	1	1	3	3	3	3
2. MULTIPLE DX										
0–19 Years	3	2.4	<1	1	1	3	3	3	3	3
20–34	70	3.5	10	1	1	3	4	8	10	14
35–49	311	3.0	7	1	1	2	4	6	8	10
50–64	202	3.7	9	1	2	3	5	6	7	16
65+	172	3.6	9	1	3	3	5	7	9	16
TOTAL SINGLE DX	219	2.1	2	1	1	1	3	4	5	9
MULTIPLE DX	758	3.4	8	1	1	3	4	6	8	14
TOTAL										
0–19 Years	4	2.7	1	1	2	3	3	5	5	5
20–34	119	3.2	8	1	1	2	4	6	9	14
35–49	409	2.8	6	1	1	2	4	6	7	9
50–64	252	3.5	6	1	1	3	4	6	7	16
65+	193	3.3	8	1	3	3	5	7	9	16
GRAND TOTAL	977	3.1	7	1	1	2	4	6	8	14

03.95: SPINAL BLOOD PATCH. Formerly included in operation group(s) 507.

Type of Patients	Observed Patients	Avg. Stay	Variance	Percentiles						
				10th	25th	50th	75th	90th	95th	99th
1. SINGLE DX										
0–19 Years	9	1.9	<1	1	1	2	2	3	3	3
20–34	88	2.4	3	1	1	2	3	5	6	8
35–49	60	2.2	2	1	1	2	2	4	4	6
50–64	19	1.8	2	1	1	1	2	4	4	7
65+	2	4.1	1	3	3	5	5	5	5	5
2. MULTIPLE DX										
0–19 Years	33	4.4	47	1	2	2	3	6	31	31
20–34	277	3.4	7	1	2	3	4	7	11	13
35–49	191	3.7	11	1	2	3	5	7	8	15
50–64	57	4.0	5	1	3	3	5	8	8	15
65+	19	6.3	13	2	4	6	8	9	15	15
TOTAL SINGLE DX	178	2.3	2	1	1	2	3	5	6	7
MULTIPLE DX	577	3.7	11	1	2	3	5	7	8	15
TOTAL										
0–19 Years	42	4.0	40	1	2	2	3	6	15	31
20–34	365	3.2	6	1	2	3	4	6	7	11
35–49	251	3.5	10	1	2	3	5	7	8	14
50–64	76	3.5	5	1	4	5	8	9	10	14
65+	21	6.2	13	2	4	5	8	9	15	15
GRAND TOTAL	755	3.4	9	1	2	3	4	7	8	14

Length of Stay by Diagnosis and Operation, United States, 1997

United States, October 1995–September 1996 Data, by Operation

04.0: PERIPH NERVE INC/DIV/EXC. Formerly included in operation group(s) 508.

Type of Patients	Observed Patients	Avg. Stay	Vari-ance	Percentiles						
				10th	25th	50th	75th	90th	95th	99th
1. SINGLE DX										
0–19 Years	30	2.2	3	1	1	1	4	5	5	7
20–34	92	3.2	8	1	1	3	5	6	6	11
35–49	172	3.0	3	1	1	3	4	6	7	8
50–64	116	3.9	4	1	3	4	5	6	6	10
65+	69	2.7	10	1	1	1	3	10	10	10
2. MULTIPLE DX										
0–19 Years	65	3.0	10	1	1	2	3	7	9	16
20–34	153	6.0	39	1	1	3	9	13	22	25
35–49	378	4.7	13	1	3	4	6	8	9	16
50–64	350	5.0	21	1	2	4	6	10	13	34
65+	310	4.5	31	1	1	3	6	9	11	35
TOTAL SINGLE DX	479	3.1	5	1	1	3	4	6	7	10
MULTIPLE DX	1256	4.8	23	1	2	4	6	9	13	27
TOTAL										
0–19 Years	95	2.7	8	1	1	2	3	6	9	16
20–34	245	5.1	31	1	1	3	7	10	21	25
35–49	550	4.1	10	1	2	4	5	7	9	13
50–64	466	4.7	17	1	2	4	6	8	13	26
65+	379	4.1	27	1	1	2	6	9	11	35
GRAND TOTAL	1735	4.3	19	1	1	4	6	8	10	25

04.07: PERIPH/CRAN NERV EXC NEC. Formerly included in operation group(s) 508.

Type of Patients	Observed Patients	Avg. Stay	Vari-ance	Percentiles						
				10th	25th	50th	75th	90th	95th	99th
1. SINGLE DX										
0–19 Years	18	1.8	2	1	1	1	2	4	5	7
20–34	42	2.3	5	1	1	1	3	6	6	11
35–49	64	1.9	1	1	1	2	2	3	4	6
50–64	32	4.6	4	1	3	5	6	6	6	10
65+	13	1.3	<1	1	1	1	1	2	3	4
2. MULTIPLE DX										
0–19 Years	35	2.4	9	1	1	1	2	5	7	16
20–34	64	4.4	42	1	1	2	5	10	25	25
35–49	120	3.7	5	2	2	4	5	6	8	9
50–64	87	4.5	45	1	1	3	4	8	14	34
65+	66	3.7	8	1	2	3	4	7	11	13
TOTAL SINGLE DX	169	2.3	3	1	1	2	3	6	6	7
MULTIPLE DX	372	3.8	19	1	1	3	5	7	10	25
TOTAL										
0–19 Years	53	2.2	7	1	1	1	2	5	6	16
20–34	106	3.8	33	1	1	2	4	8	21	25
35–49	184	3.1	4	1	1	3	5	5	7	8
50–64	119	4.6	31	1	2	3	6	6	11	34
65+	79	3.1	7	1	1	2	4	6	10	13
GRAND TOTAL	541	3.3	15	1	1	2	4	6	8	25

04.01: EXC ACOUSTIC NEUROMA. Formerly included in operation group(s) 508.

Type of Patients	Observed Patients	Avg. Stay	Vari-ance	Percentiles						
				10th	25th	50th	75th	90th	95th	99th
1. SINGLE DX										
0–19 Years	7	4.5	<1	4	4	4	5	5	7	7
20–34	35	5.2	10	3	4	5	5	6	7	33
35–49	75	4.8	2	3	4	5	6	7	7	8
50–64	55	4.4	2	3	4	5	5	6	7	8
65+	18	6.6	8	4	4	6	10	10	13	13
2. MULTIPLE DX										
0–19 Years	3	9.4	18	5	7	7	14	14	14	14
20–34	48	9.4	26	5	6	9	10	18	22	27
35–49	198	6.1	20	3	4	5	7	8	10	16
50–64	207	6.5	13	4	4	5	7	13	14	20
65+	123	8.8	62	4	5	7	9	14	35	41
TOTAL SINGLE DX	190	4.9	4	3	4	4	5	7	7	10
MULTIPLE DX	579	7.2	28	4	4	6	8	11	15	35
TOTAL										
0–19 Years	10	5.9	10	4	4	5	7	14	14	14
20–34	83	8.0	25	4	5	7	10	10	22	27
35–49	273	5.7	15	3	4	5	6	8	10	16
50–64	262	6.0	11	4	4	5	7	10	14	19
65+	141	8.6	57	4	5	6	9	13	32	41
GRAND TOTAL	769	6.6	23	4	4	5	7	10	14	35

04.1: DXTIC PX PERIPH NERV. Formerly included in operation group(s) 508, 512.

Type of Patients	Observed Patients	Avg. Stay	Vari-ance	Percentiles						
				10th	25th	50th	75th	90th	95th	99th
1. SINGLE DX										
0–19 Years	1	1.0	0	1	1	1	1	1	1	1
20–34	0									
35–49	6	1.3	2	1	1	1	1	1	5	8
50–64	5	4.0	13	1	2	3	3	10	10	10
65+	5	5.0	10	1	1	7	7	8	8	8
2. MULTIPLE DX										
0–19 Years	13	9.1	45	1	4	10	10	17	27	30
20–34	14	13.6	75	5	14	14	14	14	14	57
35–49	21	13.6	271	3	5	7	15	45	61	61
50–64	41	13.8	194	2	4	10	16	30	39	57
65+	71	11.9	54	3	7	10	16	20	27	31
TOTAL SINGLE DX	17	1.8	4	1	1	1	1	5	7	10
MULTIPLE DX	160	12.5	102	3	6	10	16	22	30	57
TOTAL										
0–19 Years	14	8.8	46	1	4	10	10	17	27	30
20–34	14	13.6	75	5	14	14	14	14	14	57
35–49	27	4.5	99	1	1	1	4	10	15	61
50–64	46	13.3	188	2	3	10	16	30	39	57
65+	76	11.5	54	3	7	8	16	20	27	31
GRAND TOTAL	177	10.0	100	1	2	8	14	20	29	57

Length of Stay by Diagnosis and Operation, United States, 1997

United States, October 1995–September 1996 Data, by Operation

04.2: DESTR PERIPH/CRAN NERVES. Formerly included in operation group(s) 509.

Type of Patients	Observed Patients	Avg. Stay	Vari-ance	10th	25th	50th	75th	90th	95th	99th
1. SINGLE DX										
0–19 Years	0									
20–34	2	1.5	<1	1	1	1	2	2	2	2
35–49	6	1.5	<1	1	1	2	2	2	2	2
50–64	9	1.7	2	1	1	1	2	2	4	4
65+	13	1.3	<1	1	1	1	2	2	2	2
2. MULTIPLE DX										
0–19 Years	3	2.3	<1	2	2	2	3	3	3	3
20–34	3	2.0	<1	2	2	2	3	3	3	3
35–49	9	2.0	<1	1	1	2	3	3	3	3
50–64	30	4.3	44	1	1	1	2	14	16	27
65+	58	1.9	3	1	1	1	2	6	6	8
TOTAL SINGLE DX	30	1.5	<1	1	1	1	2	2	4	4
MULTIPLE DX	103	2.6	15	1	1	1	2	6	8	27
TOTAL										
0–19 Years	3	2.3	<1	2	2	2	3	3	3	3
20–34	5	1.8	<1	1	1	2	2	3	3	3
35–49	15	1.8	<1	1	1	2	2	3	3	3
50–64	39	3.9	38	1	1	1	2	12	16	27
65+	71	1.8	3	1	1	1	2	6	6	8
GRAND TOTAL	133	2.4	12	1	1	1	2	5	7	27

04.3: CRAN/PERIPH NERVE SUTURE. Formerly included in operation group(s) 509.

Type of Patients	Observed Patients	Avg. Stay	Vari-ance	10th	25th	50th	75th	90th	95th	99th
1. SINGLE DX										
0–19 Years	12	1.0	<1	1	1	1	1	1	1	2
20–34	18	1.2	<1	1	1	1	1	2	2	2
35–49	3	1.0	0	1	1	1	1	1	1	1
50–64	2	1.2	<1	1	1	1	1	1	1	1
65+	1	1.0	0	1	1	1	1	1	1	1
2. MULTIPLE DX										
0–19 Years	84	3.3	16	2	2	2	4	9	11	11
20–34	163	2.3	3	1	1	2	3	4	6	9
35–49	84	2.7	6	1	1	2	3	4	6	13
50–64	44	5.0	194	1	1	1	4	7	9	90
65+	18	2.8	12	1	1	1	3	6	9	20
TOTAL SINGLE DX	36	1.1	<1	1	1	1	1	1	2	2
MULTIPLE DX	393	2.9	24	1	1	2	3	6	7	11
TOTAL										
0–19 Years	96	2.8	13	1	1	2	3	7	10	11
20–34	181	2.2	3	1	1	2	2	4	6	9
35–49	87	2.5	5	1	1	2	4	4	6	13
50–64	46	4.8	185	1	1	1	4	7	9	90
65+	19	2.7	11	1	1	1	3	6	9	20
GRAND TOTAL	429	2.6	22	1	1	2	3	5	7	11

04.4: PERIPH NERV ADHESIOLYSIS. Formerly included in operation group(s) 509.

Type of Patients	Observed Patients	Avg. Stay	Vari-ance	10th	25th	50th	75th	90th	95th	99th
1. SINGLE DX										
0–19 Years	20	1.8	2	1	1	1	2	3	6	7
20–34	91	1.9	1	1	1	1	3	3	4	7
35–49	169	2.8	2	1	1	3	4	4	4	6
50–64	87	3.1	2	1	2	3	4	6	6	6
65+	48	4.0	9	1	2	4	5	5	6	20
2. MULTIPLE DX										
0–19 Years	54	5.0	100	1	1	3	6	8	18	>99
20–34	190	3.0	20	1	1	2	3	6	10	19
35–49	384	3.0	13	1	1	2	3	6	11	19
50–64	336	3.5	11	1	1	3	4	7	9	14
65+	404	4.2	15	1	2	3	5	8	9	22
TOTAL SINGLE DX	415	2.7	3	1	1	2	4	4	5	6
MULTIPLE DX	1368	3.5	17	1	1	2	4	7	10	20
TOTAL										
0–19 Years	74	3.9	69	1	1	2	4	7	18	>99
20–34	281	2.5	12	1	1	2	3	4	7	16
35–49	553	2.9	9	1	1	2	4	4	8	17
50–64	423	3.4	9	1	2	3	4	6	8	14
65+	452	4.2	15	1	2	3	5	8	9	21
GRAND TOTAL	1783	3.3	13	1	1	2	4	6	9	18

04.41: DECOMP TRIGEMINAL ROOT. Formerly included in operation group(s) 509.

Type of Patients	Observed Patients	Avg. Stay	Vari-ance	10th	25th	50th	75th	90th	95th	99th
1. SINGLE DX										
0–19 Years	0									
20–34	12	3.8	1	2	3	4	4	6	6	6
35–49	40	4.0	<1	4	4	4	4	4	5	7
50–64	41	3.8	2	2	3	3	5	6	6	6
65+	30	4.4	15	2	3	4	5	6	9	20
2. MULTIPLE DX										
0–19 Years	0									
20–34	4	4.3	6	2	3	4	4	8	8	8
35–49	47	6.3	38	2	3	4	5	19	24	25
50–64	72	4.5	12	3	3	4	6	7	7	12
65+	133	5.3	10	2	3	5	7	9	10	21
TOTAL SINGLE DX	123	4.0	3	2	3	4	4	5	6	7
MULTIPLE DX	256	5.1	15	2	3	4	5	8	10	24
TOTAL										
0–19 Years	0									
20–34	16	3.9	2	2	3	4	4	6	6	8
35–49	87	4.6	12	3	4	4	5	6	7	25
50–64	113	4.3	9	2	3	4	5	6	8	11
65+	163	5.1	11	2	3	4	6	9	10	20
GRAND TOTAL	379	4.7	11	3	3	4	5	7	9	21

Length of Stay by Diagnosis and Operation, United States, 1997

United States, October 1995–September 1996 Data, by Operation

04.43: CARPAL TUNNEL RELEASE. Formerly included in operation group(s) 509.

Type of Patients	Observed Patients	Avg. Stay	Vari-ance	10th	25th	50th	75th	90th	95th	99th
1. SINGLE DX										
0–19 Years	0									
20–34	13	1.2	<1	1	1	1	1	2	2	2
35–49	24	1.3	<1	1	1	1	1	2	2	7
50–64	8	1.1	<1	1	1	1	1	1	3	3
65+	7	1.1	<1	1	1	1	1	2	2	2
2. MULTIPLE DX										
0–19 Years	18	5.8	269	1	1	1	4	7	9	86
20–34	71	3.2	17	1	1	2	4	6	7	16
35–49	113	3.7	19	1	1	2	4	11	15	20
50–64	121	3.2	13	1	1	2	4	7	11	20
65+	178	3.5	10	1	1	3	5	7	9	20
TOTAL SINGLE DX	52	1.2	<1	1	1	1	1	2	2	7
MULTIPLE DX	501	3.5	22	1	1	2	4	7	11	20
TOTAL										
0–19 Years	18	5.8	269	1	1	1	4	7	9	86
20–34	84	2.8	14	1	1	1	4	6	7	16
35–49	137	3.2	17	1	1	1	4	10	14	16
50–64	129	3.1	13	1	1	2	4	7	11	20
65+	185	3.4	10	1	1	3	5	7	9	20
GRAND TOTAL	553	3.3	20	1	1	2	4	7	11	20

04.49: PERIPH NERV ADHESIO NEC. Formerly included in operation group(s) 509.

Type of Patients	Observed Patients	Avg. Stay	Vari-ance	10th	25th	50th	75th	90th	95th	99th
1. SINGLE DX										
0–19 Years	16	1.3	<1	1	1	1	2	2	2	2
20–34	52	1.5	<1	1	1	1	2	3	3	4
35–49	75	1.7	<1	1	1	1	2	3	3	4
50–64	17	1.5	<1	1	1	1	2	2	2	6
65+	5	1.1	<1	1	1	1	1	1	2	2
2. MULTIPLE DX										
0–19 Years	19	3.3	6	1	1	3	4	7	7	8
20–34	84	2.4	20	1	1	1	2	4	7	16
35–49	146	2.1	5	1	1	1	2	3	5	13
50–64	82	2.7	4	1	1	2	3	5	6	10
65+	60	3.7	34	1	1	2	4	7	10	33
TOTAL SINGLE DX	165	1.6	<1	1	1	1	2	3	3	4
MULTIPLE DX	391	2.6	12	1	1	2	3	4	7	16
TOTAL										
0–19 Years	35	2.3	4	1	1	1	3	7	7	8
20–34	136	2.0	10	1	1	1	2	3	4	15
35–49	221	1.9	3	1	1	1	2	3	5	12
50–64	99	2.5	3	1	1	2	3	4	6	10
65+	65	3.6	32	1	1	2	4	7	10	33
GRAND TOTAL	556	2.2	9	1	1	1	3	4	6	14

04.5: CRAN OR PERIPH NERV GRFT. Formerly included in operation group(s) 509.

Type of Patients	Observed Patients	Avg. Stay	Vari-ance	10th	25th	50th	75th	90th	95th	99th
1. SINGLE DX										
0–19 Years	10	2.2	<1	1	1	3	3	3	3	3
20–34	8	3.2	8	1	1	2	7	7	7	7
35–49	2	2.0	0	2	2	2	2	2	2	2
50–64	0									
65+	0									
2. MULTIPLE DX										
0–19 Years	26	2.5	1	1	2	2	3	4	5	5
20–34	43	2.9	9	1	1	2	3	7	8	14
35–49	21	4.3	28	1	1	2	5	9	19	19
50–64	12	2.9	7	1	1	2	4	5	11	11
65+	1	1.0	0	1	1	1	1	1	1	1
TOTAL SINGLE DX	20	2.6	4	1	1	2	3	7	7	7
MULTIPLE DX	103	3.0	11	1	1	2	3	7	9	19
TOTAL										
0–19 Years	36	2.4	1	1	2	2	3	4	5	5
20–34	51	2.9	9	1	1	2	3	7	8	13
35–49	23	4.0	24	1	1	2	3	9	19	19
50–64	12	2.9	7	1	1	2	4	5	11	11
65+	1	1.0	0	1	1	1	1	1	1	1
GRAND TOTAL	123	2.9	9	1	1	2	3	7	8	19

04.6: PERIPH NERVES TRANSPOS. Formerly included in operation group(s) 509.

Type of Patients	Observed Patients	Avg. Stay	Vari-ance	10th	25th	50th	75th	90th	95th	99th
1. SINGLE DX										
0–19 Years	5	2.0	<1	1	1	2	3	3	3	3
20–34	12	1.6	<1	1	1	1	2	2	2	2
35–49	34	1.0	<1	1	1	1	1	1	1	2
50–64	12	1.0	<1	1	1	1	1	1	1	3
65+	3	2.0	0	2	2	2	2	2	2	2
2. MULTIPLE DX										
0–19 Years	12	1.5	<1	1	1	1	2	2	2	6
20–34	29	2.0	4	1	1	1	2	4	5	9
35–49	56	1.5	1	1	1	1	2	2	3	6
50–64	44	1.8	1	1	1	2	2	3	4	6
65+	30	3.0	8	1	1	2	3	9	9	11
TOTAL SINGLE DX	66	1.1	<1	1	1	1	1	2	2	3
MULTIPLE DX	171	1.9	3	1	1	1	2	4	5	9
TOTAL										
0–19 Years	17	1.6	<1	1	1	1	2	2	3	6
20–34	41	1.9	2	1	1	1	2	4	4	9
35–49	90	1.2	<1	1	1	1	1	2	3	4
50–64	56	1.5	<1	1	1	1	2	3	4	4
65+	33	2.9	7	1	1	2	3	9	9	11
GRAND TOTAL	237	1.6	2	1	1	1	2	3	4	9

United States, October 1995–September 1996 Data, by Operation

04.7: OTHER PERIPH NEUROPLASTY. Formerly included in operation group(s) 509.

Type of Patients	Observed Patients	Avg. Stay	Variance	Percentiles						
				10th	25th	50th	75th	90th	95th	99th
1. SINGLE DX										
0–19 Years	11	1.8	2	1	1	1	2	5	5	5
20–34	15	2.0	<1	1	1	2	2	3	3	3
35–49	18	2.2	1	2	2	2	2	4	4	4
50–64	4	1.1	<1	1	1	1	1	1	2	2
65+	5	1.2	<1	1	1	1	1	2	2	2
2. MULTIPLE DX										
0–19 Years	65	2.4	5	1	1	2	3	5	9	11
20–34	78	2.6	4	1	1	2	3	5	6	10
35–49	60	2.9	7	1	1	2	4	8	8	12
50–64	32	2.4	6	1	1	2	2	4	5	13
65+	14	1.9	<1	1	2	2	2	2	4	4
TOTAL SINGLE DX	53	1.8	1	1	1	1	2	4	4	5
MULTIPLE DX	249	2.6	5	1	1	2	3	5	8	12
TOTAL										
0–19 Years	76	2.3	4	1	1	1	3	5	6	11
20–34	93	2.6	4	1	2	2	3	5	6	10
35–49	78	2.8	6	1	2	2	4	7	8	12
50–64	36	1.9	4	1	1	1	2	4	5	13
65+	19	1.8	<1	1	2	2	2	2	4	4
GRAND TOTAL	302	2.4	5	1	1	2	3	5	7	11

04.8: PERIPHERAL NERVE INJECT. Formerly included in operation group(s) 512.

Type of Patients	Observed Patients	Avg. Stay	Variance	Percentiles						
				10th	25th	50th	75th	90th	95th	99th
1. SINGLE DX										
0–19 Years	2	3.3	<1	3	3	3	4	4	4	4
20–34	21	2.8	6	1	2	2	4	5	5	6
35–49	20	4.3	10	2	2	3	6	8	8	16
50–64	21	3.9	8	2	2	3	4	9	10	14
65+	7	5.6	24	1	2	5	7	10	17	17
2. MULTIPLE DX										
0–19 Years	12	5.9	129	1	1	5	8	11	11	93
20–34	110	6.0	66	1	2	4	6	11	17	54
35–49	257	6.9	78	1	3	4	8	16	20	65
50–64	282	7.5	75	1	3	5	8	14	22	36
65+	547	6.7	33	2	3	5	8	13	17	28
TOTAL SINGLE DX	71	3.7	8	2	2	3	5	7	9	16
MULTIPLE DX	1208	6.8	59	2	3	5	8	14	18	38
TOTAL										
0–19 Years	14	5.7	121	1	1	5	8	11	11	93
20–34	131	5.6	58	1	2	4	6	11	15	54
35–49	277	6.7	75	1	2	4	8	16	20	65
50–64	303	7.3	71	2	3	5	8	13	20	35
65+	554	6.7	33	2	3	5	8	13	17	28
GRAND TOTAL	1279	6.7	57	2	3	5	8	14	18	36

04.81: ANES INJECT PERIPH NERVE. Formerly included in operation group(s) 512.

Type of Patients	Observed Patients	Avg. Stay	Variance	Percentiles						
				10th	25th	50th	75th	90th	95th	99th
1. SINGLE DX										
0–19 Years	1	3.0	0	3	3	3	3	3	3	3
20–34	21	2.8	2	1	1	3	3	5	5	6
35–49	20	4.3	10	2	2	3	6	8	8	16
50–64	20	3.9	9	1	2	3	4	9	10	14
65+	7	5.6	24	1	2	5	7	10	17	17
2. MULTIPLE DX										
0–19 Years	12	5.9	129	1	1	5	8	11	11	93
20–34	107	6.0	67	1	2	4	6	11	17	54
35–49	251	6.8	78	2	3	3	8	16	20	65
50–64	275	7.3	71	2	3	5	8	13	18	36
65+	532	6.8	34	2	3	5	9	13	18	29
TOTAL SINGLE DX	69	3.7	8	1	2	3	5	8	9	16
MULTIPLE DX	1177	6.8	59	2	3	5	8	14	18	39
TOTAL										
0–19 Years	13	5.8	123	1	1	5	8	11	11	93
20–34	128	5.6	59	1	2	4	6	11	15	54
35–49	271	6.7	75	2	3	3	8	16	20	65
50–64	295	7.1	68	2	3	5	9	13	16	35
65+	539	6.8	34	2	3	5	9	13	18	29
GRAND TOTAL	1246	6.7	57	2	3	5	8	14	17	36

04.9: OTH PERIPH NERVE OPS. Formerly included in operation group(s) 509.

Type of Patients	Observed Patients	Avg. Stay	Variance	Percentiles						
				10th	25th	50th	75th	90th	95th	99th
1. SINGLE DX										
0–19 Years	0									
20–34	11	4.1	8	1	1	4	7	7	7	7
35–49	12	1.6	<1	1	1	1	3	3	3	3
50–64	1	1.0	0	1	1	1	1	1	1	1
65+	1	5.0	0	5	5	5	5	5	5	5
2. MULTIPLE DX										
0–19 Years	5	7.5	19	2	3	6	12	12	12	12
20–34	15	3.8	26	1	1	2	4	5	20	20
35–49	20	2.3	3	1	1	2	2	7	7	7
50–64	6	5.6	5	5	5	6	7	8	8	8
65+	5	7.1	74	1	1	2	9	22	22	22
TOTAL SINGLE DX	25	2.8	6	1	1	1	4	7	7	7
MULTIPLE DX	51	4.1	19	1	1	2	6	9	12	22
TOTAL										
0–19 Years	5	7.5	19	2	3	6	12	12	12	12
20–34	26	4.0	18	1	1	3	6	7	7	20
35–49	32	2.0	2	1	1	2	2	7	7	7
50–64	7	5.3	6	1	5	6	7	8	8	8
65+	6	6.9	66	1	1	2	9	22	22	22
GRAND TOTAL	76	3.7	15	1	1	2	5	7	12	22

Length of Stay by Diagnosis and Operation, United States, 1997

United States, October 1995–September 1996 Data, by Operation

05.0: SYMPATH NERVE DIVISION. Formerly included in operation group(s) 511.

Type of Patients	Observed Patients	Avg. Stay	Vari-ance	Percentiles						
				10th	25th	50th	75th	90th	95th	99th
1. SINGLE DX										
0–19 Years	0									
20–34	1	2.0	0	2	2	2	2	2	2	2
35–49	1	2.0	0	2	2	2	2	2	2	2
50–64	0									
65+	0									
2. MULTIPLE DX										
0–19 Years	0									
20–34	0									
35–49	0									
50–64	1	2.0	0	2	2	2	2	2	2	2
65+	1	1.0	0	1	1	1	1	1	1	1
TOTAL SINGLE DX	2	2.0	0	2	2	2	2	2	2	2
MULTIPLE DX	2	1.2	<1	1	1	1	1	2	2	2
TOTAL										
0–19 Years	0									
20–34	1	2.0	0	2	2	2	2	2	2	2
35–49	1	2.0	0	2	2	2	2	2	2	2
50–64	1	2.0	0	2	2	2	2	2	2	2
65+	1	1.0	0	1	1	1	1	1	1	1
GRAND TOTAL	4	1.6	<1	1	1	2	2	2	2	2

05.1: SYMPATH NERVE DXTIC PX. Formerly included in operation group(s) 511, 512.

Type of Patients	Observed Patients	Avg. Stay	Vari-ance	Percentiles						
				10th	25th	50th	75th	90th	95th	99th
1. SINGLE DX										
0–19 Years	0									
20–34	1	13.0	0	13	13	13	13	13	13	13
35–49	0									
50–64	0									
65+	0									
2. MULTIPLE DX										
0–19 Years	2	5.8	75	1	1	1	15	15	15	15
20–34	1	3.0	0	3	3	3	3	3	3	3
35–49	2	4.5	<1	4	4	5	5	5	5	5
50–64	2	9.3	11	7	7	7	13	13	13	13
65+	2	26.8	151	13	13	34	34	34	34	34
TOTAL SINGLE DX	1	13.0	0	13	13	13	13	13	13	13
MULTIPLE DX	9	10.2	103	1	4	7	13	34	34	34
TOTAL										
0–19 Years	2	5.8	75	1	1	1	15	15	15	15
20–34	2	7.2	39	3	3	3	13	13	13	13
35–49	2	4.5	<1	4	4	5	5	5	5	5
50–64	2	9.3	11	7	7	7	13	13	13	13
65+	2	26.8	151	13	13	34	34	34	34	34
GRAND TOTAL	10	10.4	96	3	4	7	13	34	34	34

05.2: SYMPATHECTOMY. Formerly included in operation group(s) 510.

Type of Patients	Observed Patients	Avg. Stay	Vari-ance	Percentiles						
				10th	25th	50th	75th	90th	95th	99th
1. SINGLE DX										
0–19 Years	5	2.2	<1	1	2	2	2	4	4	4
20–34	45	2.5	1	1	2	2	3	4	4	6
35–49	47	2.8	3	1	1	2	4	5	6	9
50–64	18	1.8	<1	1	1	2	2	3	4	4
65+	6	6.3	6	2	4	6	9	9	9	9
2. MULTIPLE DX										
0–19 Years	16	3.7	4	2	2	3	6	7	7	8
20–34	81	2.6	6	1	2	3	3	3	6	15
35–49	117	4.5	20	1	2	3	5	10	17	22
50–64	72	7.2	80	2	3	4	7	15	36	36
65+	124	7.6	76	2	2	4	11	15	20	36
TOTAL SINGLE DX	121	2.7	3	1	2	2	4	5	6	9
MULTIPLE DX	410	5.4	46	1	2	3	6	14	17	36
TOTAL										
0–19 Years	21	3.1	3	2	2	2	4	6	7	8
20–34	126	2.6	4	1	2	2	3	4	5	14
35–49	164	4.1	16	1	2	3	5	7	17	20
50–64	90	6.3	71	1	2	4	6	14	36	36
65+	130	7.6	74	2	2	4	11	15	20	36
GRAND TOTAL	531	4.9	39	1	2	3	5	12	15	36

05.23: LUMBAR SYMPATHECTOMY. Formerly included in operation group(s) 510.

Type of Patients	Observed Patients	Avg. Stay	Vari-ance	Percentiles						
				10th	25th	50th	75th	90th	95th	99th
1. SINGLE DX										
0–19 Years	2	3.0	3	1	1	4	4	4	4	4
20–34	14	3.0	<1	2	2	3	4	4	4	4
35–49	23	2.8	4	1	1	2	5	5	6	7
50–64	8	1.7	1	1	1	1	3	3	4	7
65+	6	6.3	6	2	4	6	9	9	9	9
2. MULTIPLE DX										
0–19 Years	3	4.6	4	3	4	4	4	8	8	8
20–34	32	2.4	4	1	1	2	3	3	4	12
35–49	57	5.0	25	1	2	3	4	17	17	17
50–64	40	9.0	106	2	4	4	7	36	36	36
65+	101	9.7	90	3	3	8	15	15	23	36
TOTAL SINGLE DX	53	2.9	3	1	1	3	4	5	6	9
MULTIPLE DX	233	6.7	64	1	2	4	8	15	17	36
TOTAL										
0–19 Years	5	4.0	4	1	3	4	4	8	8	8
20–34	46	2.5	4	1	1	2	3	4	4	12
35–49	80	4.4	20	1	2	3	5	12	17	17
50–64	48	8.1	99	1	3	4	7	26	36	36
65+	107	9.6	88	3	3	8	14	15	23	36
GRAND TOTAL	286	6.1	56	1	2	3	7	15	17	36

Length of Stay by Diagnosis and Operation, United States, 1997

United States, October 1995–September 1996 Data, by Operation

05.3: SYMPATH NERVE INJECTION. Formerly included in operation group(s) 511.

Type of Patients	Observed Patients	Avg. Stay	Variance	Percentiles						
				10th	25th	50th	75th	90th	95th	99th
1. SINGLE DX										
0–19 Years	4	4.1	4	1	4	4	5	7	7	7
20–34	21	3.9	5	1	3	4	5	5	5	11
35–49	39	4.7	2	3	5	5	5	5	5	9
50–64	10	3.5	4	1	1	4	5	5	6	8
65+	17	5.2	22	2	2	4	8	10	18	18
2. MULTIPLE DX										
0–19 Years	11	34.8	634	2	3	57	57	57	57	>99
20–34	71	8.6	30	3	7	8	15	15	15	26
35–49	195	11.0	30	4	7	13	13	13	17	26
50–64	137	6.3	29	1	3	5	7	12	19	26
65+	235	8.8	55	2	4	7	10	19	25	31
TOTAL SINGLE DX	91	4.6	3	2	4	5	5	5	7	11
MULTIPLE DX	649	9.6	66	2	4	8	13	15	22	57
TOTAL										
0–19 Years	15	31.2	657	2	3	50	57	57	57	>99
20–34	92	7.9	30	2	3	7	15	15	15	26
35–49	234	9.3	30	3	5	9	13	13	17	26
50–64	147	6.2	29	1	3	5	7	11	19	26
65+	252	8.7	54	2	4	7	10	18	25	31
GRAND TOTAL	740	8.8	60	2	4	6	13	15	20	55

05.31: ANES INJECT SYMPATH NERV. Formerly included in operation group(s) 511.

Type of Patients	Observed Patients	Avg. Stay	Variance	Percentiles						
				10th	25th	50th	75th	90th	95th	99th
1. SINGLE DX										
0–19 Years	4	4.1	4	1	4	4	5	7	7	7
20–34	19	3.9	6	1	2	4	5	9	9	11
35–49	39	4.7	2	3	5	5	5	5	5	9
50–64	9	3.3	3	1	1	3	5	5	6	6
65+	16	5.5	22	2	2	4	8	10	18	18
2. MULTIPLE DX										
0–19 Years	11	34.8	634	2	3	57	57	57	57	>99
20–34	68	8.8	30	3	4	9	15	15	15	26
35–49	190	11.0	30	4	7	13	13	13	19	26
50–64	133	6.4	30	1	3	5	7	12	19	26
65+	218	9.2	56	3	4	7	10	19	26	33
TOTAL SINGLE DX	87	4.6	3	2	4	5	5	5	6	11
MULTIPLE DX	620	9.7	67	2	4	9	13	15	22	57
TOTAL										
0–19 Years	15	31.2	657	2	3	50	57	57	57	>99
20–34	87	8.2	30	2	4	7	15	15	15	26
35–49	229	9.3	30	3	5	9	13	13	17	26
50–64	142	6.2	29	1	3	5	7	12	19	26
65+	234	9.0	55	2	4	7	10	19	25	33
GRAND TOTAL	707	8.9	61	2	4	6	13	15	21	57

05.8: OTH SYMPATH NERVE OPS. Formerly included in operation group(s) 511.

Type of Patients	Observed Patients	Avg. Stay	Variance	Percentiles						
				10th	25th	50th	75th	90th	95th	99th
1. SINGLE DX										
0–19 Years	0									
20–34	0									
35–49	0									
50–64	0									
65+	0									
2. MULTIPLE DX										
0–19 Years	2	1.2	<1	1	1	1	1	1	4	4
20–34	2	32.3	268	1	40	40	40	40	40	40
35–49	0									
50–64	0									
65+	0									
TOTAL SINGLE DX	0									
MULTIPLE DX	4	14.8	359	1	1	1	40	40	40	40
TOTAL										
0–19 Years	2	1.2	<1	1	1	1	1	1	4	4
20–34	2	32.3	268	1	40	40	40	40	40	40
35–49	0									
50–64	0									
65+	0									
GRAND TOTAL	4	14.8	359	1	1	1	40	40	40	40

05.9: OTHER NERVOUS SYSTEM OPS. Formerly included in operation group(s) 511.

Type of Patients	Observed Patients	Avg. Stay	Variance	Percentiles						
				10th	25th	50th	75th	90th	95th	99th
1. SINGLE DX										
0–19 Years	1	1.0	0	1	1	1	1	1	1	1
20–34	0									
35–49	0									
50–64	0									
65+	0									
2. MULTIPLE DX										
0–19 Years	0									
20–34	0									
35–49	0									
50–64	0									
65+	0									
TOTAL SINGLE DX	1	1.0	0	1	1	1	1	1	1	1
MULTIPLE DX	0									
TOTAL										
0–19 Years	1	1.0	0	1	1	1	1	1	1	1
20–34	0									
35–49	0									
50–64	0									
65+	0									
GRAND TOTAL	1	1.0	0	1	1	1	1	1	1	1

Length of Stay by Diagnosis and Operation, United States, 1997

United States, October 1995–September 1996 Data, by Operation

06.0: THYROID FIELD INCISION. Formerly included in operation group(s) 514.

Type of Patients	Observed Patients	Avg. Stay	Vari-ance	10th	25th	50th	75th	90th	95th	99th
1. SINGLE DX										
0–19 Years	26	3.3	3	2	2	3	4	6	6	9
20–34	25	3.6	6	1	1	3	4	6	6	8
35–49	18	2.3	4	1	1	2	2	5	8	8
50–64	15	1.9	<1	1	1	2	2	3	3	3
65+	4	2.7	4	1	2	2	4	7	7	7
2. MULTIPLE DX										
0–19 Years	50	5.8	35	1	2	5	7	10	11	28
20–34	82	3.7	15	1	1	2	4	8	16	16
35–49	69	5.0	48	1	2	3	5	11	16	34
50–64	85	5.4	32	1	2	3	7	12	16	27
65+	106	8.1	43	1	3	8	13	16	21	29
TOTAL SINGLE DX	88	2.9	4	1	1	2	4	6	8	9
MULTIPLE DX	392	5.7	37	1	2	3	8	13	16	28
TOTAL										
0–19 Years	76	4.9	25	1	2	4	6	9	10	28
20–34	107	3.7	13	1	1	2	5	8	12	16
35–49	87	4.3	38	1	1	2	4	10	14	31
50–64	100	4.9	29	1	2	3	6	10	15	27
65+	110	7.8	42	1	2	7	13	16	21	29
GRAND TOTAL	480	5.1	32	1	2	3	7	12	16	27

06.1: THYROID/PARATHY DXTIC PX. Formerly included in operation group(s) 514, 516.

Type of Patients	Observed Patients	Avg. Stay	Vari-ance	10th	25th	50th	75th	90th	95th	99th
1. SINGLE DX										
0–19 Years	4	4.7	5	1	4	4	6	7	7	7
20–34	4	1.0	0	1	1	1	1	1	1	1
35–49	14	3.0	2	1	2	4	4	4	4	7
50–64	7	2.2	<1	1	1	2	3	3	3	3
65+	5	4.0	28	1	1	1	7	16	16	16
2. MULTIPLE DX										
0–19 Years	5	2.4	<1	2	2	2	2	4	4	4
20–34	11	7.7	68	2	2	3	18	22	22	22
35–49	55	4.1	24	1	1	3	4	10	11	27
50–64	72	5.6	27	1	1	3	11	11	12	18
65+	157	8.6	65	1	3	7	12	17	30	30
TOTAL SINGLE DX	34	2.9	4	1	1	3	4	4	6	7
MULTIPLE DX	300	6.9	49	1	2	4	11	15	20	30
TOTAL										
0–19 Years	9	3.5	4	2	2	2	4	7	7	7
20–34	15	6.4	62	1	2	3	4	22	22	22
35–49	69	3.7	16	1	2	3	4	6	10	27
50–64	79	5.3	25	1	1	3	9	11	12	18
65+	162	8.5	64	1	3	7	12	17	30	30
GRAND TOTAL	334	6.4	45	1	2	4	10	14	18	30

06.09: INC THYROID FIELD NEC. Formerly included in operation group(s) 514.

Type of Patients	Observed Patients	Avg. Stay	Vari-ance	10th	25th	50th	75th	90th	95th	99th
1. SINGLE DX										
0–19 Years	24	3.4	4	2	2	3	4	6	6	9
20–34	25	3.6	6	1	1	3	6	6	8	8
35–49	16	1.8	2	1	1	2	2	2	5	8
50–64	14	1.9	<1	1	1	2	2	3	3	3
65+	3	3.4	7	1	1	4	7	7	7	7
2. MULTIPLE DX										
0–19 Years	47	5.9	36	1	1	5	7	10	13	28
20–34	77	4.1	18	1	1	3	5	9	16	20
35–49	56	4.8	54	1	2	2	4	10	19	34
50–64	64	5.0	35	1	2	3	5	10	15	27
65+	74	7.3	44	1	2	6	13	14	18	29
TOTAL SINGLE DX	82	2.8	4	1	1	2	4	6	6	9
MULTIPLE DX	318	5.4	38	1	2	3	7	13	16	29
TOTAL										
0–19 Years	71	5.0	26	1	2	4	6	9	10	28
20–34	102	4.0	15	1	1	3	6	8	13	16
35–49	72	4.0	42	1	1	2	4	10	14	34
50–64	78	4.5	31	1	2	3	6	10	15	27
65+	77	7.1	43	1	2	5	13	13	17	29
GRAND TOTAL	400	4.8	32	1	2	3	6	12	14	28

06.2: UNILAT THYROID LOBECTOMY. Formerly included in operation group(s) 513.

Type of Patients	Observed Patients	Avg. Stay	Vari-ance	10th	25th	50th	75th	90th	95th	99th
1. SINGLE DX										
0–19 Years	91	1.4	<1	1	1	1	2	2	3	4
20–34	551	1.4	<1	1	1	1	2	2	3	3
35–49	967	1.3	<1	1	1	1	1	2	2	3
50–64	526	1.4	<1	1	1	1	2	2	3	6
65+	268	1.7	2	1	1	1	2	3	3	8
2. MULTIPLE DX										
0–19 Years	52	3.6	14	1	1	1	4	10	10	10
20–34	382	1.6	1	1	1	1	2	2	3	7
35–49	991	1.6	1	1	1	1	2	2	3	6
50–64	1001	1.8	3	1	1	2	2	3	3	7
65+	952	2.6	12	1	1	2	3	4	7	16
TOTAL SINGLE DX	2403	1.4	<1	1	1	1	2	2	3	4
MULTIPLE DX	3378	1.9	5	1	1	1	2	3	4	10
TOTAL										
0–19 Years	143	2.3	7	1	1	1	2	10	10	10
20–34	933	1.5	<1	1	1	1	2	2	3	4
35–49	1958	1.5	<1	1	1	1	2	2	3	5
50–64	1527	1.7	2	1	1	1	2	3	3	6
65+	1220	2.4	9	1	1	2	2	4	6	14
GRAND TOTAL	5781	1.7	3	1	1	1	2	3	3	8

Length of Stay by Diagnosis and Operation, United States, 1997

United States, October 1995–September 1996 Data, by Operation

06.3: OTHER PART THYROIDECTOMY. Formerly included in operation group(s) 513.

Type of Patients	Observed Patients	Avg. Stay	Variance	10th	25th	50th	75th	90th	95th	99th
1. SINGLE DX										
0–19 Years	83	1.7	<1	1	1	1	2	2	2	5
20–34	380	1.6	<1	1	1	1	2	2	3	5
35–49	594	1.4	<1	1	1	1	2	2	2	3
50–64	333	1.5	<1	1	1	1	2	2	3	4
65+	142	1.7	<1	1	1	1	2	3	3	5
2. MULTIPLE DX										
0–19 Years	30	2.2	11	1	1	1	2	3	5	28
20–34	287	1.9	5	1	1	1	2	3	4	7
35–49	603	1.9	5	1	1	1	2	3	4	10
50–64	629	2.0	3	1	1	2	2	3	4	9
65+	534	3.0	17	1	1	2	3	5	8	22
TOTAL SINGLE DX	1532	1.5	<1	1	1	1	2	2	3	4
MULTIPLE DX	2083	2.2	7	1	1	2	2	3	5	12
TOTAL										
0–19 Years	113	1.8	3	1	1	1	2	3	4	7
20–34	667	1.7	1	1	1	1	2	3	4	5
35–49	1197	1.6	3	1	1	1	2	3	4	7
50–64	962	1.8	2	1	1	2	2	3	4	7
65+	676	2.7	14	1	1	2	3	4	7	22
GRAND TOTAL	3615	1.9	4	1	1	1	2	3	4	9

06.39: PART THYROIDECTOMY NEC. Formerly included in operation group(s) 513.

Type of Patients	Observed Patients	Avg. Stay	Variance	10th	25th	50th	75th	90th	95th	99th
1. SINGLE DX										
0–19 Years	65	1.7	<1	1	1	2	2	2	4	4
20–34	345	1.6	1	1	1	1	2	2	3	5
35–49	544	1.4	<1	1	1	1	2	2	3	5
50–64	303	1.5	<1	1	1	1	2	2	3	4
65+	113	1.7	<1	1	1	2	2	3	3	5
2. MULTIPLE DX										
0–19 Years	26	1.9	3	1	1	1	2	3	5	12
20–34	267	2.0	1	1	1	1	2	3	4	7
35–49	554	1.9	5	1	1	1	2	3	4	11
50–64	569	2.0	3	1	1	2	2	3	4	9
65+	469	3.0	17	1	1	2	3	5	7	22
TOTAL SINGLE DX	1370	1.5	<1	1	1	1	2	2	3	4
MULTIPLE DX	1885	2.2	7	1	1	2	2	3	5	12
TOTAL										
0–19 Years	91	1.8	1	1	1	2	2	3	4	7
20–34	612	1.8	1	1	1	1	2	3	4	5
35–49	1098	1.6	3	1	1	1	2	3	4	8
50–64	872	1.8	2	1	1	2	2	3	4	7
65+	582	2.7	14	1	1	2	3	4	7	22
GRAND TOTAL	3255	1.9	4	1	1	1	2	3	4	9

06.31: EXCISION THYROID LESION. Formerly included in operation group(s) 513.

Type of Patients	Observed Patients	Avg. Stay	Variance	10th	25th	50th	75th	90th	95th	99th
1. SINGLE DX										
0–19 Years	18	1.2	<1	1	1	1	1	1	2	5
20–34	35	1.3	<1	1	1	1	2	2	2	2
35–49	50	1.3	<1	1	1	1	2	2	2	2
50–64	30	1.2	<1	1	1	1	1	2	2	3
65+	29	1.5	2	1	1	1	2	3	4	7
2. MULTIPLE DX										
0–19 Years	4	4.0	82	1	1	1	1	28	28	28
20–34	20	1.2	<1	1	1	1	1	2	2	3
35–49	49	1.6	2	1	1	1	2	3	4	10
50–64	60	2.0	6	1	1	2	2	3	4	22
65+	65	3.2	16	1	2	2	3	7	13	24
TOTAL SINGLE DX	162	1.3	<1	1	1	1	1	2	2	3
MULTIPLE DX	198	2.0	7	1	1	1	2	3	5	18
TOTAL										
0–19 Years	22	1.7	13	1	1	1	1	1	5	28
20–34	55	1.2	<1	1	1	1	1	2	2	2
35–49	99	1.4	<1	1	1	1	2	2	3	4
50–64	90	1.7	4	1	1	1	2	2	3	5
65+	94	2.6	12	1	1	1	3	5	10	18
GRAND TOTAL	360	1.6	4	1	1	1	2	2	3	10

06.4: COMPLETE THYROIDECTOMY. Formerly included in operation group(s) 513.

Type of Patients	Observed Patients	Avg. Stay	Variance	10th	25th	50th	75th	90th	95th	99th
1. SINGLE DX										
0–19 Years	49	2.1	<1	2	2	2	2	3	3	6
20–34	238	2.0	2	1	1	2	2	3	4	11
35–49	374	1.6	<1	1	1	1	2	2	3	4
50–64	195	1.7	<1	1	1	2	2	2	3	4
65+	81	1.8	<1	1	1	2	2	3	4	5
2. MULTIPLE DX										
0–19 Years	64	2.7	3	2	2	2	3	4	6	8
20–34	401	2.2	3	1	1	2	3	4	5	8
35–49	690	2.2	2	1	1	2	3	4	6	8
50–64	553	2.5	5	1	2	2	3	4	6	12
65+	529	3.2	8	2	2	2	4	6	8	15
TOTAL SINGLE DX	937	1.7	<1	1	1	2	2	3	3	5
MULTIPLE DX	2237	2.5	5	1	1	2	3	4	6	12
TOTAL										
0–19 Years	113	2.4	2	2	2	2	3	3	5	8
20–34	639	2.1	2	1	1	2	2	4	5	8
35–49	1064	2.0	2	1	1	2	3	4	5	7
50–64	748	2.2	4	1	2	2	3	4	6	12
65+	610	3.1	7	2	2	2	4	6	8	14
GRAND TOTAL	3174	2.3	4	1	1	2	3	4	5	10

Length of Stay by Diagnosis and Operation, United States, 1997

United States, October 1995–September 1996 Data, by Operation

06.5: SUBSTERNAL THYROIDECTOMY. Formerly included in operation group(s) 513.

Type of Patients	Observed Patients	Avg. Stay	Vari-ance	10th	25th	50th	75th	90th	95th	99th
1. SINGLE DX										
0–19 Years	3	2.0	0	2	2	2	2	2	2	2
20–34	38	1.9	<1	1	1	2	2	3	3	4
35–49	52	1.8	<1	1	1	2	2	2	3	5
50–64	41	2.3	<1	1	2	2	3	3	3	5
65+	18	2.2	<1	1	2	2	2	3	3	5
2. MULTIPLE DX										
0–19 Years	5	6.1	5	2	6	6	8	8	8	8
20–34	35	4.6	7	1	2	5	7	7	7	12
35–49	88	2.4	8	1	1	2	3	4	6	16
50–64	119	2.6	5	1	1	2	3	5	7	9
65+	149	5.0	41	1	2	3	5	10	16	28
TOTAL SINGLE DX	152	2.0	<1	1	1	2	2	3	3	5
MULTIPLE DX	396	3.5	17	1	2	2	4	7	8	20
TOTAL										
0–19 Years	8	5.4	6	2	2	6	8	8	8	8
20–34	73	3.7	6	1	2	3	7	7	7	7
35–49	140	2.1	5	1	1	2	3	4	6	13
50–64	160	2.5	4	1	1	2	3	5	6	8
65+	167	4.7	38	1	2	3	4	9	16	28
GRAND TOTAL	548	3.1	14	1	1	2	3	6	8	18

06.51: PART SUBSTERN THYROIDECT. Formerly included in operation group(s) 513.

Type of Patients	Observed Patients	Avg. Stay	Vari-ance	10th	25th	50th	75th	90th	95th	99th
1. SINGLE DX										
0–19 Years	0									
20–34	21	1.9	<1	1	1	2	2	2	3	3
35–49	32	1.7	<1	1	1	2	2	2	2	3
50–64	21	2.2	<1	1	1	3	3	3	3	3
65+	14	2.1	<1	1	1	2	2	3	5	5
2. MULTIPLE DX										
0–19 Years	2	3.0	0	3	3	3	3	3	3	3
20–34	16	2.2	2	1	1	2	3	3	5	6
35–49	39	2.0	6	1	1	1	2	3	4	22
50–64	59	2.4	3	1	2	2	3	5	5	9
65+	81	4.5	47	1	2	3	4	6	16	33
TOTAL SINGLE DX	88	1.9	<1	1	1	2	2	3	3	4
MULTIPLE DX	197	2.9	19	1	1	2	3	5	6	19
TOTAL										
0–19 Years	2	3.0	0	3	3	3	3	3	3	3
20–34	37	2.1	<1	1	1	2	3	3	3	6
35–49	71	1.9	4	1	1	2	3	3	3	10
50–64	80	2.4	3	2	2	2	3	4	5	8
65+	95	4.3	44	1	2	3	4	6	16	33
GRAND TOTAL	285	2.6	14	1	1	2	3	4	5	18

06.6: LINGUAL THYROID EXCISION. Formerly included in operation group(s) 513.

Type of Patients	Observed Patients	Avg. Stay	Vari-ance	10th	25th	50th	75th	90th	95th	99th
1. SINGLE DX										
0–19 Years	3	2.0	0	2	2	2	2	2	2	2
20–34	0									
35–49	0									
50–64	0									
65+	0									
2. MULTIPLE DX										
0–19 Years	1	1.0	0	1	1	1	1	1	1	1
20–34	1	2.0	0	2	2	2	2	2	2	2
35–49	3	1.5	<1	1	1	2	2	2	2	2
50–64	1	2.0	0	2	2	2	2	2	2	2
65+	4	1.8	<1	1	1	2	2	3	3	3
TOTAL SINGLE DX	3	2.0	0	2	2	2	2	2	2	2
MULTIPLE DX	10	1.6	<1	1	1	2	2	2	2	3
TOTAL										
0–19 Years	4	1.7	<1	1	1	2	2	2	2	2
20–34	1	2.0	0	2	2	2	2	2	2	2
35–49	3	1.5	<1	1	2	1	2	2	2	2
50–64	1	2.0	0	2	2	2	2	2	2	2
65+	4	1.8	<1	1	1	2	2	3	3	3
GRAND TOTAL	13	1.7	<1	1	1	2	2	2	2	3

06.7: THYROGLOSSAL DUCT EXC. Formerly included in operation group(s) 514.

Type of Patients	Observed Patients	Avg. Stay	Vari-ance	10th	25th	50th	75th	90th	95th	99th
1. SINGLE DX										
0–19 Years	181	1.1	<1	1	1	1	1	2	2	3
20–34	28	1.4	<1	1	1	1	1	3	3	4
35–49	30	1.6	2	1	1	1	2	2	3	11
50–64	20	1.3	<1	1	1	1	1	2	3	4
65+	3	1.0	0	1	1	1	1	1	1	1
2. MULTIPLE DX										
0–19 Years	42	2.3	5	1	1	1	2	6	6	10
20–34	11	1.1	<1	1	1	1	1	1	3	3
35–49	32	1.4	1	1	1	1	1	2	3	4
50–64	16	1.5	<1	1	1	2	2	3	3	7
65+	21	2.4	6	1	1	2	3	6	7	11
TOTAL SINGLE DX	262	1.2	<1	1	1	1	1	2	2	3
MULTIPLE DX	122	1.8	3	1	1	1	2	3	6	10
TOTAL										
0–19 Years	223	1.4	<1	1	1	1	1	2	3	6
20–34	39	1.3	<1	1	1	1	1	3	3	3
35–49	62	1.4	<1	1	1	1	2	2	3	10
50–64	36	1.4	<1	1	1	1	2	2	3	4
65+	24	2.3	5	1	1	2	2	4	7	11
GRAND TOTAL	384	1.4	1	1	1	1	1	2	3	6

United States, October 1995–September 1996 Data, by Operation

06.8: PARATHYROIDECTOMY. Formerly included in operation group(s) 514.

Type of Patients	Observed Patients	Avg. Stay	Vari-ance	Percentiles						
				10th	25th	50th	75th	90th	95th	99th
1. SINGLE DX										
0-19 Years	5	2.2	1	1	1	2	3	4	4	4
20-34	37	1.8	<1	1	1	2	3	3	4	5
35-49	124	1.8	8	1	1	2	2	2	3	4
50-64	137	1.7	<1	1	1	2	2	3	3	6
65+	102	1.9	<1	1	1	2	2	3	3	5
2. MULTIPLE DX										
0-19 Years	32	8.4	48	1	2	7	13	19	19	24
20-34	272	4.8	25	1	2	3	6	11	14	21
35-49	820	3.2	13	1	1	2	4	6	9	16
50-64	1149	2.8	17	1	1	2	2	4	8	25
65+	1340	3.4	24	1	1	2	3	7	14	26
TOTAL SINGLE DX	405	1.8	4	1	1	2	2	3	3	5
MULTIPLE DX	3613	3.2	20	1	1	2	3	7	11	24
TOTAL										
0-19 Years	37	8.1	47	1	2	6	11	19	19	24
20-34	309	4.5	24	1	2	3	6	11	13	21
35-49	944	3.0	13	1	1	2	3	5	9	16
50-64	1286	2.7	16	1	1	2	2	4	7	23
65+	1442	3.3	23	1	1	2	3	7	14	25
GRAND TOTAL	4018	3.1	19	1	1	2	3	6	11	23

06.81: TOTAL PARATHYROIDECTOMY. Formerly included in operation group(s) 514.

Type of Patients	Observed Patients	Avg. Stay	Vari-ance	Percentiles						
				10th	25th	50th	75th	90th	95th	99th
1. SINGLE DX										
0-19 Years	0									
20-34	2	1.6	<1	1	1	2	2	2	2	2
35-49	13	1.4	<1	1	1	2	2	3	3	4
50-64	7	2.0	<1	1	2	2	2	3	4	4
65+	7	2.0	1	1	1	2	2	3	5	5
2. MULTIPLE DX										
0-19 Years	6	3.5	17	1	1	1	7	11	13	13
20-34	45	5.5	43	1	2	4	7	13	15	35
35-49	120	4.6	15	1	2	3	5	10	14	16
50-64	151	3.8	42	2	2	2	5	8	12	30
65+	110	4.4	28	1	2	4	8	15	15	23
TOTAL SINGLE DX	29	1.5	<1	1	1	1	2	3	3	4
MULTIPLE DX	432	4.3	33	1	2	2	4	9	15	30
TOTAL										
0-19 Years	6	3.5	17	1	1	1	7	11	13	13
20-34	47	5.4	43	1	2	4	7	13	15	35
35-49	133	3.9	14	1	2	3	5	10	14	16
50-64	158	3.7	41	1	2	3	5	8	11	30
65+	117	4.3	28	1	2	2	3	15	15	23
GRAND TOTAL	461	4.1	31	1	2	2	4	9	15	30

06.89: OTHER PARATHYROIDECTOMY. Formerly included in operation group(s) 514.

Type of Patients	Observed Patients	Avg. Stay	Vari-ance	Percentiles						
				10th	25th	50th	75th	90th	95th	99th
1. SINGLE DX										
0-19 Years	5	2.2	1	1	1	2	3	4	4	4
20-34	35	1.8	<1	1	1	2	3	3	4	5
35-49	111	1.8	10	1	1	2	2	2	3	32
50-64	130	1.7	<1	1	1	2	2	3	3	6
65+	95	1.9	<1	1	1	2	2	3	3	5
2. MULTIPLE DX										
0-19 Years	26	9.4	48	2	5	7	19	19	19	24
20-34	227	4.6	21	2	2	3	6	11	13	21
35-49	700	3.0	13	1	1	2	4	5	8	16
50-64	998	2.6	13	1	1	2	2	4	7	23
65+	1230	3.3	24	1	1	2	3	6	14	26
TOTAL SINGLE DX	376	1.8	4	1	1	2	2	3	3	6
MULTIPLE DX	3181	3.1	18	1	1	2	3	6	11	23
TOTAL										
0-19 Years	31	8.9	48	2	3	7	19	19	19	24
20-34	262	4.3	20	1	2	3	5	11	13	18
35-49	811	2.9	12	1	1	2	3	5	8	16
50-64	1128	2.5	12	1	1	2	2	4	6	21
65+	1325	3.2	23	1	1	2	3	6	13	26
GRAND TOTAL	3557	3.0	17	1	1	2	3	5	10	22

06.9: THYROID/PARATHY OPS NEC. Formerly included in operation group(s) 514.

Type of Patients	Observed Patients	Avg. Stay	Vari-ance	Percentiles						
				10th	25th	50th	75th	90th	95th	99th
1. SINGLE DX										
0-19 Years	0									
20-34	3	1.6	<1	1	1	2	2	2	2	2
35-49	2	1.5	<1	1	1	2	2	2	2	2
50-64	2	1.0	0	1	1	1	1	1	1	1
65+	1	3.0	0	3	3	3	3	3	3	3
2. MULTIPLE DX										
0-19 Years	4	2.2	<1	1	2	2	2	2	4	7
20-34	19	4.7	17	2	2	4	4	11	11	23
35-49	40	3.8	6	1	2	4	5	8	8	11
50-64	35	6.6	67	1	2	4	8	17	28	39
65+	36	5.7	58	1	2	5	5	19	24	36
TOTAL SINGLE DX	8	1.3	<1	1	1	1	2	2	3	3
MULTIPLE DX	134	4.1	24	1	2	2	4	8	13	24
TOTAL										
0-19 Years	4	2.2	<1	2	2	2	2	2	4	7
20-34	22	4.6	16	2	2	4	4	11	11	23
35-49	42	3.7	6	1	1	3	5	8	8	11
50-64	37	5.4	58	1	1	3	6	15	19	39
65+	37	5.7	57	1	2	2	5	19	24	36
GRAND TOTAL	142	4.0	24	1	2	2	4	8	12	24

United States, October 1995–September 1996 Data, by Operation

07.2: PARTIAL ADRENALECTOMY. Formerly included in operation group(s) 515.

Type of Patients	Observed Patients	Avg. Stay	Vari-ance	Percentiles 10th	25th	50th	75th	90th	95th	99th
1. SINGLE DX										
0–19 Years	28	5.1	25	2	3	4	4	8	23	23
20–34	12	3.7	5	1	2	4	5	7	7	7
35–49	22	5.2	3	3	4	6	7	7	8	9
50–64	14	3.9	2	2	3	4	5	6	6	6
65+	2	4.0	0	4	4	4	4	4	4	4
2. MULTIPLE DX										
0–19 Years	92	9.0	171	3	4	6	8	14	21	91
20–34	86	4.9	10	2	3	4	6	8	11	14
35–49	187	5.7	38	2	3	4	6	10	16	29
50–64	219	5.4	19	2	3	5	7	8	11	22
65+	181	7.8	51	3	4	6	9	12	21	35
TOTAL SINGLE DX	78	4.8	13	2	3	4	6	7	8	23
MULTIPLE DX	765	6.5	57	2	3	5	7	11	15	31
TOTAL										
0–19 Years	120	8.2	142	3	4	6	8	14	21	91
20–34	98	4.8	9	2	3	4	6	8	10	14
35–49	209	5.7	34	2	3	4	6	10	14	29
50–64	233	5.3	18	2	3	5	7	8	11	22
65+	183	7.7	51	3	4	6	9	12	21	35
GRAND TOTAL	843	6.4	53	2	3	5	7	11	14	30

07.22: UNILATERAL ADRENALECTOMY. Formerly included in operation group(s) 515.

Type of Patients	Observed Patients	Avg. Stay	Vari-ance	Percentiles 10th	25th	50th	75th	90th	95th	99th
1. SINGLE DX										
0–19 Years	18	5.4	36	2	2	3	4	12	23	23
20–34	9	3.7	6	1	2	3	7	7	7	7
35–49	15	5.6	3	3	5	6	7	7	8	9
50–64	14	3.9	2	2	3	4	5	6	6	6
65+	1	4.0	0	4	4	4	4	4	4	4
2. MULTIPLE DX										
0–19 Years	63	7.0	38	3	4	6	8	13	18	26
20–34	73	4.9	10	2	3	4	6	8	13	14
35–49	159	5.6	40	2	3	4	6	10	14	29
50–64	194	5.2	19	2	3	5	7	7	11	22
65+	156	7.4	51	3	4	6	8	12	21	60
TOTAL SINGLE DX	57	5.0	16	2	3	4	6	7	9	23
MULTIPLE DX	645	6.0	34	2	3	5	7	10	14	29
TOTAL										
0–19 Years	81	6.7	38	3	4	5	7	12	18	26
20–34	82	4.8	10	2	3	4	6	8	11	14
35–49	174	5.6	36	2	3	4	6	10	13	29
50–64	208	5.1	18	2	3	5	7	7	11	22
65+	157	7.4	51	3	4	6	8	12	21	60
GRAND TOTAL	702	5.9	32	2	3	5	7	9	14	29

07.0: ADRENAL FIELD EXPLOR. Formerly included in operation group(s) 515.

Type of Patients	Observed Patients	Avg. Stay	Vari-ance	Percentiles 10th	25th	50th	75th	90th	95th	99th
1. SINGLE DX										
0–19 Years	0									
20–34	0									
35–49	0									
50–64	0									
65+	0									
2. MULTIPLE DX										
0–19 Years	0									
20–34	0									
35–49	0									
50–64	0									
65+	0									
TOTAL SINGLE DX	0									
MULTIPLE DX	0									
TOTAL										
0–19 Years	0									
20–34	0									
35–49	0									
50–64	0									
65+	0									
GRAND TOTAL	0									

07.1: OTH ENDOCRINE DXTIC PX. Formerly included in operation group(s) 515, 516.

Type of Patients	Observed Patients	Avg. Stay	Vari-ance	Percentiles 10th	25th	50th	75th	90th	95th	99th
1. SINGLE DX										
0–19 Years	4	2.8	7	1	1	1	4	7	8	8
20–34	5	3.4	1	1	3	4	4	4	4	4
35–49	2	3.1	3	2	2	2	5	5	5	5
50–64	1	1.0	0	1	1	1	1	1	1	1
65+	1	3.0	0	3	3	3	3	3	3	3
2. MULTIPLE DX										
0–19 Years	17	7.7	7	4	8	8	8	9	11	16
20–34	9	4.0	5	1	3	4	4	6	10	10
35–49	22	5.5	20	2	3	5	7	8	9	29
50–64	63	6.7	19	3	3	6	10	14	15	17
65+	131	8.0	25	2	5	7	11	14	17	23
TOTAL SINGLE DX	13	2.6	3	1	1	2	4	4	5	8
MULTIPLE DX	242	7.2	20	2	4	6	9	14	15	18
TOTAL										
0–19 Years	21	7.3	9	4	7	8	8	9	11	16
20–34	14	3.8	4	1	3	4	4	8	10	10
35–49	24	5.4	20	2	2	5	7	8	9	29
50–64	64	6.4	19	2	3	6	10	14	15	17
65+	132	8.0	25	2	4	7	11	14	17	23
GRAND TOTAL	255	6.9	20	2	4	6	9	13	15	18

Length of Stay by Diagnosis and Operation, United States, 1997

27

United States, October 1995–September 1996 Data, by Operation

07.3: BILATERAL ADRENALECTOMY. Formerly included in operation group(s) 515.

Type of Patients	Observed Patients	Avg. Stay	Variance	10th	25th	50th	75th	90th	95th	99th
1. SINGLE DX										
0–19 Years	1	6.0	0	6	6	6	6	6	6	6
20–34	1	2.0	0	2	2	2	2	2	2	2
35–49	0									
50–64	1	7.0	0	7	7	7	7	7	7	7
65+	0									
2. MULTIPLE DX										
0–19 Years	5	7.0	39	2	2	5	10	21	21	21
20–34	7	8.3	20	3	4	7	13	13	13	14
35–49	13	6.2	38	3	3	4	8	9	13	43
50–64	8	7.0	15	1	6	6	7	14	14	14
65+	6	5.9	8	3	3	5	9	9	9	9
TOTAL SINGLE DX	3	5.6	5	2	6	6	7	7	7	7
MULTIPLE DX	39	6.7	26	3	3	6	9	13	13	21
TOTAL										
0–19 Years	6	6.9	33	2	2	6	7	21	21	21
20–34	8	8.0	21	3	3	7	13	13	13	14
35–49	13	6.2	38	3	3	4	8	9	13	43
50–64	9	7.0	13	1	6	6	7	14	14	14
65+	6	5.9	8	3	3	5	9	9	9	9
GRAND TOTAL	42	6.7	25	3	3	6	9	13	13	21

07.4: OTHER ADRENAL OPERATIONS. Formerly included in operation group(s) 515.

Type of Patients	Observed Patients	Avg. Stay	Variance	10th	25th	50th	75th	90th	95th	99th
1. SINGLE DX										
0–19 Years	0									
20–34	1	2.0	0	2	2	2	2	2	2	2
35–49	0									
50–64	0									
65+	0									
2. MULTIPLE DX										
0–19 Years	0									
20–34	0									
35–49	1	4.0	0	4	4	4	4	4	4	4
50–64	2	5.9	17	2	2	9	9	9	9	9
65+	0									
TOTAL SINGLE DX	1	2.0	0	2	2	2	2	2	2	2
MULTIPLE DX	3	5.5	13	2	2	4	9	9	9	9
TOTAL										
0–19 Years	0									
20–34	1	2.0	0	2	2	2	2	2	2	2
35–49	1	4.0	0	4	4	4	4	4	4	4
50–64	2	5.9	17	2	2	9	9	9	9	9
65+	0									
GRAND TOTAL	4	3.6	8	2	2	2	4	9	9	9

07.5: PINEAL GLAND OPERATIONS. Formerly included in operation group(s) 515.

Type of Patients	Observed Patients	Avg. Stay	Variance	10th	25th	50th	75th	90th	95th	99th
1. SINGLE DX										
0–19 Years	0									
20–34	0									
35–49	1	10.0	0	10	10	10	10	10	10	10
50–64	0									
65+	1	9.0	0	9	9	9	9	9	9	9
2. MULTIPLE DX										
0–19 Years	12	6.5	9	3	5	7	7	11	14	16
20–34	6	7.3	29	4	4	4	7	19	19	19
35–49	3	5.9	4	3	6	6	6	10	10	10
50–64	2	11.4	<1	11	11	11	12	12	12	12
65+	0									
TOTAL SINGLE DX	2	9.4	<1	9	9	9	10	10	10	10
MULTIPLE DX	23	6.9	12	3	4	7	7	11	14	19
TOTAL										
0–19 Years	12	6.5	9	3	5	7	7	11	14	16
20–34	6	7.3	29	4	4	4	11	19	19	19
35–49	4	6.4	5	6	6	6	6	10	10	10
50–64	2	11.4	<1	11	11	11	12	12	12	12
65+	1	9.0	0	9	9	9	9	9	9	9
GRAND TOTAL	25	7.0	12	3	5	7	7	11	14	19

07.6: HYPOPHYSECTOMY. Formerly included in operation group(s) 515.

Type of Patients	Observed Patients	Avg. Stay	Variance	10th	25th	50th	75th	90th	95th	99th
1. SINGLE DX										
0–19 Years	27	4.4	4	3	3	4	5	7	9	11
20–34	106	3.8	2	3	3	3	4	6	7	9
35–49	120	4.4	3	3	4	4	5	5	7	12
50–64	67	3.8	2	3	3	3	4	5	7	10
65+	30	2.9	2	2	2	3	3	4	5	8
2. MULTIPLE DX										
0–19 Years	106	9.4	73	3	5	6	10	21	36	36
20–34	278	5.7	26	3	4	4	6	8	12	16
35–49	414	5.2	12	3	3	4	6	8	11	21
50–64	400	6.6	45	3	3	4	7	13	18	31
65+	370	6.1	29	3	4	4	6	10	18	36
TOTAL SINGLE DX	350	3.9	3	3	3	3	4	6	7	9
MULTIPLE DX	1568	6.1	32	3	4	4	7	10	16	31
TOTAL										
0–19 Years	133	8.4	64	3	4	5	9	17	28	36
20–34	384	5.0	18	3	3	4	6	8	11	16
35–49	534	5.0	10	3	3	4	6	8	10	19
50–64	467	6.1	38	3	3	4	6	11	17	31
65+	400	5.8	27	3	4	4	6	9	16	34
GRAND TOTAL	1918	5.6	26	3	3	4	6	9	14	30

Length of Stay by Diagnosis and Operation, United States, 1997

28

United States, October 1995–September 1996 Data, by Operation

07.62: EXC PIT LES-TRANSSPHEN. Formerly included in operation group(s) 515.

Type of Patients	Observed Patients	Avg. Stay	Vari-ance	10th	25th	50th	75th	90th	95th	99th
1. SINGLE DX										
0–19 Years	15	4.4	4	2	3	4	5	7	7	11
20–34	75	3.5	2	3	3	3	4	5	6	9
35–49	86	4.3	3	3	3	3	5	6	7	15
50–64	46	4.3	3	3	3	4	5	7	7	12
65+	24	2.9	2	2	2	2	3	4	6	8
2. MULTIPLE DX										
0–19 Years	45	5.6	7	3	4	5	7	9	10	14
20–34	181	4.8	6	3	3	4	6	7	10	12
35–49	278	5.0	8	3	3	4	6	8	11	18
50–64	249	6.6	38	3	4	4	6	17	17	31
65+	254	5.6	19	3	4	4	6	9	15	25
TOTAL SINGLE DX	**246**	**3.8**	**3**	**3**	**3**	**3**	**4**	**6**	**7**	**10**
MULTIPLE DX	**1007**	**5.5**	**17**	**3**	**3**	**4**	**6**	**8**	**13**	**24**
TOTAL										
0–19 Years	60	5.4	7	3	4	5	7	7	10	14
20–34	256	4.3	5	3	3	4	5	7	8	12
35–49	364	4.8	6	3	3	4	5	7	9	15
50–64	295	6.3	34	3	3	4	6	13	17	31
65+	278	5.3	18	3	3	4	5	8	12	24
GRAND TOTAL	**1253**	**5.1**	**14**	**3**	**3**	**4**	**5**	**7**	**11**	**22**

07.7: OTHER HYPOPHYSIS OPS. Formerly included in operation group(s) 515.

Type of Patients	Observed Patients	Avg. Stay	Vari-ance	10th	25th	50th	75th	90th	95th	99th
1. SINGLE DX										
0–19 Years	2	2.0	2	1	1	1	4	4	4	4
20–34	3	5.2	5	3	5	5	5	10	10	10
35–49	2	2.6	<1	2	2	3	3	3	3	3
50–64	2	2.6	<1	2	2	3	3	3	3	3
65+	0									
2. MULTIPLE DX										
0–19 Years	9	6.7	35	2	2	3	14	16	16	16
20–34	5	4.7	8	1	1	7	7	7	7	7
35–49	5	8.0	24	2	4	6	9	15	15	15
50–64	11	5.8	5	4	5	5	7	8	13	13
65+	8	13.7	214	3	3	8	20	40	40	40
TOTAL SINGLE DX	**9**	**3.2**	**5**	**1**	**1**	**3**	**4**	**5**	**5**	**10**
MULTIPLE DX	**38**	**9.2**	**107**	**2**	**3**	**5**	**9**	**20**	**40**	**40**
TOTAL										
0–19 Years	11	4.5	24	1	1	3	4	14	16	16
20–34	8	4.9	6	1	3	5	7	7	10	10
35–49	7	6.7	23	2	3	4	9	15	15	15
50–64	13	5.4	5	3	4	5	7	8	8	13
65+	8	13.7	214	3	3	8	20	40	40	40
GRAND TOTAL	**47**	**7.8**	**89**	**1**	**3**	**4**	**8**	**17**	**40**	**40**

07.65: TOT EXC PIT-TRANSSPHEN. Formerly included in operation group(s) 515.

Type of Patients	Observed Patients	Avg. Stay	Vari-ance	10th	25th	50th	75th	90th	95th	99th
1. SINGLE DX										
0–19 Years	3	3.1	<1	3	3	3	5	5	5	5
20–34	23	4.2	1	3	3	4	5	6	6	7
35–49	28	4.5	2	3	3	4	5	7	7	9
50–64	17	3.4	<1	3	3	4	3	5	5	5
65+	3	3.6	<1	3	3	4	4	4	4	4
2. MULTIPLE DX										
0–19 Years	6	5.3	4	4	5	5	5	6	13	13
20–34	78	6.6	59	4	4	5	8	10	12	78
35–49	81	4.8	8	2	2	4	6	8	9	12
50–64	95	5.9	62	3	3	4	6	9	14	67
65+	80	5.5	14	3	4	5	5	8	12	21
TOTAL SINGLE DX	**74**	**3.9**	**1**	**3**	**3**	**3**	**5**	**5**	**6**	**8**
MULTIPLE DX	**340**	**5.7**	**36**	**3**	**4**	**5**	**6**	**9**	**12**	**21**
TOTAL										
0–19 Years	9	4.1	3	3	3	3	5	5	6	13
20–34	101	6.1	47	3	4	5	6	9	12	16
35–49	109	4.7	7	2	3	4	6	8	9	12
50–64	112	5.1	44	3	3	4	5	8	10	38
65+	83	5.5	14	3	4	5	5	8	12	21
GRAND TOTAL	**414**	**5.3**	**29**	**3**	**3**	**4**	**5**	**8**	**10**	**20**

07.8: THYMECTOMY. Formerly included in operation group(s) 515.

Type of Patients	Observed Patients	Avg. Stay	Vari-ance	10th	25th	50th	75th	90th	95th	99th
1. SINGLE DX										
0–19 Years	20	3.7	12	1	1	3	4	6	8	19
20–34	37	4.0	9	3	3	3	4	5	8	25
35–49	36	3.6	5	1	2	3	4	6	6	12
50–64	21	4.0	3	3	3	4	4	4	10	11
65+	5	4.8	1	3	4	5	5	7	7	7
2. MULTIPLE DX										
0–19 Years	46	7.3	57	2	3	6	8	14	21	35
20–34	83	4.1	11	2	3	3	5	6	7	19
35–49	118	5.4	41	2	3	3	5	9	18	37
50–64	124	7.2	37	3	4	6	8	13	20	37
65+	98	7.4	57	3	4	6	7	11	35	35
TOTAL SINGLE DX	**119**	**3.9**	**7**	**1**	**3**	**3**	**4**	**6**	**7**	**19**
MULTIPLE DX	**469**	**6.1**	**40**	**3**	**3**	**4**	**6**	**11**	**18**	**35**
TOTAL										
0–19 Years	66	5.8	42	1	2	4	7	11	19	35
20–34	120	4.1	11	2	3	3	5	6	7	19
35–49	154	5.2	37	2	3	3	5	7	18	37
50–64	145	6.7	34	3	4	5	8	11	18	37
65+	103	7.3	55	3	4	6	7	11	30	35
GRAND TOTAL	**588**	**5.7**	**35**	**2**	**3**	**4**	**6**	**9**	**18**	**35**

Length of Stay by Diagnosis and Operation, United States, 1997

United States, October 1995–September 1996 Data, by Operation

07.82: TOTAL EXCISION OF THYMUS. Formerly included in operation group(s) 515.

Type of Patients	Observed Patients	Avg. Stay	Variance	10th	25th	50th	75th	90th	95th	99th
1. SINGLE DX										
0–19 Years	14	5.4	17	3	3	4	6	8	8	19
20–34	25	4.2	4	3	3	4	5	5	5	19
35–49	28	3.6	5	2	3	3	5	6	6	12
50–64	10	4.0	1	4	4	4	4	4	4	10
65+	2	5.6	3	4	4	7	7	7	7	7
2. MULTIPLE DX										
0–19 Years	31	8.1	88	2	3	6	8	15	20	57
20–34	58	4.1	13	3	3	3	5	6	7	19
35–49	79	5.9	50	2	3	4	5	18	18	51
50–64	77	8.3	56	3	4	7	8	18	21	38
65+	48	6.4	27	3	4	6	6	10	11	41
TOTAL SINGLE DX	79	4.2	6	2	3	4	5	6	8	19
MULTIPLE DX	293	6.2	41	2	3	4	6	11	18	37
TOTAL										
0–19 Years	45	7.0	60	2	3	5	7	15	19	57
20–34	83	4.1	11	3	3	3	5	6	7	19
35–49	107	5.4	41	2	2	4	5	9	18	19
50–64	87	7.6	50	3	4	5	8	18	20	38
65+	50	6.4	27	3	4	6	6	10	11	41
GRAND TOTAL	372	5.9	36	2	3	4	6	10	18	35

07.9: OTHER THYMUS OPERATIONS. Formerly included in operation group(s) 515.

Type of Patients	Observed Patients	Avg. Stay	Variance	10th	25th	50th	75th	90th	95th	99th
1. SINGLE DX										
0–19 Years	0									
20–34	0									
35–49	3	1.0	0	1	1	1	1	1	1	1
50–64	0									
65+	0									
2. MULTIPLE DX										
0–19 Years	1	1.0	0	1	1	1	1	1	1	1
20–34	1	1.0	0	1	1	1	1	1	1	1
35–49	2	3.7	2	2	2	5	5	5	5	5
50–64	1	1.0	0	1	1	1	1	1	1	1
65+	0									
TOTAL SINGLE DX	3	1.0	0	1	1	1	1	1	1	1
MULTIPLE DX	5	1.6	2	1	1	1	1	5	5	5
TOTAL										
0–19 Years	1	1.0	0	1	1	1	1	1	1	1
20–34	1	1.0	0	1	1	1	1	1	1	1
35–49	5	1.6	2	1	1	1	1	5	5	5
50–64	1	1.0	0	1	1	1	1	1	1	1
65+	0									
GRAND TOTAL	8	1.4	1	1	1	1	1	2	5	5

08.0: EYELID INCISION. Formerly included in operation group(s) 518.

Type of Patients	Observed Patients	Avg. Stay	Variance	10th	25th	50th	75th	90th	95th	99th
1. SINGLE DX										
0–19 Years	15	2.8	4	1	1	2	4	6	6	6
20–34	2	5.3	3	4	4	4	7	7	7	7
35–49	2	3.5	<1	3	3	3	4	4	4	4
50–64	0									
65+	0									
2. MULTIPLE DX										
0–19 Years	28	12.2	258	1	2	4	8	43	43	43
20–34	14	3.6	6	1	1	4	9	6	6	8
35–49	11	7.9	5	4	1	9	9	9	9	9
50–64	12	1.5	2	1	1	1	1	3	4	9
65+	12	6.0	50	2	2	4	7	11	18	40
TOTAL SINGLE DX	19	3.0	4	1	1	2	4	6	6	7
MULTIPLE DX	77	6.6	85	1	1	4	9	9	43	43
TOTAL										
0–19 Years	43	9.1	193	1	2	3	8	43	43	43
20–34	16	3.7	6	1	1	4	6	6	7	8
35–49	13	7.8	5	4	9	9	9	9	9	9
50–64	12	1.5	2	1	1	1	1	3	4	9
65+	12	6.0	50	2	2	4	7	11	18	40
GRAND TOTAL	96	6.1	77	1	1	4	8	9	11	43

08.1: DXTIC PX ON EYELID. Formerly included in operation group(s) 517, 532.

Type of Patients	Observed Patients	Avg. Stay	Variance	10th	25th	50th	75th	90th	95th	99th
1. SINGLE DX										
0–19 Years	0									
20–34	0									
35–49	1	3.0	0	3	3	3	3	3	3	3
50–64	0									
65+	1	2.0	0	2	2	2	2	2	2	2
2. MULTIPLE DX										
0–19 Years	2	5.1	15	1	1	8	8	8	8	8
20–34	1	8.0	0	8	8	8	8	8	8	8
35–49	5	3.5	3	2	3	3	3	5	9	9
50–64	2	4.2	10	2	2	6	7	7	7	7
65+	6	8.1	13	4	6	6	11	14	15	15
TOTAL SINGLE DX	2	2.5	<1	2	2	3	3	3	3	3
MULTIPLE DX	16	5.7	12	2	3	6	8	11	14	15
TOTAL										
0–19 Years	2	5.1	15	1	1	8	8	8	8	8
20–34	1	8.0	0	8	8	8	8	8	8	8
35–49	6	3.5	3	2	3	3	3	5	9	9
50–64	2	4.2	10	2	2	6	7	7	7	7
65+	7	7.8	14	4	6	6	11	14	15	15
GRAND TOTAL	18	5.6	12	2	3	5	8	11	14	15

Length of Stay by Diagnosis and Operation, United States, 1997

United States, October 1995–September 1996 Data, by Operation

08.2: EXC/DESTR EYELID LESION. Formerly included in operation group(s) 517.

Type of Patients	Observed Patients	Avg. Stay	Vari-ance	10th	25th	50th	75th	90th	95th	99th
1. SINGLE DX										
0–19 Years	35	1.0	<1	1	1	1	1	1	1	2
20–34	2	2.5	<1	2	2	2	3	3	3	3
35–49	4	2.4	1	1	1	3	3	3	3	4
50–64	4	8.6	2	9	9	9	9	9	9	9
65+	4	1.4	1	1	1	1	1	4	4	4
2. MULTIPLE DX										
0–19 Years	27	2.2	3	1	1	1	3	5	6	10
20–34	19	1.9	2	1	1	1	2	4	4	6
35–49	19	5.4	10	1	2	7	8	8	8	14
50–64	19	4.2	11	1	1	6	6	8	11	>99
65+	76	7.4	64	1	1	3	15	19	19	34
TOTAL SINGLE DX	49	3.2	11	1	1	1	6	9	9	9
MULTIPLE DX	160	5.0	35	1	1	2	6	15	19	30
TOTAL										
0–19 Years	62	1.7	2	1	1	1	2	3	5	6
20–34	21	1.9	2	1	1	1	2	4	5	6
35–49	23	4.9	10	1	2	4	8	8	8	13
50–64	23	5.6	12	1	2	6	9	9	11	14
65+	80	7.2	63	1	1	3	14	19	19	34
GRAND TOTAL	209	4.6	31	1	1	2	6	11	19	22

08.3: PTOSIS/LID RETRACT REP. Formerly included in operation group(s) 518.

Type of Patients	Observed Patients	Avg. Stay	Vari-ance	10th	25th	50th	75th	90th	95th	99th
1. SINGLE DX										
0–19 Years	13	1.0	0	1	1	1	1	1	1	1
20–34	1	2.0	0	2	2	2	2	2	2	2
35–49	6	1.0	0	1	1	1	1	1	1	1
50–64	3	1.1	<1	1	1	1	1	2	2	2
65+	3	1.0	0	1	1	1	1	1	1	1
2. MULTIPLE DX										
0–19 Years	18	1.4	4	1	1	1	1	1	1	10
20–34	2	1.0	0	1	1	1	1	1	1	1
35–49	15	1.7	<1	1	1	2	2	2	2	2
50–64	28	1.9	4	1	1	2	5	5	6	10
65+	22	4.0	10	1	1	2	8	8	8	11
TOTAL SINGLE DX	26	1.0	<1	1	1	1	1	1	1	2
MULTIPLE DX	85	2.1	5	1	1	1	2	5	8	10
TOTAL										
0–19 Years	31	1.3	3	1	1	1	1	1	1	10
20–34	3	1.6	<1	1	1	2	2	2	2	2
35–49	21	1.3	<1	1	1	1	1	2	2	2
50–64	31	1.9	4	1	1	1	1	5	5	10
65+	25	3.8	10	1	1	2	8	8	8	11
GRAND TOTAL	111	1.7	3	1	1	1	2	2	6	9

08.4: ENTROPION/ECTROPION REP. Formerly included in operation group(s) 518.

Type of Patients	Observed Patients	Avg. Stay	Vari-ance	10th	25th	50th	75th	90th	95th	99th
1. SINGLE DX										
0–19 Years	2	1.0	0	1	1	1	1	1	1	1
20–34	1	1.0	0	1	1	1	1	1	1	1
35–49	2	2.0	0	2	2	2	2	2	2	2
50–64	0									
65+	4	1.5	<1	1	1	1	2	2	2	2
2. MULTIPLE DX										
0–19 Years	5	2.6	4	1	1	1	5	5	5	5
20–34	3	3.6	17	1	1	1	10	10	10	10
35–49	5	2.0	12	1	1	3	6	6	6	18
50–64	6	20.6	222	1	1	33	33	33	33	33
65+	43	10.1	113	1	2	6	15	28	28	39
TOTAL SINGLE DX	9	1.9	<1	1	2	2	2	2	2	2
MULTIPLE DX	62	8.7	116	1	1	2	12	28	33	35
TOTAL										
0–19 Years	7	2.2	4	1	1	1	5	5	5	5
20–34	4	3.4	17	1	1	1	10	10	10	10
35–49	7	2.0	4	1	1	2	2	2	2	18
50–64	6	20.6	222	1	1	33	33	33	33	33
65+	47	9.7	111	1	2	6	13	28	28	39
GRAND TOTAL	71	7.1	97	1	1	2	8	28	33	35

08.5: OTH ADJUST LID POSITION. Formerly included in operation group(s) 518.

Type of Patients	Observed Patients	Avg. Stay	Vari-ance	10th	25th	50th	75th	90th	95th	99th
1. SINGLE DX										
0–19 Years	5	1.8	3	1	1	1	1	6	6	6
20–34	5	1.7	<1	1	1	2	2	3	3	3
35–49	4	4.5	<1	4	4	5	5	5	5	5
50–64	0									
65+	2	1.4	<1	1	1	1	2	2	2	2
2. MULTIPLE DX										
0–19 Years	31	3.8	28	1	1	2	4	9	19	20
20–34	22	10.5	184	1	1	2	25	33	33	33
35–49	31	5.6	62	3	3	3	6	10	29	>99
50–64	32	7.0	58	2	2	6	7	17	26	38
65+	57	9.1	75	2	2	7	10	19	31	38
TOTAL SINGLE DX	16	2.4	3	1	1	1	4	5	6	6
MULTIPLE DX	173	7.3	89	1	2	3	8	25	33	48
TOTAL										
0–19 Years	36	3.2	22	1	1	1	3	6	19	20
20–34	27	9.3	169	1	1	2	25	33	33	33
35–49	35	5.5	58	3	3	3	5	9	29	>99
50–64	32	7.0	58	2	2	6	7	17	26	38
65+	59	8.9	75	2	2	7	10	19	31	38
GRAND TOTAL	189	6.8	83	1	2	3	7	25	33	40

United States, October 1995–September 1996 Data, by Operation

08.6: EYELID RECONST W GRAFT. Formerly included in operation group(s) 518.

Type of Patients	Observed Patients	Avg. Stay	Vari-ance	10th	25th	50th	75th	90th	95th	99th
1. SINGLE DX										
0–19 Years	2	1.8	2	1	1	1	4	4	4	4
20–34	0									
35–49	0									
50–64	0									
65+	2	1.3	<1	1	1	1	2	2	2	2
2. MULTIPLE DX										
0–19 Years	11	1.7	1	1	1	2	2	3	4	5
20–34	7	2.6	4	1	1	2	3	7	8	8
35–49	6	3.4	2	2	2	4	4	6	6	6
50–64	6	2.1	2	1	2	2	2	2	3	7
65+	16	1.9	2	1	1	1	2	4	6	6
TOTAL SINGLE DX	4	1.5	1	1	1	1	2	4	4	4
MULTIPLE DX	46	2.2	2	1	1	2	2	4	6	7
TOTAL										
0–19 Years	13	1.7	1	1	1	1	2	4	4	5
20–34	7	2.6	4	1	1	2	3	7	8	8
35–49	6	3.4	2	2	2	4	4	6	6	6
50–64	6	2.1	2	1	2	2	2	2	3	7
65+	18	1.8	2	1	1	1	2	3	6	6
GRAND TOTAL	50	2.1	2	1	1	2	2	4	6	7

08.70: LID RECONSTRUCTION NOS. Formerly included in operation group(s) 518.

Type of Patients	Observed Patients	Avg. Stay	Vari-ance	10th	25th	50th	75th	90th	95th	99th
1. SINGLE DX										
0–19 Years	6	1.3	<1	1	1	1	1	2	2	2
20–34	0									
35–49	3	1.0	<1	1	1	1	1	1	1	2
50–64	6	1.1	<1	1	1	1	1	1	2	3
65+	6	1.0	<1	1	1	1	1	1	1	2
2. MULTIPLE DX										
0–19 Years	11	1.1	<1	1	1	1	1	1	2	3
20–34	14	1.4	2	1	1	1	1	3	5	9
35–49	16	1.3	1	1	1	1	1	2	2	10
50–64	30	1.5	1	1	1	1	2	2	6	6
65+	20	1.7	5	1	1	1	1	3	3	13
TOTAL SINGLE DX	21	1.1	<1	1	1	1	1	1	2	3
MULTIPLE DX	91	1.4	1	1	1	1	1	2	3	6
TOTAL										
0–19 Years	17	1.1	<1	1	1	1	1	1	2	3
20–34	14	1.4	2	1	1	1	1	3	5	9
35–49	19	1.2	1	1	1	1	1	2	2	10
50–64	36	1.4	<1	1	1	1	1	2	3	6
65+	26	1.4	3	1	1	1	1	2	3	13
GRAND TOTAL	112	1.3	1	1	1	1	1	2	3	6

08.7: OTHER EYELID RECONST. Formerly included in operation group(s) 518.

Type of Patients	Observed Patients	Avg. Stay	Vari-ance	10th	25th	50th	75th	90th	95th	99th
1. SINGLE DX										
0–19 Years	8	1.2	<1	1	1	1	1	2	2	2
20–34	0									
35–49	3	1.0	<1	1	1	1	1	1	1	2
50–64	6	1.1	<1	1	1	1	1	1	2	3
65+	6	1.0	<1	1	1	1	1	1	1	2
2. MULTIPLE DX										
0–19 Years	11	1.1	<1	1	1	1	1	1	2	3
20–34	18	2.8	5	1	1	2	6	6	6	6
35–49	20	1.3	2	1	2	2	2	1	2	10
50–64	33	1.5	1	1	1	1	2	2	3	6
65+	24	2.5	11	1	1	1	2	6	13	16
TOTAL SINGLE DX	23	1.1	<1	1	1	1	1	1	2	3
MULTIPLE DX	106	1.6	3	1	1	1	1	3	6	9
TOTAL										
0–19 Years	19	1.1	<1	1	1	1	1	1	2	3
20–34	18	2.8	5	1	1	2	6	6	6	6
35–49	23	1.2	<1	1	1	1	1	1	2	10
50–64	39	1.4	<1	1	1	1	1	2	3	6
65+	30	1.9	8	1	1	1	2	5	6	16
GRAND TOTAL	129	1.5	2	1	1	1	1	2	6	6

08.8: OTHER REPAIR OF EYELID. Formerly included in operation group(s) 518.

Type of Patients	Observed Patients	Avg. Stay	Vari-ance	10th	25th	50th	75th	90th	95th	99th
1. SINGLE DX										
0–19 Years	55	1.2	<1	1	1	1	1	2	2	4
20–34	20	1.8	<1	1	1	1	3	3	3	3
35–49	14	1.2	<1	1	1	1	1	2	2	7
50–64	20	1.3	<1	1	1	1	2	3	5	7
65+	8	2.0	1	1	1	2	2	3	5	5
2. MULTIPLE DX										
0–19 Years	492	2.9	16	1	1	2	4	5	8	20
20–34	755	2.7	10	1	1	2	3	5	10	18
35–49	566	3.3	26	1	1	2	4	6	10	26
50–64	341	3.5	23	1	1	2	4	7	10	32
65+	895	5.6	29	2	2	4	7	11	16	28
TOTAL SINGLE DX	117	1.3	<1	1	1	1	1	2	3	4
MULTIPLE DX	3049	3.4	20	1	1	2	4	7	11	22
TOTAL										
0–19 Years	547	2.8	15	1	1	2	3	5	7	20
20–34	775	2.6	10	1	1	2	4	5	10	17
35–49	580	3.3	26	1	1	2	4	6	8	26
50–64	361	3.4	22	1	1	2	4	7	10	32
65+	903	5.6	29	2	2	4	7	11	16	27
GRAND TOTAL	3166	3.3	20	1	1	2	4	7	11	22

Length of Stay by Diagnosis and Operation, United States, 1997

United States, October 1995–September 1996 Data, by Operation

08.81: LINEAR REP EYELID LAC. Formerly included in operation group(s) 518.

Type of Patients	Observed Patients	Avg. Stay	Vari- ance	10th	25th	50th	75th	90th	95th	99th
1. SINGLE DX										
0–19 Years	38	1.3	<1	1	1	1	1	2	2	4
20–34	16	1.9	<1	1	1	2	3	3	3	3
35–49	8	1.1	<1	1	1	2	2	2	2	2
50–64	5	1.3	<1	1	1	2	2	2	2	2
65+	2	3.8	1	3	3	3	5	5	5	5
2. MULTIPLE DX										
0–19 Years	453	3.0	17	1	1	2	4	5	8	20
20–34	709	2.7	10	1	1	2	3	5	10	18
35–49	521	3.3	27	1	1	2	4	6	8	26
50–64	280	4.2	29	1	2	2	5	9	11	32
65+	850	5.7	30	1	2	4	7	12	16	28
TOTAL SINGLE DX	69	1.4	<1	1	1	1	2	3	3	4
MULTIPLE DX	2813	3.5	22	1	1	2	4	7	11	23
TOTAL										
0–19 Years	491	2.8	16	1	1	2	4	5	8	20
20–34	725	2.7	10	1	1	2	3	5	10	18
35–49	529	3.3	27	1	1	2	4	6	8	26
50–64	285	4.1	29	1	2	2	5	9	11	32
65+	852	5.7	30	1	2	4	7	12	16	28
GRAND TOTAL	2882	3.5	21	1	1	2	4	7	11	23

09.0: LACRIMAL GLAND INCISION. Formerly included in operation group(s) 519.

Type of Patients	Observed Patients	Avg. Stay	Vari- ance	10th	25th	50th	75th	90th	95th	99th
1. SINGLE DX										
0–19 Years	0									
20–34	0									
35–49	0									
50–64	0									
65+	0									
2. MULTIPLE DX										
0–19 Years	1	2.0	0	2	2	2	2	2	2	2
20–34	0									
35–49	0									
50–64	1	2.0	0	2	2	2	2	2	2	2
65+	2	20.4	85	4	25	25	25	25	25	25
TOTAL SINGLE DX	0									
MULTIPLE DX	4	12.0	133	2	2	4	25	25	25	25
TOTAL										
0–19 Years	1	2.0	0	2	2	2	2	2	2	2
20–34	0									
35–49	0									
50–64	1	2.0	0	2	2	2	2	2	2	2
65+	2	20.4	85	4	25	25	25	25	25	25
GRAND TOTAL	4	12.0	133	2	2	4	25	25	25	25

08.9: OTHER EYELID OPERATIONS. Formerly included in operation group(s) 518, 532.

Type of Patients	Observed Patients	Avg. Stay	Vari- ance	10th	25th	50th	75th	90th	95th	99th
1. SINGLE DX										
0–19 Years	0									
20–34	0									
35–49	0									
50–64	1	7.0	0	7	7	7	7	7	7	7
65+	0									
2. MULTIPLE DX										
0–19 Years	2	1.4	<1	1	1	1	1	3	3	3
20–34	2	5.5	29	1	1	6	10	10	10	10
35–49	4	5.5	91	1	1	2	4	29	29	29
50–64	0									
65+	5	9.7	111	1	1	13	13	32	32	32
TOTAL SINGLE DX	1	7.0	0	7	7	7	7	7	7	7
MULTIPLE DX	13	6.6	83	1	1	1	13	15	32	32
TOTAL										
0–19 Years	2	1.4	<1	1	1	1	1	3	3	3
20–34	2	5.5	29	1	1	6	10	10	10	10
35–49	4	5.5	91	1	1	2	4	29	29	29
50–64	1	7.0		7	7	7	7	7	7	7
65+	5	9.7	111	1	1	13	13	32	32	32
GRAND TOTAL	14	6.6	80	1	1	1	13	15	32	32

09.1: LACRIMAL SYSTEM DXTIC PX. Formerly included in operation group(s) 519, 532.

Type of Patients	Observed Patients	Avg. Stay	Vari- ance	10th	25th	50th	75th	90th	95th	99th
1. SINGLE DX										
0–19 Years	0									
20–34	1	2.0	0	2	2	2	2	2	2	2
35–49	0									
50–64	0									
65+	0									
2. MULTIPLE DX										
0–19 Years	2	9.6	1	9	9	9	11	11	11	11
20–34	1	4.0	0	4	4	4	4	4	4	4
35–49	1	4.0	0	4	4	4	4	4	4	4
50–64	1	16.0	0	16	16	16	16	16	16	16
65+	0									
TOTAL SINGLE DX	1	2.0	0	2	2	2	2	2	2	2
MULTIPLE DX	5	9.3	22	4	4	9	11	16	16	16
TOTAL										
0–19 Years	2	9.6	1	9	9	9	11	11	11	11
20–34	2	2.8	2	2	2	2	4	4	4	4
35–49	1	4.0	0	4	4	4	4	4	4	4
50–64	1	16.0	0	16	16	16	16	16	16	16
65+	0									
GRAND TOTAL	6	7.9	27	2	4	9	11	16	16	16

Length of Stay by Diagnosis and Operation, United States, 1997

United States, October 1995–September 1996 Data, by Operation

09.2: LACRIMAL GLAND LES EXC. Formerly included in operation group(s) 519.

Type of Patients	Observed Patients	Avg. Stay	Vari-ance	Percentiles						
				10th	25th	50th	75th	90th	95th	99th
1. SINGLE DX										
0–19 Years	1	8.0	0	8	8	8	8	8	8	8
20–34	0									
35–49	1	1.0	0	1	1	1	1	1	1	1
50–64	1	1.0	0	1	1	1	1	1	1	1
65+	1	1.0	0	1	1	1	1	1	1	1
2. MULTIPLE DX										
0–19 Years	2	7.3	1	7	7	7	7	10	10	10
20–34	0									
35–49	0									
50–64	0									
65+	3	6.8	<1	7	7	7	7	7	7	7
TOTAL SINGLE DX	4	4.2	13	1	1	1	8	8	8	8
MULTIPLE DX	5	6.9	<1	7	7	7	8	7	7	10
TOTAL										
0–19 Years	3	7.6	<1	7	7	7	8	8	10	10
20–34	0									
35–49	1	1.0	0	1	1	1	1	1	1	1
50–64	1	1.0	0	1	1	1	1	1	1	1
65+	4	6.7	2	7	7	7	7	7	7	7
GRAND TOTAL	9	6.5	3	5	7	7	7	7	8	8

09.3: OTHER LACRIMAL GLAND OPS. Formerly included in operation group(s) 519.

Type of Patients	Observed Patients	Avg. Stay	Vari-ance	Percentiles						
				10th	25th	50th	75th	90th	95th	99th
1. SINGLE DX										
0–19 Years	0									
20–34	0									
35–49	0									
50–64	0									
65+	0									
2. MULTIPLE DX										
0–19 Years	0									
20–34	0									
35–49	0									
50–64	0									
65+	0									
TOTAL SINGLE DX	0									
MULTIPLE DX	0									
TOTAL										
0–19 Years	0									
20–34	0									
35–49	0									
50–64	0									
65+	0									
GRAND TOTAL	0									

09.4: LACRIMAL PASSAGE MANIP. Formerly included in operation group(s) 532.

Type of Patients	Observed Patients	Avg. Stay	Vari-ance	Percentiles						
				10th	25th	50th	75th	90th	95th	99th
1. SINGLE DX										
0–19 Years	51	1.2	<1	1	1	1	1	1	2	5
20–34	0									
35–49	1	1.0	0	1	1	1	1	1	1	1
50–64	0									
65+	2	1.8	<1	1	2	2	2	2	2	2
2. MULTIPLE DX										
0–19 Years	77	4.5	18	1	2	4	5	11	14	20
20–34	6	2.1	5	1	2	1	3	4	4	12
35–49	1	2.0	0	2	2	2	2	2	2	2
50–64	1	14.0	0	14	14	14	14	14	14	14
65+	6	2.9	10	1	1	1	1	8	8	8
TOTAL SINGLE DX	54	1.3	<1	1	1	1	1	2	2	5
MULTIPLE DX	91	4.4	18	1	1	3	4	11	14	20
TOTAL										
0–19 Years	128	3.4	15	1	1	2	4	6	13	20
20–34	6	2.1	5	1	1	1	3	4	4	12
35–49	2	1.3	<1	1	1	1	2	2	2	2
50–64	1	14.0	0	14	14	14	14	14	14	14
65+	8	2.5	7	1	1	1	2	8	8	8
GRAND TOTAL	145	3.4	15	1	1	2	4	8	13	20

09.5: INC LACRIMAL SAC/PASSG. Formerly included in operation group(s) 519.

Type of Patients	Observed Patients	Avg. Stay	Vari-ance	Percentiles						
				10th	25th	50th	75th	90th	95th	99th
1. SINGLE DX										
0–19 Years	0									
20–34	1	1.0	0	1	1	1	1	1	1	1
35–49	1	3.0	0	3	3	3	3	3	3	3
50–64	1	1.0	0	1	1	1	1	1	1	1
65+	1	3.0	0	3	3	3	3	3	3	3
2. MULTIPLE DX										
0–19 Years	6	7.1	18	4	4	5	8	14	14	14
20–34	0									
35–49	1	2.0	0	2	2	2	2	2	2	2
50–64	3	3.5	7	1	1	3	6	6	6	6
65+	13	4.1	10	1	3	3	6	9	12	12
TOTAL SINGLE DX	4	1.3	<1	1	1	1	1	3	3	3
MULTIPLE DX	23	4.9	14	1	2	4	6	12	14	14
TOTAL										
0–19 Years	6	7.1	18	4	4	5	8	14	14	14
20–34	1	1.0	0	1	1	1	1	1	1	1
35–49	2	2.3	<1	2	2	2	2	2	2	2
50–64	4	3.0	7	1	1	3	6	6	6	6
65+	14	4.0	9	1	3	3	6	8	12	12
GRAND TOTAL	27	4.0	13	1	1	3	6	9	14	14

Length of Stay by Diagnosis and Operation, United States, 1997

United States, October 1995–September 1996 Data, by Operation

09.6: LACRIMAL SAC/PASSAGE EXC. Formerly included in operation group(s) 519.

Type of Patients	Observed Patients	Avg. Stay	Variance	10th	25th	50th	75th	90th	95th	99th
1. SINGLE DX										
0–19 Years	2	2.5	<1	1	1	3	3	3	3	3
20–34	0									
35–49	0									
50–64	0									
65+	0									
2. MULTIPLE DX										
0–19 Years	2	1.7	1	1	1	1	3	3	3	3
20–34	0									
35–49	0									
50–64	0									
65+	1	1.0	0	1	1	1	1	1	1	1
TOTAL SINGLE DX	2	2.5	<1	1	1	3	3	3	3	3
MULTIPLE DX	3	1.5	<1	1	1	1	1	3	3	3
TOTAL										
0–19 Years	4	2.4	<1	1	1	3	3	3	3	3
20–34	0									
35–49	0									
50–64	0									
65+	1	1.0	0	1	1	1	1	1	1	1
GRAND TOTAL	5	2.3	<1	1	1	3	3	3	3	3

09.7: CANALICULUS/PUNCTUM REP. Formerly included in operation group(s) 519.

Type of Patients	Observed Patients	Avg. Stay	Variance	10th	25th	50th	75th	90th	95th	99th
1. SINGLE DX										
0–19 Years	17	1.3	<1	1	1	1	1	2	3	3
20–34	4	1.0	0	1	1	1	1	1	1	1
35–49	1	1.0	0	1	1	1	1	1	1	1
50–64	0									
65+	0									
2. MULTIPLE DX										
0–19 Years	14	1.2	<1	1	1	1	1	2	2	2
20–34	18	2.7	74	1	1	1	1	2	2	50
35–49	7	3.0	17	1	1	2	2	12	12	12
50–64	1	1.0	0	1	1	1	1	1	1	1
65+	3	3.2	4	1	1	3	3	6	6	6
TOTAL SINGLE DX	22	1.2	<1	1	1	1	1	2	3	3
MULTIPLE DX	43	2.3	44	1	1	1	1	2	3	50
TOTAL										
0–19 Years	31	1.2	<1	1	1	1	1	2	2	3
20–34	22	2.3	58	1	1	1	1	2	2	50
35–49	8	2.7	15	1	1	1	2	12	12	12
50–64	1	1.0	0	1	1	1	1	1	1	1
65+	3	3.2	4	1	1	3	3	6	6	6
GRAND TOTAL	65	1.9	27	1	1	1	1	2	3	50

09.8: NL FISTULIZATION. Formerly included in operation group(s) 519.

Type of Patients	Observed Patients	Avg. Stay	Variance	10th	25th	50th	75th	90th	95th	99th
1. SINGLE DX										
0–19 Years	4	1.3	<1	1	1	1	2	2	2	2
20–34	2	1.5	<1	1	1	2	2	2	2	2
35–49	3	1.0	0	1	1	1	1	1	1	1
50–64	0									
65+	12	1.0	<1	1	1	1	1	1	1	2
2. MULTIPLE DX										
0–19 Years	14	2.4	6	1	1	1	3	8	8	12
20–34	5	1.4	<1	1	1	1	1	3	3	3
35–49	8	2.0	<1	2	2	2	2	3	3	3
50–64	10	4.1	50	1	1	1	1	21	21	21
65+	64	1.4	2	1	1	1	1	3	5	6
TOTAL SINGLE DX	21	1.1	<1	1	1	1	1	2	2	2
MULTIPLE DX	101	1.8	6	1	1	1	2	3	5	12
TOTAL										
0–19 Years	18	2.2	6	1	1	1	2	6	8	12
20–34	7	1.4	<1	1	1	1	2	3	3	3
35–49	11	2.0	<1	1	2	2	2	2	3	3
50–64	10	4.1	50	1	1	1	1	21	21	21
65+	76	1.4	2	1	1	1	1	2	4	6
GRAND TOTAL	122	1.7	5	1	1	1	2	3	4	12

09.9: OTH LACRIMAL SYST OPS. Formerly included in operation group(s) 519.

Type of Patients	Observed Patients	Avg. Stay	Variance	10th	25th	50th	75th	90th	95th	99th
1. SINGLE DX										
0–19 Years	0									
20–34	1	1.0	0	1	1	1	1	1	1	1
35–49	0									
50–64	0									
65+	0									
2. MULTIPLE DX										
0–19 Years	1	2.0	0	2	2	2	2	2	2	2
20–34	2	5.2	31	1	1	1	12	12	12	12
35–49	1	2.0	0	2	2	2	2	2	2	2
50–64	0									
65+	0									
TOTAL SINGLE DX	1	1.0	0	1	1	1	1	1	1	1
MULTIPLE DX	4	4.0	21	1	1	2	2	12	12	12
TOTAL										
0–19 Years	1	2.0	0	2	2	2	2	2	2	2
20–34	3	3.8	24	1	1	1	12	12	12	12
35–49	1	2.0	0	2	2	2	2	2	2	2
50–64	0									
65+	0									
GRAND TOTAL	5	3.3	18	1	1	1	2	12	12	12

Length of Stay by Diagnosis and Operation, United States, 1997

10.0: INC/RMVL FB-CONJUNCTIVA. Formerly included in operation group(s) 520.

Type of Patients	Observed Patients	Avg. Stay	Vari-ance	10th	25th	50th	75th	90th	95th	99th
1. SINGLE DX										
0–19 Years	0									
20–34	0									
35–49	1	1.0								
50–64	0									
65+	0									
2. MULTIPLE DX										
0–19 Years	4	1.4	<1	1	1	1	1	1	1	1
20–34	2	2.4	1	1	1	3	3	2	3	3
35–49	1	2.0	0	2	2	2	2	2	2	2
50–64	0									
65+	0									
TOTAL SINGLE DX	1	1.0	0	1	1	1	1	1	1	1
MULTIPLE DX	7	1.8	<1	1	1	1	3	3	4	4
TOTAL										
0–19 Years	4	1.4	<1	1	1	1	1	2	4	4
20–34	2	2.4	1	1	1	3	3	3	3	3
35–49	2	1.0	<1	1	1	1	1	1	1	2
50–64	0									
65+	0									
GRAND TOTAL	8	1.2	<1	1	1	1	1	2	3	4

10.1: CONJUNCTIVA INCISION NEC. Formerly included in operation group(s) 520.

Type of Patients	Observed Patients	Avg. Stay	Vari-ance	10th	25th	50th	75th	90th	95th	99th
1. SINGLE DX										
0–19 Years	3	3.7	<1	3	3	3	4	5	5	5
20–34	0									
35–49	2	4.8	<1	4	5	5	5	5	5	5
50–64	1	4.0	0	4	4	4	4	4	4	4
65+	0									
2. MULTIPLE DX										
0–19 Years	3	1.0	0	1	1	1	1	1	1	1
20–34	0									
35–49	2	1.0	0	1	1	1	1	1	1	1
50–64	8	5.1	4	3	3	5	7	7	8	8
65+	9	3.2	4	1	2	2	5	6	8	8
TOTAL SINGLE DX	6	4.1	<1	3	3	4	5	5	5	5
MULTIPLE DX	22	3.5	5	1	2	3	5	7	8	8
TOTAL										
0–19 Years	6	2.6	2	1	1	3	4	5	5	5
20–34	0									
35–49	4	3.5	4	1	3	5	5	5	5	5
50–64	9	5.0	3	3	3	5	7	7	8	8
65+	9	3.2	4	1	2	2	5	6	8	8
GRAND TOTAL	28	3.6	4	1	2	3	5	7	7	8

10.2: CONJUNCTIVA DXTIC PX. Formerly included in operation group(s) 520, 532.

Type of Patients	Observed Patients	Avg. Stay	Vari-ance	10th	25th	50th	75th	90th	95th	99th
1. SINGLE DX										
0–19 Years	0									
20–34	0									
35–49	0									
50–64	0									
65+	0									
2. MULTIPLE DX										
0–19 Years	10	6.5	67		2	6	6	15	15	44
20–34	0									
35–49	3	5.1	9	3	3	3	9	9	9	9
50–64	1	17.0	0	17	17	17	17	17	17	17
65+	5	11.1	23	4	7	11	15	17	17	17
TOTAL SINGLE DX	0									
MULTIPLE DX	19	7.2	49	2	3	6	9	15	17	44
TOTAL										
0–19 Years	10	6.5	67		2	6	6	15	15	44
20–34	0									
35–49	3	5.1	9	3	3	3	9	9	9	9
50–64	1	17.0	0	17	17	17	17	17	17	17
65+	5	11.1	23	4	7	11	15	17	17	17
GRAND TOTAL	19	7.2	49	2	3	6	9	15	17	44

10.3: EXC/DESTR CONJUNCT LES. Formerly included in operation group(s) 520.

Type of Patients	Observed Patients	Avg. Stay	Vari-ance	10th	25th	50th	75th	90th	95th	99th
1. SINGLE DX										
0–19 Years	0									
20–34	1	1.0	0	1	1	1	1	1	1	1
35–49	0									
50–64	0									
65+	0									
2. MULTIPLE DX										
0–19 Years	1	1.0	0	1	1	1	1	1	1	1
20–34	0									
35–49	0									
50–64	3	3.2	6	2	2	2	2	7	7	7
65+	2	4.6	15	1	1	8	8	8	8	8
TOTAL SINGLE DX	1	1.0	0	1	1	1	1	1	1	1
MULTIPLE DX	6	3.7	9	1	1	2	7	7	8	8
TOTAL										
0–19 Years	1	1.0	0	1	1	1	1	1	1	1
20–34	1	1.0	0	1	1	1	1	1	1	1
35–49	0									
50–64	3	3.2	6	2	2	2	2	7	7	7
65+	2	4.6	15	1	1	8	8	8	8	8
GRAND TOTAL	7	3.2	9	1	1	2	7	8	8	8

Length of Stay by Diagnosis and Operation, United States, 1997

United States, October 1995–September 1996 Data, by Operation

10.4: CONJUNCTIVOPLASTY. Formerly included in operation group(s) 520.

Type of Patients	Observed Patients	Avg. Stay	Variance	10th	25th	50th	75th	90th	95th	99th
1. SINGLE DX										
0–19 Years	0									
20–34	0									
35–49	0									
50–64	0									
65+	1	1.0	0					1	1	1
2. MULTIPLE DX										
0–19 Years	4	3.5	9	1	1	3	4	9	9	9
20–34	1	1.0	0	1	1	1	1	1	1	1
35–49	5	3.9	29	1	1	1	3	14	16	16
50–64	0									
65+	9	5.0	48	3	3	3	3	8	14	39
TOTAL SINGLE DX	1	1.0	0				1	1	1	1
MULTIPLE DX	19	4.7	42	1	3	3	3	8	14	39
TOTAL										
0–19 Years	4	3.5	9	1	1	3	4	9	9	9
20–34	1	1.0	0	1	1	1	1	1	1	1
35–49	5	3.9	29	1	1	1	3	14	16	16
50–64	0									
65+	10	4.9	47	3	3	3	3	8	14	39
GRAND TOTAL	20	4.6	42	1	3	3	3	8	14	39

10.6: REPAIR CONJUNCT LAC. Formerly included in operation group(s) 520.

Type of Patients	Observed Patients	Avg. Stay	Variance	10th	25th	50th	75th	90th	95th	99th
1. SINGLE DX										
0–19 Years	1	1.0	0	1	1	1	1	1	1	1
20–34	0									
35–49	0									
50–64	1	2.0	0	2	2	2	2	2	2	2
65+	0									
2. MULTIPLE DX										
0–19 Years	3	2.9	7	1	1	1	7	7	7	7
20–34	7	1.2	<1	1	1	1	1	1	4	4
35–49	5	5.2	4	1	4	5	7	7	7	7
50–64	2	1.3	<1	1	1	1	2	2	2	2
65+	2	1.5	<1	1	1	1	2	2	2	2
TOTAL SINGLE DX	2	1.8	<1	1	2	2	2	2	2	2
MULTIPLE DX	19	1.5	1	1	1	1	1	2	4	7
TOTAL										
0–19 Years	4	2.8	6	1	1	1	3	7	7	7
20–34	7	1.2	<1	1	1	1	1	1	4	4
35–49	5	5.2	4	1	4	5	7	7	7	7
50–64	3	1.3	<1	1	1	1	2	2	2	2
65+	2	1.5	<1	1	1	1	2	2	2	2
GRAND TOTAL	21	1.5	1	1	1	1	2	2	4	7

10.5: CONJUNCT/LID ADHESIO. Formerly included in operation group(s) 520.

Type of Patients	Observed Patients	Avg. Stay	Variance	10th	25th	50th	75th	90th	95th	99th
1. SINGLE DX										
0–19 Years	0									
20–34	0									
35–49	0									
50–64	0									
65+	0									
2. MULTIPLE DX										
0–19 Years	0									
20–34	0									
35–49	1	1.0	0	1	1	1	1	1	1	1
50–64	0									
65+	1	6.0	0	6	6	6	6	6	6	6
TOTAL SINGLE DX	0									
MULTIPLE DX	2	1.6	3	1	1	1	1	6	6	6
TOTAL										
0–19 Years	0									
20–34	0									
35–49	1	1.0	0	1	1	1	1	1	1	1
50–64	0									
65+	1	6.0	0	6	6	6	6	6	6	6
GRAND TOTAL	2	1.6	3	1	1	1	1	6	6	6

10.9: OTHER CONJUNCTIVAL OPS. Formerly included in operation group(s) 520.

Type of Patients	Observed Patients	Avg. Stay	Variance	10th	25th	50th	75th	90th	95th	99th
1. SINGLE DX										
0–19 Years	1	5.0	0	5	5	5	5	5	5	5
20–34	1	1.0	0	1	1	1	1	1	1	1
35–49	0									
50–64	2	1.4	<1	1	1	1	2	2	2	2
65+	3	3.9	13	1	1	1	8	8	8	8
2. MULTIPLE DX										
0–19 Years	4	5.0	23	2	2	2	6	16	16	16
20–34	2	4.2	2	3	3	5	5	5	5	5
35–49	1	7.0	0	7	7	7	7	7	7	7
50–64	7	2.3	9	1	1	1	2	7	11	11
65+	47	2.2	5	1	1	1	3	4	9	9
TOTAL SINGLE DX	7	2.7	9	1	1	1	2	8	8	8
MULTIPLE DX	61	2.4	7	1	1	1	3	6	9	11
TOTAL										
0–19 Years	5	5.0	21	2	2	2	6	16	16	16
20–34	3	1.9	3	1	1	1	3	5	5	5
35–49	1	7.0	0	7	7	7	7	7	7	7
50–64	9	2.3	8	1	1	1	2	7	11	11
65+	50	2.2	5	1	1	1	3	4	9	9
GRAND TOTAL	68	2.4	7	1	1	1	3	6	9	11

United States, October 1995–September 1996 Data, by Operation

11.0: MAGNET REMOVAL CORNEA FB. Formerly included in operation group(s) 522.

Type of Patients	Observed Patients	Avg. Stay	Variance	10th	25th	50th	75th	90th	95th	99th
1. SINGLE DX										
0–19 Years	0									
20–34	0									
35–49	1	2.0	0	2	2	2	2	2	2	2
50–64	0									
65+	0									
2. MULTIPLE DX										
0–19 Years	1	2.0	0	2	2	2	2	2	2	2
20–34	1	2.0	0	2	2	2	2	2	2	2
35–49	1	2.0	0	2	2	2	2	2	2	2
50–64	0									
65+	0									
TOTAL SINGLE DX	1	2.0	0	2	2	2	2	2	2	2
MULTIPLE DX	3	2.0	0	2	2	2	2	2	2	2
TOTAL										
0–19 Years	1	2.0	0	2	2	2	2	2	2	2
20–34	1	2.0	0	2	2	2	2	2	2	2
35–49	2	2.0	0	2	2	2	2	2	2	2
50–64	0									
65+	0									
GRAND TOTAL	4	2.0	0	2	2	2	2	2	2	2

11.1: CORNEAL INCISION. Formerly included in operation group(s) 522.

Type of Patients	Observed Patients	Avg. Stay	Variance	10th	25th	50th	75th	90th	95th	99th
1. SINGLE DX										
0–19 Years	3	1.8	<1	1	2	2	2	2	2	2
20–34	2	2.0	<1	1	1	1	3	3	3	3
35–49	0									
50–64	1	2.0	0	2	2	2	2	2	2	2
65+	0									
2. MULTIPLE DX										
0–19 Years	6	2.1	7	1	1	1	1	9	9	9
20–34	2	2.0	0	2	2	2	2	2	2	2
35–49	2	2.0	0	2	2	2	2	2	2	2
50–64	2	6.0	0	6	6	6	6	6	6	6
65+	2	1.7	<1	1	1	2	2	2	2	2
TOTAL SINGLE DX	6	1.9	<1	1	1	2	2	3	3	3
MULTIPLE DX	13	3.0	5	1	1	2	6	6	6	9
TOTAL										
0–19 Years	9	2.0	4	1	1	1	2	3	9	9
20–34	4	2.0	<1	2	2	2	2	3	3	3
35–49	2	2.0	0	2	2	2	2	2	2	2
50–64	2	5.7	1	6	6	6	6	6	6	6
65+	2	1.7	<1	1	1	2	2	2	2	2
GRAND TOTAL	19	2.7	4	1	1	2	3	6	6	9

11.2: DXTIC PX ON CORNEA. Formerly included in operation group(s) 522, 532.

Type of Patients	Observed Patients	Avg. Stay	Variance	10th	25th	50th	75th	90th	95th	99th
1. SINGLE DX										
0–19 Years	2	5.0	2	4	4	5	6	6	6	6
20–34	2	2.0	0	2	2	2	2	2	2	2
35–49	2	6.3	10	3	3	9	9	9	9	9
50–64	0									
65+	1	3.0	0	3	3	3	3	3	3	3
2. MULTIPLE DX										
0–19 Years	11	5.6	15	2	3	4	8	12	12	15
20–34	2	5.5	<1	5	5	6	6	6	6	6
35–49	5	5.4	3	5	5	5	5	8	11	11
50–64	5	9.2	21	5	5	9	9	13	21	21
65+	13	5.9	57	3	3	4	5	7	33	33
TOTAL SINGLE DX	7	5.2	9	2	3	3	9	9	9	9
MULTIPLE DX	36	6.2	28	2	3	5	7	11	13	33
TOTAL										
0–19 Years	13	5.5	14	2	3	4	8	12	12	15
20–34	4	3.8	4	2	2	4	6	6	6	6
35–49	7	5.7	5	3	5	5	9	11	11	11
50–64	5	9.2	21	5	5	9	9	13	21	21
65+	14	5.7	54	3	3	3	5	7	33	33
GRAND TOTAL	43	6.0	26	2	3	5	8	9	13	33

11.3: EXCISION OF PTERYGIUM. Formerly included in operation group(s) 522.

Type of Patients	Observed Patients	Avg. Stay	Variance	10th	25th	50th	75th	90th	95th	99th
1. SINGLE DX										
0–19 Years	0									
20–34	1	2.0	0	2	2	2	2	2	2	2
35–49	1	1.0	0	1	1	1	1	1	1	1
50–64	0									
65+	0									
2. MULTIPLE DX										
0–19 Years	1	1.0	0	1	1	1	1	1	1	1
20–34	0									
35–49	1	8.0	0	8	8	8	8	8	8	8
50–64	0									
65+	3	14.1	120	2	2	7	24	24	24	24
TOTAL SINGLE DX	2	1.4	<1	1	1	1	2	2	2	2
MULTIPLE DX	5	8.4	98	1	1	2	24	24	24	24
TOTAL										
0–19 Years	1	1.0	0	1	1	1	1	1	1	1
20–34	1	2.0	0	2	2	2	2	2	2	2
35–49	2	2.5	10	1	1	2	8	8	8	8
50–64	0									
65+	3	14.1	120	2	2	7	24	24	24	24
GRAND TOTAL	7	5.9	73	1	1	2	7	24	24	24

Length of Stay by Diagnosis and Operation, United States, 1997

United States, October 1995–September 1996 Data, by Operation

11.4: EXC/DESTR CORNEAL LESION. Formerly included in operation group(s) 522.

Type of Patients	Observed Patients	Avg. Stay	Vari-ance	10th	25th	50th	75th	90th	95th	99th
1. SINGLE DX										
0–19 Years	1	1.0	0							1
20–34	0									
35–49	0									
50–64	0									
65+	4	2.3	2	1	1	2	4	4	4	4
2. MULTIPLE DX										
0–19 Years	4	2.5	11	1	1	1	1	9	9	9
20–34	0									
35–49	4	10.0	74	1	1	14	14	21	21	21
50–64	2	2.2	<1	2	2	2	2	4	4	4
65+	8	7.1	19	1	4	7	11	11	16	16
TOTAL SINGLE DX	5	2.1	2	1	1	2	4	4	4	4
MULTIPLE DX	18	5.9	34	1	2	3	10	14	21	21
TOTAL										
0–19 Years	5	2.3	9	1	1	1	1	9	9	9
20–34	0									
35–49	4	10.0	74	1	1	14	14	21	21	21
50–64	2	2.2	<1	2	2	2	2	4	4	4
65+	12	5.5	18	1	4	4	10	11	11	16
GRAND TOTAL	23	5.2	30	1	1	2	9	14	16	21

11.5: CORNEAL REPAIR. Formerly included in operation group(s) 522.

Type of Patients	Observed Patients	Avg. Stay	Vari-ance	10th	25th	50th	75th	90th	95th	99th
1. SINGLE DX										
0–19 Years	149	2.5	3	1	1	2	3	4	6	10
20–34	66	1.8	<1	1	1	2	2	3	3	4
35–49	46	2.1	<1	1	2	2	3	3	3	4
50–64	7	1.2	<1	1	1	1	1	2	3	4
65+	8	2.8	3	1	1	3	3	6	6	6
2. MULTIPLE DX										
0–19 Years	178	2.9	6	1	1	2	4	5	7	14
20–34	94	2.2	2	1	1	2	3	4	5	7
35–49	97	2.8	2	2	2	2	4	4	5	7
50–64	44	3.0	3	1	2	3	5	5	5	6
65+	75	3.4	7	1	2	3	4	8	9	12
TOTAL SINGLE DX	276	2.1	2	1	1	2	2	4	4	6
MULTIPLE DX	488	2.8	4	1	2	2	4	5	5	11
TOTAL										
0–19 Years	327	2.8	5	1	1	2	4	5	6	14
20–34	160	2.1	2	1	1	2	3	4	4	6
35–49	143	2.6	2	1	2	2	3	4	4	6
50–64	51	2.7	3	1	2	3	3	5	5	6
65+	83	3.4	7	2	2	3	4	6	9	12
GRAND TOTAL	764	2.6	3	1	1	2	3	4	5	9

11.51: SUTURE OF CORNEAL LAC. Formerly included in operation group(s) 522.

Type of Patients	Observed Patients	Avg. Stay	Vari-ance	10th	25th	50th	75th	90th	95th	99th
1. SINGLE DX										
0–19 Years	132	2.7	3	1	2	2	4	5	6	10
20–34	57	1.8	<1	1	1	2	2	3	3	4
35–49	33	2.1	<1	1	1	2	3	3	3	4
50–64	4	1.8	<1	1	2	2	2	2	2	2
65+	1	3.0	0	3	3	3	3	3	3	3
2. MULTIPLE DX										
0–19 Years	153	3.1	6	1	2	3	4	5	7	14
20–34	73	2.1	2	1	1	2	3	4	5	6
35–49	75	2.8	2	2	2	2	3	3	4	7
50–64	26	2.3	2	1	1	2	3	3	6	6
65+	32	3.3	5	1	1	2	5	6	8	9
TOTAL SINGLE DX	227	2.2	2	1	1	2	3	4	4	6
MULTIPLE DX	359	2.7	3	1	2	2	4	4	5	9
TOTAL										
0–19 Years	285	2.9	5	1	2	2	4	5	6	14
20–34	130	2.0	1	1	1	2	2	4	4	6
35–49	108	2.6	1	1	2	2	4	4	4	6
50–64	30	2.2	2	1	1	2	3	3	6	6
65+	33	3.2	5	1	2	2	5	6	8	9
GRAND TOTAL	586	2.6	3	1	2	2	3	4	5	9

11.6: CORNEAL TRANSPLANT. Formerly included in operation group(s) 521.

Type of Patients	Observed Patients	Avg. Stay	Vari-ance	10th	25th	50th	75th	90th	95th	99th
1. SINGLE DX										
0–19 Years	9	1.3	<1	1	1	1	2	2	3	3
20–34	22	2.3	18	1	1	1	2	3	3	22
35–49	25	1.5	4	1	1	1	1	2	2	20
50–64	15	3.7	4	4	4	4	6	6	6	6
65+	41	1.2	<1	1	1	1	1	2	2	2
2. MULTIPLE DX										
0–19 Years	32	2.2	4	1	1	2	2	3	4	12
20–34	32	2.2	4	1	1	2	3	5	6	10
35–49	66	4.8	19	1	1	3	10	10	12	20
50–64	74	2.5	26	1	1	1	2	5	7	31
65+	370	2.3	14	1	1	2	2	4	7	19
TOTAL SINGLE DX	112	2.3	6	1	1	1	3	6	6	6
MULTIPLE DX	574	2.7	16	1	1	1	2	6	10	20
TOTAL										
0–19 Years	41	2.1	3	1	1	1	2	3	4	12
20–34	54	2.2	9	1	1	1	2	3	6	22
35–49	91	4.0	18	1	1	1	6	10	11	20
50–64	89	2.8	20	1	1	1	2	6	6	31
65+	411	2.3	13	1	1	1	2	4	7	19
GRAND TOTAL	686	2.6	15	1	1	1	3	6	10	20

Length of Stay by Diagnosis and Operation, United States, 1997

United States, October 1995–September 1996 Data, by Operation

11.64: PENETR KERATOPLASTY NEC. Formerly included in operation group(s) 521.

Type of Patients	Observed Patients	Avg. Stay	Vari-ance	10th	25th	50th	75th	90th	95th	99th
1. SINGLE DX										
0–19 Years	6	1.5	<1	1	1	1	2	2	3	3
20–34	20	1.3	<1	1	1	1	1	2	3	3
35–49	24	1.5	6	1	1	1	1	2	2	20
50–64	13	3.8	4	1	2	4	6	6	6	6
65+	31	1.3	<1	1	1	1	2	2	2	2
2. MULTIPLE DX										
0–19 Years	23	2.0	<1	1	1	2	2	3	3	7
20–34	24	2.2	5	1	1	1	3	6	6	10
35–49	53	4.5	18	1	1	2	10	10	12	15
50–64	51	1.2	<1	1	1	1	1	2	2	5
65+	303	2.1	13	1	1	1	2	4	7	19
TOTAL SINGLE DX	94	2.3	4	1	1	1	4	6	6	6
MULTIPLE DX	454	2.3	12	1	1	1	2	5	10	16
TOTAL										
0–19 Years	29	1.9	<1	1	1	2	2	3	3	7
20–34	44	1.9	3	1	1	1	2	3	6	10
35–49	77	3.7	17	1	1	1	6	10	11	15
50–64	64	2.1	3	1	1	1	6	6	6	6
65+	334	2.1	13	1	1	1	2	4	7	19
GRAND TOTAL	548	2.3	11	1	1	1	2	5	10	15

11.9: OTHER CORNEAL OPERATIONS. Formerly included in operation group(s) 522.

Type of Patients	Observed Patients	Avg. Stay	Vari-ance	10th	25th	50th	75th	90th	95th	99th
1. SINGLE DX										
0–19 Years	0									
20–34	0									
35–49	0									
50–64	0									
65+	0									
2. MULTIPLE DX										
0–19 Years	0									
20–34	1	5.0	0	5	5	5	5	5	5	5
35–49	0									
50–64	0									
65+	0									
TOTAL SINGLE DX	0									
MULTIPLE DX	1	5.0	0	5	5	5	5	5	5	5
TOTAL										
0–19 Years	0									
20–34	1	5.0	0	5	5	5	5	5	5	5
35–49	0									
50–64	0									
65+	0									
GRAND TOTAL	1	5.0	0	5	5	5	5	5	5	5

11.7: OTHER CORNEA RECONST. Formerly included in operation group(s) 522.

Type of Patients	Observed Patients	Avg. Stay	Vari-ance	10th	25th	50th	75th	90th	95th	99th
1. SINGLE DX										
0–19 Years	0									
20–34	0									
35–49	0									
50–64	0									
65+	1	1.0	0	1	1	1	1	1	1	1
2. MULTIPLE DX										
0–19 Years	1	1.0	0	1	1	1	1	1	1	1
20–34	1	3.0	0	3	3	3	3	3	3	3
35–49	1	1.0	0	1	1	1	1	1	1	1
50–64	2	1.0	0	1	1	1	1	1	1	1
65+	1	1.0	0	1	1	1	1	1	1	1
TOTAL SINGLE DX	1	1.0	0	1	1	1	1	1	1	1
MULTIPLE DX	6	1.2	<1	1	1	1	1	1	3	3
TOTAL										
0–19 Years	1	1.0	0	1	1	1	1	1	1	1
20–34	1	3.0	0	3	3	3	3	3	3	3
35–49	1	1.0	0	1	1	1	1	1	1	1
50–64	2	1.0	0	1	1	1	1	1	1	1
65+	2	1.0	0	1	1	1	1	1	1	1
GRAND TOTAL	7	1.2	<1	1	1	1	1	1	3	3

12.0: RMVL INOC FB ANT SEGMENT. Formerly included in operation group(s) 524.

Type of Patients	Observed Patients	Avg. Stay	Vari-ance	10th	25th	50th	75th	90th	95th	99th
1. SINGLE DX										
0–19 Years	4	2.6	<1	2	2	3	3	3	3	3
20–34	3	1.1	<1	1	1	1	1	1	2	2
35–49	2	1.6	<1	1	1	2	2	2	2	2
50–64	1	2.0	0	2	2	2	2	2	2	2
65+	0									
2. MULTIPLE DX										
0–19 Years	6	2.7	2	2	2	2	3	5	5	6
20–34	13	3.2	2	2	3	3	4	4	6	6
35–49	8	1.5	<1	1	1	1	3	3	3	6
50–64	2	2.0	3	1	1	1	1	3	3	4
65+	1	6.0	0	6	6	6	6	6	6	6
TOTAL SINGLE DX	10	1.5	<1	1	1	1	2	3	3	3
MULTIPLE DX	30	2.9	2	1	1	3	4	4	6	6
TOTAL										
0–19 Years	10	2.6	1	2	2	2	3	3	5	6
20–34	16	2.8	2	1	1	3	4	4	6	6
35–49	10	1.5	<1	1	1	1	3	3	4	4
50–64	3	2.0	<1	1	1	2	2	4	4	4
65+	1	6.0	0	6	6	6	6	6	6	6
GRAND TOTAL	40	2.6	2	1	1	3	4	4	6	6

Length of Stay by Diagnosis and Operation, United States, 1997

United States, October 1995–September 1996 Data, by Operation

12.1: IRIDOTOMY/SMP IRIDECTOMY. Formerly included in operation group(s) 524.

Type of Patients	Observed Patients	Avg. Stay	Vari-ance	10th	25th	50th	75th	90th	95th	99th
1. SINGLE DX										
0–19 Years	0									
20–34	1	2.0	0	2	2	2	2	2	2	2
35–49	4	2.4	<1	1	2	3	3	3	3	3
50–64	3	1.0	<1	1	1	1	1	1	1	2
65+	7	2.1	<1	1	1	3	3	3	3	3
2. MULTIPLE DX										
0–19 Years	8	1.2	<1	1	1	1	1	1	1	1
20–34	1	9.0	0	9	9	9	9	9	9	9
35–49	2	1.0	0	1	1	1	1	1	1	1
50–64	15	3.9	24	1	1	1	3	14	14	14
65+	54	6.6	60	1	2	4	11	29	>99	>99
TOTAL SINGLE DX	15	1.3	<1	1	1	1	1	2	3	3
MULTIPLE DX	80	5.4	39	1	1	3	9	14	22	>99
TOTAL										
0–19 Years	8	1.2	<1	1	1	1	1	1	4	5
20–34	2	7.8	7	2	9	9	9	9	9	9
35–49	6	1.3	<1	1	1	1	1	3	3	3
50–64	18	2.0	9	1	1	3	7	14	14	14
65+	61	5.6	50	1	2	3	7	19	>99	>99
GRAND TOTAL	95	3.6	26	1	1	1	3	9	14	>99

12.2: ANTERIOR SEG DXTIC PX. Formerly included in operation group(s) 524, 532.

Type of Patients	Observed Patients	Avg. Stay	Vari-ance	10th	25th	50th	75th	90th	95th	99th
1. SINGLE DX										
0–19 Years	1	4.0	0	4	4	4	4	4	4	4
20–34	0									
35–49	1	6.0	0	6	6	6	6	6	6	6
50–64	0									
65+	2	2.0	0	2	2	2	2	2	2	2
2. MULTIPLE DX										
0–19 Years	1	14.0	0	14	14	14	14	14	14	14
20–34	1	41.0	0	41	41	41	41	41	41	41
35–49	3	4.6	10	1	1	5	5	9	9	9
50–64	4	1.6	<1	1	1	1	2	3	3	3
65+	21	4.1	10	1	1	4	6	9	11	16
TOTAL SINGLE DX	4	3.5	2	2	2	4	4	6	6	6
MULTIPLE DX	30	4.3	30	1	1	3	5	9	11	41
TOTAL										
0–19 Years	2	5.5	15	4	4	4	4	14	14	14
20–34	1	41.0	0	41	41	41	41	41	41	41
35–49	4	4.9	8	1	1	5	6	9	9	9
50–64	4	1.6	<1	1	1	1	2	3	3	3
65+	23	3.9	10	1	1	3	4	9	11	16
GRAND TOTAL	34	4.2	26	1	1	3	5	9	11	41

12.3: IRIDOPLASTY/COREOPLASTY. Formerly included in operation group(s) 524.

Type of Patients	Observed Patients	Avg. Stay	Vari-ance	10th	25th	50th	75th	90th	95th	99th
1. SINGLE DX										
0–19 Years	3	1.8	1	1	1	1	3	3	3	3
20–34	0									
35–49	3	1.5	<1	1	1	1	3	3	3	3
50–64	1	3.0	0	3	3	3	3	3	3	3
65+	1	1.0	0	1	1	1	1	1	1	1
2. MULTIPLE DX										
0–19 Years	5	1.5	<1	1	1	1	1	3	3	3
20–34	2	5.6	10	3	3	8	8	8	8	8
35–49	3	7.3	11	3	8	8	8	8	8	8
50–64	4	8.0	26	2	2	12	12	12	12	12
65+	13	2.2	3	1	1	2	3	3	7	7
TOTAL SINGLE DX	8	1.6	<1	1	1	1	3	3	3	3
MULTIPLE DX	27	3.8	12	1	1	2	7	8	12	12
TOTAL										
0–19 Years	8	1.6	<1	1	1	1	3	3	3	3
20–34	2	5.6	10	3	3	8	8	8	8	8
35–49	6	4.3	11	1	1	3	8	8	8	8
50–64	5	7.6	26	2	2	12	12	12	12	12
65+	14	2.1	2	1	1	2	3	3	7	7
GRAND TOTAL	35	3.2	10	1	1	2	3	8	12	12

12.4: DESTR IRIS/CIL BODY LES. Formerly included in operation group(s) 524.

Type of Patients	Observed Patients	Avg. Stay	Vari-ance	10th	25th	50th	75th	90th	95th	99th
1. SINGLE DX										
0–19 Years	0									
20–34	0									
35–49	0									
50–64	1	1.0	0	1	1	1	1	1	1	1
65+	0									
2. MULTIPLE DX										
0–19 Years	1	1.0	0	1	1	1	1	1	1	1
20–34	0									
35–49	1	3.0	0	3	3	3	3	3	3	3
50–64	1	31.0	0	31	31	31	31	31	31	31
65+	4	2.0	3	1	1	1	3	6	7	7
TOTAL SINGLE DX	1	1.0	0	1	1	1	1	1	1	1
MULTIPLE DX	7	7.2	128	1	1	1	3	31	31	31
TOTAL										
0–19 Years	1	1.0	0	1	1	1	1	1	1	1
20–34	0									
35–49	1	3.0	0	3	3	3	3	3	3	3
50–64	2	27.8	97	1	31	31	31	31	31	31
65+	4	2.0	3	1	1	1	3	6	7	7
GRAND TOTAL	8	7.1	126	1	1	1	3	31	31	31

Length of Stay by Diagnosis and Operation, United States, 1997

United States, October 1995–September 1996 Data, by Operation

12.5: INOC CIRCULAT FACILITAT. Formerly included in operation group(s) 523.

Type of Patients	Observed Patients	Avg. Stay	Vari-ance	10th	25th	50th	75th	90th	95th	99th
1. SINGLE DX										
0–19 Years	10	1.1	<1	1	1	1	1		2	2
20–34	0									
35–49	0									
50–64	0									
65+	1	1.0	0	1	1	1	1	1	1	1
2. MULTIPLE DX										
0–19 Years	26	3.6	19	1	1	1	5	10	10	19
20–34	0									
35–49	4	3.0	<1	3	3	3	3	3	3	6
50–64	4	4.1	12	1	1	5	5	11	11	11
65+	16	2.0	3	1	1	1	3	4	6	7
TOTAL SINGLE DX	11	1.1	<1	1	1	1	1	1	2	2
MULTIPLE DX	50	3.2	12	1	1	2	4	7	10	19
TOTAL										
0–19 Years	36	2.9	14	1	1	1	2	9	10	19
20–34	0									
35–49	4	3.0	<1	3	3	3	5	3	3	6
50–64	4	4.1	12	1	1	5	5	11	11	11
65+	17	2.0	3	1	1	1	3	4	5	7
GRAND TOTAL	61	2.8	10	1	1	1	3	7	10	19

12.64: TRABECULECT AB EXTERNO. Formerly included in operation group(s) 523.

Type of Patients	Observed Patients	Avg. Stay	Vari-ance	10th	25th	50th	75th	90th	95th	99th
1. SINGLE DX										
0–19 Years	10	1.1	<1	1	1	1	1	1	2	3
20–34	6	3.2	23	1	1	1	1	16	16	16
35–49	14	2.5	3	1	1	1	4	5	6	6
50–64	22	2.9	2	1	1	4	4	4	4	4
65+	42	1.1	<1	1	1	1	1	1	2	2
2. MULTIPLE DX										
0–19 Years	15	2.0	5	1	1	1	1	7	8	8
20–34	4	1.3	<1	1	1	1	1	2	2	4
35–49	23	10.6	383	1	1	1	3	52	52	52
50–64	73	1.8	1	1	1	1	3	3	5	6
65+	411	1.5	5	1	1	1	1	2	3	14
TOTAL SINGLE DX	94	2.3	3	1	1	1	4	4	4	6
MULTIPLE DX	526	2.1	31	1	1	1	1	3	4	52
TOTAL										
0–19 Years	25	1.6	3	1	1	1	1	3	7	8
20–34	10	2.0	10	1	1	1	4	4	9	16
35–49	37	8.2	282	1	1	1	4	52	52	52
50–64	95	2.4	2	1	1	2	4	3	5	6
65+	453	1.4	5	1	1	1	1	2	3	10
GRAND TOTAL	620	2.1	24	1	1	1	2	4	4	24

12.6: SCLERAL FISTULIZATION. Formerly included in operation group(s) 523.

Type of Patients	Observed Patients	Avg. Stay	Vari-ance	10th	25th	50th	75th	90th	95th	99th
1. SINGLE DX										
0–19 Years	10	1.1	<1	1	1	1	1	1	2	3
20–34	6	3.2	23	1	1	1	1	16	16	16
35–49	16	2.3	3	1	1	1	4	5	6	6
50–64	23	2.9	2	1	1	4	4	4	4	4
65+	46	1.1	<1	1	1	1	1	1	2	2
2. MULTIPLE DX										
0–19 Years	18	2.0	5	1	1	1	1	7	8	8
20–34	8	2.8	3	1	1	3	5	5	5	5
35–49	30	8.8	302	1	1	1	3	52	52	52
50–64	86	1.9	3	1	1	1	3	3	5	5
65+	457	1.6	7	1	1	1	1	2	4	16
TOTAL SINGLE DX	101	2.3	3	1	1	1	4	4	4	6
MULTIPLE DX	599	2.2	29	1	1	1	2	3	5	24
TOTAL										
0–19 Years	28	1.6	3	1	1	1	1	3	7	8
20–34	14	2.9	6	1	1	3	5	5	16	16
35–49	46	7.1	230	1	1	1	4	52	52	52
50–64	109	2.4	3	1	1	2	4	4	4	6
65+	503	1.6	6	1	1	1	1	2	3	16
GRAND TOTAL	700	2.2	23	1	1	1	2	4	5	24

12.7: ELEVAT INOC PRESS RELIEF. Formerly included in operation group(s) 523.

Type of Patients	Observed Patients	Avg. Stay	Vari-ance	10th	25th	50th	75th	90th	95th	99th
1. SINGLE DX										
0–19 Years	1	1.0	0	1	1	1	1	1	1	1
20–34	0									
35–49	1	5.0	0	5	5	5	5	5	5	5
50–64	2	1.5	<1	1	1	2	1	2	2	2
65+	2	1.0	0	1	1	1	1	1	1	1
2. MULTIPLE DX										
0–19 Years	3	1.7	1	1	1	1	3	3	3	3
20–34	7	8.1	7	2	9	9	9	9	11	11
35–49	4	11.9	59	1	9	17	17	17	17	17
50–64	21	4.8	13	1	1	3	7	11	12	13
65+	30	4.2	13	1	1	4	6	7	7	30
TOTAL SINGLE DX	6	3.3	4	1	1	5	5	5	5	5
MULTIPLE DX	65	5.9	18	1	2	6	9	9	13	17
TOTAL										
0–19 Years	4	1.6	<1	1	1	1	3	3	3	3
20–34	7	8.1	7	2	9	9	9	9	11	11
35–49	5	9.1	46	1	5	5	17	17	17	17
50–64	23	4.7	13	1	1	3	7	11	12	13
65+	32	4.1	13	1	1	4	6	7	7	30
GRAND TOTAL	71	5.7	18	1	1	5	9	9	12	17

Length of Stay by Diagnosis and Operation, United States, 1997

United States, October 1995–September 1996 Data, by Operation

12.8: OPERATIONS ON SCLERA. Formerly included in operation group(s) 524.

Type of Patients	Observed Patients	Avg. Stay	Vari- ance	Percentiles						
				10th	25th	50th	75th	90th	95th	99th
1. SINGLE DX										
0–19 Years	28	1.8	1	1	1	1	2	3	3	6
20–34	13	1.6	<1	1	1	1	2	3	4	6
35–49	15	1.7	2	1	1	1	1	4	5	7
50–64	6	1.4	<1	1	1	1	1	3	3	4
65+	3	1.8	<1	1	2	2	2	2	2	2
2. MULTIPLE DX										
0–19 Years	33	2.5	1	1	2	2	4	4	5	5
20–34	26	2.6	4	1	1	2	3	4	5	11
35–49	31	2.8	3	1	1	2	3	5	5	7
50–64	18	2.4	<1	2	2	3	3	3	3	4
65+	62	4.0	25	1	1	2	4	9	15	31
TOTAL SINGLE DX	65	1.6	1	1	1	1	2	3	4	6
MULTIPLE DX	170	3.0	8	1	1	2	4	5	6	19
TOTAL										
0–19 Years	61	2.2	1	1	1	2	3	4	4	5
20–34	39	1.9	2	1	1	2	2	4	4	11
35–49	46	2.4	3	1	1	1	4	5	5	7
50–64	24	1.9	<1	1	1	2	3	3	3	4
65+	65	3.7	23	1	1	2	4	8	14	22
GRAND TOTAL	235	2.4	6	1	1	2	3	5	5	14

12.9: OTH ANTERIOR SEGMENT OPS. Formerly included in operation group(s) 524.

Type of Patients	Observed Patients	Avg. Stay	Vari- ance	Percentiles						
				10th	25th	50th	75th	90th	95th	99th
1. SINGLE DX										
0–19 Years	6	4.6	7	2	3	3	7	9	9	9
20–34	2	1.0	0	1	1	1	1	1	1	1
35–49	3	1.0	0	1	1	1	1	1	1	1
50–64	9	1.9	2	1	1	1	3	4	4	6
65+	4	2.8	3	1	1	2	5	5	5	5
2. MULTIPLE DX										
0–19 Years	20	6.3	12	2	2	9	9	9	10	13
20–34	13	4.9	9	1	3	4	8	8	8	15
35–49	17	4.9	22	2	2	3	6	8	21	21
50–64	20	3.2	7	1	1	2	4	6	7	14
65+	87	2.8	7	1	1	2	3	5	6	19
TOTAL SINGLE DX	24	2.6	5	1	1	2	4	7	7	9
MULTIPLE DX	157	3.7	11	1	2	2	5	8	9	19
TOTAL										
0–19 Years	26	5.9	11	2	2	6	9	9	10	13
20–34	15	4.8	9	1	3	3	8	8	8	15
35–49	20	4.5	22	2	2	3	6	6	21	21
50–64	29	2.8	5	1	1	2	4	6	7	14
65+	91	2.8	7	1	1	2	3	5	6	19
GRAND TOTAL	181	3.6	10	1	2	2	5	8	9	15

13.0: REMOVAL FB FROM LENS. Formerly included in operation group(s) 527.

Type of Patients	Observed Patients	Avg. Stay	Vari- ance	Percentiles						
				10th	25th	50th	75th	90th	95th	99th
1. SINGLE DX										
0–19 Years	0									
20–34	0									
35–49	0									
50–64	0									
65+	0									
2. MULTIPLE DX										
0–19 Years	0									
20–34	1	2.0	0	2	2	2	2	2	2	2
35–49	0									
50–64	0									
65+	2	1.5	<1	1	1	2	2	2	2	2
TOTAL SINGLE DX	0									
MULTIPLE DX	3	1.6	<1	1	1	2	2	2	2	2
TOTAL										
0–19 Years	0									
20–34	1	2.0	0	2	2	2	2	2	2	2
35–49	0									
50–64	0									
65+	2	1.5	<1	1	1	2	2	2	2	2
GRAND TOTAL	3	1.6	<1	1	1	2	2	2	2	2

13.1: INTRACAP LENS EXTRACTION. Formerly included in operation group(s) 525.

Type of Patients	Observed Patients	Avg. Stay	Vari- ance	Percentiles						
				10th	25th	50th	75th	90th	95th	99th
1. SINGLE DX										
0–19 Years	16	2.2	15	1	1	1	1	2	15	15
20–34	0									
35–49	2	3.8	4	1	1	5	5	5	5	5
50–64	2	1.8	<1	1	2	2	2	2	2	2
65+	4	1.4	<1	1	1	1	2	2	2	2
2. MULTIPLE DX										
0–19 Years	36	1.5	2	1	1	1	1	3	3	7
20–34	9	1.0	0	1	1	1	1	1	1	1
35–49	9	4.8	70	1	1	1	4	26	26	26
50–64	14	1.6	6	1	1	1	1	7	12	12
65+	37	3.5	9	1	1	3	4	7	8	16
TOTAL SINGLE DX	24	2.2	11	1	1	1	2	5	15	15
MULTIPLE DX	98	2.5	14	1	1	1	3	7	7	26
TOTAL										
0–19 Years	52	1.7	5	1	1	1	1	3	7	15
20–34	2	1.0	0	1	1	1	1	1	1	1
35–49	11	4.7	60	1	1	1	4	26	26	26
50–64	16	1.7	6	1	1	1	2	7	12	12
65+	41	3.3	9	1	1	2	4	7	8	16
GRAND TOTAL	122	2.5	13	1	1	1	2	5	7	26

Length of Stay by Diagnosis and Operation, United States, 1997

United States, October 1995–September 1996 Data, by Operation

13.2: LIN EXTRACAPS LENS EXTR. Formerly included in operation group(s) 526.

Type of Patients	Observed Patients	Avg. Stay	Variance	10th	25th	50th	75th	90th	95th	99th
1. SINGLE DX										
0–19 Years	0									
20–34	0									
35–49	0									
50–64	0									
65+	0									
2. MULTIPLE DX										
0–19 Years	0									
20–34	1	1.0	0	1	1	1	1	1	1	1
35–49	1	1.0	0	1	1	1	1	1	1	1
50–64	1	60.0	0	60	60	60	60	60	60	60
65+	4	6.6	13	3	3	10	10	10	10	10
TOTAL SINGLE DX	0									
MULTIPLE DX	7	13.9	478	1	1	3	10	60	60	60
TOTAL										
0–19 Years	0									
20–34	1	1.0	0	1	1	1	1	1	1	1
35–49	1	1.0	0	1	1	1	1	1	1	1
50–64	1	60.0	0	60	60	60	60	60	60	60
65+	4	6.6	13	3	3	10	10	60	60	60
GRAND TOTAL	7	13.9	478	1	1	3	10	60	60	60

13.3: SIMP ASP LENS EXTRACTION. Formerly included in operation group(s) 526.

Type of Patients	Observed Patients	Avg. Stay	Variance	10th	25th	50th	75th	90th	95th	99th
1. SINGLE DX										
0–19 Years	1	1.0	0	1	1	1	1	1	1	1
20–34	0									
35–49	0									
50–64	0									
65+	0									
2. MULTIPLE DX										
0–19 Years	4	1.6	<1	1	1	1	1	1	1	1
20–34	0									
35–49	1	3.0	0	3	3	3	3	3	3	3
50–64	3	5.7	4	6	6	6	7	7	7	7
65+	18	7.6	156	1	1	1	5	31	37	37
TOTAL SINGLE DX	1	1.0	0	1	1	1	1	1	1	1
MULTIPLE DX	26	5.7	95	1	1	2	6	31	31	37
TOTAL										
0–19 Years	5	1.5	<1	1	1	2	2	2	2	2
20–34	0									
35–49	1	3.0	0	3	3	3	3	3	3	3
50–64	3	5.7	4	6	6	6	7	7	7	7
65+	18	7.6	156	1	1	1	5	31	37	37
GRAND TOTAL	27	5.5	92	1	1	2	5	10	31	37

13.4: FRAG-ASP EXTRACAPS LENS. Formerly included in operation group(s) 526.

Type of Patients	Observed Patients	Avg. Stay	Variance	10th	25th	50th	75th	90th	95th	99th
1. SINGLE DX										
0–19 Years	4	1.0	0	1	1	1	1	1	1	1
20–34	1	1.0	0	1	1	1	1	1	1	1
35–49	3	1.0	0	1	1	1	1	1	1	1
50–64	5	3.1	2	3	3	4	4	4	4	4
65+	22	1.1	<1	1	1	1	1	1	1	5
2. MULTIPLE DX										
0–19 Years	10	2.5	16	1	1	1	1	10	10	18
20–34	10	1.4	<1	1	1	1	2	2	2	3
35–49	49	3.0	27	1	1	1	4	5	6	39
50–64	108	4.4	23	1	1	1	12	12	12	12
65+	573	2.9	27	1	1	1	2	7	10	23
TOTAL SINGLE DX	35	1.4	1	1	1	1	1	4	4	5
MULTIPLE DX	750	3.6	26	1	1	1	4	12	12	18
TOTAL										
0–19 Years	14	2.3	14	1	1	1	1	2	10	18
20–34	11	1.3	<1	1	1	1	2	2	2	3
35–49	52	3.0	26	1	1	1	4	5	6	39
50–64	113	4.4	23	1	1	1	12	12	12	12
65+	595	2.8	26	1	1	1	2	6	10	23
GRAND TOTAL	785	3.6	25	1	1	1	4	12	12	18

13.41: CATARACT PHACO & ASP. Formerly included in operation group(s) 526.

Type of Patients	Observed Patients	Avg. Stay	Variance	10th	25th	50th	75th	90th	95th	99th
1. SINGLE DX										
0–19 Years	3	1.0	0	1	1	1	1	1	1	1
20–34	1	1.0	0	1	1	1	1	1	1	1
35–49	3	1.0	0	1	1	1	1	1	1	1
50–64	5	3.1	2	3	3	4	4	4	4	4
65+	21	1.1	<1	1	1	1	1	1	1	5
2. MULTIPLE DX										
0–19 Years	7	1.9	8	1	1	1	1	10	10	10
20–34	7	1.6	<1	1	1	2	2	2	2	3
35–49	48	3.0	27	1	1	1	4	5	6	39
50–64	104	4.4	24	1	1	1	12	12	12	12
65+	552	3.0	28	1	1	1	3	7	10	23
TOTAL SINGLE DX	33	1.4	1	1	1	1	1	4	4	5
MULTIPLE DX	718	3.7	26	1	1	1	4	12	12	18
TOTAL										
0–19 Years	10	1.7	6	1	1	1	1	1	10	10
20–34	8	1.4	<1	1	1	1	2	2	2	3
35–49	51	3.0	26	1	1	1	4	5	6	39
50–64	109	4.4	23	1	1	1	12	12	12	12
65+	573	2.9	27	1	1	1	2	6	10	23
GRAND TOTAL	751	3.6	26	1	1	1	4	12	12	18

Length of Stay by Diagnosis and Operation, United States, 1997

United States, October 1995–September 1996 Data, by Operation

13.5: OTH EXTRACAPS LENS EXTR. Formerly included in operation group(s) 526.

Type of Patients	Observed Patients	Avg. Stay	Variance	10th	25th	50th	75th	90th	95th	99th
1. SINGLE DX										
0–19 Years	4	1.0	0	1	1			1	1	1
20–34	4	1.7	<1	1	1	2	2	2	2	2
35–49	0									
50–64	2	1.4	<1	1	1	1	1	3	3	3
65+	9	1.0	0	1	1	1	1	1	1	1
2. MULTIPLE DX										
0–19 Years	17	3.2	13	1	1	1	4	9	13	13
20–34	5	1.7	<1	1	1	1	3	3	3	3
35–49	6	3.7	24	1	1	1	3	15	16	16
50–64	38	6.3	20	1	2	8	8	10	16	16
65+	235	5.2	60	1	1	2	6	14	29	43
TOTAL SINGLE DX	19	1.2	<1	1	1	1	1	2	3	3
MULTIPLE DX	301	5.2	48	1	1	2	8	13	18	37
TOTAL										
0–19 Years	21	2.9	11	1	1	1	4	8	13	13
20–34	9	1.7	<1	1	1	1	2	3	3	3
35–49	6	3.7	24	1	1	1	3	15	16	16
50–64	40	6.0	20	1	2	8	8	10	16	16
65+	244	5.1	59	1	1	2	6	14	29	43
GRAND TOTAL	320	5.0	46	1	1	2	7	13	18	37

13.59: EXTRACAPS LENS EXTR NEC. Formerly included in operation group(s) 526.

Type of Patients	Observed Patients	Avg. Stay	Variance	10th	25th	50th	75th	90th	95th	99th
1. SINGLE DX										
0–19 Years	4	1.0	0	1	1			1	1	1
20–34	4	1.7	<1	1	1	2	2	2	2	2
35–49	0									
50–64	2	1.4	<1	1	1	1	1	3	3	3
65+	9	1.0	0	1	1	1	1	1	1	1
2. MULTIPLE DX										
0–19 Years	17	3.2	13	1	1	1	4	9	13	13
20–34	5	1.7	<1	1	1	1	3	3	3	3
35–49	6	3.7	24	1	1	1	3	15	16	16
50–64	38	6.3	20	1	2	8	8	10	16	16
65+	233	5.2	60	1	1	2	6	14	29	43
TOTAL SINGLE DX	19	1.2	<1	1	1	1	1	2	3	3
MULTIPLE DX	299	5.2	48	1	1	2	8	13	18	37
TOTAL										
0–19 Years	21	2.9	11	1	1	1	4	8	13	13
20–34	9	1.7	<1	1	1	1	2	3	3	3
35–49	6	3.7	24	1	1	1	3	15	16	16
50–64	40	6.0	20	1	2	8	8	10	16	16
65+	242	5.1	59	1	1	2	6	14	29	43
GRAND TOTAL	318	5.0	47	1	1	2	7	13	18	37

13.6: OTH CATARACT EXTRACTION. Formerly included in operation group(s) 526.

Type of Patients	Observed Patients	Avg. Stay	Variance	10th	25th	50th	75th	90th	95th	99th
1. SINGLE DX										
0–19 Years	3	1.0	0	1	1	1	1	1	1	1
20–34	0									
35–49	1	2.0	0	2	2	2	2	2	2	2
50–64	0									
65+	1	1.0	0	1	1	1	1	1	1	1
2. MULTIPLE DX										
0–19 Years	6	2.1	6	1	1	1	2	2	9	9
20–34	1	5.0	0	5	5	5	5	5	5	5
35–49	1	1.0	0	1	1	1	1	1	1	1
50–64	3	5.6	32	1	2	6	12	12	12	12
65+	46	9.3	128	1	2	6	10	20	29	64
TOTAL SINGLE DX	5	1.1	<1	1	1	1	1	1	2	2
MULTIPLE DX	57	7.8	107	1	1	6	9	19	27	64
TOTAL										
0–19 Years	9	1.5	3	1	1	1	1	2	2	9
20–34	1	5.0	0	5	5	5	5	5	5	5
35–49	2	1.1	<1	1	1	1	1	1	2	2
50–64	3	5.6	32	1	2	6	12	12	12	12
65+	47	9.2	127	1	2	6	10	20	29	64
GRAND TOTAL	62	7.0	100	1	1	4	8	19	22	64

13.7: INSERT PROSTHETIC LENS. Formerly included in operation group(s) 527.

Type of Patients	Observed Patients	Avg. Stay	Variance	10th	25th	50th	75th	90th	95th	99th
1. SINGLE DX										
0–19 Years	5	1.0	0	1	1	1	1	1	1	1
20–34	2	2.6	<1	1	3	3	3	3	3	3
35–49	4	1.8	2	1	1	1	2	2	6	6
50–64	2	1.0	0	1	1	1	1	1	1	1
65+	4	1.0	0	1	1	1	1	1	1	1
2. MULTIPLE DX										
0–19 Years	2	1.0	0	1	1	1	1	1	1	1
20–34	2	1.0	0	1	1	1	1	1	1	1
35–49	3	1.8	<1	1	2	2	2	2	2	2
50–64	10	1.2	<1	1	1	1	1	2	2	2
65+	32	3.8	31	1	1	1	3	13	18	28
TOTAL SINGLE DX	17	1.5	1	1	1	1	2	3	3	6
MULTIPLE DX	49	2.7	20	1	1	1	2	5	13	18
TOTAL										
0–19 Years	7	1.0	0	1	1	1	1	1	1	1
20–34	4	1.5	<1	1	1	1	3	3	3	3
35–49	7	1.8	1	1	1	2	2	2	6	6
50–64	12	1.2	<1	1	1	1	1	2	2	3
65+	36	3.6	30	1	1	1	3	13	18	28
GRAND TOTAL	66	2.4	16	1	1	1	2	4	13	18

Length of Stay by Diagnosis and Operation, United States, 1997

United States, October 1995–September 1996 Data, by Operation

13.8: IMPLANTED LENS REMOVAL. Formerly included in operation group(s) 527.

Type of Patients	Observed Patients	Avg. Stay	Vari-ance	10th	25th	50th	75th	90th	95th	99th
1. SINGLE DX										
0–19 Years	0									
20–34	0									
35–49	0									
50–64	0									
65+	0									
2. MULTIPLE DX										
0–19 Years	1	1.0	0	1	1	1	1	1	1	1
20–34	1	2.0	0	2	2	2	2	2	2	2
35–49	1	1.0	0	1	1	1	1	1	1	1
50–64	1	3.0	0	3	3	3	3	3	3	3
65+	11	2.5	12	1	1	1	2	5	14	14
TOTAL SINGLE DX	0									
MULTIPLE DX	15	2.3	9	1	1	1	2	5	14	14
TOTAL										
0–19 Years	1	1.0	0	1	1	1	1	1	1	1
20–34	1	2.0	0	2	2	2	2	2	2	2
35–49	1	1.0	0	1	1	1	1	1	1	1
50–64	1	3.0	0	3	3	3	3	3	3	3
65+	11	2.5	12	1	1	1	2	5	14	14
GRAND TOTAL	15	2.3	9	1	1	1	2	5	14	14

13.9: OTHER OPERATIONS ON LENS. Formerly included in operation group(s) 527.

Type of Patients	Observed Patients	Avg. Stay	Vari-ance	10th	25th	50th	75th	90th	95th	99th
1. SINGLE DX										
0–19 Years	0									
20–34	0									
35–49	0									
50–64	0									
65+	2	1.0	0	1	1	1	1	1	1	1
2. MULTIPLE DX										
0–19 Years	0									
20–34	1	19.0	0	19	19	19	19	19	19	19
35–49	3	2.7	28	1	1	1	1	1	1	19
50–64	1	1.0	0	1	1	1	1	1	1	1
65+	10	4.8	23	1	2	3	6	17	17	17
TOTAL SINGLE DX	2	1.0	0	1	1	1	1	1	1	1
MULTIPLE DX	15	4.5	38	1	1	1	3	19	19	19
TOTAL										
0–19 Years	0									
20–34	1	19.0	0	19	19	19	19	19	19	19
35–49	3	2.7	28	1	1	1	1	1	1	19
50–64	1	1.0	0	1	1	1	1	1	1	1
65+	12	4.4	22	1	1	3	6	9	17	17
GRAND TOTAL	17	4.4	37	1	1	1	3	19	19	19

14.0: RMVL OF POST SEGMENT FB. Formerly included in operation group(s) 529.

Type of Patients	Observed Patients	Avg. Stay	Vari-ance	10th	25th	50th	75th	90th	95th	99th
1. SINGLE DX										
0–19 Years	0									
20–34	2	1.0	0	1	1	1	1	1	1	1
35–49	1	1.0	0	1	1	1	1	1	1	1
50–64	0									
65+	0									
2. MULTIPLE DX										
0–19 Years	4	2.8	<1	1	3	3	3	3	4	4
20–34	2	4.0	2	3	3	5	5	5	5	5
35–49	0									
50–64	4	4.1	4	3	3	3	4	8	8	8
65+	1	4.0	0	4	4	4	4	4	4	4
TOTAL SINGLE DX	3	1.0	0	1	1	1	1	1	1	1
MULTIPLE DX	11	3.5	3	3	3	3	3	7	8	8
TOTAL										
0–19 Years	4	2.8	<1	1	3	3	3	3	4	4
20–34	4	1.2	<1	1	1	1	1	1	3	5
35–49	1	1.0	0	1	1	1	1	1	1	1
50–64	4	4.1	4	3	3	3	3	8	8	8
65+	1	4.0	0	4	4	4	4	4	4	4
GRAND TOTAL	14	1.9	2	1	1	1	3	3	5	8

14.1: DXTIC PX POSTERIOR SEG. Formerly included in operation group(s) 529, 532.

Type of Patients	Observed Patients	Avg. Stay	Vari-ance	10th	25th	50th	75th	90th	95th	99th
1. SINGLE DX										
0–19 Years	0									
20–34	1	2.0	0	2	2	2	2	2	2	2
35–49	0									
50–64	2	2.4	<1	2	2	2	3	3	3	3
65+	2	1.5	<1	1	1	2	2	2	2	2
2. MULTIPLE DX										
0–19 Years	2	2.4	1	1	1	3	3	3	3	3
20–34	2	9.4	30	4	4	14	14	14	14	14
35–49	6	7.2	39	3	3	3	9	22	22	22
50–64	6	1.4	1	1	1	1	1	1	5	5
65+	15	7.0	28	2	5	5	7	18	18	18
TOTAL SINGLE DX	5	2.0	<1	1	2	2	2	3	3	3
MULTIPLE DX	31	5.8	29	1	2	5	6	18	18	22
TOTAL										
0–19 Years	2	2.4	1	1	1	3	3	3	3	3
20–34	3	6.6	31	2	2	4	14	14	14	14
35–49	6	7.2	39	3	3	3	9	22	22	22
50–64	8	1.5	1	1	1	1	1	3	5	5
65+	17	6.7	28	2	3	5	7	18	18	18
GRAND TOTAL	36	5.5	28	1	2	5	5	14	18	22

Length of Stay by Diagnosis and Operation, United States, 1997

United States, October 1995–September 1996 Data, by Operation

14.2: RETINA-CHOROID LES DESTR. Formerly included in operation group(s) 529.

Type of Patients	Observed Patients	Avg. Stay	Vari-ance	Percentiles						
				10th	25th	50th	75th	90th	95th	99th
1. SINGLE DX										
0–19 Years	25	1.8	3	1	1	1	2	2	8	8
20–34	2	7.0	3	4	8	8	8	8	8	8
35–49	7	7.9	<1	8	8	8	8	8	8	8
50–64	6	7.9	<1	8	8	8	8	8	8	8
65+	15	5.8	8	1	4	7	8	8	8	8
2. MULTIPLE DX										
0–19 Years	85	29.1	>999	1	1	71	>99	>99	>99	>99
20–34	9	6.5	194	1	1	3	3	4	19	69
35–49	29	5.0	10	1	2	4	8	8	8	13
50–64	34	7.3	10	1	8	8	8	8	9	18
65+	54	4.6	20	1	1	3	8	9	11	16
TOTAL SINGLE DX	55	7.3	4	4	8	8	8	8	8	8
MULTIPLE DX	211	11.1	410	1	2	8	8	97	>99	>99
TOTAL										
0–19 Years	110	23.9	>999	1	1	11	>99	>99	>99	>99
20–34	11	6.8	90	1	3	8	8	8	8	69
35–49	36	6.9	6	2	8	8	8	8	8	8
50–64	40	7.5	7	3	8	8	8	8	10	18
65+	69	4.8	18	1	1	4	8	9	10	16
GRAND TOTAL	266	9.6	250	1	4	8	8	23	>99	>99

14.3: REPAIR OF RETINAL TEAR. Formerly included in operation group(s) 528.

Type of Patients	Observed Patients	Avg. Stay	Vari-ance	Percentiles						
				10th	25th	50th	75th	90th	95th	99th
1. SINGLE DX										
0–19 Years	2	1.0	<1	1	1	1	1	1	1	2
20–34	3	1.1	<1	1	1	1	1	1	1	4
35–49	1	1.0	0	1	1	1	1	1	1	1
50–64	3	5.5	12	1	1	8	8	8	8	8
65+	3	1.1	<1	1	1	1	1	1	2	2
2. MULTIPLE DX										
0–19 Years	14	4.3	140	1	2	2	5	>99	>99	>99
20–34	12	3.8	9	3	3	3	4	4	5	10
35–49	7	8.2	75	1	2	2	21	21	21	21
50–64	14	1.5	2	1	1	1	1	3	3	7
65+	18	2.1	13	1	1	1	2	2	17	17
TOTAL SINGLE DX	12	1.5	3	1	1	1	1	1	8	8
MULTIPLE DX	65	3.3	34	1	1	3	4	5	21	>99
TOTAL										
0–19 Years	16	2.1	46	1	1	1	2	5	>99	>99
20–34	15	3.0	8	1	1	3	4	4	4	10
35–49	8	7.5	72	1	1	2	10	21	21	21
50–64	17	2.6	8	1	1	1	3	8	8	8
65+	21	1.8	9	1	1	1	2	2	2	17
GRAND TOTAL	77	2.6	22	1	1	1	3	5	8	>99

14.27: CHORIORET RADIAT IMPLANT. Formerly included in operation group(s) 529.

Type of Patients	Observed Patients	Avg. Stay	Vari-ance	Percentiles						
				10th	25th	50th	75th	90th	95th	99th
1. SINGLE DX										
0–19 Years	0									
20–34	2	7.0	3	8	8	8	8	8	8	8
35–49	6	8.0	<1	8	8	8	8	8	8	8
50–64	6	7.9	<1	8	8	8	8	8	8	8
65+	10	7.3	2	4	7	8	8	8	8	8
2. MULTIPLE DX										
0–19 Years	0									
20–34	0									
35–49	7	7.6	<1	7	8	8	8	8	8	8
50–64	6	8.0	<1	8	8	8	8	8	8	8
65+	15	7.7	18	7	8	8	8	8	8	10
TOTAL SINGLE DX	24	7.9	<1	8	8	8	8	8	8	8
MULTIPLE DX	28	7.9	<1	8	8	8	8	8	8	8
TOTAL										
0–19 Years	0									
20–34	2	7.0	3	4	8	8	8	8	8	8
35–49	13	7.9	<1	8	8	8	8	8	8	8
50–64	12	8.0	<1	8	8	8	8	8	8	8
65+	25	7.5	1	5	8	8	8	8	8	10
GRAND TOTAL	52	7.9	<1	8	8	8	8	8	8	8

14.4: REP RETINA DETACH/BUCKLE. Formerly included in operation group(s) 528.

Type of Patients	Observed Patients	Avg. Stay	Vari-ance	Percentiles						
				10th	25th	50th	75th	90th	95th	99th
1. SINGLE DX										
0–19 Years	35	1.4	2	1	1	1	1	2	4	7
20–34	51	1.4	1	1	1	1	1	2	2	3
35–49	127	1.4	<1	1	1	1	2	2	2	3
50–64	171	1.4	<1	1	1	1	2	2	2	4
65+	147	1.3	<1	1	1	1	1	2	2	3
2. MULTIPLE DX										
0–19 Years	76	1.9	6	1	1	1	2	4	5	>99
20–34	94	2.1	6	1	1	1	2	4	6	10
35–49	196	1.6	3	1	1	1	1	3	4	7
50–64	372	1.6	<1	1	1	1	2	2	3	6
65+	654	1.8	3	1	1	1	2	3	7	7
TOTAL SINGLE DX	531	1.4	<1	1	1	1	2	2	2	4
MULTIPLE DX	1392	1.7	3	1	1	1	2	3	5	9
TOTAL										
0–19 Years	111	1.7	4	1	1	1	1	4	5	>99
20–34	145	1.9	4	1	1	2	2	3	6	10
35–49	323	1.5	2	1	1	1	2	2	3	6
50–64	543	1.5	<1	1	1	1	2	2	3	6
65+	801	1.7	3	1	1	1	2	3	5	7
GRAND TOTAL	1923	1.6	2	1	1	1	2	2	4	7

Length of Stay by Diagnosis and Operation, United States, 1997

United States, October 1995–September 1996 Data, by Operation

14.41: SCLERAL BUCKLING W IMPL. Formerly included in operation group(s) 528.

Type of Patients	Observed Patients	Avg. Stay	Variance	10th	25th	50th	75th	90th	95th	99th
1. SINGLE DX										
0–19 Years	7	1.0	<1	1	1	1	1	1	1	2
20–34	15	1.5	<1	1	1	1	2	2	2	2
35–49	45	1.3	<1	1	1	1	2	2	2	2
50–64	52	1.4	<1	1	1	1	2	2	2	3
65+	37	1.2	<1	1	1	1	1	2	2	3
2. MULTIPLE DX										
0–19 Years	18	1.4	1	1	1	1	1	3	5	>99
20–34	19	1.9	3	1	1	1	2	6	6	6
35–49	45	1.2	<1	1	1	1	1	2	2	4
50–64	105	1.4	<1	1	1	1	1	2	2	4
65+	202	1.5	2	1	1	1	2	2	3	6
TOTAL SINGLE DX	156	1.4	<1	1	1	1	2	2	2	2
MULTIPLE DX	389	1.5	1	1	1	1	2	2	3	6
TOTAL										
0–19 Years	25	1.2	<1	1	1	1	1	2	5	>99
20–34	34	1.7	2	1	1	1	2	3	6	6
35–49	90	1.3	<1	1	1	1	2	2	2	3
50–64	157	1.4	<1	1	1	1	2	2	2	4
65+	239	1.5	1	1	1	1	2	2	3	5
GRAND TOTAL	545	1.4	<1	1	1	1	2	2	3	6

14.5: OTH REPAIR RETINA DETACH. Formerly included in operation group(s) 528.

Type of Patients	Observed Patients	Avg. Stay	Variance	10th	25th	50th	75th	90th	95th	99th
1. SINGLE DX										
0–19 Years	3	1.0	0	1	1	1	1			1
20–34	5	1.3	<1	1	1	1	1	2	3	3
35–49	10	1.9	<1	1	2	2	2	2	2	2
50–64	19	1.7	2	1	1	1	2	4	6	6
65+	19	1.2	<1	1	1	1	1	2	2	2
2. MULTIPLE DX										
0–19 Years	20	16.8	>999	1	1	2	3	91	91	91
20–34	27	3.1	6	1	1	2	3	6	6	7
35–49	67	3.0	13	1	2	3	3	4	7	14
50–64	137	2.4	3	1	1	2	4	4	5	10
65+	116	1.7	3	1	1	1	2	3	4	7
TOTAL SINGLE DX	56	1.7	<1	1	1	2	2	2	2	4
MULTIPLE DX	367	3.1	64	1	1	2	3	4	5	18
TOTAL										
0–19 Years	23	14.8	>999	1	1	1	3	89	91	91
20–34	32	2.9	5	1	1	3	4	4	4	7
35–49	77	2.6	9	1	2	2	3	4	5	14
50–64	156	2.4	3	1	1	2	4	4	5	10
65+	135	1.6	3	1	1	1	2	3	4	7
GRAND TOTAL	423	2.8	54	1	1	2	3	4	5	14

14.49: SCLERAL BUCKLING NEC. Formerly included in operation group(s) 528.

Type of Patients	Observed Patients	Avg. Stay	Variance	10th	25th	50th	75th	90th	95th	99th
1. SINGLE DX										
0–19 Years	28	1.7	3	1	1	1	2	3	7	7
20–34	36	1.4	2	1	1	1	1	2	3	11
35–49	82	1.4	<1	1	1	1	2	2	3	3
50–64	119	1.4	<1	1	1	1	2	2	3	7
65+	110	1.3	<1	1	1	1	1	2	2	4
2. MULTIPLE DX										
0–19 Years	58	2.2	9	1	1	1	3	4	5	11
20–34	75	2.2	7	1	1	1	2	4	10	14
35–49	151	1.7	4	1	1	1	2	3	4	8
50–64	267	1.6	<1	1	1	1	2	2	3	6
65+	452	2.0	4	1	1	1	2	5	7	9
TOTAL SINGLE DX	375	1.4	<1	1	1	1	2	2	3	7
MULTIPLE DX	1003	1.8	3	1	1	1	2	3	5	10
TOTAL										
0–19 Years	86	2.0	7	1	1	1	2	4	5	11
20–34	111	2.0	6	1	1	1	2	3	8	11
35–49	233	1.6	3	1	1	1	2	3	4	6
50–64	386	1.6	<1	1	1	1	2	2	3	6
65+	562	1.9	3	1	1	1	2	3	7	9
GRAND TOTAL	1378	1.7	3	1	1	1	2	3	4	9

14.54: DETACH RETINA LASER COAG. Formerly included in operation group(s) 528.

Type of Patients	Observed Patients	Avg. Stay	Variance	10th	25th	50th	75th	90th	95th	99th
1. SINGLE DX										
0–19 Years	0									
20–34	2	1.0	0	1	1	1	1	1	1	1
35–49	1	1.0	<1	1	1	1	1	1	1	1
50–64	7	1.6	<1	1	1	1	2	3	3	3
65+	9	1.3	<1	1	1	1	2	2	2	2
2. MULTIPLE DX										
0–19 Years	7	44.5	>999	1	1	3	91	91	91	91
20–34	17	3.3	6	1	2	4	4	4	4	22
35–49	43	3.1	18	1	1	3	3	4	9	14
50–64	71	2.8	3	1	1	1	2	4	4	10
65+	51	1.7	2	1	1	1	2	3	4	7
TOTAL SINGLE DX	19	1.3	<1	1	1	1	1	2	3	3
MULTIPLE DX	189	3.9	109	1	1	3	4	4	5	89
TOTAL										
0–19 Years	7	44.5	>999	1	1	3	91	91	91	91
20–34	19	3.1	6	1	2	4	4	4	4	7
35–49	44	3.0	18	1	1	3	3	4	9	14
50–64	78	2.8	3	1	1	1	2	4	4	10
65+	60	1.7	2	1	1	1	2	3	4	7
GRAND TOTAL	208	3.7	103	1	1	2	4	4	5	89

Length of Stay by Diagnosis and Operation, United States, 1997

United States, October 1995–September 1996 Data, by Operation

14.6: RMVL PROSTH MAT POST SEG. Formerly included in operation group(s) 529.

Type of Patients	Observed Patients	Avg. Stay	Variance	10th	25th	50th	75th	90th	95th	99th
1. SINGLE DX										
0–19 Years	0									
20–34	2	1.0	0	1	1	1	1	1	1	1
35–49	1	1.0	0	1	1	1	1	1	1	1
50–64	0									
65+	0									
2. MULTIPLE DX										
0–19 Years	3	1.0	0	1	1	1	1	1	1	1
20–34	3	1.4	<1	1	1	1	2	2	2	2
35–49	3	5.9	14	1	1	8	8	8	12	12
50–64	1	3.0	0	3	3	3	3	3	3	3
65+	16	3.4	17	1	1	1	4	9	11	17
TOTAL SINGLE DX	3	1.0	0	1	1	1	1	1	1	1
MULTIPLE DX	26	3.2	13	1	1	1	4	8	11	17
TOTAL										
0–19	3	1.0	0	1	1	1	1	1	1	1
20–34	5	1.4	<1	1	1	1	2	2	2	2
35–49	4	4.6	15	1	1	1	8	8	8	12
50–64	1	3.0	0	3	3	3	3	3	3	3
65+	16	3.4	17	1	1	1	4	9	11	17
GRAND TOTAL	29	3.1	13	1	1	1	3	8	11	17

14.72: VITREOUS REMOVAL NEC. Formerly included in operation group(s) 529.

Type of Patients	Observed Patients	Avg. Stay	Variance	10th	25th	50th	75th	90th	95th	99th
1. SINGLE DX										
0–19 Years	8	1.3	<1	1	1	1	2	2	2	2
20–34	11	1.0	0	1	1	1	1	1	1	1
35–49	9	1.9	<1	1	2	2	2	2	2	3
50–64	22	1.4	<1	1	1	1	1	2	3	7
65+	26	1.5	<1	1	1	1	2	2	5	5
2. MULTIPLE DX										
0–19 Years	22	2.4	36	1	1	1	2	3	6	42
20–34	37	2.5	14	1	1	1	3	4	15	15
35–49	78	3.8	26	1	1	1	8	15	15	15
50–64	144	1.8	2	1	1	2	2	3	4	9
65+	279	1.7	2	1	1	1	2	3	5	7
TOTAL SINGLE DX	76	1.5	<1	1	1	1	2	2	3	7
MULTIPLE DX	560	2.3	10	1	1	1	2	4	9	15
TOTAL										
0–19	30	2.1	27	1	1	1	2	3	6	42
20–34	48	2.3	12	1	1	2	2	3	15	15
35–49	87	3.5	22	1	1	1	2	15	15	15
50–64	166	1.7	2	1	1	1	2	3	4	9
65+	305	1.7	2	1	1	1	2	3	5	7
GRAND TOTAL	636	2.2	9	1	1	1	2	4	7	15

14.7: OPERATIONS ON VITREOUS. Formerly included in operation group(s) 529.

Type of Patients	Observed Patients	Avg. Stay	Variance	10th	25th	50th	75th	90th	95th	99th
1. SINGLE DX										
0–19 Years	34	1.3	<1	1	1	1	1	2	2	5
20–34	27	1.5	2	1	1	1	1	2	3	6
35–49	29	1.7	<1	1	1	2	2	2	2	3
50–64	72	1.3	<1	1	1	1	1	2	2	7
65+	132	1.4	1	1	1	1	1	2	3	5
2. MULTIPLE DX										
0–19 Years	136	2.4	15	1	1	1	3	3	6	26
20–34	187	3.2	22	1	1	1	4	7	9	15
35–49	325	3.2	28	1	1	1	2	9	15	30
50–64	625	2.0	8	1	1	1	2	4	7	20
65+	1208	1.9	8	1	1	1	2	4	6	10
TOTAL SINGLE DX	294	1.4	<1	1	1	1	2	2	3	6
MULTIPLE DX	2481	2.3	14	1	1	1	2	5	7	20
TOTAL										
0–19	170	2.2	12	1	1	1	3	3	5	26
20–34	214	3.1	21	1	1	1	3	7	9	15
35–49	354	3.0	25	1	1	1	2	9	15	27
50–64	697	1.9	7	1	1	1	2	3	5	20
65+	1340	1.9	7	1	1	1	2	4	5	10
GRAND TOTAL	2775	2.2	12	1	1	1	2	4	7	20

14.74: MECH VITRECTOMY NEC. Formerly included in operation group(s) 529.

Type of Patients	Observed Patients	Avg. Stay	Variance	10th	25th	50th	75th	90th	95th	99th
1. SINGLE DX										
0–19 Years	13	1.5	<1	1	1	1	2	2	5	5
20–34	14	1.8	3	1	1	1	1	6	6	6
35–49	15	1.3	<1	1	1	1	2	2	2	5
50–64	46	1.3	<1	1	1	1	1	2	2	2
65+	97	1.4	1	1	1	1	1	2	4	7
2. MULTIPLE DX										
0–19 Years	89	2.4	13	1	1	1	3	3	4	26
20–34	135	3.5	27	1	1	1	7	7	7	18
35–49	225	2.9	30	1	1	1	2	6	19	30
50–64	438	1.5	2	1	1	1	1	2	4	8
65+	831	1.9	10	1	1	1	2	3	5	11
TOTAL SINGLE DX	185	1.4	1	1	1	1	1	2	3	6
MULTIPLE DX	1718	2.1	14	1	1	1	2	4	7	20
TOTAL										
0–19	102	2.3	12	1	1	1	3	3	4	26
20–34	149	3.4	25	1	1	1	7	7	9	18
35–49	240	2.8	29	1	1	1	2	5	16	30
50–64	484	1.4	2	1	1	1	1	3	4	7
65+	928	1.8	9	1	1	1	2	3	5	10
GRAND TOTAL	1903	2.1	12	1	1	1	2	4	7	18

United States, October 1995–September 1996 Data, by Operation

14.9: OTHER POST SEGMENT OPS. Formerly included in operation group(s) 529.

Type of Patients	Observed Patients	Avg. Stay	Vari-ance	10th	25th	50th	Percentiles 75th	90th	95th	99th
1. SINGLE DX										
0–19 Years	5	1.0	0	1	1	1	1	1	1	1
20–34	1	2.0	0	2	2	2	2	2	2	2
35–49	2	1.0	0	1	1	1	1	1	1	1
50–64	8	1.0	0	1	1	1	1	1	1	1
65+	20	1.0	<1	1	1	1	1	1	1	2
2. MULTIPLE DX										
0–19 Years	13	1.9	3	1	1	1	2	4	7	7
20–34	28	1.7	2	1	1	1	2	3	3	10
35–49	44	2.3	9	1	1	2	2	2	13	13
50–64	71	1.4	1	1	1	1	1	3	5	5
65+	137	1.8	2	1	1	1	2	4	5	7
TOTAL SINGLE DX	36	1.0	<1	1	1	1	1	1	1	2
MULTIPLE DX	293	1.8	3	1	1	1	2	4	5	13
TOTAL										
0–19 Years	18	1.7	3	1	1	1	2	4	7	7
20–34	29	1.7	2	1	1	1	2	3	3	10
35–49	46	2.3	9	1	1	2	2	2	13	13
50–64	79	1.4	1	1	1	1	1	3	5	5
65+	157	1.8	2	1	1	1	2	4	5	7
GRAND TOTAL	329	1.8	3	1	1	1	2	4	5	13

15.0: EXOC MUSC-TEND DXTIC PX. Formerly included in operation group(s) 530, 532.

Type of Patients	Observed Patients	Avg. Stay	Vari-ance	10th	25th	50th	Percentiles 75th	90th	95th	99th
1. SINGLE DX										
0–19 Years	0									
20–34	0									
35–49	0									
50–64	0									
65+	0									
2. MULTIPLE DX										
0–19 Years	0									
20–34	0									
35–49	1	13.0	0	13	13	13	13	13	13	13
50–64	0									
65+	0									
TOTAL SINGLE DX	0									
MULTIPLE DX	1	13.0	0	13	13	13	13	13	13	13
TOTAL										
0–19 Years	0									
20–34	0									
35–49	1	13.0	0	13	13	13	13	13	13	13
50–64	0									
65+	0									
GRAND TOTAL	1	13.0	0	13	13	13	13	13	13	13

15.1: 1 EXOC MUSC OPS W DETACH. Formerly included in operation group(s) 530.

Type of Patients	Observed Patients	Avg. Stay	Vari-ance	10th	25th	50th	Percentiles 75th	90th	95th	99th
1. SINGLE DX										
0–19 Years	10	1.8	3	1	1	1	1	5	5	5
20–34	2	1.0	0	1	1	1	1	1	1	1
35–49	0									
50–64	1	1.0	0	1	1	1	1	1	1	1
65+	0									
2. MULTIPLE DX										
0–19 Years	29	1.2	<1	1	1	1	1	2	2	4
20–34	1	4.0	0	4	4	4	4	4	4	4
35–49	4	1.6	1	1	1	1	1	4	4	4
50–64	1	9.0	0	9	9	9	9	9	9	9
65+	4	2.9	3	1	2	3	3	7	7	7
TOTAL SINGLE DX	13	1.6	2	1	1	1	1	5	5	5
MULTIPLE DX	39	1.7	3	1	1	1	1	4	4	9
TOTAL										
0–19 Years	39	1.3	<1	1	1	1	1	2	4	5
20–34	3	2.2	2	1	1	1	4	4	4	4
35–49	4	1.6	1	1	1	1	1	4	4	4
50–64	2	6.9	14	1	1	9	9	9	9	9
65+	4	2.9	3	1	2	3	3	7	7	7
GRAND TOTAL	52	1.7	3	1	1	1	1	4	5	9

15.2: OTH OPS ON 1 EXOC MUSCLE. Formerly included in operation group(s) 530.

Type of Patients	Observed Patients	Avg. Stay	Vari-ance	10th	25th	50th	Percentiles 75th	90th	95th	99th
1. SINGLE DX										
0–19 Years	0									
20–34	0									
35–49	1	1.0	0	1	1	1	1	1	1	1
50–64	0									
65+	0									
2. MULTIPLE DX										
0–19 Years	2	1.0	0	1	1	1	1	1	1	1
20–34	0									
35–49	0									
50–64	1	2.0	0	2	2	2	2	2	2	2
65+	0									
TOTAL SINGLE DX	1	1.0	0	1	1	1	1	1	1	1
MULTIPLE DX	3	1.6	<1	1	1	2	2	2	2	2
TOTAL										
0–19 Years	2	1.0	0	1	1	1	1	1	1	1
20–34	0									
35–49	0									
50–64	2	1.9	<1	1	2	2	2	2	2	2
65+	0									
GRAND TOTAL	4	1.6	<1	1	1	2	2	2	2	2

Length of Stay by Diagnosis and Operation, United States, 1997

United States, October 1995–September 1996 Data, by Operation

15.3: TEMP DETACH >1 EXOC MUSC. Formerly included in operation group(s) 530.

Type of Patients	Observed Patients	Avg. Stay	Vari- ance	Percentiles						
				10th	25th	50th	75th	90th	95th	99th
1. SINGLE DX										
0–19 Years	119	1.0	0	1	1	1	1	1	1	1
20–34	3	1.0	0	1	1	1	1	1	1	1
35–49	2	1.0	0	1	1	1	1	1	1	1
50–64	0									
65+	0									
2. MULTIPLE DX										
0–19 Years	107	1.1	<1	1	1	1	1	1	2	4
20–34	2	1.0	0	1	1	1	1	1	1	1
35–49	3	2.8	10	1	1	1	7	7	7	7
50–64	3	3.2	4	1	1	5	5	5	5	5
65+	3	5.9	8	1	4	8	8	8	8	8
TOTAL SINGLE DX	124	1.0	0	1	1	1	1	1	1	1
MULTIPLE DX	118	1.4	1	1	1	1	1	2	4	8
TOTAL										
0–19 Years	226	1.1	<1	1	1	1	1	1	1	2
20–34	5	1.0	0	1	1	1	1	1	1	1
35–49	5	1.7	4	1	1	1	1	7	7	7
50–64	3	3.2	4	1	1	5	5	5	5	5
65+	3	5.9	8	1	4	8	8	8	8	8
GRAND TOTAL	242	1.2	<1	1	1	1	1	1	2	5

15.4: OTH OPS ON >1 EXOC MUSC. Formerly included in operation group(s) 530.

Type of Patients	Observed Patients	Avg. Stay	Vari- ance	Percentiles						
				10th	25th	50th	75th	90th	95th	99th
1. SINGLE DX										
0–19 Years	1	1.0	0	1	1	1	1	1	1	1
20–34	0									
35–49	0									
50–64	1	1.0	0	1	1	1	1	1	1	1
65+	0									
2. MULTIPLE DX										
0–19 Years	4	1.7	<1	1	1	2	2	2	2	3
20–34	0									
35–49	1	1.0	0	1	1	1	1	1	1	1
50–64	0									
65+	1	3.0	0	3	3	3	3	3	3	3
TOTAL SINGLE DX	2	1.0	0	1	1	1	1	1	1	1
MULTIPLE DX	6	1.8	<1	1	1	2	2	3	3	3
TOTAL										
0–19 Years	5	1.7	<1	1	1	2	2	2	3	3
20–34	0									
35–49	1	1.0	0	1	1	1	1	1	1	1
50–64	1	1.0	0	1	1	1	1	1	1	1
65+	1	3.0	0	3	3	3	3	3	3	3
GRAND TOTAL	8	1.5	<1	1	1	1	2	3	3	3

15.5: EXOC MUSC TRANSPOSITION. Formerly included in operation group(s) 530.

Type of Patients	Observed Patients	Avg. Stay	Vari- ance	Percentiles						
				10th	25th	50th	75th	90th	95th	99th
1. SINGLE DX										
0–19 Years	0									
20–34	1	8.0	0	8	8	8	8	8	8	8
35–49	1	8.0	0	8	8	8	8	8	8	8
50–64	0									
65+	0									
2. MULTIPLE DX										
0–19 Years	2	1.0	0	1	1	1	1	1	1	1
20–34	0									
35–49	3	2.0	5	1	1	1	1	6	6	6
50–64	0									
65+	0									
TOTAL SINGLE DX	2	8.0	0	8	8	8	8	8	8	8
MULTIPLE DX	5	1.4	2	1	1	1	1	1	6	6
TOTAL										
0–19 Years	2	1.0	0	1	1	1	1	1	1	1
20–34	1	8.0	0	8	8	8	8	8	8	8
35–49	4	7.7	2	8	8	8	8	8	8	8
50–64	0									
65+	0									
GRAND TOTAL	7	7.8	2	8	8	8	8	8	8	8

15.6: REV EXOC MUSCLE SURGERY. Formerly included in operation group(s) 530.

Type of Patients	Observed Patients	Avg. Stay	Vari- ance	Percentiles						
				10th	25th	50th	75th	90th	95th	99th
1. SINGLE DX										
0–19 Years	2	1.0	0	1	1	1	1	1	1	1
20–34	0									
35–49	1	1.0	0	1	1	1	1	1	1	1
50–64	0									
65+	0									
2. MULTIPLE DX										
0–19 Years	7	1.0	0	1	1	1	1	1	1	1
20–34	0									
35–49	0									
50–64	0									
65+	0									
TOTAL SINGLE DX	3	1.0	0	1	1	1	1	1	1	1
MULTIPLE DX	7	1.0	0	1	1	1	1	1	1	1
TOTAL										
0–19 Years	9	1.0	0	1	1	1	1	1	1	1
20–34	0									
35–49	1	1.0	0	1	1	1	1	1	1	1
50–64	0									
65+	0									
GRAND TOTAL	10	1.0	0	1	1	1	1	1	1	1

Length of Stay by Diagnosis and Operation, United States, 1997

United States, October 1995–September 1996 Data, by Operation

15.7: EXOC MUSCLE INJURY REP. Formerly included in operation group(s) 530.

Type of Patients	Observed Patients	Avg. Stay	Vari-ance	Percentiles						
				10th	25th	50th	75th	90th	95th	99th
1. SINGLE DX										
0–19 Years	1	1.0	0	1	1	1	1	1	1	1
20–34	1	3.0	0	3	3	3	3	3	3	3
35–49	1	2.0	0	2	2	2	2	2	2	2
50–64	0									
65+	0									
2. MULTIPLE DX										
0–19 Years	4	2.1	2	1	1	1	4	4	4	4
20–34	12	2.6	1	1	1	3	4	4	4	5
35–49	5	2.4	2	1	2	3	3	3	7	7
50–64	2	7.6	66	1	1	14	14	14	14	14
65+	1	7.0	0	7	7	7	7	7	7	7
TOTAL SINGLE DX	3	1.7	<1	1	1	1	2	3	3	3
MULTIPLE DX	24	2.6	3	1	1	3	3	4	4	14
TOTAL										
0–19 Years	5	1.8	2	1	1	1	1	4	4	4
20–34	13	2.6	1	1	1	3	3	4	4	4
35–49	6	2.3	2	1	2	2	3	3	7	7
50–64	2	7.6	66	1	1	14	14	14	14	14
65+	1	7.0	0	7	7	7	7	7	7	7
GRAND TOTAL	27	2.6	3	1	1	3	3	4	4	7

16.0: ORBITOTOMY. Formerly included in operation group(s) 531.

Type of Patients	Observed Patients	Avg. Stay	Vari-ance	Percentiles						
				10th	25th	50th	75th	90th	95th	99th
1. SINGLE DX										
0–19 Years	31	2.3	2	1	1	2	3	4	4	7
20–34	20	1.4	<1	1	1	1	2	4	3	5
35–49	15	2.4	2	1	1	1	3	4	4	10
50–64	5	1.1	<1	1	1	1	1	1	2	2
65+	3	2.4	3	1	1	2	5	5	5	5
2. MULTIPLE DX										
0–19 Years	127	4.8	20	1	1	4	7	11	14	18
20–34	65	2.8	4	1	2	2	4	5	7	11
35–49	60	3.6	10	1	2	2	4	9	9	14
50–64	54	3.9	15	1	3	3	5	7	7	14
65+	42	3.5	6	1	2	3	4	8	9	11
TOTAL SINGLE DX	74	2.0	2	1	1	1	3	4	4	7
MULTIPLE DX	348	3.8	12	1	2	2	5	8	11	14
TOTAL										
0–19 Years	158	4.5	18	1	1	3	6	11	14	18
20–34	85	2.7	4	1	2	2	3	5	7	11
35–49	75	3.4	9	1	2	2	3	9	9	14
50–64	59	3.7	14	1	1	3	5	7	7	14
65+	45	3.4	6	1	2	3	4	7	9	11
GRAND TOTAL	422	3.6	11	1	1	2	5	7	10	14

15.9: OTH EXOC MUSC-TEND OPS. Formerly included in operation group(s) 530.

Type of Patients	Observed Patients	Avg. Stay	Vari-ance	Percentiles						
				10th	25th	50th	75th	90th	95th	99th
1. SINGLE DX										
0–19 Years	1	1.0	0	1	1	1	1	1	1	1
20–34	0									
35–49	1	3.0	0	3	3	3	3	3	3	3
50–64	0									
65+	0									
2. MULTIPLE DX										
0–19 Years	1	4.0	0	4	4	4	4	4	4	4
20–34	1	4.0	0	4	4	4	4	4	4	4
35–49	3	5.7	23	4	4	4	4	18	18	18
50–64	2	4.5	<1	4	4	5	5	5	5	5
65+	5	9.5	11	7	8	9	9	17	17	17
TOTAL SINGLE DX	2	2.0	2	1	1	3	3	3	3	3
MULTIPLE DX	12	6.0	13	4	4	4	7	9	17	18
TOTAL										
0–19 Years	2	3.1	3	1	1	4	4	4	4	4
20–34	1	4.0	0	4	4	4	4	4	4	4
35–49	4	5.5	21	3	4	5	5	18	18	18
50–64	2	4.5	<1	4	4	5	5	5	5	5
65+	5	9.5	11	7	8	9	9	17	17	17
GRAND TOTAL	14	5.8	13	4	4	4	7	9	17	18

16.09: ORBITOTOMY NEC. Formerly included in operation group(s) 531.

Type of Patients	Observed Patients	Avg. Stay	Vari-ance	Percentiles						
				10th	25th	50th	75th	90th	95th	99th
1. SINGLE DX										
0–19 Years	13	2.7	4	1	1	2	4	7	7	7
20–34	15	1.8	<1	1	1	2	2	3	4	5
35–49	11	2.2	3	1	1	1	4	4	4	10
50–64	4	1.0	0	1	1	1	1	1	1	1
65+	3	2.4	3	1	1	2	5	5	5	5
2. MULTIPLE DX										
0–19 Years	112	5.0	21	1	1	4	7	11	14	18
20–34	53	2.9	4	1	2	2	3	7	7	12
35–49	48	3.8	10	1	2	2	4	9	9	14
50–64	48	4.1	7	1	3	3	7	8	9	12
65+	40	3.6	7	1	3	3	4	8	9	11
TOTAL SINGLE DX	46	2.1	3	1	1	1	3	4	5	7
MULTIPLE DX	301	3.9	12	1	2	3	5	9	11	14
TOTAL										
0–19 Years	125	4.9	21	1	1	4	7	11	14	18
20–34	68	2.9	4	1	2	2	3	7	7	12
35–49	59	3.7	10	1	2	2	3	9	9	14
50–64	52	4.0	8	1	1	3	7	7	7	12
65+	43	3.5	7	1	3	3	4	7	9	11
GRAND TOTAL	347	3.8	12	1	2	2	5	9	11	14

Length of Stay by Diagnosis and Operation, United States, 1997

United States, October 1995–September 1996 Data, by Operation

16.1: RMVL PENETR FB EYE NOS. Formerly included in operation group(s) 531.

Type of Patients	Observed Patients	Avg. Stay	Vari-ance	10th	25th	50th	75th	90th	95th	99th
1. SINGLE DX										
0–19 Years	4	1.3	<1	1	1	1	1	3	3	3
20–34	0									
35–49	0									
50–64	0									
65+	0									
2. MULTIPLE DX										
0–19 Years	7	2.6	9	1	1	1	3	5	12	12
20–34	6	2.0	2	1	1	1	3	4	4	7
35–49	3	2.5	<1	1	2	3	3	3	3	3
50–64	1	7.0	0	7	7	7	7	7	7	7
65+	1	8.0	0	8	8	8	8	8	8	8
TOTAL SINGLE DX	4	1.3	<1	1	1	1	1	3	3	3
MULTIPLE DX	18	2.4	6	1	1	1	3	5	7	12
TOTAL										
0–19 Years	11	2.3	8	1	1	1	2	5	10	12
20–34	6	2.0	2	1	2	1	3	4	4	7
35–49	3	2.5	<1	1	1	3	3	3	3	3
50–64	1	7.0	0	7	7	7	7	7	7	7
65+	1	8.0	0	8	8	8	8	8	8	8
GRAND TOTAL	22	2.3	5	1	1	1	3	5	7	12

16.2: ORBIT & EYEBALL DXTIC PX. Formerly included in operation group(s) 531, 532.

Type of Patients	Observed Patients	Avg. Stay	Vari-ance	10th	25th	50th	75th	90th	95th	99th
1. SINGLE DX										
0–19 Years	8	3.8	8	1	2	3	4	6	12	12
20–34	0									
35–49	2	1.4	<1	1	1	1	2	2	2	2
50–64	1	1.0	0	1	1	1	1	1	1	1
65+	2	1.6	<1	1	1	2	2	2	2	2
2. MULTIPLE DX										
0–19 Years	17	4.9	45	1	1	2	6	23	23	23
20–34	3	5.6	4	5	5	5	5	9	9	15
35–49	9	6.0	40	1	1	4	9	18	22	22
50–64	9	3.2	4	1	1	4	4	7	7	7
65+	21	4.5	26	1	1	2	4	16	16	18
TOTAL SINGLE DX	13	2.9	7	1	1	2	4	6	6	12
MULTIPLE DX	59	4.9	26	1	1	4	5	9	18	23
TOTAL										
0–19 Years	25	4.7	39	1	1	2	6	12	23	23
20–34	3	5.6	4	5	5	5	5	9	9	15
35–49	11	5.5	38	1	1	2	9	18	22	22
50–64	10	3.0	25	1	1	2	4	7	7	7
65+	23	4.3	25	1	1	2	5	16	16	18
GRAND TOTAL	72	4.7	24	1	1	4	5	9	16	23

16.3: EVISCERATION OF EYEBALL. Formerly included in operation group(s) 531.

Type of Patients	Observed Patients	Avg. Stay	Vari-ance	10th	25th	50th	75th	90th	95th	99th
1. SINGLE DX										
0–19 Years	2	1.0	0	1	1	1	1	1	1	1
20–34	3	1.6	<1	1	1	2	2	2	2	2
35–49	1	1.0	0	1	1	1	1	1	1	1
50–64	0									
65+	1	1.0	0	1	1	1	1	1	1	1
2. MULTIPLE DX										
0–19 Years	1	1.0	0	1	1	1	1	1	1	1
20–34	8	2.3	7	2	2	2	2	2	2	15
35–49	15	5.5	33	1	1	3	14	14	14	20
50–64	12	1.9	1	1	1	2	2	3	5	5
65+	51	4.4	10	1	2	4	7	8	10	11
TOTAL SINGLE DX	7	1.3	<1	1	1	1	2	2	2	2
MULTIPLE DX	87	3.7	17	1	1	2	4	11	14	14
TOTAL										
0–19 Years	3	1.0	0	1	1	1	1	1	1	1
20–34	11	2.3	6	2	2	2	2	2	2	15
35–49	16	5.4	33	1	1	3	14	14	14	20
50–64	12	1.9	1	1	1	2	2	3	5	5
65+	52	4.3	10	1	2	4	7	8	10	11
GRAND TOTAL	94	3.7	17	1	1	2	4	11	14	14

16.4: ENUCLEATION OF EYEBALL. Formerly included in operation group(s) 531.

Type of Patients	Observed Patients	Avg. Stay	Vari-ance	10th	25th	50th	75th	90th	95th	99th
1. SINGLE DX										
0–19 Years	30	1.5	<1	1	1	1	2	3	3	3
20–34	9	1.4	<1	1	1	1	2	3	4	4
35–49	14	1.8	5	1	1	1	1	2	9	9
50–64	12	1.6	2	1	1	2	2	3	3	8
65+	7	2.8	14	1	2	2	2	3	17	17
2. MULTIPLE DX										
0–19 Years	45	2.8	51	1	1	1	2	5	6	13
20–34	73	3.1	13	1	1	1	4	11	11	14
35–49	55	5.2	24	1	1	4	10	10	16	25
50–64	48	3.0	7	1	1	3	3	5	8	11
65+	173	3.4	17	1	1	2	4	8	12	23
TOTAL SINGLE DX	72	1.8	4	1	1	1	2	3	3	17
MULTIPLE DX	394	3.6	19	1	1	2	4	10	11	16
TOTAL										
0–19 Years	75	2.3	31	1	1	1	2	4	6	13
20–34	82	3.0	12	1	1	1	3	11	11	14
35–49	69	4.9	23	1	1	4	7	10	16	16
50–64	60	2.8	6	1	1	3	3	5	8	11
65+	180	3.3	16	1	1	2	4	8	12	23
GRAND TOTAL	466	3.4	17	1	1	2	4	10	11	16

Length of Stay by Diagnosis and Operation, United States, 1997

United States, October 1995–September 1996 Data, by Operation

16.5: EXENTERATION OF ORBIT. Formerly included in operation group(s) 531.

Type of Patients	Observed Patients	Avg. Stay	Variance	10th	25th	50th	75th	90th	95th	99th
1. SINGLE DX										
0–19 Years	3	1.8	<1	1	2	2	2	2	2	2
20–34	0									
35–49	1	1.0	0	1	1	1	1	1	1	1
50–64	1	1.0	0	1	1	1	1	1	1	1
65+	3	4.2	3	2	2	5	6	6	6	6
2. MULTIPLE DX										
0–19 Years	3	5.1	<1	5	5	5	5	5	6	6
20–34	3	6.0	9	3	3	8	9	9	9	9
35–49	2	5.6	4	4	4	7	7	7	7	7
50–64	7	8.7	29	2	5	8	9	18	18	18
65+	24	3.9	9	1	2	3	5	7	11	13
TOTAL SINGLE DX	8	2.6	3	1	1	2	5	6	6	6
MULTIPLE DX	39	5.1	15	1	2	5	7	9	13	18
TOTAL										
0–19 Years	6	3.8	3	2	2	5	5	5	6	6
20–34	3	6.0	9	3	3	8	9	9	9	9
35–49	3	3.9	8	1	1	4	7	7	7	7
50–64	8	8.4	30	2	5	8	9	18	18	18
65+	27	3.9	9	1	2	3	5	7	11	13
GRAND TOTAL	47	4.8	14	1	2	4	6	9	12	18

16.6: 2ND PX POST RMVL EYEBALL. Formerly included in operation group(s) 531.

Type of Patients	Observed Patients	Avg. Stay	Variance	10th	25th	50th	75th	90th	95th	99th
1. SINGLE DX										
0–19 Years	0									
20–34	4	2.3	2	1	1	1	4	4	4	4
35–49	1	1.0	0	1	1	1	1	1	1	1
50–64	2	1.2	<1	1	1	1	1	1	1	1
65+	1	1.0	0	1	1	1	1	1	1	1
2. MULTIPLE DX										
0–19 Years	9	1.4	2	1	1	1	1	2	3	8
20–34	11	1.7	2	1	1	1	2	3	3	10
35–49	10	1.3	<1	1	1	1	2	2	3	5
50–64	6	3.1	19	1	1	1	4	15	15	15
65+	14	3.1	10	1	1	1	5	8	10	10
TOTAL SINGLE DX	8	1.8	2	1	1	1	2	4	4	4
MULTIPLE DX	50	2.0	7	1	1	1	2	4	8	15
TOTAL										
0–19 Years	9	1.4	2	1	1	1	1	2	3	8
20–34	15	1.8	2	1	1	1	3	3	4	10
35–49	11	1.3	<1	1	1	1	1	2	3	5
50–64	8	2.9	17	1	1	1	4	4	15	15
65+	15	3.0	10	1	1	1	5	8	10	10
GRAND TOTAL	58	2.0	6	1	1	1	2	4	6	15

16.7: OCULAR/ORBITAL IMPL RMVL. Formerly included in operation group(s) 531.

Type of Patients	Observed Patients	Avg. Stay	Variance	10th	25th	50th	75th	90th	95th	99th
1. SINGLE DX										
0–19 Years	1	1.0	0	1	1	1	1	1	1	1
20–34	2	4.9	<1	5	5	5	5	5	5	5
35–49	1	1.0	0	1	1	1	1	1	1	1
50–64	0									
65+	1	1.0	0	1	1	1	1	1	1	1
2. MULTIPLE DX										
0–19 Years	4	1.7	<1	1	1	2	2	2	2	2
20–34	4	3.1	4	1	1	3	3	7	7	7
35–49	2	5.0	<1	5	5	5	5	5	5	5
50–64	3	12.5	40	1	5	16	16	16	16	16
65+	9	3.8	15	1	1	2	8	8	12	12
TOTAL SINGLE DX	5	3.9	3	1	1	5	5	5	5	5
MULTIPLE DX	22	4.8	11	1	3	5	5	8	16	16
TOTAL										
0–19 Years	5	1.5	<1	1	1	1	2	2	2	2
20–34	6	4.5	2	5	5	5	5	5	5	7
35–49	3	4.7	1	5	5	5	5	5	5	5
50–64	3	12.5	40	1	5	16	16	16	16	16
65+	10	3.6	14	1	1	1	8	8	12	12
GRAND TOTAL	27	4.6	9	1	3	5	5	5	12	16

16.8: EYEBALL/ORBIT INJ REPAIR. Formerly included in operation group(s) 531.

Type of Patients	Observed Patients	Avg. Stay	Variance	10th	25th	50th	75th	90th	95th	99th
1. SINGLE DX										
0–19 Years	54	3.6	3	1	3	4	4	6	6	8
20–34	36	3.7	6	1	1	4	7	7	7	11
35–49	28	1.6	0	1	1	1	2	3	3	6
50–64	1	1.0	0	1	1	1	1	1	1	1
65+	9	2.2	2	1	1	2	4	4	4	4
2. MULTIPLE DX										
0–19 Years	84	6.8	41	2	2	4	17	17	17	17
20–34	115	4.4	18	1	2	3	5	13	13	16
35–49	84	2.7	6	1	1	2	3	5	6	12
50–64	44	3.0	3	2	2	3	4	5	7	8
65+	105	4.6	28	1	2	3	5	11	13	26
TOTAL SINGLE DX	128	3.0	4	1	1	3	4	6	7	7
MULTIPLE DX	432	4.1	19	1	2	3	4	12	13	17
TOTAL										
0–19 Years	138	5.0	22	1	2	4	5	17	17	17
20–34	151	4.2	14	1	1	3	5	13	13	15
35–49	112	2.3	4	1	1	2	3	5	6	12
50–64	45	2.9	3	2	2	3	3	4	7	8
65+	114	4.4	26	1	2	3	5	10	13	26
GRAND TOTAL	560	3.7	14	1	1	3	4	7	13	17

Length of Stay by Diagnosis and Operation, United States, 1997

United States, October 1995–September 1996 Data, by Operation

16.82: REPAIR EYEBALL RUPTURE. Formerly included in operation group(s) 531.

Type of Patients	Observed Patients	Avg. Stay	Variance	10th	25th	50th	75th	90th	95th	99th
1. SINGLE DX										
0–19 Years	27	3.4	2	1	3	4	4	5	5	7
20–34	24	4.4	8	1	2	4	7	7	7	11
35–49	17	2.4	<1	1	2	2	3	3	5	5
50–64	1	1.0	0	1	1	1	1	1	1	1
65+	7	2.5	2	1	1	3	4	4	4	4
2. MULTIPLE DX										
0–19 Years	50	7.9	47	2	2	4	17	17	17	17
20–34	75	3.1	3	1	2	3	3	5	5	9
35–49	49	2.9	9	1	1	2	3	6	9	12
50–64	31	3.0	3	2	2	2	4	6	7	8
65+	76	4.0	25	1	2	3	5	6	11	26
TOTAL SINGLE DX	76	3.5	4	1	2	3	5	7	7	7
MULTIPLE DX	281	4.0	19	1	2	3	4	8	17	17
TOTAL										
0–19 Years	77	5.7	30	1	2	4	5	17	17	17
20–34	99	3.5	5	1	2	3	5	7	7	9
35–49	66	2.7	7	1	1	2	3	5	7	12
50–64	32	3.0	3	2	2	2	4	6	7	8
65+	83	3.9	23	1	2	3	5	6	11	26
GRAND TOTAL	357	3.9	15	1	2	3	4	7	12	17

16.89: EYE/ORBIT INJ REPAIR NEC. Formerly included in operation group(s) 531.

Type of Patients	Observed Patients	Avg. Stay	Variance	10th	25th	50th	75th	90th	95th	99th
1. SINGLE DX										
0–19 Years	23	4.0	3	1	4	4	6	6	6	8
20–34	12	2.6	2	1	1	2	4	4	4	6
35–49	11	1.2	<1	1	1	1	1	1	3	6
50–64	0									
65+	2	1.0	0	1	1	1	1	1	1	1
2. MULTIPLE DX										
0–19 Years	30	3.7	10	1	2	3	5	6	14	14
20–34	33	6.5	33	1	1	4	13	13	13	16
35–49	29	2.3	3	1	1	2	3	4	4	13
50–64	12	2.9	2	1	2	3	3	3	5	8
65+	27	6.4	33	1	2	3	13	13	19	19
TOTAL SINGLE DX	48	2.5	3	1	1	1	4	6	6	7
MULTIPLE DX	131	4.3	19	1	1	3	4	13	13	16
TOTAL										
0–19 Years	53	3.9	5	1	2	4	5	6	7	14
20–34	45	5.4	27	1	1	4	13	13	13	16
35–49	40	1.8	2	1	2	1	3	4	4	6
50–64	12	2.9	2	1	1	3	3	3	5	8
65+	29	6.1	33	1	1	3	10	13	19	19
GRAND TOTAL	179	3.7	14	1	1	3	4	13	13	16

16.9: OTHER EYE & ORBIT OPS. Formerly included in operation group(s) 531.

Type of Patients	Observed Patients	Avg. Stay	Variance	10th	25th	50th	75th	90th	95th	99th
1. SINGLE DX										
0–19 Years	31	2.8	4	1	2	2	4	8	8	9
20–34	8	1.9	2	1	1	1	2	4	4	10
35–49	9	2.7	<1	2	2	3	3	3	3	5
50–64	6	3.0	1	1	2	4	4	4	4	4
65+	8	1.3	<1	1	1	1	1	2	4	4
2. MULTIPLE DX										
0–19 Years	53	5.0	61	1	1	4	6	7	11	24
20–34	31	4.2	12	1	1	4	5	11	11	12
35–49	52	4.8	39	1	1	3	5	8	17	33
50–64	26	4.8	23	1	2	3	6	16	16	20
65+	34	3.3	11	1	1	2	6	7	11	14
TOTAL SINGLE DX	62	2.5	3	1	1	2	3	4	5	8
MULTIPLE DX	196	4.6	37	1	1	3	5	10	14	30
TOTAL										
0–19 Years	84	4.4	47	1	1	3	5	7	11	24
20–34	39	3.6	11	1	1	2	4	11	11	12
35–49	61	4.2	29	1	2	3	5	6	12	33
50–64	32	4.5	20	1	2	3	6	14	16	20
65+	42	2.8	9	1	1	2	3	7	10	14
GRAND TOTAL	258	4.1	29	1	1	3	5	7	11	24

18.0: EXTERNAL EAR INCISION. Formerly included in operation group(s) 533, 539.

Type of Patients	Observed Patients	Avg. Stay	Variance	10th	25th	50th	75th	90th	95th	99th
1. SINGLE DX										
0–19 Years	57	3.5	6	1	2	4	4	5	6	16
20–34	8	3.9	4	2	2	3	6	6	6	10
35–49	3	3.6	7	3	3	3	3	3	14	14
50–64	1	2.0	0	2	2	2	2	2	2	2
65+	0									
2. MULTIPLE DX										
0–19 Years	87	4.6	11	2	2	4	6	8	9	24
20–34	31	4.8	28	1	2	4	5	7	15	28
35–49	25	4.1	2	3	3	4	5	5	7	13
50–64	13	6.5	118	1	1	2	6	21	21	54
65+	29	8.0	34	3	4	5	9	19	21	21
TOTAL SINGLE DX	69	3.6	5	1	2	3	4	6	6	16
MULTIPLE DX	185	4.9	22	1	3	4	5	8	10	24
TOTAL										
0–19 Years	144	4.2	9	1	2	4	5	6	9	20
20–34	39	4.6	21	1	2	4	5	6	10	28
35–49	28	4.0	3	3	3	3	5	5	7	14
50–64	14	6.4	115	1	1	2	4	21	21	54
65+	29	8.0	34	3	4	5	9	19	21	21
GRAND TOTAL	254	4.5	18	1	2	4	5	7	9	24

Length of Stay by Diagnosis and Operation, United States, 1997

United States, October 1995–September 1996 Data, by Operation

18.09: EXTERNAL EAR INC NEC. Formerly included in operation group(s) 533.

Type of Patients	Observed Patients	Avg. Stay	Variance	10th	25th	50th	75th	90th	95th	99th
1. SINGLE DX										
0–19 Years	54	3.5	6	1	2	4	4	5	6	16
20–34	8	3.9	4	2	2	3	6	6	6	10
35–49	3	3.6	7	3	3	3	3	3	14	14
50–64	1	2.0	0	2	2	2	2	2	2	2
65+	0									
2. MULTIPLE DX										
0–19 Years	80	4.4	11	1	2	4	6	6	8	24
20–34	28	4.8	30	1	2	4	5	7	15	28
35–49	23	4.2	3	3	3	4	5	5	7	13
50–64	13	6.5	118	1	1	4	6	21	21	54
65+	26	8.5	34	4	4	6	10	19	21	21
TOTAL SINGLE DX	66	3.6	6	1	2	3	4	6	6	16
MULTIPLE DX	170	4.8	24	1	2	4	5	7	10	24
TOTAL										
0–19 Years	134	4.1	9	1	2	4	5	6	7	20
20–34	36	4.6	22	1	2	4	5	6	10	28
35–49	26	4.1	4	3	3	4	5	5	7	14
50–64	14	6.4	115	1	1	4	6	21	21	54
65+	26	8.5	34	4	4	6	10	19	21	21
GRAND TOTAL	236	4.5	19	1	2	4	5	6	10	24

18.2: EXC/DESTR EXT EAR LESION. Formerly included in operation group(s) 533.

Type of Patients	Observed Patients	Avg. Stay	Variance	10th	25th	50th	75th	90th	95th	99th
1. SINGLE DX										
0–19 Years	23	1.3	<1	1	1	1	1	2	3	4
20–34	6	1.6	3	1	1	1	1	5	5	8
35–49	4	1.2	<1	1	1	1	1	2	2	2
50–64	2	1.0	0	1	1	1	1	1	1	1
65+	3	1.4	<1	1	1	1	2	2	2	2
2. MULTIPLE DX										
0–19 Years	207	2.2	3	1	1	2	3	3	5	7
20–34	27	5.3	32	2	2	4	5	7	22	29
35–49	13	4.0	12	1	2	3	6	8	8	20
50–64	22	3.1	8	1	1	2	4	6	9	16
65+	83	7.4	37	2	4	6	10	15	20	25
TOTAL SINGLE DX	38	1.3	1	1	1	1	1	2	3	8
MULTIPLE DX	352	3.1	13	1	1	2	3	6	9	21
TOTAL										
0–19 Years	230	2.1	3	1	1	2	2	3	5	7
20–34	33	4.0	25	1	1	3	5	7	8	29
35–49	17	3.7	12	1	2	3	5	8	8	20
50–64	24	3.0	8	1	1	2	4	6	9	16
65+	86	7.2	37	2	2	6	10	14	20	25
GRAND TOTAL	390	2.9	11	1	1	2	3	6	8	20

18.1: EXTERNAL EAR DXTIC PX. Formerly included in operation group(s) 533, 539.

Type of Patients	Observed Patients	Avg. Stay	Variance	10th	25th	50th	75th	90th	95th	99th
1. SINGLE DX										
0–19 Years	4	2.4	<1	2	2	2	3	3	3	3
20–34	0									
35–49	1	4.0	0	4	4	4	4	4	4	4
50–64	0									
65+	1	6.0	0	6	6	6	6	6	6	6
2. MULTIPLE DX										
0–19 Years	17	3.8	5	2	3	3	4	7	11	12
20–34	7	1.8	8	1	1	1	1	3	3	20
35–49	4	9.6	63	4	6	6	23	23	23	23
50–64	7	3.9	3	2	2	5	5	6	6	6
65+	36	5.5	33	1	2	4	7	10	19	31
TOTAL SINGLE DX	6	3.0	1	2	2	3	3	4	6	6
MULTIPLE DX	71	4.3	23	1	1	3	5	9	14	24
TOTAL										
0–19 Years	21	3.5	4	2	3	3	3	6	7	12
20–34	7	1.8	8	1	1	1	1	3	3	20
35–49	5	8.2	52	4	4	6	5	23	23	23
50–64	7	3.9	3	2	2	5	5	6	6	6
65+	37	5.6	33	1	2	4	7	10	19	31
GRAND TOTAL	77	4.2	22	1	1	3	5	8	14	24

18.29: DESTR EXT EAR LES NEC. Formerly included in operation group(s) 533.

Type of Patients	Observed Patients	Avg. Stay	Variance	10th	25th	50th	75th	90th	95th	99th
1. SINGLE DX										
0–19 Years	15	1.3	<1	1	1	1	1	2	3	4
20–34	5	1.6	3	1	1	1	1	5	8	8
35–49	3	1.0	0	1	1	1	1	1	1	1
50–64	2	1.0	0	1	1	1	1	1	1	1
65+	3	1.4	<1	1	1	1	2	2	2	2
2. MULTIPLE DX										
0–19 Years	193	2.2	3	1	1	2	3	3	5	7
20–34	24	5.5	33	2	3	5	6	7	22	29
35–49	13	4.0	12	2	2	3	6	8	8	20
50–64	19	3.3	8	1	2	2	4	6	9	16
65+	80	7.9	41	1	2	7	13	16	22	25
TOTAL SINGLE DX	28	1.4	1	1	1	1	1	2	3	8
MULTIPLE DX	329	3.1	13	1	1	2	3	6	10	22
TOTAL										
0–19 Years	208	2.1	3	1	1	2	2	3	5	7
20–34	29	4.1	26	1	1	3	5	7	10	29
35–49	16	3.8	12	1	1	3	5	8	8	20
50–64	21	3.1	8	1	1	2	4	6	9	16
65+	83	7.7	41	2	2	6	13	15	22	25
GRAND TOTAL	357	2.9	12	1	1	2	3	6	8	20

Length of Stay by Diagnosis and Operation, United States, 1997

United States, October 1995–September 1996 Data, by Operation

18.3: OTHER EXTERNAL EAR EXC. Formerly included in operation group(s) 533.

Type of Patients	Observed Patients	Avg. Stay	Variance	10th	25th	50th	75th	90th	95th	99th
1. SINGLE DX										
0–19 Years	0									
20–34	0									
35–49	1	1.0	0	1	1	1	1	1	1	1
50–64	3	4.4	1	2	5	5	5	5	5	5
65+	6	2.4	9	1	1	1	2	9	9	9
2. MULTIPLE DX										
0–19 Years	1	8.0	0	8	8	8	8	8	8	8
20–34	1	8.0	0	8	8	8	8	8	8	8
35–49	4	3.0	1	2	2	3	4	5	5	5
50–64	14	2.5	11	1	2	2	2	3	6	32
65+	43	4.6	26	1	2	3	6	9	13	34
TOTAL SINGLE DX	10	3.6	5	1	1	5	5	5	5	9
MULTIPLE DX	63	4.0	19	1	2	2	6	8	9	32
TOTAL										
0–19 Years	1	8.0	0	8	8	8	8	8	8	8
20–34	1	8.0	0	8	8	8	8	8	8	8
35–49	5	2.4	2	1	1	2	3	4	5	5
50–64	17	3.0	9	2	2	2	3	5	6	6
65+	49	4.3	25	1	2	3	6	9	13	34
GRAND TOTAL	73	3.9	16	1	2	2	5	8	9	32

18.4: SUTURE EXT EAR LAC. Formerly included in operation group(s) 533.

Type of Patients	Observed Patients	Avg. Stay	Variance	10th	25th	50th	75th	90th	95th	99th
1. SINGLE DX										
0–19 Years	8	1.9	2	1	1	1	3	3	6	6
20–34	8	1.6	<1	1	1	2	2	2	4	4
35–49	5	1.4	<1	1	1	1	2	2	2	2
50–64	2	2.0	0	2	2	2	2	2	2	2
65+	2	1.7	1	1	1	1	3	3	3	3
2. MULTIPLE DX										
0–19 Years	101	2.5	3	1	1	2	3	5	6	8
20–34	143	2.4	4	1	1	1	3	5	6	11
35–49	95	2.4	2	1	1	2	4	4	6	6
50–64	69	3.6	6	1	2	3	4	7	7	12
65+	106	5.9	10	2	3	5	8	9	13	15
TOTAL SINGLE DX	25	1.7	1	1	1	1	2	3	3	6
MULTIPLE DX	514	3.1	6	1	1	2	4	6	8	12
TOTAL										
0–19 Years	109	2.4	3	1	1	2	3	5	6	8
20–34	151	2.3	4	1	1	1	3	5	6	11
35–49	100	2.4	2	1	1	2	4	4	6	6
50–64	71	3.6	6	2	2	3	4	7	7	12
65+	108	5.9	10	2	3	5	8	9	13	15
GRAND TOTAL	539	3.0	6	1	1	2	4	6	8	12

18.5: CORRECTION PROMINENT EAR. Formerly included in operation group(s) 533.

Type of Patients	Observed Patients	Avg. Stay	Variance	10th	25th	50th	75th	90th	95th	99th
1. SINGLE DX										
0–19 Years	6	1.0	0	1	1	1	1	1	1	1
20–34	0									
35–49	0									
50–64	0									
65+	0									
2. MULTIPLE DX										
0–19 Years	10	1.0	0	1	1	1	1	1	1	1
20–34	0									
35–49	0									
50–64	0									
65+	0									
TOTAL SINGLE DX	6	1.0	0	1	1	1	1	1	1	1
MULTIPLE DX	10	1.0	0	1	1	1	1	1	1	1
TOTAL										
0–19 Years	16	1.0	0	1	1	1	1	1	1	1
20–34	0									
35–49	0									
50–64	0									
65+	0									
GRAND TOTAL	16	1.0	0	1	1	1	1	1	1	1

18.6: EXT AUDIT CANAL RECONST. Formerly included in operation group(s) 533.

Type of Patients	Observed Patients	Avg. Stay	Variance	10th	25th	50th	75th	90th	95th	99th
1. SINGLE DX										
0–19 Years	37	1.6	<1	1	1	1	2	3	3	4
20–34	4	1.1	<1	1	1	1	1	1	2	2
35–49	1	2.0	0	2	2	2	2	2	2	2
50–64	3	2.3	4	1	1	1	5	5	5	5
65+	3	2.2	5	1	1	1	1	6	6	6
2. MULTIPLE DX										
0–19 Years	56	1.7	4	1	1	1	1	3	5	11
20–34	9	1.7	<1	1	1	2	2	3	3	3
35–49	5	4.7	20	1	1	3	11	11	11	11
50–64	6	3.8	7	1	1	1	7	7	7	7
65+	6	9.6	250	1	1	1	11	43	43	43
TOTAL SINGLE DX	48	1.5	<1	1	1	1	2	3	3	5
MULTIPLE DX	82	2.6	23	1	1	1	2	6	11	11
TOTAL										
0–19 Years	93	1.6	3	1	1	1	1	3	4	11
20–34	13	1.3	<1	1	1	1	2	3	2	3
35–49	6	4.6	20	1	1	3	11	11	11	11
50–64	9	3.3	6	1	3	3	5	7	7	7
65+	9	7.9	203	1	1	1	6	43	43	43
GRAND TOTAL	130	2.1	14	1	1	1	2	4	7	11

Length of Stay by Diagnosis and Operation, United States, 1997

United States, October 1995–September 1996 Data, by Operation

18.7: OTH PLASTIC REP EXT EAR. Formerly included in operation group(s) 533.

Type of Patients	Observed Patients	Vari-ance	Avg. Stay	10th	25th	50th	75th	90th	95th	99th
1. SINGLE DX										
0–19 Years	182	2	2.0	1	1	2	3	4	4	6
20–34	24	1	1.6	1	1	1	3	3	4	6
35–49	7	1	2.3	1	2	2	3	4	4	4
50–64	2	<1	1.0	1	1	1	1	1	1	1
65+	1	0	1.0	1	1	1	1	1	1	1
2. MULTIPLE DX										
0–19 Years	144	6	2.6	1	1	2	3	5	5	15
20–34	60	11	2.9	1	1	2	3	6	10	21
35–49	29	12	4.1	1	1	4	5	8	10	20
50–64	17	16	4.7	1	2	2	9	9	13	16
65+	31	14	4.4	1	2	3	5	7	13	16
TOTAL SINGLE DX	216	1	1.7	1	1	1	2	3	4	5
MULTIPLE DX	281	9	3.0	1	1	2	4	5	9	17
TOTAL										
0–19 Years	326	4	2.3	1	1	2	3	4	5	8
20–34	84	9	2.6	1	1	2	5	5	9	17
35–49	36	10	3.8	1	1	3	5	8	10	20
50–64	19	16	4.4	1	2	3	9	9	13	16
65+	32	14	4.3	2	3	3	5	7	13	16
GRAND TOTAL	497	5	2.3	1	1	1	3	4	5	13

18.79: PLASTIC REP EXT EAR NEC. Formerly included in operation group(s) 533.

Type of Patients	Observed Patients	Vari-ance	Avg. Stay	10th	25th	50th	75th	90th	95th	99th
1. SINGLE DX										
0–19 Years	46	1	1.9	1	1	1	3	3	4	5
20–34	12	<1	1.3	1	1	1	1	3	3	5
35–49	1	0	1.0	1	1	1	1	1	1	3
50–64	2	<1	1.0	1	1	1	1	1	1	1
65+	0									
2. MULTIPLE DX										
0–19 Years	75	10	2.7	1	1	2	4	5	5	23
20–34	36	18	3.5	1	1	2	3	9	13	21
35–49	16	11	5.0	2	3	5	5	8	8	20
50–64	14	16	5.0	2	2	2	9	9	13	16
65+	28	15	4.4	1	2	3	5	7	16	16
TOTAL SINGLE DX	61	<1	1.3	1	1	1	1	2	3	5
MULTIPLE DX	169	14	3.5	1	1	2	5	8	11	21
TOTAL										
0–19 Years	121	7	2.4	1	1	1	3	5	5	16
20–34	48	15	3.1	1	1	2	2	7	11	21
35–49	17	11	4.8	1	2	5	5	8	8	20
50–64	16	16	4.4	1	2	2	5	9	13	16
65+	28	15	4.4	1	2	3	5	7	16	16
GRAND TOTAL	230	8	2.3	1	1	1	2	5	8	16

18.71: CONSTRUCTION EAR AURICLE. Formerly included in operation group(s) 533.

Type of Patients	Observed Patients	Vari-ance	Avg. Stay	10th	25th	50th	75th	90th	95th	99th
1. SINGLE DX										
0–19 Years	129	1	2.0	1	1	2	3	3	4	6
20–34	8	2	1.6	1	1	1	2	4	4	6
35–49	5	<1	2.3	2	2	2	3	3	3	3
50–64	0									
65+	1	0	1.0	1	1	1	1	1	1	1
2. MULTIPLE DX										
0–19 Years	63	2	2.4	1	1	2	3	4	5	6
20–34	15	2	2.4	1	1	3	3	4	5	9
35–49	7	3	1.9	1	1	1	1	5	7	7
50–64	1	0	1.0	1	1	1	1	1	1	1
65+	3	3	4.3	3	3	4	4	7	7	7
TOTAL SINGLE DX	143	2	2.0	1	1	2	2	3	4	6
MULTIPLE DX	89	2	2.4	1	1	2	3	4	5	7
TOTAL										
0–19 Years	192	1	2.1	1	1	2	3	4	4	6
20–34	23	2	2.2	1	1	2	3	4	5	9
35–49	12	2	2.0	1	2	2	2	5	5	7
50–64	1	0	1.0	1	1	1	1	1	1	1
65+	4	3	3.5	3	3	3	4	7	7	7
GRAND TOTAL	232	2	2.1	1	1	2	3	4	4	6

18.9: OTHER EXT EAR OPERATIONS. Formerly included in operation group(s) 533.

Type of Patients	Observed Patients	Vari-ance	Avg. Stay	10th	25th	50th	75th	90th	95th	99th
1. SINGLE DX										
0–19 Years	1	0	1.0	1	1	1	1	1	1	1
20–34	0									
35–49	0									
50–64	0									
65+	0									
2. MULTIPLE DX										
0–19 Years	1	0	4.0	4	4	4	4	4	4	4
20–34	3	9	5.2	3	3	3	9	9	9	9
35–49	0									
50–64	0									
65+	1	0	2.0	2	2	2	2	2	2	2
TOTAL SINGLE DX	1	0	1.0	1	1	1	1	1	1	1
MULTIPLE DX	5	8	4.9	3	3	3	9	9	9	9
TOTAL										
0–19 Years	2	1	1.4	1	1	2	1	4	4	4
20–34	3	9	5.2	3	3	3	9	9	9	9
35–49	0									
50–64	0									
65+	1	0	2.0	2	2	2	2	2	2	2
GRAND TOTAL	6	9	3.9	1	1	3	4	9	9	9

Length of Stay by Diagnosis and Operation, United States, 1997

United States, October 1995–September 1996 Data, by Operation

19.0: STAPES MOBILIZATION. Formerly included in operation group(s) 534.

Type of Patients	Observed Patients	Avg. Stay	Vari- ance	10th	25th	50th	75th	90th	95th	99th
1. SINGLE DX										
0–19 Years	0									
20–34	0									
35–49	0									
50–64	0									
65+	0									
2. MULTIPLE DX										
0–19 Years	2	1.0	0	1	1	1	1	1	1	1
20–34	1	1.0	0	1	1	1	1	1	1	1
35–49	3	1.0	0	1	1	1	1	1	1	1
50–64	0									
65+	0									
TOTAL SINGLE DX	0									
MULTIPLE DX	6	1.0	0	1	1	1	1	1	1	1
TOTAL										
0–19 Years	2	1.0	0	1	1	1	1	1	1	1
20–34	1	1.0	0	1	1	1	1	1	1	1
35–49	3	1.0	0	1	1	1	1	1	1	1
50–64	0									
65+	0									
GRAND TOTAL	6	1.0	0	1	1	1	1	1	1	1

19.1: STAPEDECTOMY. Formerly included in operation group(s) 534.

Type of Patients	Observed Patients	Avg. Stay	Vari- ance	10th	25th	50th	75th	90th	95th	99th
1. SINGLE DX										
0–19 Years	3	1.2	<1	1	1	1	1	2	2	2
20–34	33	1.0	<1	1	1	1	1	1	2	2
35–49	50	1.0	<1	1	1	1	1	1	1	2
50–64	36	1.2	<1	1	1	1	1	2	2	4
65+	14	1.1	<1	1	1	1	1	1	2	3
2. MULTIPLE DX										
0–19 Years	14	1.7	4	1	1	1	1	2	8	8
20–34	22	1.0	<1	1	1	1	1	1	1	2
35–49	67	1.2	<1	1	1	1	1	2	2	2
50–64	44	2.5	5	1	1	1	5	5	7	7
65+	34	1.3	<1	1	1	1	1	2	2	7
TOTAL SINGLE DX	136	1.1	<1	1	1	1	1	1	2	2
MULTIPLE DX	181	1.6	2	1	1	1	1	3	5	7
TOTAL										
0–19 Years	17	1.6	3	1	1	1	1	2	8	8
20–34	55	1.0	<1	1	1	1	1	1	1	2
35–49	117	1.1	<1	1	1	1	1	2	2	2
50–64	80	2.1	4	1	1	1	2	5	7	7
65+	48	1.2	<1	1	1	1	1	2	2	6
GRAND TOTAL	317	1.4	1	1	1	1	1	2	5	7

19.19: STAPEDECTOMY NEC. Formerly included in operation group(s) 534.

Type of Patients	Observed Patients	Avg. Stay	Vari- ance	10th	25th	50th	75th	90th	95th	99th
1. SINGLE DX										
0–19 Years	3	1.2	<1	1	1	1	1	2	2	2
20–34	27	1.0	<1	1	1	1	1	1	1	2
35–49	35	1.0	<1	1	1	1	1	1	1	2
50–64	27	1.2	<1	1	1	1	1	2	2	4
65+	10	1.1	<1	1	1	1	1	1	1	3
2. MULTIPLE DX										
0–19 Years	10	2.2	6	1	1	1	2	8	8	8
20–34	16	1.0	0	1	1	1	1	1	1	1
35–49	38	1.1	<1	1	1	1	1	2	2	2
50–64	31	3.1	6	1	1	1	5	7	7	7
65+	25	1.2	<1	1	1	1	1	2	2	6
TOTAL SINGLE DX	102	1.1	<1	1	1	1	1	1	1	2
MULTIPLE DX	120	2.0	4	1	1	1	1	5	7	7
TOTAL										
0–19 Years	13	2.0	5	1	1	1	2	8	8	8
20–34	43	1.0	<1	1	1	1	1	1	1	2
35–49	73	1.1	<1	1	1	1	1	2	2	2
50–64	58	2.5	5	1	1	1	5	7	7	7
65+	35	1.1	<1	1	1	1	1	2	2	6
GRAND TOTAL	222	1.5	2	1	1	1	1	2	5	7

19.2: STAPEDECTOMY REVISION. Formerly included in operation group(s) 534.

Type of Patients	Observed Patients	Avg. Stay	Vari- ance	10th	25th	50th	75th	90th	95th	99th
1. SINGLE DX										
0–19 Years	0									
20–34	0									
35–49	4	1.0	0	1	1	1	1	1	1	1
50–64	0									
65+	2	1.1	<1	1	1	1	1	1	2	2
2. MULTIPLE DX										
0–19 Years	1	1.0	0	1	1	1	1	1	1	1
20–34	5	1.1	<1	1	1	1	1	2	2	2
35–49	7	1.3	<1	1	1	1	2	2	3	3
50–64	6	1.5	<1	1	1	1	2	2	4	4
65+	10	1.1	<1	1	1	1	1	2	2	2
TOTAL SINGLE DX	6	1.0	<1	1	1	1	1	1	1	2
MULTIPLE DX	29	1.2	<1	1	1	1	1	2	2	4
TOTAL										
0–19 Years	1	1.0	0	1	1	1	1	1	1	1
20–34	5	1.1	<1	1	1	1	1	2	2	2
35–49	11	1.2	<1	1	1	1	2	2	3	3
50–64	6	1.5	<1	1	1	1	1	1	4	4
65+	12	1.1	<1	1	1	1	1	2	2	2
GRAND TOTAL	35	1.2	<1	1	1	1	1	2	2	4

Length of Stay by Diagnosis and Operation, United States, 1997

United States, October 1995–September 1996 Data, by Operation

19.3: OSSICULAR CHAIN OPS NEC. Formerly included in operation group(s) 534.

Type of Patients	Observed Patients	Avg. Stay	Variance	10th	25th	50th	75th	90th	95th	99th
1. SINGLE DX										
0–19 Years	4	1.0	0	1	1	1	1	1	1	1
20–34	2	1.0	0	1	1	1	1	1	1	1
35–49	0									
50–64	0									
65+	0									
2. MULTIPLE DX										
0–19 Years	10	1.0	0	1	1	1	1	1	1	1
20–34	0									
35–49	4	1.4	1	1	1	1	1	4	4	4
50–64	3	1.0	0	1	1	1	1	1	1	1
65+	3	1.3	<1	1	1	1	2	2	2	2
TOTAL SINGLE DX	6	1.0	0	1	1	1	1	1	1	1
MULTIPLE DX	20	1.1	<1	1	1	1	1	1	1	4
TOTAL										
0–19 Years	14	1.0	0	1	1	1	1	1	1	1
20–34	2	1.0	0	1	1	1	1	1	1	1
35–49	4	1.4	1	1	1	1	1	4	4	4
50–64	3	1.0	0	1	1	1	1	1	1	1
65+	3	1.3	<1	1	1	1	2	2	2	2
GRAND TOTAL	26	1.0	<1	1	1	1	1	1	1	2

19.4: MYRINGOPLASTY. Formerly included in operation group(s) 535.

Type of Patients	Observed Patients	Avg. Stay	Variance	10th	25th	50th	75th	90th	95th	99th
1. SINGLE DX										
0–19 Years	89	1.0	0	1	1	1	1	1	1	1
20–34	7	1.0	0	1	1	1	1	1	1	1
35–49	11	2.1	3	1	1	1	5	5	5	5
50–64	9	1.7	3	1	1	1	1	6	6	6
65+	2	1.0	0	1	1	1	1	1	1	1
2. MULTIPLE DX										
0–19 Years	180	1.6	6	1	1	1	1	2	7	10
20–34	20	1.1	<1	1	1	1	1	2	2	3
35–49	31	3.3	10	1	1	2	5	10	10	10
50–64	18	1.5	<1	1	1	1	2	4	4	4
65+	22	2.7	6	1	1	1	4	4	5	15
TOTAL SINGLE DX	118	1.1	<1	1	1	1	1	1	1	6
MULTIPLE DX	271	1.9	6	1	1	1	1	5	7	10
TOTAL										
0–19 Years	269	1.4	4	1	1	1	1	1	4	8
20–34	27	1.1	<1	1	1	1	1	2	2	2
35–49	42	3.1	9	1	1	1	5	10	10	10
50–64	27	1.6	2	1	1	1	2	2	5	6
65+	24	2.6	6	1	1	1	4	4	5	15
GRAND TOTAL	389	1.6	4	1	1	1	1	3	5	10

19.5: OTHER TYMPANOPLASTY. Formerly included in operation group(s) 535.

Type of Patients	Observed Patients	Avg. Stay	Variance	10th	25th	50th	75th	90th	95th	99th
1. SINGLE DX										
0–19 Years	9	1.0	0	1	1	1	1	1	1	1
20–34	6	1.1	<1	1	1	1	1	1	2	1
35–49	6	1.0	0	1	1	1	1	1	1	1
50–64	2	1.0	0	1	1	1	1	1	1	2
65+	3	1.3	<1	2	1	1	2	2	2	2
2. MULTIPLE DX										
0–19 Years	43	1.2	<1	1	1	1	1	2	2	3
20–34	25	1.0	0	1	1	1	1	1	1	1
35–49	16	1.0	<1	1	1	1	1	1	1	2
50–64	17	1.3	<1	1	1	1	1	2	2	6
65+	12	1.6	1	1	1	1	1	4	4	4
TOTAL SINGLE DX	26	1.0	<1	1	1	1	1	1	1	2
MULTIPLE DX	113	1.1	<1	1	1	1	1	1	2	3
TOTAL										
0–19 Years	52	1.1	<1	1	1	1	1	2	2	3
20–34	31	1.0	<1	1	1	1	1	1	1	2
35–49	22	1.0	<1	1	1	1	1	1	1	2
50–64	19	1.3	<1	1	1	1	1	2	2	6
65+	15	1.5	1	1	1	1	1	4	4	4
GRAND TOTAL	139	1.1	<1	1	1	1	1	1	2	3

19.6: TYMPANOPLASTY REVISION. Formerly included in operation group(s) 538.

Type of Patients	Observed Patients	Avg. Stay	Variance	10th	25th	50th	75th	90th	95th	99th
1. SINGLE DX										
0–19 Years	10	1.0	0	1	1	1	1	1	1	1
20–34	2	1.0	0	1	1	1	1	1	1	1
35–49	3	1.0	0	1	1	1	1	1	1	1
50–64	1	2.0	0	2	2	2	2	2	2	2
65+	0									
2. MULTIPLE DX										
0–19 Years	21	1.5	1	1	1	1	1	3	6	6
20–34	6	1.8	2	1	1	1	2	2	6	6
35–49	17	1.8	3	1	1	1	2	3	8	8
50–64	5	1.6	<1	1	1	1	3	3	3	3
65+	8	1.7	2	1	1	2	1	5	5	5
TOTAL SINGLE DX	16	1.2	<1	1	1	1	1	2	2	2
MULTIPLE DX	57	1.7	2	1	1	1	2	3	6	8
TOTAL										
0–19 Years	31	1.3	1	1	1	1	1	2	3	6
20–34	8	1.6	2	1	1	1	2	2	6	6
35–49	20	1.8	3	1	1	1	2	3	8	8
50–64	6	1.8	<1	1	2	2	3	3	3	3
65+	8	1.7	2	1	1	1	1	5	5	5
GRAND TOTAL	73	1.6	2	1	1	1	2	3	5	8

Length of Stay by Diagnosis and Operation, United States, 1997

United States, October 1995–September 1996 Data, by Operation

19.9: MIDDLE EAR REPAIR NEC. Formerly included in operation group(s) 538.

Type of Patients	Observed Patients	Avg. Stay	Variance	10th	25th	50th	75th	90th	95th	99th
1. SINGLE DX										
0–19 Years	0									
20–34	2	3.2	6	2	2	2	2	8	8	8
35–49	0									
50–64	3	1.5	2	1	1	1	1	5	5	5
65+	0									
2. MULTIPLE DX										
0–19 Years	3	2.3	<1	1	2	2	3	3	3	3
20–34	3	19.6	44	2	22	22	22	22	22	22
35–49	7	8.3	64	3	3	3	20	20	20	20
50–64	4	6.0	24	2	3	3	13	13	13	13
65+	7	4.4	7	1	1	5	5	8	8	9
TOTAL SINGLE DX	5	2.2	4	1	1	1	2	5	8	8
MULTIPLE DX	24	8.3	66	1	2	4	20	22	22	22
TOTAL										
0–19 Years	3	2.3	<1	1	2	2	3	3	3	3
20–34	5	15.4	88	2	2	22	22	22	22	22
35–49	7	8.3	64	3	3	3	20	20	20	20
50–64	7	3.6	17	1	1	2	4	13	13	13
65+	7	4.4	7	1	1	5	5	8	8	9
GRAND TOTAL	29	7.4	61	1	2	3	8	22	22	22

20.01: MYRINGOTOMY W INTUBATION. Formerly included in operation group(s) 536.

Type of Patients	Observed Patients	Avg. Stay	Variance	10th	25th	50th	75th	90th	95th	99th
1. SINGLE DX										
0–19 Years	164	2.0	3	1	1	1	3	4	6	9
20–34	0									
35–49	4	1.4	<1	1	1	1	2	2	2	2
50–64	1	1.0	0	1	1	1	1	1	1	1
65+	1	4.0	0	4	4	4	4	4	4	4
2. MULTIPLE DX										
0–19 Years	1789	3.1	27	1	1	2	3	6	9	40
20–34	48	5.3	22	1	1	5	8	11	13	24
35–49	57	8.3	49	1	2	8	13	17	22	>99
50–64	60	3.1	21	1	1	1	5	7	11	21
65+	115	9.6	110	1	2	8	15	22	28	45
TOTAL SINGLE DX	170	2.0	3	1	1	1	3	4	6	9
MULTIPLE DX	2069	3.4	30	1	1	2	4	7	11	40
TOTAL										
0–19 Years	1953	3.0	25	1	1	2	3	6	8	40
20–34	48	5.3	22	1	2	5	8	11	13	24
35–49	61	8.1	49	1	2	7	12	17	22	>99
50–64	61	3.1	20	1	1	1	5	7	11	21
65+	116	9.6	110	1	2	7	15	22	28	45
GRAND TOTAL	2239	3.3	28	1	1	2	4	7	10	32

20.0: MYRINGOTOMY. Formerly included in operation group(s) 536.

Type of Patients	Observed Patients	Avg. Stay	Variance	10th	25th	50th	75th	90th	95th	99th
1. SINGLE DX										
0–19 Years	182	2.1	3	1	1	1	3	4	6	9
20–34	1	1.0	0	1	1	1	1	1	1	1
35–49	6	2.2	3	1	1	2	2	6	6	6
50–64	2	1.0	0	1	1	1	1	1	1	1
65+	2	2.2	3	1	1	1	4	4	4	4
2. MULTIPLE DX										
0–19 Years	1917	3.3	28	1	1	2	4	6	9	40
20–34	53	5.0	22	1	1	4	8	11	15	24
35–49	66	7.9	48	1	2	7	12	17	21	>99
50–64	71	3.2	20	1	1	1	5	7	11	21
65+	134	9.4	99	1	2	7	13	21	24	45
TOTAL SINGLE DX	193	2.0	3	1	1	1	3	4	6	9
MULTIPLE DX	2241	3.5	31	1	1	2	4	7	11	39
TOTAL										
0–19 Years	2099	3.2	26	1	1	2	4	6	9	40
20–34	54	4.9	22	1	1	4	8	11	15	24
35–49	72	7.6	47	1	2	6	12	17	21	30
50–64	73	3.2	20	1	1	1	5	7	11	21
65+	136	9.4	99	1	2	7	13	21	24	45
GRAND TOTAL	2434	3.4	29	1	2	2	4	7	11	33

20.1: TYMPANOSTOMY TUBE RMVL. Formerly included in operation group(s) 538.

Type of Patients	Observed Patients	Avg. Stay	Variance	10th	25th	50th	75th	90th	95th	99th
1. SINGLE DX										
0–19 Years	13	2.3	3	1	1	2	3	7	7	7
20–34	0									
35–49	0									
50–64	0									
65+	0									
2. MULTIPLE DX										
0–19 Years	57	5.8	32	1	2	4	7	13	17	21
20–34	1	10.0	0	10	10	10	10	10	10	10
35–49	4	2.8	14	1	2	2	2	2	16	16
50–64	1	4.0	0	4	4	4	4	4	4	4
65+	1	22.0	0	22	22	22	22	22	22	22
TOTAL SINGLE DX	13	2.3	3	1	1	2	3	7	7	7
MULTIPLE DX	64	5.8	33	1	2	4	7	14	17	22
TOTAL										
0–19 Years	70	5.2	29	1	2	3	7	12	17	21
20–34	1	10.0	0	10	10	10	10	10	10	10
35–49	4	2.8	14	1	2	2	4	4	16	16
50–64	1	4.0	0	4	4	4	4	4	4	4
65+	1	22.0	0	22	22	22	22	22	22	22
GRAND TOTAL	77	5.3	30	1	2	3	7	12	17	22

Length of Stay by Diagnosis and Operation, United States, 1997

United States, October 1995–September 1996 Data, by Operation

20.4: MASTOIDECTOMY. Formerly included in operation group(s) 537.

Type of Patients	Observed Patients	Avg. Stay	Variance	10th	25th	50th	75th	90th	95th	99th
1. SINGLE DX										
0–19 Years	142	1.7	3	1	1	1	1	4	5	9
20–34	54	1.3	<1	1	1	1	1	2	3	8
35–49	34	1.2	<1	1	1	1	1	2	2	4
50–64	31	1.2	<1	1	1	1	1	2	2	8
65+	20	2.5	7	1	1	1	2	6	12	12
2. MULTIPLE DX										
0–19 Years	375	2.8	15	1	1	1	3	7	9	17
20–34	119	2.0	7	1	1	1	2	4	6	14
35–49	181	2.6	15	1	1	1	2	8	8	20
50–64	142	2.3	11	1	1	1	4	5	8	17
65+	151	4.9	100	1	1	2	4	13	17	37
TOTAL SINGLE DX	281	1.5	2	1	1	1	1	3	4	8
MULTIPLE DX	968	2.8	22	1	1	1	3	7	9	20
TOTAL										
0–19 Years	517	2.5	12	1	1	1	3	7	9	16
20–34	173	1.8	6	1	1	1	2	3	5	14
35–49	215	2.5	13	1	1	1	2	7	8	20
50–64	173	2.1	10	1	1	1	2	3	7	17
65+	171	4.6	91	1	1	2	4	13	15	37
GRAND TOTAL	1249	2.6	18	1	1	1	2	6	9	19

20.42: RADICAL MASTOIDECTOMY. Formerly included in operation group(s) 537.

Type of Patients	Observed Patients	Avg. Stay	Variance	10th	25th	50th	75th	90th	95th	99th
1. SINGLE DX										
0–19 Years	84	1.4	1	1	1	1	1	2	3	8
20–34	29	1.2	<1	1	1	1	1	1	4	4
35–49	12	1.0	0	1	1	1	1	1	1	1
50–64	15	1.0	<1	1	1	1	1	1	1	2
65+	10	2.5	13	1	1	1	1	12	12	12
2. MULTIPLE DX										
0–19 Years	175	2.2	10	1	1	1	2	5	8	12
20–34	64	1.5	2	1	1	1	1	2	4	6
35–49	95	2.5	10	1	1	1	3	9	9	11
50–64	66	1.6	4	1	1	1	3	3	4	17
65+	69	3.1	20	1	1	2	3	5	14	20
TOTAL SINGLE DX	150	1.3	1	1	1	1	1	2	3	8
MULTIPLE DX	469	2.2	9	1	1	1	2	5	9	14
TOTAL										
0–19 Years	259	1.9	8	1	1	1	1	3	7	12
20–34	93	1.4	2	1	1	1	1	2	4	6
35–49	107	2.4	9	1	1	1	3	9	9	11
50–64	81	1.5	3	1	1	1	1	2	3	7
65+	79	3.0	19	1	1	2	3	5	14	20
GRAND TOTAL	619	2.0	8	1	1	1	2	4	8	13

20.2: MASTOID & MID EAR INC. Formerly included in operation group(s) 538.

Type of Patients	Observed Patients	Avg. Stay	Variance	10th	25th	50th	75th	90th	95th	99th
1. SINGLE DX										
0–19 Years	6	5.4	8	2	4	5	6	10	10	10
20–34	4	1.2	<1	1	1	1	1	2	2	2
35–49	3	1.3	<1	1	1	1	2	2	2	2
50–64	4	3.7	21	1	1	1	11	11	11	11
65+	0									
2. MULTIPLE DX										
0–19 Years	24	3.9	8	1	1	3	6	7	9	14
20–34	7	2.6	5	1	1	1	3	6	8	8
35–49	17	4.1	5	1	2	5	5	7	7	14
50–64	11	9.1	48	2	4	7	20	20	20	20
65+	8	2.3	5	1	1	1	2	7	7	7
TOTAL SINGLE DX	17	3.4	12	1	1	1	5	10	11	11
MULTIPLE DX	63	4.7	18	1	1	4	6	7	14	20
TOTAL										
0–19 Years	30	4.2	9	1	1	4	6	7	10	14
20–34	11	2.1	4	1	1	1	2	6	6	8
35–49	20	3.8	5	1	2	3	5	7	7	14
50–64	11	7.6	46	1	4	7	11	20	20	20
65+	8	2.3	5	1	1	1	2	7	7	7
GRAND TOTAL	80	4.4	17	1	1	3	6	7	11	20

20.3: MID & INNER EAR DXTIC PX. Formerly included in operation group(s) 538, 539.

Type of Patients	Observed Patients	Avg. Stay	Variance	10th	25th	50th	75th	90th	95th	99th
1. SINGLE DX										
0–19 Years	1	1.0	0	1	1	1	1	1	1	1
20–34	0									
35–49	0									
50–64	0									
65+										
2. MULTIPLE DX										
0–19 Years	10	5.2	13	1	1	6	9	10	13	13
20–34	2	3.5	6	2	2	2	7	7	7	7
35–49	2	5.0	0	5	5	5	5	5	5	5
50–64	1	4.0	0	4	4	4	4	4	4	4
65+	4	3.1	4	1	1	2	5	5	5	5
TOTAL SINGLE DX	1	1.0	0	1	1	1	1	1	1	1
MULTIPLE DX	19	4.7	11	1	2	4	6	10	10	13
TOTAL										
0–19 Years	11	5.1	13	2	1	6	9	10	13	13
20–34	2	3.5	6	2	2	2	7	7	7	7
35–49	2	5.0	0	5	5	5	5	5	5	5
50–64	1	4.0	0	4	4	4	4	4	4	4
65+	4	3.1	4	1	1	2	5	5	5	5
GRAND TOTAL	20	4.7	11	1	2	4	6	10	10	13

Length of Stay by Diagnosis and Operation, United States, 1997

United States, October 1995–September 1996 Data, by Operation

20.49: MASTOIDECTOMY NEC. Formerly included in operation group(s) 537.

Type of Patients	Observed Patients	Avg. Stay	Vari-ance	Percentiles						
				10th	25th	50th	75th	90th	95th	99th
1. SINGLE DX										
0–19 Years	47	1.9	4	1	1	1	2	4	6	8
20–34	17	1.2	<1	1	1	1	1	2	2	3
35–49	17	1.2	<1	1	1	1	1	2	2	5
50–64	16	1.3	1	1	1	1	1	2	2	8
65+	9	2.3	3	1	1	2	2	6	6	6
2. MULTIPLE DX										
0–19 Years	133	3.3	21	1	1	1	4	8	12	27
20–34	47	1.8	4	1	1	1	2	3	5	6
35–49	66	2.6	24	1	1	1	2	3	13	27
50–64	61	3.1	18	1	1	1	3	7	15	17
65+	58	4.6	83	1	1	1	4	15	23	37
TOTAL SINGLE DX	106	1.6	2	1	1	1	1	3	4	8
MULTIPLE DX	365	3.1	26	1	1	1	3	7	13	27
TOTAL										
0–19 Years	180	3.0	17	1	1	1	3	8	10	23
20–34	64	1.6	3	1	1	1	1	3	5	6
35–49	83	2.3	19	1	1	1	2	3	13	27
50–64	77	2.6	14	1	1	1	3	7	12	17
65+	67	4.3	73	1	1	1	4	9	15	37
GRAND TOTAL	471	2.8	21	1	1	1	2	7	10	27

20.6: FENESTRATION INNER EAR. Formerly included in operation group(s) 538.

Type of Patients	Observed Patients	Avg. Stay	Vari-ance	Percentiles						
				10th	25th	50th	75th	90th	95th	99th
1. SINGLE DX										
0–19 Years	0									
20–34	0									
35–49	0									
50–64	0									
65+	0									
2. MULTIPLE DX										
0–19 Years	1	3.0	0	3	3	3	3	3	3	3
20–34	0									
35–49	0									
50–64	1	6.0	0	6	6	6	6	6	6	6
65+	0									
TOTAL SINGLE DX	0									
MULTIPLE DX	2	4.6	4	3	3	6	6	6	6	6
TOTAL										
0–19 Years	1	3.0	0	3	3	3	3	3	3	3
20–34	0									
35–49	0									
50–64	1	6.0	0	6	6	6	6	6	6	6
65+	0									
GRAND TOTAL	2	4.6	4	3	3	6	6	6	6	6

20.5: OTH MIDDLE EAR EXCISION. Formerly included in operation group(s) 538.

Type of Patients	Observed Patients	Avg. Stay	Vari-ance	Percentiles						
				10th	25th	50th	75th	90th	95th	99th
1. SINGLE DX										
0–19 Years	13	1.1	<1	1	1	1	1	1	1	7
20–34	2	2.5	<1	1	2	3	3	3	3	3
35–49	9	2.5	5	2	2	1	3	5	7	9
50–64	6	1.2	<1	1	1	1	1	1	1	4
65+	2	2.0	1	1	1	1	1	3	3	3
2. MULTIPLE DX										
0–19 Years	50	3.0	29	1	1	1	3	7	8	36
20–34	14	2.7	6	1	1	1	4	7	8	8
35–49	16	3.2	21	1	1	1	4	9	9	23
50–64	14	2.7	22	1	1	1	4	4	9	35
65+	13	4.1	3	1	2	5	5	6	6	7
TOTAL SINGLE DX	32	1.5	2	1	1	1	1	3	5	9
MULTIPLE DX	107	3.0	20	1	1	1	4	7	9	35
TOTAL										
0–19 Years	63	2.5	22	1	1	1	1	6	8	36
20–34	16	2.7	6	1	1	1	4	7	9	8
35–49	25	3.0	16	1	1	1	3	9	9	23
50–64	20	2.3	17	1	1	1	3	4	6	35
65+	15	3.9	3	2	2	5	5	6	6	7
GRAND TOTAL	139	2.7	17	1	1	1	3	6	8	23

20.7: INC/EXC/DESTR INNER EAR. Formerly included in operation group(s) 538.

Type of Patients	Observed Patients	Avg. Stay	Vari-ance	Percentiles						
				10th	25th	50th	75th	90th	95th	99th
1. SINGLE DX										
0–19 Years	1	1.0	0	1	1	1	1	1	1	1
20–34	5	2.1	2	1	1	2	4	4	4	4
35–49	29	2.4	1	1	1	3	3	4	4	4
50–64	11	1.9	<1	1	1	2	2	3	4	5
65+	16	1.7	1	1	1	1	2	4	4	4
2. MULTIPLE DX										
0–19 Years	8	4.1	11	1	2	4	4	12	12	13
20–34	11	4.9	208	1	1	4	3	4	8	70
35–49	31	2.0	2	1	1	2	2	3	5	8
50–64	34	3.4	36	1	1	2	3	4	15	33
65+	35	3.1	3	1	2	3	3	6	6	10
TOTAL SINGLE DX	62	2.2	1	1	1	2	3	4	4	4
MULTIPLE DX	119	3.1	32	1	1	2	3	4	6	33
TOTAL										
0–19 Years	9	3.8	11	1	1	4	4	12	12	13
20–34	16	3.7	118	1	1	2	3	4	4	70
35–49	60	2.2	1	1	1	3	3	4	4	5
50–64	45	3.1	30	1	1	2	3	4	5	33
65+	51	2.5	3	1	1	3	3	4	6	10
GRAND TOTAL	181	2.7	20	1	1	2	3	4	4	33

Length of Stay by Diagnosis and Operation, United States, 1997

United States, October 1995–September 1996 Data, by Operation

20.8: EUSTACHIAN TUBE OPS. Formerly included in operation group(s) 538.

Type of Patients	Observed Patients	Avg. Stay	Variance	10th	25th	50th	75th	90th	95th	99th
1. SINGLE DX										
0–19 Years	1	4.0	0	4	4	4	4	4	4	4
20–34	0									
35–49	0									
50–64	0									
65+	0									
2. MULTIPLE DX										
0–19 Years	3	8.4	15	1	9	9	10	10	10	10
20–34	0									
35–49	0									
50–64	1	8.0	0	8	8	8	8	8	8	8
65+	0									
TOTAL SINGLE DX	1	4.0	0	4	4	4	4	4	4	4
MULTIPLE DX	4	8.2	6	8	8	8	9	10	10	10
TOTAL										
0–19 Years	4	6.4	12	4	4	4	9	10	10	10
20–34	0									
35–49	0									
50–64	1	8.0	0	8	8	8	8	8	8	8
65+	0									
GRAND TOTAL	5	6.9	8	4	4	8	9	10	10	10

21.0: CONTROL OF EPISTAXIS. Formerly included in operation group(s) 543, 556.

Type of Patients	Observed Patients	Avg. Stay	Variance	10th	25th	50th	75th	90th	95th	99th
1. SINGLE DX										
0–19 Years	22	2.2	1	1	1	2	4	4	4	4
20–34	69	2.0	1	1	1	2	4	4	5	6
35–49	119	3.1	2	1	2	3	4	5	6	6
50–64	122	2.6	2	1	1	2	3	5	5	6
65+	111	2.3	2	1	1	2	3	5	5	7
2. MULTIPLE DX										
0–19 Years	126	3.8	16	1	1	3	5	8	12	25
20–34	203	4.0	12	1	2	3	6	8	8	>99
35–49	579	3.8	7	1	2	3	5	6	9	14
50–64	1120	4.2	11	1	2	4	5	7	9	17
65+	2639	4.3	18	1	2	3	5	9	11	21
TOTAL SINGLE DX	443	2.6	2	1	1	2	4	5	5	6
MULTIPLE DX	4667	4.2	14	1	2	3	5	7	10	21
TOTAL										
0–19 Years	148	3.6	14	1	1	2	4	7	12	25
20–34	272	3.5	10	1	1	3	5	6	14	>99
35–49	698	3.6	6	1	2	3	5	6	7	14
50–64	1242	4.1	10	1	2	4	5	7	9	17
65+	2750	4.2	18	1	2	3	5	8	11	21
GRAND TOTAL	5110	4.0	13	1	2	3	5	7	10	20

20.9: OTHER ME & IE OPS. Formerly included in operation group(s) 538.

Type of Patients	Observed Patients	Avg. Stay	Variance	10th	25th	50th	75th	90th	95th	99th
1. SINGLE DX										
0–19 Years	103	1.1	<1	1	1	1	1	2	2	3
20–34	15	1.3	<1	1	1	1	1	2	2	5
35–49	30	1.1	<1	1	1	1	1	1	3	3
50–64	16	1.5	<1	1	1	1	2	3	3	3
65+	9	1.4	<1	1	1	1	1	3	3	3
2. MULTIPLE DX										
0–19 Years	110	1.8	3	1	1	1	2	4	6	7
20–34	27	1.7	2	1	1	1	2	3	5	8
35–49	50	2.2	3	1	1	2	3	4	5	8
50–64	42	1.7	2	1	1	2	3	4	5	7
65+	41	3.5	18	1	1	2	5	6	12	21
TOTAL SINGLE DX	173	1.2	<1	1	1	1	1	2	2	3
MULTIPLE DX	270	2.0	4	1	1	1	2	5	5	8
TOTAL										
0–19 Years	213	1.5	2	1	1	1	1	3	4	6
20–34	42	1.5	2	1	1	1	1	2	5	8
35–49	80	1.8	2	1	1	1	2	2	5	7
50–64	58	1.7	2	1	1	1	2	3	5	5
65+	50	3.2	16	1	1	2	4	5	8	21
GRAND TOTAL	443	1.7	3	1	1	1	2	3	5	7

21.01: ANT NAS PACK FOR EPISTX. Formerly included in operation group(s) 556.

Type of Patients	Observed Patients	Avg. Stay	Variance	10th	25th	50th	75th	90th	95th	99th
1. SINGLE DX										
0–19 Years	9	2.0	<1	1	1	2	2	4	4	4
20–34	16	1.9	<1	1	1	1	2	4	4	4
35–49	24	1.9	<1	1	1	2	2	5	5	5
50–64	18	1.9	2	1	1	2	2	5	5	5
65+	24	2.2	2	1	1	2	3	5	5	5
2. MULTIPLE DX										
0–19 Years	47	4.5	18	1	1	3	6	12	12	12
20–34	76	3.8	8	1	2	3	6	6	6	18
35–49	159	3.6	10	1	1	3	4	6	8	17
50–64	306	4.1	9	1	2	4	4	7	9	16
65+	850	4.3	18	1	2	3	5	9	12	21
TOTAL SINGLE DX	91	2.0	1	1	1	2	2	4	5	5
MULTIPLE DX	1438	4.1	14	1	2	3	5	8	10	21
TOTAL										
0–19 Years	56	3.8	14	1	1	2	5	12	12	12
20–34	92	3.6	8	1	1	3	6	6	6	18
35–49	183	3.3	9	1	1	3	4	6	7	17
50–64	324	4.0	9	1	2	4	4	6	9	15
65+	874	4.2	18	1	2	3	5	9	11	21
GRAND TOTAL	1529	4.0	14	1	2	3	5	8	10	21

United States, October 1995–September 1996 Data, by Operation

21.02: POST NAS PACK FOR EPISTX. Formerly included in operation group(s) 543.

Type of Patients	Observed Patients	Avg. Stay	Vari-ance	Percentiles						
				10th	25th	50th	75th	90th	95th	99th
1. SINGLE DX										
0–19 Years	2	3.8	<1	4	4	4	4	4	4	4
20–34	28	2.6	2	1	2	2	3	3	3	7
35–49	51	3.9	2	2	3	4	5	6	6	6
50–64	47	2.7	2	1	2	2	3	5	5	6
65+	51	2.7	3	1	1	2	4	5	6	7
2. MULTIPLE DX										
0–19 Years	13	4.3	33	1	1	3	3	8	25	25
20–34	52	3.4	5	1	2	3	4	5	6	8
35–49	209	4.1	3	2	3	4	5	6	7	11
50–64	373	3.8	5	2	2	3	5	7	7	12
65+	845	4.0	10	1	2	3	5	7	9	19
TOTAL SINGLE DX	179	3.3	2	1	2	3	4	5	6	6
MULTIPLE DX	1492	4.0	8	1	2	3	5	6	8	14
TOTAL										
0–19 Years	15	4.2	26	1	2	3	4	8	9	25
20–34	80	3.1	4	1	2	3	4	5	6	8
35–49	260	4.0	3	1	3	4	5	6	6	9
50–64	420	3.8	5	2	2	3	5	7	7	10
65+	896	3.9	10	1	2	3	5	6	9	18
GRAND TOTAL	1671	3.9	7	1	2	3	5	6	8	13

21.03: CAUT TO CNTRL EPISTAXIS. Formerly included in operation group(s) 543.

Type of Patients	Observed Patients	Avg. Stay	Vari-ance	Percentiles						
				10th	25th	50th	75th	90th	95th	99th
1. SINGLE DX										
0–19 Years	8	1.2	<1	1	1	1	1	2	2	3
20–34	13	1.5	<1	1	1	1	2	2	3	4
35–49	24	2.3	1	1	1	3	3	4	4	4
50–64	33	2.7	2	1	1	3	4	4	5	6
65+	28	1.8	1	1	1	1	2	3	5	7
2. MULTIPLE DX										
0–19 Years	48	2.8	13	1	1	2	2	6	7	>99
20–34	51	3.9	12	1	2	4	6	>99	>99	>99
35–49	141	3.5	11	1	2	3	4	7	9	14
50–64	276	4.4	13	1	2	4	6	7	10	18
65+	669	4.9	29	1	2	3	6	10	16	25
TOTAL SINGLE DX	106	2.1	2	1	1	2	3	4	4	6
MULTIPLE DX	1185	4.5	21	1	2	3	5	9	13	29
TOTAL										
0–19 Years	56	2.7	12	1	1	2	2	6	7	30
20–34	64	3.3	10	1	1	2	5	>99	>99	>99
35–49	165	3.2	9	1	2	4	4	6	9	14
50–64	309	4.3	13	1	2	4	6	7	10	18
65+	697	4.8	29	1	2	3	6	10	16	25
GRAND TOTAL	1291	4.3	20	1	2	3	5	8	12	28

21.1: INCISION OF NOSE. Formerly included in operation group(s) 542.

Type of Patients	Observed Patients	Avg. Stay	Vari-ance	Percentiles						
				10th	25th	50th	75th	90th	95th	99th
1. SINGLE DX										
0–19 Years	9	2.0	<1	1	2	2	2	3	3	3
20–34	7	2.0	<1	1	2	2	2	3	3	3
35–49	5	3.6	7	1	2	3	3	3	7	7
50–64	5	4.0	<1	4	4	4	4	4	5	5
65+	2	1.6	<1	1	1	2	2	2	2	2
2. MULTIPLE DX										
0–19 Years	22	4.4	14	1	1	3	8	11	11	>99
20–34	7	5.4	162	2	3	3	3	6	6	77
35–49	11	4.3	5	2	3	4	6	7	7	12
50–64	8	4.3	5	2	2	5	5	8	8	8
65+	10	12.7	54	2	5	14	20	20	20	20
TOTAL SINGLE DX	28	3.0	2	2	2	2	4	4	7	7
MULTIPLE DX	58	5.9	43	1	2	4	8	14	20	77
TOTAL										
0–19 Years	31	3.7	11	1	2	3	4	11	11	>99
20–34	14	4.6	127	2	2	3	3	6	7	77
35–49	16	4.1	6	2	2	4	6	7	7	12
50–64	13	4.1	2	2	4	4	5	5	8	8
65+	12	12.2	57	2	5	14	20	20	20	20
GRAND TOTAL	86	4.9	31	1	2	3	5	11	20	20

21.2: NASAL DIAGNOSTIC PX. Formerly included in operation group(s) 542, 556.

Type of Patients	Observed Patients	Avg. Stay	Vari-ance	Percentiles						
				10th	25th	50th	75th	90th	95th	99th
1. SINGLE DX										
0–19 Years	9	1.6	<1	1	1	1	3	3	3	3
20–34	2	5.0	0	5	5	5	5	5	5	5
35–49	4	4.1	16	1	1	2	9	9	9	9
50–64	1	2.0	0	2	2	2	2	2	2	2
65+	1	2.0	0	2	2	2	2	2	2	2
2. MULTIPLE DX										
0–19 Years	39	5.1	18	1	3	3	7	10	14	17
20–34	19	5.2	36	2	2	3	7	8	15	37
35–49	32	6.5	227	2	2	2	4	8	10	80
50–64	28	8.4	115	3	4	5	7	19	20	63
65+	91	7.3	49	2	3	5	8	16	18	42
TOTAL SINGLE DX	17	2.6	4	1	1	2	3	5	5	9
MULTIPLE DX	209	6.5	83	2	2	4	7	14	18	63
TOTAL										
0–19 Years	48	4.5	16	1	2	3	6	10	13	17
20–34	21	5.1	30	2	2	3	5	8	15	37
35–49	36	6.4	219	2	3	2	4	8	10	80
50–64	29	8.1	111	2	3	5	7	19	20	63
65+	92	7.2	49	2	3	5	8	16	18	42
GRAND TOTAL	226	6.2	79	2	2	4	7	13	17	42

Length of Stay by Diagnosis and Operation, United States, 1997

United States, October 1995–September 1996 Data, by Operation

21.3: NASAL LESION DESTR/EXC. Formerly included in operation group(s) 542.

Type of Patients	Observed Patients	Avg. Stay	Variance	Percentiles						
				10th	25th	50th	75th	90th	95th	99th
1. SINGLE DX										
0–19 Years	25	1.3	<1	1	1	1	1	2	2	5
20–34	6	1.5	<1	1	1	1	2	2	2	2
35–49	6	1.0	<1	1	1	1	1	1	1	2
50–64	7	1.7	2	1	1	1	2	5	5	5
65+	12	2.5	1	1	2	3	3	3	3	7
2. MULTIPLE DX										
0–19 Years	55	4.3	19	1	1	2	6	9	14	21
20–34	20	5.0	53	1	1	3	6	6	27	27
35–49	36	5.5	139	1	1	2	4	10	13	56
50–64	45	4.0	37	1	1	1	3	9	25	25
65+	138	4.4	18	1	1	3	7	10	15	20
TOTAL SINGLE DX	56	1.5	1	1	1	1	2	3	3	6
MULTIPLE DX	294	4.5	42	1	1	2	6	9	14	27
TOTAL										
0–19 Years	80	3.3	16	1	1	1	5	8	11	21
20–34	26	4.4	46	1	1	3	5	6	15	27
35–49	42	4.4	110	1	1	1	3	7	12	56
50–64	52	3.6	33	1	1	1	3	8	8	25
65+	150	4.2	17	1	1	3	6	9	14	20
GRAND TOTAL	350	3.9	36	1	1	2	5	8	14	27

21.4: RESECTION OF NOSE. Formerly included in operation group(s) 542.

Type of Patients	Observed Patients	Avg. Stay	Variance	Percentiles						
				10th	25th	50th	75th	90th	95th	99th
1. SINGLE DX										
0–19 Years	0									
20–34	1	5.0	0	5	5	5	5	5	5	5
35–49	0									
50–64	2	2.4	<1	1	2	3	3	5	5	5
65+	3	3.0	2	2	2	2	5	5	5	5
2. MULTIPLE DX										
0–19 Years	0									
20–34	0									
35–49	2	6.8	44	2	2	2	13	13	13	13
50–64	6	1.5	1	1	1	1	1	4	5	5
65+	17	3.2	4	2	2	3	6	4	6	10
TOTAL SINGLE DX	6	3.4	2	1	2	3	5	5	5	5
MULTIPLE DX	25	2.6	5	1	1	2	4	4	5	13
TOTAL										
0–19 Years	0									
20–34	1	5.0	0	5	5	5	5	5	5	5
35–49	8	6.8	44	2	2	2	13	13	13	13
50–64	8	1.6	1	1	1	1	3	4	5	5
65+	20	3.1	4	2	2	3	4	4	6	10
GRAND TOTAL	31	2.8	4	1	1	2	4	5	5	13

21.5: SUBMUC NAS SEPTUM RESECT. Formerly included in operation group(s) 540.

Type of Patients	Observed Patients	Avg. Stay	Variance	Percentiles						
				10th	25th	50th	75th	90th	95th	99th
1. SINGLE DX										
0–19 Years	4	1.0	0	1	1	1	1	1	1	1
20–34	4	3.5	1	1	4	4	4	4	4	4
35–49	4	1.0	0	1	1	1	1	1	1	1
50–64	1	2.0	0	2	2	2	2	2	2	2
65+	3	1.8	<1	1	2	2	2	2	2	2
2. MULTIPLE DX										
0–19 Years	44	3.3	24	1	1	1	5	5	15	24
20–34	91	1.8	5	1	1	1	2	3	4	8
35–49	172	2.0	7	1	1	1	2	4	4	13
50–64	105	1.6	3	1	1	1	2	2	3	9
65+	66	3.1	6	1	1	3	5	5	7	12
TOTAL SINGLE DX	16	2.4	2	1	1	2	4	4	4	4
MULTIPLE DX	478	2.0	7	1	1	1	2	4	5	15
TOTAL										
0–19 Years	48	3.1	23	1	1	1	4	5	15	24
20–34	95	1.9	4	1	1	1	3	4	4	5
35–49	176	2.0	7	1	1	1	2	2	3	13
50–64	106	1.6	3	1	1	1	2	2	3	9
65+	69	3.1	6	1	1	3	5	5	7	12
GRAND TOTAL	494	2.0	7	1	1	1	2	4	5	15

21.6: TURBINECTOMY. Formerly included in operation group(s) 542.

Type of Patients	Observed Patients	Avg. Stay	Variance	Percentiles						
				10th	25th	50th	75th	90th	95th	99th
1. SINGLE DX										
0–19 Years	6	1.5	<1	1	1	1	2	3	3	3
20–34	6	1.1	<1	1	1	1	1	1	2	2
35–49	5	2.0	4	1	1	1	2	7	7	7
50–64	5	2.3	<1	1	1	3	3	3	7	7
65+	1	1.0	0	1	1	1	1	1	1	1
2. MULTIPLE DX										
0–19 Years	49	2.4	5	1	1	1	2	8	8	8
20–34	56	2.7	4	1	2	2	3	6	6	7
35–49	98	2.2	6	1	1	1	2	4	6	18
50–64	58	2.2	9	1	1	1	3	6	8	16
65+	30	3.4	21	1	1	3	3	6	18	23
TOTAL SINGLE DX	23	1.5	<1	1	1	1	2	3	3	3
MULTIPLE DX	291	2.4	7	1	1	1	2	6	7	16
TOTAL										
0–19 Years	55	2.2	4	1	1	1	2	7	8	8
20–34	62	2.6	4	1	1	1	3	6	6	7
35–49	103	2.2	6	1	1	1	2	4	6	18
50–64	63	2.2	8	1	1	1	2	4	8	16
65+	31	3.0	18	1	1	3	3	4	14	23
GRAND TOTAL	314	2.3	6	1	1	1	2	5	7	16

Length of Stay by Diagnosis and Operation, United States, 1997

United States, October 1995–September 1996 Data, by Operation

21.69: TURBINECTOMY NEC. Formerly included in operation group(s) 542.

Type of Patients	Observed Patients	Avg. Stay	Vari-ance	10th	25th	50th	75th	90th	95th	99th
1. SINGLE DX										
0–19 Years	5	1.4	<1	1	1	1	1	3	3	3
20–34	6	1.1	<1	1	1	1	1	1	2	2
35–49	4	2.5	6	1	1	2	2	7	7	7
50–64	4	2.5	<1	1	2	3	3	3	3	3
65+	1	1.0	0	1	1	1	1	1	1	1
2. MULTIPLE DX										
0–19 Years	35	2.6	6	1	1	2	3	8	8	8
20–34	38	2.7	4	1	1	2	3	6	7	7
35–49	62	2.1	2	1	2	1	2	4	5	7
50–64	39	1.8	6	1	1	1	2	2	4	16
65+	21	3.6	23	1	1	2	3	4	18	23
TOTAL SINGLE DX	20	1.5	<1	1	1	1	1	3	3	3
MULTIPLE DX	195	2.4	6	1	1	2	2	6	7	11
TOTAL										
0–19 Years	40	2.3	5	1	1	1	2	8	8	8
20–34	44	2.5	4	1	1	2	2	6	7	7
35–49	66	2.1	2	1	1	1	3	4	5	7
50–64	43	1.9	5	1	1	2	2	3	4	16
65+	22	3.1	20	1	1	2	3	3	18	23
GRAND TOTAL	215	2.3	5	1	1	1	2	4	7	10

21.7: NASAL FRACTURE REDUCTION. Formerly included in operation group(s) 543.

Type of Patients	Observed Patients	Avg. Stay	Vari-ance	10th	25th	50th	75th	90th	95th	99th
1. SINGLE DX										
0–19 Years	19	1.0	0	1	1	1	1	1	1	1
20–34	15	1.6	1	1	1	1	2	2	2	6
35–49	7	1.4	<1	1	1	2	2	2	2	2
50–64	3	1.0	0	1	1	1	1	1	1	1
65+	1	1.0	0	1	1	1	1	1	1	1
2. MULTIPLE DX										
0–19 Years	125	2.9	6	1	1	2	4	6	9	11
20–34	186	3.4	8	1	1	2	5	7	9	14
35–49	113	3.4	7	1	2	3	4	4	9	11
50–64	56	5.8	31	1	1	2	8	15	15	17
65+	88	6.8	32	2	4	6	10	10	12	22
TOTAL SINGLE DX	45	1.2	<1	1	1	1	1	2	2	6
MULTIPLE DX	568	4.1	15	1	2	3	6	9	11	15
TOTAL										
0–19 Years	144	2.6	5	1	1	2	4	6	8	11
20–34	201	3.3	8	1	1	2	5	7	9	14
35–49	120	3.3	6	1	2	3	4	7	9	11
50–64	59	5.5	31	1	1	3	8	15	15	17
65+	89	6.7	32	2	4	6	10	10	12	22
GRAND TOTAL	613	3.9	15	1	1	2	5	9	10	15

21.71: CLSD REDUCTION NASAL FX. Formerly included in operation group(s) 543.

Type of Patients	Observed Patients	Avg. Stay	Vari-ance	10th	25th	50th	75th	90th	95th	99th
1. SINGLE DX										
0–19 Years	12	1.0	0	1	1	1	1	1	1	1
20–34	8	1.7	1	1	1	1	2	2	6	6
35–49	2	1.8	<1	2	2	2	2	2	2	2
50–64	2	1.0	0	1	1	1	1	1	1	1
65+	1	1.0	0	1	1	1	1	1	1	1
2. MULTIPLE DX										
0–19 Years	65	3.1	6	1	1	2	4	7	9	12
20–34	86	3.6	11	1	2	2	4	9	10	13
35–49	50	3.7	6	1	2	3	4	9	10	10
50–64	26	5.2	14	1	2	5	7	8	17	17
65+	63	6.4	64	2	3	5	7	12	14	74
TOTAL SINGLE DX	25	1.3	<1	1	1	1	1	2	2	6
MULTIPLE DX	290	3.9	17	1	2	3	5	9	10	14
TOTAL										
0–19 Years	77	2.7	6	1	1	2	4	6	9	11
20–34	94	3.4	10	1	2	3	4	9	10	13
35–49	52	3.6	6	1	2	3	4	9	10	10
50–64	28	4.9	14	1	2	5	6	8	17	17
65+	64	6.3	64	2	3	5	7	12	14	74
GRAND TOTAL	315	3.7	16	1	1	3	4	9	10	14

21.72: OPEN REDUCTION NASAL FX. Formerly included in operation group(s) 543.

Type of Patients	Observed Patients	Avg. Stay	Vari-ance	10th	25th	50th	75th	90th	95th	99th
1. SINGLE DX										
0–19 Years	7	1.0	0	1	1	1	1	1	1	1
20–34	7	1.1	<1	1	1	1	1	1	2	2
35–49	5	1.3	<1	1	1	1	2	2	2	2
50–64	1	1.0	0	1	1	1	1	1	1	1
65+	0									
2. MULTIPLE DX										
0–19 Years	60	2.7	5	1	1	2	4	6	8	9
20–34	100	3.3	7	1	2	2	5	6	7	14
35–49	63	3.2	7	1	1	2	4	7	8	11
50–64	30	5.9	36	1	1	2	15	15	15	15
65+	25	7.0	12	3	6	6	10	10	10	22
TOTAL SINGLE DX	20	1.1	<1	1	1	1	1	1	2	2
MULTIPLE DX	278	4.2	14	1	2	3	6	10	15	15
TOTAL										
0–19 Years	67	2.5	5	1	1	2	3	6	8	9
20–34	107	3.3	7	1	2	2	5	6	7	14
35–49	68	3.0	6	1	1	2	4	7	8	11
50–64	31	5.7	35	1	1	2	15	15	15	11
65+	25	7.0	12	3	6	6	10	10	10	22
GRAND TOTAL	298	4.0	14	1	1	2	6	10	14	15

Length of Stay by Diagnosis and Operation, United States, 1997

United States, October 1995–September 1996 Data, by Operation

21.8: NASAL REP & PLASTIC OPS. Formerly included in operation group(s) 541.

Type of Patients	Observed Patients	Avg. Stay	Vari-ance	Percentiles						
				10th	25th	50th	75th	90th	95th	99th
1. SINGLE DX										
0–19 Years	86	1.5	<1	1	1	1	2	2	3	7
20–34	52	1.9	3	1	1	1	2	6	7	7
35–49	44	1.4	<1	1	1	1	1	2	3	5
50–64	19	1.1	<1	1	1	1	1	1	2	4
65+	15	1.1	<1	1	1	1	1	1	2	3
2. MULTIPLE DX										
0–19 Years	402	2.5	20	1	1	1	2	4	7	31
20–34	486	2.0	7	1	1	1	2	3	5	14
35–49	610	2.5	6	1	1	2	3	6	7	10
50–64	426	2.4	7	1	1	2	3	5	7	12
65+	451	3.5	14	1	1	2	4	7	10	18
TOTAL SINGLE DX	216	1.5	1	1	1	1	1	2	4	7
MULTIPLE DX	2375	2.5	10	1	1	1	3	6	7	15
TOTAL										
0–19 Years	488	2.3	17	1	1	1	2	3	6	24
20–34	538	2.0	7	1	1	1	3	6	5	14
35–49	654	2.5	6	1	1	1	3	6	7	10
50–64	445	2.3	6	1	1	1	2	5	7	12
65+	466	3.4	14	1	1	2	4	7	10	17
GRAND TOTAL	2591	2.4	9	1	1	1	2	5	7	15

21.88: SEPTOPLASTY NEC. Formerly included in operation group(s) 541.

Type of Patients	Observed Patients	Avg. Stay	Vari-ance	Percentiles						
				10th	25th	50th	75th	90th	95th	99th
1. SINGLE DX										
0–19 Years	16	1.4	2	1	1	1	1	2	7	7
20–34	14	1.3	<1	1	1	1	2	2	2	2
35–49	17	1.3	<1	1	1	1	2	2	2	2
50–64	8	1.1	<1	1	1	1	1	1	1	2
65+	2	1.0	0	1	1	1	1	1	1	1
2. MULTIPLE DX										
0–19 Years	73	2.4	23	1	1	1	2	3	7	31
20–34	232	1.6	3	1	1	1	2	3	3	11
35–49	411	2.1	4	1	1	1	2	4	7	11
50–64	284	2.2	7	1	1	1	2	5	7	12
65+	167	3.0	12	1	1	2	3	7	11	17
TOTAL SINGLE DX	57	1.3	<1	1	1	1	1	2	2	7
MULTIPLE DX	1167	2.1	7	1	1	1	2	4	7	14
TOTAL										
0–19 Years	89	2.2	18	1	1	1	1	3	7	31
20–34	246	1.6	3	1	1	1	2	3	3	11
35–49	428	2.0	4	1	1	1	2	4	7	11
50–64	292	2.1	6	1	1	1	2	4	7	12
65+	169	3.0	12	1	1	2	3	7	11	17
GRAND TOTAL	1224	2.0	6	1	1	1	2	4	6	13

21.81: NASAL LACERATION SUTURE. Formerly included in operation group(s) 541.

Type of Patients	Observed Patients	Avg. Stay	Vari-ance	Percentiles						
				10th	25th	50th	75th	90th	95th	99th
1. SINGLE DX										
0–19 Years	7	1.2	<1	1	1	1	1	2	2	2
20–34	0									
35–49	0									
50–64	0									
65+										
2. MULTIPLE DX										
0–19 Years	68	2.4	11	1	1	2	3	5	5	5
20–34	124	1.9	3	1	1	1	2	3	4	8
35–49	70	4.6	6	1	2	6	4	7	7	7
50–64	55	3.1	7	1	1	3	4	7	9	11
65+	142	4.3	14	1	2	3	5	8	10	29
TOTAL SINGLE DX	7	1.2	<1	1	1	1	1	2	2	2
MULTIPLE DX	459	3.1	8	1	1	2	5	7	7	12
TOTAL										
0–19 Years	75	2.3	10	1	1	1	3	5	5	5
20–34	124	1.9	3	1	1	1	2	3	4	8
35–49	70	4.6	6	1	2	6	4	7	7	7
50–64	55	3.1	7	1	1	3	4	7	9	11
65+	142	4.3	14	1	2	3	5	8	10	29
GRAND TOTAL	466	3.1	8	1	1	2	4	7	7	11

21.9: OTHER NASAL OPERATIONS. Formerly included in operation group(s) 543.

Type of Patients	Observed Patients	Avg. Stay	Vari-ance	Percentiles						
				10th	25th	50th	75th	90th	95th	99th
1. SINGLE DX										
0–19 Years	6	6.3	29	2	2	4	15	15	15	15
20–34	0									
35–49	0									
50–64	0									
65+	0									
2. MULTIPLE DX										
0–19 Years	23	3.6	4	1	2	4	4	8	8	8
20–34	3	2.2	10	1	1	1	1	11	11	11
35–49	7	3.1	4	1	1	3	5	6	6	6
50–64	3	10.4	103	1	1	6	21	21	21	21
65+	3	4.4	<1	4	4	4	4	6	6	6
TOTAL SINGLE DX	6	6.3	29	2	2	4	15	15	15	15
MULTIPLE DX	39	3.8	10	1	1	4	4	8	8	21
TOTAL										
0–19 Years	29	4.3	12	1	2	4	4	8	15	15
20–34	3	2.2	10	1	1	1	1	11	11	11
35–49	7	3.1	4	1	1	3	5	6	6	6
50–64	3	10.4	103	1	4	6	21	21	21	21
65+	3	4.4	<1	4	4	4	4	6	6	6
GRAND TOTAL	45	4.3	15	1	2	4	4	8	15	21

Length of Stay by Diagnosis and Operation, United States, 1997

United States, October 1995–September 1996 Data, by Operation

22.0: NASAL SINUS ASP & LAVAGE. Formerly included in operation group(s) 545.

Type of Patients	Observed Patients	Avg. Stay	Vari-ance	Percentiles						
				10th	25th	50th	75th	90th	95th	99th
1. SINGLE DX										
0–19 Years	4	1.8	2	1	1	1	2	4	4	4
20–34	3	2.2	<1	2	2	2	2	3	3	3
35–49	2	9.4	4	10	10	10	10	10	10	10
50–64	3	4.9	9	1	1	7	7	7	7	7
65+	0									
2. MULTIPLE DX										
0–19 Years	63	5.0	17	1	1	4	7	11	13	16
20–34	37	6.7	15	3	5	6	9	12	14	14
35–49	44	5.8	33	2	2	4	5	17	19	21
50–64	26	5.6	29	2	2	4	7	14	15	17
65+	26	7.2	13	3	5	7	10	12	12	16
TOTAL SINGLE DX	12	4.6	14	1	1	3	10	10	10	10
MULTIPLE DX	196	5.8	22	1	3	5	7	12	15	21
TOTAL										
0–19 Years	67	4.9	17	1	1	4	6	10	13	16
20–34	40	6.5	16	2	4	6	7	12	14	14
35–49	46	6.1	32	2	2	5	6	17	19	21
50–64	29	5.5	28	2	2	4	7	14	15	17
65+	26	7.2	13	3	5	7	10	12	12	16
GRAND TOTAL	208	5.8	22	1	2	5	7	12	14	21

22.1: NASAL SINUS DXTIC PX. Formerly included in operation group(s) 545, 556.

Type of Patients	Observed Patients	Avg. Stay	Vari-ance	Percentiles						
				10th	25th	50th	75th	90th	95th	99th
1. SINGLE DX										
0–19 Years	10	2.4	2	1	1	2	3	5	5	5
20–34	4	1.4	1	1	1	1	1	4	4	4
35–49	5	1.3	<1	1	1	1	2	2	2	2
50–64	3	2.6	2	2	2	2	2	5	5	5
65+	5	2.0	1	1	1	2	2	4	4	4
2. MULTIPLE DX										
0–19 Years	71	8.1	222	1	1	3	6	30	36	84
20–34	29	8.5	107	2	3	6	8	19	35	54
35–49	29	8.7	164	1	2	3	6	41	41	41
50–64	38	6.4	16	2	4	5	7	11	17	21
65+	71	7.8	60	1	3	5	9	23	24	34
TOTAL SINGLE DX	27	2.0	2	1	1	2	2	4	5	5
MULTIPLE DX	238	7.9	119	1	2	5	8	21	36	41
TOTAL										
0–19 Years	81	7.4	198	1	1	3	5	19	36	84
20–34	33	7.4	97	1	2	6	8	11	21	54
35–49	34	8.0	153	1	1	3	6	41	41	41
50–64	41	6.2	16	2	4	5	8	11	17	21
65+	76	7.6	59	1	3	5	9	23	24	34
GRAND TOTAL	265	7.4	112	1	2	4	7	18	34	41

22.2: INTRANASAL ANTROTOMY. Formerly included in operation group(s) 545.

Type of Patients	Observed Patients	Avg. Stay	Vari-ance	Percentiles						
				10th	25th	50th	75th	90th	95th	99th
1. SINGLE DX										
0–19 Years	15	1.5	<1	1	1	1	2	2	4	4
20–34	5	1.1	<1	1	1	1	1	1	1	3
35–49	1	4.0	0	4	4	4	4	4	4	4
50–64	1	1.0	0	1	1	1	1	1	1	1
65+	0									
2. MULTIPLE DX										
0–19 Years	78	4.9	35	1	1	3	6	11	17	29
20–34	39	4.2	25	1	1	3	6	12	18	18
35–49	39	3.7	22	1	1	1	4	10	17	19
50–64	31	2.8	14	1	1	1	3	7	11	21
65+	30	4.4	11	1	3	3	5	10	12	13
TOTAL SINGLE DX	22	1.3	<1	1	1	1	1	2	4	4
MULTIPLE DX	217	3.9	24	1	1	2	4	11	17	25
TOTAL										
0–19 Years	93	4.4	31	1	1	2	5	11	14	29
20–34	44	3.1	18	1	1	1	3	9	14	18
35–49	40	3.7	21	1	1	1	4	10	17	19
50–64	32	2.8	14	1	1	1	3	7	11	21
65+	30	4.4	11	1	3	3	5	10	12	13
GRAND TOTAL	239	3.6	21	1	1	1	4	9	14	21

22.3: EXT MAXILLARY ANTROTOMY. Formerly included in operation group(s) 544.

Type of Patients	Observed Patients	Avg. Stay	Vari-ance	Percentiles						
				10th	25th	50th	75th	90th	95th	99th
1. SINGLE DX										
0–19 Years	2	1.7	<1	1	1	2	2	2	2	2
20–34	13	2.0	2	1	1	1	3	4	5	5
35–49	7	1.1	<1	1	1	1	1	1	2	2
50–64	11	1.8	<1	1	1	1	3	3	3	4
65+	1	2.0	0	2	2	2	2	2	2	2
2. MULTIPLE DX										
0–19 Years	30	6.9	48	1	2	5	8	20	20	43
20–34	46	4.6	32	1	2	5	4	17	20	20
35–49	88	6.6	60	1	1	3	9	18	22	36
50–64	76	4.6	31	1	1	4	4	8	16	40
65+	65	4.6	29	2	2	2	6	13	14	35
TOTAL SINGLE DX	34	1.8	1	1	1	1	2	3	4	5
MULTIPLE DX	305	5.5	43	1	1	3	6	18	20	36
TOTAL										
0–19 Years	32	6.3	45	1	2	5	8	16	20	43
20–34	59	4.1	27	1	1	2	4	9	20	20
35–49	95	6.3	58	1	1	3	7	18	22	36
50–64	87	4.4	29	1	2	3	4	8	16	31
65+	66	4.5	29	1	2	2	6	11	14	35
GRAND TOTAL	339	5.1	40	1	1	3	6	17	19	35

Length of Stay by Diagnosis and Operation, United States, 1997

United States, October 1995–September 1996 Data, by Operation

22.42: FRONTAL SINUSECTOMY. Formerly included in operation group(s) 545.

Type of Patients	Observed Patients	Avg. Stay	Variance	Percentiles						
				10th	25th	50th	75th	90th	95th	99th
1. SINGLE DX										
0–19 Years	6	3.4	3	1	1	4	5	5	5	5
20–34	8	3.0	5	1	1	3	5	5	7	7
35–49	15	2.1	2	1	1	2	3	4	4	4
50–64	5	3.4	2	2	2	3	5	6	6	6
65+	5	2.7	2	2	2	2	4	6	6	6
2. MULTIPLE DX										
0–19 Years	12	5.1	13	1	2	4	7	8	8	18
20–34	43	3.8	10	1	2	3	4	9	12	16
35–49	70	2.7	6	1	1	2	3	7	8	12
50–64	55	5.9	23	2	2	4	8	11	11	34
65+	43	4.5	21	1	2	3	6	9	17	29
TOTAL SINGLE DX	39	2.8	3	1	1	3	4	5	6	7
MULTIPLE DX	223	4.0	15	1	1	3	5	8	11	17
TOTAL										
0–19 Years	18	4.4	9	1	2	4	7	8	8	18
20–34	51	3.7	10	1	2	3	3	8	12	16
35–49	85	2.6	6	1	1	2	3	7	8	12
50–64	60	5.8	23	2	2	4	8	11	11	34
65+	48	4.3	19	1	2	3	6	7	11	29
GRAND TOTAL	262	3.9	14	1	1	3	4	8	11	16

22.5: OTHER NASAL SINUSOTOMY. Formerly included in operation group(s) 545.

Type of Patients	Observed Patients	Avg. Stay	Variance	Percentiles						
				10th	25th	50th	75th	90th	95th	99th
1. SINGLE DX										
0–19 Years	3	3.0	<1	2	3	3	3	3	5	5
20–34	5	4.4	15	1	1	2	9	9	9	9
35–49	4	2.8	6	1	1	3	3	9	9	9
50–64	1	1.0	0	1	1	1	1	1	1	1
65+	1	2.0	0	2	2	2	2	2	2	2
2. MULTIPLE DX										
0–19 Years	34	6.2	29	1	3	4	8	13	20	23
20–34	35	8.7	117	1	2	4	10	19	40	40
35–49	55	4.7	27	1	1	3	5	13	15	22
50–64	38	5.5	20	1	2	4	8	12	12	29
65+	39	9.0	99	2	2	4	14	22	22	61
TOTAL SINGLE DX	14	3.6	10	1	1	3	5	9	9	9
MULTIPLE DX	201	6.5	58	1	2	4	8	17	22	40
TOTAL										
0–19 Years	37	6.0	28	1	3	4	8	13	17	23
20–34	40	8.0	104	1	1	4	9	19	38	40
35–49	59	4.6	26	1	1	3	5	11	15	22
50–64	39	5.4	20	1	2	4	8	12	12	29
65+	40	8.9	98	1	2	4	14	22	22	61
GRAND TOTAL	215	6.3	56	1	2	4	8	17	22	40

22.39: EXT MAX ANTROTOMY NEC. Formerly included in operation group(s) 544.

Type of Patients	Observed Patients	Avg. Stay	Variance	Percentiles						
				10th	25th	50th	75th	90th	95th	99th
1. SINGLE DX										
0–19 Years	2	1.7	<1	1	1	2	2	2	2	2
20–34	12	1.9	2	1	1	1	1	4	5	5
35–49	6	1.0	0	1	1	1	1	1	1	1
50–64	9	1.9	<1	1	1	1	3	3	3	4
65+	0									
2. MULTIPLE DX										
0–19 Years	19	4.7	11	1	2	4	8	8	12	12
20–34	34	5.1	36	2	2	3	5	20	12	20
35–49	68	5.1	52	1	1	3	6	11	25	36
50–64	54	4.5	21	1	1	4	6	9	16	27
65+	46	4.6	34	1	2	2	7	13	17	35
TOTAL SINGLE DX	29	1.7	1	1	1	1	2	3	4	5
MULTIPLE DX	221	4.8	34	1	1	3	6	10	20	35
TOTAL										
0–19 Years	21	4.2	11	1	1	3	8	8	8	12
20–34	46	4.4	30	1	2	2	4	9	20	20
35–49	74	4.8	49	1	1	3	6	11	25	36
50–64	63	4.2	19	1	1	2	6	9	16	27
65+	46	4.6	34	1	2	2	7	13	17	35
GRAND TOTAL	250	4.5	31	1	1	3	5	9	19	30

22.4: FRONT SINUSOT & SINUSECT. Formerly included in operation group(s) 545.

Type of Patients	Observed Patients	Avg. Stay	Variance	Percentiles						
				10th	25th	50th	75th	90th	95th	99th
1. SINGLE DX										
0–19 Years	7	3.3	3	1	1	4	5	5	5	5
20–34	12	2.6	3	2	2	2	3	7	7	7
35–49	24	2.3	3	1	1	1	3	4	6	7
50–64	9	3.6	3	2	2	3	5	6	7	7
65+	8	2.2	1	1	2	2	3	4	4	6
2. MULTIPLE DX										
0–19 Years	35	6.6	35	1	2	5	8	11	18	30
20–34	78	3.5	11	1	1	3	4	6	12	17
35–49	97	3.3	12	1	1	3	6	8	12	14
50–64	74	5.7	23	2	2	4	8	11	11	25
65+	66	4.8	22	1	2	3	6	11	17	19
TOTAL SINGLE DX	60	2.7	3	1	1	2	4	5	6	7
MULTIPLE DX	350	4.2	18	1	1	3	6	9	12	18
TOTAL										
0–19 Years	42	5.9	30	1	2	5	7	11	18	30
20–34	90	3.4	11	1	1	3	4	6	12	17
35–49	121	3.2	11	1	1	3	6	8	12	14
50–64	83	5.6	22	2	2	4	8	11	11	25
65+	74	4.4	19	1	2	3	6	11	13	19
GRAND TOTAL	410	4.1	16	1	1	3	5	9	12	18

United States, October 1995–September 1996 Data, by Operation

22.6: OTHER NASAL SINUSECTOMY. Formerly included in operation group(s) 545.

Type of Patients	Observed Patients	Avg. Stay	Vari- ance	Percentiles						
				10th	25th	50th	75th	90th	95th	99th
1. SINGLE DX										
0–19 Years	88	2.1	5	1	1	1	2	7	8	9
20–34	39	2.3	6	1	1	1	3	4	10	11
35–49	48	2.0	2	1	1	1	3	4	5	7
50–64	45	3.6	28	1	1	2	3	6	25	25
65+	19	4.2	15	1	2	3	4	13	13	13
2. MULTIPLE DX										
0–19 Years	559	5.0	31	1	1	3	7	13	16	27
20–34	363	4.6	43	1	1	2	6	10	14	39
35–49	502	4.6	38	1	1	2	6	10	15	29
50–64	439	3.4	17	1	1	2	4	8	10	22
65+	417	5.2	46	1	1	2	7	12	16	31
TOTAL SINGLE DX	239	2.5	10	1	1	1	3	5	8	13
MULTIPLE DX	2280	4.5	34	1	1	2	6	11	15	27
TOTAL										
0–19 Years	647	4.7	29	1	1	2	6	12	16	27
20–34	402	4.4	40	1	1	2	6	10	14	24
35–49	550	4.4	36	1	1	2	6	10	13	28
50–64	484	3.4	18	1	1	2	4	8	10	23
65+	436	5.2	45	1	2	2	7	12	16	31
GRAND TOTAL	2519	4.4	32	1	1	2	6	10	14	27

22.63: ETHMOIDECTOMY. Formerly included in operation group(s) 545.

Type of Patients	Observed Patients	Avg. Stay	Vari- ance	Percentiles						
				10th	25th	50th	75th	90th	95th	99th
1. SINGLE DX										
0–19 Years	64	1.8	5	1	1	1	1	7	8	9
20–34	27	2.5	8	1	1	1	3	5	11	11
35–49	23	2.0	2	1	1	1	2	5	5	6
50–64	22	4.0	38	1	1	3	3	7	25	25
65+	7	6.5	27	1	2	5	13	13	13	13
2. MULTIPLE DX										
0–19 Years	436	4.8	28	1	1	2	7	12	15	27
20–34	263	4.4	50	1	1	2	5	10	15	39
35–49	355	3.8	16	1	1	2	6	10	11	21
50–64	297	3.5	18	1	1	2	4	8	11	21
65+	246	5.3	60	1	1	2	7	14	16	31
TOTAL SINGLE DX	143	2.5	13	1	1	1	3	6	8	25
MULTIPLE DX	1597	4.2	30	1	1	2	6	10	14	26
TOTAL										
0–19 Years	500	4.4	26	1	1	2	6	12	14	27
20–34	290	4.3	47	1	1	2	5	10	14	39
35–49	378	3.7	16	1	1	2	5	10	11	21
50–64	319	3.5	19	1	1	2	4	8	11	25
65+	253	5.3	59	1	1	2	7	14	16	31
GRAND TOTAL	1740	4.1	29	1	1	2	5	10	13	25

22.62: EXC MAX SINUS LESION NEC. Formerly included in operation group(s) 545.

Type of Patients	Observed Patients	Avg. Stay	Vari- ance	Percentiles						
				10th	25th	50th	75th	90th	95th	99th
1. SINGLE DX										
0–19 Years	9	4.9	7	3	3	3	8	9	9	9
20–34	7	3.4	3	1	1	4	4	4	7	7
35–49	15	2.0	<1	1	1	2	3	3	3	4
50–64	17	2.4	2	1	2	2	3	4	4	4
65+	8	2.5	<1	2	2	2	3	3	4	4
2. MULTIPLE DX										
0–19 Years	76	7.5	48	1	2	5	10	21	21	21
20–34	53	4.8	20	1	2	4	6	9	9	24
35–49	84	7.3	68	1	1	4	9	24	27	28
50–64	78	3.7	9	1	1	3	5	8	9	14
65+	105	4.1	16	2	2	3	5	9	11	20
TOTAL SINGLE DX	56	2.7	3	1	1	3	3	4	7	9
MULTIPLE DX	396	5.7	38	1	2	4	7	12	21	27
TOTAL										
0–19 Years	85	7.4	46	1	2	5	10	21	21	21
20–34	60	4.7	18	1	2	4	6	9	9	20
35–49	99	6.2	58	1	1	3	7	23	27	28
50–64	95	3.5	15	1	2	3	5	7	8	14
65+	113	4.1	15	2	2	2	5	9	11	20
GRAND TOTAL	452	5.4	34	1	2	3	7	11	21	27

22.7: NASAL SINUS REPAIR. Formerly included in operation group(s) 545.

Type of Patients	Observed Patients	Avg. Stay	Vari- ance	Percentiles						
				10th	25th	50th	75th	90th	95th	99th
1. SINGLE DX										
0–19 Years	3	1.1	<1	1	1	1	1	2	2	2
20–34	7	1.9	<1	1	1	2	3	3	3	3
35–49	9	3.2	0	1	1	4	4	7	7	7
50–64	1	3.0	0	3	3	3	3	3	3	3
65+	0									
2. MULTIPLE DX										
0–19 Years	11	3.2	7	1	1	2	5	5	9	14
20–34	10	6.1	14	1	3	5	10	10	11	11
35–49	27	3.6	9	2	2	2	3	7	9	17
50–64	8	2.8	5	2	2	3	3	4	4	9
65+	9	4.6	14	2	3	3	6	10	17	17
TOTAL SINGLE DX	20	2.3	2	1	1	2	3	4	5	7
MULTIPLE DX	65	4.1	11	1	2	3	5	10	10	17
TOTAL										
0–19 Years	14	2.7	6	1	1	2	4	5	5	14
20–34	17	4.9	14	1	2	3	10	10	10	11
35–49	36	3.5	9	2	2	2	3	4	9	17
50–64	9	2.9	4	2	2	2	3	4	9	9
65+	9	4.6	14	2	3	3	6	10	17	17
GRAND TOTAL	85	3.8	10	1	2	3	5	10	10	17

Length of Stay by Diagnosis and Operation, United States, 1997

United States, October 1995–September 1996 Data, by Operation

22.9: OTHER NASAL SINUS OPS. Formerly included in operation group(s) 545.

Type of Patients	Observed Patients	Avg. Stay	Variance	Percentiles						
				10th	25th	50th	75th	90th	95th	99th
1. SINGLE DX										
0–19 Years	2	3.0	0	3	3	3	3	3	3	3
20–34	0									
35–49	0									
50–64	0									
65+	1	15.0	0	15	15	15	15	15	15	15
2. MULTIPLE DX										
0–19 Years	15	4.6	23	1	1	4	8	14	14	14
20–34	4	21.4	715	1	4	4	26	64	64	64
35–49	4	3.9	25	1	3	3	3	3	23	23
50–64	6	9.3	21	1	3	12	12	12	12	12
65+	3	2.8	5	1	1	2	6	6	6	6
TOTAL SINGLE DX	3	5.0	22	3	3	3	3	15	15	15
MULTIPLE DX	32	7.3	98	1	1	4	12	14	14	64
TOTAL										
0–19 Years	17	4.4	20	1	1	3	4	14	14	14
20–34	4	21.4	715	1	4	4	26	64	64	64
35–49	4	3.9	25	1	3	3	3	3	23	23
50–64	6	9.3	21	1	3	12	12	12	12	12
65+	4	7.3	42	1	2	6	15	15	15	15
GRAND TOTAL	35	7.1	90	1	2	4	12	14	15	64

23.09: TOOTH EXTRACTION NEC. Formerly included in operation group(s) 546.

Type of Patients	Observed Patients	Avg. Stay	Variance	Percentiles						
				10th	25th	50th	75th	90th	95th	99th
1. SINGLE DX										
0–19 Years	16	1.7	<1	1	1	2	2	3	3	3
20–34	11	2.5	5	2	2	2	3	3	7	7
35–49	10	4.5	5	2	3	4	6	7	9	9
50–64	1	1.0	0	1	1	1	1	1	1	1
65+	2	3.4	<1	3	3	3	4	4	4	4
2. MULTIPLE DX										
0–19 Years	231	3.4	36	1	1	2	3	5	12	34
20–34	169	7.4	115	1	4	4	7	14	26	59
35–49	206	7.5	94	2	3	4	8	15	28	65
50–64	122	9.0	55	2	4	8	11	16	20	37
65+	198	8.9	59	2	5	6	11	22	25	44
TOTAL SINGLE DX	40	2.7	3	1	2	2	3	5	7	9
MULTIPLE DX	926	7.1	76	1	2	4	8	16	22	45
TOTAL										
0–19 Years	247	3.3	34	1	2	2	3	5	12	34
20–34	180	7.1	110	1	2	4	7	14	26	59
35–49	216	7.5	92	2	3	4	8	15	25	65
50–64	123	9.0	55	2	4	7	11	16	20	37
65+	200	8.9	59	2	5	6	11	22	25	44
GRAND TOTAL	966	7.0	74	1	2	4	8	15	22	45

23.0: FORCEPS TOOTH EXTRACTION. Formerly included in operation group(s) 546.

Type of Patients	Observed Patients	Avg. Stay	Variance	Percentiles						
				10th	25th	50th	75th	90th	95th	99th
1. SINGLE DX										
0–19 Years	22	1.5	<1	1	1	1	2	3	3	6
20–34	11	2.5	2	2	2	2	3	3	7	7
35–49	10	4.5	5	3	3	4	6	7	9	9
50–64	1	1.0	0	1	1	1	1	1	1	1
65+	2	3.4	<1	3	3	3	4	4	4	4
2. MULTIPLE DX										
0–19 Years	283	3.1	27	1	1	2	3	4	9	31
20–34	172	7.3	114	1	2	4	7	14	26	59
35–49	207	7.6	94	2	3	7	8	15	28	65
50–64	125	8.9	54	2	4	7	11	16	20	37
65+	198	8.9	59	2	5	6	11	22	25	44
TOTAL SINGLE DX	46	2.2	3	1	1	2	3	4	6	9
MULTIPLE DX	985	6.7	71	1	2	4	8	15	22	42
TOTAL										
0–19 Years	305	3.0	26	1	1	2	3	4	8	31
20–34	183	7.0	109	1	2	4	7	14	26	59
35–49	217	7.5	92	2	3	8	8	15	25	65
50–64	126	8.9	54	2	4	7	11	16	20	37
65+	200	8.9	59	2	5	6	11	22	25	44
GRAND TOTAL	1031	6.6	70	1	2	4	7	15	22	40

23.1: SURG REMOVAL OF TOOTH. Formerly included in operation group(s) 546.

Type of Patients	Observed Patients	Avg. Stay	Variance	Percentiles						
				10th	25th	50th	75th	90th	95th	99th
1. SINGLE DX										
0–19 Years	24	1.6	<1	1	1	1	2	3	3	3
20–34	18	1.8	1	1	1	2	2	4	4	5
35–49	7	2.3	7	1	1	1	2	7	10	10
50–64	6	2.5	2	1	2	2	2	4	4	4
65+	4	4.6	37	1	1	2	2	15	15	15
2. MULTIPLE DX										
0–19 Years	256	2.7	13	1	1	2	3	5	8	13
20–34	252	5.4	35	1	2	4	7	10	16	32
35–49	266	6.6	109	1	2	3	6	14	22	69
50–64	185	5.9	58	2	2	4	6	12	17	43
65+	331	5.9	50	2	2	4	7	11	14	49
TOTAL SINGLE DX	59	2.0	4	1	1	1	2	4	4	15
MULTIPLE DX	1290	5.3	55	1	2	3	6	11	16	46
TOTAL										
0–19 Years	280	2.7	12	1	2	2	3	5	7	13
20–34	270	5.3	34	1	2	3	7	10	15	32
35–49	273	6.5	107	2	2	3	8	14	22	69
50–64	191	5.9	57	1	2	4	6	12	17	42
65+	335	5.9	50	2	2	4	7	11	15	49
GRAND TOTAL	1349	5.2	54	1	2	3	6	10	16	46

Length of Stay by Diagnosis and Operation, United States, 1997

United States, October 1995–September 1996 Data, by Operation

23.19: SURG TOOTH EXTRACT NEC. Formerly included in operation group(s) 546.

Type of Patients	Observed Patients	Avg. Stay	Vari-ance	10th	25th	50th	75th	90th	95th	99th
1. SINGLE DX										
0–19 Years	24	1.6	<1	1	1	1	2	3	3	3
20–34	18	1.8	1	1	1	2	2	4	4	5
35–49	7	2.3	7	1	1	1	2	7	10	10
50–64	6	2.5	2	1	1	2	4	4	4	4
65+	4	4.6	37	1	1	2	2	15	15	15
2. MULTIPLE DX										
0–19 Years	253	2.7	13	1	1	2	3	5	8	13
20–34	250	5.5	36	1	2	4	7	10	16	32
35–49	259	6.6	109	1	2	3	6	14	22	69
50–64	183	5.9	58	1	2	4	6	12	17	43
65+	327	5.8	50	2	2	4	7	11	14	49
TOTAL SINGLE DX	59	2.0	4	1	1	1	2	4	4	15
MULTIPLE DX	1272	5.3	55	1	2	3	6	11	16	46
TOTAL										
0–19 Years	277	2.7	12	1	1	2	3	5	7	13
20–34	268	5.3	35	1	2	3	7	10	15	32
35–49	266	6.5	107	1	2	3	6	14	22	69
50–64	189	5.9	58	1	2	4	6	12	17	42
65+	331	5.8	50	2	2	4	7	11	14	49
GRAND TOTAL	1331	5.2	54	1	2	3	6	10	16	46

23.2: TOOTH RESTOR BY FILLING. Formerly included in operation group(s) 547.

Type of Patients	Observed Patients	Avg. Stay	Vari-ance	10th	25th	50th	75th	90th	95th	99th
1. SINGLE DX										
0–19 Years	4	1.2	<1	1	1	1	1	2	2	2
20–34	0									
35–49	0									
50–64	0									
65+	0									
2. MULTIPLE DX										
0–19 Years	56	9.6	37	1	2	13	13	13	13	19
20–34	6	7.0	110	1	1	2	4	28	28	28
35–49	1	23.0	0	23	23	23	23	23	23	23
50–64	0									
65+	1	5.0	0	5	5	5	5	5	5	5
TOTAL SINGLE DX	4	1.2	<1	1	1	1	1	2	2	2
MULTIPLE DX	64	9.5	41	1	2	13	13	13	13	28
TOTAL										
0–19 Years	60	9.4	38	1	1	13	13	13	13	19
20–34	6	7.0	110	1	1	2	4	28	28	28
35–49	1	23.0	0	23	23	23	23	23	23	23
50–64	0									
65+	1	5.0	0	5	5	5	5	5	5	5
GRAND TOTAL	68	9.3	41	1	1	13	13	13	13	28

23.3: TOOTH RESTOR BY INLAY. Formerly included in operation group(s) 547.

Type of Patients	Observed Patients	Avg. Stay	Vari-ance	10th	25th	50th	75th	90th	95th	99th
1. SINGLE DX										
0–19 Years	0									
20–34	0									
35–49	0									
50–64	0									
65+	0									
2. MULTIPLE DX										
0–19 Years	1	2.0	0	2	2	2	2	2	2	2
20–34	1	1.0	0	1	1	1	1	1	1	1
35–49	0									
50–64	0									
65+	0									
TOTAL SINGLE DX	0									
MULTIPLE DX	2	1.7	0	1	1	2	2	2	2	2
TOTAL										
0–19 Years	1	2.0	0	2	2	2	2	2	2	2
20–34	1	1.0	0	1	1	1	1	1	1	1
35–49	0									
50–64	0									
65+	0									
GRAND TOTAL	2	1.7	0	1	1	2	2	2	2	2

23.4: OTHER DENTAL RESTORATION. Formerly included in operation group(s) 547.

Type of Patients	Observed Patients	Avg. Stay	Vari-ance	10th	25th	50th	75th	90th	95th	99th
1. SINGLE DX										
0–19 Years	4	1.1	<1	1	1	1	1	1	2	2
20–34	1	1.0	0	1	1	1	1	1	1	1
35–49	0									
50–64	0									
65+	0									
2. MULTIPLE DX										
0–19 Years	60	2.1	7	1	1	1	2	4	10	12
20–34	8	2.2	12	1	1	1	1	4	4	19
35–49	4	6.6	79	1	1	1	20	20	20	20
50–64	4	2.7	7	1	1	1	6	6	8	8
65+	2	4.8	1	4	4	4	6	6	6	6
TOTAL SINGLE DX	5	1.1	<1	1	1	1	1	1	2	2
MULTIPLE DX	78	2.4	11	1	1	1	2	6	12	20
TOTAL										
0–19 Years	64	2.0	7	1	1	1	2	3	10	12
20–34	9	2.2	11	1	1	1	1	4	4	19
35–49	4	6.6	79	1	1	1	20	20	20	20
50–64	4	2.7	7	1	1	1	6	6	8	8
65+	2	4.8	1	4	4	4	6	6	6	6
GRAND TOTAL	83	2.3	11	1	1	1	2	6	12	20

United States, October 1995–September 1996 Data, by Operation

23.5: TOOTH IMPLANTATION. Formerly included in operation group(s) 547.

Type of Patients	Observed Patients	Avg. Stay	Vari-ance	Percentiles						
				10th	25th	50th	75th	90th	95th	99th
1. SINGLE DX										
0–19 Years	0									
20–34	0									
35–49	0									
50–64	0									
65+	0									
2. MULTIPLE DX										
0–19 Years	7	2.2	4	1	1	2	2	7	7	7
20–34	1	3.0	0	3	3	3	3	3	3	3
35–49	2	1.6	<1	1	1	2	2	2	2	2
50–64	0									
65+	0									
TOTAL SINGLE DX	0									
MULTIPLE DX	10	2.2	3	1	1	2	2	7	7	7
TOTAL										
0–19 Years	7	2.2	4	1	1	2	2	7	7	7
20–34	1	3.0	0	3	3	3	3	3	3	3
35–49	2	1.6	<1	1	1	2	2	2	2	2
50–64	0									
65+	0									
GRAND TOTAL	10	2.2	3	1	1	2	2	7	7	7

23.6: PROSTHETIC DENTAL IMPL. Formerly included in operation group(s) 547.

Type of Patients	Observed Patients	Avg. Stay	Vari-ance	Percentiles						
				10th	25th	50th	75th	90th	95th	99th
1. SINGLE DX										
0–19 Years	0									
20–34	0									
35–49	1	1.0	0	1	1	1	1	1	1	1
50–64	0									
65+	1	1.0	0	1	1	1	1	1	1	1
2. MULTIPLE DX										
0–19 Years	1	2.0	0	2	2	2	2	2	2	2
20–34	1	1.0	0	1	1	1	1	1	1	1
35–49	5	1.8	1	1	1	1	3	3	3	3
50–64	3	1.1	<1	1	1	1	1	1	3	3
65+	0									
TOTAL SINGLE DX	2	1.0	0	1	1	1	1	1	1	1
MULTIPLE DX	10	1.2	<1	1	1	1	1	2	3	3
TOTAL										
0–19 Years	1	2.0	0	2	2	2	2	2	2	2
20–34	6	1.0	0	1	1	1	1	1	1	1
35–49	6	1.4	<1	1	1	1	1	1	3	3
50–64	3	1.1	<1	1	1	1	1	1	3	3
65+	1	1.0	0	1	1	1	1	1	1	1
GRAND TOTAL	12	1.2	<1	1	1	1	1	1	3	3

23.7: ROOT CANAL TX & APICOECT. Formerly included in operation group(s) 548.

Type of Patients	Observed Patients	Avg. Stay	Vari-ance	Percentiles						
				10th	25th	50th	75th	90th	95th	99th
1. SINGLE DX										
0–19 Years	1	2.0	0	2	2	2	2	2	2	2
20–34	0									
35–49	0									
50–64	0									
65+	0									
2. MULTIPLE DX										
0–19 Years	20	5.4	40	1	2	5	6	6	14	35
20–34	9	6.6	46	2	2	4	8	13	23	26
35–49	4	6.9	47	1	2	3	15	15	15	15
50–64	1	2.0	0	2	2	2	2	2	2	2
65+	4	6.1	49	3	3	3	4	22	22	22
TOTAL SINGLE DX	1	2.0	0	2	2	2	2	2	2	2
MULTIPLE DX	38	5.6	41	1	2	4	6	13	22	35
TOTAL										
0–19 Years	21	4.8	35	1	2	5	5	6	14	35
20–34	9	6.6	46	2	2	4	8	13	23	26
35–49	4	6.9	47	1	2	3	15	15	15	15
50–64	1	2.0	0	2	2	2	2	2	2	2
65+	4	6.1	49	3	3	3	4	22	22	22
GRAND TOTAL	39	5.2	37	1	2	3	5	8	19	35

24.0: GUM OR ALVEOLAR INCISION. Formerly included in operation group(s) 548.

Type of Patients	Observed Patients	Avg. Stay	Vari-ance	Percentiles						
				10th	25th	50th	75th	90th	95th	99th
1. SINGLE DX										
0–19 Years	12	2.1	2	1	1	2	3	5	5	5
20–34	14	2.6	1	1	2	2	3	4	5	5
35–49	6	2.6	<1	2	2	2	3	4	4	4
50–64	0									
65+	0									
2. MULTIPLE DX										
0–19 Years	52	3.3	4	1	2	3	4	5	9	9
20–34	65	3.2	4	1	2	3	4	6	9	9
35–49	38	4.0	5	2	3	3	4	6	12	13
50–64	23	4.1	25	1	1	3	6	8	25	25
65+	23	6.2	67	3	3	3	6	10	27	36
TOTAL SINGLE DX	32	2.4	1	1	2	2	3	4	5	5
MULTIPLE DX	201	3.7	11	1	2	3	4	6	9	13
TOTAL										
0–19 Years	64	3.1	4	1	2	3	4	5	8	9
20–34	79	3.1	4	1	2	3	4	5	9	9
35–49	44	3.9	5	2	3	3	4	6	7	13
50–64	23	4.1	25	1	1	3	6	8	9	25
65+	23	6.2	67	3	3	3	6	10	27	36
GRAND TOTAL	233	3.5	10	1	2	3	4	6	9	13

Length of Stay by Diagnosis and Operation, United States, 1997

United States, October 1995–September 1996 Data, by Operation

24.1: TOOTH & GUM DXTIC PX. Formerly included in operation group(s) 548, 556.

Type of Patients	Observed Patients	Avg. Stay	Variance	10th	25th	50th	75th	90th	95th	99th
1. SINGLE DX										
0–19 Years	1	3.0	0	3	3	3	3	3	3	3
20–34	0									
35–49	0									
50–64	0									
65+	0									
2. MULTIPLE DX										
0–19 Years	5	6.9	15	1	7	7	7	11	11	17
20–34	1	10.0	0	10	10	10	10	10	10	10
35–49	5	8.6	60	1	6	6	8	25	25	25
50–64	3	22.5	141	4	8	30	30	30	30	30
65+	15	11.0	102	3	6	9	11	19	19	49
TOTAL SINGLE DX	1	3.0	0	3	3	3	3	3	3	3
MULTIPLE DX	29	13.2	125	4	6	8	19	30	30	49
TOTAL										
0–19 Years	6	6.6	15	1	3	7	7	11	11	17
20–34	1	10.0	0	10	10	10	10	10	10	10
35–49	5	8.6	60	1	6	6	8	25	25	25
50–64	3	22.5	141	4	8	30	30	30	30	30
65+	15	11.0	102	3	6	9	11	19	19	49
GRAND TOTAL	30	13.1	125	3	6	8	19	30	30	49

24.2: GINGIVOPLASTY. Formerly included in operation group(s) 548.

Type of Patients	Observed Patients	Avg. Stay	Variance	10th	25th	50th	75th	90th	95th	99th
1. SINGLE DX										
0–19 Years	2	1.0	0	1	1	1	1	1	1	1
20–34	0									
35–49	0									
50–64	0									
65+	0									
2. MULTIPLE DX										
0–19 Years	11	5.4	106	1	1	1	6	7	36	36
20–34	5	3.7	2	2	2	5	5	5	5	5
35–49	1	26.0	0	26	26	26	26	26	26	26
50–64	1	1.0	0	1	1	1	1	1	1	1
65+	0									
TOTAL SINGLE DX	2	1.0	0	1	1	1	1	1	1	1
MULTIPLE DX	18	5.1	74	1	1	2	5	7	36	36
TOTAL										
0–19 Years	13	5.0	97	1	1	1	6	7	36	36
20–34	5	3.7	2	2	2	5	5	5	5	5
35–49	1	26.0	0	26	26	26	26	26	26	26
50–64	1	1.0	0	1	1	1	1	1	1	1
65+	0									
GRAND TOTAL	20	4.9	71	1	1	2	5	7	26	36

24.3: OTHER OPERATIONS ON GUMS. Formerly included in operation group(s) 548.

Type of Patients	Observed Patients	Avg. Stay	Variance	10th	25th	50th	75th	90th	95th	99th
1. SINGLE DX										
0–19 Years	0									
20–34	0									
35–49	2	3.2	2		1	4	4	4	4	4
50–64	0									
65+	0									
2. MULTIPLE DX										
0–19 Years	27	2.0	2	1	1	1	2	4	4	5
20–34	17	2.2	5	1	1	2	2	3	10	10
35–49	17	3.1	9	1	1	2	4	6	6	17
50–64	8	3.9	8	1	2	3	8	8	8	8
65+	17	6.6	31	1	3	5	8	18	18	22
TOTAL SINGLE DX	2	3.2	2	1	1	4	4	4	4	4
MULTIPLE DX	86	2.8	9	1	1	2	4	6	8	18
TOTAL										
0–19 Years	27	2.0	2	1	1	1	2	4	4	5
20–34	17	2.2	5	1	1	2	2	3	10	10
35–49	19	3.1	8	1	1	3	4	6	6	17
50–64	8	3.9	8	1	2	3	8	8	8	8
65+	17	6.6	31	1	3	5	8	18	18	22
GRAND TOTAL	88	2.9	9	1	1	2	4	6	8	18

24.4: EXC OF DENTAL LES OF JAW. Formerly included in operation group(s) 548.

Type of Patients	Observed Patients	Avg. Stay	Variance	10th	25th	50th	75th	90th	95th	99th
1. SINGLE DX										
0–19 Years	12	1.6	<1	1	1	2	2	2	2	3
20–34	9	1.4	<1	1	1	1	1	2	2	3
35–49	8	1.9	2	1	1	1	4	4	4	4
50–64	2	2.0	2	1	1	3	3	3	3	3
65+	2	2.1	1	1	1	3	3	3	3	3
2. MULTIPLE DX										
0–19 Years	40	2.8	13	1	1	3	3	5	9	20
20–34	16	3.7	10	1	2	3	6	6	14	14
35–49	24	2.4	6	2	2	1	2	6	8	12
50–64	24	6.8	48	2	2	4	13	13	13	39
65+	29	5.8	58	1	2	4	6	9	11	54
TOTAL SINGLE DX	33	1.6	<1	1	1	1	2	3	4	4
MULTIPLE DX	133	4.3	29	1	1	3	6	9	13	31
TOTAL										
0–19 Years	52	2.4	9	1	1	2	2	4	6	20
20–34	25	3.2	9	1	1	2	4	6	6	14
35–49	32	2.2	5	1	1	1	4	6	7	9
50–64	26	6.7	48	1	2	4	13	13	13	39
65+	31	5.7	56	1	2	4	6	9	11	54
GRAND TOTAL	166	3.8	25	1	1	2	4	9	13	31

Length of Stay by Diagnosis and Operation, United States, 1997

United States, October 1995–September 1996 Data, by Operation

24.5: ALVEOLOPLASTY. Formerly included in operation group(s) 548.

Type of Patients	Observed Patients	Avg. Stay	Variance	10th	25th	50th	75th	90th	95th	99th
1. SINGLE DX										
0–19 Years	48	1.4	2	1	1	1	1	2	3	9
20–34	2	1.0	0	1	1	1	1			1
35–49	8	4.1	26	1	1	1	11	13	13	13
50–64	2	2.5	<1	2	2	3	3	3	3	3
65+	2	1.0	0	1	1	1	1	1	1	1
2. MULTIPLE DX										
0–19 Years	162	1.6	<1	1	1	1	2	3	3	4
20–34	28	3.9	14	1	2	2	4	11	14	17
35–49	67	9.8	192	1	2	5	8	32	33	59
50–64	76	5.9	95	1	2	3	6	13	14	82
65+	100	7.0	56	1	2	5	9	17	22	36
TOTAL SINGLE DX	62	1.7	5	1	1	1	1	2	3	13
MULTIPLE DX	433	4.4	64	1	1	2	4	9	14	42
TOTAL										
0–19 Years	210	1.5	<1	1	1	1	2	2	3	4
20–34	30	3.7	14	1	1	2	4	8	14	17
35–49	75	9.2	179	1	2	4	8	32	32	59
50–64	78	5.9	94	1	2	3	6	13	14	82
65+	102	7.0	56	1	2	4	9	17	22	36
GRAND TOTAL	495	4.0	56	1	1	2	3	8	14	36

24.6: EXPOSURE OF TOOTH. Formerly included in operation group(s) 547.

Type of Patients	Observed Patients	Avg. Stay	Variance	10th	25th	50th	75th	90th	95th	99th
1. SINGLE DX										
0–19 Years	0									
20–34	0									
35–49	0									
50–64	0									
65+	0									
2. MULTIPLE DX										
0–19 Years	1	4.0	0	4	4	4	4	4	4	4
20–34	0									
35–49	0									
50–64	0									
65+	0									
TOTAL SINGLE DX	0									
MULTIPLE DX	1	4.0	0	4	4	4	4	4	4	4
TOTAL										
0–19 Years	1	4.0	0	4	4	4	4	4	4	4
20–34	0									
35–49	0									
50–64	0									
65+	0									
GRAND TOTAL	1	4.0	0	4	4	4	4	4	4	4

24.7: APPL ORTHODONT APPLIANCE. Formerly included in operation group(s) 547.

Type of Patients	Observed Patients	Avg. Stay	Variance	10th	25th	50th	75th	90th	95th	99th
1. SINGLE DX										
0–19 Years	8	1.4	<1	1	1	1	1	3	3	3
20–34	2	1.8	<1	1	2	2	2	2	2	2
35–49	1	1.0	0	1	1	1	1	1	1	1
50–64	1	1.0	0	1	1	1	1	1	1	1
65+	0									
2. MULTIPLE DX										
0–19 Years	10	8.6	40	2	4	4	13	14	22	22
20–34	4	3.2	5	1	1	3	5	7	7	7
35–49	7	1.9	<1	1	1	1	3	3	3	3
50–64	2	6.2	29	1	1	10	10	10	10	10
65+	3	3.3	21	1	1	1	4	15	15	15
TOTAL SINGLE DX	12	1.5	<1	1	1	1	2	3	3	3
MULTIPLE DX	26	4.5	24	1	1	2	4	13	14	22
TOTAL										
0–19 Years	18	4.5	30	1	1	2	4	13	14	22
20–34	6	2.6	3	1	1	2	3	5	7	7
35–49	8	1.8	<1	1	1	2	2	2	3	3
50–64	3	4.8	26	1	1	1	10	10	10	10
65+	3	3.3	21	1	1	1	4	15	15	15
GRAND TOTAL	38	3.4	18	1	1	2	3	11	13	22

24.8: OTHER ORTHODONTIC OP. Formerly included in operation group(s) 547.

Type of Patients	Observed Patients	Avg. Stay	Variance	10th	25th	50th	75th	90th	95th	99th
1. SINGLE DX										
0–19 Years	4	1.2	<1	1	1	1	1	2	2	2
20–34	0									
35–49	0									
50–64	0									
65+	0									
2. MULTIPLE DX										
0–19 Years	0									
20–34	5	31.1	234	7	13	41	41	41	41	41
35–49	2	37.5	13	35	35	38	40	40	40	40
50–64	2	5.1	<1	5	5	5	5	5	7	7
65+	0									
TOTAL SINGLE DX	4	1.2	<1	1	1	1	1	2	2	2
MULTIPLE DX	9	21.0	301	5	5	13	41	41	41	41
TOTAL										
0–19 Years	4	1.2	<1	1	1	1	1	2	2	2
20–34	5	31.1	234	7	13	41	41	41	41	41
35–49	2	37.5	13	35	35	38	40	40	40	40
50–64	2	5.1	<1	5	5	5	5	5	7	7
65+	0									
GRAND TOTAL	13	15.2	294	1	1	5	41	41	41	41

Length of Stay by Diagnosis and Operation, United States, 1997

United States, October 1995–September 1996 Data, by Operation

24.9: OTHER DENTAL OPERATION. Formerly included in operation group(s) 548.

Type of Patients	Observed Patients	Avg. Stay	Vari-ance	Percentiles						
				10th	25th	50th	75th	90th	95th	99th
1. SINGLE DX										
0–19 Years	2	1.0	0	1	1	1	1	1	1	1
20–34	1	4.0	0	4	4	4	4	4	4	4
35–49	1	2.0	0	2	2	2	2	2	2	2
50–64	3	2.4	<1	2	2	2	3	3	3	3
65+	1	2.0	0	2	2	2	2	2	2	2
2. MULTIPLE DX										
0–19 Years	4	2.0	<1	1	1	2	3	3	3	3
20–34	5	1.2	<1	1	1	1	1	2	2	2
35–49	5	1.6	<1	1	1	1	2	3	3	3
50–64	12	2.0	1	1	2	2	2	2	6	3
65+	11	4.5	16	1	2	3	8	8	14	14
TOTAL SINGLE DX	8	2.4	1	1	2	2	3	4	4	4
MULTIPLE DX	37	2.2	5	1	1	2	2	3	8	14
TOTAL										
0–19 Years	6	1.8	<1	1	1	1	3	3	3	3
20–34	6	1.5	1	1	1	1	2	4	4	4
35–49	6	1.6	<1	1	1	1	2	3	3	3
50–64	15	2.1	1	1	2	2	2	3	3	6
65+	12	4.3	15	1	2	3	8	8	14	14
GRAND TOTAL	45	2.2	4	1	1	2	2	4	6	14

25.0: DXTIC PX ON TONGUE. Formerly included in operation group(s) 551, 556.

Type of Patients	Observed Patients	Avg. Stay	Vari-ance	Percentiles						
				10th	25th	50th	75th	90th	95th	99th
1. SINGLE DX										
0–19 Years	1	1.0	0	1	1	1	1	1	1	1
20–34	2	3.4	<1	2	2	4	4	4	4	4
35–49	7	2.1	5	1	1	1	1	7	7	7
50–64	5	4.4	48	1	1	1	1	17	18	18
65+	1	2.0	0	2	2	2	2	2	2	2
2. MULTIPLE DX										
0–19 Years	2	7.9	9	6	6	6	12	12	12	12
20–34	10	5.5	19	1	2	5	8	10	13	16
35–49	31	5.9	18	1	4	6	7	11	15	17
50–64	38	7.3	42	3	4	4	8	19	21	41
65+	66	6.0	35	2	2	3	9	15	20	26
TOTAL SINGLE DX	16	2.6	12	1	1	1	2	7	7	18
MULTIPLE DX	147	6.5	34	2	3	4	8	15	20	25
TOTAL										
0–19 Years	3	6.0	17	1	1	6	6	12	12	12
20–34	12	4.9	15	2	2	4	7	10	13	16
35–49	38	5.0	17	1	1	4	7	10	14	17
50–64	43	7.2	43	2	3	4	8	19	21	41
65+	67	6.0	35	2	2	3	9	15	20	26
GRAND TOTAL	163	6.2	34	2	2	4	8	13	20	25

25.1: EXC/DESTR TONGUE LES. Formerly included in operation group(s) 551.

Type of Patients	Observed Patients	Avg. Stay	Vari-ance	Percentiles						
				10th	25th	50th	75th	90th	95th	99th
1. SINGLE DX										
0–19 Years	18	1.0	<1	1	1	1	1	1	1	1
20–34	4	2.7	4	1	1	2	3	6	6	6
35–49	12	1.8	7	1	1	1	1	3	4	17
50–64	13	2.2	2	1	1	2	2	3	5	8
65+	13	2.4	7	1	1	1	3	7	7	11
2. MULTIPLE DX										
0–19 Years	18	8.6	173	1	2	2	6	39	39	39
20–34	1	1.0	0	1	1	1	1	1	1	1
35–49	23	6.2	46	1	1	3	11	11	27	27
50–64	32	2.8	11	1	1	1	3	9	10	17
65+	81	7.4	77	1	1	4	10	20	34	34
TOTAL SINGLE DX	60	1.8	4	1	1	1	2	3	7	11
MULTIPLE DX	155	5.9	66	1	1	2	7	14	27	39
TOTAL										
0–19 Years	36	3.8	75	1	1	1	2	6	29	39
20–34	5	1.9	3	1	1	1	2	6	6	6
35–49	35	4.4	34	1	1	2	4	11	11	27
50–64	45	2.7	9	1	1	1	3	8	9	17
65+	94	6.1	64	1	1	3	7	14	27	34
GRAND TOTAL	215	4.4	48	1	1	1	4	11	20	38

25.2: PARTIAL GLOSSECTOMY. Formerly included in operation group(s) 551.

Type of Patients	Observed Patients	Avg. Stay	Vari-ance	Percentiles						
				10th	25th	50th	75th	90th	95th	99th
1. SINGLE DX										
0–19 Years	4	2.5	4	1	1	1	5	5	5	5
20–34	9	2.4	<1	2	2	2	2	4	4	5
35–49	20	2.2	3	1	1	3	2	5	5	10
50–64	24	3.0	5	1	2	3	4	4	7	14
65+	8	2.7	2	1	1	3	3	5	5	5
2. MULTIPLE DX										
0–19 Years	39	4.8	11	1	2	4	7	10	10	11
20–34	7	6.2	7	2	4	8	8	8	11	11
35–49	49	6.8	69	1	2	3	8	17	31	31
50–64	104	7.3	35	1	3	6	14	14	14	19
65+	190	7.0	46	1	2	5	9	17	21	36
TOTAL SINGLE DX	65	2.5	3	1	2	2	3	4	5	8
MULTIPLE DX	389	6.8	43	1	2	5	9	14	19	31
TOTAL										
0–19 Years	43	4.6	10	1	2	4	7	9	10	11
20–34	16	3.1	4	2	2	2	4	7	8	8
35–49	69	5.6	56	1	1	2	5	16	31	31
50–64	128	6.4	32	1	2	4	10	14	14	17
65+	198	6.9	45	1	2	5	9	16	21	30
GRAND TOTAL	454	6.0	38	1	2	4	8	14	17	31

Length of Stay by Diagnosis and Operation, United States, 1997

United States, October 1995–September 1996 Data, by Operation

25.5: REPAIR OF TONGUE. Formerly included in operation group(s) 551.

Type of Patients	Observed Patients	Avg. Stay	Variance	10th	25th	50th	75th	90th	95th	99th
1. SINGLE DX										
0–19 Years	28	1.4	<1	1	1	1	1	3	3	3
20–34	0									
35–49	0									
50–64	1	1.0	0	1	1	1	1	1	1	1
65+	1	6.0	0	6	6	6	6	6	6	6
2. MULTIPLE DX										
0–19 Years	57	7.1	133	1	1	2	9	26	28	56
20–34	51	3.0	4	1	2	3	4	5	8	9
35–49	34	4.3	11	1	2	3	5	9	9	21
50–64	20	4.3	22	2	3	3	6	6	6	7
65+	19	5.2	14	1	2	7	8	9	9	19
TOTAL SINGLE DX	30	1.4	<1	1	1	1	1	3	3	3
MULTIPLE DX	181	4.7	45	1	2	3	5	8	13	32
TOTAL										
0–19 Years	85	4.9	89	1	1	1	3	13	28	56
20–34	51	3.0	4	1	1	3	4	5	8	9
35–49	34	4.3	11	1	2	3	5	9	9	21
50–64	21	4.3	22	2	3	3	6	6	6	7
65+	20	5.3	14	1	2	7	8	9	9	19
GRAND TOTAL	211	4.2	40	1	1	3	4	8	10	30

25.9: OTHER TONGUE OPERATIONS. Formerly included in operation group(s) 551, 556.

Type of Patients	Observed Patients	Avg. Stay	Variance	10th	25th	50th	75th	90th	95th	99th
1. SINGLE DX										
0–19 Years	8	1.8	<1	1	2	2	2	2	2	2
20–34	0									
35–49	1	2.0	0	2	2	2	2	2	2	2
50–64	1	4.0	0	4	4	4	4	4	4	4
65+	2	2.0	0	2	2	2	2	2	2	2
2. MULTIPLE DX										
0–19 Years	265	2.2	3	1	1	2	2	4	4	9
20–34	3	3.5	6	2	3	3	3	3	11	11
35–49	5	4.5	1	2	5	5	5	5	5	5
50–64	8	5.0	26	1	1	3	6	16	16	16
65+	7	6.3	18	2	2	9	10	11	11	11
TOTAL SINGLE DX	12	1.9	<1	1	1	2	2	2	2	4
MULTIPLE DX	288	2.3	4	1	1	2	3	4	5	13
TOTAL										
0–19 Years	273	2.2	3	1	1	2	2	4	4	9
20–34	3	3.5	6	2	3	3	3	3	11	11
35–49	6	4.2	2	2	3	5	5	5	5	5
50–64	9	4.9	22	1	2	3	6	16	16	16
65+	9	5.3	17	1	2	3	10	11	11	11
GRAND TOTAL	300	2.3	3	1	1	2	3	4	5	11

25.3: COMPLETE GLOSSECTOMY. Formerly included in operation group(s) 551.

Type of Patients	Observed Patients	Avg. Stay	Variance	10th	25th	50th	75th	90th	95th	99th
1. SINGLE DX										
0–19 Years	0									
20–34	0									
35–49	0									
50–64	0									
65+	0									
2. MULTIPLE DX										
0–19 Years	0									
20–34	1	10.0	0	10	10	10	10	10	10	10
35–49	6	14.1	30	3	10	18	18	18	18	18
50–64	5	13.6	10	11	11	13	13	15	23	23
65+	8	16.7	77	1	12	15	24	24	31	31
TOTAL SINGLE DX	0									
MULTIPLE DX	20	14.8	42	8	11	14	18	24	24	31
TOTAL										
0–19 Years	0									
20–34	1	10.0	0	10	10	10	10	10	10	10
35–49	6	14.1	30	3	10	18	18	18	18	18
50–64	5	13.6	10	11	11	13	13	15	23	23
65+	8	16.7	77	1	12	15	24	24	31	31
GRAND TOTAL	20	14.8	42	8	11	14	18	24	24	31

25.4: RADICAL GLOSSECTOMY. Formerly included in operation group(s) 551.

Type of Patients	Observed Patients	Avg. Stay	Variance	10th	25th	50th	75th	90th	95th	99th
1. SINGLE DX										
0–19 Years	0									
20–34	0									
35–49	0									
50–64	0									
65+	0									
2. MULTIPLE DX										
0–19 Years	1	13.0	0	13	13	13	13	13	13	13
20–34	0									
35–49	3	11.0	71	5	5	9	23	23	23	23
50–64	5	35.2	>999	1	1	26	91	91	91	91
65+	5	13.1	41	8	8	9	21	23	23	23
TOTAL SINGLE DX	0									
MULTIPLE DX	14	20.3	654	1	8	9	23	91	91	91
TOTAL										
0–19 Years	1	13.0	0	13	13	13	13	13	13	13
20–34	0									
35–49	3	11.0	71	5	5	9	23	23	23	23
50–64	5	35.2	>999	1	1	26	91	91	91	91
65+	5	13.1	41	8	8	9	21	23	23	23
GRAND TOTAL	14	20.3	654	1	8	9	23	91	91	91

Length of Stay by Diagnosis and Operation, United States, 1997

United States, October 1995–September 1996 Data, by Operation

26.0: INC SALIVARY GLAND/DUCT. Formerly included in operation group(s) 549.

Type of Patients	Observed Patients	Avg. Stay	Variance	10th	25th	50th	75th	90th	95th	99th
1. SINGLE DX										
0–19 Years	14	4.1	2	2	2	5	5	5	5	6
20–34	3	3.1	5	1	1	3	3	7	7	7
35–49	5	2.7	2	2	2	3	2	6	6	6
50–64	1	6.0	0	6	6	6	6	6	6	6
65+	1	6.0	0	6	6	6	6	6	6	6
2. MULTIPLE DX										
0–19 Years	13	3.5	2	2	3	3	4	5	6	7
20–34	18	6.7	18	2	3	4	11	13	13	13
35–49	27	5.1	12	2	2	5	8	8	14	16
50–64	23	4.6	8	1	4	4	6	6	8	16
65+	59	8.2	73	1	2	5	12	24	29	31
TOTAL SINGLE DX	**24**	**3.8**	**2**	**2**	**2**	**5**	**5**	**5**	**6**	**6**
MULTIPLE DX	**140**	**5.8**	**29**	**2**	**3**	**4**	**6**	**12**	**16**	**31**
TOTAL										
0–19 Years	27	3.9	2	2	3	5	5	5	5	6
20–34	21	6.4	18	2	3	4	11	11	13	13
35–49	32	4.3	10	2	2	2	6	8	8	16
50–64	24	4.6	8	1	4	4	6	6	8	16
65+	60	8.2	72	1	2	5	12	24	29	31
GRAND TOTAL	**164**	**5.2**	**23**	**2**	**2**	**4**	**6**	**11**	**14**	**29**

26.1: SALIVARY GLAND DXTIC PX. Formerly included in operation group(s) 549, 556.

Type of Patients	Observed Patients	Avg. Stay	Variance	10th	25th	50th	75th	90th	95th	99th
1. SINGLE DX										
0–19 Years	3	2.3	3	1	2	2	2	5	5	5
20–34	3	6.7	8	8	8	8	8	8	8	8
35–49	2	3.7	5	2	1	5	5	5	5	5
50–64	4	2.8	2	1	1	3	4	4	4	4
65+	1	1.0	0	1	1	1	1	1	1	1
2. MULTIPLE DX										
0–19 Years	6	3.3	5	1	1	4	5	6	6	6
20–34	9	3.8	6	2	3	3	3	8	10	10
35–49	13	5.4	6	1	4	6	7	8	8	8
50–64	25	9.4	100	3	3	5	11	27	35	35
65+	73	10.4	59	2	4	8	15	22	23	28
TOTAL SINGLE DX	**13**	**4.0**	**7**	**1**	**1**	**4**	**5**	**8**	**8**	**8**
MULTIPLE DX	**126**	**9.1**	**62**	**2**	**3**	**6**	**12**	**22**	**24**	**35**
TOTAL										
0–19 Years	9	3.0	4	1	1	2	5	6	6	6
20–34	12	4.8	8	2	3	3	8	8	10	10
35–49	15	5.2	6	1	4	5	7	8	8	8
50–64	29	7.9	85	1	3	4	9	15	35	35
65+	74	10.3	60	2	4	8	14	22	23	28
GRAND TOTAL	**139**	**8.5**	**59**	**1**	**3**	**6**	**11**	**22**	**23**	**35**

26.2: EXC OF SG LESION. Formerly included in operation group(s) 549.

Type of Patients	Observed Patients	Avg. Stay	Variance	10th	25th	50th	75th	90th	95th	99th
1. SINGLE DX										
0–19 Years	31	1.3	<1	1	1	1	1	2	3	6
20–34	25	1.1	<1	1	1	1	1	1	1	3
35–49	30	1.1	<1	1	1	1	1	1	2	3
50–64	23	1.1	<1	1	1	1	1	1	1	3
65+	22	1.1	<1	1	1	1	1	2	2	3
2. MULTIPLE DX										
0–19 Years	10	1.5	3	1	1	1	1	2	5	10
20–34	14	1.6	2	1	1	1	2	2	3	10
35–49	20	1.5	<1	1	1	1	2	2	3	4
50–64	35	2.3	3	1	1	2	2	5	6	8
65+	72	2.0	4	1	1	1	2	4	7	8
TOTAL SINGLE DX	**131**	**1.2**	**<1**	**1**	**1**	**1**	**1**	**2**	**2**	**3**
MULTIPLE DX	**151**	**1.9**	**3**	**1**	**1**	**1**	**2**	**4**	**5**	**8**
TOTAL										
0–19 Years	41	1.4	1	1	1	1	1	2	3	7
20–34	39	1.2	<1	1	1	1	1	2	2	3
35–49	50	1.3	<1	1	1	1	1	2	3	4
50–64	58	1.6	2	1	1	1	2	3	4	7
65+	94	1.7	3	1	1	1	2	3	4	8
GRAND TOTAL	**282**	**1.5**	**2**	**1**	**1**	**1**	**1**	**2**	**3**	**7**

26.29: SALIVARY LES EXC NEC. Formerly included in operation group(s) 549.

Type of Patients	Observed Patients	Avg. Stay	Variance	10th	25th	50th	75th	90th	95th	99th
1. SINGLE DX										
0–19 Years	28	1.3	<1	1	1	1	1	3	3	6
20–34	25	1.1	<1	1	1	1	1	1	1	3
35–49	30	1.1	<1	1	1	1	1	2	2	3
50–64	23	1.1	<1	1	1	1	1	1	1	3
65+	22	1.1	<1	1	1	1	1	2	2	3
2. MULTIPLE DX										
0–19 Years	10	1.5	3	1	1	1	1	2	5	10
20–34	12	1.6	2	1	1	1	2	2	3	10
35–49	20	1.5	<1	1	1	1	2	2	3	4
50–64	35	2.3	3	1	1	2	2	5	6	8
65+	69	2.0	4	1	1	1	2	4	7	8
TOTAL SINGLE DX	**128**	**1.2**	**<1**	**1**	**1**	**1**	**1**	**2**	**2**	**3**
MULTIPLE DX	**146**	**1.9**	**3**	**1**	**1**	**1**	**2**	**4**	**5**	**8**
TOTAL										
0–19 Years	38	1.4	1	1	1	1	1	2	3	7
20–34	37	1.2	<1	1	1	1	1	2	2	3
35–49	50	1.3	<1	1	1	1	1	2	3	4
50–64	58	1.6	2	1	1	1	2	3	4	7
65+	91	1.6	3	1	1	1	2	3	4	8
GRAND TOTAL	**274**	**1.5**	**1**	**1**	**1**	**1**	**1**	**2**	**3**	**7**

United States, October 1995–September 1996 Data, by Operation

26.3: SIALOADENECTOMY. Formerly included in operation group(s) 549.

Type of Patients	Observed Patients	Avg. Stay	Vari-ance	10th	25th	50th	75th	90th	95th	99th
1. SINGLE DX										
0–19 Years	64	1.9	1	1	1	2	2	3	4	5
20–34	184	1.5	<1	1	1	1	2	2	3	4
35–49	359	1.5	<1	1	1	1	2	2	3	5
50–64	311	1.5	<1	1	1	1	2	2	3	4
65+	241	1.6	<1	1	1	1	2	2	3	4
2. MULTIPLE DX										
0–19 Years	89	2.9	11	1	1	2	3	7	11	17
20–34	140	2.1	2	1	1	1	3	3	5	7
35–49	335	1.7	2	1	1	1	2	3	4	8
50–64	542	2.1	7	1	1	2	2	3	5	11
65+	914	2.6	13	1	1	2	3	4	7	13
TOTAL SINGLE DX	1159	1.5	<1	1	1	1	2	2	3	4
MULTIPLE DX	2020	2.3	9	1	1	2	2	4	6	12
TOTAL										
0–19 Years	153	2.5	8	1	1	2	2	6	8	16
20–34	324	1.8	1	1	1	1	2	3	4	6
35–49	694	1.6	2	1	1	1	2	3	3	6
50–64	853	1.9	5	1	1	2	2	3	4	11
65+	1155	2.4	11	1	1	2	3	4	6	12
GRAND TOTAL	3179	2.0	6	1	1	1	2	3	5	11

26.30: SIALOADENECTOMY NOS. Formerly included in operation group(s) 549.

Type of Patients	Observed Patients	Avg. Stay	Vari-ance	10th	25th	50th	75th	90th	95th	99th
1. SINGLE DX										
0–19 Years	18	1.9	1	1	1	2	2	2	4	4
20–34	31	1.3	<1	1	1	1	2	2	2	2
35–49	52	1.4	<1	1	1	1	2	2	3	5
50–64	40	1.5	<1	1	1	1	2	2	3	3
65+	30	1.3	<1	1	1	1	2	2	2	3
2. MULTIPLE DX										
0–19 Years	20	2.2	5	1	1	1	2	6	8	8
20–34	24	1.9	2	1	1	1	2	3	4	7
35–49	37	1.6	1	1	1	1	2	3	5	6
50–64	64	2.7	13	1	1	2	2	11	11	20
65+	120	3.2	33	1	1	2	3	5	9	48
TOTAL SINGLE DX	171	1.4	<1	1	1	1	2	2	3	4
MULTIPLE DX	265	2.5	16	1	1	1	2	5	8	20
TOTAL										
0–19 Years	38	2.1	4	1	1	1	2	4	4	8
20–34	55	1.5	<1	1	1	1	2	2	3	5
35–49	89	1.5	<1	1	1	1	2	2	4	6
50–64	104	2.1	8	1	1	2	2	3	11	11
65+	150	2.9	28	1	1	2	3	4	8	30
GRAND TOTAL	436	2.1	10	1	1	1	2	3	5	11

26.31: PARTIAL SIALOADENECTOMY. Formerly included in operation group(s) 549.

Type of Patients	Observed Patients	Avg. Stay	Vari-ance	10th	25th	50th	75th	90th	95th	99th
1. SINGLE DX										
0–19 Years	30	1.6	<1	1	1	1	2	2	3	5
20–34	86	1.4	<1	1	1	1	2	2	3	6
35–49	189	1.4	<1	1	1	1	2	2	3	6
50–64	164	1.5	<1	1	1	1	2	2	3	4
65+	119	1.6	<1	1	1	1	2	3	3	4
2. MULTIPLE DX										
0–19 Years	19	4.1	14	1	1	2	6	11	11	11
20–34	46	2.0	1	1	1	2	2	2	4	6
35–49	170	1.7	3	1	1	1	2	2	3	9
50–64	262	1.9	7	1	1	1	2	3	3	8
65+	393	2.2	13	1	1	2	2	3	5	11
TOTAL SINGLE DX	588	1.5	<1	1	1	1	2	2	3	4
MULTIPLE DX	890	2.0	9	1	1	1	2	3	4	11
TOTAL										
0–19 Years	49	2.4	7	1	1	2	2	6	11	11
20–34	132	1.6	<1	1	1	1	2	2	3	4
35–49	359	1.5	2	1	1	1	2	3	3	7
50–64	426	1.7	5	1	1	1	2	3	3	7
65+	512	2.1	11	1	1	2	2	3	4	11
GRAND TOTAL	1478	1.8	5	1	1	1	2	3	3	8

26.32: COMPLETE SIALOADENECTOMY. Formerly included in operation group(s) 549.

Type of Patients	Observed Patients	Avg. Stay	Vari-ance	10th	25th	50th	75th	90th	95th	99th
1. SINGLE DX										
0–19 Years	16	2.4	2	1	2	2	3	4	4	8
20–34	67	1.7	<1	1	1	2	2	2	3	4
35–49	118	1.6	<1	1	1	1	2	2	3	5
50–64	107	1.5	<1	1	1	1	2	2	3	5
65+	92	1.7	<1	1	1	1	2	3	3	4
2. MULTIPLE DX										
0–19 Years	50	3.0	13	1	1	2	3	7	10	17
20–34	70	2.2	2	1	1	2	3	4	5	7
35–49	128	1.9	3	1	1	1	2	3	5	7
50–64	216	2.2	5	1	1	2	2	3	6	11
65+	401	2.7	9	1	1	2	3	5	8	12
TOTAL SINGLE DX	400	1.6	<1	1	1	1	2	3	3	5
MULTIPLE DX	865	2.5	7	1	1	2	3	4	7	12
TOTAL										
0–19 Years	66	2.9	11	1	1	2	3	7	10	17
20–34	137	2.0	1	1	1	2	2	3	5	7
35–49	246	1.8	2	1	1	1	2	3	4	6
50–64	323	2.0	4	1	1	2	2	3	4	8
65+	493	2.6	8	1	1	2	3	4	7	12
GRAND TOTAL	1265	2.2	5	1	1	2	2	4	6	11

Length of Stay by Diagnosis and Operation, United States, 1997

United States, October 1995–September 1996 Data, by Operation

26.4: SG & DUCT REPAIR. Formerly included in operation group(s) 549.

Type of Patients	Observed Patients	Avg. Stay	Vari-ance	10th	25th	50th	75th	90th	95th	99th
1. SINGLE DX										
0–19 Years	3	2.3	<1	2	2	2	3	3	3	3
20–34	0									
35–49	1	3.0	0	3	3	3	3	3	3	3
50–64	0									
65+	2	11.9	68	1	1	17	17	17	17	17
2. MULTIPLE DX										
0–19 Years	15	1.7	2	1	1	2	2	2	2	12
20–34	5	2.0	2	1	1	1	4	4	4	12
35–49	2	14.3	261	2	2	2	31	31	31	31
50–64	3	24.8	853	1	1	3	52	52	52	52
65+	4	3.5	<1	3	3	3	4	4	6	6
TOTAL SINGLE DX	6	7.5	57	1	2	3	17	17	17	17
MULTIPLE DX	29	3.2	52	1	1	2	2	4	4	52
TOTAL										
0–19 Years	18	1.7	2	1	1	2	2	2	2	12
20–34	5	2.0	2	1	1	1	4	4	4	4
35–49	3	11.6	214	2	2	3	31	31	31	31
50–64	3	24.8	853	1	1	3	52	52	52	52
65+	6	6.0	33	3	3	3	4	17	17	17
GRAND TOTAL	35	3.6	53	1	1	2	2	4	17	52

27.0: DRAIN FACE & MOUTH FLOOR. Formerly included in operation group(s) 551.

Type of Patients	Observed Patients	Avg. Stay	Vari-ance	10th	25th	50th	75th	90th	95th	99th
1. SINGLE DX										
0–19 Years	91	3.7	5	1	2	3	5	6	7	16
20–34	111	3.5	3	2	2	3	5	6	6	8
35–49	68	3.8	4	2	3	3	5	6	7	11
50–64	24	3.1	4	1	1	3	5	6	7	8
65+	6	5.3	3	3	3	7	7	7	7	7
2. MULTIPLE DX										
0–19 Years	304	4.3	12	2	3	4	5	7	9	16
20–34	496	4.2	5	2	3	4	5	6	8	12
35–49	420	5.1	34	2	3	4	6	8	13	26
50–64	165	5.0	40	2	2	3	5	12	13	21
65+	143	6.3	57	2	3	5	7	12	17	35
TOTAL SINGLE DX	300	3.6	4	1	2	3	5	6	7	11
MULTIPLE DX	1528	4.7	22	2	3	4	5	8	11	19
TOTAL										
0–19 Years	395	4.2	11	2	3	3	5	7	9	16
20–34	607	4.0	5	2	3	4	5	6	8	11
35–49	488	4.9	31	2	3	4	6	8	12	26
50–64	189	4.8	36	2	2	3	5	10	13	21
65+	149	6.3	55	2	3	5	7	12	17	27
GRAND TOTAL	1828	4.5	19	2	3	4	5	7	10	18

26.9: OTH SALIVARY OPERATIONS. Formerly included in operation group(s) 549.

Type of Patients	Observed Patients	Avg. Stay	Vari-ance	10th	25th	50th	75th	90th	95th	99th
1. SINGLE DX										
0–19 Years	2	3.0	0	3	3	3	3	3	3	3
20–34	0									
35–49	2	8.9	<1	9	9	9	9	9	9	9
50–64	1	3.0	0	3	3	3	3	3	3	3
65+	1	8.0	0	8	8	8	8	8	8	8
2. MULTIPLE DX										
0–19 Years	7	5.2	14	1	2	2	9	9	9	9
20–34	3	2.8	2	2	2	2	4	5	5	5
35–49	3	2.2	<1	2	2	2	2	3	3	4
50–64	4	3.0	1	2	3	3	3	5	5	5
65+	16	9.7	135	3	3	6	9	12	46	46
TOTAL SINGLE DX	6	8.3	4	3	9	9	9	9	9	9
MULTIPLE DX	33	6.1	72	2	2	3	9	9	12	46
TOTAL										
0–19 Years	9	4.9	12	1	2	3	9	9	9	9
20–34	3	2.8	2	2	2	2	4	5	5	5
35–49	5	6.5	11	2	2	3	3	5	5	5
50–64	5	3.0	<1	2	3	3	3	5	5	5
65+	17	9.7	132	3	3	6	9	12	46	46
GRAND TOTAL	39	6.8	51	2	3	6	9	9	9	46

27.1: INCISION OF PALATE. Formerly included in operation group(s) 551.

Type of Patients	Observed Patients	Avg. Stay	Vari-ance	10th	25th	50th	75th	90th	95th	99th
1. SINGLE DX										
0–19 Years	0									
20–34	2	1.3	<1	1	1	1	2	2	2	2
35–49	1	4.0	0	4	4	4	4	4	4	4
50–64	1	3.0	0	3	3	3	3	3	3	3
65+	0									
2. MULTIPLE DX										
0–19 Years	4	9.0	66	1	4	4	20	20	20	20
20–34	3	2.4	<1	2	2	3	3	3	3	3
35–49	7	3.4	4	1	1	4	5	5	7	7
50–64	4	3.3	3	2	2	3	3	7	7	7
65+	2	3.4	<1	3	3	3	4	4	4	4
TOTAL SINGLE DX	4	2.5	<1	1	2	3	3	3	4	4
MULTIPLE DX	20	4.8	27	1	2	3	5	7	20	20
TOTAL										
0–19 Years	4	9.0	66	1	4	4	20	20	20	20
20–34	5	1.7	<1	1	1	2	2	3	3	3
35–49	8	3.4	4	1	3	4	5	5	7	7
50–64	5	3.1	<1	3	3	3	3	4	4	4
65+	2	3.4	<1	3	3	3	4	4	4	4
GRAND TOTAL	24	3.8	17	1	2	3	4	5	20	20

Length of Stay by Diagnosis and Operation, United States, 1997

United States, October 1995–September 1996 Data, by Operation

27.2: ORAL CAVITY DXTIC PX. Formerly included in operation group(s) 551, 556.

Type of Patients	Observed Patients	Avg. Stay	Vari-ance	Percentiles						
				10th	25th	50th	75th	90th	95th	99th
1. SINGLE DX										
0–19 Years	1	1.0	0	1	1	1	1			1
20–34	3	2.7	2	1	1	3	4	4	4	4
35–49	1	1.0	0	1	1	1	1	1	1	1
50–64	2	3.6	1	1	4	4	4	4	4	4
65+	2	5.1	4	6	6	6	6	6	6	6
2. MULTIPLE DX										
0–19 Years	18	3.8	28	2	2	2	3	8	11	38
20–34	20	6.7	19	3	4	5	9	16	16	17
35–49	52	10.9	114	3	4	8	14	26	32	49
50–64	42	6.9	86	3	4	5	6	13	15	34
65+	81	9.6	89	1	4	7	10	17	28	51
TOTAL SINGLE DX	9	3.7	4	1	1	4	6	6	6	6
MULTIPLE DX	213	8.7	90	2	3	6	10	14	29	51
TOTAL										
0–19 Years	19	3.8	27	2	2	2	3	8	11	38
20–34	23	6.1	18	3	4	4	8	11	16	17
35–49	53	10.9	114	2	4	8	14	26	32	49
50–64	44	6.7	81	3	4	5	6	13	15	34
65+	83	9.5	87	1	4	7	10	17	28	51
GRAND TOTAL	222	8.5	87	2	3	6	10	14	29	51

27.3: EXC BONY PALATE LES/TISS. Formerly included in operation group(s) 551.

Type of Patients	Observed Patients	Avg. Stay	Vari-ance	Percentiles						
				10th	25th	50th	75th	90th	95th	99th
1. SINGLE DX										
0–19 Years	4	3.1	10	1	1	2	2	9	9	9
20–34	1	2.0	0	2	2	2	2	2	2	2
35–49	9	1.3	<1	1	1	1	1	1	5	6
50–64	5	2.2	<1	1	1	2	3	3	3	3
65+	8	1.7	3	1	1	1	1	4	8	8
2. MULTIPLE DX										
0–19 Years	5	1.9	<1	1	1	2	3	3	3	3
20–34	9	3.4	6	1	2	3	5	8	8	8
35–49	16	2.9	6	1	2	2	2	7	9	11
50–64	21	3.2	8	1	2	2	3	7	9	15
65+	47	4.0	7	1	3	4	4	7	9	17
TOTAL SINGLE DX	27	1.8	3	1	1	1	2	3	8	9
MULTIPLE DX	98	3.5	7	1	2	3	4	7	9	15
TOTAL										
0–19 Years	9	2.5	6	1	1	2	3	9	9	9
20–34	10	3.3	5	2	2	2	5	8	8	8
35–49	25	2.2	5	1	1	1	2	5	7	11
50–64	26	3.0	7	1	2	2	3	5	9	15
65+	55	3.6	7	1	3	4	4	7	8	13
GRAND TOTAL	125	3.1	6	1	1	2	4	6	8	13

27.4: OTHER EXCISION OF MOUTH. Formerly included in operation group(s) 551.

Type of Patients	Observed Patients	Avg. Stay	Vari-ance	Percentiles						
				10th	25th	50th	75th	90th	95th	99th
1. SINGLE DX										
0–19 Years	36	1.8	<1	1	1	2	2	2	2	3
20–34	15	1.5	<1	1	1	1	2	2	4	4
35–49	19	1.9	<1	1	1	1	2	3	3	6
50–64	28	2.8	5	1	1	2	5	6	6	10
65+	39	3.0	7	1	1	2	4	9	9	9
2. MULTIPLE DX										
0–19 Years	71	3.3	13	1	1	3	4	5	9	28
20–34	41	4.8	18	1	2	3	7	9	9	26
35–49	75	5.2	59	1	1	3	7	12	14	44
50–64	169	6.6	40	1	2	5	9	13	18	33
65+	332	5.3	29	1	2	3	7	12	15	22
TOTAL SINGLE DX	137	2.0	2	1	1	2	2	3	5	9
MULTIPLE DX	688	5.2	32	1	2	3	7	12	15	28
TOTAL										
0–19 Years	107	2.4	6	1	1	2	2	4	5	12
20–34	56	3.9	16	1	1	2	6	8	9	26
35–49	94	4.6	50	1	1	2	5	11	14	44
50–64	197	5.9	36	1	2	4	9	13	16	33
65+	371	5.1	27	1	1	3	7	11	15	22
GRAND TOTAL	825	4.3	26	1	1	2	6	10	14	24

27.49: EXCISION OF MOUTH NEC. Formerly included in operation group(s) 551.

Type of Patients	Observed Patients	Avg. Stay	Vari-ance	Percentiles						
				10th	25th	50th	75th	90th	95th	99th
1. SINGLE DX										
0–19 Years	18	2.0	<1	2	2	2	2	2	2	3
20–34	12	1.4	<1	1	1	1	1	3	4	4
35–49	13	2.1	<1	1	2	2	2	3	3	6
50–64	20	3.2	6	1	1	2	3	6	8	10
65+	28	2.6	5	2	2	2	3	6	8	9
2. MULTIPLE DX										
0–19 Years	22	4.2	14	1	2	4	5	5	13	28
20–34	8	6.0	8	1	6	6	8	9	9	9
35–49	49	6.8	84	1	2	4	8	14	15	68
50–64	139	6.7	43	1	2	5	10	14	18	33
65+	236	5.5	34	1	1	3	7	13	17	27
TOTAL SINGLE DX	91	2.1	2	1	2	2	2	3	5	8
MULTIPLE DX	454	5.9	40	1	2	4	8	13	16	33
TOTAL										
0–19 Years	40	2.4	4	2	2	2	2	4	5	13
20–34	20	4.0	10	1	1	2	8	8	9	9
35–49	62	5.8	70	1	2	3	8	14	14	44
50–64	159	6.2	39	1	2	5	8	13	18	33
65+	264	5.2	32	1	1	3	7	12	16	27
GRAND TOTAL	545	4.7	31	1	2	2	6	11	14	28

Length of Stay by Diagnosis and Operation, United States, 1997

82

United States, October 1995–September 1996 Data, by Operation

27.5: PLASTIC REPAIR OF MOUTH. Formerly included in operation group(s) 551.

Type of Patients	Observed Patients	Avg. Stay	Vari-ance	10th	25th	50th	75th	90th	95th	99th
1. SINGLE DX										
0–19 Years	623	1.4	<1	1	1	1	2	2	3	4
20–34	27	2.6	5	1	1	2	3	7	7	7
35–49	10	2.1	1	1	1	2	3	4	4	4
50–64	4	1.6	2	1	1	1	1	5	5	5
65+	7	3.4	3	2	2	2	6	6	6	6
2. MULTIPLE DX										
0–19 Years	996	2.1	14	1	1	1	2	3	5	15
20–34	412	2.3	6	1	1	2	3	4	5	12
35–49	334	3.0	15	1	1	2	3	6	8	16
50–64	189	3.6	19	1	1	2	5	7	12	39
65+	307	5.2	19	1	2	4	6	9	10	26
TOTAL SINGLE DX	671	1.5	<1	1	1	1	2	2	3	6
MULTIPLE DX	2238	2.7	15	1	1	2	3	6	8	16
TOTAL										
0–19 Years	1619	1.9	9	1	1	1	2	3	4	12
20–34	439	2.3	6	1	1	2	3	4	6	12
35–49	344	2.9	15	1	1	2	3	6	8	16
50–64	193	3.6	18	1	1	2	5	7	11	39
65+	314	5.1	19	1	2	4	6	9	10	26
GRAND TOTAL	2909	2.4	12	1	1	1	2	5	7	15

27.54: REPAIR OF CLEFT LIP. Formerly included in operation group(s) 551.

Type of Patients	Observed Patients	Avg. Stay	Vari-ance	10th	25th	50th	75th	90th	95th	99th
1. SINGLE DX										
0–19 Years	546	1.5	<1	1	1	1	2	2	3	4
20–34	5	1.5	<1	1	1	1	2	2	3	2
35–49	0									
50–64	0									
65+	0									
2. MULTIPLE DX										
0–19 Years	589	1.8	5	1	1	2	2	3	3	14
20–34	6	2.2	2	1	1	2	3	3	6	6
35–49	1	3.0	0	3	3	3	3	3	3	3
50–64	1	1.0	0	1	1	1	1	1	1	1
65+	0									
TOTAL SINGLE DX	551	1.5	<1	1	1	1	2	2	3	4
MULTIPLE DX	597	1.8	5	1	1	2	2	3	3	14
TOTAL										
0–19 Years	1135	1.6	3	1	1	1	2	2	3	11
20–34	11	2.0	2	1	1	2	3	3	6	6
35–49	1	3.0	0	3	3	3	3	3	3	3
50–64	1	1.0	0	1	1	1	1	1	1	1
65+	0									
GRAND TOTAL	1148	1.6	3	1	1	1	2	2	3	11

27.51: SUTURE OF LIP LACERATION. Formerly included in operation group(s) 551.

Type of Patients	Observed Patients	Avg. Stay	Vari-ance	10th	25th	50th	75th	90th	95th	99th
1. SINGLE DX										
0–19 Years	18	1.2	<1	1	1	1	1	1	3	3
20–34	11	1.2	<1	1	1	1	1	2	3	3
35–49	3	1.3	<1	1	1	2	2	2	2	2
50–64	1	1.0	0	1	1	1	1	1	1	1
65+	2	3.3	5	2	2	2	6	6	6	6
2. MULTIPLE DX										
0–19 Years	243	2.1	4	1	1	2	2	4	5	10
20–34	325	2.3	7	1	1	2	3	4	5	12
35–49	263	3.0	18	1	1	2	3	6	8	16
50–64	137	3.4	22	1	1	2	4	7	12	32
65+	234	4.7	17	1	2	4	6	9	10	21
TOTAL SINGLE DX	35	1.2	<1	1	1	1	1	2	3	3
MULTIPLE DX	1202	2.8	12	1	1	2	3	6	8	16
TOTAL										
0–19 Years	261	2.0	3	1	1	2	2	4	5	8
20–34	336	2.2	6	1	1	2	3	4	5	12
35–49	266	3.0	18	1	1	2	3	6	9	16
50–64	138	3.4	22	1	1	2	4	7	12	32
65+	236	4.7	17	2	2	4	6	9	10	21
GRAND TOTAL	1237	2.8	12	1	1	2	3	6	8	16

27.59: MOUTH REPAIR NEC. Formerly included in operation group(s) 551.

Type of Patients	Observed Patients	Avg. Stay	Vari-ance	10th	25th	50th	75th	90th	95th	99th
1. SINGLE DX										
0–19 Years	32	1.1	<1	1	1	1	1	1	2	5
20–34	3	2.3	<1	2	2	2	3	3	3	3
35–49	2	2.8	2	2	2	2	4	4	4	4
50–64	1	1.0	0	1	1	1	1	1	1	1
65+	0									
2. MULTIPLE DX										
0–19 Years	74	4.8	127	1	1	2	3	8	15	52
20–34	43	2.8	5	1	1	2	3	6	8	9
35–49	33	2.6	6	1	1	2	4	4	5	11
50–64	20	3.5	5	1	1	4	5	7	9	9
65+	22	6.3	11	2	6	6	6	10	10	26
TOTAL SINGLE DX	38	1.2	<1	1	1	1	1	1	2	5
MULTIPLE DX	192	4.3	54	1	1	2	6	8	10	46
TOTAL										
0–19 Years	106	3.4	83	1	1	1	2	7	13	52
20–34	46	2.8	5	1	1	2	3	6	8	9
35–49	35	2.6	6	1	1	2	3	4	5	11
50–64	21	3.3	5	1	1	3	5	7	9	9
65+	22	6.3	11	2	6	6	6	10	10	26
GRAND TOTAL	230	3.7	46	1	1	2	5	7	10	46

© 1997 by HCIA Inc.

Length of Stay by Diagnosis and Operation, United States, 1997

83

United States, October 1995–September 1996 Data, by Operation

27.6: PALATOPLASTY. Formerly included in operation group(s) 550.

Type of Patients	Observed Patients	Avg. Stay	Vari-ance	Percentiles						
				10th	25th	50th	75th	90th	95th	99th
1. SINGLE DX										
0–19 Years	813	1.6	<1	1	1	1	2	3	3	4
20–34	17	1.8	1	1	1	1	3	3	3	6
35–49	16	1.6	<1	1	1	1	2	3	3	3
50–64	10	2.2	4	1	1	2	2	7	7	7
65+	1	2.0	0	2	2	2	2	2	2	2
2. MULTIPLE DX										
0–19 Years	1619	1.9	2	1	1	2	2	3	4	6
20–34	50	3.1	11	1	2	2	3	5	8	13
35–49	53	2.1	8	1	1	2	2	4	4	7
50–64	30	3.1	7	1	1	3	4	7	9	11
65+	21	3.2	9	2	2	2	4	8	12	13
TOTAL SINGLE DX	857	1.6	<1	1	1	1	2	3	3	4
MULTIPLE DX	1773	2.0	2	1	1	2	2	3	4	7
TOTAL										
0–19 Years	2432	1.8	2	1	1	2	2	3	4	5
20–34	67	2.8	9	1	1	2	3	5	7	13
35–49	69	2.0	7	1	1	2	2	4	4	7
50–64	40	2.9	6	1	1	2	4	7	7	11
65+	22	3.1	9	2	1	2	4	8	12	13
GRAND TOTAL	2630	1.9	2	1	1	2	2	3	4	6

27.62: CLEFT PALATE CORRECTION. Formerly included in operation group(s) 550.

Type of Patients	Observed Patients	Avg. Stay	Vari-ance	Percentiles						
				10th	25th	50th	75th	90th	95th	99th
1. SINGLE DX										
0–19 Years	544	1.7	<1	1	1	2	2	3	3	4
20–34	10	2.3	1	1	2	2	3	3	3	4
35–49	4	1.2	<1	1	1	1	1	2	2	2
50–64	1	1.0	0	1	1	1	1	1	1	1
65+	0									
2. MULTIPLE DX										
0–19 Years	1075	2.1	2	1	1	2	2	4	4	6
20–34	12	2.4	3	1	1	2	3	5	7	7
35–49	6	2.0	3	1	1	1	2	6	6	6
50–64	4	2.1	3	1	1	2	2	5	5	5
65+	1	2.0	0	2	2	2	2	2	2	2
TOTAL SINGLE DX	559	1.7	<1	1	1	2	2	3	3	4
MULTIPLE DX	1098	2.1	2	1	1	2	2	4	4	6
TOTAL										
0–19 Years	1619	2.0	2	1	1	2	2	3	4	5
20–34	22	2.3	2	1	2	2	3	4	5	7
35–49	10	1.6	2	1	1	1	2	6	6	6
50–64	5	1.8	2	1	1	2	2	5	5	5
65+	1	2.0	0	2	2	2	2	2	2	2
GRAND TOTAL	1657	2.0	2	1	1	2	2	3	4	5

27.63: REV CLEFT PALATE REPAIR. Formerly included in operation group(s) 550.

Type of Patients	Observed Patients	Avg. Stay	Vari-ance	Percentiles						
				10th	25th	50th	75th	90th	95th	99th
1. SINGLE DX										
0–19 Years	152	1.4	<1	1	1	1	2	2	3	3
20–34	5	1.9	4	1	1	1	2	6	6	6
35–49	4	2.4	<1	2	2	2	3	3	3	3
50–64	3	1.3	<1	1	1	1	2	2	2	2
65+	0									
2. MULTIPLE DX										
0–19 Years	413	1.7	<1	1	1	1	2	3	3	5
20–34	11	4.0	13	1	1	3	3	8	13	13
35–49	10	1.9	<1	2	2	2	2	2	3	3
50–64	2	2.6	4	1	1	4	4	4	4	4
65+	2	1.6	<1	1	1	2	2	2	2	2
TOTAL SINGLE DX	164	1.5	<1	1	1	1	2	3	3	3
MULTIPLE DX	438	1.7	1	1	1	1	2	3	3	5
TOTAL										
0–19 Years	565	1.6	<1	1	1	1	2	3	3	4
20–34	16	3.7	12	1	1	3	3	8	13	13
35–49	14	2.0	<1	2	2	2	2	4	4	4
50–64	5	1.7	1	1	1	2	2	2	2	2
65+	2	1.6	<1	1	1	2	2	2	2	2
GRAND TOTAL	602	1.6	<1	1	1	1	2	3	3	5

27.69: OTHER PLASTIC REP PALATE. Formerly included in operation group(s) 550.

Type of Patients	Observed Patients	Avg. Stay	Vari-ance	Percentiles						
				10th	25th	50th	75th	90th	95th	99th
1. SINGLE DX										
0–19 Years	77	1.6	<1	1	1	1	2	2	3	3
20–34	0									
35–49	8	1.2	<1	1	1	2	1	2	2	2
50–64	6	2.7	5	2	2	2	2	7	7	7
65+	1	2.0	0	2	2	2	2	2	2	2
2. MULTIPLE DX										
0–19 Years	116	1.9	5	1	1	1	2	3	4	10
20–34	20	2.9	19	2	2	2	2	3	7	36
35–49	33	2.0	12	1	1	1	2	4	4	30
50–64	23	2.9	7	1	1	2	3	5	9	11
65+	12	2.9	8	2	1	2	3	5	12	12
TOTAL SINGLE DX	92	1.6	<1	1	1	1	2	2	3	4
MULTIPLE DX	204	2.1	7	1	1	1	2	3	5	11
TOTAL										
0–19 Years	193	1.8	4	1	1	1	2	3	3	10
20–34	20	2.9	19	2	2	2	2	4	7	36
35–49	41	1.9	10	1	1	1	2	4	9	30
50–64	29	2.8	6	2	1	2	3	7	9	11
65+	13	2.8	7	2	2	2	3	5	12	12
GRAND TOTAL	296	1.9	6	1	1	1	2	3	4	10

Length of Stay by Diagnosis and Operation, United States, 1997

United States, October 1995–September 1996 Data, by Operation

27.7: OPERATIONS ON UVULA. Formerly included in operation group(s) 551.

Type of Patients	Observed Patients	Avg. Stay	Vari- ance	Percentiles						
				10th	25th	50th	75th	90th	95th	99th
1. SINGLE DX										
0–19 Years	1	1.0	0	1	1	1	1	1	1	1
20–34	3	3.5	1	2	4	4	4	4	4	4
35–49	5	1.5	<1	1	1	2	2	2	2	2
50–64	5	2.0	<1	1	1	2	3	3	3	3
65+	0									
2. MULTIPLE DX										
0–19 Years	14	6.0	17	1	2	8	8	8	9	19
20–34	17	2.0	2	1	1	2	2	3	4	10
35–49	34	1.4	<1	1	1	1	2	2	2	4
50–64	38	2.4	10	1	1	1	2	4	4	18
65+	14	5.6	51	1	1	3	4	19	19	19
TOTAL SINGLE DX	14	2.4	2	1	1	2	4	4	4	4
MULTIPLE DX	117	2.7	11	1	1	2	2	7	8	19
TOTAL										
0–19 Years	15	5.8	17	1	1	7	8	8	9	19
20–34	20	2.3	2	1	1	2	2	4	4	10
35–49	39	1.4	<1	1	1	1	2	2	2	3
50–64	43	2.4	9	1	1	2	3	4	4	18
65+	14	5.6	51	1	1	3	4	19	19	19
GRAND TOTAL	131	2.7	10	1	1	2	2	6	8	19

28.0: TONSIL/PERITONSILLAR I&D. Formerly included in operation group(s) 555.

Type of Patients	Observed Patients	Avg. Stay	Vari- ance	Percentiles						
				10th	25th	50th	75th	90th	95th	99th
1. SINGLE DX										
0–19 Years	345	2.3	1	1	1	2	3	4	4	6
20–34	304	2.2	1	1	1	2	3	3	4	5
35–49	119	2.1	1	1	1	2	2	4	4	8
50–64	29	1.9	<1	1	1	2	2	3	4	4
65+	5	2.0	1	1	1	2	3	4	4	4
2. MULTIPLE DX										
0–19 Years	448	4.2	60	1	2	3	5	7	9	27
20–34	322	2.7	4	1	1	2	3	5	8	10
35–49	202	3.4	13	1	2	2	4	6	9	24
50–64	56	2.8	6	1	1	2	3	5	8	14
65+	59	8.0	92	2	2	4	8	32	32	32
TOTAL SINGLE DX	802	2.2	1	1	1	2	3	4	4	6
MULTIPLE DX	1087	3.6	30	1	2	2	4	6	8	24
TOTAL										
0–19 Years	793	3.3	33	1	2	2	4	6	7	15
20–34	626	2.5	3	1	1	2	3	4	6	9
35–49	321	2.8	8	1	1	2	3	5	7	24
50–64	85	2.4	4	1	1	2	3	4	6	14
65+	64	7.7	89	2	2	3	4	32	32	32
GRAND TOTAL	1889	3.0	18	1	1	2	3	5	7	14

27.9: OTH OPS ON MOUTH & FACE. Formerly included in operation group(s) 551, 556.

Type of Patients	Observed Patients	Avg. Stay	Vari- ance	Percentiles						
				10th	25th	50th	75th	90th	95th	99th
1. SINGLE DX										
0–19 Years	12	1.3	<1	1	1	1	1	2	2	5
20–34	7	3.9	<1	3	3	4	4	5	6	6
35–49	3	2.3	<1	2	2	2	3	3	3	3
50–64	4	3.3	3	1	2	4	5	5	5	5
65+	0									
2. MULTIPLE DX										
0–19 Years	32	3.1	7	1	2	2	3	6	9	15
20–34	30	4.0	4	1	2	5	5	6	6	13
35–49	27	4.6	15	3	2	3	6	10	15	15
50–64	17	5.8	24	3	3	6	9	13	19	21
65+	20	9.7	51	2	4	6	19	19	19	22
TOTAL SINGLE DX	26	2.6	2	1	1	2	4	5	5	6
MULTIPLE DX	126	4.7	19	1	2	3	5	10	15	19
TOTAL										
0–19 Years	44	2.7	6	1	1	2	3	5	6	15
20–34	37	4.0	4	2	2	4	5	6	6	7
35–49	30	4.4	14	2	2	3	6	10	15	15
50–64	21	5.5	22	2	3	3	5	13	19	21
65+	20	9.7	51	2	4	6	19	19	19	22
GRAND TOTAL	152	4.4	17	1	2	3	5	9	15	19

28.1: TONSIL ADENOID DXTIC PX. Formerly included in operation group(s) 555, 556.

Type of Patients	Observed Patients	Avg. Stay	Vari- ance	Percentiles						
				10th	25th	50th	75th	90th	95th	99th
1. SINGLE DX										
0–19 Years	6	2.0	<1	1	2	2	2	3	3	3
20–34	7	2.1	<1	1	1	2	2	3	3	3
35–49	5	2.7	7	1	1	1	1	7	7	7
50–64	5	1.2	<1	1	1	1	2	2	2	2
65+	1	2.0	0	2	2	2	2	2	2	2
2. MULTIPLE DX										
0–19 Years	9	6.5	18	3	3	6	10	10	11	19
20–34	12	3.2	3	2	2	3	3	7	7	7
35–49	19	3.2	25	1	1	2	4	4	8	33
50–64	32	5.6	26	1	3	4	8	9	16	31
65+	36	5.9	24	1	3	5	7	11	17	25
TOTAL SINGLE DX	24	2.1	2	1	1	2	3	3	3	7
MULTIPLE DX	108	5.1	22	1	2	4	7	9	12	31
TOTAL										
0–19 Years	15	4.3	15	1	2	3	6	10	10	19
20–34	19	2.7	2	1	1	3	3	4	7	7
35–49	24	3.1	21	1	1	2	4	7	7	33
50–64	37	5.4	26	1	3	4	8	9	16	31
65+	37	5.9	24	1	3	5	7	11	17	25
GRAND TOTAL	132	4.5	20	1	2	3	7	9	11	25

Length of Stay by Diagnosis and Operation, United States, 1997

United States, October 1995–September 1996 Data, by Operation

28.2: TONSILLECTOMY. Formerly included in operation group(s) 552.

Type of Patients	Observed Patients	Avg. Stay	Vari-ance	10th	25th	50th	75th	90th	95th	99th
1. SINGLE DX										
0–19 Years	445	1.2	<1	1	1	1	1	2	2	4
20–34	221	1.4	<1	1	1	1	1	2	3	4
35–49	51	1.8	<1	1	1	2	2	2	3	5
50–64	12	3.9	5	1	2	6	6	6	6	6
65+	1	3.0	0	3	3	3	3	3	3	3
2. MULTIPLE DX										
0–19 Years	547	1.9	8	1	1	1	2	4	5	10
20–34	318	1.9	3	1	1	1	2	3	5	12
35–49	232	2.0	5	1	1	1	2	4	5	14
50–64	98	3.4	19	1	1	2	3	7	13	26
65+	45	6.5	33	3	3	3	14	14	14	23
TOTAL SINGLE DX	730	1.4	<1	1	1	1	2	2	3	6
MULTIPLE DX	1240	2.1	8	1	1	1	2	4	6	14
TOTAL										
0–19 Years	992	1.6	5	1	1	1	2	3	4	8
20–34	539	1.7	3	1	1	1	2	3	4	9
35–49	283	1.9	3	1	1	2	2	3	5	10
50–64	110	3.5	16	1	1	2	3	6	11	26
65+	46	6.4	33	3	3	3	14	14	14	23
GRAND TOTAL	1970	1.8	5	1	1	1	2	3	4	12

28.3: T&A. Formerly included in operation group(s) 553.

Type of Patients	Observed Patients	Avg. Stay	Vari-ance	10th	25th	50th	75th	90th	95th	99th
1. SINGLE DX										
0–19 Years	967	1.2	<1	1	1	1	1	2	2	4
20–34	16	1.2	<1	1	1	1	1	2	2	2
35–49	6	1.6	<1	1	1	2	2	2	2	2
50–64	1	3.0	0	3	3	3	3	3	3	3
65+	0									
2. MULTIPLE DX										
0–19 Years	3869	1.9	7	1	1	1	2	3	5	12
20–34	70	2.3	4	1	1	1	3	4	5	10
35–49	15	2.0	<1	1	2	2	3	3	3	3
50–64	3	3.9	5	3	3	6	6	6	6	6
65+	0									
TOTAL SINGLE DX	990	1.2	<1	1	1	1	1	2	2	4
MULTIPLE DX	3957	1.9	7	1	1	1	2	3	5	12
TOTAL										
0–19 Years	4836	1.7	6	1	1	1	2	3	5	11
20–34	86	2.1	3	1	1	1	3	4	5	10
35–49	21	1.9	<1	2	2	2	3	3	3	6
50–64	4	3.6	4	3	3	3	6	6	6	6
65+	0									
GRAND TOTAL	4947	1.8	6	1	1	1	2	3	5	11

28.4: EXCISION OF TONSIL TAG. Formerly included in operation group(s) 555.

Type of Patients	Observed Patients	Avg. Stay	Vari-ance	10th	25th	50th	75th	90th	95th	99th
1. SINGLE DX										
0–19 Years	0									
20–34	0									
35–49	1	1.0	0	1	1	1	1	1	1	1
50–64	0									
65+	0									
2. MULTIPLE DX										
0–19 Years	2	9.8	52	2	2	16	16	16	16	16
20–34	0									
35–49	0									
50–64	2	2.3	4	1	1	1	4	4	4	4
65+	2	1.0	0	1	1	1	1	1	1	1
TOTAL SINGLE DX	1	1.0	0	1	1	1	1	1	1	1
MULTIPLE DX	6	7.4	51	1	2	2	16	16	16	16
TOTAL										
0–19 Years	2	9.8	52	2	2	16	16	16	16	16
20–34	0									
35–49	1	1.0	0	1	1	1	1	1	1	1
50–64	2	2.3	4	1	1	1	4	4	4	4
65+	2	1.0	0	1	1	1	1	1	1	1
GRAND TOTAL	7	2.9	23	1	1	1	16	16	16	16

28.5: EXCISION LINGUAL TONSIL. Formerly included in operation group(s) 555.

Type of Patients	Observed Patients	Avg. Stay	Vari-ance	10th	25th	50th	75th	90th	95th	99th
1. SINGLE DX										
0–19 Years	0									
20–34	0									
35–49	1	1.0	0	1	1	1	1	1	1	1
50–64	1	1.0	0	1	1	1	1	1	1	1
65+	0									
2. MULTIPLE DX										
0–19 Years	2	3.3	<1	3	3	3	4	4	4	4
20–34	4	1.5	<1	1	1	1	2	2	3	3
35–49	10	2.7	2	1	2	3	3	4	7	7
50–64	4	1.7	1	1	1	1	2	2	4	4
65+	0									
TOTAL SINGLE DX	2	1.0	0	1	1	1	1	1	1	1
MULTIPLE DX	20	2.4	2	1	1	2	3	4	4	7
TOTAL										
0–19 Years	2	3.3	<1	3	3	3	4	4	4	4
20–34	4	1.5	<1	1	1	1	2	2	3	3
35–49	11	2.5	2	1	1	2	3	4	7	7
50–64	5	1.6	1	1	1	1	2	2	4	4
65+	0									
GRAND TOTAL	22	2.3	2	1	1	2	3	4	4	7

Length of Stay by Diagnosis and Operation, United States, 1997

United States, October 1995–September 1996 Data, by Operation

28.6: ADENOIDECTOMY. Formerly included in operation group(s) 554.

Type of Patients	Observed Patients	Avg. Stay	Vari-ance	Percentiles						
				10th	25th	50th	75th	90th	95th	99th
1. SINGLE DX										
0–19 Years	45	1.3	<1	1	1	1	1	2	3	4
20–34	0									
35–49	0									
50–64	0									
65+	0									
2. MULTIPLE DX										
0–19 Years	338	3.0	27	1	1	1	2	8	11	30
20–34	5	2.5	5	1	1	1	2	6	6	6
35–49	7	2.7	8	1	1	2	3	3	11	11
50–64	1	2.0	0	2	2	2	2	2	2	2
65+	1	4.0	0	4	4	4	4	4	4	4
TOTAL SINGLE DX	45	1.3	<1	1	1	1	1	2	3	4
MULTIPLE DX	352	3.0	27	1	1	1	2	8	11	30
TOTAL										
0–19 Years	383	2.9	25	1	1	1	2	7	11	24
20–34	5	2.5	5	1	1	1	2	6	6	6
35–49	7	2.7	8	1	1	2	3	3	11	11
50–64	1	2.0	0	2	2	2	2	2	2	2
65+	1	4.0	0	4	4	4	4	4	4	4
GRAND TOTAL	397	2.8	25	1	1	1	2	7	11	24

28.9: OTHER TONSIL/ADENOID OPS. Formerly included in operation group(s) 555.

Type of Patients	Observed Patients	Avg. Stay	Vari-ance	Percentiles						
				10th	25th	50th	75th	90th	95th	99th
1. SINGLE DX										
0–19 Years	9	1.5	<1	1	1	1	2	3	3	3
20–34	1	2.0	0	2	2	2	2	3	3	3
35–49	4	1.2	<1	1	1	1	1	2	3	3
50–64	3	4.3	23	2	2	3	3	15	15	15
65+	0									
2. MULTIPLE DX										
0–19 Years	19	5.3	284	1	1	2	3	4	6	97
20–34	8	2.3	<1	2	2	2	2	4	5	5
35–49	10	2.0	7	1	1	1	1	3	8	11
50–64	11	6.7	16	2	4	6	10	13	14	16
65+	10	8.9	30	3	4	8	10	18	20	20
TOTAL SINGLE DX	17	1.6	3	1	1	1	2	3	3	15
MULTIPLE DX	58	5.0	144	1	1	2	4	10	13	97
TOTAL										
0–19 Years	28	4.4	221	1	1	1	3	4	6	97
20–34	9	2.3	<1	2	2	2	2	4	5	5
35–49	14	1.5	3	1	1	1	1	2	3	11
50–64	14	6.3	17	2	4	4	8	13	14	16
65+	10	8.9	30	3	4	8	10	18	20	20
GRAND TOTAL	75	4.1	106	1	1	2	3	8	13	97

28.7: HEMOR CONTROL POST T&A. Formerly included in operation group(s) 555.

Type of Patients	Observed Patients	Avg. Stay	Vari-ance	Percentiles						
				10th	25th	50th	75th	90th	95th	99th
1. SINGLE DX										
0–19 Years	374	1.2	<1	1	1	1	1	2	2	4
20–34	76	1.3	<1	1	1	1	2	2	3	3
35–49	28	1.3	<1	1	1	1	2	2	2	4
50–64	5	1.0	0	1	1	1	1	1	1	1
65+	0									
2. MULTIPLE DX										
0–19 Years	244	1.8	1	1	1	1	2	3	4	7
20–34	78	1.7	2	1	1	1	2	3	4	9
35–49	30	1.6	<1	1	1	1	2	2	3	4
50–64	11	6.5	69	1	1	1	20	20	20	20
65+	2	2.4	<1	2	2	2	2	4	4	4
TOTAL SINGLE DX	483	1.2	<1	1	1	1	1	2	2	4
MULTIPLE DX	365	2.2	8	1	1	1	2	3	5	20
TOTAL										
0–19 Years	618	1.4	<1	1	1	1	1	2	3	5
20–34	154	1.5	<1	1	1	1	2	2	3	5
35–49	58	1.4	<1	1	1	1	2	2	3	4
50–64	16	6.2	67	1	1	2	20	20	20	20
65+	2	2.4	<1	2	2	2	2	4	4	4
GRAND TOTAL	848	1.6	4	1	1	1	2	2	3	8

29.0: PHARYNGOTOMY. Formerly included in operation group(s) 555.

Type of Patients	Observed Patients	Avg. Stay	Vari-ance	Percentiles						
				10th	25th	50th	75th	90th	95th	99th
1. SINGLE DX										
0–19 Years	5	5.1	7	1	4	4	7	8	8	8
20–34	5	5.8	11	2	2	5	9	8	9	9
35–49	2	2.7	<1	2	2	3	3	3	3	3
50–64	0									
65+	0									
2. MULTIPLE DX										
0–19 Years	7	4.5	3	1	5	5	6	6	6	6
20–34	13	4.6	32	2	2	4	5	5	28	28
35–49	7	5.3	7	1	4	4	8	9	10	10
50–64	3	30.5	>999	4	4	6	91	91	91	91
65+	9	8.2	49	3	3	6	9	25	25	25
TOTAL SINGLE DX	12	5.1	9	2	2	4	9	9	9	9
MULTIPLE DX	39	5.7	86	2	2	4	5	8	15	28
TOTAL										
0–19 Years	12	4.8	5	1	4	5	7	8	8	8
20–34	18	5.1	23	2	3	4	6	9	9	28
35–49	9	4.1	6	2	3	3	5	9	9	9
50–64	3	30.5	>999	4	4	6	91	91	91	91
65+	9	8.2	49	3	3	6	9	25	25	25
GRAND TOTAL	51	5.5	55	2	2	4	6	9	9	28

Length of Stay by Diagnosis and Operation, United States, 1997

United States, October 1995–September 1996 Data, by Operation

29.1: PHARYNGEAL DXTIC PX. Formerly included in operation group(s) 555, 556.

Type of Patients	Observed Patients	Avg. Stay	Vari-ance	10th	25th	50th	75th	90th	95th	99th
1. SINGLE DX										
0–19 Years	42	4.4	17	1	1	3	10	10	10	21
20–34	10	2.7	<1	2	2	3	3	3	4	4
35–49	19	3.0	3	2	2	3	5	5	5	10
50–64	10	1.7	1	1	1	1	2	3	5	5
65+	6	1.8	1	1	1	1	3	4	4	4
2. MULTIPLE DX										
0–19 Years	191	5.7	38	1	2	4	8	10	17	34
20–34	59	4.3	22	1	2	4	4	13	14	28
35–49	84	5.7	21	1	3	5	7	11	14	24
50–64	124	5.7	44	1	2	4	7	11	13	42
65+	219	6.2	29	1	3	6	8	12	16	30
TOTAL SINGLE DX	87	3.3	8	1	1	3	4	10	10	10
MULTIPLE DX	677	5.8	34	1	2	4	8	11	15	30
TOTAL										
0–19 Years	233	5.5	35	1	2	4	8	10	15	33
20–34	69	3.9	18	1	2	2	3	10	14	17
35–49	103	4.8	17	1	2	4	5	10	12	24
50–64	134	5.5	43	1	2	4	7	11	13	42
65+	225	6.1	29	1	3	6	8	12	16	30
GRAND TOTAL	764	5.4	31	1	2	4	7	11	14	28

29.2: EXC BRANCHIAL CLEFT CYST. Formerly included in operation group(s) 555.

Type of Patients	Observed Patients	Avg. Stay	Vari-ance	10th	25th	50th	75th	90th	95th	99th
1. SINGLE DX										
0–19 Years	59	1.2	<1	1	1	1	1	2	3	4
20–34	30	1.2	<1	1	1	1	1	2	2	3
35–49	17	1.1	<1	1	1	1	1	1	2	3
50–64	5	1.0	<1	1	1	1	1	1	1	2
65+	4	1.5	<1	1	1	1	2	2	2	2
2. MULTIPLE DX										
0–19 Years	23	1.9	2	1	1	1	3	4	5	6
20–34	15	1.6	<1	1	1	1	3	3	3	3
35–49	16	1.8	3	1	1	1	2	3	7	10
50–64	11	1.8	2	1	1	2	2	2	2	8
65+	8	1.7	5	1	1	1	1	2	5	11
TOTAL SINGLE DX	115	1.2	<1	1	1	1	1	2	2	3
MULTIPLE DX	73	1.7	2	1	1	1	2	3	4	8
TOTAL										
0–19 Years	82	1.4	1	1	1	1	1	3	4	6
20–34	45	1.4	<1	1	1	1	1	3	3	3
35–49	33	1.3	<1	1	1	1	1	2	2	7
50–64	16	1.5	1	1	1	2	1	2	2	8
65+	12	1.6	4	1	1	1	1	2	5	11
GRAND TOTAL	188	1.4	1	1	1	1	1	2	3	6

29.3: EXC/DESTR PHARYNGEAL LES. Formerly included in operation group(s) 555.

Type of Patients	Observed Patients	Avg. Stay	Vari-ance	10th	25th	50th	75th	90th	95th	99th
1. SINGLE DX										
0–19 Years	18	3.7	18	1	1	2	4	15	15	15
20–34	7	5.8	6	3	4	6	9	9	9	9
35–49	11	2.1	1	1	2	3	4	6	6	6
50–64	17	2.8	2	1	1	3	4	4	6	7
65+	34	2.3	3	1	2	2	2	4	6	7
2. MULTIPLE DX										
0–19 Years	36	6.1	24	2	2	5	9	9	17	22
20–34	11	7.2	75	2	2	2	9	24	24	24
35–49	42	3.9	38	1	2	2	4	7	10	32
50–64	98	7.9	78	2	2	5	11	20	20	47
65+	320	6.0	62	1	2	3	7	14	22	41
TOTAL SINGLE DX	87	2.7	5	1	1	2	3	5	6	15
MULTIPLE DX	507	6.2	61	1	2	3	7	16	22	37
TOTAL										
0–19 Years	54	5.5	23	1	2	4	7	9	16	22
20–34	18	7.0	67	2	2	2	9	24	24	24
35–49	53	3.6	32	1	2	2	4	7	10	21
50–64	115	7.1	70	1	2	4	8	20	20	47
65+	354	5.4	54	1	2	3	6	13	21	31
GRAND TOTAL	594	5.6	54	1	2	3	7	15	20	31

29.11: PHARYNGOSCOPY. Formerly included in operation group(s) 556.

Type of Patients	Observed Patients	Avg. Stay	Vari-ance	10th	25th	50th	75th	90th	95th	99th
1. SINGLE DX										
0–19 Years	36	2.3	2	1	1	2	3	3	4	12
20–34	7	2.7	<1	2	2	3	3	4	4	4
35–49	16	3.4	2	2	2	3	5	5	5	5
50–64	5	1.7	<1	1	1	1	3	3	3	3
65+	4	2.0	2	1	1	1	3	4	4	4
2. MULTIPLE DX										
0–19 Years	173	4.8	37	1	2	3	6	10	15	34
20–34	48	3.1	9	1	2	2	3	6	9	17
35–49	55	5.4	19	1	3	4	6	12	14	24
50–64	72	4.9	18	1	3	4	6	12	12	15
65+	147	6.4	20	2	3	6	8	10	13	30
TOTAL SINGLE DX	68	2.7	2	1	2	3	3	5	5	5
MULTIPLE DX	495	5.2	25	1	2	4	7	10	13	25
TOTAL										
0–19 Years	209	4.4	33	1	1	3	5	9	12	34
20–34	55	3.0	7	1	2	2	3	5	9	15
35–49	71	4.5	12	2	2	4	5	11	12	24
50–64	77	4.8	18	1	2	4	5	12	13	15
65+	151	6.3	20	2	3	6	8	10	13	30
GRAND TOTAL	563	4.8	23	1	2	3	6	9	13	25

Length of Stay by Diagnosis and Operation, United States, 1997

United States, October 1995–September 1996 Data, by Operation

29.4: PLASTIC OP ON PHARYNX. Formerly included in operation group(s) 555.

Type of Patients	Observed Patients	Avg. Stay	Vari-ance	10th	25th	50th	75th	90th	95th	99th
1. SINGLE DX										
0–19 Years	105	1.8	1	1	1	2	2	3	3	7
20–34	26	1.5	<1	1	1	1	2	3	3	4
35–49	89	1.3	<1	1	1	1	1	2	3	3
50–64	53	1.3	<1	1	1	1	2	2	2	3
65+	9	2.2	3	1	1	2	2	7	7	7
2. MULTIPLE DX										
0–19 Years	200	3.0	36	1	1	2	3	3	7	46
20–34	257	1.7	5	1	1	1	2	3	3	5
35–49	691	1.5	<1	1	1	1	2	2	3	5
50–64	454	2.1	4	1	1	2	2	4	6	9
65+	116	2.2	9	1	1	1	2	3	6	15
TOTAL SINGLE DX	282	1.5	<1	1	1	1	2	3	3	6
MULTIPLE DX	1718	1.9	8	1	1	1	2	3	4	9
TOTAL										
0–19 Years	305	2.7	27	1	1	2	3	3	6	46
20–34	283	1.7	4	1	1	1	2	3	3	5
35–49	780	1.5	<1	1	1	1	2	2	3	5
50–64	507	2.0	3	1	1	2	2	3	6	9
65+	125	2.2	8	1	1	1	2	3	7	15
GRAND TOTAL	2000	1.9	7	1	1	1	2	3	4	9

29.5: OTHER PHARYNGEAL REPAIR. Formerly included in operation group(s) 555.

Type of Patients	Observed Patients	Avg. Stay	Vari-ance	10th	25th	50th	75th	90th	95th	99th
1. SINGLE DX										
0–19 Years	15	2.6	3	1	1	3	3	5	5	9
20–34	4	2.9	2	1	1	4	4	4	4	4
35–49	1	5.0	0	5	5	5	5	5	5	5
50–64	2	1.2	<1	1	1	1	1	2	2	2
65+	1	2.0	0	2	2	2	2	2	2	2
2. MULTIPLE DX										
0–19 Years	22	6.6	131	1	1	2	7	39	39	39
20–34	5	5.0	15	2	2	2	8	8	15	15
35–49	17	6.4	27	1	3	8	8	8	8	36
50–64	17	5.3	17	1	3	3	6	13	13	14
65+	23	8.4	58	2	2	7	10	13	21	41
TOTAL SINGLE DX	23	2.9	3	1	1	3	5	5	5	9
MULTIPLE DX	84	6.9	72	1	2	4	8	13	36	39
TOTAL										
0–19 Years	37	4.9	78	1	1	2	5	9	39	39
20–34	9	3.9	9	1	2	4	4	8	8	15
35–49	18	6.1	22	1	3	5	8	8	8	36
50–64	19	4.8	17	1	3	3	6	13	13	14
65+	24	8.3	58	2	2	7	10	13	21	41
GRAND TOTAL	107	5.7	56	1	2	3	7	10	14	39

29.9: OTHER PHARYNGEAL OPS. Formerly included in operation group(s) 555.

Type of Patients	Observed Patients	Avg. Stay	Vari-ance	10th	25th	50th	75th	90th	95th	99th
1. SINGLE DX										
0–19 Years	7	1.6	1	1	1	1	2	4	4	4
20–34	0									
35–49	1	2.0	0	2	2	2	2	2	2	2
50–64	0									
65+	1	2.0	0	2	2	2	2	2	2	2
2. MULTIPLE DX										
0–19 Years	15	6.4	60	1	2	2	8	20	20	20
20–34	0									
35–49	1	1.0	0	1	1	1	1	1	1	1
50–64	5	5.0	25	2	2	3	4	14	14	14
65+	3	3.5	12	1	1	3	8	8	8	8
TOTAL SINGLE DX	9	1.6	1	1	1	1	2	4	4	4
MULTIPLE DX	24	6.0	54	1	2	2	7	20	20	20
TOTAL										
0–19 Years	22	4.7	45	1	1	2	3	20	20	20
20–34	0									
35–49	2	1.6	<1	1	1	2	4	2	2	2
50–64	5	5.0	25	2	2	3	4	14	14	14
65+	4	3.1	9	1	1	3	3	8	8	8
GRAND TOTAL	33	4.6	41	1	1	2	3	20	20	20

30.0: EXC/DESTR LES LARYNX. Formerly included in operation group(s) 557.

Type of Patients	Observed Patients	Avg. Stay	Vari-ance	10th	25th	50th	75th	90th	95th	99th
1. SINGLE DX										
0–19 Years	201	1.8	2	1	1	1	2	4	5	6
20–34	16	1.1	<1	1	1	1	1	1	2	2
35–49	14	1.0	<1	1	1	1	1	1	1	2
50–64	15	1.4	<1	1	1	1	1	2	5	5
65+	10	1.3	<1	1	1	1	1	1	4	5
2. MULTIPLE DX										
0–19 Years	361	5.7	119	1	1	3	6	11	16	58
20–34	19	4.3	52	1	1	2	4	9	32	32
35–49	68	2.7	15	1	1	2	3	3	5	19
50–64	112	3.7	22	1	1	3	4	6	15	22
65+	154	4.8	30	1	1	3	6	10	19	26
TOTAL SINGLE DX	256	1.7	2	1	1	1	2	4	5	6
MULTIPLE DX	714	4.8	74	1	1	2	5	10	14	37
TOTAL										
0–19 Years	562	4.2	78	1	1	2	4	8	12	37
20–34	35	2.8	30	1	1	1	3	4	9	32
35–49	82	2.5	14	1	2	2	3	3	5	19
50–64	127	3.5	20	1	2	2	4	9	15	22
65+	164	4.5	29	1	1	2	6	10	15	26
GRAND TOTAL	970	3.9	56	1	1	2	4	8	13	32

United States, October 1995–September 1996 Data, by Operation

30.09: EXC/DESTR LARYNX LES NEC. Formerly included in operation group(s) 557.

Type of Patients	Observed Patients	Avg. Stay	Variance	Percentiles						
				10th	25th	50th	75th	90th	95th	99th
1. SINGLE DX										
0–19 Years	197	1.8	2	1	1	1	2	4	5	6
20–34	16	1.1	<1	1	1	1	1	1	1	2
35–49	14	1.0	<1	1	1	1	1	1	1	2
50–64	15	1.4	<1	1	1	1	1	2	5	5
65+	10	1.3	<1	1	1	1	1	1	4	5
2. MULTIPLE DX										
0–19 Years	356	5.8	121	1	1	3	6	11	17	58
20–34	18	4.4	54	1	1	2	4	3	32	32
35–49	68	2.7	15	1	1	2	3	3	5	5
50–64	111	3.2	14	1	1	2	4	9	14	15
65+	152	4.7	30	1	1	2	6	10	17	26
TOTAL SINGLE DX	252	1.7	2	1	1	1	2	4	5	6
MULTIPLE DX	705	4.7	73	1	1	2	5	10	14	37
TOTAL										
0–19 Years	553	4.2	79	1	1	2	4	8	12	37
20–34	34	2.8	31	1	1	1	2	4	9	32
35–49	82	2.5	14	1	1	2	3	3	5	19
50–64	126	3.1	13	1	1	2	3	7	14	15
65+	162	4.4	28	1	1	2	6	10	14	26
GRAND TOTAL	957	3.9	55	1	1	2	4	8	12	32

30.2: PARTIAL LARYNGECTOMY NEC. Formerly included in operation group(s) 558.

Type of Patients	Observed Patients	Avg. Stay	Variance	Percentiles						
				10th	25th	50th	75th	90th	95th	99th
1. SINGLE DX										
0–19 Years	10	4.9	80	1	1	1	3	16	38	38
20–34	2	3.0	6	1	5	5	5	5	5	5
35–49	6	7.3	26	2	5	7	7	8	22	22
50–64	10	6.6	17	1	2	7	9	12	12	15
65+	6	7.4	41	1	5	5	7	9	26	26
2. MULTIPLE DX										
0–19 Years	46	11.4	153	2	2	9	15	23	50	50
20–34	9	5.8	7	1	4	7	7	10	10	10
35–49	21	4.1	14	2	2	5	7	10	10	10
50–64	70	9.3	51	1	3	7	14	17	23	31
65+	61	9.0	116	1	3	7	10	17	35	57
TOTAL SINGLE DX	34	6.1	45	1	1	5	7	12	16	38
MULTIPLE DX	207	8.7	86	1	2	7	11	18	23	50
TOTAL										
0–19 Years	56	10.2	146	1	2	5	15	20	38	50
20–34	11	5.6	7	1	2	5	7	10	10	10
35–49	27	4.6	17	2	2	2	7	10	11	22
50–64	80	9.0	48	1	3	7	14	16	23	31
65+	67	8.9	112	1	3	7	10	17	26	57
GRAND TOTAL	241	8.4	82	1	2	7	10	17	23	50

30.1: HEMILARYNGECTOMY. Formerly included in operation group(s) 558.

Type of Patients	Observed Patients	Avg. Stay	Variance	Percentiles						
				10th	25th	50th	75th	90th	95th	99th
1. SINGLE DX										
0–19 Years	0									
20–34	1	5.0	0	5	5	5	5	5	5	5
35–49	1	11.0	0	11	11	11	11	11	11	11
50–64	1	4.0	0	4	4	4	4	4	4	4
65+	5	4.6	2	4	4	4	4	7	8	8
2. MULTIPLE DX										
0–19 Years	1	9.0	0	9	9	9	9	9	9	9
20–34	0									
35–49	2	3.8	6	2	2	2	6	6	6	6
50–64	14	8.6	3	7	8	8	9	11	11	18
65+	31	10.9	28	6	7	10	14	21	21	26
TOTAL SINGLE DX	8	5.0	3	4	4	4	5	7	11	11
MULTIPLE DX	48	9.4	14	7	8	9	9	14	14	26
TOTAL										
0–19 Years	1	9.0	0	9	9	9	9	9	9	9
20–34	1	5.0	0	5	5	5	5	5	5	5
35–49	3	6.3	18	2	2	6	11	11	11	11
50–64	15	8.5	3	7	8	8	11	14	14	18
65+	36	9.1	28	4	7	8	12	14	21	26
GRAND TOTAL	56	8.6	15	4	7	8	9	13	14	26

30.3: COMPLETE LARYNGECTOMY. Formerly included in operation group(s) 559.

Type of Patients	Observed Patients	Avg. Stay	Variance	Percentiles						
				10th	25th	50th	75th	90th	95th	99th
1. SINGLE DX										
0–19 Years	0									
20–34	1	8.0	0	8	8	8	8	8	8	8
35–49	8	6.9	2	5	5	7	7	9	10	10
50–64	25	8.4	10	3	6	9	11	11	14	14
65+	12	7.6	2	7	7	8	8	9	11	12
2. MULTIPLE DX										
0–19 Years	4	20.8	46	17	18	18	18	33	37	37
20–34	3	8.5	26	7	7	7	7	7	25	25
35–49	41	15.1	92	6	8	10	18	33	36	36
50–64	203	13.4	71	6	9	11	15	20	31	42
65+	269	13.3	45	7	9	12	15	22	26	38
TOTAL SINGLE DX	46	8.0	7	5	6	8	9	11	14	14
MULTIPLE DX	520	13.5	62	7	9	12	15	22	31	42
TOTAL										
0–19 Years	4	20.8	46	17	18	18	18	33	37	37
20–34	4	8.4	23	7	7	7	7	8	25	25
35–49	49	13.9	88	5	8	10	17	31	36	36
50–64	228	12.6	65	6	8	10	15	18	31	42
65+	281	12.9	44	7	9	11	15	22	26	38
GRAND TOTAL	566	12.9	59	6	8	11	15	21	30	42

Length of Stay by Diagnosis and Operation, United States, 1997

United States, October 1995–September 1996 Data, by Operation

30.4: RADICAL LARYNGECTOMY. Formerly included in operation group(s) 559.

Type of Patients	Observed Patients	Avg. Stay	Vari-ance	10th	25th	50th	75th	90th	95th	99th
1. SINGLE DX										
0–19 Years	0									
20–34	0									
35–49	4	11.8	107	6	11	11	11	11	11	68
50–64	29	10.0	11	6	7	11	11	14	17	19
65+	8	8.4	5	7	7	8	9	12	12	12
2. MULTIPLE DX										
0–19 Years	0									
20–34	2	12.7	9	7	14	14	14	14	14	14
35–49	96	11.8	61	7	8	9	12	21	27	54
50–64	356	14.2	62	7	9	12	17	24	28	43
65+	344	13.0	70	7	8	11	15	21	29	63
TOTAL SINGLE DX	41	10.2	32	6	8	11	11	12	17	19
MULTIPLE DX	798	13.5	65	7	8	11	16	23	29	50
TOTAL										
0–19 Years	0									
20–34	2	12.7	9	7	14	14	14	14	14	14
35–49	100	11.8	65	7	8	9	12	21	27	54
50–64	385	14.0	60	7	9	12	17	24	28	43
65+	352	12.9	69	7	8	11	15	20	29	63
GRAND TOTAL	839	13.3	64	7	8	11	16	22	28	50

31.1: TEMPORARY TRACHEOSTOMY. Formerly included in operation group(s) 560.

Type of Patients	Observed Patients	Avg. Stay	Vari-ance	10th	25th	50th	75th	90th	95th	99th
1. SINGLE DX										
0–19 Years	19	13.0	78	5	7	14	18	49	>99	>99
20–34	27	5.9	7	3	5	6	7	8	13	13
35–49	44	7.1	15	3	4	7	8	11	12	26
50–64	46	7.2	96	3	4	6	8	10	11	90
65+	36	15.2	216	4	6	7	18	37	40	73
2. MULTIPLE DX										
0–19 Years	731	30.1	522	8	14	27	57	>99	>99	>99
20–34	923	28.1	431	6	12	24	40	62	86	>99
35–49	1391	28.1	433	5	12	24	43	65	83	>99
50–64	2176	34.0	780	5	11	28	50	95	95	>99
65+	3830	33.6	412	10	18	32	47	68	88	>99
TOTAL SINGLE DX	172	9.1	95	3	5	7	9	17	32	>99
MULTIPLE DX	9051	31.9	526	7	14	28	47	76	95	>99
TOTAL										
0–19 Years	750	29.7	518	8	13	25	57	>99	>99	>99
20–34	950	27.5	432	6	11	23	39	61	86	>99
35–49	1435	27.6	434	5	11	24	42	65	83	>99
50–64	2222	33.4	781	5	10	27	49	95	95	>99
65+	3866	33.5	414	9	18	31	47	68	87	>99
GRAND TOTAL	9223	31.5	528	6	14	28	46	76	95	>99

31.0: INJECTION OF LARYNX. Formerly included in operation group(s) 561.

Type of Patients	Observed Patients	Avg. Stay	Vari-ance	10th	25th	50th	75th	90th	95th	99th
1. SINGLE DX										
0–19 Years	1	1.0	0	1	1	1	1	1	1	1
20–34	1	1.0	0	1	1	1	1	1	1	1
35–49	0									
50–64	0									
65+	0									
2. MULTIPLE DX										
0–19 Years	1	1.0	0	1	1	1	1	1	1	1
20–34	0									
35–49	6	4.9	47	2	2	2	3	24	24	24
50–64	6	5.8	52	1	1	2	9	18	18	18
65+	26	6.2	30	1	1	6	9	9	11	26
TOTAL SINGLE DX	2	1.0	0	1	1	1	1	1	1	1
MULTIPLE DX	39	5.7	40	1	1	2	9	18	18	26
TOTAL										
0–19 Years	2	1.0	0	1	1	1	1	1	1	1
20–34	1	1.0	0	1	1	1	1	1	1	1
35–49	6	4.9	47	2	2	2	3	24	24	24
50–64	6	5.8	52	1	1	1	9	18	18	18
65+	26	6.2	30	1	1	6	9	9	11	26
GRAND TOTAL	41	5.6	39	1	1	2	9	18	18	26

31.2: PERMANENT TRACHEOSTOMY. Formerly included in operation group(s) 560.

Type of Patients	Observed Patients	Avg. Stay	Vari-ance	10th	25th	50th	75th	90th	95th	99th
1. SINGLE DX										
0–19 Years	6	5.8	33	3	3	4	4	19	19	19
20–34	6	13.4	585	4	4	5	8	12	90	90
35–49	7	8.8	234	1	2	3	3	30	50	50
50–64	16	7.7	40	2	4	5	8	23	23	23
65+	13	16.0	251	4	5	8	25	40	46	58
2. MULTIPLE DX										
0–19 Years	260	30.4	514	8	14	27	63	>99	>99	>99
20–34	176	27.7	311	8	17	27	44	81	>99	>99
35–49	351	26.2	373	6	11	23	42	55	91	>99
50–64	645	24.7	444	4	8	20	35	58	81	>99
65+	1299	31.5	413	7	17	30	47	77	>99	>99
TOTAL SINGLE DX	48	10.0	186	3	3	5	8	25	40	58
MULTIPLE DX	2731	28.7	427	6	13	26	44	75	>99	>99
TOTAL										
0–19 Years	266	29.7	517	8	13	23	59	>99	>99	>99
20–34	182	27.4	321	8	16	27	44	81	>99	>99
35–49	358	26.0	375	6	11	23	42	55	91	>99
50–64	661	24.4	442	4	8	20	35	57	81	>99
65+	1312	31.4	413	7	17	30	46	76	>99	>99
GRAND TOTAL	2779	28.5	429	6	13	26	43	74	>99	>99

Length of Stay by Diagnosis and Operation, United States, 1997

31.29: OTHER PERM TRACHEOSTOMY. Formerly included in operation group(s) 560.

Type of Patients	Observed Patients	Avg. Stay	Variance	10th	25th	50th	75th	90th	95th	99th
1. SINGLE DX										
0–19 Years	6	5.8	33	3	3	4	4	19	19	19
20–34	5	16.8	778	5	5	8	12	90	90	90
35–49	7	8.8	234	1	2	3	3	30	50	50
50–64	16	7.7	40	2	4	5	8	23	23	23
65+	13	16.0	251	4	5	8	25	40	46	58
2. MULTIPLE DX										
0–19 Years	259	30.4	514	8	14	27	63	>99	>99	>99
20–34	176	27.7	311	8	17	27	44	81	>99	>99
35–49	347	26.3	374	6	11	23	42	55	85	>99
50–64	642	24.7	445	4	8	20	35	58	81	>99
65+	1286	31.6	413	7	18	30	47	78	>99	>99
TOTAL SINGLE DX	47	10.2	191	2	3	5	9	25	40	58
MULTIPLE DX	2710	28.8	428	6	13	26	44	75	>99	>99
TOTAL										
0–19 Years	265	29.7	518	8	13	23	59	>99	>99	>99
20–34	181	27.5	319	8	16	27	44	81	>99	>99
35–49	354	26.1	376	6	11	23	41	55	85	>99
50–64	658	24.4	443	4	8	20	35	57	81	>99
65+	1299	31.5	413	7	17	30	47	77	>99	>99
GRAND TOTAL	2757	28.5	429	6	13	26	43	74	>99	>99

31.4: LARYNX/TRACHEA DXTIC PX. Formerly included in operation group(s) 557, 558, 581.

Type of Patients	Observed Patients	Avg. Stay	Variance	10th	25th	50th	75th	90th	95th	99th
1. SINGLE DX										
0–19 Years	1077	2.0	3	1	1	2	2	3	5	11
20–34	71	1.7	<1	1	1	1	2	3	3	4
35–49	90	2.5	5	1	1	2	3	4	6	13
50–64	66	2.9	7	1	2	2	3	4	8	14
65+	40	2.3	2	1	2	2	3	4	5	8
2. MULTIPLE DX										
0–19 Years	3457	3.4	33	1	1	3	3	6	10	24
20–34	278	5.2	91	1	2	3	4	6	13	58
35–49	507	4.4	21	1	2	3	5	9	13	23
50–64	695	7.2	165	1	2	3	7	15	21	79
65+	1305	7.4	51	2	3	6	9	15	18	32
TOTAL SINGLE DX	1344	2.1	4	1	1	2	2	4	5	11
MULTIPLE DX	6242	4.9	63	1	2	3	5	11	15	51
TOTAL										
0–19 Years	4534	3.1	27	1	1	2	3	6	9	23
20–34	349	4.6	76	1	1	2	4	10	11	58
35–49	597	4.0	19	1	2	3	5	8	12	21
50–64	761	6.8	152	1	2	3	7	15	20	79
65+	1345	7.2	50	2	3	6	9	15	18	32
GRAND TOTAL	7586	4.5	55	1	1	2	5	10	14	38

31.3: INC LARYNX/TRACHEA NEC. Formerly included in operation group(s) 561.

Type of Patients	Observed Patients	Avg. Stay	Variance	10th	25th	50th	75th	90th	95th	99th
1. SINGLE DX										
0–19 Years	1	1.0	0	1	1	1	1	1	1	1
20–34	1	2.0	0	2	2	2	2	2	2	2
35–49	1	1.0	0	1	1	1	1	1	1	1
50–64	4	2.5	2	2	2	2	2	6	6	6
65+	1	4.0	0	4	4	4	4	4	4	4
2. MULTIPLE DX										
0–19 Years	19	8.5	89	1	1	3	15	25	27	27
20–34	7	4.1	7	2	1	4	4	5	13	13
35–49	6	4.0	9	1	1	3	7	9	9	9
50–64	9	8.9	54	1	1	10	14	24	24	24
65+	14	5.8	24	1	1	5	8	11	17	17
TOTAL SINGLE DX	8	2.4	2	1	2	2	2	4	6	6
MULTIPLE DX	55	6.6	52	1	2	4	9	15	25	27
TOTAL										
0–19 Years	20	8.4	89	1	1	3	15	25	27	27
20–34	8	4.1	6	2	2	4	4	5	13	13
35–49	7	3.7	9	2	1	3	7	9	9	9
50–64	13	6.2	41	2	2	2	10	14	24	24
65+	15	5.6	22	1	2	5	8	11	17	17
GRAND TOTAL	63	6.2	49	1	2	4	8	15	25	27

31.42: LARYNGOSCOPY/TRACHEOSCOP. Formerly included in operation group(s) 581.

Type of Patients	Observed Patients	Avg. Stay	Variance	10th	25th	50th	75th	90th	95th	99th
1. SINGLE DX										
0–19 Years	1045	2.0	3	1	1	2	2	3	5	11
20–34	68	1.7	<1	1	1	1	2	3	3	4
35–49	81	2.6	5	1	2	2	3	4	4	13
50–64	42	3.1	8	1	2	3	3	4	8	14
65+	27	2.4	2	1	2	2	3	4	4	13
2. MULTIPLE DX										
0–19 Years	3330	3.4	33	1	1	2	3	6	10	24
20–34	265	5.2	92	1	2	3	4	10	12	58
35–49	430	4.1	21	1	2	3	5	8	13	23
50–64	498	5.3	60	1	2	2	6	12	17	51
65+	1037	7.5	50	2	3	6	9	15	19	36
TOTAL SINGLE DX	1263	2.1	3	1	1	2	2	4	5	11
MULTIPLE DX	5560	4.5	45	1	2	2	5	10	14	35
TOTAL										
0–19 Years	4375	3.1	27	1	1	2	3	6	9	22
20–34	333	4.6	78	1	1	2	4	10	11	58
35–49	511	3.8	19	1	1	3	4	7	12	21
50–64	540	5.1	56	1	2	2	6	12	17	51
65+	1064	7.3	49	2	3	6	9	15	18	35
GRAND TOTAL	6823	4.1	39	1	1	2	4	9	13	30

Length of Stay by Diagnosis and Operation, United States, 1997

United States, October 1995–September 1996 Data, by Operation

31.43: CLSD (ENDO) BX LARYNX. Formerly included in operation group(s) 557.

Type of Patients	Observed Patients	Avg. Stay	Variance	10th	25th	50th	75th	90th	95th	99th
1. SINGLE DX										
0–19 Years	5	1.6	1	1	1	1	2	2	5	5
20–34	2	2.9	3	1	1	4	4	4	4	4
35–49	8	2.0	8	1	1	1	1	3	11	11
50–64	22	2.3	4	1	1	2	3	3	6	12
65+	11	2.1	3	1	1	1	4	5	5	5
2. MULTIPLE DX										
0–19 Years	14	8.2	49	1	1	7	13	13	23	23
20–34	10	3.2	4	1	1	3	5	7	4	7
35–49	60	5.9	21	1	3	6	7	10	14	25
50–64	156	14.9	521	1	2	6	15	79	79	79
65+	211	6.3	48	1	2	5	9	13	15	32
TOTAL SINGLE DX	48	2.1	5	1	1	1	3	4	6	11
MULTIPLE DX	451	10.0	271	1	2	5	11	17	32	79
TOTAL										
0–19 Years	19	5.8	42	1	1	2	13	13	23	23
20–34	12	3.2	4	1	1	3	5	7	7	7
35–49	68	5.0	20	1	1	4	6	10	12	25
50–64	178	13.4	478	1	2	5	15	24	79	79
65+	222	6.1	47	1	2	4	8	13	15	28
GRAND TOTAL	499	9.1	248	1	2	5	9	15	27	79

31.6: REPAIR OF LARYNX. Formerly included in operation group(s) 561.

Type of Patients	Observed Patients	Avg. Stay	Variance	10th	25th	50th	75th	90th	95th	99th
1. SINGLE DX										
0–19 Years	47	3.7	18	1	2	2	4	6	10	25
20–34	9	1.2	<1	1	1	1	1	2	2	2
35–49	14	1.6	1	1	1	1	2	4	4	4
50–64	3	4.6	16	1	1	2	9	9	9	9
65+	11	1.9	3	1	1	2	2	2	2	13
2. MULTIPLE DX										
0–19 Years	175	9.8	102	1	3	7	14	20	26	47
20–34	15	3.4	8	1	1	2	5	5	11	11
35–49	39	5.1	88	1	1	1	4	14	34	43
50–64	59	2.9	13	1	1	1	3	6	9	21
65+	74	3.5	31	1	1	1	4	7	13	33
TOTAL SINGLE DX	84	2.9	13	1	1	2	4	5	9	17
MULTIPLE DX	362	7.1	81	1	1	4	9	17	22	43
TOTAL										
0–19 Years	222	8.6	91	1	2	6	12	19	24	47
20–34	24	2.3	5	1	1	1	2	5	5	11
35–49	53	4.3	71	1	1	1	4	8	21	43
50–64	62	2.9	13	1	1	2	3	6	9	21
65+	85	3.1	24	1	1	2	4	7	11	33
GRAND TOTAL	446	6.2	70	1	1	3	8	16	21	41

31.5: LOC EXC/DESTR LARYNX LES. Formerly included in operation group(s) 558.

Type of Patients	Observed Patients	Avg. Stay	Variance	10th	25th	50th	75th	90th	95th	99th
1. SINGLE DX										
0–19 Years	24	4.3	26	1	1	2	7	8	22	22
20–34	2	6.0	5	2	7	7	7	7	7	7
35–49	7	1.6	1	1	1	1	2	4	4	4
50–64	3	4.7	2	3	3	5	5	7	7	7
65+	5	2.8	5	1	1	1	6	6	6	6
2. MULTIPLE DX										
0–19 Years	180	4.3	38	1	1	2	4	11	21	23
20–34	27	9.5	91	1	3	7	20	20	55	>99
35–49	64	7.6	66	1	1	6	9	17	24	24
50–64	43	10.8	68	2	4	7	22	22	22	22
65+	71	9.9	69	1	3	7	19	19	19	51
TOTAL SINGLE DX	41	3.6	18	1	1	2	4	7	10	22
MULTIPLE DX	385	6.6	59	1	1	3	9	19	22	>99
TOTAL										
0–19 Years	204	4.3	37	1	1	2	4	11	21	>99
20–34	29	9.4	88	1	3	7	13	20	55	>99
35–49	71	6.8	62	1	1	5	9	15	24	24
50–64	46	10.6	66	2	4	7	22	22	22	22
65+	76	9.6	68	1	3	6	19	19	19	51
GRAND TOTAL	426	6.3	57	1	1	3	8	19	22	69

31.69: OTHER LARYNGEAL REPAIR. Formerly included in operation group(s) 561.

Type of Patients	Observed Patients	Avg. Stay	Variance	10th	25th	50th	75th	90th	95th	99th
1. SINGLE DX										
0–19 Years	44	3.5	19	1	2	2	4	6	10	27
20–34	8	1.2	<1	1	1	1	1	2	2	2
35–49	13	1.6	1	1	1	2	2	4	4	4
50–64	2	1.6	<1	1	1	1	2	2	2	2
65+	10	1.8	6	1	1	1	2	2	2	13
2. MULTIPLE DX										
0–19 Years	171	9.9	103	1	3	7	14	20	26	47
20–34	11	2.9	3	1	1	2	5	5	5	11
35–49	34	4.4	86	1	1	1	4	5	34	43
50–64	56	2.5	9	1	1	1	3	6	6	21
65+	66	3.3	31	1	1	3	3	7	11	33
TOTAL SINGLE DX	77	2.8	14	1	1	2	3	4	9	17
MULTIPLE DX	338	7.1	83	1	1	4	9	17	22	43
TOTAL										
0–19 Years	215	8.6	93	1	2	6	12	19	24	47
20–34	19	2.1	2	1	1	1	2	5	5	5
35–49	47	3.8	68	1	1	1	4	5	8	43
50–64	58	2.5	9	1	1	1	3	6	6	21
65+	76	3.0	26	1	1	2	2	6	11	33
GRAND TOTAL	415	6.3	73	1	1	3	8	16	21	42

United States, October 1995–September 1996 Data, by Operation

31.7: REPAIR OF TRACHEA. Formerly included in operation group(s) 561.

Type of Patients	Observed Patients	Avg. Stay	Vari-ance	Percentiles						
				10th	25th	50th	75th	90th	95th	99th
1. SINGLE DX										
0–19 Years	68	5.7	27	1	1	4	9	11	14	26
20–34	4	3.2	6	2	3	3	3	5	5	5
35–49	5	2.8	6	1	1	1	4	7	7	7
50–64	5	1.9	<1	1	1	2	2	3	4	4
65+	5	2.5	2	1	1	3	3	4	4	4
2. MULTIPLE DX										
0–19 Years	411	16.0	306	1	3	11	22	43	63	>99
20–34	63	7.9	155	1	2	2	13	20	25	70
35–49	71	9.1	213	3	3	4	7	16	57	65
50–64	104	7.9	61	1	2	8	11	12	17	37
65+	172	8.0	82	1	2	5	12	16	21	88
TOTAL SINGLE DX	87	5.2	24	1	1	4	8	11	12	26
MULTIPLE DX	821	12.3	234	1	2	7	16	31	51	83
TOTAL										
0–19 Years	479	14.4	278	3	3	9	19	40	58	>99
20–34	67	7.5	145	1	1	2	9	20	25	70
35–49	76	8.8	204	1	2	4	7	16	57	65
50–64	109	7.7	60	1	2	8	11	12	17	37
65+	177	7.9	81	2	2	5	12	16	21	48
GRAND TOTAL	908	11.6	217	1	2	7	15	29	48	83

31.74: REVISION OF TRACHEOSTOMY. Formerly included in operation group(s) 561.

Type of Patients	Observed Patients	Avg. Stay	Vari-ance	Percentiles						
				10th	25th	50th	75th	90th	95th	99th
1. SINGLE DX										
0–19 Years	7	5.0	59	1	1	2	2	21	21	21
20–34	2	2.7	<1	2	2	3	3	3	3	3
35–49	2	1.0	0	1	1	1	1	1	1	1
50–64	3	1.8	<1	1	1	2	2	2	4	4
65+	4	2.8	1	1	3	3	4	4	4	4
2. MULTIPLE DX										
0–19 Years	63	11.4	254	1	2	5	16	23	58	80
20–34	29	3.9	51	1	3	3	13	13	14	15
35–49	47	9.6	262	1	3	4	7	16	65	65
50–64	61	7.9	38	1	3	9	11	12	17	32
65+	118	7.0	92	1	2	3	9	16	21	31
TOTAL SINGLE DX	18	3.2	25	1	1	2	3	4	21	21
MULTIPLE DX	318	8.2	142	1	2	4	11	17	23	65
TOTAL										
0–19 Years	70	10.7	236	2	2	4	15	23	58	80
20–34	31	3.8	47	1	1	2	3	13	14	15
35–49	49	9.3	255	1	2	3	7	16	57	65
50–64	64	7.7	38	1	2	9	11	12	17	32
65+	122	6.9	90	1	2	3	9	16	21	31
GRAND TOTAL	336	7.9	137	1	2	4	11	16	23	65

31.73: TRACH FISTULA CLOSE NEC. Formerly included in operation group(s) 561.

Type of Patients	Observed Patients	Avg. Stay	Vari-ance	Percentiles						
				10th	25th	50th	75th	90th	95th	99th
1. SINGLE DX										
0–19 Years	33	7.0	22	1	1	8	11	12	14	15
20–34	1	2.0	0	2	2	2	2	2	2	2
35–49	0									
50–64	0									
65+	1	1.0	0	1	1	1	1	1	1	1
2. MULTIPLE DX										
0–19 Years	185	20.6	345	1	9	16	30	43	72	>99
20–34	6	23.0	503	1	16	16	16	70	70	70
35–49	3	3.8	<1	3	4	4	4	4	4	4
50–64	14	7.7	110	1	1	2	15	15	37	37
65+	17	10.0	118	2	4	8	19	42	>99	>99
TOTAL SINGLE DX	35	6.9	22	1	1	8	11	12	14	15
MULTIPLE DX	225	19.8	342	1	8	15	28	43	72	>99
TOTAL										
0–19 Years	218	18.7	322	1	8	13	27	43	71	>99
20–34	7	22.4	501	1	16	16	16	70	70	70
35–49	3	3.8	<1	3	1	4	4	4	4	4
50–64	14	7.7	110	1	1	2	15	15	37	37
65+	18	9.7	116	1	4	6	19	42	>99	>99
GRAND TOTAL	260	18.2	319	1	5	12	27	43	71	>99

31.9: OTHER LARYNX/TRACHEA OPS. Formerly included in operation group(s) 561.

Type of Patients	Observed Patients	Avg. Stay	Vari-ance	Percentiles						
				10th	25th	50th	75th	90th	95th	99th
1. SINGLE DX										
0–19 Years	20	2.9	6	1	1	2	5	8	8	8
20–34	8	1.3	<1	1	1	1	1	2	5	5
35–49	5	1.1	<1	1	1	1	1	1	1	2
50–64	6	4.9	37	1	1	2	14	14	14	14
65+	2	1.6	<1	1	2	2	2	2	2	2
2. MULTIPLE DX										
0–19 Years	119	6.9	76	1	2	3	10	18	26	30
20–34	15	10.0	326	1	1	2	5	49	49	57
35–49	50	3.3	27	1	1	1	5	7	8	12
50–64	57	7.3	76	1	2	2	11	23	23	25
65+	84	7.6	74	1	2	4	8	24	24	34
TOTAL SINGLE DX	41	2.6	10	1	1	1	2	8	8	14
MULTIPLE DX	325	6.5	77	1	1	3	8	21	24	47
TOTAL										
0–19 Years	139	6.2	66	1	1	2	8	18	23	30
20–34	23	7.5	245	1	1	1	3	49	49	57
35–49	55	3.0	24	1	1	1	5	7	8	12
50–64	63	7.1	73	1	1	2	11	22	23	25
65+	86	7.5	74	2	2	4	8	24	24	34
GRAND TOTAL	366	6.0	70	1	1	2	8	18	24	41

Length of Stay by Diagnosis and Operation, United States, 1997

United States, October 1995–September 1996 Data, by Operation

32.0: LOC EXC/DESTR BRONCH LES. Formerly included in operation group(s) 562.

Type of Patients	Observed Patients	Avg. Stay	Vari-ance	10th	25th	50th	75th	90th	95th	99th
1. SINGLE DX										
0–19 Years	18	3.3	2	2	3	3	4	5	7	7
20–34	4	6.6	2	5	5	7	8	8	8	8
35–49	6	3.9	2	2	4	4	4	4	4	10
50–64	6	2.0	4	1	1	1	2	7	7	7
65+	0									
2. MULTIPLE DX										
0–19 Years	50	4.5	11	1	2	4	7	>99	>99	>99
20–34	10	3.8	5	1	2	4	5	7	7	7
35–49	28	5.1	19	1	3	5	6	12	16	19
50–64	61	5.6	20	1	2	5	9	11	13	22
65+	64	4.8	13	1	2	4	7	9	13	19
TOTAL SINGLE DX	34	3.7	3	2	3	4	4	7	7	10
MULTIPLE DX	213	5.0	15	1	2	4	7	11	14	>99
TOTAL										
0–19 Years	68	4.1	8	1	2	3	7	11	>99	>99
20–34	14	4.7	5	1	4	5	7	7	8	8
35–49	34	4.5	11	1	3	4	5	7	12	19
50–64	67	5.3	19	1	2	4	7	11	13	22
65+	64	4.8	13	1	2	4	7	9	13	19
GRAND TOTAL	247	4.7	13	1	2	4	6	11	13	>99

32.2: LOC EXC/DESTR LUNG LES. Formerly included in operation group(s) 564.

Type of Patients	Observed Patients	Avg. Stay	Vari-ance	10th	25th	50th	75th	90th	95th	99th
1. SINGLE DX										
0–19 Years	71	4.1	3	2	3	5	5	5	7	11
20–34	83	5.7	11	2	3	5	8	10	11	15
35–49	131	4.1	8	2	2	3	6	8	9	16
50–64	157	4.3	7	1	2	3	6	7	9	12
65+	145	4.8	12	2	3	3	5	11	11	16
2. MULTIPLE DX										
0–19 Years	308	8.1	43	3	4	6	10	13	18	32
20–34	625	8.0	50	2	4	6	10	16	22	38
35–49	959	7.6	45	2	3	6	10	15	21	36
50–64	1786	7.8	63	2	3	5	9	16	22	41
65+	2380	8.2	58	2	4	6	10	16	22	40
TOTAL SINGLE DX	587	4.5	8	2	3	4	5	8	11	13
MULTIPLE DX	6058	7.9	55	2	4	6	10	16	21	38
TOTAL										
0–19 Years	379	7.2	37	3	4	6	10	12	15	27
20–34	708	7.7	47	2	4	6	9	16	21	34
35–49	1090	7.3	43	2	3	5	9	15	20	36
50–64	1943	7.6	61	2	3	5	9	16	21	40
65+	2525	7.9	56	2	4	6	9	15	22	39
GRAND TOTAL	6645	7.7	52	2	4	6	9	15	21	37

32.1: OTHER BRONCHIAL EXCISION. Formerly included in operation group(s) 563.

Type of Patients	Observed Patients	Avg. Stay	Vari-ance	10th	25th	50th	75th	90th	95th	99th
1. SINGLE DX										
0–19 Years	1	8.0	0	8	8	8	8	8	8	8
20–34	0									
35–49	4	4.7	<1	4	4	5	5	5	5	5
50–64	0									
65+	1	10.0	0	10	10	10	10	10	10	10
2. MULTIPLE DX										
0–19 Years	0									
20–34	3	5.2	<1	4	5	5	6	6	6	6
35–49	6	7.7	29	2	2	9	15	15	15	15
50–64	4	9.2	<1	9	9	9	9	9	9	15
65+	4	22.9	19	24	24	24	24	24	24	24
TOTAL SINGLE DX	6	5.8	4	4	5	5	5	10	10	10
MULTIPLE DX	17	15.8	64	9	9	10	24	24	24	24
TOTAL										
0–19 Years	1	8.0	0	8	8	8	8	8	8	8
20–34	3	5.2	<1	4	5	5	6	6	6	6
35–49	10	6.1	16	2	4	5	9	15	15	15
50–64	4	9.2	<1	9	9	9	9	9	9	15
65+	5	22.5	23	24	24	24	24	24	24	24
GRAND TOTAL	23	14.9	67	5	9	9	24	24	24	24

32.21: EMPHYSEM BLEB PLICATION. Formerly included in operation group(s) 564.

Type of Patients	Observed Patients	Avg. Stay	Vari-ance	10th	25th	50th	75th	90th	95th	99th
1. SINGLE DX										
0–19 Years	9	4.6	5	1	5	5	5	5	8	11
20–34	7	6.8	2	5	5	7	8	8	10	10
35–49	2	5.5	6	4	4	4	9	9	9	9
50–64	3	9.2	<1	9	9	9	9	10	10	10
65+	5	5.0	11	3	3	3	5	11	11	11
2. MULTIPLE DX										
0–19 Years	24	8.0	17	3	4	7	12	14	15	15
20–34	103	8.5	26	3	5	9	12	16	18	23
35–49	78	10.8	43	4	7	11	12	22	23	30
50–64	68	15.3	271	5	7	11	18	23	48	98
65+	79	18.0	221	7	9	13	22	33	60	70
TOTAL SINGLE DX	26	5.7	7	2	5	5	8	9	10	11
MULTIPLE DX	352	12.1	123	4	6	10	14	22	25	70
TOTAL										
0–19 Years	33	6.3	13	2	4	5	7	13	14	15
20–34	110	8.4	25	3	4	8	11	16	18	23
35–49	80	10.7	43	4	5	10	12	22	23	30
50–64	71	14.8	251	6	8	10	18	23	46	98
65+	84	17.3	219	5	8	12	21	32	60	70
GRAND TOTAL	378	11.4	115	3	5	9	13	21	24	70

Length of Stay by Diagnosis and Operation, United States, 1997

United States, October 1995–September 1996 Data, by Operation

32.22: LUNG VOLUME RED SURGERY. Formerly included in operation group(s) 564.

Type of Patients	Observed Patients	Avg. Stay	Vari-ance	10th	25th	50th	75th	90th	95th	99th
1. SINGLE DX										
0–19 Years	1	2.0	0	2	2	2	2	2	2	2
20–34	1	4.0	0	4	4	4	4	4	4	4
35–49	5	6.6	4	4	5	6	9	9	9	9
50–64	16	6.1	5	3	4	7	8	8	9	10
65+	19	6.6	9	4	4	6	7	11	12	16
2. MULTIPLE DX										
0–19 Years	0									
20–34	2	15.5	4	16	16	16	16	16	16	16
35–49	24	10.2	39	5	6	7	16	16	23	31
50–64	216	14.9	103	6	8	12	19	27	36	49
65+	232	14.5	134	6	8	11	17	28	35	>99
TOTAL SINGLE DX	42	6.2	7	4	4	6	7	9	11	16
MULTIPLE DX	474	14.4	113	6	8	12	17	27	34	63
TOTAL										
0–19 Years	1	2.0	0	2	2	2	2	2	2	2
20–34	3	14.0	18	4	16	16	16	16	16	16
35–49	29	9.8	37	5	5	7	13	16	23	31
50–64	232	14.3	102	6	7	12	18	27	32	49
65+	251	13.9	129	6	7	11	16	27	34	>99
GRAND TOTAL	516	13.8	110	5	7	11	16	24	33	63

32.29: LOC EXC LUNG LES NEC. Formerly included in operation group(s) 564.

Type of Patients	Observed Patients	Avg. Stay	Vari-ance	10th	25th	50th	75th	90th	95th	99th
1. SINGLE DX										
0–19 Years	54	4.1	3	3	3	4	5	5	7	8
20–34	60	5.7	12	2	3	5	8	11	11	15
35–49	111	4.1	8	2	2	3	5	7	9	16
50–64	126	4.1	6	1	2	3	5	7	8	12
65+	110	4.7	12	2	3	3	5	11	11	12
2. MULTIPLE DX										
0–19 Years	249	8.2	45	3	4	6	10	13	18	32
20–34	457	7.8	54	2	4	6	9	16	23	48
35–49	799	7.5	44	2	3	6	9	15	20	36
50–64	1404	7.0	47	2	3	5	9	14	20	37
65+	1944	7.6	43	2	4	6	9	15	20	35
TOTAL SINGLE DX	461	4.4	8	2	3	4	5	8	11	13
MULTIPLE DX	4853	7.4	45	2	4	5	9	15	20	36
TOTAL										
0–19 Years	303	7.4	39	3	4	6	10	12	16	27
20–34	517	7.6	50	2	4	6	9	16	21	38
35–49	910	7.2	42	2	3	5	8	15	19	36
50–64	1530	6.8	45	2	3	5	8	13	19	37
65+	2054	7.4	41	2	4	6	9	14	19	35
GRAND TOTAL	5314	7.2	43	2	4	5	8	14	19	36

32.28: ENDO EXC/DESTR LUNG LES. Formerly included in operation group(s) 564.

Type of Patients	Observed Patients	Avg. Stay	Vari-ance	10th	25th	50th	75th	90th	95th	99th
1. SINGLE DX										
0–19 Years	7	2.7	1	2	2	2	4	5	5	5
20–34	15	5.5	9	3	3	5	6	9	13	16
35–49	13	2.6	<1	2	2	3	3	4	4	4
50–64	12	2.3	<1	1	2	2	3	3	4	4
65+	11	2.9	2	2	2	2	3	6	6	6
2. MULTIPLE DX										
0–19 Years	35	6.8	35	2	3	5	9	12	15	34
20–34	63	7.9	50	2	3	6	10	19	25	25
35–49	58	5.3	35	2	2	5	7	14	14	28
50–64	98	7.6	45	2	3	5	10	19	19	20
65+	125	5.5	28	2	2	4	6	10	12	27
TOTAL SINGLE DX	58	3.5	6	2	2	3	4	6	9	16
MULTIPLE DX	379	6.4	39	2	2	4	8	14	19	28
TOTAL										
0–19 Years	42	6.2	32	2	3	4	9	12	15	34
20–34	78	7.4	43	3	5	5	9	17	25	25
35–49	71	5.1	34	2	2	2	7	14	14	28
50–64	110	7.1	43	2	3	4	9	19	19	20
65+	136	5.3	27	2	2	4	6	10	12	27
GRAND TOTAL	437	6.1	36	2	2	4	8	14	19	27

32.3: SEGMENTAL LUNG RESECTION. Formerly included in operation group(s) 564.

Type of Patients	Observed Patients	Avg. Stay	Vari-ance	10th	25th	50th	75th	90th	95th	99th
1. SINGLE DX										
0–19 Years	21	4.8	6	3	3	4	6	8	12	12
20–34	11	3.9	3	2	2	4	5	6	7	8
35–49	20	6.9	18	4	4	6	11	13	17	17
50–64	54	6.7	7	4	4	6	9	9	10	14
65+	47	7.0	31	3	5	7	8	9	12	38
2. MULTIPLE DX										
0–19 Years	74	10.7	92	4	4	7	14	23	36	39
20–34	86	12.8	122	4	5	8	17	30	30	53
35–49	229	7.8	41	4	4	6	9	13	16	32
50–64	617	9.0	48	4	5	7	11	16	21	42
65+	1216	10.2	71	5	6	8	11	17	24	48
TOTAL SINGLE DX	153	6.3	14	3	4	6	8	9	12	17
MULTIPLE DX	2222	9.8	67	4	5	7	11	17	24	47
TOTAL										
0–19 Years	95	9.5	80	3	3	6	12	19	32	39
20–34	97	12.2	119	4	5	8	15	30	30	53
35–49	249	7.7	39	3	4	6	9	13	16	32
50–64	671	8.8	45	4	5	7	10	16	20	42
65+	1263	10.1	70	5	6	8	11	16	23	48
GRAND TOTAL	2375	9.5	64	4	5	7	11	16	24	46

Length of Stay by Diagnosis and Operation, United States, 1997

United States, October 1995–September 1996 Data, by Operation

32.4: LOBECTOMY OF LUNG. Formerly included in operation group(s) 565.

Type of Patients	Observed Patients	Avg. Stay	Vari-ance	10th	25th	50th	75th	90th	95th	99th
1. SINGLE DX										
0–19 Years	44	4.8	3	4	4	4	5	7	8	11
20–34	19	9.2	4	5	10	10	10	10	10	10
35–49	51	5.6	2	4	5	5	6	7	8	10
50–64	143	6.5	7	4	5	6	7	12	12	14
65+	124	6.5	4	4	5	6	7	10	10	12
2. MULTIPLE DX										
0–19 Years	105	11.6	86	4	5	9	14	22	35	55
20–34	114	8.8	41	4	5	6	10	16	21	35
35–49	580	9.7	62	4	5	7	11	17	25	37
50–64	2246	9.1	44	4	5	7	10	15	20	43
65+	4468	9.5	42	4	6	8	11	17	22	35
TOTAL SINGLE DX	381	6.4	6	4	5	6	7	10	11	12
MULTIPLE DX	7513	9.4	45	4	5	7	11	16	22	37
TOTAL										
0–19 Years	149	8.3	57	4	4	5	10	17	24	48
20–34	133	9.0	26	5	5	9	10	13	17	32
35–49	631	9.3	57	4	5	6	10	15	24	37
50–64	2389	8.9	41	4	5	7	10	15	20	42
65+	4592	9.5	42	4	6	8	11	17	22	35
GRAND TOTAL	7894	9.2	43	4	5	7	11	16	21	37

32.6: RAD DISSECT THOR STRUCT. Formerly included in operation group(s) 567.

Type of Patients	Observed Patients	Avg. Stay	Vari-ance	10th	25th	50th	75th	90th	95th	99th
1. SINGLE DX										
0–19 Years	0									
20–34	0									
35–49	2	13.4	17	8	8	16	16	16	16	16
50–64	1	5.0	0	5	5	5	5	5	5	5
65+	1	9.0	0	9	9	9	9	9	9	9
2. MULTIPLE DX										
0–19 Years	0									
20–34	1	2.0	0	2	2	2	2	2	2	2
35–49	7	8.0	3	5	8	8	8	11	11	11
50–64	14	25.7	305	7	7	25	43	43	43	43
65+	29	11.6	74	6	8	10	13	16	23	61
TOTAL SINGLE DX	4	9.4	23	5	5	8	16	16	16	16
MULTIPLE DX	51	17.5	227	6	7	10	25	43	43	43
TOTAL										
0–19 Years	0									
20–34	1	2.0	0	2	2	2	2	2	2	2
35–49	9	8.3	5	5	8	8	8	11	11	16
50–64	15	25.3	307	7	7	25	43	43	43	43
65+	30	11.6	73	6	8	10	13	16	23	61
GRAND TOTAL	55	17.3	224	6	7	10	23	43	43	43

32.5: COMPLETE PNEUMONECTOMY. Formerly included in operation group(s) 565.

Type of Patients	Observed Patients	Avg. Stay	Vari-ance	10th	25th	50th	75th	90th	95th	99th
1. SINGLE DX										
0–19 Years	1	14.0	0	14	14	14	14	14	14	14
20–34	2	3.8	2	3	3	3	5	5	5	5
35–49	5	4.9	<1	4	4	5	5	7	7	7
50–64	27	5.4	1	4	5	5	6	6	7	10
65+	4	6.5	3	5	6	6	9	9	9	9
2. MULTIPLE DX										
0–19 Years	17	13.2	85	7	7	10	15	28	28	60
20–34	17	8.4	12	5	6	8	9	12	19	19
35–49	132	10.0	81	5	5	7	10	15	30	47
50–64	481	8.9	40	5	5	7	10	16	22	29
65+	569	10.9	117	5	6	7	12	19	30	57
TOTAL SINGLE DX	39	5.8	4	4	5	5	6	7	10	14
MULTIPLE DX	1216	10.0	82	5	6	7	11	18	23	57
TOTAL										
0–19 Years	18	13.3	77	7	7	10	14	28	28	60
20–34	19	8.1	12	5	6	8	9	12	17	19
35–49	137	9.9	79	5	5	7	10	15	30	47
50–64	508	8.6	38	5	5	7	10	15	21	27
65+	573	10.9	116	5	6	7	12	19	29	57
GRAND TOTAL	1255	9.9	80	5	5	7	11	17	23	57

32.9: OTHER EXCISION OF LUNG. Formerly included in operation group(s) 567.

Type of Patients	Observed Patients	Avg. Stay	Vari-ance	10th	25th	50th	75th	90th	95th	99th
1. SINGLE DX										
0–19 Years	0									
20–34	1	9.0	0	9	9	9	9	9	9	9
35–49	0									
50–64	0									
2. MULTIPLE DX										
0–19 Years	2	2.9	1	2	2	2	4	4	4	4
20–34	2	11.6	9	9	9	14	14	14	14	14
35–49	4	11.1	103	2	2	3	24	24	24	24
50–64	9	8.2	33	3	5	6	8	18	23	23
65+	9	11.4	34	5	6	10	15	19	22	22
TOTAL SINGLE DX	1	9.0	0	9	9	9	9	9	9	9
MULTIPLE DX	26	9.7	45	2	5	8	14	22	24	24
TOTAL										
0–19 Years	2	2.9	1	2	2	2	4	4	4	4
20–34	3	9.3	2	9	9	9	9	9	14	14
35–49	4	11.1	103	2	2	3	24	24	24	24
50–64	9	8.2	33	3	5	6	8	18	23	23
65+	9	11.4	34	5	6	10	15	19	22	22
GRAND TOTAL	27	9.5	33	3	5	9	10	19	23	24

Length of Stay by Diagnosis and Operation, United States, 1997

United States, October 1995–September 1996 Data, by Operation

33.0: INCISION OF BRONCHUS. Formerly included in operation group(s) 562.

Type of Patients	Observed Patients	Avg. Stay	Variance	10th	25th	50th	75th	90th	95th	99th
1. SINGLE DX										
0–19 Years	1	1.0	0	1	1	1	1	1	1	1
20–34	0									
35–49	0									
50–64	0									
65+	1	4.0	0	4	4	4	4	4	4	4
2. MULTIPLE DX										
0–19 Years	1	2.0	0	2	2	2	2	2	2	2
20–34	0									
35–49	1	10.0	0	10	10	10	10	10	10	10
50–64	1	5.0	0	5	5	5	5	5	5	5
65+	1	7.0	0	7	7	7	7	7	7	7
TOTAL SINGLE DX	2	2.8	3	1	1	4	4	4	4	4
MULTIPLE DX	4	4.9	9	2	2	5	7	10	10	10
TOTAL										
0–19 Years	2	1.7	<1	1	1	2	2	2	2	2
20–34	0									
35–49	1	10.0	0	10	10	10	10	10	10	10
50–64	1	5.0	0	5	5	5	5	5	5	5
65+	2	5.6	3	4	4	7	7	7	7	7
GRAND TOTAL	6	4.3	8	1	2	4	7	7	10	10

33.1: INCISION OF LUNG. Formerly included in operation group(s) 567.

Type of Patients	Observed Patients	Avg. Stay	Variance	10th	25th	50th	75th	90th	95th	99th
1. SINGLE DX										
0–19 Years	7	4.9	17	1	2	3	7	11	13	13
20–34	3	4.7	14	1	1	5	9	9	9	9
35–49	7	4.0	9	2	2	2	6	8	10	10
50–64	2	6.8	9	3	3	9	9	9	9	9
65+	1	8.0	0	8	8	8	8	8	8	8
2. MULTIPLE DX										
0–19 Years	28	10.6	134	2	5	6	13	18	26	56
20–34	15	19.5	144	5	10	20	31	31	31	41
35–49	23	14.9	6	15	15	15	15	15	15	20
50–64	35	12.3	90	2	4	10	17	26	27	40
65+	40	14.9	95	4	9	14	21	24	34	49
TOTAL SINGLE DX	20	5.0	12	2	2	3	8	9	10	13
MULTIPLE DX	141	14.3	53	5	11	15	15	20	26	43
TOTAL										
0–19 Years	35	10.0	125	2	5	6	13	18	26	56
20–34	18	17.3	152	5	7	11	31	31	31	41
35–49	30	14.4	12	15	15	15	15	15	15	20
50–64	37	11.8	85	4	4	9	17	26	27	40
65+	41	14.7	94	4	9	14	21	24	34	49
GRAND TOTAL	161	13.7	55	5	10	15	15	20	26	43

33.2: BRONCHIAL/LUNG DXTIC PX. Formerly included in operation group(s) 562, 564, 566, 581.

Type of Patients	Observed Patients	Avg. Stay	Variance	10th	25th	50th	75th	90th	95th	99th
1. SINGLE DX										
0–19 Years	537	2.1	5	1	1	1	2	4	7	11
20–34	160	4.1	10	1	2	3	6	8	10	16
35–49	302	4.4	14	1	2	3	6	9	11	19
50–64	311	4.9	12	1	2	5	7	9	11	17
65+	303	4.8	27	1	2	3	6	10	13	24
2. MULTIPLE DX										
0–19 Years	2823	8.2	109	1	2	5	10	18	28	67
20–34	2995	9.4	60	3	4	7	12	19	24	41
35–49	6854	9.7	76	3	5	7	12	19	27	46
50–64	10700	8.7	53	2	4	7	11	16	21	39
65+	23778	9.9	57	3	5	8	13	18	23	39
TOTAL SINGLE DX	1613	3.7	13	1	1	2	5	8	10	16
MULTIPLE DX	47150	9.5	63	2	4	8	12	18	24	40
TOTAL										
0–19 Years	3360	7.0	94	1	2	4	8	16	25	55
20–34	3155	9.1	58	1	4	7	12	19	24	40
35–49	7156	9.5	75	3	4	7	12	18	27	46
50–64	11011	8.6	52	2	4	7	11	16	21	38
65+	24081	9.9	57	3	5	8	13	18	23	38
GRAND TOTAL	48763	9.3	62	2	4	7	12	18	23	40

33.22: FIBER-OPTIC BRONCHOSCOPY. Formerly included in operation group(s) 566.

Type of Patients	Observed Patients	Avg. Stay	Variance	10th	25th	50th	75th	90th	95th	99th
1. SINGLE DX										
0–19 Years	108	2.0	3	1	1	1	2	4	5	9
20–34	24	5.0	21	1	2	4	5	16	16	16
35–49	20	3.9	10	1	2	3	5	8	11	12
50–64	20	4.8	13	1	2	3	6	9	8	19
65+	27	4.3	8	1	2	4	6	9	10	12
2. MULTIPLE DX										
0–19 Years	657	7.5	81	1	2	5	9	16	28	49
20–34	300	9.5	57	3	5	7	12	19	24	39
35–49	608	8.2	47	3	4	6	10	15	20	41
50–64	822	8.6	47	2	4	6	10	15	22	35
65+	1723	10.8	70	2	5	9	14	23	30	36
TOTAL SINGLE DX	199	3.0	9	1	1	2	4	7	8	16
MULTIPLE DX	4110	9.3	63	2	4	7	11	18	26	39
TOTAL										
0–19 Years	765	6.6	72	1	2	4	8	15	25	48
20–34	324	9.2	55	3	5	7	12	18	24	39
35–49	628	8.1	46	3	5	6	9	15	20	40
50–64	842	8.5	47	2	4	7	9	15	22	35
65+	1750	10.7	70	2	5	9	14	23	30	36
GRAND TOTAL	4309	9.0	62	2	4	7	11	18	25	39

Length of Stay by Diagnosis and Operation, United States, 1997

United States, October 1995–September 1996 Data, by Operation

33.23: OTHER BRONCHOSCOPY. Formerly included in operation group(s) 566.

Type of Patients	Observed Patients	Avg. Stay	Vari-ance	10th	25th	50th	75th	90th	95th	99th
1. SINGLE DX										
0–19 Years	342	1.8	3	1	1	1	2	3	5	11
20–34	16	3.0	5	1	1	2	5	5	8	8
35–49	27	6.6	47	1	1	5	8	11	19	31
50–64	25	4.3	11	1	2	4	5	10	10	16
65+	13	11.4	336	1	1	5	11	55	55	55
2. MULTIPLE DX										
0–19 Years	1068	6.6	79	1	2	4	7	15	24	53
20–34	255	9.3	59	2	4	7	12	18	26	44
35–49	448	8.9	70	3	4	7	10	15	25	51
50–64	446	10.0	88	2	4	7	12	21	29	55
65+	873	10.0	81	2	4	8	12	20	27	46
TOTAL SINGLE DX	**423**	**2.2**	**11**	**1**	**1**	**1**	**2**	**4**	**7**	**12**
MULTIPLE DX	**3090**	**8.6**	**80**	**1**	**3**	**6**	**11**	**18**	**27**	**51**
TOTAL										
0–19 Years	1410	5.1	60	1	1	2	5	12	19	49
20–34	271	8.9	58	2	4	7	12	18	24	44
35–49	475	8.8	69	3	4	7	10	15	25	51
50–64	471	9.7	86	2	4	7	12	21	28	55
65+	886	10.0	82	2	4	8	12	20	27	46
GRAND TOTAL	**3513**	**7.6**	**75**	**1**	**2**	**5**	**10**	**16**	**25**	**51**

33.24: CLSD (ENDO) BRONCHUS BX. Formerly included in operation group(s) 562.

Type of Patients	Observed Patients	Avg. Stay	Vari-ance	10th	25th	50th	75th	90th	95th	99th
1. SINGLE DX										
0–19 Years	56	3.1	9	1	1	2	4	7	8	15
20–34	45	4.3	8	1	2	4	6	8	8	14
35–49	80	5.6	12	1	3	5	7	9	11	17
50–64	99	6.1	16	2	3	5	8	11	15	18
65+	89	6.7	23	2	4	5	9	12	17	24
2. MULTIPLE DX										
0–19 Years	679	8.2	79	1	3	6	10	17	22	39
20–34	1207	9.2	44	3	5	7	12	19	21	37
35–49	2793	9.5	60	3	5	7	12	18	25	39
50–64	4343	8.7	39	3	5	7	11	16	20	32
65+	10187	10.1	52	3	6	8	13	18	23	39
TOTAL SINGLE DX	**369**	**5.3**	**16**	**1**	**2**	**4**	**8**	**11**	**12**	**18**
MULTIPLE DX	**19209**	**9.6**	**51**	**3**	**5**	**8**	**12**	**18**	**22**	**37**
TOTAL										
0–19 Years	735	7.7	75	1	2	5	10	16	22	39
20–34	1252	9.0	44	3	5	7	12	18	21	36
35–49	2873	9.4	60	3	5	7	11	18	24	39
50–64	4442	8.6	39	3	4	7	11	16	20	32
65+	10276	10.1	52	3	6	8	13	18	23	39
GRAND TOTAL	**19578**	**9.5**	**51**	**3**	**5**	**8**	**12**	**18**	**22**	**37**

33.26: CLOSED LUNG BIOPSY. Formerly included in operation group(s) 564.

Type of Patients	Observed Patients	Avg. Stay	Vari-ance	10th	25th	50th	75th	90th	95th	99th
1. SINGLE DX										
0–19 Years	4	4.3	5	3	4	4	4	4	12	12
20–34	8	3.8	10	1	1	3	6	8	11	11
35–49	14	2.9	5	1	1	3	3	5	9	11
50–64	25	4.4	4	1	2	5	5	7	7	8
65+	39	2.8	10	1	1	1	3	9	12	13
2. MULTIPLE DX										
0–19 Years	18	8.5	53	2	4	6	10	24	24	24
20–34	69	7.5	31	2	4	6	9	14	16	35
35–49	300	6.7	37	1	3	5	8	13	17	35
50–64	934	7.0	32	2	3	6	10	13	16	28
65+	2697	7.7	39	2	3	6	10	14	18	31
TOTAL SINGLE DX	**90**	**3.8**	**6**	**1**	**1**	**4**	**5**	**7**	**8**	**12**
MULTIPLE DX	**4018**	**7.5**	**37**	**2**	**3**	**6**	**10**	**14**	**18**	**31**
TOTAL										
0–19 Years	22	7.2	41	2	4	6	6	22	24	24
20–34	77	7.2	30	2	4	6	9	14	15	35
35–49	314	6.5	36	1	2	5	8	12	17	35
50–64	959	6.9	31	2	3	5	9	13	16	28
65+	2736	7.7	39	2	3	6	10	14	18	31
GRAND TOTAL	**4108**	**7.4**	**36**	**2**	**3**	**6**	**10**	**14**	**17**	**31**

33.27: ENDO LUNG BX (CLOSED). Formerly included in operation group(s) 564.

Type of Patients	Observed Patients	Avg. Stay	Vari-ance	10th	25th	50th	75th	90th	95th	99th
1. SINGLE DX										
0–19 Years	6	2.3	2	1	2	2	2	4	7	7
20–34	38	4.8	8	2	2	4	7	10	10	11
35–49	70	3.9	11	1	2	4	5	10	10	13
50–64	53	5.0	13	1	2	5	7	9	10	22
65+	67	4.8	25	3	3	3	5	9	13	23
2. MULTIPLE DX										
0–19 Years	126	7.5	38	2	4	6	8	14	18	37
20–34	965	10.6	80	2	5	8	13	21	32	43
35–49	2110	11.0	102	3	5	8	13	21	29	65
50–64	3200	9.2	59	3	4	8	11	17	22	42
65+	6888	10.4	60	3	6	9	13	19	23	39
TOTAL SINGLE DX	**234**	**4.5**	**16**	**1**	**2**	**3**	**6**	**9**	**11**	**17**
MULTIPLE DX	**13289**	**10.2**	**68**	**3**	**5**	**8**	**13**	**19**	**24**	**42**
TOTAL										
0–19 Years	132	7.3	38	2	4	6	8	14	18	37
20–34	1003	10.3	79	2	5	8	13	20	32	43
35–49	2180	10.6	100	3	5	8	13	21	29	64
50–64	3253	9.1	58	3	4	7	11	17	22	42
65+	6955	10.3	60	3	5	9	13	19	23	38
GRAND TOTAL	**13523**	**10.1**	**67**	**3**	**5**	**8**	**13**	**19**	**24**	**42**

Length of Stay by Diagnosis and Operation, United States, 1997

United States, October 1995–September 1996 Data, by Operation

33.28: OPEN BIOPSY OF LUNG. Formerly included in operation group(s) 564.

Type of Patients	Observed Patients	Avg. Stay	Variance	10th	25th	50th	75th	90th	95th	99th
1. SINGLE DX										
0–19 Years	18	5.3	12	2	2	3	9	9	9	11
20–34	27	3.3	7	2	2	3	6	6	8	15
35–49	90	4.2	12	1	2	3	6	8	12	19
50–64	89	3.6	5	1	2	3	5	5	8	12
65+	66	3.1	6	1	2	2	3	6	8	14
2. MULTIPLE DX										
0–19 Years	187	17.2	325	2	6	11	25	45	67	79
20–34	173	7.3	56	2	3	4	10	18	23	39
35–49	559	10.3	117	2	3	6	14	28	30	49
50–64	900	8.9	99	2	3	5	10	21	30	51
65+	1299	9.5	77	2	3	7	14	21	26	48
TOTAL SINGLE DX	290	3.8	9	1	2	3	5	8	9	15
MULTIPLE DX	3118	9.8	110	2	3	6	13	23	30	51
TOTAL										
0–19 Years	205	15.9	305	2	4	9	24	37	67	79
20–34	200	6.8	51	2	3	4	8	15	23	35
35–49	649	9.2	104	2	3	5	11	25	30	49
50–64	989	8.6	94	2	3	5	10	21	29	51
65+	1365	9.2	76	2	3	6	13	21	25	48
GRAND TOTAL	3408	9.3	104	2	3	5	12	22	29	51

33.3: SURG COLLAPSE OF LUNG. Formerly included in operation group(s) 567.

Type of Patients	Observed Patients	Avg. Stay	Variance	10th	25th	50th	75th	90th	95th	99th
1. SINGLE DX										
0–19 Years	8	3.7	1	2	3	4	4	5	5	5
20–34	28	5.4	50	2	2	3	4	9	33	33
35–49	5	3.0	<1	2	2	3	3	3	5	5
50–64	9	2.1	2	1	1	1	3	3	4	6
65+	1	7.0	0	7	7	7	7	7	7	7
2. MULTIPLE DX										
0–19 Years	25	4.4	114	1	1	2	4	6	11	90
20–34	32	6.4	25	3	3	5	7	13	13	34
35–49	33	7.0	44	2	4	5	8	20	22	31
50–64	79	12.3	185	3	4	8	13	37	45	62
65+	98	17.9	233	4	7	16	22	28	69	69
TOTAL SINGLE DX	51	3.8	24	1	2	3	4	7	9	33
MULTIPLE DX	267	12.0	177	2	4	7	15	23	38	69
TOTAL										
0–19 Years	33	4.2	86	1	1	3	4	6	11	90
20–34	60	5.9	36	2	3	4	7	12	13	33
35–49	38	6.4	39	2	3	4	8	12	22	29
50–64	88	9.9	161	1	3	5	8	31	45	48
65+	99	17.8	232	4	7	15	22	28	69	69
GRAND TOTAL	318	10.3	157	2	3	6	13	22	37	69

33.4: LUNG AND BRONCHUS REPAIR. Formerly included in operation group(s) 563, 567.

Type of Patients	Observed Patients	Avg. Stay	Variance	10th	25th	50th	75th	90th	95th	99th
1. SINGLE DX										
0–19 Years	2	2.8	2	1	1	4	4	4	4	4
20–34	4	8.0	<1	8	8	8	8	8	8	12
35–49	3	5.4	<1	5	5	5	6	6	6	6
50–64	1	4.0	0	4	4	4	4	4	4	4
65+	0									
2. MULTIPLE DX										
0–19 Years	23	14.0	142	4	5	10	15	36	39	39
20–34	38	14.1	179	5	5	9	14	35	50	50
35–49	25	14.0	164	4	6	11	17	26	41	67
50–64	15	13.0	98	4	5	14	14	24	39	43
65+	21	26.4	>999	5	5	12	26	97	97	97
TOTAL SINGLE DX	10	7.2	4	4	8	8	8	8	8	12
MULTIPLE DX	122	16.3	341	4	5	10	17	37	50	97
TOTAL										
0–19 Years	25	12.3	137	3	4	9	14	36	39	39
20–34	42	11.5	113	5	7	8	10	24	40	50
35–49	28	13.2	154	4	6	10	17	26	41	67
50–64	16	12.8	97	4	5	14	14	24	39	43
65+	21	26.4	>999	5	5	12	26	97	97	97
GRAND TOTAL	132	14.3	281	4	5	8	14	33	43	97

33.5: LUNG TRANSPLANTION. Formerly included in operation group(s) 567.

Type of Patients	Observed Patients	Avg. Stay	Variance	10th	25th	50th	75th	90th	95th	99th
1. SINGLE DX										
0–19 Years	1	21.0	0	21	21	21	21	21	21	21
20–34	1	30.0	0	30	30	30	30	30	30	30
35–49	3	12.9	41	8	9	9	21	21	21	21
50–64	4	12.5	69	5	7	8	22	22	22	22
65+	0									
2. MULTIPLE DX										
0–19 Years	12	32.1	249	18	25	25	39	62	62	62
20–34	23	25.4	347	9	14	18	24	58	79	79
35–49	37	25.5	267	11	14	22	31	45	62	>99
50–64	78	18.8	179	9	11	16	26	86	>99	>99
65+	2	10.8	3	9	9	12	12	12	12	12
TOTAL SINGLE DX	9	16.7	74	7	8	21	22	30	30	30
MULTIPLE DX	152	23.1	253	9	13	18	30	58	90	>99
TOTAL										
0–19 Years	13	31.2	237	18	24	25	36	62	62	62
20–34	24	25.6	329	9	15	18	29	58	79	79
35–49	40	24.8	262	11	13	21	31	45	62	>99
50–64	82	18.5	176	8	11	16	25	86	>99	>99
65+	2	10.8	3	9	9	12	12	12	12	12
GRAND TOTAL	161	22.8	246	9	13	18	29	56	90	>99

United States, October 1995–September 1996 Data, by Operation

33.6: HEART-LUNG TRANSPLANT. Formerly included in operation group(s) 572.

Type of Patients	Observed Patients	Avg. Stay	Variance	Percentiles						
				10th	25th	50th	75th	90th	95th	99th
1. SINGLE DX										
0–19 Years	0									
20–34	0									
35–49	1	1.0	0	1	1	1	1	1	1	1
50–64	0									
65+	0									
2. MULTIPLE DX										
0–19 Years	1	26.0	0	26	26	26	26	26	26	26
20–34	3	40.2	188	17	37	50	50	50	50	50
35–49	4	27.0	135	35	>99	>99	>99	>99	>99	>99
50–64	0									
65+	0									
TOTAL SINGLE DX	1	1.0	0	1	1	1	1	1	1	1
MULTIPLE DX	8	33.3	180	33	>99	>99	>99	>99	>99	>99
TOTAL										
0–19 Years	1	26.0	0	26	26	26	26	26	26	26
20–34	3	40.2	188	17	37	50	50	50	50	50
35–49	5	17.8	257	33	>99	>99	>99	>99	>99	>99
50–64	0									
65+	0									
GRAND TOTAL	9	27.5	311	26	50	>99	>99	>99	>99	>99

33.9: OTHER BRONCHIAL LUNG OPS. Formerly included in operation group(s) 563, 567.

Type of Patients	Observed Patients	Avg. Stay	Variance	Percentiles						
				10th	25th	50th	75th	90th	95th	99th
1. SINGLE DX										
0–19 Years	6	4.0	5	1	2	5	6	6	6	6
20–34	10	5.6	10	1	3	5	10	10	10	10
35–49	2	5.4	<1	5	5	5	6	6	6	6
50–64	3	4.9	1	5	5	5	5	5	7	7
65+	1	1.0	0	1	1	1	1	1	1	1
2. MULTIPLE DX										
0–19 Years	40	9.3	73	1	3	6	16	22	26	40
20–34	18	6.0	27	1	2	4	9	11	19	21
35–49	41	9.0	149	4	4	5	12	17	42	42
50–64	77	9.0	87	2	4	5	10	22	25	50
65+	108	8.3	39	2	4	6	12	16	22	31
TOTAL SINGLE DX	22	4.8	6	1	2	5	6	7	10	10
MULTIPLE DX	284	8.9	75	2	4	6	12	18	25	42
TOTAL										
0–19 Years	46	8.5	66	1	3	6	14	17	22	40
20–34	28	5.8	19	1	3	5	9	10	12	21
35–49	43	10.0	145	4	4	5	12	17	42	42
50–64	80	8.6	81	2	4	5	10	20	25	50
65+	109	8.2	39	2	4	6	12	16	22	31
GRAND TOTAL	306	8.5	70	2	4	6	11	17	23	42

34.0: INC CHEST WALL & PLEURA. Formerly included in operation group(s) 568.

Type of Patients	Observed Patients	Avg. Stay	Variance	Percentiles						
				10th	25th	50th	75th	90th	95th	99th
1. SINGLE DX										
0–19 Years	445	4.2	9	2	2	3	5	8	11	14
20–34	1151	3.7	5	2	2	3	4	7	8	12
35–49	471	4.5	8	2	3	3	5	7	10	12
50–64	169	4.1	7	2	3	4	5	7	8	14
65+	92	4.5	6	1	3	5	6	6	7	14
2. MULTIPLE DX										
0–19 Years	1487	9.6	158	3	4	6	10	16	25	88
20–34	2699	6.0	28	2	3	4	7	11	16	27
35–49	3129	7.0	36	2	3	5	9	13	17	34
50–64	3265	7.9	38	2	4	6	10	15	18	30
65+	6280	8.6	50	2	4	7	11	17	22	33
TOTAL SINGLE DX	2328	4.0	7	2	2	3	5	7	10	13
MULTIPLE DX	16860	7.8	52	2	4	6	9	15	20	34
TOTAL										
0–19 Years	1932	8.5	131	2	3	6	9	15	21	88
20–34	3850	5.3	22	2	3	4	6	10	13	23
35–49	3600	6.7	33	2	3	5	8	12	16	29
50–64	3434	7.7	37	2	4	6	9	15	18	30
65+	6372	8.6	49	2	4	7	11	17	22	33
GRAND TOTAL	19188	7.3	48	2	3	5	9	14	19	33

34.01: INCISION OF CHEST WALL. Formerly included in operation group(s) 568.

Type of Patients	Observed Patients	Avg. Stay	Variance	Percentiles						
				10th	25th	50th	75th	90th	95th	99th
1. SINGLE DX										
0–19 Years	10	3.9	9	1	2	4	4	10	10	10
20–34	11	3.4	8	1	2	2	5	7	12	12
35–49	4	2.4	2	1	1	2	4	4	5	5
50–64	2	3.4	<1	3	3	3	3	5	5	5
65+	7	2.2	1	1	1	2	3	4	4	4
2. MULTIPLE DX										
0–19 Years	34	5.9	14	1	1	8	8	11	12	>99
20–34	27	6.3	17	1	4	6	8	12	12	21
35–49	66	5.2	18	1	1	4	7	10	12	22
50–64	106	6.4	48	1	2	4	8	16	22	25
65+	176	6.5	30	1	2	5	11	15	16	22
TOTAL SINGLE DX	34	3.2	7	1	2	2	4	6	10	12
MULTIPLE DX	409	6.2	31	1	2	5	9	13	16	23
TOTAL										
0–19 Years	44	5.4	14	1	1	6	8	11	12	>99
20–34	38	5.1	15	2	2	4	7	12	12	21
35–49	70	5.0	18	1	1	4	7	9	12	22
50–64	108	6.3	47	1	2	4	7	15	18	25
65+	183	6.4	30	1	2	4	11	15	16	22
GRAND TOTAL	443	6.0	30	2	2	4	8	12	16	23

Length of Stay by Diagnosis and Operation, United States, 1997

United States, October 1995–September 1996 Data, by Operation

34.02: EXPLORATORY THORACOTOMY. Formerly included in operation group(s) 568.

Type of Patients	Observed Patients	Avg. Stay	Variance	10th	25th	50th	75th	90th	95th	99th
1. SINGLE DX										
0–19 Years	1	4.0	0	4	4	4	4	4	4	4
20–34	3	7.2	3	3	8	8	8	8	8	8
35–49	5	5.9	6	2	4	7	8	8	8	8
50–64	17	5.8	3	4	4	5	7	8	8	12
65+	5	5.6	<1	4	5	6	6	6	6	6
2. MULTIPLE DX										
0–19 Years	26	13.3	52	4	6	15	16	26	28	28
20–34	34	10.1	81	2	2	6	19	19	25	38
35–49	47	11.3	161	3	4	6	14	26	45	63
50–64	131	6.9	56	1	4	5	7	12	18	34
65+	215	7.6	34	2	4	6	9	15	21	32
TOTAL SINGLE DX	31	6.1	4	4	4	6	8	8	8	12
MULTIPLE DX	453	8.3	61	2	4	6	10	18	23	34
TOTAL										
0–19 Years	27	13.2	52	4	6	15	16	26	28	28
20–34	37	9.6	68	2	2	8	17	19	25	38
35–49	52	10.9	150	2	4	6	13	26	45	63
50–64	148	6.8	53	3	4	5	7	12	18	34
65+	220	7.6	33	2	4	6	9	15	21	29
GRAND TOTAL	484	8.2	58	2	4	6	10	17	21	34

34.09: OTHER PLEURAL INCISION. Formerly included in operation group(s) 568.

Type of Patients	Observed Patients	Avg. Stay	Variance	10th	25th	50th	75th	90th	95th	99th
1. SINGLE DX										
0–19 Years	56	4.9	15	2	3	4	6	9	10	13
20–34	122	3.1	6	1	2	2	4	6	8	13
35–49	51	4.7	16	2	2	4	5	8	12	24
50–64	22	4.1	6	2	3	3	5	8	10	14
65+	13	4.7	4	1	3	6	6	6	6	6
2. MULTIPLE DX										
0–19 Years	194	9.0	47	3	6	7	11	18	22	48
20–34	315	6.6	26	3	4	6	8	11	13	25
35–49	385	6.9	27	3	4	5	8	14	17	25
50–64	416	9.0	34	3	6	9	10	15	17	35
65+	728	8.6	53	2	4	7	11	17	22	40
TOTAL SINGLE DX	264	3.8	9	1	2	3	5	6	9	13
MULTIPLE DX	2038	8.1	39	3	4	7	9	15	19	33
TOTAL										
0–19 Years	250	8.4	44	3	5	6	10	15	22	34
20–34	437	5.4	22	2	3	4	7	11	11	21
35–49	436	6.7	26	3	3	5	8	13	16	25
50–64	438	8.9	34	3	5	9	10	15	17	35
65+	741	8.5	53	2	4	7	11	17	22	40
GRAND TOTAL	2302	7.6	38	2	4	6	9	14	18	30

34.04: INSERT INTERCOSTAL CATH. Formerly included in operation group(s) 568.

Type of Patients	Observed Patients	Avg. Stay	Variance	10th	25th	50th	75th	90th	95th	99th
1. SINGLE DX										
0–19 Years	377	4.1	8	2	2	3	5	8	11	14
20–34	1015	3.8	5	2	2	3	4	7	8	12
35–49	410	4.5	7	2	3	4	5	10	10	11
50–64	125	4.1	7	2	3	4	4	6	7	16
65+	66	4.6	6	2	3	5	5	7	8	14
2. MULTIPLE DX										
0–19 Years	1224	9.7	184	3	4	6	10	16	27	88
20–34	2319	5.8	27	2	3	4	7	11	16	27
35–49	2594	7.0	36	2	3	5	9	13	17	34
50–64	2554	7.6	35	2	3	6	10	15	18	29
65+	5065	8.7	48	3	4	7	11	17	22	33
TOTAL SINGLE DX	1993	4.0	6	2	2	3	5	7	10	14
MULTIPLE DX	13756	7.7	54	2	4	6	9	15	20	34
TOTAL										
0–19 Years	1601	8.5	150	2	3	5	9	15	20	88
20–34	3334	5.2	21	2	3	4	6	9	13	22
35–49	3004	6.6	33	2	3	5	8	12	16	31
50–64	2679	7.4	34	2	3	6	10	15	18	29
65+	5131	8.6	48	3	4	7	11	17	22	33
GRAND TOTAL	15749	7.2	49	2	3	5	9	14	18	33

34.1: INCISION OF MEDIASTINUM. Formerly included in operation group(s) 569.

Type of Patients	Observed Patients	Avg. Stay	Variance	10th	25th	50th	75th	90th	95th	99th
1. SINGLE DX										
0–19 Years	2	3.1	6	1	1	5	5	5	5	5
20–34	5	1.8	3	1	1	1	2	6	6	6
35–49	6	2.4	3	1	1	2	3	7	7	7
50–64	6	1.3	<1	1	1	1	1	2	2	2
65+	1	1.0	0	1	1	1	1	1	1	1
2. MULTIPLE DX										
0–19 Years	9	9.3	49	3	3	13	13	17	20	31
20–34	31	8.5	55	2	2	7	12	16	29	29
35–49	50	13.4	67	5	5	18	20	20	21	26
50–64	85	7.2	71	1	1	4	9	17	26	29
65+	115	7.6	67	1	1	4	12	18	23	36
TOTAL SINGLE DX	20	1.9	2	1	1	1	2	5	6	7
MULTIPLE DX	290	9.0	72	1	2	6	16	20	22	31
TOTAL										
0–19 Years	11	8.7	48	2	3	5	13	17	20	31
20–34	36	8.0	54	2	2	6	12	16	29	29
35–49	56	12.9	70	1	5	13	20	20	21	26
50–64	91	6.9	69	1	1	4	9	17	19	29
65+	116	7.6	67	1	1	4	12	18	23	36
GRAND TOTAL	310	8.8	71	1	2	6	15	20	22	31

Length of Stay by Diagnosis and Operation, United States, 1997

United States, October 1995–September 1996 Data, by Operation

34.2: THORAX DXTIC PROCEDURES. Formerly included in operation group(s) 569, 581.

Type of Patients	Observed Patients	Avg. Stay	Vari-ance	10th	25th	50th	75th	90th	95th	99th
1. SINGLE DX										
0–19 Years	35	5.5	11	1	2	5	9	10	10	10
20–34	70	2.9	11	1	1	2	3	7	9	19
35–49	100	8.5	24	1	2	12	12	12	12	12
50–64	82	3.1	29	1	1	1	3	5	8	33
65+	65	4.2	31	1	1	2	4	7	22	22
2. MULTIPLE DX										
0–19 Years	106	8.8	103	1	4	8	10	13	25	62
20–34	282	8.2	61	1	3	7	10	16	20	43
35–49	495	7.2	63	1	2	5	9	17	22	40
50–64	1022	7.6	61	1	2	5	10	16	23	42
65+	2039	8.2	56	1	3	6	11	18	23	36
TOTAL SINGLE DX	352	6.6	29	1	1	5	12	12	12	22
MULTIPLE DX	3944	7.9	60	1	3	6	10	17	23	38
TOTAL										
0–19 Years	141	8.0	82	1	3	7	10	12	16	62
20–34	352	7.3	57	1	2	6	9	15	19	43
35–49	595	7.7	48	1	2	7	12	12	17	40
50–64	1104	7.3	60	1	2	5	10	16	23	42
65+	2104	8.0	56	1	3	6	10	18	23	36
GRAND TOTAL	4296	7.7	56	1	2	6	11	16	22	36

34.22: MEDIASTINOSCOPY. Formerly included in operation group(s) 569.

Type of Patients	Observed Patients	Avg. Stay	Vari-ance	10th	25th	50th	75th	90th	95th	99th
1. SINGLE DX										
0–19 Years	0									
20–34	14	1.4	<1	1	1	1	1	3	4	4
35–49	37	1.4	2	1	1	1	1	3	4	13
50–64	26	3.3	60	1	1	1	1	3	33	33
65+	16	1.2	<1	1	1	1	1	1	3	6
2. MULTIPLE DX										
0–19 Years	4	6.2	16	4	4	4	5	12	16	16
20–34	61	7.2	88	1	1	5	8	16	18	49
35–49	143	5.7	56	1	2	5	8	14	21	35
50–64	323	7.0	87	1	3	3	10	16	28	46
65+	475	6.8	56	1	4	4	9	18	21	37
TOTAL SINGLE DX	93	1.9	17	1	1	1	1	3	4	33
MULTIPLE DX	1006	6.7	69	1	1	3	9	16	22	46
TOTAL										
0–19 Years	4	6.2	16	4	4	4	5	12	16	16
20–34	75	6.0	76	1	1	3	8	14	17	49
35–49	180	4.5	44	1	1	3	6	12	16	35
50–64	349	6.7	85	1	1	3	9	15	28	46
65+	491	6.5	55	1	1	4	9	17	21	37
GRAND TOTAL	1099	6.1	65	1	1	3	9	16	21	46

34.21: TRANSPLEURA THORACOSCOPY. Formerly included in operation group(s) 569.

Type of Patients	Observed Patients	Avg. Stay	Vari-ance	10th	25th	50th	75th	90th	95th	99th
1. SINGLE DX										
0–19 Years	9	4.1	6	1	2	4	5	8	10	10
20–34	8	5.7	16	2	3	7	7	11	14	14
35–49	25	4.6	18	2	2	3	5	14	14	19
50–64	21	3.4	4	1	2	3	4	7	7	9
65+	16	9.7	63	2	3	7	22	22	22	22
2. MULTIPLE DX										
0–19 Years	41	10.3	128	3	6	8	11	14	18	62
20–34	62	9.8	52	3	7	8	11	18	20	40
35–49	120	7.5	61	1	3	5	9	16	21	42
50–64	242	9.3	58	2	3	8	14	19	23	31
65+	456	9.5	71	2	4	7	12	21	29	36
TOTAL SINGLE DX	79	5.7	31	2	2	3	7	14	22	22
MULTIPLE DX	921	9.2	67	2	3	7	12	19	25	36
TOTAL										
0–19 Years	50	9.1	111	2	4	7	10	14	18	62
20–34	70	9.5	51	3	6	8	11	18	20	40
35–49	145	7.1	56	1	3	5	9	15	21	30
50–64	263	9.0	57	2	3	7	14	18	23	31
65+	472	9.5	70	2	4	7	12	22	28	36
GRAND TOTAL	1000	9.0	65	2	3	7	11	19	25	36

34.24: PLEURAL BIOPSY. Formerly included in operation group(s) 569.

Type of Patients	Observed Patients	Avg. Stay	Vari-ance	10th	25th	50th	75th	90th	95th	99th
1. SINGLE DX										
0–19 Years	2	6.4	5	4	4	8	8	8	8	8
20–34	4	8.4	22	5	6	6	8	18	18	18
35–49	9	11.7	3	12	12	12	12	12	12	12
50–64	15	3.1	8	1	1	1	4	8	10	10
65+	18	2.9	2	1	2	3	4	4	5	5
2. MULTIPLE DX										
0–19 Years	8	6.3	11	1	1	7	9	9	9	9
20–34	37	10.3	76	4	5	8	14	19	21	56
35–49	99	6.5	42	1	2	5	9	14	19	32
50–64	201	7.0	29	2	3	5	9	14	18	30
65+	596	8.2	48	2	3	6	11	17	22	33
TOTAL SINGLE DX	48	10.7	10	4	12	12	12	12	12	12
MULTIPLE DX	941	7.8	44	2	3	6	10	16	21	32
TOTAL										
0–19 Years	10	6.3	9	1	4	7	9	9	9	9
20–34	41	10.1	71	4	5	8	14	19	21	56
35–49	108	10.1	21	2	8	12	12	15	21	23
50–64	216	6.8	28	2	3	5	9	14	17	30
65+	614	8.1	47	2	3	6	11	17	22	33
GRAND TOTAL	989	8.5	37	2	4	8	12	14	19	31

Length of Stay by Diagnosis and Operation, United States, 1997

United States, October 1995–September 1996 Data, by Operation

34.4: EXC/DESTR CHEST WALL LES. Formerly included in operation group(s) 569.

Type of Patients	Observed Patients	Avg. Stay	Variance	10th	25th	50th	75th	90th	95th	99th
1. SINGLE DX										
0–19 Years	34	3.4	3	1	2	3	5	6	6	7
20–34	22	3.3	7	1	1	3	5	7	8	11
35–49	21	2.9	4	1	1	2	4	7	7	7
50–64	21	3.1	6	1	1	2	5	8	8	8
65+	11	3.8	4	2	2	3	6	6	7	7
2. MULTIPLE DX										
0–19 Years	52	6.6	95	1	3	5	9	9	11	53
20–34	23	8.3	39	1	3	5	15	17	20	20
35–49	84	5.0	34	2	2	3	6	9	14	46
50–64	121	7.2	48	1	3	5	9	14	17	40
65+	165	9.4	48	2	3	8	17	18	18	29
TOTAL SINGLE DX	109	3.2	5	1	1	3	5	7	7	9
MULTIPLE DX	445	7.3	51	2	3	5	9	17	18	40
TOTAL										
0–19 Years	86	5.3	59	1	3	4	6	9	9	53
20–34	45	6.1	31	1	2	4	7	17	17	20
35–49	105	4.6	29	2	2	3	6	9	13	36
50–64	142	6.7	45	1	2	5	9	14	17	40
65+	176	9.2	47	2	3	8	17	18	18	29
GRAND TOTAL	554	6.6	45	1	2	5	9	18	18	36

34.5: PLEURECTOMY. Formerly included in operation group(s) 569.

Type of Patients	Observed Patients	Avg. Stay	Variance	10th	25th	50th	75th	90th	95th	99th
1. SINGLE DX										
0–19 Years	12	8.7	10	5	7	8	10	14	14	14
20–34	27	7.3	11	3	4	9	9	11	12	16
35–49	25	7.9	8	4	5	10	10	18	12	12
50–64	15	7.7	25	4	4	7	12	18	19	19
65+	10	6.2	4	3	4	7	8	8	9	9
2. MULTIPLE DX										
0–19 Years	260	13.6	83	6	8	11	16	24	31	54
20–34	276	12.6	68	5	7	10	16	20	26	47
35–49	512	15.1	89	5	10	13	19	27	36	40
50–64	483	12.0	76	5	6	12	15	23	30	40
65+	677	14.1	86	5	7	12	19	25	31	45
TOTAL SINGLE DX	89	7.7	13	4	4	7	10	12	14	19
MULTIPLE DX	2208	13.6	83	5	7	12	17	24	31	44
TOTAL										
0–19 Years	272	13.4	81	6	8	11	15	24	31	44
20–34	303	12.1	65	5	7	10	15	20	26	47
35–49	537	14.6	87	5	9	12	18	26	36	40
50–64	498	11.8	74	5	6	12	15	23	29	40
65+	687	14.0	86	5	7	12	19	25	31	45
GRAND TOTAL	2297	13.3	81	5	7	11	17	24	31	44

34.26: OPEN MEDIASTINAL BIOPSY. Formerly included in operation group(s) 569.

Type of Patients	Observed Patients	Avg. Stay	Variance	10th	25th	50th	75th	90th	95th	99th
1. SINGLE DX										
0–19 Years	14	6.7	13	1	4	8	10	10	10	10
20–34	30	2.5	12	1	2	2	2	10	10	19
35–49	23	2.0	3	1	1	1	3	5	5	5
50–64	12	2.1	1	1	1	2	2	4	5	5
65+	6	1.5	2	1	1	1	2	5	5	5
2. MULTIPLE DX										
0–19 Years	33	7.0	71	1	1	4	9	25	26	35
20–34	85	6.9	48	1	2	5	8	15	24	36
35–49	66	8.2	40	1	4	6	11	17	17	33
50–64	126	6.6	46	1	3	5	8	14	27	29
65+	203	6.1	47	1	2	5	8	11	18	30
TOTAL SINGLE DX	85	2.9	10	1	1	2	4	8	10	12
MULTIPLE DX	513	6.7	48	1	2	5	9	15	20	34
TOTAL										
0–19 Years	47	6.9	53	1	1	5	10	12	25	35
20–34	115	5.8	43	1	1	4	7	14	19	36
35–49	89	6.6	38	1	2	5	10	17	17	25
50–64	138	6.3	44	1	2	5	7	13	27	29
65+	209	5.9	46	1	1	4	7	11	17	30
GRAND TOTAL	598	6.2	44	1	2	5	8	13	18	30

34.3: DESTR MEDIASTINUM LES. Formerly included in operation group(s) 569.

Type of Patients	Observed Patients	Avg. Stay	Variance	10th	25th	50th	75th	90th	95th	99th
1. SINGLE DX										
0–19 Years	55	4.4	5	2	3	4	5	7	8	13
20–34	20	3.1	2	2	2	3	4	4	5	7
35–49	19	3.0	1	1	2	3	4	4	5	6
50–64	20	5.1	10	3	4	4	5	11	15	15
65+	8	2.9	6	1	2	2	3	9	9	9
2. MULTIPLE DX										
0–19 Years	76	8.3	87	2	4	5	10	22	22	65
20–34	69	6.9	37	3	4	5	7	12	29	31
35–49	86	4.7	10	2	3	4	5	9	9	14
50–64	83	6.2	12	2	3	5	8	9	12	20
65+	90	8.4	54	3	4	6	10	15	18	49
TOTAL SINGLE DX	122	3.8	4	2	3	3	4	7	8	13
MULTIPLE DX	404	6.9	43	2	4	5	8	14	15	31
TOTAL										
0–19 Years	131	6.8	59	2	3	5	7	12	22	35
20–34	89	6.3	33	2	3	5	7	10	14	31
35–49	105	4.1	7	2	3	4	5	6	9	14
50–64	103	6.1	12	3	4	5	8	10	13	20
65+	98	8.0	52	2	4	6	9	15	15	49
GRAND TOTAL	526	6.2	35	2	3	4	7	12	15	31

Length of Stay by Diagnosis and Operation, United States, 1997

United States, October 1995–September 1996 Data, by Operation

34.51: DECORTICATION OF LUNG. Formerly included in operation group(s) 569.

Type of Patients	Observed Patients	Avg. Stay	Vari-ance	Percentiles						
				10th	25th	50th	75th	90th	95th	99th
1. SINGLE DX										
0–19 Years	8	8.1	3	6	7	7	10	10	10	11
20–34	12	8.4	8	4	6	9	9	12	14	16
35–49	14	7.6	5	5	5	9	10	12	10	10
50–64	9	11.3	23	4	8	12	12	19	19	19
65+	5	6.9	3	4	5	7	8	9	9	9
2. MULTIPLE DX										
0–19 Years	221	14.8	90	7	10	12	17	24	31	54
20–34	225	13.2	57	6	9	12	17	21	26	45
35–49	431	16.4	92	7	10	14	20	30	36	44
50–64	398	12.4	76	5	6	10	15	24	31	40
65+	532	14.5	88	5	7	13	19	25	31	47
TOTAL SINGLE DX	48	8.5	10	5	6	9	10	12	12	19
MULTIPLE DX	1807	14.3	84	5	8	12	18	25	33	44
TOTAL										
0–19 Years	229	14.5	88	7	10	11	17	24	31	54
20–34	237	13.0	56	6	9	11	17	20	26	44
35–49	445	15.9	91	6	10	14	19	28	36	44
50–64	407	12.3	75	5	6	10	15	24	30	40
65+	537	14.4	88	5	7	13	19	25	31	47
GRAND TOTAL	1855	14.1	83	5	8	12	18	25	32	44

34.6: SCARIFICATION OF PLEURA. Formerly included in operation group(s) 569.

Type of Patients	Observed Patients	Avg. Stay	Vari-ance	Percentiles						
				10th	25th	50th	75th	90th	95th	99th
1. SINGLE DX										
0–19 Years	15	4.9	12	2	2	5	7	9	9	17
20–34	32	6.6	11	3	4	6	10	11	11	12
35–49	13	7.5	19	2	4	6	10	10	11	19
50–64	6	16.3	170	4	6	13	33	33	33	33
65+	5	6.3	12	3	3	6	7	13	13	13
2. MULTIPLE DX										
0–19 Years	45	10.0	55	4	5	8	12	16	25	36
20–34	111	7.6	52	3	5	5	8	12	19	43
35–49	98	9.9	49	4	5	8	12	19	23	36
50–64	183	10.3	65	3	5	8	14	18	27	46
65+	376	10.7	68	3	5	10	13	20	24	41
TOTAL SINGLE DX	71	6.7	26	2	3	6	9	11	13	33
MULTIPLE DX	813	9.8	62	3	5	8	12	18	24	42
TOTAL										
0–19 Years	60	8.4	47	2	4	7	10	16	20	36
20–34	143	7.5	46	3	5	5	8	12	17	43
35–49	111	9.6	47	4	5	8	11	18	23	36
50–64	189	10.4	67	3	5	8	14	18	27	43
65+	381	10.6	67	3	5	9	13	20	24	41
GRAND TOTAL	884	9.6	60	3	5	8	12	17	23	41

34.59: OTHER PLEURAL EXCISION. Formerly included in operation group(s) 569.

Type of Patients	Observed Patients	Avg. Stay	Vari-ance	Percentiles						
				10th	25th	50th	75th	90th	95th	99th
1. SINGLE DX										
0–19 Years	4	10.7	26	2	4	4	14	14	14	14
20–34	15	6.4	11	3	4	4	11	11	11	12
35–49	11	8.5	13	3	4	10	10	12	12	16
50–64	6	4.6	7	4	4	4	4	7	7	18
65+	5	5.4	4	3	4	6	6	8	8	8
2. MULTIPLE DX										
0–19 Years	39	8.7	27	4	6	8	8	15	19	29
20–34	51	9.2	112	3	4	5	8	20	30	52
35–49	81	10.1	47	3	5	10	15	17	22	34
50–64	85	9.8	66	3	3	8	14	18	20	40
65+	145	13.0	79	4	6	13	22	25	26	42
TOTAL SINGLE DX	41	6.8	14	3	4	4	10	12	14	16
MULTIPLE DX	401	10.7	67	3	5	8	15	22	25	42
TOTAL										
0–19 Years	43	8.8	27	4	6	8	9	15	19	29
20–34	66	8.5	90	3	4	5	9	15	21	52
35–49	92	9.9	44	3	5	10	13	17	22	34
50–64	91	9.1	61	3	3	7	14	18	20	40
65+	150	12.9	78	4	6	9	22	25	26	42
GRAND TOTAL	442	10.3	63	3	5	8	14	22	25	40

34.7: REPAIR OF CHEST WALL. Formerly included in operation group(s) 569.

Type of Patients	Observed Patients	Avg. Stay	Vari-ance	Percentiles						
				10th	25th	50th	75th	90th	95th	99th
1. SINGLE DX										
0–19 Years	344	3.7	1	2	3	4	4	5	5	7
20–34	20	3.1	3	1	1	4	5	5	5	5
35–49	8	1.4	<1	1	1	1	1	3	3	3
50–64	2	7.4	4	2	8	8	8	8	8	8
65+	6	3.1	3	1	2	3	3	6	6	6
2. MULTIPLE DX										
0–19 Years	274	4.4	8	3	3	4	5	6	7	15
20–34	54	5.0	16	1	1	4	8	8	11	14
35–49	59	5.9	28	2	3	4	6	13	13	22
50–64	104	15.2	282	2	3	7	18	51	51	51
65+	138	8.7	92	2	4	7	10	17	25	54
TOTAL SINGLE DX	380	3.6	2	2	3	4	4	5	6	7
MULTIPLE DX	629	6.8	74	2	3	4	6	12	19	51
TOTAL										
0–19 Years	618	4.0	5	3	3	4	5	5	6	9
20–34	74	4.6	14	1	1	4	7	8	10	14
35–49	67	5.3	26	1	3	4	6	13	13	22
50–64	106	14.9	275	2	4	7	17	51	51	51
65+	144	8.6	90	2	4	7	10	17	25	54
GRAND TOTAL	1009	5.6	50	2	3	4	5	8	14	51

Length of Stay by Diagnosis and Operation, United States, 1997

United States, October 1995–September 1996 Data, by Operation

34.74: PECTUS DEFORMITY REPAIR. Formerly included in operation group(s) 569.

Type of Patients	Observed Patients	Avg. Stay	Vari-ance	10th	25th	50th	75th	90th	95th	99th
1. SINGLE DX										
0–19 Years	340	3.7	1	2	3	4	4	5	5	7
20–34	11	4.4		3	4	4	5	5	5	5
35–49		3.0	<1	3	3	3	3	3	3	3
50–64	0									
65+	0									
2. MULTIPLE DX										
0–19 Years	247	4.2	1	3	4	4	5	6	6	7
20–34	16	5.1	5	3	4	4	6	8	12	12
35–49	1	6.0	0	6	6	6	6	6	6	6
50–64	0									
65+	0									
TOTAL SINGLE DX	352	3.7	1	2	3	4	4	5	5	7
MULTIPLE DX	264	4.3	1	3	4	4	5	6	6	8
TOTAL										
0–19 Years	587	3.9	1	3	3	4	5	5	6	7
20–34	27	4.7	3	3	4	4	5	6	8	12
35–49	2	5.7	<1	6	6	6	6	6	6	6
50–64	0									
65+	0									
GRAND TOTAL	616	4.0	1	3	3	4	5	5	6	7

34.9: OTHER OPS ON THORAX. Formerly included in operation group(s) 569, 580, 581.

Type of Patients	Observed Patients	Avg. Stay	Vari-ance	10th	25th	50th	75th	90th	95th	99th
1. SINGLE DX										
0–19 Years	21	4.0	8	2	3	3	4	6	12	17
20–34	49	4.3	14	1	2	3	4	10	11	23
35–49	47	5.3	40	2	2	3	7	10	13	36
50–64	37	6.1	31	2	3	6	6	15	15	28
65+	71	4.8	16	1	1	4	7	10	13	17
2. MULTIPLE DX										
0–19 Years	654	8.3	65	3	4	6	10	15	20	60
20–34	872	8.2	42	2	4	7	11	17	20	31
35–49	2227	8.4	55	2	4	7	11	15	19	40
50–64	4434	7.9	41	2	4	6	10	15	20	31
65+	15897	8.7	42	3	4	7	11	16	21	32
TOTAL SINGLE DX	225	4.9	21	1	2	3	6	10	13	28
MULTIPLE DX	24084	8.5	44	2	4	7	11	16	21	33
TOTAL										
0–19 Years	675	8.1	63	3	4	6	10	14	20	60
20–34	921	8.0	42	2	3	6	10	17	20	30
35–49	2274	8.3	55	2	4	7	11	15	19	40
50–64	4471	7.8	41	2	4	7	10	15	20	31
65+	15968	8.7	42	3	4	7	11	16	21	32
GRAND TOTAL	24309	8.4	44	2	4	7	11	16	21	32

34.8: OPERATIONS ON DIAPHRAGM. Formerly included in operation group(s) 569.

Type of Patients	Observed Patients	Avg. Stay	Vari-ance	10th	25th	50th	75th	90th	95th	99th
1. SINGLE DX										
0–19 Years	3	4.2	5	1	1	6	6	6	6	6
20–34	3	8.4	17	2	3	11	11	11	11	11
35–49	4	5.0	4	3	3	4	7	7	7	7
50–64	0									
65+	0									
2. MULTIPLE DX										
0–19 Years	80	9.5	79	3	5	6	11	19	22	36
20–34	191	9.4	61	4	5	7	10	19	27	38
35–49	85	7.7	74	4	5	4	7	18	23	53
50–64	32	13.2	170	4	5	8	20	26	32	75
65+	34	10.6	101	5	5	7	10	22	35	52
TOTAL SINGLE DX	10	6.5	14	2	3	6	11	11	11	11
MULTIPLE DX	422	9.1	79	4	4	6	10	20	26	53
TOTAL										
0–19 Years	83	9.3	77	3	5	6	11	19	22	36
20–34	194	9.4	59	4	5	7	10	19	27	38
35–49	89	7.7	73	4	5	4	7	18	23	53
50–64	32	13.2	170	4	5	8	20	26	32	75
65+	34	10.6	101	5	5	7	10	22	35	52
GRAND TOTAL	432	9.0	78	4	4	6	10	20	26	53

34.91: THORACENTESIS. Formerly included in operation group(s) 580.

Type of Patients	Observed Patients	Avg. Stay	Vari-ance	10th	25th	50th	75th	90th	95th	99th
1. SINGLE DX										
0–19 Years	19	3.9	9	2	3	3	4	6	12	17
20–34	38	4.2	16	1	2	3	4	10	11	23
35–49	41	4.4	14	2	2	3	5	10	11	20
50–64	32	5.9	31	2	3	6	6	12	15	28
65+	67	4.8	16	1	1	4	7	10	13	17
2. MULTIPLE DX										
0–19 Years	627	8.1	60	3	4	6	10	14	20	60
20–34	839	7.8	39	2	4	6	10	15	20	31
35–49	2109	8.4	56	2	4	7	11	15	20	40
50–64	4175	7.9	42	2	4	7	10	15	20	31
65+	15299	8.7	42	3	4	7	11	16	21	32
TOTAL SINGLE DX	197	4.6	17	1	2	3	6	10	13	23
MULTIPLE DX	23049	8.4	44	2	4	7	11	16	21	33
TOTAL										
0–19 Years	646	7.9	59	3	4	6	10	14	20	60
20–34	877	7.6	38	2	3	6	10	15	20	30
35–49	2150	8.3	56	2	4	7	11	15	20	40
50–64	4207	7.8	42	2	4	6	10	15	20	31
65+	15366	8.7	42	3	4	7	11	16	21	32
GRAND TOTAL	23246	8.4	44	2	4	7	11	16	21	32

Length of Stay by Diagnosis and Operation, United States, 1997

United States, October 1995–September 1996 Data, by Operation

34.92: INJECT INTO THOR CAVIT. Formerly included in operation group(s) 581.

Type of Patients	Observed Patients	Avg. Stay	Variance	10th	25th	50th	75th	90th	95th	99th
1. SINGLE DX										
0–19 Years	2	5.4	<1	5	5	5	5	7	7	7
20–34	11	4.9	6	2	2	4	8	8	9	9
35–49	5	13.8	184	5	5	8	36	36	36	36
50–64	5	7.8	30	3	3	7	15	15	15	15
65+	3	6.9	4	5	5	6	9	9	9	9
2. MULTIPLE DX										
0–19 Years	19	11.3	203	3	4	5	14	23	65	65
20–34	24	13.7	55	3	6	20	20	20	20	22
35–49	107	8.1	30	4	4	6	12	15	17	25
50–64	245	8.0	25	3	5	7	9	15	18	27
65+	578	8.9	40	3	4	7	11	18	20	35
TOTAL SINGLE DX	26	7.7	58	2	4	5	8	15	36	36
MULTIPLE DX	973	8.9	41	3	4	7	11	18	20	32
TOTAL										
0–19 Years	21	10.8	187	4	4	5	14	21	25	65
20–34	35	12.8	57	2	4	15	20	20	20	22
35–49	112	8.3	35	4	4	6	12	15	17	35
50–64	250	8.0	25	3	5	7	9	15	18	27
65+	581	8.9	40	3	4	7	11	18	20	35
GRAND TOTAL	999	8.8	41	3	4	7	11	18	20	32

35.0: CLOSED HEART VALVOTOMY. Formerly included in operation group(s) 579.

Type of Patients	Observed Patients	Avg. Stay	Variance	10th	25th	50th	75th	90th	95th	99th
1. SINGLE DX										
0–19 Years	11	1.6	2	1	1	1	1	4	4	8
20–34	1	1.0	0	1	1	1	1	1	1	1
35–49	1	5.0	0	5	5	5	5	5	5	5
50–64	0									
65+	0									
2. MULTIPLE DX										
0–19 Years	30	5.6	34	1	1	4	7	15	17	32
20–34	2	8.8	7	7	7	7	11	11	11	11
35–49	1	2.0	0	2	2	2	2	2	2	2
50–64	4	5.9	16	2	2	5	9	11	11	11
65+	4	9.9	72	2	7	8	8	27	27	27
TOTAL SINGLE DX	13	1.6	2	1	1	1	1	4	5	8
MULTIPLE DX	41	5.9	35	1	1	5	9	15	17	27
TOTAL										
0–19 Years	41	4.3	27	1	1	1	5	15	16	18
20–34	3	3.2	15	1	1	1	7	11	11	11
35–49	2	3.8	4	2	2	5	5	5	5	5
50–64	4	5.9	16	2	2	5	9	11	11	11
65+	4	9.9	72	2	7	8	8	27	27	27
GRAND TOTAL	54	4.5	28	1	1	1	6	11	16	27

35.1: OPEN HEART VALVULOPLASTY. Formerly included in operation group(s) 572.

Type of Patients	Observed Patients	Avg. Stay	Variance	10th	25th	50th	75th	90th	95th	99th
1. SINGLE DX										
0–19 Years	48	3.6	2	2	3	4	4	6	6	7
20–34	7	5.7	6	1	4	6	7	9	9	9
35–49	15	5.3	4	3	5	5	5	8	9	12
50–64	7	6.0	10	1	5	6	6	7	14	14
65+	3	6.1	2	6	6	6	6	6	6	16
2. MULTIPLE DX										
0–19 Years	569	8.0	110	3	4	5	7	15	29	63
20–34	84	6.8	30	4	4	5	8	8	12	41
35–49	186	7.6	32	4	4	6	8	15	20	37
50–64	306	9.5	54	5	6	8	11	15	19	35
65+	393	11.3	62	5	6	9	12	19	26	38
TOTAL SINGLE DX	80	5.0	4	3	4	5	6	6	7	12
MULTIPLE DX	1538	9.1	77	4	5	6	10	17	24	48
TOTAL										
0–19 Years	617	7.8	105	3	4	5	7	14	27	63
20–34	91	6.8	29	4	4	5	8	8	12	41
35–49	201	7.5	30	4	5	5	8	13	19	37
50–64	313	9.4	54	5	6	8	11	15	18	35
65+	396	10.9	60	5	6	9	12	19	26	38
GRAND TOTAL	1618	8.9	74	4	5	6	10	16	23	43

35.11: OPN AORTIC VALVULOPLASTY. Formerly included in operation group(s) 572.

Type of Patients	Observed Patients	Avg. Stay	Variance	10th	25th	50th	75th	90th	95th	99th
1. SINGLE DX										
0–19 Years	35	3.7	2	2	3	4	4	5	6	7
20–34	2	3.1	2	1	1	4	4	4	4	4
35–49	2	4.2	2	3	3	5	5	5	5	5
50–64	0									
65+	3	6.1	2	6	6	6	6	6	6	16
2. MULTIPLE DX										
0–19 Years	222	7.6	102	3	3	5	7	15	21	73
20–34	37	6.5	7	4	4	7	8	8	8	18
35–49	34	8.6	67	4	4	5	8	19	37	37
50–64	53	11.1	202	5	5	8	10	18	25	90
65+	50	9.6	44	6	6	6	11	18	21	37
TOTAL SINGLE DX	42	5.0	3	3	4	6	6	6	6	7
MULTIPLE DX	396	8.2	87	3	4	6	8	16	21	48
TOTAL										
0–19 Years	257	7.2	94	3	3	4	7	14	21	73
20–34	39	6.4	7	4	4	7	8	8	8	18
35–49	36	8.4	66	4	4	5	8	19	37	37
50–64	53	11.1	202	5	5	8	10	18	25	90
65+	53	8.6	35	6	6	6	8	17	18	34
GRAND TOTAL	438	7.8	78	3	4	6	8	15	20	37

Length of Stay by Diagnosis and Operation, United States, 1997

United States, October 1995–September 1996 Data, by Operation

35.12: OPN MITRAL VALVULOPLASTY. Formerly included in operation group(s) 572.

Type of Patients	Observed Patients	Avg. Stay	Variance	Percentiles						
				10th	25th	50th	75th	90th	95th	99th
1. SINGLE DX										
0–19 Years	8	3.5	<1	3	3	3	4	4	6	6
20–34	5	7.1	2	5	6	7	8	9	9	9
35–49	13	5.4	4	5	5	5	5	8	9	9
50–64	7	6.0	10	1	5	6	6	7	12	14
65+	0									
2. MULTIPLE DX										
0–19 Years	196	7.9	99	3	4	5	7	13	30	55
20–34	43	5.6	4	3	5	5	6	10	10	12
35–49	146	7.3	21	4	5	6	8	13	17	24
50–64	246	9.2	29	5	6	8	11	13	17	31
65+	328	11.7	66	5	7	9	12	20	30	38
TOTAL SINGLE DX	33	5.1	5	3	3	5	6	8	9	14
MULTIPLE DX	959	9.5	61	4	5	7	11	17	25	41
TOTAL										
0–19 Years	204	7.8	97	3	4	5	7	11	30	55
20–34	48	5.7	4	4	5	5	6	9	10	12
35–49	159	7.1	20	4	5	5	8	13	17	24
50–64	253	9.1	29	5	6	8	11	13	16	31
65+	328	11.7	66	5	7	9	12	20	30	38
GRAND TOTAL	992	9.3	60	4	5	7	11	17	24	40

35.2: HEART VALVE REPLACEMENT. Formerly included in operation group(s) 570.

Type of Patients	Observed Patients	Avg. Stay	Variance	Percentiles						
				10th	25th	50th	75th	90th	95th	99th
1. SINGLE DX										
0–19 Years	28	5.5	16	3	3	5	5	8	18	18
20–34	42	5.8	4	4	4	6	6	8	10	14
35–49	86	5.5	7	4	4	4	6	9	12	15
50–64	81	7.7	58	5	5	6	7	9	12	67
65+	51	11.6	16	6	7	14	14	14	14	21
2. MULTIPLE DX										
0–19 Years	479	8.9	94	4	5	6	9	17	29	50
20–34	449	9.2	57	4	5	6	10	18	23	48
35–49	1455	10.2	55	5	6	8	13	18	24	37
50–64	3469	10.5	70	5	6	8	12	19	24	49
65+	8681	12.4	83	6	7	10	14	22	30	55
TOTAL SINGLE DX	288	7.9	30	4	5	6	9	14	14	22
MULTIPLE DX	14533	11.5	78	5	6	9	13	21	28	50
TOTAL										
0–19 Years	507	8.8	92	4	5	6	9	17	29	50
20–34	491	8.9	53	4	5	6	10	16	22	48
35–49	1541	9.9	53	4	6	8	13	17	23	37
50–64	3550	10.4	70	5	6	8	12	19	24	49
65+	8732	12.4	82	6	7	10	14	22	30	55
GRAND TOTAL	14821	11.4	77	5	6	9	13	20	28	50

35.21: REPL AORTIC VALVE-TISSUE. Formerly included in operation group(s) 570.

Type of Patients	Observed Patients	Avg. Stay	Variance	Percentiles						
				10th	25th	50th	75th	90th	95th	99th
1. SINGLE DX										
0–19 Years	10	4.0	<1	3	3	4	5	5	5	5
20–34	7	4.4	<1	3	3	4	6	6	6	6
35–49	12	4.7	2	4	4	4	5	6	10	10
50–64	3	6.3	1	5	5	7	7	7	7	7
65+	10	6.3	<1	5	6	7	7	7	7	7
2. MULTIPLE DX										
0–19 Years	141	8.2	74	4	4	5	8	12	34	39
20–34	72	7.9	27	4	5	6	8	15	20	27
35–49	142	10.8	23	5	7	13	13	13	16	27
50–64	233	10.9	65	4	5	7	14	21	21	38
65+	1735	11.3	64	6	7	9	13	19	24	47
TOTAL SINGLE DX	42	5.0	2	3	4	5	6	7	7	10
MULTIPLE DX	2323	10.9	61	5	6	9	13	19	24	44
TOTAL										
0–19 Years	151	8.0	71	4	4	5	7	12	34	39
20–34	79	7.6	26	4	5	6	8	15	20	27
35–49	154	10.5	23	4	6	13	13	13	16	27
50–64	236	10.9	65	4	6	7	14	21	21	38
65+	1745	11.3	64	6	7	9	13	19	24	47
GRAND TOTAL	2365	10.8	60	5	6	9	13	19	24	44

35.22: REPL AORTIC VALVE NEC. Formerly included in operation group(s) 570.

Type of Patients	Observed Patients	Avg. Stay	Variance	Percentiles						
				10th	25th	50th	75th	90th	95th	99th
1. SINGLE DX										
0–19 Years	7	6.6	4	4	5	6	8	8	11	11
20–34	24	5.8	3	4	5	6	7	7	9	14
35–49	50	5.5	9	4	4	4	6	9	15	15
50–64	58	7.0	9	5	5	7	8	9	11	22
65+	35	12.1	10	7	10	14	14	14	14	14
2. MULTIPLE DX										
0–19 Years	98	8.0	36	3	5	6	9	17	17	35
20–34	205	8.8	37	4	5	7	11	16	23	34
35–49	752	9.6	50	5	6	8	11	17	23	37
50–64	2021	9.1	32	5	6	7	10	15	19	30
65+	4659	12.2	81	6	7	9	14	22	32	56
TOTAL SINGLE DX	174	8.3	17	4	5	7	14	14	14	16
MULTIPLE DX	7735	10.9	65	5	6	8	13	19	26	44
TOTAL										
0–19 Years	105	8.0	35	3	5	6	9	17	17	35
20–34	229	8.5	35	4	5	6	10	15	21	34
35–49	802	9.3	48	5	5	7	13	17	23	37
50–64	2079	9.1	32	5	6	7	10	15	19	30
65+	4694	12.2	80	6	7	9	14	22	32	56
GRAND TOTAL	7909	10.9	64	5	6	8	13	19	26	44

Length of Stay by Diagnosis and Operation, United States, 1997

35.23: REPL MITRAL VALVE W TISS. Formerly included in operation group(s) 570.

Type of Patients	Observed Patients	Avg. Stay	Vari-ance	10th	25th	50th	75th	90th	95th	99th
1. SINGLE DX										
0–19 Years	1	5.0	0	5	5	5	5	5	5	5
20–34	0									
35–49	1	4.0	0	4	4	4	4	4	4	4
50–64	0									
65+	1	14.0	0	14	14	14	14	14	14	14
2. MULTIPLE DX										
0–19 Years	5	9.9	32	5	5	8	13	18	18	18
20–34	18	18.7	245	5	6	10	21	48	48	48
35–49	25	12.1	42	6	7	9	15	21	21	35
50–64	78	20.5	475	6	8	10	21	51	85	85
65+	472	13.6	122	5	6	11	16	25	33	57
TOTAL SINGLE DX	3	10.2	25	4	5	14	14	14	14	14
MULTIPLE DX	598	14.4	164	5	7	10	16	26	46	61
TOTAL										
0–19 Years	6	9.0	29	5	5	5	13	18	18	18
20–34	18	18.7	245	5	6	10	21	48	48	48
35–49	26	12.0	43	6	7	9	15	21	21	35
50–64	78	20.5	475	6	8	10	21	51	85	85
65+	473	13.6	122	5	6	11	16	25	33	57
GRAND TOTAL	601	14.4	163	5	7	10	16	26	46	61

35.3: TISS ADJ TO HRT VALV OPS. Formerly included in operation group(s) 572.

Type of Patients	Observed Patients	Avg. Stay	Vari-ance	10th	25th	50th	75th	90th	95th	99th
1. SINGLE DX										
0–19 Years	28	3.2	<1	2	3	3	4	4	4	5
20–34	2	8.2	71	3	3	3	17	17	17	17
35–49	2	5.8	9	4	4	4	10	10	10	10
50–64	5	5.1	1	3	5	5	6	7	7	7
65+	1	6.0	0	6	6	6	6	6	6	6
2. MULTIPLE DX										
0–19 Years	126	5.8	21	3	4	4	6	11	14	27
20–34	37	6.1	8	4	4	5	8	9	12	17
35–49	100	9.3	185	4	5	6	7	14	26	86
50–64	222	10.0	42	5	6	7	12	17	20	37
65+	349	12.8	84	5	7	11	15	22	33	56
TOTAL SINGLE DX	38	3.8	4	2	3	3	4	6	6	10
MULTIPLE DX	834	10.3	80	4	5	7	12	19	25	48
TOTAL										
0–19 Years	154	5.3	19	3	3	4	6	10	12	27
20–34	39	6.2	9	4	4	5	8	10	14	17
35–49	102	9.3	182	4	5	6	7	13	26	86
50–64	227	9.9	41	5	6	7	12	17	20	37
65+	350	12.8	84	5	7	11	15	22	33	56
GRAND TOTAL	872	10.1	78	4	5	7	12	18	24	48

35.24: REPL MITRAL VALVE NEC. Formerly included in operation group(s) 570.

Type of Patients	Observed Patients	Avg. Stay	Vari-ance	10th	25th	50th	75th	90th	95th	99th
1. SINGLE DX										
0–19 Years	5	3.8	<1	3	3	3	5	5	5	5
20–34	9	7.1	4	5	6	6	10	10	10	10
35–49	19	6.1	2	4	5	6	7	9	9	9
50–64	20	8.7	121	6	6	6	6	12	22	67
65+	5	14.8	64	4	5	21	21	21	21	21
2. MULTIPLE DX										
0–19 Years	86	11.0	100	5	6	7	12	23	33	58
20–34	115	9.5	72	5	5	7	10	18	24	55
35–49	509	10.7	80	4	6	8	12	20	30	42
50–64	1116	12.5	103	5	7	9	14	23	33	60
65+	1779	13.6	91	6	8	10	16	24	33	52
TOTAL SINGLE DX	58	8.0	76	5	6	6	6	10	21	67
MULTIPLE DX	3605	12.6	94	5	7	10	15	23	33	54
TOTAL										
0–19 Years	91	10.6	97	5	5	7	11	22	33	58
20–34	124	9.2	65	5	5	7	10	15	24	55
35–49	528	10.6	78	4	6	8	11	20	30	42
50–64	1136	12.3	104	6	6	9	13	23	32	60
65+	1784	13.6	91	6	8	10	16	24	33	52
GRAND TOTAL	3663	12.5	94	5	7	9	14	23	33	55

35.33: ANNULOPLASTY. Formerly included in operation group(s) 572.

Type of Patients	Observed Patients	Avg. Stay	Vari-ance	10th	25th	50th	75th	90th	95th	99th
1. SINGLE DX										
0–19 Years	3	2.7	1	2	2	2	4	4	4	4
20–34	1	3.0	0	3	3	3	3	3	3	3
35–49	2	5.8	9	4	4	4	10	10	10	10
50–64	5	5.1	1	3	5	5	6	7	7	7
65+	1	6.0	0	6	6	6	6	6	6	6
2. MULTIPLE DX										
0–19 Years	26	7.2	44	2	4	5	8	16	17	27
20–34	28	5.8	7	4	4	5	6	10	12	14
35–49	96	9.4	189	4	5	6	7	14	26	86
50–64	214	9.6	42	5	6	7	11	18	20	37
65+	342	12.8	85	5	7	11	15	23	33	56
TOTAL SINGLE DX	12	4.7	4	2	3	5	6	6	7	10
MULTIPLE DX	706	11.1	88	5	6	8	12	20	27	56
TOTAL										
0–19 Years	29	6.9	42	2	4	5	8	14	17	27
20–34	29	5.7	7	3	4	5	6	10	12	14
35–49	98	9.3	186	4	5	6	7	14	26	86
50–64	219	9.5	41	5	6	7	11	17	20	37
65+	343	12.8	85	5	7	11	15	22	33	56
GRAND TOTAL	718	11.0	87	5	6	8	12	20	27	56

Length of Stay by Diagnosis and Operation, United States, 1997

United States, October 1995–September 1996 Data, by Operation

35.4: SEPTAL DEFECT PRODUCTION. Formerly included in operation group(s) 572.

Type of Patients	Observed Patients	Avg. Stay	Variance	Percentiles						
				10th	25th	50th	75th	90th	95th	99th
1. SINGLE DX										
0–19 Years	2	5.1	3	4	4	4	7	7	7	7
20–34	0									
35–49	0									
50–64	0									
65+	0									
2. MULTIPLE DX										
0–19 Years	158	13.5	117	5	6	9	18	30	41	>99
20–34	2	5.0	22	1	1	1	10	10	10	10
35–49	1	15.0	0	15	15	15	15	15	15	15
50–64	0									
65+	1	2.0	0	2	2	2	2	2	2	2
TOTAL SINGLE DX	2	5.1	3	4	4	4	7	7	7	7
MULTIPLE DX	162	13.3	116	5	6	9	17	30	41	>99
TOTAL										
0–19 Years	160	13.4	117	5	6	9	18	30	41	>99
20–34	2	5.0	22	1	1	1	10	10	10	10
35–49	1	15.0	0	15	15	15	15	15	15	15
50–64	0									
65+	1	2.0	0	2	2	2	2	2	2	2
GRAND TOTAL	164	13.2	115	4	6	9	17	30	41	>99

35.5: PROSTH REP HEART SEPTA. Formerly included in operation group(s) 572, 579.

Type of Patients	Observed Patients	Avg. Stay	Variance	Percentiles						
				10th	25th	50th	75th	90th	95th	99th
1. SINGLE DX										
0–19 Years	158	3.5	2	2	3	3	4	5	6	9
20–34	10	3.6	<1	3	3	3	4	5	5	5
35–49	9	4.5	2	4	4	4	4	7	7	7
50–64	3	4.4	1	2	4	4	4	7	7	7
65+	1	6.0	0	6	6	6	6	6	6	6
2. MULTIPLE DX										
0–19 Years	1160	8.7	80	3	4	6	9	18	26	51
20–34	39	7.1	25	3	5	7	7	11	11	38
35–49	30	5.5	11	1	4	6	6	8	15	17
50–64	29	10.0	112	4	9	6	8	21	37	52
65+	33	13.7	88	6	9	10	17	30	32	48
TOTAL SINGLE DX	181	3.6	2	2	3	3	4	5	6	7
MULTIPLE DX	1291	8.7	79	3	4	6	9	18	26	51
TOTAL										
0–19 Years	1318	8.2	74	3	4	5	9	17	24	49
20–34	49	6.5	23	3	4	7	7	9	11	38
35–49	39	5.1	8	2	4	4	7	7	9	17
50–64	32	9.5	104	4	4	7	7	21	37	52
65+	34	13.5	87	6	9	10	17	30	32	48
GRAND TOTAL	1472	8.2	73	3	4	6	9	17	24	49

35.53: PROSTH REP VSD. Formerly included in operation group(s) 572.

Type of Patients	Observed Patients	Avg. Stay	Variance	Percentiles						
				10th	25th	50th	75th	90th	95th	99th
1. SINGLE DX										
0–19 Years	79	3.5	2	2	3	3	4	5	6	8
20–34	3	3.3	<1	3	3	3	4	4	4	4
35–49	1	7.0	0	7	7	7	7	7	7	7
50–64	1	4.0	0	4	4	4	4	6	6	7
65+	1	6.0	0	6	6	6	6	6	6	6
2. MULTIPLE DX										
0–19 Years	788	8.8	77	3	4	6	9	18	26	51
20–34	12	6.3	4	3	5	7	7	10	10	14
35–49	8	7.6	23	3	4	6	9	15	17	17
50–64	9	19.0	225	6	7	16	21	37	52	52
65+	18	16.8	72	6	9	17	20	30	32	32
TOTAL SINGLE DX	85	3.6	2	2	3	3	4	6	7	8
MULTIPLE DX	835	8.9	77	3	4	6	9	18	26	51
TOTAL										
0–19 Years	867	8.4	73	3	4	6	9	17	24	49
20–34	15	5.9	5	3	4	7	7	7	8	14
35–49	9	7.4	15	3	6	6	9	15	17	17
50–64	10	17.5	222	4	7	11	21	37	52	52
65+	19	16.2	74	6	9	16	20	30	32	32
GRAND TOTAL	920	8.5	74	3	4	6	9	17	24	49

35.6: TISS GRFT REP HRT SEPTA. Formerly included in operation group(s) 572.

Type of Patients	Observed Patients	Avg. Stay	Variance	Percentiles						
				10th	25th	50th	75th	90th	95th	99th
1. SINGLE DX										
0–19 Years	173	3.5	1	2	3	3	4	5	5	8
20–34	24	3.3	<1	2	3	3	4	5	5	6
35–49	14	4.4	<1	3	4	5	5	5	6	6
50–64	2	4.0	0	4	4	5	5	4	4	4
65+	1	2.0	0	2	2	2	2	2	2	2
2. MULTIPLE DX										
0–19 Years	688	7.4	60	3	4	5	8	14	20	43
20–34	64	5.4	5	3	4	5	7	8	9	13
35–49	70	6.3	18	3	4	5	7	13	18	18
50–64	55	7.4	24	4	5	6	7	14	16	26
65+	47	9.7	51	5	6	8	10	15	24	44
TOTAL SINGLE DX	214	3.6	1	2	3	3	4	5	5	7
MULTIPLE DX	924	7.3	52	3	4	5	8	14	20	43
TOTAL										
0–19 Years	861	6.6	50	3	3	4	7	13	19	43
20–34	88	4.9	4	3	3	4	6	9	9	13
35–49	84	5.9	15	3	4	5	6	11	18	18
50–64	57	7.3	24	4	5	6	7	14	16	26
65+	48	9.6	52	5	6	8	10	15	24	44
GRAND TOTAL	1138	6.6	44	3	4	5	7	13	18	38

Length of Stay by Diagnosis and Operation, United States, 1997

United States, October 1995–September 1996 Data, by Operation

35.61: REPAIR ASD W TISS GRAFT. Formerly included in operation group(s) 572.

Type of Patients	Observed Patients	Avg. Stay	Vari-ance	Percentiles						
				10th	25th	50th	75th	90th	95th	99th
1. SINGLE DX										
0–19 Years	151	3.4	<1	2	3	3	4	5	5	6
20–34	23	3.3	<1	2	3	3	4	5	5	6
35–49	14	4.4	<1	3	4	5	5	5	5	6
50–64	2	4.0	0	4	4	4	4	4	4	4
65+	1	2.0	0	2	2	2	2	2	2	2
2. MULTIPLE DX										
0–19 Years	288	5.9	50	3	3	4	5	11	20	26
20–34	58	5.2	4	3	4	5	6	8	9	13
35–49	66	6.3	18	3	4	5	6	11	18	18
50–64	48	6.5	9	4	5	6	6	10	14	16
65+	36	8.4	11	5	6	8	9	14	15	21
TOTAL SINGLE DX	191	3.5	<1	2	3	3	4	5	5	6
MULTIPLE DX	496	6.1	36	3	3	5	6	10	18	24
TOTAL										
0–19 Years	439	5.1	35	3	3	4	5	7	15	24
20–34	81	4.7	4	3	3	4	5	7	9	13
35–49	80	5.9	15	3	4	5	6	11	18	18
50–64	50	6.4	9	4	5	6	6	10	14	16
65+	37	8.3	12	5	6	8	9	14	15	21
GRAND TOTAL	687	5.3	28	3	3	4	6	8	14	22

35.7: HEART SEPTA REP NEC/NOS. Formerly included in operation group(s) 572.

Type of Patients	Observed Patients	Avg. Stay	Vari-ance	Percentiles						
				10th	25th	50th	75th	90th	95th	99th
1. SINGLE DX										
0–19 Years	381	3.2	1	2	3	3	4	5	5	6
20–34	25	4.1	<1	3	4	4	5	5	6	6
35–49	22	4.1	1	3	3	4	5	5	5	6
50–64	3	4.6	1	4	4	4	6	6	6	6
65+	1	2.0	0	2	2	2	2	2	2	2
2. MULTIPLE DX										
0–19 Years	940	6.6	77	3	3	4	6	11	15	57
20–34	83	5.0	4	3	4	4	6	7	9	12
35–49	99	6.2	63	4	4	5	6	9	11	17
50–64	97	7.4	19	4	5	6	10	11	15	22
65+	78	14.3	369	5	6	8	13	25	85	85
TOTAL SINGLE DX	432	3.3	1	2	3	3	4	5	5	6
MULTIPLE DX	1297	6.9	84	3	3	5	7	11	16	61
TOTAL										
0–19 Years	1321	5.6	57	2	3	4	5	9	14	50
20–34	108	4.8	3	3	4	4	5	7	9	12
35–49	121	5.7	49	3	4	5	6	9	11	17
50–64	100	7.4	19	4	5	6	10	11	15	22
65+	79	14.2	368	5	6	8	13	25	85	85
GRAND TOTAL	1729	6.0	65	3	3	4	6	10	14	53

35.71: REPAIR ASD NEC. Formerly included in operation group(s) 572.

Type of Patients	Observed Patients	Avg. Stay	Vari-ance	Percentiles						
				10th	25th	50th	75th	90th	95th	99th
1. SINGLE DX										
0–19 Years	327	3.2	<1	2	3	3	4	4	5	6
20–34	22	4.2	<1	3	4	4	5	5	6	6
35–49	18	3.9	<1	3	3	4	5	5	5	6
50–64	3	4.6	1	4	4	4	6	6	6	6
65+	1	2.0	0	2	2	2	2	2	2	2
2. MULTIPLE DX										
0–19 Years	542	4.9	26	2	3	4	5	7	9	30
20–34	67	4.8	3	3	4	4	6	7	9	9
35–49	91	6.2	70	4	4	5	6	9	11	84
50–64	87	6.9	18	4	5	6	9	11	15	21
65+	61	14.9	429	5	5	8	13	27	85	85
TOTAL SINGLE DX	371	3.3	1	2	3	3	4	5	5	6
MULTIPLE DX	848	5.7	55	3	3	4	6	9	12	42
TOTAL										
0–19 Years	869	4.3	18	2	3	3	5	6	8	18
20–34	89	4.6	3	3	4	4	5	6	8	9
35–49	109	5.7	57	3	4	4	6	7	11	17
50–64	90	6.8	18	4	5	6	9	11	15	21
65+	62	14.8	427	5	5	8	13	27	85	85
GRAND TOTAL	1219	4.9	39	2	3	4	5	7	10	27

35.72: REPAIR VSD NEC. Formerly included in operation group(s) 572.

Type of Patients	Observed Patients	Avg. Stay	Vari-ance	Percentiles						
				10th	25th	50th	75th	90th	95th	99th
1. SINGLE DX										
0–19 Years	44	3.8	2	3	3	4	4	5	5	14
20–34	3	3.3	<1	3	3	4	4	4	4	4
35–49	3	4.8	<1	3	5	5	5	5	5	5
50–64	0									
65+	0									
2. MULTIPLE DX										
0–19 Years	268	8.2	102	3	4	5	8	14	28	61
20–34	12	5.9	4	3	5	5	8	9	10	10
35–49	7	6.3	2	5	6	6	6	7	11	11
50–64	5	10.9	12	10	10	10	10	11	22	22
65+	17	11.0	28	5	7	11	14	18	18	25
TOTAL SINGLE DX	50	3.9	2	3	3	4	4	5	5	14
MULTIPLE DX	309	8.3	93	3	4	5	8	14	28	61
TOTAL										
0–19 Years	312	7.7	92	3	4	5	7	14	28	61
20–34	15	5.4	5	3	4	5	7	9	10	10
35–49	10	5.7	2	5	5	5	6	7	11	11
50–64	5	10.9	12	10	10	10	10	11	22	22
65+	17	11.0	28	5	7	11	14	18	18	25
GRAND TOTAL	359	7.8	84	3	4	5	8	14	27	61

United States, October 1995–September 1996 Data, by Operation

35.8: TOT REP CONG CARD ANOM. Formerly included in operation group(s) 572.

Type of Patients	Observed Patients	Avg. Stay	Vari-ance	10th	25th	50th	75th	90th	95th	99th
1. SINGLE DX										
0–19 Years	102	6.1	6	4	5	5	7	9	11	15
20–34	1	4.0	0	4	4	4	4	4	4	4
35–49	0									
50–64	0									
65+	0									
2. MULTIPLE DX										
0–19 Years	984	13.8	169	5	7	10	16	27	39	88
20–34	7	7.0	7	4	5	7	10	11	11	11
35–49	7	9.1	18	6	6	6	13	16	16	16
50–64	5	13.5	67	7	7	8	22	24	24	24
65+	4	6.8	6	5	5	6	10	10	10	10
TOTAL SINGLE DX	103	6.1	6	4	4	5	7	9	11	14
MULTIPLE DX	1007	13.7	168	5	7	10	15	27	38	88
TOTAL										
0–19 Years	1086	13.1	160	5	6	9	15	26	37	88
20–34	8	6.1	6	4	4	5	8	10	11	11
35–49	7	9.1	18	6	6	6	13	16	16	16
50–64	5	13.5	67	7	7	8	22	24	24	24
65+	4	6.8	6	5	5	6	10	10	10	10
GRAND TOTAL	1110	13.0	158	5	6	9	14	26	37	88

35.81: TOT REP TETRALOGY FALLOT. Formerly included in operation group(s) 572.

Type of Patients	Observed Patients	Avg. Stay	Vari-ance	10th	25th	50th	75th	90th	95th	99th
1. SINGLE DX										
0–19 Years	89	6.0	5	4	5	5	7	9	11	13
20–34	1	4.0	0	4	4	4	4	4	4	4
35–49	0									
50–64	0									
65+	0									
2. MULTIPLE DX										
0–19 Years	598	11.9	165	5	6	8	12	23	31	90
20–34	5	8.1	5	5	7	8	10	11	11	11
35–49	6	9.5	18	6	6	6	13	16	16	16
50–64	3	12.4	70	7	7	8	24	24	24	24
65+	1	5.0	0	5	5	5	5	5	5	5
TOTAL SINGLE DX	90	6.0	5	4	5	5	7	9	11	13
MULTIPLE DX	613	11.8	163	5	6	8	12	23	29	88
TOTAL										
0–19 Years	687	11.2	149	5	6	7	11	20	28	88
20–34	6	6.6	7	4	4	5	8	11	11	11
35–49	6	9.5	18	6	6	6	13	16	16	16
50–64	3	12.4	70	7	7	8	24	24	24	24
65+	1	5.0	0	5	5	5	5	5	5	5
GRAND TOTAL	703	11.1	147	5	6	7	11	20	28	88

35.9: VALVES & SEPTA OPS NEC. Formerly included in operation group(s) 572.

Type of Patients	Observed Patients	Avg. Stay	Vari-ance	10th	25th	50th	75th	90th	95th	99th
1. SINGLE DX										
0–19 Years	172	2.0	5	1	1	1	2	5	7	12
20–34	10	1.5	1	1	1	1	2	3	3	6
35–49	16	1.5	<1	1	1	1	2	2	3	3
50–64	6	1.0	0	1	1	1	1	1	1	1
65+	2	4.2	12	1	1	7	7	7	7	7
2. MULTIPLE DX										
0–19 Years	1023	8.6	86	1	3	6	10	19	27	50
20–34	42	6.7	40	1	1	6	8	14	17	37
35–49	62	4.7	32	1	1	2	6	12	21	27
50–64	84	5.7	22	1	2	5	7	13	16	20
65+	189	8.5	55	1	3	7	12	17	22	41
TOTAL SINGLE DX	206	1.9	5	1	1	1	2	5	7	11
MULTIPLE DX	1400	8.2	77	1	2	6	10	18	26	43
TOTAL										
0–19 Years	1195	7.6	80	1	1	5	9	17	26	44
20–34	52	5.7	37	1	1	5	8	14	17	37
35–49	78	4.0	26	1	1	2	4	10	17	27
50–64	90	5.4	22	1	1	4	7	13	16	20
65+	191	8.5	55	1	3	7	12	17	22	41
GRAND TOTAL	1606	7.4	72	1	1	5	9	16	25	42

35.94: CREAT CONDUIT ATRIUM-PA. Formerly included in operation group(s) 572.

Type of Patients	Observed Patients	Avg. Stay	Vari-ance	10th	25th	50th	75th	90th	95th	99th
1. SINGLE DX										
0–19 Years	20	7.7	9	4	6	7	10	11	12	14
20–34	0									
35–49	0									
50–64	0									
65+	0									
2. MULTIPLE DX										
0–19 Years	449	11.5	71	5	7	9	13	24	29	44
20–34	10	9.5	59	5	6	6	10	14	37	37
35–49	1	17.0	0	17	17	17	17	17	17	17
50–64	0									
65+	0									
TOTAL SINGLE DX	20	7.7	9	4	6	7	10	11	12	14
MULTIPLE DX	460	11.4	70	5	7	9	13	24	29	44
TOTAL										
0–19 Years	469	11.4	69	5	7	9	12	24	29	44
20–34	10	9.5	59	5	6	6	10	14	37	37
35–49	1	17.0	0	17	17	17	17	17	17	17
50–64	0									
65+	0									
GRAND TOTAL	480	11.3	69	5	6	8	12	24	29	44

Length of Stay by Diagnosis and Operation, United States, 1997

United States, October 1995–September 1996 Data, by Operation

35.96: PERC VALVULOPLASTY. Formerly included in operation group(s) 572.

Type of Patients	Observed Patients	Avg. Stay	Vari-ance	10th	25th	50th	75th	90th	95th	99th
1. SINGLE DX										
0–19 Years	141	1.4	1	1	1	1	1	2	3	7
20–34	9	1.3	<1	1	1	1	1	2	3	3
35–49	16	1.5	<1	1	1	1	2	2	3	3
50–64	6	1.0	0	1	1	1	1	1	1	1
65+	1	1.0	0	1	1	1	1	1	1	1
2. MULTIPLE DX										
0–19 Years	242	3.3	39	1	1	1	2	9	13	24
20–34	13	2.4	7	1	1	1	2	8	9	10
35–49	51	3.2	19	1	1	2	3	6	12	21
50–64	65	3.4	15	1	1	2	3	10	13	16
65+	165	7.2	36	1	2	6	10	16	19	28
TOTAL SINGLE DX	173	1.4	1	1	1	1	1	2	3	7
MULTIPLE DX	536	4.2	37	1	1	2	5	11	16	24
TOTAL										
0–19 Years	383	2.7	28	1	1	1	2	6	9	23
20–34	22	2.0	5	1	1	1	2	5	8	10
35–49	67	2.7	14	1	1	2	2	4	10	21
50–64	71	3.2	14	1	1	2	3	10	13	16
65+	166	7.1	36	1	2	6	10	16	19	28
GRAND TOTAL	709	3.5	29	1	1	1	3	8	14	24

36.0: RMVL CORONARY ART OBSTR. Formerly included in operation group(s) 573, 579.

Type of Patients	Observed Patients	Avg. Stay	Vari-ance	10th	25th	50th	75th	90th	95th	99th
1. SINGLE DX										
0–19 Years	9	1.0	0	1	1	1	1	1	1	1
20–34	24	2.9	4	1	2	2	4	6	7	12
35–49	544	2.6	6	1	1	2	3	5	7	11
50–64	1202	2.4	4	1	1	2	3	5	7	9
65+	1035	2.3	3	1	1	2	3	5	5	8
2. MULTIPLE DX										
0–19 Years	70	5.5	108	1	1	1	2	14	15	71
20–34	614	3.9	9	1	2	3	5	7	9	14
35–49	14811	3.5	7	1	2	3	5	7	8	12
50–64	38620	3.7	9	1	2	3	5	7	9	14
65+	48675	4.2	15	1	2	3	6	8	11	18
TOTAL SINGLE DX	2814	2.4	4	1	1	2	3	5	6	9
MULTIPLE DX	102790	3.9	12	1	2	3	5	8	10	16
TOTAL										
0–19 Years	79	5.1	100	1	1	1	6	13	15	71
20–34	638	3.8	9	1	2	3	5	7	9	14
35–49	15355	3.5	7	1	1	3	5	7	8	12
50–64	39822	3.7	9	1	2	3	5	7	9	14
65+	49710	4.2	15	1	2	3	6	8	11	18
GRAND TOTAL	105604	3.9	11	1	2	3	5	8	10	16

36.01: 1 PTCA/ATHERECT W/O TL. Formerly included in operation group(s) 573.

Type of Patients	Observed Patients	Avg. Stay	Vari-ance	10th	25th	50th	75th	90th	95th	99th
1. SINGLE DX										
0–19 Years	7	1.0	0	1	1	1	1	1	1	1
20–34	19	4.3	5	2	3	4	5	5	7	12
35–49	461	2.6	6	1	1	2	3	5	7	11
50–64	1018	2.4	4	1	1	2	3	5	6	9
65+	909	2.2	3	1	1	2	3	4	5	8
2. MULTIPLE DX										
0–19 Years	54	4.4	129	1	1	1	3	6	15	71
20–34	512	3.7	7	1	2	3	5	7	8	12
35–49	12496	3.5	7	1	1	3	5	7	8	12
50–64	32287	3.6	9	1	2	3	5	7	9	14
65+	40321	4.2	14	1	2	3	5	8	11	18
TOTAL SINGLE DX	2414	2.4	4	1	1	2	3	5	6	9
MULTIPLE DX	85670	3.8	11	1	2	3	5	8	10	15
TOTAL										
0–19 Years	61	4.0	116	1	1	1	2	6	15	71
20–34	531	3.7	7	1	2	3	5	7	8	12
35–49	12957	3.4	7	1	1	3	5	7	8	12
50–64	33305	3.6	9	1	2	3	5	7	9	14
65+	41230	4.1	14	1	2	3	5	8	11	18
GRAND TOTAL	88084	3.8	11	1	2	3	5	7	9	15

36.02: 1 PTCA/ATHERECT W TL. Formerly included in operation group(s) 573.

Type of Patients	Observed Patients	Avg. Stay	Vari-ance	10th	25th	50th	75th	90th	95th	99th
1. SINGLE DX										
0–19 Years	0									
20–34	1	5.0	0	5	5	5	5	5	5	5
35–49	17	4.3	3	3	3	5	5	6	7	9
50–64	25	5.3	6	1	4	5	7	9	9	9
65+	18	2.8	5	1	1	2	4	7	7	7
2. MULTIPLE DX										
0–19 Years	2	12.9	7	7	14	14	14	14	14	14
20–34	32	3.7	3	3	3	3	4	6	7	8
35–49	517	4.8	10	2	3	5	6	7	9	14
50–64	1196	4.9	20	2	3	4	6	8	10	16
65+	1323	5.7	21	1	3	5	7	10	13	22
TOTAL SINGLE DX	61	4.2	6	1	2	4	5	8	9	9
MULTIPLE DX	3070	5.2	18	2	3	5	6	9	12	18
TOTAL										
0–19 Years	2	12.9	7	7	14	14	14	14	14	14
20–34	33	3.7	3	3	3	3	4	6	7	8
35–49	534	4.8	10	2	3	5	6	7	9	14
50–64	1221	4.9	20	2	3	5	6	8	10	16
65+	1341	5.6	20	1	3	5	7	10	13	22
GRAND TOTAL	3131	5.2	18	2	3	5	6	9	11	18

Length of Stay by Diagnosis and Operation, United States, 1997

United States, October 1995–September 1996 Data, by Operation

36.05: PTCA/ATHERECT>1 VESSEL. Formerly included in operation group(s) 573.

Type of Patients	Observed Patients	Avg. Stay	Vari-ance	10th	25th	50th	75th	90th	95th	99th
1. SINGLE DX										
0–19 Years	0									
20–34	3	1.0	0	1	1	1	1	1	1	1
35–49	48	2.5	4	1	1	2	3	5	8	9
50–64	131	2.5	3	1	1	2	3	5	6	8
65+	89	2.4	3	1	1	2	4	4	6	6
2. MULTIPLE DX										
0–19 Years	5	4.1	18	1	1	1	5	11	11	11
20–34	55	5.7	20	1	2	5	7	14	14	14
35–49	1417	3.3	6	1	1	3	5	7	8	11
50–64	4195	3.9	10	1	2	3	6	8	10	15
65+	5960	4.3	16	1	2	3	6	9	12	19
TOTAL SINGLE DX	271	2.4	3	1	1	2	3	5	6	8
MULTIPLE DX	11632	4.0	12	1	1	3	5	8	10	17
TOTAL										
0–19 Years	5	4.1	18	1	1	1	5	11	11	11
20–34	58	5.1	20	1	1	5	6	14	14	14
35–49	1465	3.3	6	1	1	3	4	7	8	11
50–64	4326	3.8	10	1	2	3	6	8	10	15
65+	6049	4.3	16	1	2	3	6	9	12	19
GRAND TOTAL	11903	4.0	12	1	1	3	5	8	10	17

36.1: HRT REVASC BYPASS ANAST. Formerly included in operation group(s) 574.

Type of Patients	Observed Patients	Avg. Stay	Vari-ance	10th	25th	50th	75th	90th	95th	99th
1. SINGLE DX										
0–19 Years	1	3.0	0	3	3	3	3	3	3	3
20–34	6	5.2	2	3	5	6	6	6	7	7
35–49	118	6.2	5	4	5	6	7	9	10	15
50–64	359	6.9	15	4	5	6	8	10	13	23
65+	268	7.5	9	5	6	7	8	11	16	16
2. MULTIPLE DX										
0–19 Years	6	17.9	558	3	3	6	53	59	59	59
20–34	204	8.0	20	4	5	7	9	12	17	29
35–49	7456	7.5	19	4	5	7	9	11	14	23
50–64	28669	8.3	24	4	5	7	10	13	17	28
65+	43500	10.1	43	5	6	8	12	16	21	36
TOTAL SINGLE DX	752	7.1	11	4	5	7	8	10	14	16
MULTIPLE DX	79835	9.2	35	5	6	8	11	15	19	33
TOTAL										
0–19 Years	7	16.0	509	3	3	3	9	59	59	59
20–34	210	7.9	20	4	5	7	9	12	17	29
35–49	7574	7.5	18	4	5	7	9	11	14	23
50–64	29028	8.3	24	5	5	7	10	13	17	28
65+	43768	10.1	43	5	6	8	12	16	21	36
GRAND TOTAL	80587	9.2	34	5	6	8	11	15	19	32

36.06: INSERT CORONARY STENT. Formerly included in operation group(s) 573.

Type of Patients	Observed Patients	Avg. Stay	Vari-ance	10th	25th	50th	75th	90th	95th	99th
1. SINGLE DX										
0–19 Years	1	1.0	0	1	1	1	1	1	1	1
20–34	1	2.0	0	2	2	2	2	2	2	2
35–49	15	2.7	2	2	2	2	3	5	6	6
50–64	20	2.5	4	1	1	2	3	5	7	7
65+	13	3.0	4	1	1	2	4	6	7	7
2. MULTIPLE DX										
0–19 Years	3	6.7	23	2	2	6	13	13	13	13
20–34	10	3.0	3	2	2	2	5	5	5	8
35–49	320	4.3	7	2	2	4	5	7	8	14
50–64	825	4.3	13	1	2	3	5	9	10	17
65+	927	4.8	15	2	2	4	6	9	12	20
TOTAL SINGLE DX	50	2.5	2	1	2	2	2	5	6	7
MULTIPLE DX	2085	4.5	12	1	2	4	6	9	10	18
TOTAL										
0–19 Years	4	6.0	24	1	2	6	13	13	13	13
20–34	11	2.4	2	2	2	2	5	5	5	8
35–49	335	4.2	7	2	2	4	5	7	9	14
50–64	845	4.3	13	1	2	3	5	9	10	17
65+	940	4.7	15	2	2	4	6	9	12	20
GRAND TOTAL	2135	4.4	12	1	2	4	6	9	10	18

36.11: AO-COR BYPASS-1 COR ART. Formerly included in operation group(s) 574.

Type of Patients	Observed Patients	Avg. Stay	Vari-ance	10th	25th	50th	75th	90th	95th	99th
1. SINGLE DX										
0–19 Years	0									
20–34	2	3.7	1	3	3	3	5	5	5	5
35–49	26	6.0	4	4	5	6	6	9	9	15
50–64	51	7.3	7	4	5	6	8	10	13	13
65+	24	7.4	8	5	5	6	11	11	12	14
2. MULTIPLE DX										
0–19 Years	4	8.6	191	3	3	3	6	9	53	53
20–34	32	7.2	29	4	4	7	8	11	12	35
35–49	1109	7.2	18	4	5	6	8	11	14	20
50–64	3260	8.8	29	5	6	8	10	16	19	27
65+	3522	9.7	38	5	6	8	11	16	22	32
TOTAL SINGLE DX	103	6.9	7	4	5	6	9	11	12	14
MULTIPLE DX	7927	9.0	32	4	5	7	11	16	19	31
TOTAL										
0–19 Years	4	8.6	191	3	3	3	6	9	53	53
20–34	34	7.0	28	3	4	7	8	10	12	35
35–49	1135	7.2	18	4	5	6	8	11	14	20
50–64	3311	8.8	28	5	5	7	10	16	19	27
65+	3546	9.7	37	5	6	8	11	16	22	32
GRAND TOTAL	8030	8.9	31	5	5	7	10	16	19	30

Length of Stay by Diagnosis and Operation, United States, 1997

United States, October 1995–September 1996 Data, by Operation

36.12: AO-COR BYPASS-2 COR ART. Formerly included in operation group(s) 574.

Type of Patients	Observed Patients	Avg. Stay	Variance	10th	25th	50th	75th	90th	95th	99th
1. SINGLE DX										
0–19 Years	0									
20–34	4	6.0	<1	5	6	6	6	7	7	7
35–49	30	5.7	4	3	4	6	7	9	9	10
50–64	83	6.8	7	4	5	6	8	12	12	14
65+	59	6.3	5	4	5	6	7	8	10	16
2. MULTIPLE DX										
0–19 Years	0									
20–34	55	8.1	11	5	6	7	9	12	17	17
35–49	1972	7.6	21	4	5	7	9	12	14	25
50–64	7539	8.2	21	5	5	7	10	13	15	26
65+	10971	9.8	34	5	6	8	12	15	20	32
TOTAL SINGLE DX	176	6.4	6	4	5	6	7	9	12	14
MULTIPLE DX	20537	9.0	29	5	6	8	11	14	18	30
TOTAL										
0–19 Years	0									
20–34	59	8.0	11	5	6	7	9	12	17	17
35–49	2002	7.6	21	4	5	6	9	12	14	25
50–64	7622	8.2	21	4	5	7	10	13	15	26
65+	11030	9.8	34	5	6	8	12	15	20	32
GRAND TOTAL	20713	8.9	28	5	6	8	11	14	18	30

36.14: AO-COR BYPASS-4+ COR ART. Formerly included in operation group(s) 574.

Type of Patients	Observed Patients	Avg. Stay	Variance	10th	25th	50th	75th	90th	95th	99th
1. SINGLE DX										
0–19 Years	0									
20–34	0									
35–49	19	7.3	5	5	6	7	9	9	11	16
50–64	83	7.8	38	3	5	6	8	16	16	39
65+	61	7.5	3	5	6	8	8	8	11	15
2. MULTIPLE DX										
0–19 Years	0									
20–34	28	7.8	14	4	4	7	9	15	15	16
35–49	1197	7.8	18	4	5	7	9	12	14	20
50–64	5582	8.5	26	5	6	7	10	14	17	26
65+	10258	10.6	56	5	6	8	12	18	23	42
TOTAL SINGLE DX	163	7.6	19	4	5	8	8	10	16	39
MULTIPLE DX	17065	9.7	44	5	6	8	11	16	20	36
TOTAL										
0–19 Years	0									
20–34	28	7.8	14	4	4	7	9	15	15	16
35–49	1216	7.8	18	4	5	7	9	11	14	20
50–64	5665	8.5	26	5	6	7	10	14	17	27
65+	10319	10.6	56	5	6	8	12	18	23	41
GRAND TOTAL	17228	9.6	44	5	6	8	11	16	20	36

36.13: AO-COR BYPASS-3 COR ART. Formerly included in operation group(s) 574.

Type of Patients	Observed Patients	Avg. Stay	Variance	10th	25th	50th	75th	90th	95th	99th
1. SINGLE DX										
0–19 Years	0									
20–34	0									
35–49	21	7.0	4	5	5	7	7	11	11	11
50–64	94	6.4	9	4	5	6	7	10	11	23
65+	95	8.2	13	5	6	7	8	16	16	16
2. MULTIPLE DX										
0–19 Years	0									
20–34	45	10.1	55	5	6	8	10	19	29	50
35–49	1836	7.5	17	4	5	7	9	11	13	24
50–64	8290	8.5	25	5	6	7	10	13	17	30
65+	14047	10.3	43	5	6	9	12	17	21	37
TOTAL SINGLE DX	210	7.4	11	4	5	7	8	12	16	16
MULTIPLE DX	24218	9.4	35	5	6	8	11	15	19	34
TOTAL										
0–19 Years	0									
20–34	45	10.1	55	5	6	8	10	19	29	50
35–49	1857	7.5	17	4	5	7	9	11	13	24
50–64	8384	8.5	25	5	6	7	10	13	17	30
65+	14142	10.3	42	5	6	9	12	16	21	37
GRAND TOTAL	24428	9.4	35	5	6	8	11	15	19	34

36.15: 1 INT MAM-COR ART BYPASS. Formerly included in operation group(s) 574.

Type of Patients	Observed Patients	Avg. Stay	Variance	10th	25th	50th	75th	90th	95th	99th
1. SINGLE DX										
0–19 Years	0									
20–34	0									
35–49	18	5.7	3	3	4	6	7	8	9	9
50–64	38	6.5	4	4	5	6	8	9	10	11
65+	28	5.5	5	3	4	5	7	8	10	12
2. MULTIPLE DX										
0–19 Years	1	3.0	0	3	3	3	3	3	3	3
20–34	30	7.4	12	4	4	6	9	13	13	19
35–49	1094	7.3	19	4	5	7	8	11	13	21
50–64	3502	7.7	22	4	5	7	8	12	15	24
65+	4332	9.3	39	5	6	8	11	15	19	35
TOTAL SINGLE DX	84	6.1	4	4	5	6	8	9	10	11
MULTIPLE DX	8959	8.4	30	4	5	7	10	13	17	31
TOTAL										
0–19 Years	1	3.0	0	3	3	3	3	3	3	3
20–34	30	7.4	12	4	4	6	9	13	13	19
35–49	1112	7.3	19	4	5	7	8	11	13	21
50–64	3540	7.7	22	4	5	7	9	12	15	24
65+	4360	9.3	39	5	6	8	11	15	19	35
GRAND TOTAL	9043	8.4	30	4	5	7	10	13	17	31

Length of Stay by Diagnosis and Operation, United States, 1997

United States, October 1995–September 1996 Data, by Operation

36.16: 2 INT MAM-COR ART BYPASS. Formerly included in operation group(s) 574.

Type of Patients	Observed Patients	Avg. Stay	Variance	Percentiles						
				10th	25th	50th	75th	90th	95th	99th
1. SINGLE DX										
0–19 Years	0									
20–34	0									
35–49	4	5.0	<1	4	4	5	6	6	6	6
50–64	10	5.3	1	3	4	6	6	6	7	7
65+	1	5.0	0	5	5	5	5	5	5	5
2. MULTIPLE DX										
0–19 Years	0									
20–34	14	5.7	1	5	5	5	6	8	8	9
35–49	231	6.5	8	5	5	6	7	10	11	19
50–64	470	7.0	15	4	5	6	8	11	13	17
65+	325	9.5	30	5	6	8	12	15	18	39
TOTAL SINGLE DX	15	5.2	1	4	4	6	6	6	6	7
MULTIPLE DX	1040	7.7	20	4	5	6	9	12	15	24
TOTAL										
0–19 Years	0									
20–34	14	5.7	1	5	5	5	6	8	8	9
35–49	235	6.5	8	4	5	6	7	10	11	19
50–64	480	7.0	15	4	5	6	8	11	13	17
65+	326	9.5	30	5	6	8	12	15	18	39
GRAND TOTAL	1055	7.7	20	4	5	6	9	12	15	24

36.3: HEART REVASC NEC. Formerly included in operation group(s) 579.

Type of Patients	Observed Patients	Avg. Stay	Variance	Percentiles						
				10th	25th	50th	75th	90th	95th	99th
1. SINGLE DX										
0–19 Years	0									
20–34	0									
35–49	0									
50–64	0									
65+	1	1.0	0	1	1	1	1	1	1	1
2. MULTIPLE DX										
0–19 Years	1	5.0	0	5	5	5	5	5	5	5
20–34	1	6.0	0	6	6	6	6	6	6	6
35–49	6	7.8	22	4	5	5	9	16	16	16
50–64	37	11.0	116	2	5	9	15	17	17	89
65+	34	8.2	41	2	4	6	9	18	22	29
TOTAL SINGLE DX	1	1.0	0	1	1	1	1	1	1	1
MULTIPLE DX	79	9.4	76	2	4	7	15	17	19	34
TOTAL										
0–19 Years	1	5.0	0	5	5	5	5	5	5	5
20–34	1	6.0	0	6	6	6	6	6	6	6
35–49	6	7.8	22	4	5	5	9	16	16	16
50–64	37	11.0	116	2	5	9	15	17	17	89
65+	35	8.0	41	2	4	6	9	18	22	29
GRAND TOTAL	80	9.3	76	2	4	7	15	17	19	34

36.2: ARTERIAL IMPLANT REVASC. Formerly included in operation group(s) 579.

Type of Patients	Observed Patients	Avg. Stay	Variance	Percentiles						
				10th	25th	50th	75th	90th	95th	99th
1. SINGLE DX										
0–19 Years	0									
20–34	0									
35–49	0									
50–64	0									
65+	0									
2. MULTIPLE DX										
0–19 Years	2	4.9	1	4	4	4	6	6	6	6
20–34	0									
35–49	2	8.7	1	8	8	8	10	10	10	10
50–64	2	6.0	1	5	5	7	7	7	7	7
65+	0									
TOTAL SINGLE DX	0									
MULTIPLE DX	6	6.6	4	4	5	7	8	10	10	10
TOTAL										
0–19 Years	2	4.9	1	4	4	4	6	6	6	6
20–34	0									
35–49	2	8.7	1	8	8	8	10	10	10	10
50–64	2	6.0	1	5	5	7	7	7	7	7
65+	0									
GRAND TOTAL	6	6.6	4	4	5	7	8	10	10	10

36.9: OTHER HEART VESSEL OPS. Formerly included in operation group(s) 579.

Type of Patients	Observed Patients	Avg. Stay	Variance	Percentiles						
				10th	25th	50th	75th	90th	95th	99th
1. SINGLE DX										
0–19 Years	12	2.6	2	1	1	3	4	4	4	4
20–34	1	3.0	0	3	3	3	3	3	3	3
35–49	2	3.4	<1	3	3	3	4	4	4	4
50–64	0									
65+	1	6.0	0	6	6	6	6	6	6	6
2. MULTIPLE DX										
0–19 Years	34	12.6	113	4	5	11	15	24	32	>99
20–34	7	6.5	11	4	4	4	8	12	13	13
35–49	16	11.3	105	3	6	7	16	25	25	50
50–64	49	9.2	35	5	6	7	11	21	22	34
65+	59	12.2	57	6	8	10	14	22	30	42
TOTAL SINGLE DX	16	2.7	2	1	1	3	4	4	4	6
MULTIPLE DX	165	11.2	69	4	6	9	13	22	30	54
TOTAL										
0–19 Years	46	8.0	87	1	3	4	12	21	24	54
20–34	8	6.2	11	4	4	4	8	12	13	13
35–49	18	10.7	101	3	5	7	14	16	25	50
50–64	49	9.2	35	5	6	7	11	21	22	34
65+	60	12.2	57	6	8	10	14	22	30	42
GRAND TOTAL	181	9.7	67	3	4	7	12	21	24	50

Length of Stay by Diagnosis and Operation, United States, 1997

United States, October 1995–September 1996 Data, by Operation

37.0: PERICARDIOCENTESIS. Formerly included in operation group(s) 579.

Type of Patients	Observed Patients	Avg. Stay	Vari-ance	10th	25th	50th	75th	90th	95th	99th
1. SINGLE DX										
0–19 Years	19	4.0	9	1	2	3	6	6	7	16
20–34	2	13.5	14	15	15	15	15	15	15	15
35–49	10	3.2	16	1	1	2	3	4	15	15
50–64	4	4.0	4	2	2	3	6	6	6	6
65+	6	9.7	44	1	2	15	15	15	15	15
2. MULTIPLE DX										
0–19 Years	128	7.1	166	2	2	4	6	11	24	93
20–34	80	6.4	39	1	2	5	8	11	17	36
35–49	166	7.2	55	2	2	5	9	17	28	35
50–64	252	6.5	32	2	3	4	9	12	17	25
65+	327	8.4	41	3	5	7	9	14	18	38
TOTAL SINGLE DX	41	5.1	24	1	1	3	6	15	15	16
MULTIPLE DX	953	7.4	64	2	3	5	9	14	19	38
TOTAL										
0–19	147	6.8	150	2	2	4	6	10	24	93
20–34	82	6.6	40	1	2	5	8	15	17	36
35–49	176	6.9	53	2	2	4	8	17	27	34
50–64	256	6.5	31	2	3	4	9	12	16	25
65+	333	8.4	41	3	5	7	10	15	18	38
GRAND TOTAL	994	7.3	63	2	3	5	9	14	19	38

37.12: PERICARDIOTOMY. Formerly included in operation group(s) 579.

Type of Patients	Observed Patients	Avg. Stay	Vari-ance	10th	25th	50th	75th	90th	95th	99th
1. SINGLE DX										
0–19 Years	7	3.3	8	1	1	3	5	9	9	9
20–34	9	3.9	6	2	2	3	4	10	10	10
35–49	9	6.0	14	3	3	5	8	12	12	12
50–64	12	9.1	46	3	4	5	18	18	18	18
65+	6	6.5	12	2	4	6	7	13	13	13
2. MULTIPLE DX										
0–19 Years	106	9.6	69	3	5	6	12	20	31	47
20–34	181	9.0	59	4	6	7	11	17	22	43
35–49	360	9.3	74	3	4	8	11	17	21	44
50–64	541	9.6	51	3	5	8	13	17	21	40
65+	654	11.7	70	4	6	10	15	21	29	39
TOTAL SINGLE DX	43	6.5	30	1	3	4	8	18	18	18
MULTIPLE DX	1842	10.1	65	3	5	8	12	18	26	43
TOTAL										
0–19	113	9.2	68	3	4	6	10	20	31	47
20–34	190	8.9	59	3	6	7	9	17	22	43
35–49	369	9.3	74	3	4	8	11	17	23	44
50–64	553	9.6	51	3	5	8	13	18	21	39
65+	660	11.6	70	4	6	10	15	21	29	39
GRAND TOTAL	1885	10.0	65	3	5	8	12	18	26	42

37.1: CARDIOTOMY & PERICARDIOT. Formerly included in operation group(s) 579.

Type of Patients	Observed Patients	Avg. Stay	Vari-ance	10th	25th	50th	75th	90th	95th	99th
1. SINGLE DX										
0–19 Years	7	3.3	8	1	1	3	6	9	9	9
20–34	9	3.9	6	2	2	3	4	10	10	10
35–49	9	6.0	14	3	3	4	8	12	12	12
50–64	13	9.0	45	3	4	5	18	18	18	18
65+	6	6.5	12	2	4	6	7	13	13	13
2. MULTIPLE DX										
0–19 Years	124	9.1	67	3	5	6	10	20	31	46
20–34	187	9.0	58	4	6	7	9	17	22	43
35–49	374	9.2	71	3	4	8	11	17	22	44
50–64	568	9.6	50	3	5	8	13	17	21	39
65+	723	11.6	74	4	6	9	14	21	29	45
TOTAL SINGLE DX	44	6.5	29	1	3	4	8	18	18	18
MULTIPLE DX	1976	10.1	65	3	5	8	12	18	26	44
TOTAL										
0–19	131	8.8	65	3	4	6	10	18	31	46
20–34	196	8.9	57	3	6	7	9	17	22	43
35–49	383	9.2	70	3	4	8	11	17	22	44
50–64	581	9.6	50	3	5	8	13	18	21	39
65+	729	11.5	74	4	6	9	14	21	29	45
GRAND TOTAL	2020	10.0	65	3	5	8	12	18	26	44

37.2: DXTIC PX HRT/PERICARDIUM. Formerly included in operation group(s) 575, 581, 579.

Type of Patients	Observed Patients	Avg. Stay	Vari-ance	10th	25th	50th	75th	90th	95th	99th
1. SINGLE DX										
0–19 Years	556	1.5	2	1	1	1	1	3	4	6
20–34	465	2.1	11	1	1	1	3	4	6	8
35–49	2081	2.4	3	1	1	2	3	6	6	7
50–64	2007	2.1	3	1	1	1	3	4	6	8
65+	1133	2.5	6	1	1	2	3	5	8	11
2. MULTIPLE DX										
0–19 Years	2498	3.4	33	1	1	1	3	8	13	33
20–34	2485	4.1	33	1	1	3	5	8	10	37
35–49	22912	3.5	9	2	2	3	5	7	8	14
50–64	48282	4.0	11	2	2	3	5	7	9	16
65+	69109	4.9	17	1	2	4	6	9	12	20
TOTAL SINGLE DX	6242	2.2	4	1	1	1	3	5	6	8
MULTIPLE DX	145286	4.4	14	1	2	3	6	8	11	18
TOTAL										
0–19	3054	3.1	29	1	1	1	3	7	11	32
20–34	2950	3.8	30	1	1	2	4	7	9	37
35–49	24993	3.4	8	1	2	3	4	6	9	14
50–64	50289	3.9	11	1	2	3	5	7	9	16
65+	70242	4.9	16	1	2	4	6	9	12	20
GRAND TOTAL	151528	4.3	14	1	2	3	6	8	11	18

Length of Stay by Diagnosis and Operation, United States, 1997

United States, October 1995–September 1996 Data, by Operation

37.21: RT HEART CARDIAC CATH. Formerly included in operation group(s) 575.

Type of Patients	Observed Patients	Avg. Stay	Vari-ance	Percentiles						
				10th	25th	50th	75th	90th	95th	99th
1. SINGLE DX										
0–19 Years	59	1.7	6	1	1	1	1	4	5	19
20–34	16	5.9	305	1	1	2	3	7	7	89
35–49	21	2.3	1	1	2	2	3	4	4	4
50–64	22	2.1	2	1	1	2	4	4	4	4
65+	10	1.9	<1	1	1	2	2	4	4	4
2. MULTIPLE DX										
0–19 Years	276	4.3	53	1	1	1	4	11	15	37
20–34	117	9.9	165	1	2	5	9	37	44	44
35–49	420	5.9	33	1	2	4	8	12	17	34
50–64	780	6.4	43	1	3	6	7	13	16	27
65+	912	7.3	41	1	3	6	10	15	19	36
TOTAL SINGLE DX	128	2.3	34	1	1	1	2	4	5	19
MULTIPLE DX	2505	6.6	48	1	2	5	8	14	18	37
TOTAL										
0–19 Years	335	3.9	46	1	1	1	4	10	14	37
20–34	133	9.5	177	1	2	4	9	37	37	44
35–49	441	5.7	33	1	2	4	8	12	17	33
50–64	802	6.3	43	1	3	5	7	13	16	27
65+	922	7.2	41	1	3	6	10	14	19	36
GRAND TOTAL	2633	6.5	49	1	2	5	8	13	18	37

37.22: LEFT HEART CARDIAC CATH. Formerly included in operation group(s) 575.

Type of Patients	Observed Patients	Avg. Stay	Vari-ance	Percentiles						
				10th	25th	50th	75th	90th	95th	99th
1. SINGLE DX										
0–19 Years	26	2.0	2	1	1	1	3	5	5	5
20–34	209	2.2	2	1	1	2	3	5	5	8
35–49	1627	2.2	2	1	1	2	3	4	5	7
50–64	1594	2.2	3	1	1	2	3	4	5	7
65+	823	2.3	5	1	1	2	3	5	6	10
2. MULTIPLE DX										
0–19 Years	111	3.0	16	1	1	2	3	6	9	20
20–34	1435	3.3	6	1	2	3	4	6	8	12
35–49	17902	3.2	6	1	2	3	5	6	7	12
50–64	36344	3.7	8	1	2	3	5	7	8	14
65+	46543	4.5	12	1	2	4	6	8	11	17
TOTAL SINGLE DX	4279	2.2	3	1	1	2	3	4	5	8
MULTIPLE DX	102335	4.0	10	1	2	3	5	7	9	15
TOTAL										
0–19 Years	137	2.8	14	1	1	2	3	6	8	20
20–34	1644	3.1	6	1	2	3	4	6	8	11
35–49	19529	3.1	6	1	2	3	5	7	7	11
50–64	37938	3.6	8	1	2	3	5	7	8	13
65+	47366	4.5	12	1	2	4	6	8	11	17
GRAND TOTAL	106614	3.9	10	1	2	3	5	7	9	15

37.23: RT/LEFT HEART CARD CATH. Formerly included in operation group(s) 575.

Type of Patients	Observed Patients	Avg. Stay	Vari-ance	Percentiles						
				10th	25th	50th	75th	90th	95th	99th
1. SINGLE DX										
0–19 Years	294	1.3	1	1	1	1	1	2	3	6
20–34	55	2.8	6	1	1	1	2	7	8	8
35–49	217	3.2	6	1	1	2	6	8	8	8
50–64	233	2.1	3	1	1	1	3	4	5	8
65+	196	3.1	8	1	2	2	4	8	8	10
2. MULTIPLE DX										
0–19 Years	1685	3.0	30	1	1	1	2	7	13	32
20–34	524	4.0	13	2	2	3	5	7	11	16
35–49	3649	4.3	12	1	2	3	6	8	11	18
50–64	9299	4.8	17	1	2	4	6	9	11	19
65+	18366	5.7	21	2	3	5	8	11	14	22
TOTAL SINGLE DX	995	2.6	5	1	1	1	4	6	6	8
MULTIPLE DX	33523	5.1	20	1	2	4	7	10	13	21
TOTAL										
0–19 Years	1979	2.8	26	1	1	1	2	6	11	31
20–34	579	3.9	12	1	2	3	5	8	11	16
35–49	3866	4.2	11	1	2	3	6	8	10	18
50–64	9532	4.7	17	1	2	5	8	9	11	19
65+	18562	5.7	21	1	3	5	8	11	14	22
GRAND TOTAL	34518	5.0	20	1	2	4	7	10	13	21

37.25: CARDIAC BIOPSY. Formerly included in operation group(s) 579.

Type of Patients	Observed Patients	Avg. Stay	Vari-ance	Percentiles						
				10th	25th	50th	75th	90th	95th	99th
1. SINGLE DX										
0–19 Years	28	2.3	3	1	1	1	4	6	6	7
20–34	4	1.3	<1	1	1	1	1	3	3	3
35–49	8	2.0	5	1	1	1	1	7	7	7
50–64	11	3.6	7	2	2	2	6	6	6	12
65+	2	1.5	<1	1	1	1	2	2	2	2
2. MULTIPLE DX										
0–19 Years	165	6.1	57	1	2	5	7	11	18	43
20–34	76	13.3	335	1	2	4	11	51	51	51
35–49	164	7.7	61	1	2	6	10	19	29	31
50–64	259	5.8	54	1	2	4	7	13	15	28
65+	58	5.6	23	1	2	3	8	12	12	24
TOTAL SINGLE DX	53	2.5	5	1	1	1	4	6	6	7
MULTIPLE DX	722	7.0	87	1	2	4	8	13	23	51
TOTAL										
0–19 Years	193	5.8	54	1	2	4	6	11	16	43
20–34	80	12.8	328	1	1	3	11	51	51	51
35–49	172	7.2	59	1	2	5	10	17	29	31
50–64	270	5.6	51	1	2	4	7	12	15	28
65+	60	5.4	22	1	2	3	8	12	12	24
GRAND TOTAL	775	6.7	83	1	2	4	8	13	21	51

Length of Stay by Diagnosis and Operation, United States, 1997

United States, October 1995–September 1996 Data, by Operation

37.26: CARD EPS/RECORD STUDIES. Formerly included in operation group(s) 581.

Type of Patients	Observed Patients	Avg. Stay	Variance	10th	25th	50th	75th	90th	95th	99th
1. SINGLE DX										
0–19 Years	143	1.6	2	1	1	1	1	4	6	6
20–34	170	1.5	1	1	1	1	1	3	6	6
35–49	200	1.7	2	1	1	1	2	3	4	6
50–64	140	2.0	4	1	1	1	2	4	6	11
65+	99	3.4	12	1	1	2	6	6	9	21
2. MULTIPLE DX										
0–19 Years	239	3.6	24	1	1	2	4	7	10	32
20–34	304	3.0	10	1	1	2	4	6	9	14
35–49	734	4.2	15	1	1	3	6	11	13	13
50–64	1521	4.5	17	1	1	3	6	10	13	18
65+	3096	6.3	32	1	3	5	8	12	15	26
TOTAL SINGLE DX	752	1.9	3	1	1	1	2	4	6	9
MULTIPLE DX	5894	5.3	26	1	2	4	7	11	14	22
TOTAL										
0–19 Years	382	2.8	15	1	1	1	3	6	8	23
20–34	474	2.5	7	1	1	1	3	6	7	12
35–49	934	3.6	13	1	1	2	5	8	13	13
50–64	1661	4.3	16	1	1	3	6	9	12	18
65+	3195	6.2	31	1	3	5	8	12	15	26
GRAND TOTAL	6646	4.9	24	1	1	4	7	10	14	22

37.3: PERICARDIECT/EXC HRT LES. Formerly included in operation group(s) 578, 579.

Type of Patients	Observed Patients	Avg. Stay	Variance	10th	25th	50th	75th	90th	95th	99th
1. SINGLE DX										
0–19 Years	260	1.4	<1	1	1	1	1	2	3	6
20–34	198	1.4	1	1	1	1	1	2	3	6
35–49	222	1.4	<1	1	1	1	1	3	3	5
50–64	125	1.4	<1	1	1	1	2	2	3	5
65+	80	1.4	1	1	1	1	1	2	4	6
2. MULTIPLE DX										
0–19 Years	404	3.2	33	1	1	1	3	7	12	34
20–34	326	3.9	43	1	1	1	4	10	18	32
35–49	515	4.3	39	1	1	2	6	9	15	26
50–64	799	6.5	46	1	1	5	8	17	18	33
65+	1099	5.8	39	1	2	4	8	13	18	30
TOTAL SINGLE DX	885	1.4	<1	1	1	1	1	2	3	5
MULTIPLE DX	3143	5.1	42	1	1	2	7	12	18	32
TOTAL										
0–19 Years	664	2.6	23	1	1	1	2	5	8	23
20–34	524	3.1	32	1	1	1	2	6	12	32
35–49	737	3.4	29	1	1	1	7	15	18	19
50–64	924	5.6	42	1	1	3	8	13	18	33
65+	1179	5.5	37	1	1	3	8	13	17	30
GRAND TOTAL	4028	4.2	35	1	1	2	5	11	16	30

37.31: PERICARDIECTOMY. Formerly included in operation group(s) 579.

Type of Patients	Observed Patients	Avg. Stay	Variance	10th	25th	50th	75th	90th	95th	99th
1. SINGLE DX										
0–19 Years	4	5.6	5	3	5	5	7	9	9	9
20–34	4	6.1	4	4	5	6	6	9	9	9
35–49	9	3.5	3	1	2	4	5	5	6	6
50–64	1	7.0	0	7	7	7	7	7	7	7
65+	0									
2. MULTIPLE DX										
0–19 Years	22	11.4	141	2	2	9	16	23	39	59
20–34	36	13.8	124	5	5	10	22	32	32	42
35–49	54	11.1	90	3	7	10	14	17	17	68
50–64	104	12.9	55	4	6	12	18	20	24	33
65+	110	11.8	59	4	7	9	15	22	24	43
TOTAL SINGLE DX	18	4.5	5	1	3	5	5	7	9	9
MULTIPLE DX	326	12.3	79	4	6	10	18	23	27	42
TOTAL										
0–19 Years	26	10.9	132	2	2	9	16	23	39	59
20–34	40	13.4	121	5	5	9	21	32	32	42
35–49	63	10.4	87	3	5	8	13	17	24	68
50–64	105	12.9	55	4	6	12	18	20	24	33
65+	110	11.8	59	4	7	9	15	22	24	43
GRAND TOTAL	344	12.1	78	4	5	9	17	23	27	42

37.33: HEART LES EXC/DESTR NEC. Formerly included in operation group(s) 579.

Type of Patients	Observed Patients	Avg. Stay	Variance	10th	25th	50th	75th	90th	95th	99th
1. SINGLE DX										
0–19 Years	25	3.3	3	1	2	3	4	6	7	9
20–34	8	2.7	3	1	1	2	4	5	5	5
35–49	7	2.6	4	1	1	1	5	5	5	5
50–64	3	2.7	7	1	1	2	2	7	7	7
65+	5	1.4	2	1	1	1	1	1	6	9
2. MULTIPLE DX										
0–19 Years	80	6.6	44	2	3	5	7	13	21	37
20–34	30	8.5	59	3	4	4	12	17	26	50
35–49	52	9.3	93	4	6	7	10	15	18	70
50–64	121	10.6	60	4	6	8	13	21	33	35
65+	142	10.5	45	3	6	8	14	19	21	33
TOTAL SINGLE DX	48	2.5	3	1	1	2	4	5	6	9
MULTIPLE DX	425	9.3	60	3	5	7	12	18	23	35
TOTAL										
0–19 Years	105	6.0	38	2	3	4	6	12	20	37
20–34	38	7.6	55	2	4	4	12	16	18	50
35–49	59	8.7	88	3	5	7	9	13	18	70
50–64	124	10.5	60	4	6	8	13	21	33	35
65+	147	9.2	49	1	4	7	14	18	21	32
GRAND TOTAL	473	8.5	58	2	4	7	11	17	21	35

Length of Stay by Diagnosis and Operation, United States, 1997

United States, October 1995–September 1996 Data, by Operation

37.34: CATH ABLATION HEART LES. Formerly included in operation group(s) 578.

Type of Patients	Observed Patients	Avg. Stay	Vari- ance	Percentiles						
				10th	25th	50th	75th	90th	95th	99th
1. SINGLE DX										
0–19 Years	231	1.2	<1	1	1	1	1	2	2	4
20–34	185	1.3	<1	1	1	1	1	2	3	5
35–49	206	1.4	<1	1	1	1	1	3	3	3
50–64	121	1.4	<1	1	1	1	2	2	3	5
65+	75	1.3	<1	1	1	1	1	2	4	5
2. MULTIPLE DX										
0–19 Years	294	1.9	13	1	1	1	1	3	6	20
20–34	258	1.8	5	1	1	1	2	3	6	10
35–49	394	2.2	6	1	1	1	2	4	7	15
50–64	494	3.1	12	1	1	2	5	6	8	16
65+	759	3.8	15	1	1	2	5	9	11	18
TOTAL SINGLE DX	818	1.3	<1	1	1	1	1	2	3	4
MULTIPLE DX	2199	2.8	12	1	1	1	3	6	9	16
TOTAL										
0–19 Years	525	1.6	8	1	1	1	1	2	4	9
20–34	443	1.6	4	1	1	1	1	2	4	10
35–49	600	1.9	4	1	1	1	2	4	5	13
50–64	615	2.7	9	1	1	2	3	6	7	14
65+	834	3.6	14	1	1	2	5	8	11	17
GRAND TOTAL	3017	2.4	9	1	1	1	2	6	8	14

37.4: REP HEART & PERICARDIUM. Formerly included in operation group(s) 579.

Type of Patients	Observed Patients	Avg. Stay	Vari- ance	Percentiles						
				10th	25th	50th	75th	90th	95th	99th
1. SINGLE DX										
0–19 Years	1	4.0	0	4	4	4	4	4	4	4
20–34	2	9.5	5	8	8	8	12	12	12	12
35–49	2	2.9	3	2	2	2	5	5	5	5
50–64	0									
65+	0									
2. MULTIPLE DX										
0–19 Years	23	8.7	13	4	9	9	9	9	9	25
20–34	50	10.5	51	5	7	7	11	24	30	34
35–49	38	7.9	53	4	4	5	9	14	27	>99
50–64	19	11.5	54	4	5	9	21	24	24	26
65+	20	7.3	13	6	6	7	7	8	12	29
TOTAL SINGLE DX	5	6.2	15	2	2	5	8	12	12	12
MULTIPLE DX	150	8.8	32	4	6	7	9	13	24	34
TOTAL										
0–19 Years	24	8.7	13	4	9	9	9	9	9	25
20–34	52	10.5	50	5	7	7	11	22	30	34
35–49	40	7.8	52	4	4	5	9	14	27	>99
50–64	19	11.5	54	4	5	9	21	24	24	26
65+	20	7.3	13	6	6	7	7	8	12	29
GRAND TOTAL	155	8.8	31	4	6	7	9	13	24	34

37.5: HEART TRANSPLANTATION. Formerly included in operation group(s) 572.

Type of Patients	Observed Patients	Avg. Stay	Vari- ance	Percentiles						
				10th	25th	50th	75th	90th	95th	99th
1. SINGLE DX										
0–19 Years	3	35.1	596	11	12	56	56	56	56	56
20–34	0									
35–49	0									
50–64	1	13.0	0	13	13	13	13	13	13	13
65+	0									
2. MULTIPLE DX										
0–19 Years	107	30.0	486	7	13	26	45	66	94	>99
20–34	24	52.5	708	13	31	69	81	>99	>99	>99
35–49	86	29.3	457	10	16	22	47	91	>99	>99
50–64	212	30.7	574	8	13	25	59	>99	>99	>99
65+	18	44.9	644	10	20	56	66	92	>99	>99
TOTAL SINGLE DX	4	31.5	560	11	12	13	56	56	56	56
MULTIPLE DX	447	32.0	564	8	14	26	57	90	>99	>99
TOTAL										
0–19 Years	110	30.1	486	7	12	26	46	63	94	>99
20–34	24	52.5	708	13	31	69	81	>99	>99	>99
35–49	86	29.3	457	10	16	22	47	91	>99	>99
50–64	213	30.6	573	8	13	25	59	>99	>99	>99
65+	18	44.9	644	10	20	56	66	92	>99	>99
GRAND TOTAL	451	32.0	564	8	13	26	57	90	>99	>99

37.6: IMPL HEART ASSIST SYST. Formerly included in operation group(s) 571.

Type of Patients	Observed Patients	Avg. Stay	Vari- ance	Percentiles						
				10th	25th	50th	75th	90th	95th	99th
1. SINGLE DX										
0–19 Years	0									
20–34	3	4.9	1	4	4	5	6	6	6	6
35–49	5	3.1	<1	1	3	3	3	4	5	5
50–64	8	3.6	6	1	1	4	6	6	8	8
65+	5	6.3	18	3	3	5	10	14	14	14
2. MULTIPLE DX										
0–19 Years	0									
20–34	18	7.3	10	4	5	6	9	10	13	18
35–49	289	8.5	68	3	4	7	10	13	22	41
50–64	848	8.1	65	2	4	6	10	15	21	44
65+	1164	9.6	75	3	5	7	12	19	24	39
TOTAL SINGLE DX	21	4.1	7	1	3	4	5	6	10	14
MULTIPLE DX	2319	8.9	70	2	4	7	11	17	22	41
TOTAL										
0–19 Years	0									
20–34	21	7.1	10	4	5	6	9	10	13	18
35–49	294	8.4	67	3	4	6	10	12	22	41
50–64	856	8.1	64	2	4	6	10	15	21	44
65+	1169	9.6	75	3	5	7	12	19	24	39
GRAND TOTAL	2340	8.9	70	2	4	7	11	17	22	41

Length of Stay by Diagnosis and Operation, United States, 1997

United States, October 1995–September 1996 Data, by Operation

37.61: PULSATION BALLOON IMPL. Formerly included in operation group(s) 571.

Type of Patients	Observed Patients	Avg. Stay	Vari-ance	10th	25th	50th	75th	90th	95th	99th
1. SINGLE DX										
0–19 Years	0									
20–34	2	4.9	1	4	4	4	6	6	6	6
35–49	4	2.9	<1	1	3	3	3	3	5	5
50–64	8	3.6	6	1	1	4	6	6	8	8
65+	4	4.9	7	3	3	3	5	10	10	10
2. MULTIPLE DX										
0–19 Years	0									
20–34	16	7.2	8	4	5	6	9	10	13	14
35–49	276	8.2	49	3	4	7	10	12	22	41
50–64	831	8.1	62	2	4	6	10	15	21	44
65+	1142	9.6	75	3	5	7	12	19	24	39
TOTAL SINGLE DX	18	3.7	5	1	3	3	5	6	8	10
MULTIPLE DX	2265	8.8	67	2	4	7	11	17	22	41
TOTAL										
0–19 Years	0									
20–34	18	7.0	7	4	4	6	9	10	13	14
35–49	280	8.1	49	3	4	6	10	12	22	41
50–64	839	8.0	62	2	4	6	10	15	21	44
65+	1146	9.6	75	3	5	7	12	19	24	39
GRAND TOTAL	2283	8.8	66	2	4	7	11	17	22	41

37.71: INSERT TV LEAD-VENTRICLE. Formerly included in operation group(s) 577.

Type of Patients	Observed Patients	Avg. Stay	Vari-ance	10th	25th	50th	75th	90th	95th	99th
1. SINGLE DX										
0–19 Years	2	1.5	<1	1	1	2	2	2	2	2
20–34	0									
35–49	4	4.0	6	1	1	6	6	6	6	6
50–64	6	1.6	<1	1	1	1	2	3	3	3
65+	22	3.2	7	1	1	2	5	9	9	9
2. MULTIPLE DX										
0–19 Years	6	3.1	4	2	2	2	4	7	7	7
20–34	4	4.5	9	1	2	6	8	8	8	8
35–49	14	9.2	37	2	4	9	13	20	20	20
50–64	103	6.3	29	2	3	4	10	13	13	21
65+	1326	6.7	39	2	3	5	9	13	17	28
TOTAL SINGLE DX	34	3.1	6	1	1	2	5	6	9	9
MULTIPLE DX	1453	6.7	38	2	3	5	9	13	17	27
TOTAL										
0–19 Years	8	3.0	4	2	2	2	3	7	7	7
20–34	4	4.5	9	1	2	6	8	8	8	8
35–49	18	7.8	34	2	2	6	10	20	20	20
50–64	109	6.2	29	1	3	4	10	13	13	21
65+	1348	6.7	39	2	3	5	9	13	17	28
GRAND TOTAL	1487	6.6	38	1	3	5	9	13	17	27

37.7: CARDIAC PACER LEAD OP. Formerly included in operation group(s) 577, 581.

Type of Patients	Observed Patients	Avg. Stay	Vari-ance	10th	25th	50th	75th	90th	95th	99th
1. SINGLE DX										
0–19 Years	32	2.3	4	1	1	1	3	4	8	8
20–34	33	1.7	1	1	1	1	3	3	3	5
35–49	69	2.6	2	1	2	3	3	3	6	8
50–64	114	2.9	4	1	1	2	5	6	6	8
65+	492	2.1	2	1	1	2	3	3	5	7
2. MULTIPLE DX										
0–19 Years	150	5.7	32	1	2	3	8	14	14	27
20–34	139	4.5	15	1	2	4	6	8	10	22
35–49	436	5.1	25	1	2	4	6	12	19	19
50–64	1787	5.3	22	1	2	4	7	12	14	22
65+	14134	5.7	27	1	2	4	7	11	15	25
TOTAL SINGLE DX	740	2.2	2	1	1	2	3	4	5	8
MULTIPLE DX	16646	5.7	26	1	2	4	7	11	15	24
TOTAL										
0–19 Years	182	5.1	29	1	2	3	7	14	14	27
20–34	172	4.0	14	1	1	3	6	7	9	21
35–49	505	4.7	22	1	2	3	5	10	11	19
50–64	1901	5.2	21	1	2	4	7	11	13	22
65+	14626	5.6	26	1	2	4	7	11	15	24
GRAND TOTAL	17386	5.5	26	1	2	4	7	11	15	24

37.72: INSERT TV LEAD-ATR&VENT. Formerly included in operation group(s) 577.

Type of Patients	Observed Patients	Avg. Stay	Vari-ance	10th	25th	50th	75th	90th	95th	99th
1. SINGLE DX										
0–19 Years	15	1.6	<1	1	1	1	2	3	3	3
20–34	23	1.4	<1	1	1	1	2	3	3	4
35–49	51	2.4	4	1	1	2	3	4	6	8
50–64	79	3.0	4	1	1	3	5	6	6	6
65+	347	2.1	2	1	1	2	3	3	4	7
2. MULTIPLE DX										
0–19 Years	42	3.1	9	1	1	2	4	8	9	12
20–34	63	4.0	6	1	2	4	5	7	8	12
35–49	285	4.2	12	1	2	3	5	9	11	16
50–64	1239	5.2	21	1	2	4	7	10	15	21
65+	10349	5.5	24	1	2	4	7	11	14	24
TOTAL SINGLE DX	515	2.2	2	1	1	2	3	4	5	7
MULTIPLE DX	11978	5.5	24	1	2	4	7	11	14	24
TOTAL										
0–19 Years	57	2.6	6	1	1	2	3	5	9	12
20–34	86	3.4	6	1	1	3	5	7	7	11
35–49	336	4.0	11	1	2	3	5	9	10	16
50–64	1318	5.0	20	1	2	4	7	10	14	21
65+	10696	5.4	24	1	2	4	7	11	14	24
GRAND TOTAL	12493	5.3	23	1	2	4	7	11	14	23

Length of Stay by Diagnosis and Operation

United States, October 1995–September 1996 Data, by Operation

37.75: REVISION PACEMAKER LEAD. Formerly included in operation group(s) 577.

Type of Patients	Observed Patients	Avg. Stay	Vari-ance	10th	25th	50th	75th	90th	95th	99th
1. SINGLE DX										
0–19 Years	2	2.8	9	1	1	1	6	6	6	6
20–34	3	3.0	<1	1	3	3	3	3	5	5
35–49	2	1.0	0	1	1	1	1	1	1	1
50–64	13	1.0	0	1	1	1	1	1	1	1
65+	33	1.7	<1	1	1	1	3	3	3	4
2. MULTIPLE DX										
0–19 Years	12	6.0	52	1	1	3	3	20	20	20
20–34	14	3.6	8	1	2	3	6	6	6	6
35–49	25	2.0	5	1	1	1	3	4	4	16
50–64	70	3.2	6	1	1	3	4	7	10	12
65+	374	4.3	17	1	2	3	5	9	15	15
TOTAL SINGLE DX	53	1.7	1	1	1	1	3	3	3	5
MULTIPLE DX	495	4.1	16	1	2	3	5	8	15	16
TOTAL										
0–19 Years	14	5.8	50	1	1	3	6	20	20	20
20–34	17	3.5	3	1	2	3	5	6	6	6
35–49	27	2.0	5	1	1	1	3	4	4	16
50–64	83	3.0	6	1	1	3	4	5	10	12
65+	407	4.2	17	1	2	3	5	9	15	15
GRAND TOTAL	548	3.9	15	1	1	3	5	8	15	16

37.76: REPLACE TRANSVENOUS LEAD. Formerly included in operation group(s) 577.

Type of Patients	Observed Patients	Avg. Stay	Vari-ance	10th	25th	50th	75th	90th	95th	99th
1. SINGLE DX										
0–19 Years	5	3.3	8	1	1	3	7	7	7	7
20–34	7	1.9	1	1	1	1	3	3	3	3
35–49	5	1.0	0	1	1	1	1	1	1	1
50–64	10	2.2	6	1	1	1	2	8	8	8
65+	68	2.1	3	1	1	2	2	4	7	8
2. MULTIPLE DX										
0–19 Years	34	2.6	2	1	2	3	3	4	5	6
20–34	26	3.0	8	1	1	2	5	9	9	9
35–49	34	2.4	3	1	1	2	4	5	5	7
50–64	113	3.0	10	1	1	3	4	7	8	13
65+	683	3.5	14	1	1	2	4	8	11	17
TOTAL SINGLE DX	95	2.1	3	1	1	2	2	4	7	8
MULTIPLE DX	890	3.4	12	1	1	2	4	7	11	17
TOTAL										
0–19 Years	39	2.6	2	1	1	3	3	5	6	7
20–34	33	2.9	7	1	1	2	3	8	9	9
35–49	39	2.3	3	1	1	2	3	5	5	7
50–64	123	3.0	10	1	1	2	3	7	8	13
65+	751	3.4	13	1	1	2	4	7	11	17
GRAND TOTAL	985	3.3	12	1	1	2	4	7	11	17

37.78: INSERT TEMP TV PACER. Formerly included in operation group(s) 577.

Type of Patients	Observed Patients	Avg. Stay	Vari-ance	10th	25th	50th	75th	90th	95th	99th
1. SINGLE DX										
0–19 Years	1	4.0	0	4	4	4	4	4	4	4
20–34										
35–49	3	2.9	<1	2	3	3	3	3	3	3
50–64	2	8.6	4	7	7	10	10	10	10	10
65+	9	5.0	6	3	3	5	7	8	9	9
2. MULTIPLE DX										
0–19 Years	14	12.9	15	7	14	14	14	14	20	21
20–34	20	7.0	23	3	5	6	7	11	22	22
35–49	58	10.5	53	2	4	9	19	19	19	19
50–64	210	6.8	24	2	4	6	8	12	15	26
65+	1098	8.3	32	3	4	7	11	17	18	27
TOTAL SINGLE DX	15	3.3	2	2	3	3	3	4	7	10
MULTIPLE DX	1400	8.2	32	3	4	7	11	17	19	26
TOTAL										
0–19 Years	15	12.5	18	4	14	14	14	14	20	21
20–34	20	7.0	23	3	5	6	7	11	22	22
35–49	61	8.1	48	2	4	6	14	19	19	19
50–64	212	6.8	24	2	4	6	8	12	15	26
65+	1107	8.3	32	3	4	7	11	17	18	27
GRAND TOTAL	1415	8.1	32	3	4	7	11	17	19	26

37.8: CARDIAC PACEMAKER DEV OP. Formerly included in operation group(s) 577.

Type of Patients	Observed Patients	Avg. Stay	Vari-ance	10th	25th	50th	75th	90th	95th	99th
1. SINGLE DX										
0–19 Years	56	2.4	4	1	1	2	3	6	6	9
20–34	36	2.1	3	1	1	1	3	3	6	7
35–49	42	2.0	4	1	1	1	2	4	8	8
50–64	122	1.8	3	1	1	1	2	3	7	7
65+	677	1.9	3	1	1	1	2	4	6	8
2. MULTIPLE DX										
0–19 Years	348	4.4	37	1	1	2	5	12	15	42
20–34	216	4.7	21	1	1	3	7	10	12	21
35–49	475	5.3	46	1	2	4	7	9	14	47
50–64	1946	5.3	23	1	2	4	7	10	14	24
65+	19089	5.8	31	1	2	4	8	12	15	27
TOTAL SINGLE DX	933	1.9	3	1	1	1	2	4	6	8
MULTIPLE DX	22074	5.7	31	1	2	4	7	12	15	27
TOTAL										
0–19 Years	404	4.0	32	1	1	2	4	9	15	32
20–34	252	4.1	18	1	1	3	6	8	12	19
35–49	517	4.9	42	1	2	3	7	9	13	47
50–64	2068	5.0	23	1	2	4	7	10	14	24
65+	19766	5.7	30	1	2	4	7	12	15	26
GRAND TOTAL	23007	5.6	30	1	2	4	7	12	15	26

Length of Stay by Diagnosis and Operation, United States, 1997

United States, October 1995–September 1996 Data, by Operation

37.80: INSERT PACEMAKER DEV NOS. Formerly included in operation group(s) 577.

Type of Patients	Observed Patients	Avg. Stay	Vari-ance	10th	25th	50th	75th	90th	95th	99th
1. SINGLE DX										
0–19 Years	8	1.6	<1	1	1	2	2	2	2	4
20–34	1	3.0	0	3	3	3	3	3	3	3
35–49	5	2.6	4	1	1	3	3	6	6	6
50–64	4	1.0	0	1	1	1	1	1	1	1
65+	26	2.1	4	1	1	1	3	6	7	10
2. MULTIPLE DX										
0–19 Years	21	3.8	10	1	1	3	5	8	12	12
20–34	6	5.1	21	1	3	3	7	15	15	15
35–49	11	29.7	441	3	5	47	47	47	47	47
50–64	70	5.1	20	1	1	3	8	9	13	21
65+	785	5.9	23	1	2	5	9	12	14	22
TOTAL SINGLE DX	44	1.9	2	1	1	1	2	3	6	7
MULTIPLE DX	893	6.1	35	1	2	5	9	12	15	47
TOTAL										
0–19 Years	29	2.8	7	1	1	2	3	7	8	12
20–34	7	4.8	19	3	3	3	7	15	15	15
35–49	16	21.7	465	1	3	6	47	47	47	47
50–64	74	5.0	20	1	1	3	8	9	9	21
65+	811	5.8	23	1	2	5	9	11	13	22
GRAND TOTAL	937	5.9	34	1	2	4	8	11	15	47

37.81: INSERT SINGLE CHAMB DEV. Formerly included in operation group(s) 577.

Type of Patients	Observed Patients	Avg. Stay	Vari-ance	10th	25th	50th	75th	90th	95th	99th
1. SINGLE DX										
0–19 Years	5	2.2	1	2	2	2	2	3	3	3
20–34	1	1.0	0	1	1	1	1	1	1	1
35–49	2	1.5	<1	1	1	1	2	2	2	2
50–64	8	2.8	5	1	2	2	2	6	9	9
65+	69	1.8	2	1	1	1	3	4	5	8
2. MULTIPLE DX										
0–19 Years	20	7.3	44	1	2	5	13	13	13	29
20–34	10	3.7	14	1	2	3	4	6	14	15
35–49	42	4.3	13	2	2	3	5	8	8	23
50–64	227	5.9	25	2	3	5	7	10	14	21
65+	3656	7.0	40	2	3	5	9	14	19	28
TOTAL SINGLE DX	85	1.9	2	1	1	1	2	4	5	8
MULTIPLE DX	3955	6.9	39	2	3	5	8	14	18	28
TOTAL										
0–19 Years	25	4.7	28	1	2	2	5	13	13	29
20–34	11	3.6	13	1	2	3	4	6	14	15
35–49	44	4.2	13	2	2	3	5	8	8	23
50–64	235	5.9	24	2	3	5	7	10	14	21
65+	3725	6.9	40	2	3	5	9	14	18	28
GRAND TOTAL	4040	6.8	38	2	3	5	8	14	18	28

37.82: INSERT RATE-RESPON DEV. Formerly included in operation group(s) 577.

Type of Patients	Observed Patients	Avg. Stay	Vari-ance	10th	25th	50th	75th	90th	95th	99th
1. SINGLE DX										
0–19 Years	9	1.6	2	1	1	1	1	5	5	7
20–34	0									
35–49	3	1.5	<1	1	1	1	2	2	2	2
50–64	14	1.4	<1	1	1	1	1	3	3	3
65+	63	2.2	3	1	1	2	3	5	7	8
2. MULTIPLE DX										
0–19 Years	35	7.5	116	1	1	2	5	32	32	42
20–34	17	5.9	32	1	2	2	12	12	12	26
35–49	51	5.3	22	1	2	3	8	13	17	17
50–64	295	7.9	44	2	3	7	9	16	24	27
65+	3606	6.8	31	1	3	6	9	14	17	25
TOTAL SINGLE DX	89	1.9	2	1	1	1	2	3	6	8
MULTIPLE DX	4004	6.9	33	1	3	6	9	14	17	26
TOTAL										
0–19 Years	44	6.3	99	1	1	2	5	25	32	42
20–34	17	5.9	32	1	2	2	12	12	12	26
35–49	54	5.1	22	1	2	3	7	13	17	17
50–64	309	7.1	43	1	3	6	8	15	21	26
65+	3669	6.7	31	1	3	6	9	14	17	25
GRAND TOTAL	4093	6.7	33	1	3	5	9	14	17	26

37.83: INSERT DUAL-CHAMBER DEV. Formerly included in operation group(s) 577.

Type of Patients	Observed Patients	Avg. Stay	Vari-ance	10th	25th	50th	75th	90th	95th	99th
1. SINGLE DX										
0–19 Years	17	3.0	4	1	1	3	6	6	6	6
20–34	17	1.7	4	1	1	1	1	3	4	16
35–49	15	3.1	6	1	1	2	4	8	8	8
50–64	46	2.1	5	1	1	1	2	7	7	11
65+	216	2.7	5	1	1	2	3	6	6	8
2. MULTIPLE DX										
0–19 Years	79	5.1	28	1	2	3	6	15	16	>99
20–34	66	4.9	14	1	2	3	8	8	8	19
35–49	234	5.1	22	1	2	4	7	9	10	20
50–64	976	5.1	20	1	2	4	7	10	14	22
65+	7227	5.9	29	1	2	5	8	12	15	28
TOTAL SINGLE DX	311	2.5	5	1	1	1	3	6	6	8
MULTIPLE DX	8582	5.8	28	1	2	4	7	11	15	27
TOTAL										
0–19 Years	96	4.6	23	1	2	3	6	15	15	>99
20–34	83	3.9	13	1	1	3	7	8	9	19
35–49	249	5.0	21	2	2	4	7	9	10	20
50–64	1022	4.9	20	1	2	4	6	10	14	21
65+	7443	5.8	28	2	2	4	7	11	15	27
GRAND TOTAL	8893	5.6	27	1	2	4	7	11	15	27

Length of Stay by Diagnosis and Operation, United States, 1997

United States, October 1995–September 1996 Data, by Operation

37.85: REPL W 1-CHAMBER DEVICE. Formerly included in operation group(s) 577.

Type of Patients	Observed Patients	Avg. Stay	Vari-ance	Percentiles						
				10th	25th	50th	75th	90th	95th	99th
1. SINGLE DX										
0–19 Years	3	1.5	<1	1	1	1	2	2	2	2
20–34	1	7.0	0	7	7	7	7	7	7	7
35–49	1	1.0	0	1	1	1	1	1	1	1
50–64	10	1.6	<1	1	1	1	2	4	4	4
65+	75	1.2	<1	1	1	1	1	2	2	5
2. MULTIPLE DX										
0–19 Years	27	1.9	<1	1	1	2	2	3	4	4
20–34	15	3.5	5	1	1	3	6	7	7	7
35–49	11	5.4	12	1	2	7	7	10	10	14
50–64	70	2.2	4	1	1	2	3	5	6	12
65+	952	3.5	19	1	1	2	4	8	10	22
TOTAL SINGLE DX	90	1.3	<1	1	1	1	1	2	2	7
MULTIPLE DX	1075	3.4	17	1	1	2	4	7	10	21
TOTAL										
0–19 Years	30	1.9	<1	1	1	2	2	3	3	4
20–34	16	3.9	6	1	1	4	6	7	7	7
35–49	12	5.2	13	1	2	7	7	10	10	14
50–64	80	2.2	3	1	1	2	3	5	5	8
65+	1027	3.2	17	1	1	2	4	7	10	21
GRAND TOTAL	1165	3.1	16	1	1	2	3	7	10	19

37.86: REPL W RATE-RESPON DEV. Formerly included in operation group(s) 577.

Type of Patients	Observed Patients	Avg. Stay	Vari-ance	Percentiles						
				10th	25th	50th	75th	90th	95th	99th
1. SINGLE DX										
0–19 Years	4	1.4	<1	1	1	1	2	2	2	2
20–34	3	1.0	0	1	1	1	1	1	1	1
35–49	1	1.0	0	1	1	1	1	1	1	1
50–64	10	1.8	1	1	1	1	3	3	5	5
65+	76	1.3	<1	1	1	1	1	2	3	5
2. MULTIPLE DX										
0–19 Years	36	3.1	9	1	1	2	4	9	9	11
20–34	24	2.7	14	1	1	1	3	5	5	27
35–49	20	2.7	11	1	2	2	4	5	7	27
50–64	53	3.0	6	1	1	3	4	5	7	14
65+	887	3.5	14	1	1	2	4	7	10	19
TOTAL SINGLE DX	94	1.4	<1	1	1	1	1	2	3	5
MULTIPLE DX	1020	3.4	13	1	1	2	4	7	9	19
TOTAL										
0–19 Years	40	2.9	8	1	1	2	3	9	9	11
20–34	27	2.5	12	1	1	1	3	5	5	27
35–49	21	2.7	11	1	1	2	3	5	7	27
50–64	63	2.9	5	1	1	3	3	5	7	14
65+	963	3.3	13	1	1	2	4	7	9	19
GRAND TOTAL	1114	3.2	12	1	1	2	4	7	9	18

37.87: REPL W DUAL-CHAMB DEVICE. Formerly included in operation group(s) 577.

Type of Patients	Observed Patients	Avg. Stay	Vari-ance	Percentiles						
				10th	25th	50th	75th	90th	95th	99th
1. SINGLE DX										
0–19 Years	9	4.3	11	1	2	2	9	9	9	9
20–34	13	2.2	1	1	1	3	3	3	4	4
35–49	13	1.1	<1	1	1	1	1	1	1	1
50–64	28	1.5	<1	1	1	1	2	2	3	5
65+	148	1.4	1	1	1	1	2	2	3	5
2. MULTIPLE DX										
0–19 Years	120	3.3	21	1	1	2	4	7	11	21
20–34	67	3.9	28	1	1	3	6	9	15	22
35–49	87	2.6	5	1	1	2	3	5	7	9
50–64	219	3.9	6	1	2	5	5	7	7	12
65+	1777	3.8	22	1	1	2	5	9	13	24
TOTAL SINGLE DX	211	1.5	2	1	1	1	2	3	3	6
MULTIPLE DX	2270	3.8	20	1	1	2	5	8	12	21
TOTAL										
0–19 Years	129	3.4	20	1	1	2	4	7	11	21
20–34	80	3.4	20	1	1	2	4	7	10	22
35–49	100	2.1	4	1	2	2	3	4	6	9
50–64	247	3.8	6	1	2	5	5	7	7	11
65+	1925	3.6	21	1	1	2	4	9	12	24
GRAND TOTAL	2481	3.6	18	1	1	2	5	8	11	21

37.9: HRT/PERICARDIUM OPS NEC. Formerly included in operation group(s) 576, 579, 584.

Type of Patients	Observed Patients	Avg. Stay	Vari-ance	Percentiles						
				10th	25th	50th	75th	90th	95th	99th
1. SINGLE DX										
0–19 Years	13	2.1	<1	2	2	2	2	3	3	4
20–34	9	1.8	2	1	1	1	3	3	5	5
35–49	22	2.5	2	1	1	2	3	3	5	8
50–64	37	3.7	27	1	1	1	1	8	21	21
65+	51	1.5	2	1	1	1	1	2	5	8
2. MULTIPLE DX										
0–19 Years	51	7.0	40	1	2	7	8	14	24	28
20–34	103	8.4	229	1	2	4	9	15	20	91
35–49	444	7.7	90	1	3	5	9	16	22	56
50–64	1389	8.6	47	1	3	7	12	16	20	35
65+	2620	8.5	59	1	3	7	12	18	23	34
TOTAL SINGLE DX	132	2.1	5	1	1	2	2	3	5	8
MULTIPLE DX	4607	8.4	61	1	3	7	12	17	23	35
TOTAL										
0–19 Years	64	4.5	25	1	2	3	7	10	14	28
20–34	112	7.9	217	1	2	3	8	15	20	91
35–49	466	7.4	86	1	2	5	9	15	20	56
50–64	1426	8.5	47	1	3	7	13	16	20	35
65+	2671	8.2	59	1	2	6	12	18	23	34
GRAND TOTAL	4739	8.1	60	1	2	6	11	16	23	35

Length of Stay by Diagnosis and Operation, United States, 1997

United States, October 1995–September 1996 Data, by Operation

37.94: IMPL/REPL AICD TOT SYST. Formerly included in operation group(s) 576.

Type of Patients	Observed Patients	Avg. Stay	Vari-ance	10th	25th	50th	75th	90th	95th	99th
1. SINGLE DX										
0–19 Years	10	2.1	<1	2	2	2	2	3	3	4
20–34	3	1.9	1	1	1	1	3	3	3	3
35–49	10	3.1	1	2	2	3	3	5	5	8
50–64	19	5.0	39	1	1	2	6	21	21	21
65+	16	1.7	4	1	1	1	1	2	8	8
2. MULTIPLE DX										
0–19 Years	26	7.1	21	2	3	7	10	13	14	26
20–34	76	9.8	286	2	2	5	10	16	16	91
35–49	329	7.7	49	2	3	6	10	15	19	33
50–64	1059	9.9	46	3	6	9	13	17	20	35
65+	1899	9.8	59	2	5	8	13	19	24	37
TOTAL SINGLE DX	58	2.4	7	1	1	2	2	3	8	21
MULTIPLE DX	3389	9.7	58	2	5	8	13	17	23	36
TOTAL										
0–19 Years	36	3.7	12	2	2	2	3	7	11	16
20–34	79	9.5	277	2	2	4	10	15	20	91
35–49	339	7.4	48	2	3	6	10	15	19	33
50–64	1078	9.9	46	3	6	9	13	17	20	35
65+	1915	9.6	60	2	4	8	13	19	24	36
GRAND TOTAL	3447	9.3	58	2	4	8	13	17	22	36

38.0: INCISION OF VESSEL. Formerly included in operation group(s) 590.

Type of Patients	Observed Patients	Avg. Stay	Vari-ance	10th	25th	50th	75th	90th	95th	99th
1. SINGLE DX										
0–19 Years	5	3.0	5	1	1	2	6	6	6	6
20–34	11	4.5	11	1	1	4	7	8	13	13
35–49	27	4.3	10	1	1	4	6	9	11	12
50–64	36	3.9	4	3	3	4	5	7	8	9
65+	36	4.9	11	1	2	4	8	8	10	17
2. MULTIPLE DX										
0–19 Years	56	9.6	120	2	4	7	9	17	40	63
20–34	136	10.4	98	1	3	7	13	28	28	40
35–49	445	7.2	46	2	3	5	9	15	20	32
50–64	1033	7.6	53	2	3	6	10	15	20	42
65+	3275	8.2	52	2	4	6	10	16	21	36
TOTAL SINGLE DX	115	4.3	8	1	2	4	6	8	9	13
MULTIPLE DX	4945	8.1	55	2	4	6	10	16	22	40
TOTAL										
0–19 Years	61	9.2	116	2	4	7	8	17	40	63
20–34	147	10.2	96	1	3	7	13	28	28	40
35–49	472	7.0	45	2	3	5	9	14	20	32
50–64	1069	7.5	52	2	3	5	10	15	20	42
65+	3311	8.2	52	2	4	6	10	16	21	36
GRAND TOTAL	5060	8.0	54	2	3	6	10	16	22	40

37.98: REPL AICD GENERATOR ONLY. Formerly included in operation group(s) 584.

Type of Patients	Observed Patients	Avg. Stay	Vari-ance	10th	25th	50th	75th	90th	95th	99th
1. SINGLE DX										
0–19 Years	2	1.0	0	1	1	1	1	1	1	1
20–34	2	1.4	<1	1	1	1	2	2	2	2
35–49	10	1.4	1	1	1	1	2	2	2	6
50–64	11	1.1	<1	1	1	1	1	2	2	2
65+	25	1.2	<1	1	1	1	1	2	2	3
2. MULTIPLE DX										
0–19 Years	8	1.0	0	1	1	1	1	1	1	1
20–34	13	2.3	3	1	1	1	4	6	6	6
35–49	57	1.8	3	1	1	1	2	4	5	12
50–64	182	3.4	19	1	1	2	6	8	8	9
65+	479	4.3	40	1	1	2	4	13	23	23
TOTAL SINGLE DX	50	1.2	<1	1	1	1	1	2	2	3
MULTIPLE DX	739	3.9	32	1	1	2	4	8	23	23
TOTAL										
0–19 Years	10	1.0	0	1	1	1	1	1	1	1
20–34	15	2.2	3	1	1	1	3	5	6	6
35–49	67	1.8	3	1	1	1	4	4	5	6
50–64	193	3.3	19	1	1	1	6	8	8	9
65+	504	4.1	38	1	1	2	3	11	23	23
GRAND TOTAL	789	3.7	31	1	1	1	3	8	23	23

38.03: UPPER LIMB VESSEL INC. Formerly included in operation group(s) 590.

Type of Patients	Observed Patients	Avg. Stay	Vari-ance	10th	25th	50th	75th	90th	95th	99th
1. SINGLE DX										
0–19 Years	2	1.0	0	1	1	1	1	1	1	1
20–34	5	3.0	7	1	1	2	4	8	8	8
35–49	7	3.5	8	1	2	2	4	9	9	9
50–64	5	2.5	5	1	1	1	4	5	7	7
65+	7	3.1	3	1	1	4	4	5	7	7
2. MULTIPLE DX										
0–19 Years	16	8.6	155	2	3	4	7	41	41	47
20–34	63	9.6	127	1	1	3	13	28	28	28
35–49	157	5.5	22	1	2	4	7	13	14	24
50–64	283	6.5	49	2	2	4	8	15	15	34
65+	882	7.5	54	2	3	5	9	16	16	46
TOTAL SINGLE DX	26	2.9	5	1	1	2	4	5	8	9
MULTIPLE DX	1401	7.2	56	1	3	5	9	15	18	41
TOTAL										
0–19 Years	18	8.1	149	1	2	4	5	17	41	47
20–34	68	9.4	124	1	1	3	13	28	28	28
35–49	164	5.5	22	1	2	4	7	13	14	24
50–64	288	6.5	48	1	2	4	8	15	15	34
65+	889	7.5	54	2	3	5	9	16	16	46
GRAND TOTAL	1427	7.2	55	1	3	5	9	15	18	41

Length of Stay by Diagnosis and Operation

United States, 1997

United States, October 1995–September 1996 Data, by Operation

38.08: LOWER LIMB ARTERY INC. Formerly included in operation group(s) 590.

Type of Patients	Observed Patients	Avg. Stay	Vari-ance	10th	25th	50th	75th	90th	95th	99th
1. SINGLE DX										
0–19 Years	3	3.5	5	1	2	2	6	6	6	6
20–34	3	4.8	6	1	4	4	7	7	7	7
35–49	16	3.6	5	1	1	3	6	6	8	8
50–64	25	3.9	3	2	3	4	5	6	7	8
65+	24	5.6	12	1	4	5	8	8	13	17
2. MULTIPLE DX										
0–19 Years	15	7.9	99	2	4	7	7	13	13	63
20–34	46	11.9	69	4	7	9	15	26	30	33
35–49	206	8.3	57	2	4	6	10	18	20	30
50–64	584	7.8	39	2	4	6	10	15	18	68
65+	2043	8.2	41	2	4	7	11	15	20	33
TOTAL SINGLE DX	71	4.2	7	1	3	4	6	8	8	13
MULTIPLE DX	2894	8.2	43	2	4	7	10	16	20	33
TOTAL										
0–19 Years	18	7.5	91	1	4	7	7	13	13	63
20–34	49	11.7	69	4	7	9	14	26	30	33
35–49	222	7.9	54	2	4	6	10	17	20	28
50–64	609	7.6	38	2	4	6	10	15	18	68
65+	2067	8.2	41	2	4	7	10	15	20	33
GRAND TOTAL	2965	8.1	43	2	4	7	10	15	20	33

38.12: HEAD/NK ENDARTERECT NEC. Formerly included in operation group(s) 586.

Type of Patients	Observed Patients	Avg. Stay	Vari-ance	10th	25th	50th	75th	90th	95th	99th
1. SINGLE DX										
0–19 Years	0									
20–34	0									
35–49	79	2.3	2	1	1	2	3	3	4	8
50–64	806	2.3	3	1	1	2	3	4	5	8
65+	2176	2.2	2	1	1	2	2	3	5	8
2. MULTIPLE DX										
0–19 Years	1	1.0	0	1	1	1	1	1	1	1
20–34	8	2.4	14	1	1	1	2	4	15	15
35–49	632	3.4	12	1	2	2	4	8	9	14
50–64	7991	3.4	14	1	2	2	4	7	10	17
65+	30507	3.6	14	1	2	2	4	7	10	20
TOTAL SINGLE DX	3061	2.2	2	1	1	2	3	3	5	8
MULTIPLE DX	39139	3.6	14	1	2	2	4	7	10	19
TOTAL										
0–19 Years	1	1.0	0	1	1	1	1	1	1	1
20–34	8	2.4	14	1	1	1	2	4	15	15
35–49	711	3.3	11	1	2	2	4	7	9	13
50–64	8797	3.3	13	1	2	2	4	7	10	16
65+	32683	3.5	14	1	2	2	4	7	10	19
GRAND TOTAL	42200	3.5	13	1	2	2	4	7	10	18

38.1: ENDARTERECTOMY. Formerly included in operation group(s) 586, 590.

Type of Patients	Observed Patients	Avg. Stay	Vari-ance	10th	25th	50th	75th	90th	95th	99th
1. SINGLE DX										
0–19 Years	0									
20–34	6	4.2	5	2	2	4	7	7	7	7
35–49	100	2.4	2	1	1	2	3	4	4	8
50–64	858	2.4	4	1	1	2	4	4	5	9
65+	2224	2.2	2	1	1	2	2	4	5	8
2. MULTIPLE DX										
0–19 Years	5	14.7	200	1	1	13	35	35	35	35
20–34	35	6.3	42	1	1	5	8	14	15	35
35–49	842	4.4	21	1	2	3	5	9	14	21
50–64	8777	3.7	17	1	2	2	4	8	10	20
65+	32124	3.8	16	1	2	2	4	8	11	20
TOTAL SINGLE DX	3188	2.3	3	1	1	2	3	4	5	9
MULTIPLE DX	41783	3.8	16	1	2	2	4	8	11	20
TOTAL										
0–19 Years	5	14.7	200	1	1	13	35	35	35	35
20–34	41	6.1	38	1	2	5	8	14	15	35
35–49	942	4.2	19	1	2	3	5	9	13	21
50–64	9635	3.6	16	1	2	2	4	7	10	20
65+	34348	3.7	15	1	2	2	4	8	11	20
GRAND TOTAL	44971	3.7	15	1	2	2	4	8	11	20

38.16: ABDOMINAL ENDARTERECTOMY. Formerly included in operation group(s) 590.

Type of Patients	Observed Patients	Avg. Stay	Vari-ance	10th	25th	50th	75th	90th	95th	99th
1. SINGLE DX										
0–19 Years	0									
20–34	1	2.0	0	2	2	2	2	2	2	2
35–49	2	1.5	2	1	1	1	1	4	4	4
50–64	5	2.4	1	2	2	2	2	4	4	10
65+	7	3.6	8	2	2	2	4	9	9	9
2. MULTIPLE DX										
0–19 Years	1	6.0	0	6	6	6	6	6	6	6
20–34	4	6.8	9	4	4	7	7	12	12	12
35–49	34	9.2	44	3	4	7	12	21	21	39
50–64	121	8.7	39	3	5	7	10	18	22	29
65+	230	9.6	60	3	5	7	11	23	27	34
TOTAL SINGLE DX	15	2.9	5	2	2	2	2	4	5	9
MULTIPLE DX	390	9.2	50	3	4	7	11	21	27	29
TOTAL										
0–19 Years	1	6.0	0	6	6	6	6	6	6	6
20–34	5	6.1	11	2	4	6	7	12	12	12
35–49	36	8.8	45	3	4	6	12	18	21	39
50–64	126	7.9	39	2	4	6	10	18	21	29
65+	237	9.0	58	2	4	7	10	21	27	34
GRAND TOTAL	405	8.5	49	2	4	7	10	18	27	29

Length of Stay by Diagnosis and Operation, United States, 1997

United States, October 1995–September 1996 Data, by Operation

38.18: LOWER LIMB ENDARTERECT. Formerly included in operation group(s) 590.

Type of Patients	Observed Patients	Avg. Stay	Vari-ance	10th	25th	50th	75th	90th	95th	99th
1. SINGLE DX										
0–19 Years	0									
20–34	2	2.0	0	2	2	2	2	2	2	2
35–49	13	2.8	2	1	1	3	4	4	4	4
50–64	39	2.0	2	1	1	1	3	4	4	8
65+	38	2.9	8	2	2	2	3	5	5	16
2. MULTIPLE DX										
0–19 Years	1	13.0	0	13	13	13	13	13	13	13
20–34	12	9.4	65	4	5	7	9	13	35	35
35–49	127	7.0	39	2	3	5	9	17	17	33
50–64	538	6.0	32	1	3	5	7	12	15	30
65+	1221	6.7	28	2	3	5	8	13	16	28
TOTAL SINGLE DX	92	2.4	4	1	1	2	3	4	5	9
MULTIPLE DX	1899	6.5	30	2	3	5	8	13	17	30
TOTAL										
0–19 Years	1	13.0	0	13	13	13	13	13	13	13
20–34	14	8.2	61	2	4	7	9	13	35	35
35–49	140	6.7	37	2	3	5	8	17	17	33
50–64	577	5.6	31	1	2	4	7	11	15	30
65+	1259	6.5	27	2	3	5	8	13	16	28
GRAND TOTAL	1991	6.2	30	2	3	5	8	12	17	29

38.2: DXTIC PX ON BLOOD VESSEL. Formerly included in operation group(s) 590, 596.

Type of Patients	Observed Patients	Avg. Stay	Vari-ance	10th	25th	50th	75th	90th	95th	99th
1. SINGLE DX										
0–19 Years	0									
20–34	2	9.7	5	6	6	11	11	11	11	11
35–49	6	4.2	8	3	3	3	4	7	7	14
50–64	11	3.0	<1	3	3	3	3	3	3	6
65+	22	4.7	1	4	5	5	5	5	6	8
2. MULTIPLE DX										
0–19 Years	1	1.0	0	1	1	1	1	1	1	1
20–34	8	9.6	54	4	4	7	8	24	24	24
35–49	63	7.9	35	2	4	6	11	13	19	39
50–64	315	4.2	36	1	1	2	5	9	12	26
65+	1550	8.3	52	3	4	7	10	15	18	36
TOTAL SINGLE DX	41	4.2	3	3	3	5	5	5	6	11
MULTIPLE DX	1937	7.4	51	1	3	6	9	14	17	34
TOTAL										
0–19 Years	1	1.0	0	1	1	1	1	1	1	1
20–34	10	9.6	42	4	6	7	11	24	24	24
35–49	69	7.4	33	3	3	6	10	13	17	39
50–64	326	4.1	33	1	1	3	5	9	12	25
65+	1572	8.2	50	3	4	6	10	14	18	35
GRAND TOTAL	1978	7.2	49	2	3	6	9	14	17	33

38.21: BLOOD VESSEL BIOPSY. Formerly included in operation group(s) 590.

Type of Patients	Observed Patients	Avg. Stay	Vari-ance	10th	25th	50th	75th	90th	95th	99th
1. SINGLE DX										
0–19 Years	0									
20–34	2	9.7	5	6	6	11	11	11	11	11
35–49	4	5.7	12	3	3	4	7	7	14	14
50–64	11	3.0	<1	3	3	3	3	3	3	6
65+	21	4.7	1	3	5	5	5	5	6	8
2. MULTIPLE DX										
0–19 Years	1	1.0	0	1	1	1	1	1	1	1
20–34	8	9.6	54	4	4	7	8	24	24	24
35–49	59	7.8	36	2	4	6	9	15	19	39
50–64	310	4.2	36	1	1	2	5	9	12	26
65+	1542	8.4	52	3	4	7	10	15	19	36
TOTAL SINGLE DX	38	4.2	3	3	3	5	5	5	6	11
MULTIPLE DX	1920	7.4	51	3	3	6	9	14	17	34
TOTAL										
0–19 Years	1	1.0	0	1	1	1	1	1	1	1
20–34	10	9.6	42	4	6	7	11	24	24	24
35–49	63	7.6	34	3	4	6	9	14	19	39
50–64	321	4.1	33	1	1	3	5	9	12	25
65+	1563	8.2	50	3	4	6	10	15	18	35
GRAND TOTAL	1958	7.3	49	1	3	6	9	14	17	33

38.3: VESSEL RESECT W ANAST. Formerly included in operation group(s) 590.

Type of Patients	Observed Patients	Avg. Stay	Vari-ance	10th	25th	50th	75th	90th	95th	99th
1. SINGLE DX										
0–19 Years	41	4.3	4	3	3	4	4	6	8	14
20–34	7	2.9	2	1	2	3	3	5	7	7
35–49	3	5.8	<1	5	5	6	6	6	6	6
50–64	13	4.7	13	1	2	5	6	7	7	18
65+	7	3.2	6	1	1	2	6	7	7	7
2. MULTIPLE DX										
0–19 Years	268	8.8	76	3	4	6	10	19	24	57
20–34	41	8.5	56	2	5	7	9	14	28	38
35–49	65	7.6	49	2	3	6	8	13	23	46
50–64	141	9.1	72	1	3	6	12	19	28	43
65+	389	9.0	51	3	5	7	11	16	21	37
TOTAL SINGLE DX	71	4.2	6	2	3	4	5	7	8	14
MULTIPLE DX	904	8.8	64	3	4	7	10	17	24	46
TOTAL										
0–19 Years	309	8.3	70	3	4	5	9	17	24	53
20–34	48	7.5	51	2	3	6	9	14	20	38
35–49	68	7.5	48	2	3	6	8	13	23	46
50–64	154	8.8	70	1	3	6	11	18	28	43
65+	396	9.0	51	3	5	7	10	16	21	37
GRAND TOTAL	975	8.5	61	3	4	7	10	17	24	46

Length of Stay by Diagnosis and Operation, United States, 1997

United States, October 1995–September 1996 Data, by Operation

38.34: AORTA RESECTION & ANAST. Formerly included in operation group(s) 590.

Type of Patients	Observed Patients	Avg. Stay	Variance	10th	25th	50th	75th	90th	95th	99th
1. SINGLE DX										
0–19 Years	35	4.4	4	3	3	4	4	6	9	14
20–34	0									
35–49										
50–64	5	6.8	16	5	5	6	6	18	18	18
65+	2	6.6	<1	6	6	7	7	7	7	7
2. MULTIPLE DX										
0–19 Years	242	8.9	79	3	4	6	10	19	24	57
20–34	3	6.7	5	4	5	8	8	8	8	8
35–49	11	9.8	31	4	6	10	12	12	24	24
50–64	54	12.1	62	6	7	9	17	28	28	44
65+	192	10.5	44	6	7	9	11	17	22	37
TOTAL SINGLE DX	42	4.7	6	3	3	4	5	7	9	18
MULTIPLE DX	502	9.7	67	3	5	7	11	19	24	51
TOTAL										
0–19 Years	277	8.4	74	3	4	5	9	17	24	57
20–34	3	6.7	5	4	4	8	8	8	8	8
35–49	11	9.8	31	4	6	10	12	12	24	24
50–64	59	11.7	61	5	7	9	17	28	28	44
65+	194	10.4	44	6	7	9	11	17	22	37
GRAND TOTAL	544	9.4	64	3	5	7	11	18	24	51

38.4: VESSEL RESECT W REPL. Formerly included in operation group(s) 587, 590.

Type of Patients	Observed Patients	Avg. Stay	Variance	10th	25th	50th	75th	90th	95th	99th
1. SINGLE DX										
0–19 Years	19	4.4	5	1	3	5	6	6	8	8
20–34	10	3.4	7	1	2	3	4	6	12	12
35–49	20	5.2	8	2	4	4	6	10	12	12
50–64	64	5.8	4	4	4	6	6	7	8	13
65+	116	5.6	6	2	4	6	7	8	9	12
2. MULTIPLE DX										
0–19 Years	204	9.5	153	3	4	5	11	16	34	68
20–34	151	8.9	71	3	5	7	12	17	22	53
35–49	309	9.8	76	3	6	7	10	23	29	38
50–64	2285	9.1	53	4	6	8	10	16	21	41
65+	9335	10.5	74	5	6	8	11	18	25	52
TOTAL SINGLE DX	229	5.5	6	2	4	6	7	8	9	12
MULTIPLE DX	12284	10.2	72	5	6	8	11	17	25	50
TOTAL										
0–19 Years	223	9.0	142	3	4	5	9	14	30	68
20–34	161	8.7	69	2	4	6	12	16	22	53
35–49	329	9.6	74	3	5	7	10	23	29	37
50–64	2349	9.0	52	4	6	7	10	16	21	39
65+	9451	10.4	73	5	6	8	11	18	25	51
GRAND TOTAL	12513	10.0	71	5	6	8	11	17	24	49

38.44: ABD AORTA RESECT W REPL. Formerly included in operation group(s) 587.

Type of Patients	Observed Patients	Avg. Stay	Variance	10th	25th	50th	75th	90th	95th	99th
1. SINGLE DX										
0–19 Years	2	4.5	<1	4	4	4	5	5	5	5
20–34	0									
35–49	2	10.2	9	6	6	12	12	12	12	12
50–64	45	6.3	2	5	6	6	6	7	8	13
65+	84	6.7	3	5	6	6	7	8	9	13
2. MULTIPLE DX										
0–19 Years	12	15.2	280	4	5	7	18	34	55	55
20–34	12	11.8	147	4	6	7	10	27	53	53
35–49	82	9.4	49	5	6	7	10	18	25	38
50–64	1681	9.1	44	5	6	7	10	15	19	37
65+	7731	10.6	69	6	7	8	11	17	24	51
TOTAL SINGLE DX	133	6.5	3	5	6	6	7	8	9	13
MULTIPLE DX	9518	10.3	65	5	6	8	11	17	23	48
TOTAL										
0–19 Years	14	13.1	243	4	5	7	8	34	55	55
20–34	12	11.8	147	4	6	7	10	27	53	53
35–49	84	9.4	48	5	6	7	10	18	25	38
50–64	1726	9.0	42	5	6	7	10	15	19	37
65+	7815	10.5	68	6	7	8	11	17	24	51
GRAND TOTAL	9651	10.2	63	5	6	8	11	17	23	48

38.45: THOR VESS RESECT W REPL. Formerly included in operation group(s) 587.

Type of Patients	Observed Patients	Avg. Stay	Variance	10th	25th	50th	75th	90th	95th	99th
1. SINGLE DX										
0–19 Years	13	4.3	4	1	3	5	6	6	6	6
20–34	1	6.0	0	6	6	6	6	6	6	6
35–49	4	5.0	3	4	4	4	5	6	10	10
50–64	3	3.9	3	2	2	5	5	5	5	5
65+	1	7.0	0	7	7	7	7	7	7	7
2. MULTIPLE DX										
0–19 Years	156	9.3	159	3	4	5	10	14	30	90
20–34	56	8.2	34	4	5	6	9	13	23	32
35–49	103	12.7	89	5	6	9	16	25	29	43
50–64	213	15.1	131	6	7	11	19	30	37	54
65+	474	14.8	168	4	7	10	18	31	45	66
TOTAL SINGLE DX	22	4.5	4	2	4	5	6	6	6	10
MULTIPLE DX	1002	13.2	150	4	6	9	16	28	38	64
TOTAL										
0–19 Years	169	9.0	150	3	4	5	9	13	27	90
20–34	57	8.2	34	4	5	6	9	13	23	32
35–49	107	12.1	86	4	6	9	15	25	28	43
50–64	216	15.0	131	6	7	11	19	30	37	54
65+	475	14.8	167	4	7	10	18	31	45	66
GRAND TOTAL	1024	13.0	149	4	6	9	15	28	37	64

Length of Stay by Diagnosis and Operation, United States, 1997

United States, October 1995–September 1996 Data, by Operation

38.46: ABD ARTERY RESECT W REPL. Formerly included in operation group(s) 590.

Type of Patients	Observed Patients	Avg. Stay	Vari-ance	10th	25th	50th	75th	90th	95th	99th
1. SINGLE DX										
0–19 Years	0									
20–34	1	3.0	0	3	3	3	3	3	3	3
35–49	2	5.5	5	4	4	6	7	7	7	7
50–64	2	5.7	<1	5	5	6	6	6	6	6
65+	10	5.3	4	3	3	6	7	8	8	8
2. MULTIPLE DX										
0–19 Years	0									
20–34	1	7.0	0	7	7	7	7	7	7	7
35–49	11	6.3	2	5	5	6	7	8	9	9
50–64	91	9.2	73	2	5	6	10	29	29	37
65+	337	11.1	92	5	6	8	13	19	34	55
TOTAL SINGLE DX	15	5.3	4	3	3	6	7	8	8	8
MULTIPLE DX	440	10.5	86	5	6	7	11	20	29	50
TOTAL										
0–19 Years	0									
20–34	2	5.0	8	3	3	5	7	7	7	7
35–49	13	6.3	2	5	5	6	7	8	9	9
50–64	93	9.2	73	2	5	6	9	29	29	37
65+	347	11.0	91	5	6	8	13	19	34	55
GRAND TOTAL	455	10.4	85	5	6	7	11	20	29	50

38.5: LIG&STRIP VARICOSE VEINS. Formerly included in operation group(s) 582.

Type of Patients	Observed Patients	Avg. Stay	Vari-ance	10th	25th	50th	75th	90th	95th	99th
1. SINGLE DX										
0–19 Years	0									
20–34	55	1.8	2	1	1	1	2	4	4	9
35–49	149	1.7	4	1	1	1	2	3	4	15
50–64	103	1.5	<1	1	1	1	2	2	3	5
65+	44	1.7	1	1	1	1	2	3	3	6
2. MULTIPLE DX										
0–19 Years	2	1.3	<1	1	1	1	1	3	3	3
20–34	49	3.5	10	1	1	2	7	8	8	12
35–49	192	2.9	15	1	1	2	3	7	10	18
50–64	213	2.4	9	1	1	1	2	6	7	16
65+	198	5.2	36	1	1	3	7	12	19	24
TOTAL SINGLE DX	351	1.7	2	1	1	1	2	3	4	9
MULTIPLE DX	654	3.3	18	1	1	2	4	8	12	24
TOTAL										
0–19 Years	2	1.3	<1	1	1	1	1	3	3	3
20–34	104	2.7	7	1	1	1	4	8	8	11
35–49	341	2.4	11	1	1	1	2	5	9	17
50–64	316	2.1	6	1	1	1	2	4	7	14
65+	242	4.7	33	1	1	2	6	12	17	24
GRAND TOTAL	1005	2.8	13	1	1	1	3	7	9	19

38.48: LEG ARTERY RESECT W REPL. Formerly included in operation group(s) 590.

Type of Patients	Observed Patients	Avg. Stay	Vari-ance	10th	25th	50th	75th	90th	95th	99th
1. SINGLE DX										
0–19 Years	1	2.0	0	2	2	2	2	2	2	2
20–34	1	3.0	0	3	3	3	3	3	3	3
35–49	5	3.3	2	2	2	3	4	5	5	5
50–64	9	3.1	1	2	2	3	4	5	5	5
65+	19	2.8	3	1	2	3	3	5	7	9
2. MULTIPLE DX										
0–19 Years	16	8.3	28	2	4	7	14	14	14	24
20–34	29	11.1	248	2	5	5	9	22	53	70
35–49	50	8.2	89	2	3	6	12	17	17	30
50–64	193	5.6	31	1	3	4	8	10	15	38
65+	650	6.8	35	2	3	5	8	14	20	28
TOTAL SINGLE DX	35	2.9	3	1	2	3	3	5	6	9
MULTIPLE DX	938	6.8	45	2	3	5	8	14	18	32
TOTAL										
0–19 Years	17	8.2	28	2	4	7	14	14	14	24
20–34	30	10.9	244	2	5	5	9	22	53	70
35–49	55	8.0	86	2	3	5	10	17	17	30
50–64	202	5.5	31	1	3	4	7	9	15	38
65+	669	6.6	34	2	3	5	8	14	19	27
GRAND TOTAL	973	6.6	43	2	3	5	8	14	18	32

38.59: LOWER LIMB VV LIG&STRIP. Formerly included in operation group(s) 582.

Type of Patients	Observed Patients	Avg. Stay	Vari-ance	10th	25th	50th	75th	90th	95th	99th
1. SINGLE DX										
0–19 Years	0									
20–34	54	1.8	2	1	1	1	2	4	4	9
35–49	146	1.7	4	1	1	1	2	3	4	15
50–64	101	1.5	<1	1	1	1	2	2	3	5
65+	44	1.7	1	1	1	1	2	3	3	6
2. MULTIPLE DX										
0–19 Years	0									
20–34	46	3.5	9	1	1	2	7	8	8	11
35–49	182	2.9	14	1	1	2	3	7	10	18
50–64	207	2.3	8	1	1	1	2	6	7	16
65+	190	4.7	36	1	1	2	5	12	19	24
TOTAL SINGLE DX	345	1.7	2	1	1	1	2	3	4	9
MULTIPLE DX	625	3.1	17	1	1	1	3	8	10	24
TOTAL										
0–19 Years	0									
20–34	100	2.6	7	1	1	1	4	8	8	11
35–49	328	2.4	10	1	1	1	2	5	9	17
50–64	308	2.1	6	1	1	1	2	4	6	14
65+	234	4.3	32	1	1	2	5	10	18	24
GRAND TOTAL	970	2.6	12	1	1	1	3	6	9	19

Length of Stay by Diagnosis and Operation, United States, 1997

United States, October 1995–September 1996 Data, by Operation

38.6: OTHER VESSEL EXCISION. Formerly included in operation group(s) 590.

Type of Patients	Observed Patients	Avg. Stay	Variance	10th	25th	50th	75th	90th	95th	99th
1. SINGLE DX										
0–19 Years	74	4.1	8	2	3	4	5	6	7	11
20–34	34	2.9	6	1	2	2	4	6	7	14
35–49	31	4.2	4	3	3	3	5	8	8	11
50–64	20	3.6	8	1	2	2	4	7	9	13
65+	11	5.4	94	1	1	1	4	30	30	30
2. MULTIPLE DX										
0–19 Years	278	9.7	185	3	4	6	9	19	37	90
20–34	118	9.0	71	1	3	5	15	26	26	31
35–49	188	7.3	41	2	3	6	9	14	19	31
50–64	312	9.1	64	2	3	7	12	21	30	34
65+	667	9.0	52	2	4	7	10	18	23	35
TOTAL SINGLE DX	170	3.9	11	1	2	3	5	6	8	14
MULTIPLE DX	1563	8.9	80	2	4	6	11	18	26	48
TOTAL										
0–19 Years	352	8.3	148	2	3	5	7	15	34	90
20–34	152	7.9	64	1	2	5	11	22	26	30
35–49	219	7.0	37	2	3	5	9	14	17	30
50–64	332	8.9	63	2	3	6	12	20	29	34
65+	678	8.9	53	2	4	7	10	18	23	35
GRAND TOTAL	1733	8.4	76	2	3	6	10	17	25	43

38.68: LOWER LIMB ARTERY EXC. Formerly included in operation group(s) 590.

Type of Patients	Observed Patients	Avg. Stay	Variance	10th	25th	50th	75th	90th	95th	99th
1. SINGLE DX										
0–19 Years	3	3.1	9	1	1	1	7	7	7	7
20–34	3	1.8	<1	1	1	3	2	7	7	7
35–49	3	4.0	4	3	3	3	4	8	8	8
50–64	6	2.3	4	1	1	2	2	7	7	7
65+	2	2.6	3	1	1	4	4	4	4	4
2. MULTIPLE DX										
0–19 Years	7	4.4	14	2	2	2	8	11	13	13
20–34	8	6.5	37	2	5	5	7	11	25	25
35–49	30	8.8	30	3	4	8	14	14	14	31
50–64	100	6.7	41	1	2	4	10	15	15	25
65+	261	6.8	36	2	3	5	9	12	19	27
TOTAL SINGLE DX	16	2.8	5	1	1	2	3	7	7	8
MULTIPLE DX	406	6.9	37	2	3	5	9	15	17	27
TOTAL										
0–19 Years	10	4.1	13	1	2	2	7	8	11	13
20–34	10	5.3	32	2	2	3	5	11	25	25
35–49	33	8.5	30	3	4	8	14	14	14	31
50–64	106	6.6	41	1	2	4	10	15	15	25
65+	263	6.7	36	2	3	5	9	12	19	27
GRAND TOTAL	422	6.8	37	2	3	5	9	15	17	27

38.64: EXCISION OF AORTA. Formerly included in operation group(s) 590.

Type of Patients	Observed Patients	Avg. Stay	Variance	10th	25th	50th	75th	90th	95th	99th
1. SINGLE DX										
0–19 Years	36	3.6	3	2	2	3	5	6	7	8
20–34	0									
35–49	0									
50–64	2	6.0	0	6	6	6	6	6	6	6
65+	1	6.0	0	6	6	6	6	6	6	6
2. MULTIPLE DX										
0–19 Years	206	8.6	118	3	4	6	8	15	34	92
20–34	6	10.7	115	3	5	6	10	33	33	33
35–49	3	8.6	23	4	4	10	14	14	14	14
50–64	53	11.1	57	5	6	8	17	22	29	34
65+	161	10.6	46	6	7	9	12	17	23	62
TOTAL SINGLE DX	39	3.7	3	2	2	3	5	6	7	8
MULTIPLE DX	429	9.6	87	3	5	7	10	18	27	62
TOTAL										
0–19 Years	242	7.9	105	2	4	5	7	14	27	92
20–34	6	10.7	115	3	5	6	10	33	33	33
35–49	3	8.6	23	4	4	10	14	14	14	14
50–64	55	10.9	57	5	6	8	17	22	29	34
65+	162	10.6	45	6	7	9	12	17	23	62
GRAND TOTAL	468	9.1	83	3	4	7	10	17	25	61

38.7: INTERRUPTION VENA CAVA. Formerly included in operation group(s) 588.

Type of Patients	Observed Patients	Avg. Stay	Variance	10th	25th	50th	75th	90th	95th	99th
1. SINGLE DX										
0–19 Years	1	10.0	0	10	10	10	10	10	10	10
20–34	14	6.3	17	2	2	6	9	11	16	17
35–49	31	6.6	9	3	6	7	7	12	14	14
50–64	26	4.5	6	2	3	4	5	9	10	12
65+	45	10.0	62	2	5	11	11	16	27	46
2. MULTIPLE DX										
0–19 Years	32	16.2	378	3	5	10	19	32	53	91
20–34	233	11.7	108	4	6	9	12	23	34	67
35–49	698	24.5	627	3	6	11	63	63	63	77
50–64	1413	10.5	89	3	5	8	13	21	28	55
65+	4399	11.1	87	3	6	9	14	22	29	50
TOTAL SINGLE DX	117	7.2	29	2	4	6	10	11	14	27
MULTIPLE DX	6775	13.1	199	3	6	9	14	26	55	64
TOTAL										
0–19 Years	33	15.9	364	3	5	10	19	32	53	91
20–34	247	11.3	104	3	6	9	11	22	34	67
35–49	729	23.5	610	3	6	10	51	63	63	77
50–64	1439	10.4	88	3	6	8	13	20	28	55
65+	4444	11.1	87	3	6	9	13	22	29	49
GRAND TOTAL	6892	13.0	196	3	6	9	14	26	51	63

Length of Stay by Diagnosis and Operation, United States, 1997

United States, October 1995–September 1996 Data, by Operation

38.8: OTHER SURG VESSEL OCCL. Formerly included in operation group(s) 590.

Type of Patients	Observed Patients	Avg. Stay	Vari-ance	Percentiles						
				10th	25th	50th	75th	90th	95th	99th
1. SINGLE DX										
0–19 Years	465	2.0	2	1	1	2	2	4	4	11
20–34	92	2.5	3	1	1	2	4	5	5	8
35–49	92	2.9	10	1	1	2	3	5	10	13
50–64	49	2.0	4	1	1	1	2	4	5	11
65+	20	1.8	1	1	1	1	3	3	4	5
2. MULTIPLE DX										
0–19 Years	1119	13.1	481	1	2	4	16	81	>99	>99
20–34	315	5.8	83	1	1	3	7	11	18	46
35–49	403	6.1	45	1	2	3	8	15	20	35
50–64	429	6.6	46	1	2	5	9	14	20	36
65+	511	8.4	90	1	3	6	10	21	30	55
TOTAL SINGLE DX	718	2.2	3	1	1	2	3	4	5	11
MULTIPLE DX	2777	9.6	261	1	2	4	10	29	78	>99
TOTAL										
0–19 Years	1584	9.7	358	1	1	3	9	57	99	>99
20–34	407	5.2	69	1	1	3	6	10	18	46
35–49	495	5.6	41	1	2	3	7	14	19	31
50–64	478	6.1	44	1	2	4	9	13	19	36
65+	531	8.2	89	1	3	5	10	20	30	55
GRAND TOTAL	3495	8.0	214	1	2	3	8	22	63	>99

38.85: OCCL THORACIC VESS NEC. Formerly included in operation group(s) 590.

Type of Patients	Observed Patients	Avg. Stay	Vari-ance	Percentiles						
				10th	25th	50th	75th	90th	95th	99th
1. SINGLE DX										
0–19 Years	399	2.0	2	1	1	2	2	4	4	11
20–34	4	4.0	1	2	4	4	4	6	6	6
35–49	5	4.2	82	1	1	1	1	27	27	27
50–64	1	1.0	0	1	1	1	1	3	3	1
65+	1	3.0	0	3	3	3	3	3	3	3
2. MULTIPLE DX										
0–19 Years	919	14.7	559	1	2	4	22	92	>99	>99
20–34	57	8.9	238	1	1	5	10	16	21	90
35–49	33	6.5	27	3	4	4	8	14	19	26
50–64	37	7.3	82	1	1	5	9	19	28	55
65+	46	9.0	75	2	4	5	10	25	25	>99
TOTAL SINGLE DX	410	2.0	3	1	1	2	2	4	4	11
MULTIPLE DX	1092	13.7	500	1	2	4	18	82	>99	>99
TOTAL										
0–19 Years	1318	10.6	414	1	1	3	11	70	>99	>99
20–34	61	8.6	223	1	1	5	9	16	21	90
35–49	38	6.3	30	2	4	4	7	14	20	26
50–64	38	7.2	82	1	1	5	9	19	28	55
65+	47	9.0	75	2	3	5	10	25	25	>99
GRAND TOTAL	1502	10.3	382	1	1	3	10	64	>99	>99

38.82: OCCL HEAD/NECK VESS NEC. Formerly included in operation group(s) 590.

Type of Patients	Observed Patients	Avg. Stay	Vari-ance	Percentiles						
				10th	25th	50th	75th	90th	95th	99th
1. SINGLE DX										
0–19 Years	19	3.0	4	1	2	2	3	8	8	8
20–34	28	2.8	4	1	1	2	4	5	5	13
35–49	21	2.2	1	1	1	2	2	4	4	5
50–64	20	1.5	1	1	1	1	3	4	4	7
65+	5	2.4	2	1	1	3	3	4	4	4
2. MULTIPLE DX										
0–19 Years	34	4.4	54	1	3	3	3	8	9	53
20–34	68	4.7	33	1	2	3	5	9	16	38
35–49	75	4.9	22	1	2	3	7	11	16	>99
50–64	117	4.6	21	2	2	3	5	12	15	21
65+	107	6.3	72	1	2	3	7	13	22	41
TOTAL SINGLE DX	93	2.3	3	1	1	2	3	4	5	8
MULTIPLE DX	401	5.1	41	1	2	3	6	11	15	38
TOTAL										
0–19 Years	53	4.1	42	1	2	3	3	8	9	53
20–34	96	4.0	23	1	1	3	4	9	11	28
35–49	96	4.2	18	1	2	3	5	11	16	20
50–64	137	3.9	18	1	1	2	4	9	15	21
65+	112	6.2	70	1	2	3	7	13	22	41
GRAND TOTAL	494	4.4	34	1	2	3	5	9	14	30

38.86: SURG OCCL ABD ARTERY NEC. Formerly included in operation group(s) 590.

Type of Patients	Observed Patients	Avg. Stay	Vari-ance	Percentiles						
				10th	25th	50th	75th	90th	95th	99th
1. SINGLE DX										
0–19 Years	1	1.0	0	1	1	1	1	1	1	1
20–34	5	4.4	6	1	4	4	5	8	8	8
35–49	6	3.6	4	2	2	4	6	6	6	6
50–64	6	2.3	10	1	1	1	2	11	11	11
65+	1	2.0	0	2	2	2	2	2	2	2
2. MULTIPLE DX										
0–19 Years	33	5.8	43	1	2	3	7	12	16	28
20–34	58	8.2	128	1	2	4	8	18	46	46
35–49	106	7.7	86	1	1	4	10	20	29	42
50–64	117	9.0	54	2	5	9	9	17	21	44
65+	199	10.9	120	2	4	7	12	27	34	>99
TOTAL SINGLE DX	19	2.9	8	1	1	1	4	8	11	11
MULTIPLE DX	513	8.9	92	1	3	6	10	20	31	55
TOTAL										
0–19 Years	34	5.8	42	1	2	3	7	11	16	28
20–34	63	8.0	121	1	2	4	8	18	46	46
35–49	112	7.5	84	1	1	4	10	19	28	42
50–64	123	8.4	54	1	3	9	9	15	21	36
65+	200	10.9	120	2	4	7	12	27	34	>99
GRAND TOTAL	532	8.7	90	1	3	6	10	20	30	55

Length of Stay by Diagnosis and Operation, United States, 1997

United States, October 1995–September 1996 Data, by Operation

38.9: PUNCTURE OF VESSEL. Formerly included in operation group(s) 590, 595, 596.

Type of Patients	Observed Patients	Avg. Stay	Variance	Percentiles						
				10th	25th	50th	75th	90th	95th	99th
1. SINGLE DX										
0–19 Years	765	5.3	21	1	2	4	7	11	14	23
20–34	385	5.7	23	1	2	4	7	14	17	22
35–49	345	5.1	23	1	2	4	6	11	15	22
50–64	191	4.4	18	1	2	3	5	8	11	22
65+	183	5.5	22	1	2	5	7	9	13	36
2. MULTIPLE DX										
0–19 Years	11544	14.5	270	2	4	9	18	37	57	>99
20–34	4969	8.9	63	2	4	7	11	17	23	42
35–49	9469	8.8	65	2	4	7	11	18	23	43
50–64	9877	8.8	64	2	4	7	11	18	24	41
65+	20963	10.5	67	3	5	8	14	21	25	42
TOTAL SINGLE DX	1869	5.3	22	1	2	4	7	11	15	23
MULTIPLE DX	56822	10.6	116	2	4	7	13	22	30	64
TOTAL										
0–19 Years	12309	13.9	260	2	4	8	17	35	55	98
20–34	5354	8.7	61	2	4	7	11	17	22	41
35–49	9814	8.6	64	2	4	7	11	17	23	43
50–64	10068	8.7	64	2	4	6	11	18	24	41
65+	21146	10.4	67	3	5	8	13	21	25	42
GRAND TOTAL	58691	10.4	114	2	4	7	13	22	30	63

38.92: UMBILICAL VEIN CATH. Formerly included in operation group(s) 590.

Type of Patients	Observed Patients	Avg. Stay	Variance	Percentiles						
				10th	25th	50th	75th	90th	95th	99th
1. SINGLE DX										
0–19 Years	21	2.6	9	1	2	2	3	3	4	5
20–34	0									
35–49	0									
50–64	0									
65+	0									
2. MULTIPLE DX										
0–19 Years	1570	13.7	220	2	4	8	21	29	46	91
20–34	2	6.8	86	1	1	1	16	16	16	16
35–49	2	6.0	0	6	6	6	6	6	6	6
50–64	1	2.0	0	2	2	2	2	2	2	2
65+	3	11.6	21	9	10	10	10	22	22	22
TOTAL SINGLE DX	21	2.6	9	1	2	2	3	3	4	5
MULTIPLE DX	1578	13.7	219	2	4	8	21	29	46	91
TOTAL										
0–19 Years	1591	13.5	218	2	4	8	21	29	46	91
20–34	2	6.8	86	1	1	1	16	16	16	16
35–49	2	6.0	0	6	6	6	6	6	6	6
50–64	1	2.0	0	2	2	2	2	2	2	2
65+	3	11.6	21	9	10	10	10	22	22	22
GRAND TOTAL	1599	13.5	218	2	4	8	21	29	46	91

38.91: ARTERIAL CATHETERIZATION. Formerly included in operation group(s) 590.

Type of Patients	Observed Patients	Avg. Stay	Variance	Percentiles						
				10th	25th	50th	75th	90th	95th	99th
1. SINGLE DX										
0–19 Years	90	4.4	9	2	3	4	6	7	10	15
20–34	20	3.6	8	1	2	3	4	7	10	14
35–49	19	5.1	8	2	3	5	6	8	8	18
50–64	12	4.4	15	1	2	4	6	6	14	15
65+	11	3.3	4	1	1	4	5	5	7	7
2. MULTIPLE DX										
0–19 Years	4599	17.7	360	3	5	10	23	53	69	>99
20–34	236	7.4	63	2	3	5	9	15	27	37
35–49	424	6.4	44	2	4	5	7	12	17	32
50–64	616	7.8	35	2	4	6	10	15	19	27
65+	1016	8.6	40	3	5	7	11	16	21	34
TOTAL SINGLE DX	152	4.4	9	1	3	4	6	7	10	15
MULTIPLE DX	6891	14.9	289	3	5	9	18	42	59	>99
TOTAL										
0–19 Years	4689	17.5	357	3	5	10	23	52	68	>99
20–34	256	7.2	61	2	3	5	9	14	27	37
35–49	443	6.4	42	2	3	5	7	12	17	32
50–64	628	7.8	35	2	4	6	10	15	19	27
65+	1027	8.6	40	3	5	7	11	16	21	34
GRAND TOTAL	7043	14.7	286	3	5	8	17	41	59	>99

38.93: VENOUS CATHETER NEC. Formerly included in operation group(s) 595.

Type of Patients	Observed Patients	Avg. Stay	Variance	Percentiles						
				10th	25th	50th	75th	90th	95th	99th
1. SINGLE DX										
0–19 Years	545	5.8	24	1	3	5	7	13	14	26
20–34	312	5.9	24	2	3	4	7	14	17	20
35–49	260	5.5	26	1	2	5	7	13	15	23
50–64	124	4.5	18	2	2	5	5	8	13	22
65+	97	6.3	22	2	3	6	7	9	13	36
2. MULTIPLE DX										
0–19 Years	4383	12.2	195	2	4	8	14	28	42	88
20–34	3845	9.6	67	3	4	7	13	18	23	44
35–49	7251	9.1	65	3	4	7	12	18	24	42
50–64	6742	9.2	62	3	4	7	11	19	24	40
65+	14375	11.2	70	4	6	9	14	21	27	40
TOTAL SINGLE DX	1338	5.7	24	1	2	5	7	13	15	23
MULTIPLE DX	36596	10.3	83	3	5	8	13	21	27	47
TOTAL										
0–19 Years	4928	11.5	180	2	4	7	14	27	38	86
20–34	4157	9.3	64	3	4	7	12	18	23	43
35–49	7511	9.0	64	2	4	7	12	18	24	42
50–64	6866	9.1	61	3	4	7	11	18	24	39
65+	14472	11.2	70	4	6	9	14	22	27	42
GRAND TOTAL	37934	10.1	82	3	4	8	13	21	27	46

Length of Stay by Diagnosis and Operation, United States, 1997

United States, October 1995–September 1996 Data, by Operation

38.94: VENOUS CUTDOWN. Formerly included in operation group(s) 590.

Type of Patients	Observed Patients	Avg. Stay	Vari-ance	10th	25th	50th	75th	90th	95th	99th
1. SINGLE DX										
0–19 Years	22	6.9	16	2	4	9	9	10	11	22
20–34	3	6.0	<1	6	6	6	6	6	6	6
35–49	4	6.1	5	2	5	8	8	8	8	8
50–64	4	4.2	2	2	4	4	5	6	6	6
65+	1	10.0	0	10	10	10	10	10	10	10
2. MULTIPLE DX										
0–19 Years	198	12.7	305	2	4	7	14	24	57	>99
20–34	49	7.4	56	2	3	5	8	19	24	44
35–49	73	9.1	58	3	4	7	11	19	28	36
50–64	86	8.6	73	2	2	5	13	18	25	>99
65+	146	10.3	58	4	6	8	13	22	24	38
TOTAL SINGLE DX	34	6.5	10	2	5	6	9	10	10	22
MULTIPLE DX	552	10.8	171	2	4	7	12	23	33	90
TOTAL										
0–19 Years	220	12.3	285	2	4	7	13	23	48	>99
20–34	52	7.2	47	2	4	6	7	16	24	44
35–49	77	8.9	55	3	4	7	11	19	28	36
50–64	90	8.5	72	2	2	5	12	18	25	>99
65+	147	10.3	57	4	6	8	13	22	24	38
GRAND TOTAL	586	10.5	162	2	4	7	12	23	31	90

38.98: ARTERIAL PUNCTURE NEC. Formerly included in operation group(s) 590.

Type of Patients	Observed Patients	Avg. Stay	Vari-ance	10th	25th	50th	75th	90th	95th	99th
1. SINGLE DX										
0–19 Years	43	2.7	2	1	2	2	3	4	7	7
20–34	30	2.8	2	1	2	2	3	5	6	7
35–49	33	2.5	4	1	1	2	3	6	6	9
50–64	24	4.2	5	1	2	5	5	7	8	9
65+	35	2.8	2	1	2	3	3	5	6	7
2. MULTIPLE DX										
0–19 Years	344	6.7	78	2	2	4	7	13	25	48
20–34	149	4.3	13	1	2	3	6	9	11	20
35–49	302	5.3	42	1	2	4	7	10	13	26
50–64	509	5.3	13	2	3	4	7	10	12	17
65+	1724	6.2	21	2	3	5	8	11	14	21
TOTAL SINGLE DX	165	2.9	3	1	2	2	4	6	7	9
MULTIPLE DX	3028	5.9	29	2	3	5	7	11	14	27
TOTAL										
0–19 Years	387	6.3	72	2	2	4	7	12	23	48
20–34	179	4.1	11	1	2	3	5	9	10	16
35–49	335	5.1	39	1	2	4	6	9	13	23
50–64	533	5.2	13	2	3	4	7	9	12	17
65+	1759	6.1	21	2	3	5	8	11	14	21
GRAND TOTAL	3193	5.8	28	2	3	4	7	11	14	26

38.95: VENOUS CATH FOR RD. Formerly included in operation group(s) 595.

Type of Patients	Observed Patients	Avg. Stay	Vari-ance	10th	25th	50th	75th	90th	95th	99th
1. SINGLE DX										
0–19 Years	12	4.0	23	1	1	2	4	13	13	15
20–34	17	6.3	52	1	3	5	5	27	27	27
35–49	28	2.7	6	1	1	2	3	7	7	10
50–64	25	3.8	34	1	1	2	5	8	10	37
65+	38	4.6	28	1	1	2	7	9	16	27
2. MULTIPLE DX										
0–19 Years	219	10.1	100	1	3	7	12	27	29	48
20–34	654	6.3	31	2	3	5	8	13	16	30
35–49	1327	7.7	63	1	3	6	10	16	20	46
50–64	1806	8.0	84	1	3	5	9	16	29	46
65+	3522	9.3	68	2	3	7	13	19	24	39
TOTAL SINGLE DX	120	4.1	27	1	1	2	5	8	13	27
MULTIPLE DX	7528	8.5	70	2	3	6	11	18	24	43
TOTAL										
0–19 Years	231	9.9	98	1	2	7	12	27	29	48
20–34	671	6.3	31	2	3	5	8	13	16	30
35–49	1355	7.6	62	1	3	5	10	15	20	46
50–64	1831	7.9	83	1	3	5	9	16	29	46
65+	3560	9.3	68	2	3	7	13	19	24	39
GRAND TOTAL	7648	8.4	70	1	3	6	11	18	24	43

38.99: VENOUS PUNCTURE NEC. Formerly included in operation group(s) 596.

Type of Patients	Observed Patients	Avg. Stay	Vari-ance	10th	25th	50th	75th	90th	95th	99th
1. SINGLE DX										
0–19 Years	32	4.3	13	1	2	3	5	11	11	17
20–34	3	4.0	10	2	2	3	8	8	8	8
35–49	1	3.0	0	3	3	3	3	3	3	3
50–64	2	6.9	81	1	1	1	15	15	15	15
65+	1	1.0	0	1	1	1	1	1	1	1
2. MULTIPLE DX										
0–19 Years	231	6.7	52	2	3	4	7	14	22	29
20–34	34	4.1	37	1	1	3	4	7	11	36
35–49	90	7.9	144	2	3	5	7	14	19	65
50–64	117	8.5	136	2	4	5	8	13	53	53
65+	177	6.3	23	2	3	5	8	13	17	22
TOTAL SINGLE DX	39	4.2	14	1	2	3	5	8	11	17
MULTIPLE DX	649	7.2	85	2	3	5	7	13	19	60
TOTAL										
0–19 Years	263	6.4	48	2	3	4	7	14	22	29
20–34	37	4.1	34	1	1	3	4	8	8	36
35–49	91	7.9	143	2	3	5	7	14	19	62
50–64	119	8.5	135	2	4	5	8	13	53	53
65+	178	6.3	23	2	3	5	8	13	17	22
GRAND TOTAL	688	7.1	83	2	3	5	7	13	19	57

Length of Stay by Diagnosis and Operation, United States, 1997

United States, October 1995–September 1996 Data, by Operation

39.0: SYSTEMIC TO PA SHUNT. Formerly included in operation group(s) 583.

Type of Patients	Observed Patients	Avg. Stay	Vari-ance	10th	25th	50th	75th	90th	95th	99th
1. SINGLE DX										
0–19 Years	32	6.0	9	3	4	5	7	11	13	15
20–34	1	5.0	0	5	5	5	5	5	5	5
35–49	2	3.0	0	3	3	3	3	3	3	3
50–64	0									
65+	0									
2. MULTIPLE DX										
0–19 Years	508	17.9	339	5	7	11	20	44	72	94
20–34	2	6.1	28	5	3	7	12	12	12	12
35–49	1	7.0		7	7	7	7	7	7	7
50–64	4	5.7	9	3	3	4	10	10	10	10
65+	2	27.2	559	8	8	8	48	48	48	48
TOTAL SINGLE DX	35	5.9	8	3	4	5	7	9	13	15
MULTIPLE DX	517	17.8	338	5	7	11	20	44	72	94
TOTAL										
0–19 Years	540	17.4	331	4	6	10	20	43	72	94
20–34	4	5.2	5	3	5	5	5	5	12	12
35–49	2	5.5	5	3	3	7	7	7	7	7
50–64	4	5.7	9	3	3	4	10	10	10	10
65+	2	27.2	559	8	8	8	48	48	48	48
GRAND TOTAL	552	17.2	329	4	6	10	20	43	72	94

39.2: OTHER SHUNT/VASC BYPASS. Formerly included in operation group(s) 583, 585.

Type of Patients	Observed Patients	Avg. Stay	Vari-ance	10th	25th	50th	75th	90th	95th	99th
1. SINGLE DX										
0–19 Years	37	4.3	7	1	3	4	6	7	8	14
20–34	69	4.6	27	1	1	3	6	7	14	31
35–49	201	2.5	7	1	1	3	3	5	7	10
50–64	430	3.7	12	2	2	3	4	6	10	15
65+	425	4.5	14	2	2	3	6	9	9	18
2. MULTIPLE DX										
0–19 Years	599	9.8	70	3	5	7	12	19	32	39
20–34	1018	7.6	84	1	3	6	9	16	25	44
35–49	3803	7.5	49	2	3	6	9	15	21	34
50–64	11548	8.3	65	2	3	6	10	18	24	36
65+	24035	9.1	70	3	4	7	11	18	25	42
TOTAL SINGLE DX	1162	3.7	12	1	2	3	4	7	9	18
MULTIPLE DX	41003	8.7	67	2	4	6	10	18	24	40
TOTAL										
0–19 Years	636	9.5	69	3	5	7	11	19	32	39
20–34	1087	7.4	81	2	2	5	9	16	25	43
35–49	4004	7.1	47	1	3	5	8	15	21	34
50–64	11978	8.1	63	2	3	6	10	18	23	36
65+	24460	9.0	69	3	4	7	11	18	24	42
GRAND TOTAL	42165	8.5	66	2	4	6	10	17	24	40

39.1: INTRA-ABD VENOUS SHUNT. Formerly included in operation group(s) 583.

Type of Patients	Observed Patients	Avg. Stay	Vari-ance	10th	25th	50th	75th	90th	95th	99th
1. SINGLE DX										
0–19 Years	2	4.6	<1	4	4	5	5	5	5	5
20–34	1	3.0	0	3	3	3	3	3	3	3
35–49	4	8.6	44	1	1	13	15	15	15	15
50–64	1	1.0	0	1	1	1	1	1	1	1
65+	2	4.4	<1	4	4	4	5	5	5	5
2. MULTIPLE DX										
0–19 Years	36	11.4	116	2	6	9	12	28	35	49
20–34	40	12.6	195	3	5	9	17	17	38	91
35–49	303	9.1	74	2	3	6	12	20	30	41
50–64	314	9.6	100	2	4	9	11	20	27	54
65+	258	11.0	60	4	5	9	17	20	24	35
TOTAL SINGLE DX	10	6.7	32	1	1	5	13	15	15	15
MULTIPLE DX	951	9.9	83	2	4	8	13	20	28	49
TOTAL										
0–19 Years	38	11.0	112	3	5	8	12	28	35	49
20–34	41	12.5	194	3	5	9	17	17	37	91
35–49	307	9.1	74	2	3	6	12	20	30	41
50–64	315	9.6	100	2	4	6	11	20	27	54
65+	260	10.9	60	2	5	9	17	20	24	35
GRAND TOTAL	961	9.9	82	2	4	8	13	20	28	49

39.21: CAVAL-PA ANASTOMOSIS. Formerly included in operation group(s) 583.

Type of Patients	Observed Patients	Avg. Stay	Vari-ance	10th	25th	50th	75th	90th	95th	99th
1. SINGLE DX										
0–19 Years	15	5.1	2	3	4	5	6	7	8	8
20–34	0									
35–49	0									
50–64	0									
65+	0									
2. MULTIPLE DX										
0–19 Years	388	9.9	68	4	5	7	11	19	35	39
20–34	5	12.6	119	5	5	6	27	27	27	27
35–49	2	8.7	<1	8	8	9	9	9	9	9
50–64	0									
65+	1	24.0	0	24	24	24	24	24	24	24
TOTAL SINGLE DX	15	5.1	2	3	4	5	6	7	8	8
MULTIPLE DX	396	10.0	68	4	5	7	11	19	35	39
TOTAL										
0–19 Years	403	9.7	66	4	5	7	11	19	35	39
20–34	5	12.6	119	5	5	6	27	27	37	27
35–49	2	8.7	<1	8	8	9	9	9	9	9
50–64	0									
65+	1	24.0	0	24	24	24	24	24	24	24
GRAND TOTAL	411	9.7	66	4	5	7	11	19	35	39

Length of Stay by Diagnosis and Operation, United States, 1997

United States, October 1995–September 1996 Data, by Operation

39.22: AORTA-SCL-CAROTID BYPASS. Formerly included in operation group(s) 583.

Type of Patients	Observed Patients	Avg. Stay	Vari-ance	10th	25th	50th	75th	90th	95th	99th
1. SINGLE DX										
0–19 Years	0									
20–34	4	5.5	2	4	6	6	6	6	6	6
35–49	10	3.4	5	1	2	2	6	8	8	8
50–64	20	2.5	2	1	1	2	3	4	5	5
65+	13	3.1	6	2	2	3	3	4	6	14
2. MULTIPLE DX										
0–19 Years	5	6.0	7	3	3	6	7	11	11	11
20–34	4	4.4	5	2	3	4	4	8	8	8
35–49	62	5.5	22	1	3	3	9	9	11	22
50–64	269	5.6	28	2	2	3	9	14	14	17
65+	344	6.1	49	2	2	3	6	15	26	28
TOTAL SINGLE DX	47	3.9	5	1	2	3	6	6	6	8
MULTIPLE DX	684	5.8	37	2	2	3	7	14	17	28
TOTAL										
0–19 Years	5	6.0	7	3	3	6	7	11	11	11
20–34	8	5.4	2	3	6	6	6	6	6	8
35–49	72	5.4	21	1	3	3	9	9	11	22
50–64	289	5.4	27	2	2	3	8	14	14	17
65+	357	6.0	49	2	2	3	6	15	26	28
GRAND TOTAL	731	5.7	35	2	2	3	7	13	16	28

39.27: ARTERIOVENOSTOMY FOR RD. Formerly included in operation group(s) 585.

Type of Patients	Observed Patients	Avg. Stay	Vari-ance	10th	25th	50th	75th	90th	95th	99th
1. SINGLE DX										
0–19 Years	13	2.0	7	1	1	1	2	3	3	13
20–34	44	3.8	46	1	1	1	2	7	31	31
35–49	86	1.6	6	1	1	1	1	2	4	21
50–64	94	5.0	27	1	1	2	8	11	12	25
65+	96	3.2	14	1	1	1	3	11	13	14
2. MULTIPLE DX										
0–19 Years	130	9.2	69	1	2	7	15	19	19	32
20–34	836	6.9	76	1	2	5	9	15	18	44
35–49	1863	8.1	66	1	2	6	11	18	23	38
50–64	3178	8.0	71	1	3	6	11	17	24	51
65+	5493	10.2	116	1	3	7	13	22	31	53
TOTAL SINGLE DX	333	2.5	15	1	1	1	2	6	11	25
MULTIPLE DX	11500	8.9	92	1	2	6	12	19	27	51
TOTAL										
0–19 Years	143	8.9	69	1	2	7	15	19	19	32
20–34	880	6.8	75	1	2	5	9	15	18	44
35–49	1949	7.3	64	1	2	5	10	16	22	37
50–64	3272	7.9	70	1	2	5	11	17	24	51
65+	5589	10.1	116	1	3	7	13	22	31	53
GRAND TOTAL	11833	8.6	90	1	2	6	11	19	27	50

39.25: AORTA-ILIAC-FEMORAL BYP. Formerly included in operation group(s) 583.

Type of Patients	Observed Patients	Avg. Stay	Vari-ance	10th	25th	50th	75th	90th	95th	99th
1. SINGLE DX										
0–19 Years	1	2.0	0	2	2	2	2	2	2	2
20–34	2	3.5	<1	3	3	4	4	4	4	4
35–49	27	4.7	6	2	2	5	5	10	10	10
50–64	66	7.5	60	3	5	6	7	9	14	44
65+	19	5.8	5	4	5	5	7	8	8	16
2. MULTIPLE DX										
0–19 Years	2	5.0	0	5	5	5	5	5	5	5
20–34	29	19.3	160	5	7	14	32	32	32	32
35–49	618	8.1	31	4	5	7	8	12	19	30
50–64	2220	8.5	38	4	5	7	9	14	18	36
65+	2824	10.2	54	5	6	8	11	18	24	40
TOTAL SINGLE DX	115	5.9	27	2	4	5	6	9	10	44
MULTIPLE DX	5693	9.3	47	4	6	7	10	16	22	36
TOTAL										
0–19 Years	3	4.3	2	2	5	5	5	5	5	5
20–34	31	18.9	162	4	7	14	32	32	32	32
35–49	645	7.8	29	4	5	6	8	11	19	30
50–64	2286	8.5	38	4	5	7	9	14	18	36
65+	2843	10.2	54	5	6	8	11	18	24	40
GRAND TOTAL	5808	9.2	47	4	6	7	10	16	22	36

39.29: VASC SHUNT & BYPASS NEC. Formerly included in operation group(s) 583.

Type of Patients	Observed Patients	Avg. Stay	Vari-ance	10th	25th	50th	75th	90th	95th	99th
1. SINGLE DX										
0–19 Years	4	5.4	29	1	1	4	5	14	14	14
20–34	16	5.1	17	2	2	3	6	14	14	14
35–49	77	3.5	3	2	3	3	4	5	6	10
50–64	248	3.2	3	2	3	3	3	4	6	10
65+	295	4.7	15	2	3	4	6	9	9	18
2. MULTIPLE DX										
0–19 Years	36	8.7	38	3	4	7	10	16	21	38
20–34	124	7.5	54	2	3	5	9	15	19	40
35–49	1189	6.8	37	2	3	6	7	12	18	30
50–64	5709	8.4	72	2	3	5	10	19	30	33
65+	15090	8.6	56	3	4	6	10	17	23	37
TOTAL SINGLE DX	640	3.9	8	2	2	3	4	7	9	18
MULTIPLE DX	22148	8.4	60	3	4	6	10	17	23	35
TOTAL										
0–19 Years	40	8.4	38	3	4	7	10	14	21	38
20–34	140	7.3	51	2	3	5	9	14	17	32
35–49	1266	6.6	36	2	3	6	7	12	17	30
50–64	5957	8.0	69	2	3	5	9	19	28	33
65+	15385	8.5	55	3	4	6	10	17	22	37
GRAND TOTAL	22788	8.2	58	2	4	6	10	17	23	34

Length of Stay by Diagnosis and Operation, United States, 1997

United States, October 1995–September 1996 Data, by Operation

39.3: SUTURE OF VESSEL. Formerly included in operation group(s) 590.

Type of Patients	Observed Patients	Avg. Stay	Variance	10th	25th	50th	75th	90th	95th	99th
1. SINGLE DX										
0–19 Years	15	3.0	2	1	2	3	4	5	5	6
20–34	24	1.7	<1	1	1	1	1	2	3	4
35–49	14	1.3	<1	1	1	1	2	2	2	4
50–64	8	2.0	2	1	1	1	3	3	6	6
65+	5	2.6	10	1	1	1	4	9	9	9
2. MULTIPLE DX										
0–19 Years	154	5.7	69	1	2	4	6	12	20	42
20–34	386	4.7	60	1	1	3	5	10	16	36
35–49	263	4.8	26	2	2	3	6	15	15	22
50–64	215	6.8	78	1	2	5	9	13	18	42
65+	415	8.0	63	1	3	6	10	15	22	50
TOTAL SINGLE DX	66	2.0	2	1	1	1	3	4	5	6
MULTIPLE DX	1433	6.0	59	1	2	4	7	13	17	38
TOTAL										
0–19 Years	169	5.4	62	2	2	4	5	11	18	33
20–34	410	4.6	58	1	1	3	5	9	16	36
35–49	277	4.6	25	2	2	3	5	13	15	20
50–64	223	6.7	77	1	2	5	8	12	17	42
65+	420	7.9	62	1	3	6	10	15	22	50
GRAND TOTAL	1499	5.8	57	1	2	3	7	13	17	38

39.4: VASCULAR PX REVISION. Formerly included in operation group(s) 585, 590.

Type of Patients	Observed Patients	Avg. Stay	Variance	10th	25th	50th	75th	90th	95th	99th
1. SINGLE DX										
0–19 Years	9	3.2	4	1	1	3	5	5	5	7
20–34	10	1.6	<1	1	1	2	2	5	3	3
35–49	41	3.0	5	1	1	3	4	6	8	8
50–64	92	8.4	80	1	3	4	7	25	25	25
65+	86	3.9	23	1	1	3	5	7	9	41
2. MULTIPLE DX										
0–19 Years	212	6.5	57	1	2	4	8	16	25	39
20–34	1077	5.1	36	1	1	3	5	12	16	31
35–49	3082	4.6	30	1	1	3	6	10	15	27
50–64	5714	5.6	46	1	2	4	7	13	18	37
65+	9503	5.9	50	1	2	4	7	14	18	36
TOTAL SINGLE DX	238	5.2	43	1	1	3	5	10	25	25
MULTIPLE DX	19588	5.5	45	1	2	3	7	13	18	34
TOTAL										
0–19 Years	221	6.4	56	1	2	4	8	16	25	39
20–34	1087	5.1	36	1	1	3	7	12	16	31
35–49	3123	4.5	30	1	1	3	6	10	15	27
50–64	5806	5.7	47	1	2	4	7	13	18	37
65+	9589	5.9	50	1	2	4	7	13	18	36
GRAND TOTAL	19826	5.5	45	1	2	3	7	13	18	34

39.31: SUTURE OF ARTERY. Formerly included in operation group(s) 590.

Type of Patients	Observed Patients	Avg. Stay	Variance	10th	25th	50th	75th	90th	95th	99th
1. SINGLE DX										
0–19 Years	12	3.0	2	1	2	3	4	5	5	6
20–34	18	1.4	<1	1	1	1	1	2	3	4
35–49	10	1.2	<1	1	1	1	1	2	2	2
50–64	6	2.2	3	1	1	1	3	3	6	6
65+	3	3.1	15	1	1	1	4	9	9	9
2. MULTIPLE DX										
0–19 Years	120	5.6	74	1	2	4	5	12	18	44
20–34	297	4.5	54	1	1	3	5	9	14	24
35–49	197	4.9	24	2	2	3	6	15	15	19
50–64	182	6.4	51	1	2	5	9	16	16	42
65+	350	7.5	55	1	3	6	10	15	19	34
TOTAL SINGLE DX	49	2.0	2	1	1	1	2	5	5	9
MULTIPLE DX	1146	5.7	51	1	2	3	7	13	16	34
TOTAL										
0–19 Years	132	5.4	68	1	2	4	5	11	17	42
20–34	315	4.4	52	1	1	3	5	9	14	22
35–49	207	4.7	24	2	2	3	5	15	15	19
50–64	188	6.3	50	1	2	5	8	15	16	42
65+	353	7.5	55	1	3	6	10	15	19	34
GRAND TOTAL	1195	5.6	50	1	2	3	7	13	16	33

39.42: REV AV SHUNT FOR RD. Formerly included in operation group(s) 585.

Type of Patients	Observed Patients	Avg. Stay	Variance	10th	25th	50th	75th	90th	95th	99th
1. SINGLE DX										
0–19 Years	1	5.0	0	5	5	5	5	5	5	5
20–34	4	1.5	<1	1	1	1	2	2	2	2
35–49	5	2.5	2	1	2	2	4	4	4	4
50–64	12	1.8	<1	1	1	2	3	4	3	3
65+	14	3.2	18	1	1	1	3	14	14	15
2. MULTIPLE DX										
0–19 Years	42	5.3	31	1	1	2	7	16	16	16
20–34	348	4.4	23	1	1	3	6	12	12	22
35–49	878	3.7	22	1	1	3	4	9	12	24
50–64	1371	4.5	34	1	1	3	5	10	15	29
65+	2168	4.9	41	1	3	3	6	11	17	35
TOTAL SINGLE DX	36	2.6	7	1	1	2	3	5	5	15
MULTIPLE DX	4807	4.4	33	1	1	2	5	10	15	29
TOTAL										
0–19 Years	43	5.3	30	1	1	3	6	16	16	16
20–34	352	4.4	22	1	1	3	6	12	12	22
35–49	883	3.7	21	1	1	3	4	9	12	24
50–64	1383	4.4	34	1	1	3	5	10	15	29
65+	2182	4.9	41	1	3	3	6	11	17	35
GRAND TOTAL	4843	4.4	33	1	1	2	5	10	15	29

Length of Stay by Diagnosis and Operation, United States, 1997

United States, October 1995–September 1996 Data, by Operation

39.43: RMVL AV SHUNT FOR RD. Formerly included in operation group(s) 585.

Type of Patients	Observed Patients	Avg. Stay	Vari-ance	10th	25th	50th	75th	90th	95th	99th
1. SINGLE DX										
0–19 Years	1	1.0	0	1	1	1	1	1	1	1
20–34	0									
35–49	2	2.7	10	1	1	5	5	8	8	8
50–64	1	5.0	0	5	5	5	5	5	5	5
65+	2	7.0	0	7	7	7	7	7	7	7
2. MULTIPLE DX										
0–19 Years	12	8.0	25	2	3	9	13	13	13	14
20–34	119	7.2	25	2	4	6	10	13	17	22
35–49	343	8.1	58	2	3	6	9	18	22	35
50–64	428	10.1	106	1	4	7	14	22	32	63
65+	478	9.8	137	2	3	6	11	22	33	47
TOTAL SINGLE DX	**6**	**3.1**	**9**	**1**	**1**	**1**	**7**	**8**	**8**	**8**
MULTIPLE DX	**1380**	**9.3**	**96**	**2**	**3**	**6**	**11**	**20**	**30**	**47**
TOTAL										
0–19 Years	13	7.2	27	1	2	7	13	13	13	14
20–34	119	7.2	25	2	4	6	10	13	17	22
35–49	345	8.0	58	2	3	6	9	18	22	35
50–64	429	10.1	106	1	4	7	14	22	32	63
65+	480	9.8	136	2	3	6	11	22	33	47
GRAND TOTAL	**1386**	**9.2**	**96**	**2**	**3**	**6**	**11**	**20**	**30**	**47**

39.49: VASCULAR PX REVISION NEC. Formerly included in operation group(s) 590.

Type of Patients	Observed Patients	Avg. Stay	Vari-ance	10th	25th	50th	75th	90th	95th	99th
1. SINGLE DX										
0–19 Years	7	3.2	4	1	1	3	5	5	7	7
20–34	6	1.8	<1	1	1	2	2	3	3	3
35–49	33	3.1	5	1	1	3	4	6	7	8
50–64	77	9.2	84	3	3	5	12	25	25	25
65+	70	3.9	24	1	2	3	5	7	9	41
2. MULTIPLE DX										
0–19 Years	158	6.8	68	1	2	4	8	21	25	44
20–34	608	5.1	46	1	1	3	6	13	16	41
35–49	1854	4.4	27	1	1	2	6	10	14	26
50–64	3898	5.5	41	1	2	4	7	12	17	34
65+	6806	5.9	46	1	2	4	8	14	18	32
TOTAL SINGLE DX	**193**	**5.6**	**48**	**1**	**2**	**3**	**5**	**12**	**25**	**25**
MULTIPLE DX	**13324**	**5.5**	**42**	**1**	**2**	**3**	**7**	**13**	**17**	**31**
TOTAL										
0–19 Years	165	6.7	66	1	2	4	8	21	25	44
20–34	614	5.1	46	1	1	3	6	12	16	41
35–49	1887	4.4	26	1	1	2	6	10	14	26
50–64	3975	5.6	42	1	2	4	7	13	18	33
65+	6876	5.9	46	1	2	4	8	13	18	32
GRAND TOTAL	**13517**	**5.5**	**42**	**1**	**2**	**3**	**7**	**13**	**17**	**31**

39.5: OTHER VESSEL REPAIR. Formerly included in operation group(s) 589, 590.

Type of Patients	Observed Patients	Avg. Stay	Vari-ance	10th	25th	50th	75th	90th	95th	99th
1. SINGLE DX										
0–19 Years	119	2.1	4	1	1	1	2	5	7	10
20–34	123	4.6	16	1	1	4	6	11	11	15
35–49	272	6.5	16	1	4	8	8	10	13	21
50–64	360	3.1	11	1	1	2	4	6	10	18
65+	295	3.2	12	1	1	2	5	8	10	14
2. MULTIPLE DX										
0–19 Years	782	5.1	62	1	1	2	5	13	20	37
20–34	692	8.3	57	1	3	7	10	18	23	33
35–49	2252	7.4	74	1	2	5	9	18	24	43
50–64	5128	6.1	70	1	1	3	8	14	20	42
65+	9386	6.3	61	1	1	4	8	14	20	38
TOTAL SINGLE DX	**1169**	**4.2**	**15**	**1**	**1**	**3**	**7**	**9**	**11**	**20**
MULTIPLE DX	**18240**	**6.4**	**65**	**1**	**1**	**4**	**8**	**15**	**21**	**40**
TOTAL										
0–19 Years	901	4.6	55	1	1	2	5	10	19	36
20–34	815	7.7	52	1	3	6	10	17	21	33
35–49	2524	7.3	65	1	2	5	9	17	23	40
50–64	5488	5.9	66	1	1	3	7	14	20	41
65+	9681	6.2	59	1	1	4	8	14	20	38
GRAND TOTAL	**19409**	**6.2**	**62**	**1**	**1**	**4**	**8**	**14**	**20**	**38**

39.50: PTA/ATHERECTOMY OTH VSL. Formerly included in operation group(s) 590.

Type of Patients	Observed Patients	Avg. Stay	Vari-ance	10th	25th	50th	75th	90th	95th	99th
1. SINGLE DX										
0–19 Years	51	1.3	<1	1	1	1	1	2	2	7
20–34	24	4.4	16	1	1	2	7	11	11	11
35–49	91	2.6	5	1	1	2	4	5	7	11
50–64	178	1.7	2	1	1	1	2	3	4	10
65+	196	2.7	11	1	1	1	3	10	10	10
2. MULTIPLE DX										
0–19 Years	350	3.6	43	1	1	1	3	8	18	33
20–34	177	5.9	31	1	2	4	9	14	20	23
35–49	915	4.1	25	1	1	2	6	11	14	23
50–64	2838	3.9	25	1	1	2	5	9	12	23
65+	6243	5.1	39	1	1	3	7	12	16	38
TOTAL SINGLE DX	**540**	**2.2**	**6**	**1**	**1**	**1**	**2**	**5**	**10**	**11**
MULTIPLE DX	**10523**	**4.6**	**34**	**1**	**1**	**2**	**6**	**11**	**15**	**32**
TOTAL										
0–19 Years	401	3.2	37	1	1	1	2	7	16	33
20–34	201	5.7	29	1	1	4	9	11	19	23
35–49	1006	4.0	24	1	1	2	5	10	14	22
50–64	3016	3.7	24	1	1	2	4	9	12	23
65+	6439	5.0	39	1	1	3	7	12	16	38
GRAND TOTAL	**11063**	**4.5**	**33**	**1**	**1**	**2**	**6**	**11**	**15**	**31**

Length of Stay by Diagnosis and Operation, United States, 1997

United States, October 1995–September 1996 Data, by Operation

39.51: CLIPPING OF ANEURYSM. Formerly included in operation group(s) 589.

Type of Patients	Observed Patients	Avg. Stay	Variance	10th	25th	50th	75th	90th	95th	99th
1. SINGLE DX										
0–19 Years	7	6.4	7	3	3	7	9	9	10	10
20–34	56	8.2	19	4	5	7	10	13	15	26
35–49	124	8.2	12	4	8	8	8	12	15	21
50–64	93	5.8	17	3	3	5	6	12	17	22
65+	26	7.1	23	4	5	5	8	13	14	27
2. MULTIPLE DX										
0–19 Years	14	10.4	42	8	8	8	8	19	25	45
20–34	152	11.8	74	5	7	10	15	20	25	37
35–49	761	13.5	120	4	5	10	19	28	35	57
50–64	933	14.3	174	4	7	10	19	26	40	94
65+	529	16.4	161	5	7	13	22	33	41	78
TOTAL SINGLE DX	306	7.5	15	3	5	8	8	12	15	21
MULTIPLE DX	2389	14.3	147	4	6	10	19	28	38	65
TOTAL										
0–19 Years	21	9.6	37	7	8	8	8	16	25	45
20–34	208	11.1	65	4	6	9	13	20	25	36
35–49	885	11.9	93	4	5	8	15	23	32	51
50–64	1026	13.3	163	3	5	10	17	25	37	85
65+	555	15.9	158	5	7	13	21	32	41	78
GRAND TOTAL	2695	13.0	130	4	6	9	17	25	35	60

39.53: AV FISTULA REPAIR. Formerly included in operation group(s) 590.

Type of Patients	Observed Patients	Avg. Stay	Variance	10th	25th	50th	75th	90th	95th	99th
1. SINGLE DX										
0–19 Years	12	2.2	1	1	1	3	3	3	3	4
20–34	20	3.2	3	1	1	4	5	5	5	8
35–49	14	3.3	7	1	1	2	7	8	8	8
50–64	12	2.4	3	1	1	2	3	4	4	8
65+	9	2.2	2	1	1	2	4	4	4	4
2. MULTIPLE DX										
0–19 Years	27	5.5	55	1	1	3	5	15	29	29
20–34	43	7.3	23	1	4	6	13	14	14	22
35–49	87	5.6	27	1	2	5	6	12	15	61
50–64	175	6.1	45	1	2	4	9	11	17	22
65+	217	8.1	114	1	2	4	10	19	20	50
TOTAL SINGLE DX	67	2.7	3	1	1	2	4	5	7	8
MULTIPLE DX	549	6.7	65	1	2	5	9	14	19	45
TOTAL										
0–19 Years	39	4.2	36	1	1	3	4	5	20	29
20–34	63	5.8	20	1	2	5	7	14	14	16
35–49	101	5.4	26	1	2	5	6	10	14	61
50–64	187	5.9	44	1	2	4	9	11	17	22
65+	226	7.9	112	1	2	4	10	19	20	50
GRAND TOTAL	616	6.3	60	1	2	4	8	14	19	38

39.52: ANEURYSM REPAIR NEC. Formerly included in operation group(s) 590.

Type of Patients	Observed Patients	Avg. Stay	Variance	10th	25th	50th	75th	90th	95th	99th
1. SINGLE DX										
0–19 Years	4	3.0	4	1	1	2	5	5	5	5
20–34	6	5.9	4	4	6	6	6	6	9	13
35–49	12	5.5	10	3	4	4	6	11	12	12
50–64	30	5.2	12	3	3	5	6	8	8	21
65+	17	4.8	2	3	5	5	5	6	7	8
2. MULTIPLE DX										
0–19 Years	15	7.8	91	1	3	4	9	18	41	41
20–34	39	7.8	36	2	6	8	8	10	12	33
35–49	123	7.5	66	2	3	6	8	15	29	38
50–64	404	6.7	48	1	2	5	8	14	18	30
65+	1039	8.9	99	2	4	7	11	16	25	52
TOTAL SINGLE DX	69	5.0	6	2	4	5	6	7	8	13
MULTIPLE DX	1620	8.2	80	2	3	6	10	15	23	41
TOTAL										
0–19 Years	19	6.1	65	1	1	4	6	18	18	41
20–34	45	7.6	32	2	6	6	8	10	12	33
35–49	135	7.3	63	2	3	5	8	15	29	38
50–64	434	6.6	46	1	2	5	8	14	18	30
65+	1056	8.8	96	2	4	7	11	16	25	52
GRAND TOTAL	1689	8.0	77	2	3	6	10	15	22	39

39.56: REP VESS W TISS PATCH. Formerly included in operation group(s) 590.

Type of Patients	Observed Patients	Avg. Stay	Variance	10th	25th	50th	75th	90th	95th	99th
1. SINGLE DX										
0–19 Years	9	4.0	3	1	3	5	5	5	6	6
20–34	8	3.0	2	1	3	4	4	4	4	4
35–49	5	3.6	16	2	2	2	3	14	14	14
50–64	5	2.5	<1	2	2	3	3	3	3	3
65+	8	2.3	2	2	2	2	2	3	3	7
2. MULTIPLE DX										
0–19 Years	113	8.9	124	3	4	5	8	19	27	82
20–34	113	8.1	63	2	3	5	10	20	20	37
35–49	80	7.4	23	3	5	7	7	12	18	31
50–64	76	5.9	41	1	2	5	9	10	14	38
65+	121	6.8	41	1	2	5	9	14	22	28
TOTAL SINGLE DX	32	3.1	4	1	2	2	4	5	6	14
MULTIPLE DX	503	7.5	63	2	3	5	8	16	20	38
TOTAL										
0–19 Years	122	8.7	119	3	4	5	7	19	27	82
20–34	121	7.9	62	2	3	4	10	20	20	37
35–49	85	7.3	41	2	5	7	7	14	18	31
50–64	78	5.9	41	1	1	5	9	10	14	38
65+	129	6.3	39	2	2	4	8	14	20	28
GRAND TOTAL	535	7.3	61	2	3	5	8	16	20	38

Length of Stay by Diagnosis and Operation, United States, 1997

United States, October 1995–September 1996 Data, by Operation

39.57: REP VESS W SYNTH PATCH. Formerly included in operation group(s) 590.

Type of Patients	Observed Patients	Avg. Stay	Vari-ance	10th	25th	50th	75th	90th	95th	99th
1. SINGLE DX										
0–19 Years	3	3.1	<1	3	3	3	3	4	4	4
20–34	0									
35–49	5	4.6	8	1	3	3	8	8	8	8
50–64	5	1.7	<1	1	1	2	2	2	2	2
65+	13	3.5	8	1	2	2	5	5	12	12
2. MULTIPLE DX										
0–19 Years	53	8.5	44	3	5	5	14	22	25	>99
20–34	42	11.2	73	4	4	9	15	29	29	29
35–49	45	7.2	86	2	3	4	6	15	38	38
50–64	145	6.1	51	2	2	4	7	14	15	24
65+	275	7.4	51	1	2	5	10	15	25	30
TOTAL SINGLE DX	26	3.3	7	1	2	3	4	8	8	12
MULTIPLE DX	560	7.4	58	2	3	5	9	15	25	38
TOTAL										
0–19	56	8.3	43	3	4	5	14	22	25	>99
20–34	42	11.2	73	4	4	9	15	29	29	29
35–49	50	7.0	80	2	3	4	7	15	38	38
50–64	150	6.0	50	2	2	4	7	14	15	24
65+	288	7.3	50	1	2	5	10	15	24	30
GRAND TOTAL	586	7.3	56	2	3	5	9	15	24	38

39.6: OPEN HEART AUXILIARY PX. Formerly included in operation group(s) 590.

Type of Patients	Observed Patients	Avg. Stay	Vari-ance	10th	25th	50th	75th	90th	95th	99th
1. SINGLE DX										
0–19 Years	0									
20–34	0									
35–49	0									
50–64	1	4.0	0	4	4	4	4	4	4	4
65+	0									
2. MULTIPLE DX										
0–19 Years	123	24.2	286	6	11	21	34	50	58	85
20–34	7	17.9	487	5	5	5	29	34	87	87
35–49	7	7.6	23	6	6	6	7	23	>99	>99
50–64	24	9.1	25	4	5	8	14	16	20	22
65+	29	11.1	120	4	4	7	15	20	43	56
TOTAL SINGLE DX	1	4.0	0	4	4	4	4	4	4	4
MULTIPLE DX	190	20.3	278	4	7	16	30	39	58	85
TOTAL										
0–19	123	24.2	286	6	11	21	34	50	58	85
20–34	7	17.9	487	5	5	5	29	34	87	87
35–49	7	7.6	23	6	6	6	7	23	>99	>99
50–64	25	8.9	25	4	5	7	14	14	20	22
65+	29	11.1	120	4	4	7	15	20	43	56
GRAND TOTAL	191	20.2	278	4	7	16	29	39	58	85

39.59: REPAIR OF VESSEL NEC. Formerly included in operation group(s) 590.

Type of Patients	Observed Patients	Avg. Stay	Vari-ance	10th	25th	50th	75th	90th	95th	99th
1. SINGLE DX										
0–19 Years	29	3.0	8	1	1	2	3	10	10	10
20–34	7	1.2	<1	1	1	1	1	1	3	3
35–49	20	3.1	4	1	1	3	4	5	8	10
50–64	37	3.2	27	1	1	2	3	5	6	30
65+	24	2.2	4	1	1	1	2	6	6	8
2. MULTIPLE DX										
0–19 Years	181	3.8	40	1	1	1	4	8	16	33
20–34	100	6.6	47	1	2	5	7	17	17	34
35–49	219	4.6	30	1	1	3	6	10	16	28
50–64	527	4.9	38	1	1	3	6	12	16	28
65+	898	5.2	27	1	2	3	7	12	15	25
TOTAL SINGLE DX	117	2.4	10	1	1	1	3	5	6	10
MULTIPLE DX	1925	4.9	33	1	1	3	6	11	16	28
TOTAL										
0–19	210	3.7	37	1	1	1	4	8	15	33
20–34	107	5.4	41	1	2	4	7	14	17	34
35–49	239	4.5	29	1	1	3	5	10	15	25
50–64	564	4.8	38	1	1	2	6	11	16	30
65+	922	5.1	26	1	2	3	7	12	14	25
GRAND TOTAL	2042	4.8	32	1	1	3	6	11	15	28

39.8: VASCULAR BODY OPERATIONS. Formerly included in operation group(s) 590.

Type of Patients	Observed Patients	Avg. Stay	Vari-ance	10th	25th	50th	75th	90th	95th	99th
1. SINGLE DX										
0–19 Years	3	1.4	<1	1	1	1	2	2	2	2
20–34	7	2.4	1	1	2	2	3	3	5	5
35–49	8	3.7	3	1	3	5	5	5	5	5
50–64	5	2.6	<1	2	2	2	3	4	4	4
65+	5	1.9	<1	1	2	2	2	2	2	2
2. MULTIPLE DX										
0–19 Years	2	2.0	0	2	2	2	2	2	2	2
20–34	9	4.6	7	1	3	5	6	8	9	9
35–49	11	3.4	1	2	3	4	4	4	4	6
50–64	12	2.5	1	2	2	2	3	3	6	6
65+	28	3.5	9	2	2	3	4	7	8	18
TOTAL SINGLE DX	28	2.7	2	1	2	2	4	5	5	5
MULTIPLE DX	62	3.5	5	2	2	3	4	6	7	18
TOTAL										
0–19	5	1.5	<1	1	1	2	2	2	2	2
20–34	16	3.6	5	1	2	3	6	8	8	9
35–49	19	3.5	2	2	3	4	4	5	5	6
50–64	17	2.6	1	2	2	2	3	4	4	6
65+	33	3.3	8	1	2	3	4	7	8	18
GRAND TOTAL	90	3.3	4	1	2	3	4	5	7	9

Length of Stay by Diagnosis and Operation, United States, 1997

United States, October 1995–September 1996 Data, by Operation

39.9: OTHER VESSEL OPERATIONS. Formerly included in operation group(s) 585, 590, 596.

Type of Patients	Observed Patients	Avg. Stay	Vari- ance	Percentiles						
				10th	25th	50th	75th	90th	95th	99th
1. SINGLE DX										
0–19 Years	47	1.8	2	1	1	1	3	3	3	7
20–34	82	1.5	6	1	1	1	2	3	3	9
35–49	105	2.5	4	1	1	2	3	6	8	9
50–64	94	4.3	30	1	1	2	5	10	10	40
65+	108	2.9	6	1	1	2	4	6	8	12
2. MULTIPLE DX										
0–19 Years	549	6.4	98	1	2	4	7	12	20	54
20–34	3640	4.7	30	1	2	3	6	9	14	24
35–49	7916	5.0	26	1	2	4	6	9	13	26
50–64	11383	5.2	27	1	3	4	6	10	14	25
65+	19483	6.0	32	2	3	4	7	12	16	30
TOTAL SINGLE DX	436	2.3	9	1	1	1	3	5	7	12
MULTIPLE DX	42971	5.5	30	1	2	4	7	11	15	28
TOTAL										
0–19 Years	596	5.7	86	1	2	3	6	11	17	52
20–34	3722	4.6	30	1	2	3	6	9	13	24
35–49	8021	5.0	26	1	2	4	6	9	13	26
50–64	11477	5.2	27	1	2	4	6	10	14	25
65+	19591	6.0	32	2	3	4	7	12	16	30
GRAND TOTAL	43407	5.4	30	1	2	4	7	11	15	28

39.95: HEMODIALYSIS. Formerly included in operation group(s) 584.

Type of Patients	Observed Patients	Avg. Stay	Vari- ance	Percentiles						
				10th	25th	50th	75th	90th	95th	99th
1. SINGLE DX										
0–19 Years	13	1.8	4	1	1	1	2	3	3	12
20–34	53	1.8	2	1	1	1	2	4	5	7
35–49	70	2.0	3	1	1	1	2	4	6	8
50–64	72	5.0	35	1	1	4	6	10	10	40
65+	89	2.9	6	1	1	2	4	5	8	12
2. MULTIPLE DX										
0–19 Years	431	5.4	55	1	2	3	7	10	14	26
20–34	3444	4.6	29	1	2	3	6	9	13	22
35–49	7549	4.9	25	1	2	4	6	9	13	26
50–64	10847	5.1	24	1	2	4	6	10	13	24
65+	18592	5.9	31	2	3	4	7	12	15	29
TOTAL SINGLE DX	297	2.9	12	1	1	2	4	6	8	12
MULTIPLE DX	40863	5.4	28	1	2	4	7	11	14	26
TOTAL										
0–19 Years	444	5.2	54	1	2	3	6	10	14	26
20–34	3497	4.6	29	1	2	3	6	9	13	22
35–49	7619	4.9	25	1	2	4	6	9	13	26
50–64	10919	5.1	24	1	3	4	6	10	13	24
65+	18681	5.9	31	2	3	4	7	12	15	29
GRAND TOTAL	41160	5.3	28	1	2	4	7	10	14	26

39.93: INSERT VESS-VESS CANNULA. Formerly included in operation group(s) 585.

Type of Patients	Observed Patients	Avg. Stay	Vari- ance	Percentiles						
				10th	25th	50th	75th	90th	95th	99th
1. SINGLE DX										
0–19 Years	1	1.0	0	1	1	1	1	1	1	1
20–34	7	2.0	4	1	1	1	2	4	4	9
35–49	12	2.9	11	1	1	1	3	9	9	11
50–64	10	3.0	12	1	1	1	7	9	10	10
65+	8	3.6	14	1	1	2	6	8	13	13
2. MULTIPLE DX										
0–19 Years	40	16.5	380	2	4	6	29	39	52	88
20–34	94	8.1	59	1	4	5	12	17	18	33
35–49	208	7.4	56	2	3	5	8	15	21	38
50–64	350	9.2	113	3	3	7	11	19	28	57
65+	555	9.5	61	2	4	8	13	18	25	36
TOTAL SINGLE DX	38	2.7	9	1	1	1	2	9	9	13
MULTIPLE DX	1247	9.1	85	1	3	7	12	19	26	43
TOTAL										
0–19 Years	41	15.7	372	1	3	6	29	39	52	88
20–34	101	7.8	58	1	3	4	12	17	18	33
35–49	220	7.2	55	1	3	5	7	15	21	38
50–64	360	9.1	112	1	2	7	11	19	28	57
65+	563	9.5	61	2	4	8	13	18	25	36
GRAND TOTAL	1285	9.0	84	1	3	7	12	18	26	43

39.97: OTHER PERFUSION. Formerly included in operation group(s) 590.

Type of Patients	Observed Patients	Avg. Stay	Vari- ance	Percentiles						
				10th	25th	50th	75th	90th	95th	99th
1. SINGLE DX										
0–19 Years	2	2.0	2	1	1	2	3	3	3	3
20–34	0									
35–49	9	5.6	4	4	4	6	6	8	8	13
50–64	3	4.6	14	2	2	2	5	11	11	11
65+	3	2.3	<1	2	2	2	3	3	3	3
2. MULTIPLE DX										
0–19 Years	2	5.1	9	1	1	7	7	7	7	7
20–34	13	5.3	11	1	3	7	8	9	11	11
35–49	47	5.3	14	2	2	6	8	7	11	23
50–64	86	5.9	9	2	3	6	8	10	11	17
65+	165	5.6	18	3	3	4	6	8	13	25
TOTAL SINGLE DX	17	5.0	6	2	4	4	6	8	8	13
MULTIPLE DX	313	5.6	15	2	3	5	6	9	11	24
TOTAL										
0–19 Years	4	4.3	9	1	1	7	7	7	7	7
20–34	13	5.3	11	1	3	7	8	9	11	11
35–49	56	5.3	12	1	4	6	8	7	10	23
50–64	89	5.9	18	2	4	6	8	10	10	17
65+	168	5.5	18	3	3	4	6	8	13	25
GRAND TOTAL	330	5.5	15	2	3	5	6	9	11	23

Length of Stay by Diagnosis and Operation, United States, 1997

United States, October 1995–September 1996 Data, by Operation

39.98: HEMORRHAGE CONTROL NOS. Formerly included in operation group(s) 590.

Type of Patients	Observed Patients	Avg. Stay	Vari-ance	Percentiles						
				10th	25th	50th	75th	90th	95th	99th
1. SINGLE DX										
0–19 Years	10	1.6	<1	1	1	1	3	3	3	3
20–34	18	1.3	7	1	1	1	2	3	3	26
35–49	12	2.0	6	1	1	2	2	5	5	5
50–64	3	1.0	0	1	1	1	1	1	1	1
65+	7	3.1	9	1	1	2	3	10	10	10
2. MULTIPLE DX										
0–19 Years	26	4.9	59	1	1	2	5	13	31	31
20–34	68	4.2	22	1	2	3	4	9	10	33
35–49	79	6.0	62	1	2	3	7	18	21	38
50–64	55	4.1	23	1	1	2	6	7	11	23
65+	109	5.8	34	2	3	3	8	15	15	34
TOTAL SINGLE DX	50	1.5	5	1	1	1	1	2	3	5
MULTIPLE DX	337	5.2	40	1	2	3	6	12	21	33
TOTAL										
0–19 Years	36	2.7	23	1	1	1	3	4	6	31
20–34	86	2.2	13	1	1	1	2	4	7	26
35–49	91	5.2	52	1	2	2	6	14	21	38
50–64	58	3.8	22	1	1	2	6	6	10	23
65+	116	5.7	33	1	3	3	8	15	15	34
GRAND TOTAL	387	3.7	29	1	1	2	4	8	15	26

40.1: LYMPHATIC DXTIC PX. Formerly included in operation group(s) 591, 596.

Type of Patients	Observed Patients	Avg. Stay	Vari-ance	Percentiles						
				10th	25th	50th	75th	90th	95th	99th
1. SINGLE DX										
0–19 Years	107	4.1	11	1	2	3	5	7	13	13
20–34	76	2.7	5	1	1	2	4	5	6	13
35–49	91	2.6	6	1	1	2	3	5	6	16
50–64	67	2.5	9	1	1	1	3	6	8	16
65+	44	2.7	9	1	1	1	3	7	10	14
2. MULTIPLE DX										
0–19 Years	284	8.3	89	1	3	5	10	18	31	48
20–34	406	8.4	55	2	4	7	10	21	24	34
35–49	707	8.9	65	2	3	7	12	19	21	38
50–64	1074	7.7	49	1	3	6	10	17	22	36
65+	1895	9.0	90	1	3	7	11	19	25	54
TOTAL SINGLE DX	385	3.0	8	1	1	2	4	6	8	14
MULTIPLE DX	4366	8.6	73	1	3	7	11	18	23	42
TOTAL										
0–19 Years	391	7.3	74	1	2	5	9	16	25	47
20–34	482	7.8	52	1	3	7	9	18	21	33
35–49	798	7.9	61	1	2	6	11	18	21	37
50–64	1141	7.4	48	1	2	6	10	16	21	34
65+	1939	8.9	90	1	3	6	11	19	24	54
GRAND TOTAL	4751	8.1	70	1	3	6	10	18	22	41

40.0: INC LYMPHATIC STRUCTURE. Formerly included in operation group(s) 591.

Type of Patients	Observed Patients	Avg. Stay	Vari-ance	Percentiles						
				10th	25th	50th	75th	90th	95th	99th
1. SINGLE DX										
0–19 Years	67	3.4	5	1	2	3	5	5	6	9
20–34	5	4.4	5	1	1	5	5	7	7	7
35–49	1	1.0	0	1	1	1	1	1	1	1
50–64	0									
65+	1	6.0	0	6	6	6	6	6	6	6
2. MULTIPLE DX										
0–19 Years	100	4.6	6	2	2	4	6	8	9	12
20–34	24	5.2	41	1	1	3	7	14	23	28
35–49	20	4.2	14	2	2	2	5	11	11	15
50–64	24	4.2	9	1	2	3	6	9	9	13
65+	39	6.6	18	2	4	6	7	15	15	20
TOTAL SINGLE DX	74	3.4	5	1	2	3	5	6	7	9
MULTIPLE DX	207	5.0	14	2	2	4	6	9	14	15
TOTAL										
0–19 Years	167	4.0	6	2	2	4	5	7	8	11
20–34	29	5.1	36	1	1	3	7	14	23	28
35–49	21	4.2	14	1	2	2	5	11	11	15
50–64	24	4.2	9	1	2	3	6	9	9	13
65+	40	6.6	18	2	4	6	7	15	15	20
GRAND TOTAL	281	4.5	12	1	2	4	6	8	11	15

40.11: LYMPHATIC STRUCT BIOPSY. Formerly included in operation group(s) 591.

Type of Patients	Observed Patients	Avg. Stay	Vari-ance	Percentiles						
				10th	25th	50th	75th	90th	95th	99th
1. SINGLE DX										
0–19 Years	103	4.1	11	1	2	3	5	7	13	13
20–34	74	2.7	5	1	1	2	4	5	6	13
35–49	89	2.6	6	1	1	2	3	5	6	16
50–64	67	2.5	9	1	1	1	3	6	8	16
65+	44	2.7	9	1	1	1	3	7	10	14
2. MULTIPLE DX										
0–19 Years	270	8.6	94	1	4	6	10	19	31	48
20–34	401	8.5	55	2	4	7	10	21	24	34
35–49	704	8.9	65	2	3	7	12	19	21	38
50–64	1069	7.8	49	1	3	6	10	17	22	36
65+	1885	9.0	91	1	3	7	11	19	25	54
TOTAL SINGLE DX	377	3.0	8	1	1	2	4	6	8	14
MULTIPLE DX	4329	8.6	73	1	3	7	11	19	23	42
TOTAL										
0–19 Years	373	7.5	78	1	2	5	9	16	27	48
20–34	475	7.8	53	1	3	7	9	18	21	33
35–49	793	7.9	61	1	2	6	11	18	21	37
50–64	1136	7.4	48	1	2	6	10	16	21	34
65+	1929	8.9	90	1	3	6	11	19	24	54
GRAND TOTAL	4706	8.1	70	1	3	6	10	18	22	41

Length of Stay by Diagnosis and Operation, United States, 1997

United States, October 1995–September 1996 Data, by Operation

40.2: SMP EXC LYMPHATIC STRUCT. Formerly included in operation group(s) 591.

Type of Patients	Observed Patients	Avg. Stay	Vari-ance	10th	25th	50th	75th	90th	95th	99th
1. SINGLE DX										
0–19 Years	241	3.0	9	1	1	2	4	6	9	18
20–34	73	2.2	3	1	1	2	3	5	6	8
35–49	134	1.8	5	1	1	1	2	3	6	16
50–64	143	2.2	3	1	1	1	4	5	5	7
65+	95	2.2	3	1	1	2	3	5	6	10
2. MULTIPLE DX										
0–19 Years	218	5.9	41	1	2	4	8	14	18	36
20–34	189	7.2	104	1	2	5	7	11	21	56
35–49	363	5.8	41	1	1	4	8	13	17	36
50–64	577	4.4	26	1	1	3	5	10	14	22
65+	919	6.3	48	1	1	4	9	14	20	33
TOTAL SINGLE DX	686	2.4	6	1	1	1	3	5	6	13
MULTIPLE DX	2266	5.7	45	1	1	4	7	13	17	33
TOTAL										
0–19 Years	459	4.3	25	1	1	3	5	10	15	26
20–34	262	5.7	79	1	2	3	7	10	15	39
35–49	497	4.6	33	1	1	3	6	11	14	33
50–64	720	4.0	22	1	1	3	5	9	13	21
65+	1014	5.9	45	1	1	4	8	14	19	33
GRAND TOTAL	2952	4.9	37	1	1	3	6	11	15	32

40.23: EXC AXILLARY LYMPH NODE. Formerly included in operation group(s) 591.

Type of Patients	Observed Patients	Avg. Stay	Vari-ance	10th	25th	50th	75th	90th	95th	99th
1. SINGLE DX										
0–19 Years	10	1.8	4	1	1	1	2	3	3	10
20–34	7	2.7	3	1	1	2	5	5	5	5
35–49	65	1.3	<1	1	1	1	1	2	2	3
50–64	78	1.5	<1	1	1	1	2	2	3	4
65+	39	1.6	4	1	1	1	2	2	2	14
2. MULTIPLE DX										
0–19 Years	11	4.2	18	1	2	3	7	9	15	16
20–34	37	9.1	201	1	2	3	7	21	39	95
35–49	96	4.5	37	1	1	2	8	13	13	29
50–64	162	2.7	19	1	1	1	2	8	9	21
65+	246	5.2	41	1	1	2	9	13	14	23
TOTAL SINGLE DX	199	1.4	2	1	1	1	2	2	3	5
MULTIPLE DX	552	4.4	42	1	1	2	7	10	14	29
TOTAL										
0–19 Years	21	3.0	12	1	1	1	3	9	10	16
20–34	44	8.3	180	1	1	3	9	21	39	39
35–49	161	3.1	24	1	1	1	3	8	10	25
50–64	240	2.4	14	1	1	2	6	8	13	21
65+	285	4.8	38	1	1	2	9	13	14	22
GRAND TOTAL	751	3.7	34	1	1	1	4	9	13	25

40.21: EXC DEEP CERVICAL NODE. Formerly included in operation group(s) 591.

Type of Patients	Observed Patients	Avg. Stay	Vari-ance	10th	25th	50th	75th	90th	95th	99th
1. SINGLE DX										
0–19 Years	29	5.6	39	1	1	2	10	18	18	21
20–34	15	2.7	5	1	1	2	3	8	8	8
35–49	10	1.8	1	1	1	1	3	4	4	4
50–64	8	1.6	2	1	1	1	1	3	6	6
65+	6	1.8	2	1	1	1	2	5	5	5
2. MULTIPLE DX										
0–19 Years	41	6.0	26	1	2	4	8	15	18	24
20–34	31	7.3	30	1	1	8	10	13	20	23
35–49	63	5.6	42	1	3	3	6	11	17	36
50–64	79	7.5	35	1	3	6	11	15	17	28
65+	126	10.4	78	1	3	8	15	24	29	35
TOTAL SINGLE DX	68	3.3	18	1	1	1	4	8	18	18
MULTIPLE DX	340	7.7	50	1	3	5	10	17	22	35
TOTAL										
0–19 Years	70	5.8	31	1	1	4	8	16	18	21
20–34	46	6.1	27	1	1	6	9	11	13	23
35–49	73	5.2	40	1	3	4	6	10	17	36
50–64	87	6.8	34	1	2	4	10	15	15	28
65+	132	10.1	78	1	3	8	14	24	27	35
GRAND TOTAL	408	7.0	48	1	2	4	10	17	21	35

40.24: EXC INGUINAL LYMPH NODE. Formerly included in operation group(s) 591.

Type of Patients	Observed Patients	Avg. Stay	Vari-ance	10th	25th	50th	75th	90th	95th	99th
1. SINGLE DX										
0–19 Years	11	2.1	3	1	1	1	3	6	6	6
20–34	15	1.6	3	1	1	1	1	4	4	9
35–49	25	2.6	5	1	1	2	4	5	6	13
50–64	17	1.9	3	1	1	1	2	3	5	11
65+	14	2.2	3	1	1	2	2	4	7	7
2. MULTIPLE DX										
0–19 Years	19	5.9	33	1	2	3	9	15	15	20
20–34	46	8.1	141	1	2	5	8	11	39	56
35–49	60	6.1	44	1	2	5	6	12	16	40
50–64	100	5.0	31	1	2	3	6	13	16	22
65+	210	6.0	42	1	2	4	7	11	18	33
TOTAL SINGLE DX	82	2.0	3	1	1	1	2	4	6	9
MULTIPLE DX	435	5.9	47	1	2	4	7	13	16	33
TOTAL										
0–19 Years	30	5.0	29	1	1	3	6	15	15	20
20–34	61	4.8	80	1	2	2	5	9	11	56
35–49	85	5.1	35	1	2	4	5	10	15	40
50–64	117	4.3	26	1	1	3	5	13	16	22
65+	224	5.8	41	1	2	4	7	11	16	33
GRAND TOTAL	517	5.1	41	1	1	3	6	11	16	33

Length of Stay by Diagnosis and Operation, United States, 1997

United States, October 1995–September 1996 Data, by Operation

40.29: SMP EXC LYMPHATIC NEC. Formerly included in operation group(s) 591.

Type of Patients	Observed Patients	Avg. Stay	Vari-ance	10th	25th	50th	75th	90th	95th	99th
1. SINGLE DX										
0–19 Years	190	2.9	5	1	1	2	4	6	8	11
20–34	36	2.6	2	1	2	2	3	4	5	7
35–49	33	3.0	16	1	1	1	3	7	16	16
50–64	40	3.4	4	1	2	2	5	5	5	8
65+	36	2.7	2	1	2	2	3	4	6	8
2. MULTIPLE DX										
0–19 Years	146	5.9	48	1	2	4	7	13	26	41
20–34	74	6.3	86	2	3	5	7	8	11	32
35–49	143	7.2	39	1	3	5	11	14	19	33
50–64	233	4.5	20	1	2	4	5	9	12	19
65+	335	6.2	42	1	2	4	8	15	18	30
TOTAL SINGLE DX	335	2.9	6	1	1	2	4	6	7	12
MULTIPLE DX	931	5.8	41	1	2	4	7	12	16	32
TOTAL										
0–19 Years	336	4.0	24	1	1	3	5	8	12	26
20–34	110	5.4	68	2	2	4	7	7	9	32
35–49	176	6.2	37	1	1	5	8	14	17	26
50–64	273	4.3	17	1	2	4	5	8	11	18
65+	371	5.7	38	1	2	4	7	13	17	30
GRAND TOTAL	1266	4.9	32	1	2	4	6	10	14	27

40.4: RAD EXC CERV LYMPH NODE. Formerly included in operation group(s) 592.

Type of Patients	Observed Patients	Avg. Stay	Vari-ance	10th	25th	50th	75th	90th	95th	99th
1. SINGLE DX										
0–19 Years	16	2.7	4	1	1	2	3	4	8	8
20–34	23	2.2	2	1	1	2	3	4	5	5
35–49	57	2.4	3	1	1	2	3	5	5	7
50–64	66	3.5	8	1	2	3	5	7	9	16
65+	50	2.5	4	1	1	2	3	4	5	9
2. MULTIPLE DX										
0–19 Years	28	3.3	16	1	2	2	4	6	6	35
20–34	66	3.6	7	1	2	3	4	7	9	11
35–49	338	5.0	26	2	2	3	6	10	15	21
50–64	758	5.3	31	2	3	4	6	10	17	32
65+	1044	5.1	20	2	3	4	6	10	12	23
TOTAL SINGLE DX	212	2.7	5	1	1	2	3	5	6	11
MULTIPLE DX	2234	5.1	24	2	2	4	6	10	14	24
TOTAL										
0–19 Years	44	3.1	13	1	2	3	4	6	8	13
20–34	89	3.3	6	1	2	3	4	7	8	11
35–49	395	4.4	22	1	2	3	5	9	13	21
50–64	824	5.2	29	2	2	4	6	10	17	30
65+	1094	4.9	19	2	2	4	6	10	12	23
GRAND TOTAL	2446	4.8	23	1	2	3	6	9	13	23

40.3: REGIONAL LYMPH NODE EXC. Formerly included in operation group(s) 592.

Type of Patients	Observed Patients	Avg. Stay	Vari-ance	10th	25th	50th	75th	90th	95th	99th
1. SINGLE DX										
0–19 Years	6	4.0	6	2	2	2	6	9	9	9
20–34	32	3.4	5	2	2	2	5	6	6	12
35–49	71	1.7	3	1	1	1	2	3	5	14
50–64	99	1.5	<1	1	1	1	2	3	3	5
65+	112	1.5	1	1	1	1	2	3	4	7
2. MULTIPLE DX										
0–19 Years	29	5.6	5	3	5	6	6	9	9	13
20–34	114	5.7	18	2	4	5	7	8	12	21
35–49	228	3.8	18	1	1	5	5	8	12	20
50–64	426	3.1	9	1	1	2	4	6	7	15
65+	686	4.0	28	1	1	2	4	8	13	28
TOTAL SINGLE DX	320	1.8	2	1	1	1	2	3	5	9
MULTIPLE DX	1483	3.8	19	1	1	2	5	7	10	23
TOTAL										
0–19 Years	35	5.4	5	2	5	5	6	9	9	13
20–34	146	5.3	16	2	3	5	6	8	11	21
35–49	299	3.2	15	1	1	2	4	7	11	19
50–64	525	2.8	8	1	1	2	4	5	7	15
65+	798	3.6	25	1	1	2	4	7	11	28
GRAND TOTAL	1803	3.4	16	1	1	2	4	7	9	21

40.41: UNILAT RAD NECK DISSECT. Formerly included in operation group(s) 592.

Type of Patients	Observed Patients	Avg. Stay	Vari-ance	10th	25th	50th	75th	90th	95th	99th
1. SINGLE DX										
0–19 Years	13	2.4	4	1	1	2	2	3	8	8
20–34	22	2.2	2	1	1	2	3	4	5	5
35–49	54	2.4	3	1	1	2	3	5	5	7
50–64	61	3.4	8	1	2	3	5	6	8	16
65+	48	2.5	4	1	1	2	4	4	6	9
2. MULTIPLE DX										
0–19 Years	20	4.8	31	1	2	3	6	6	13	35
20–34	62	3.6	8	1	2	3	5	7	9	11
35–49	300	4.7	21	1	2	3	6	9	13	21
50–64	673	4.7	20	2	2	4	5	8	12	26
65+	950	5.0	20	2	3	4	6	10	12	23
TOTAL SINGLE DX	198	2.6	4	1	1	2	3	5	6	11
MULTIPLE DX	2005	4.8	20	2	2	4	6	9	12	23
TOTAL										
0–19 Years	33	3.8	21	1	2	3	5	6	9	35
20–34	84	3.3	7	1	2	2	4	7	8	11
35–49	354	4.1	18	1	2	3	5	8	12	21
50–64	734	4.6	20	2	2	4	5	9	12	24
65+	998	4.8	19	2	2	4	6	9	12	22
GRAND TOTAL	2203	4.6	19	2	2	3	5	8	12	22

Length of Stay by Diagnosis and Operation, United States, 1997

United States, October 1995–September 1996 Data, by Operation

40.5: OTH RAD NODE DISSECTION. Formerly included in operation group(s) 592.

Type of Patients	Observed Patients	Avg. Stay	Variance	10th	25th	50th	75th	90th	95th	99th
1. SINGLE DX										
0–19 Years	6	7.3	13	4	4	8	8	8	19	19
20–34	23	4.0	13	2	4	5	5	6	7	8
35–49	26	2.7	4	1	1	2	4	6	7	8
50–64	38	2.5	3	1	1	2	2	5	5	6
65+	50	1.7	2	1	1	1	2	4	5	8
2. MULTIPLE DX										
0–19 Years	9	4.9	4	3	3	5	6	7	8	8
20–34	94	5.2	11	2	4	5	6	9	11	15
35–49	156	4.7	21	1	2	4	6	8	12	26
50–64	232	4.2	11	1	2	4	5	8	11	16
65+	393	4.7	27	1	2	4	5	9	18	23
TOTAL SINGLE DX	143	2.7	5	1	1	2	5	6	7	8
MULTIPLE DX	884	4.6	19	1	2	4	5	9	12	20
TOTAL										
0–19 Years	15	6.2	10	3	4	6	8	8	8	19
20–34	117	4.9	9	2	3	5	6	8	10	13
35–49	182	4.4	19	1	2	4	6	8	10	26
50–64	270	4.0	10	1	2	4	5	8	11	15
65+	443	4.3	24	1	1	3	4	8	15	22
GRAND TOTAL	1027	4.3	17	1	2	4	5	8	11	19

40.9: LYMPHATIC STRUCT OPS NEC. Formerly included in operation group(s) 596.

Type of Patients	Observed Patients	Avg. Stay	Variance	10th	25th	50th	75th	90th	95th	99th
1. SINGLE DX										
0–19 Years	9	3.6	8	1	1	2	7	7	10	10
20–34	2	2.8	6	1	1	1	5	5	5	5
35–49	0									
50–64	1	3.0	0	3	3	3	3	3	3	3
65+	1	3.0	0	3	3	3	3	3	3	3
2. MULTIPLE DX										
0–19 Years	14	19.3	506	5	8	14	14	76	76	78
20–34	6	4.7	7	2	5	5	8	8	8	8
35–49	14	4.8	3	2	5	5	6	6	7	9
50–64	17	9.2	216	1	2	3	12	12	63	63
65+	20	4.8	21	3	3	3	5	8	12	25
TOTAL SINGLE DX	13	3.4	7	1	1	3	5	7	10	10
MULTIPLE DX	71	9.4	215	2	3	5	9	14	35	78
TOTAL										
0–19 Years	23	15.5	428	2	5	9	14	44	76	78
20–34	8	4.3	7	1	2	3	7	6	8	8
35–49	14	4.8	3	2	5	5	6	6	7	9
50–64	18	8.9	205	1	2	3	12	12	63	63
65+	21	4.7	20	3	3	3	5	8	12	25
GRAND TOTAL	84	8.8	195	2	3	5	8	14	25	78

40.6: THORACIC DUCT OPERATIONS. Formerly included in operation group(s) 596.

Type of Patients	Observed Patients	Avg. Stay	Variance	10th	25th	50th	75th	90th	95th	99th
1. SINGLE DX										
0–19 Years	0									
20–34	0									
35–49	0									
50–64	0									
65+										
2. MULTIPLE DX										
0–19 Years	9	15.3	50	6	7	17	21	23	23	25
20–34	3	7.5	5	6	6	9	9	9	9	9
35–49	4	15.2	150	5	5	13	33	33	33	33
50–64	4	21.5	86	7	7	26	26	26	31	31
65+	5	19.5	318	3	6	17	17	60	60	60
TOTAL SINGLE DX	0									
MULTIPLE DX	25	15.4	113	6	7	13	21	26	31	60
TOTAL										
0–19 Years	9	15.3	50	6	7	17	21	23	23	25
20–34	3	7.5	5	6	6	9	9	9	9	9
35–49	4	15.2	150	5	5	13	33	33	33	33
50–64	4	21.5	86	7	7	26	26	26	31	31
65+	5	19.5	318	3	6	17	17	60	60	60
GRAND TOTAL	25	15.4	113	6	7	13	21	26	31	60

41.0: BONE MARROW TRANSPLANT. Formerly included in operation group(s) 593.

Type of Patients	Observed Patients	Avg. Stay	Variance	10th	25th	50th	75th	90th	95th	99th
1. SINGLE DX										
0–19 Years	22	31.8	417	1	20	29	37	56	77	99
20–34	14	38.1	761	19	22	29	43	99	99	99
35–49	20	17.1	74	6	6	18	24	27	28	29
50–64	11	26.5	81	13	21	29	32	39	39	41
65+	0									
2. MULTIPLE DX										
0–19 Years	592	36.0	238	20	28	35	44	58	71	>99
20–34	345	29.6	182	17	21	26	37	45	58	74
35–49	816	25.3	148	17	20	22	29	38	51	94
50–64	506	24.9	103	16	21	23	28	38	43	67
65+	26	28.3	212	12	20	22	50	50	50	50
TOTAL SINGLE DX	67	28.7	398	6	19	27	32	43	77	99
MULTIPLE DX	2285	29.5	200	18	21	26	36	48	61	>99
TOTAL										
0–19 Years	614	35.9	242	20	27	34	44	58	71	>99
20–34	359	30.0	210	17	21	27	38	45	61	85
35–49	836	25.2	148	17	20	22	29	38	50	84
50–64	517	25.0	102	16	21	23	28	38	43	67
65+	26	28.3	212	12	20	22	50	50	50	50
GRAND TOTAL	2352	29.5	205	17	21	26	36	48	61	>99

Length of Stay by Diagnosis and Operation, United States, 1997

United States, October 1995–September 1996 Data, by Operation

41.01: AUTOLOG MARROW TRANSPL. Formerly included in operation group(s) 593.

Type of Patients	Observed Patients	Avg. Stay	Vari-ance	10th	25th	50th	75th	90th	95th	99th
1. SINGLE DX										
0–19 Years	10	26.8	168	1	25	32	36	37	37	37
20–34	1	17.0	0	17	17	17	17	17	17	17
35–49	4	24.4	16	18	23	27	27	27	27	27
50–64	2	33.3	8	32	32	32	32	39	39	39
65+	0									
2. MULTIPLE DX										
0–19 Years	149	36.0	200	21	26	33	42	58	62	83
20–34	71	28.5	173	18	22	25	31	42	65	85
35–49	208	25.1	96	19	21	23	27	34	40	74
50–64	148	27.5	101	19	22	25	31	48	49	75
65+	7	38.3	212	20	21	50	50	50	50	50
TOTAL SINGLE DX	17	28.1	105	17	27	32	34	37	39	39
MULTIPLE DX	583	30.4	170	20	22	26	35	50	60	83
TOTAL										
0–19 Years	159	35.7	201	21	26	33	42	58	62	83
20–34	72	28.4	172	18	22	25	31	42	65	85
35–49	212	25.1	95	19	21	23	27	34	40	74
50–64	150	27.7	99	19	22	25	32	46	49	75
65+	7	38.3	212	20	21	50	50	50	50	50
GRAND TOTAL	600	30.3	168	20	22	26	35	50	59	83

41.03: ALLO MARROW TRANSPL NEC. Formerly included in operation group(s) 593.

Type of Patients	Observed Patients	Avg. Stay	Vari-ance	10th	25th	50th	75th	90th	95th	99th
1. SINGLE DX										
0–19 Years	8	30.5	260	17	17	28	43	56	56	56
20–34	7	45.0	892	27	27	31	43	99	99	99
35–49	5	16.1	179	2	4	26	28	28	28	28
50–64	2	31.7	30	29	29	29	29	41	41	41
65+	0									
2. MULTIPLE DX										
0–19 Years	245	39.0	240	26	31	38	46	68	89	>99
20–34	109	38.6	147	27	31	37	43	58	65	93
35–49	144	36.0	218	25	29	34	41	78	>99	>99
50–64	58	29.9	278	1	22	32	38	45	50	69
65+	4	11.3	128	1	1	7	12	32	32	32
TOTAL SINGLE DX	22	35.8	590	17	27	29	43	56	99	99
MULTIPLE DX	560	37.5	231	25	30	36	43	64	80	>99
TOTAL										
0–19 Years	253	38.8	241	26	30	38	46	68	89	>99
20–34	116	39.2	220	27	31	37	43	61	65	99
35–49	149	35.7	224	25	29	34	41	78	84	>99
50–64	60	30.0	264	1	24	32	38	43	50	69
65+	4	11.3	128	1	1	7	12	32	32	32
GRAND TOTAL	582	37.4	245	25	30	36	43	64	80	>99

41.04: STEM CELL TRANSPLANT. Formerly included in operation group(s) 593.

Type of Patients	Observed Patients	Avg. Stay	Vari-ance	10th	25th	50th	75th	90th	95th	99th
1. SINGLE DX										
0–19 Years	1	2.0	0	2	2	2	2	2	2	2
20–34	6	21.1	9	19	19	20	22	28	28	28
35–49	11	15.7	56	6	6	16	22	24	24	29
50–64	7	17.4	33	9	13	21	21	22	22	22
65+	0									
2. MULTIPLE DX										
0–19 Years	109	26.2	191	1	20	27	33	43	47	53
20–34	144	21.7	70	15	18	21	24	30	39	51
35–49	422	20.9	57	14	18	21	24	28	31	47
50–64	284	22.3	57	15	19	22	25	29	35	43
65+	14	21.7	42	18	19	21	25	32	32	32
TOTAL SINGLE DX	25	16.9	48	6	9	19	22	24	24	29
MULTIPLE DX	973	22.3	85	14	19	21	25	31	38	48
TOTAL										
0–19 Years	110	26.2	191	1	20	27	33	42	47	53
20–34	150	21.7	68	15	18	21	24	30	39	51
35–49	433	20.8	58	14	18	21	24	28	30	47
50–64	291	22.2	57	14	19	22	25	29	35	43
65+	14	21.7	42	18	19	21	25	32	32	32
GRAND TOTAL	998	22.2	84	13	19	21	25	31	38	48

41.1: PUNCTURE OF SPLEEN. Formerly included in operation group(s) 594.

Type of Patients	Observed Patients	Avg. Stay	Vari-ance	10th	25th	50th	75th	90th	95th	99th
1. SINGLE DX										
0–19 Years	0									
20–34	0									
35–49	1	12.0	0	12	12	12	12	12	12	12
50–64	1	2.0	0	2	2	2	2	2	2	2
65+	0									
2. MULTIPLE DX										
0–19 Years	2	4.5	44	2	2	2	2	17	17	17
20–34	5	21.5	898	2	2	6	18	74	74	74
35–49	10	9.7	35	1	1	12	16	16	16	20
50–64	11	11.5	67	3	8	11	15	15	38	38
65+	10	14.3	38	3	10	16	18	21	25	25
TOTAL SINGLE DX	2	11.4	6	12	12	12	12	12	12	12
MULTIPLE DX	38	11.8	122	1	4	11	16	18	21	74
TOTAL										
0–19 Years	2	4.5	44	2	2	2	2	17	17	17
20–34	5	21.5	898	2	2	6	18	74	74	74
35–49	11	10.2	28	2	7	12	12	16	16	20
50–64	12	11.3	67	3	6	11	15	15	38	38
65+	10	14.3	38	3	10	16	18	21	25	25
GRAND TOTAL	40	11.8	109	1	7	12	15	18	21	74

United States, October 1995–September 1996 Data, by Operation

41.2: SPLENOTOMY. Formerly included in operation group(s) 594.

Type of Patients	Observed Patients	Avg. Stay	Vari-ance	10th	25th	50th	75th	90th	95th	99th
1. SINGLE DX										
0–19 Years	1	11.0	0	11	11	11	11	11	11	11
20–34	1	4.0	0	4	4	4	4	4	4	4
35–49	0									
50–64	1	3.0	0	3	3	3	3	3	3	3
65+	0									
2. MULTIPLE DX										
0–19 Years	3	6.5	46	1	3	1	14	14	14	14
20–34	8	7.7	29	4	4	4	10	15	22	22
35–49	3	16.5	176	6	6	6	31	31	31	31
50–64	4	31.3	421	6	6	45	47	47	47	47
65+	2	9.7	51	4	4	4	16	16	16	16
TOTAL SINGLE DX	3	5.7	14	3	3	4	11	11	11	11
MULTIPLE DX	20	14.7	237	3	4	6	16	47	47	47
TOTAL										
0–19 Years	4	7.3	40	1	1	11	13	14	14	14
20–34	9	7.3	27	3	4	4	10	15	15	22
35–49	3	16.5	176	6	6	6	31	31	31	31
50–64	5	27.8	458	6	6	45	47	47	47	47
65+	2	9.7	51	4	4	4	16	16	16	16
GRAND TOTAL	23	13.8	221	3	4	6	15	45	47	47

41.31: BONE MARROW BIOPSY. Formerly included in operation group(s) 594.

Type of Patients	Observed Patients	Avg. Stay	Vari-ance	10th	25th	50th	75th	90th	95th	99th
1. SINGLE DX										
0–19 Years	441	4.3	12	1	2	3	6	8	10	19
20–34	105	4.7	82	1	2	3	5	9	10	83
35–49	110	4.1	16	1	2	3	5	8	12	18
50–64	84	6.6	36	1	2	4	7	18	18	18
65+	95	5.1	37	1	2	3	5	9	17	29
2. MULTIPLE DX										
0–19 Years	1616	9.5	98	2	3	6	12	22	29	48
20–34	1197	9.8	88	3	4	7	12	22	29	49
35–49	2100	9.3	79	3	4	6	10	21	28	45
50–64	2765	9.4	103	2	4	7	11	21	28	48
65+	8374	9.0	56	3	4	7	11	17	23	40
TOTAL SINGLE DX	835	4.7	27	1	2	3	6	9	16	20
MULTIPLE DX	16052	9.2	75	3	4	7	11	19	26	43
TOTAL										
0–19 Years	2057	8.5	86	2	3	6	10	20	27	47
20–34	1302	9.4	89	2	4	7	11	21	27	49
35–49	2210	9.1	77	3	4	6	10	21	28	44
50–64	2849	9.3	101	2	4	6	11	20	28	47
65+	8469	9.0	56	3	4	7	11	17	23	40
GRAND TOTAL	16887	9.0	73	2	4	7	11	18	25	42

41.3: MARROW & SPLEEN DXTIC PX. Formerly included in operation group(s) 594, 596.

Type of Patients	Observed Patients	Avg. Stay	Vari-ance	10th	25th	50th	75th	90th	95th	99th
1. SINGLE DX										
0–19 Years	441	4.3	12	1	2	3	6	8	10	19
20–34	105	4.7	82	1	2	3	5	9	10	83
35–49	110	4.1	16	1	2	3	5	8	12	18
50–64	84	6.6	36	1	2	4	7	18	18	18
65+	96	5.2	37	1	2	3	6	9	17	29
2. MULTIPLE DX										
0–19 Years	1620	9.5	98	2	3	6	12	22	29	48
20–34	1202	9.8	87	3	4	7	12	22	29	49
35–49	2107	9.3	79	3	4	6	10	21	28	45
50–64	2772	9.4	103	2	4	7	11	21	28	48
65+	8399	9.0	56	3	4	7	11	17	23	40
TOTAL SINGLE DX	836	4.7	27	1	2	3	6	9	15	20
MULTIPLE DX	16100	9.2	75	3	4	7	11	19	26	43
TOTAL										
0–19 Years	2061	8.5	86	2	3	6	10	20	27	47
20–34	1307	9.4	89	2	4	7	11	21	27	49
35–49	2217	9.1	77	3	4	6	10	21	28	44
50–64	2856	9.2	101	2	4	6	11	20	28	47
65+	8495	9.0	56	3	4	7	11	17	23	40
GRAND TOTAL	16936	9.0	73	2	4	7	11	18	25	42

41.4: EXC/DESTR SPLENIC TISSUE. Formerly included in operation group(s) 594.

Type of Patients	Observed Patients	Avg. Stay	Vari-ance	10th	25th	50th	75th	90th	95th	99th
1. SINGLE DX										
0–19 Years	18	2.4	<1	2	2	2	2	4	4	5
20–34	2	3.2	<1	3	3	3	3	4	4	4
35–49	1	2.0	0	2	2	2	2	2	2	2
50–64	1	4.0	0	4	4	4	4	4	4	4
65+	0									
2. MULTIPLE DX										
0–19 Years	42	6.4	50	2	4	4	6	9	20	40
20–34	16	6.5	20	3	4	6	6	10	22	22
35–49	14	7.9	10	7	7	7	7	14	14	19
50–64	8	13.3	165	7	7	8	11	43	43	54
65+	4	5.7	3	5	5	5	5	8	12	12
TOTAL SINGLE DX	22	2.5	<1	2	2	2	3	4	4	5
MULTIPLE DX	84	7.5	49	3	4	6	7	11	20	43
TOTAL										
0–19 Years	60	4.6	31	2	2	4	5	8	9	40
20–34	18	5.7	17	3	3	5	6	10	22	22
35–49	15	7.7	11	5	7	7	7	14	14	19
50–64	9	12.9	161	7	7	8	11	43	43	54
65+	4	5.7	3	5	5	5	5	8	12	12
GRAND TOTAL	106	6.0	40	2	2	5	7	9	14	40

Length of Stay by Diagnosis and Operation, United States, 1997

United States, October 1995–September 1996 Data, by Operation

41.91: DONOR MARROW ASPIRATION. Formerly included in operation group(s) 594.

Type of Patients	Observed Patients	Avg. Stay	Variance	Percentiles 10th	25th	50th	75th	90th	95th	99th
1. SINGLE DX										
0–19 Years	93	1.2	<1	1	1	1	1	1	2	7
20–34	60	1.1	<1	1	1	1	1	1	2	2
35–49	57	1.1	<1	1	1	1	1	1	2	2
50–64	20	2.0	15	1	1	1	1	2	18	18
65+	1	1.0	0	1	1	1	1	1	1	1
2. MULTIPLE DX										
0–19 Years	76	2.5	7	1	1	1	3	6	8	15
20–34	32	2.2	5	1	1	1	3	5	5	18
35–49	78	2.6	23	1	1	1	1	5	14	26
50–64	65	5.2	106	1	1	1	1	24	28	48
65+	4	6.5	68	1	1	1	8	21	21	21
TOTAL SINGLE DX	231	1.2	1	1	1	1	1	1	2	5
MULTIPLE DX	255	3.1	33	1	1	1	3	5	15	28
TOTAL										
0–19 Years	169	1.6	3	1	1	1	1	3	5	8
20–34	92	1.4	2	1	1	1	1	3	3	5
35–49	135	1.7	10	1	1	1	1	2	4	21
50–64	85	4.3	82	1	1	1	1	18	28	38
65+	5	5.4	58	1	1	1	8	21	21	21
GRAND TOTAL	486	2.0	15	1	1	1	1	3	5	24

42.0: ESOPHAGOTOMY. Formerly included in operation group(s) 597.

Type of Patients	Observed Patients	Avg. Stay	Variance	Percentiles 10th	25th	50th	75th	90th	95th	99th
1. SINGLE DX										
0–19 Years	3	1.0	0	1	1	1	1	1	1	1
20–34	1	7.0	0	7	7	7	7	7	7	7
35–49	0									
50–64	0									
65+	1	21.0	0	21	21	21	21	21	21	21
2. MULTIPLE DX										
0–19 Years	2	3.5	6	1	5	5	>99	>99	>99	>99
20–34	0									
35–49	4	20.9	269	1	1	28	36	36	36	36
50–64	0									
65+	15	19.3	150	10	13	21	21	27	27	>99
TOTAL SINGLE DX	5	5.6	64	1	1	1	7	21	21	21
MULTIPLE DX	21	19.0	165	5	12	21	23	36	85	>99
TOTAL										
0–19 Years	5	2.0	3	1	1	1	5	>99	>99	>99
20–34	1	7.0	0	7	7	7	7	7	7	7
35–49	4	20.9	269	1	1	28	36	36	36	36
50–64	0									
65+	16	19.3	147	10	13	21	21	27	27	>99
GRAND TOTAL	26	17.9	169	3	12	21	23	28	85	>99

41.5: TOTAL SPLENECTOMY. Formerly included in operation group(s) 594.

Type of Patients	Observed Patients	Avg. Stay	Variance	Percentiles 10th	25th	50th	75th	90th	95th	99th
1. SINGLE DX										
0–19 Years	272	3.8	4	2	3	3	5	6	6	16
20–34	193	4.8	10	3	3	4	5	7	8	16
35–49	114	4.6	4	3	3	4	5	7	8	11
50–64	68	4.3	3	2	4	4	6	6	8	10
65+	36	5.2	4	3	4	5	6	8	10	13
2. MULTIPLE DX										
0–19 Years	532	7.6	111	2	4	5	6	14	23	67
20–34	866	8.3	93	3	4	6	8	14	23	55
35–49	883	9.1	85	3	5	6	9	16	27	49
50–64	814	9.0	54	4	5	7	10	18	23	37
65+	967	14.4	377	4	5	8	15	27	44	99
TOTAL SINGLE DX	683	4.3	6	2	3	4	5	6	8	14
MULTIPLE DX	4062	9.9	154	3	5	6	10	19	28	92
TOTAL										
0–19 Years	804	6.3	80	2	3	4	6	10	18	45
20–34	1059	7.7	79	3	4	5	7	13	20	50
35–49	997	8.6	78	3	5	6	9	15	25	49
50–64	882	8.5	51	3	5	6	10	16	23	37
65+	1003	14.1	370	4	5	8	15	27	41	99
GRAND TOTAL	4745	9.1	136	3	4	6	9	17	26	85

41.9: OTH SPLEEN & MARROW OPS. Formerly included in operation group(s) 594.

Type of Patients	Observed Patients	Avg. Stay	Variance	Percentiles 10th	25th	50th	75th	90th	95th	99th
1. SINGLE DX										
0–19 Years	121	1.7	2	1	1	1	1	4	5	7
20–34	68	1.3	<1	1	1	1	1	2	4	5
35–49	57	1.1	<1	1	1	1	1	1	2	2
50–64	20	2.0	15	1	1	1	1	2	18	18
65+	1	1.0	0	1	1	1	1	1	1	1
2. MULTIPLE DX										
0–19 Years	186	5.4	24	1	2	5	6	10	15	30
20–34	143	7.2	60	1	4	5	8	14	19	35
35–49	138	5.6	53	1	1	5	7	12	17	41
50–64	81	6.3	98	1	1	1	6	22	28	38
65+	25	11.6	89	2	7	9	13	22	28	46
TOTAL SINGLE DX	267	1.5	2	1	1	1	1	3	4	6
MULTIPLE DX	573	6.2	52	1	1	5	7	13	19	38
TOTAL										
0–19 Years	307	3.6	17	1	1	2	5	7	10	25
20–34	211	5.1	47	1	1	4	6	10	17	35
35–49	195	3.8	37	1	1	1	5	9	13	26
50–64	101	5.3	81	1	1	1	4	19	28	38
65+	26	11.1	90	1	6	9	13	21	28	46
GRAND TOTAL	840	4.3	37	1	1	1	6	9	14	34

United States, October 1995–September 1996 Data, by Operation

42.1: ESOPHAGOSTOMY. Formerly included in operation group(s) 597.

Type of Patients	Observed Patients	Avg. Stay	Variance	Percentiles						
				10th	25th	50th	75th	90th	95th	99th
1. SINGLE DX										
0–19 Years	2	1.5	<1	1	1	2	2	2	2	2
20–34	0									
35–49	0									
50–64	1	3.0	0	3	3	3	3	3	3	3
65+	0									
2. MULTIPLE DX										
0–19 Years	6	24.1	299	16	16	16	20	61	61	61
20–34	3	28.0	933	4	4	4	65	65	65	65
35–49	2	14.5	24	9	9	18	18	18	18	18
50–64	8	17.4	419	3	3	8	17	42	71	71
65+	8	16.0	59	7	8	13	23	25	28	28
TOTAL SINGLE DX	3	2.1	<1	1	1	2	3	3	3	3
MULTIPLE DX	27	20.0	357	4	7	15	23	61	65	71
TOTAL										
0–19 Years	8	20.3	322	2	16	16	16	61	61	61
20–34	3	28.0	933	4	4	4	65	65	65	65
35–49	2	14.5	24	9	9	18	18	18	18	18
50–64	9	15.9	394	3	3	8	17	42	71	71
65+	8	16.0	59	7	8	13	23	25	28	28
GRAND TOTAL	30	19.1	355	3	7	14	23	61	65	71

42.23: ESOPHAGOSCOPY NEC. Formerly included in operation group(s) 598.

Type of Patients	Observed Patients	Avg. Stay	Variance	Percentiles						
				10th	25th	50th	75th	90th	95th	99th
1. SINGLE DX										
0–19 Years	524	1.2	<1	1	1	1	1	2	2	3
20–34	22	2.3	1	1	1	3	3	3	5	6
35–49	39	2.4	4	1	1	1	4	5	6	9
50–64	22	1.5	1	1	1	1	2	3	3	7
65+	21	2.3	5	1	1	1	3	6	6	11
2. MULTIPLE DX										
0–19 Years	284	3.0	17	1	1	1	3	7	9	23
20–34	101	5.1	21	1	2	4	6	12	13	26
35–49	180	8.4	74	1	3	5	11	22	27	32
50–64	324	5.0	19	1	1	4	6	10	15	18
65+	820	6.7	41	1	3	6	8	12	17	36
TOTAL SINGLE DX	628	1.3	<1	1	1	1	1	2	3	6
MULTIPLE DX	1709	5.8	37	1	2	4	7	12	16	32
TOTAL										
0–19 Years	808	1.7	6	1	1	1	1	3	4	16
20–34	123	4.3	17	1	2	3	5	9	13	20
35–49	219	6.9	64	1	1	4	9	16	27	32
50–64	346	4.8	19	1	1	4	6	10	14	18
65+	841	6.6	41	1	3	6	8	12	17	35
GRAND TOTAL	2337	4.4	30	1	1	2	6	10	15	27

42.2: ESOPHAGEAL DXTIC PX. Formerly included in operation group(s) 597, 598, 631.

Type of Patients	Observed Patients	Avg. Stay	Variance	Percentiles						
				10th	25th	50th	75th	90th	95th	99th
1. SINGLE DX										
0–19 Years	689	1.4	1	1	1	1	1	3	3	6
20–34	23	2.3	1	1	1	3	3	3	5	6
35–49	42	2.4	4	1	1	1	4	5	6	9
50–64	25	1.5	4	1	1	1	2	3	3	7
65+	25	2.4	5	1	1	1	3	6	6	11
2. MULTIPLE DX										
0–19 Years	764	4.2	26	1	1	3	5	10	16	29
20–34	124	5.3	24	1	2	4	7	13	14	26
35–49	223	10.2	164	1	2	5	12	27	52	52
50–64	409	5.4	24	1	2	4	7	12	16	23
65+	1012	7.1	45	2	3	6	9	13	19	36
TOTAL SINGLE DX	804	1.5	1	1	1	1	1	3	4	6
MULTIPLE DX	2532	6.0	47	1	2	4	7	13	18	35
TOTAL										
0–19 Years	1453	2.9	16	1	1	1	3	6	10	21
20–34	147	4.6	20	1	2	3	6	10	13	21
35–49	265	8.6	141	1	1	4	10	23	32	52
50–64	434	5.2	23	1	1	4	7	11	16	23
65+	1037	7.0	45	2	3	6	9	13	18	36
GRAND TOTAL	3336	4.8	38	1	2	3	6	10	16	32

42.29: ESOPHAGEAL DXTIC PX NEC. Formerly included in operation group(s) 631.

Type of Patients	Observed Patients	Avg. Stay	Variance	Percentiles						
				10th	25th	50th	75th	90th	95th	99th
1. SINGLE DX										
0–19 Years	158	2.1	2	1	1	2	3	4	5	8
20–34	0									
35–49	0									
50–64	0									
65+	0									
2. MULTIPLE DX										
0–19 Years	448	4.7	26	1	2	3	6	10	16	26
20–34	3	4.5	31	1	1	1	13	13	13	13
35–49	3	3.3	24	1	1	4	4	14	14	14
50–64	2	6.4	<1	6	6	6	7	7	7	7
65+	5	8.0	18	2	5	7	13	13	13	13
TOTAL SINGLE DX	158	2.1	2	1	1	2	3	4	5	8
MULTIPLE DX	461	4.7	26	1	2	3	6	10	16	26
TOTAL										
0–19 Years	606	4.0	21	1	1	3	5	9	13	21
20–34	3	4.5	31	1	1	1	13	13	13	13
35–49	3	3.3	24	1	1	4	4	14	14	14
50–64	2	6.4	<1	6	6	6	7	7	7	7
65+	5	8.0	18	2	5	7	13	13	13	13
GRAND TOTAL	619	4.0	21	1	1	3	5	9	13	21

Length of Stay by Diagnosis and Operation, United States, 1997

United States, October 1995–September 1996 Data, by Operation

42.3: EXC/DESTR ESOPH LES/TISS. Formerly included in operation group(s) 597.

Type of Patients	Observed Patients	Avg. Stay	Vari-ance	10th	25th	50th	75th	90th	95th	99th
1. SINGLE DX										
0–19 Years	25	3.0	12	1	1	2	5	5	5	23
20–34	7	5.3	9	1	2	6	8	8	8	8
35–49	27	3.6	5	2	2	3	4	8	8	11
50–64	38	2.9	3	1	2	2	4	5	6	7
65+	35	3.9	4	2	2	3	5	7	8	10
2. MULTIPLE DX										
0–19 Years	144	4.9	38	1	1	3	6	9	13	31
20–34	182	6.1	69	2	4	4	6	9	14	55
35–49	1296	5.3	23	2	3	4	7	10	13	24
50–64	1338	5.5	19	2	3	4	6	10	13	24
65+	1744	5.9	24	2	3	5	7	11	15	25
TOTAL SINGLE DX	132	3.4	7	1	2	3	4	7	8	11
MULTIPLE DX	4704	5.6	25	2	3	4	7	10	14	25
TOTAL										
0–19 Years	169	4.6	34	1	1	3	5	9	12	31
20–34	189	6.1	68	2	4	4	6	8	13	55
35–49	1323	5.3	23	2	3	4	7	10	13	24
50–64	1376	5.5	19	2	3	4	6	10	13	24
65+	1779	5.9	24	2	3	5	7	11	15	25
GRAND TOTAL	4836	5.6	25	2	3	4	6	10	14	25

42.33: ENDO EXC/DESTR ESOPH LES. Formerly included in operation group(s) 597.

Type of Patients	Observed Patients	Avg. Stay	Vari-ance	10th	25th	50th	75th	90th	95th	99th
1. SINGLE DX										
0–19 Years	15	2.8	16	1	1	1	5	5	5	23
20–34	3	2.0	<1	1	1	2	3	3	3	3
35–49	19	4.0	7	1	2	3	4	8	8	11
50–64	16	3.3	4	1	2	3	5	6	6	7
65+	15	3.0	2	1	2	3	4	5	6	6
2. MULTIPLE DX										
0–19 Years	130	4.6	38	1	1	3	5	9	12	31
20–34	174	5.8	53	2	4	4	6	8	13	31
35–49	1259	5.3	23	2	3	4	7	10	13	24
50–64	1270	5.5	18	2	3	4	6	10	13	24
65+	1465	5.8	22	2	3	5	7	10	14	25
TOTAL SINGLE DX	68	3.2	9	1	1	2	4	5	8	23
MULTIPLE DX	4298	5.5	24	2	3	4	6	10	13	25
TOTAL										
0–19 Years	145	4.3	36	1	1	2	5	9	12	31
20–34	177	5.7	53	2	4	4	6	8	13	31
35–49	1278	5.3	23	2	3	4	7	10	13	24
50–64	1286	5.5	18	2	3	4	6	10	13	24
65+	1480	5.8	22	2	3	5	7	10	14	25
GRAND TOTAL	4366	5.5	24	2	3	4	6	10	13	25

42.31: EXC ESOPH DIVERTICULUM. Formerly included in operation group(s) 597.

Type of Patients	Observed Patients	Avg. Stay	Vari-ance	10th	25th	50th	75th	90th	95th	99th
1. SINGLE DX										
0–19 Years	0									
20–34	2	6.7	8	1	8	8	8	8	8	8
35–49	6	2.8	2	2	2	2	3	5	6	6
50–64	20	2.6	2	1	2	2	3	4	6	7
65+	20	4.4	5	2	3	4	6	8	8	10
2. MULTIPLE DX										
0–19 Years	3	12.5	62	8	8	8	16	27	27	27
20–34	1	3.0	0	3	3	3	3	3	3	3
35–49	17	5.5	25	2	3	4	7	8	11	32
50–64	48	5.2	46	2	4	3	7	8	12	43
65+	251	6.7	34	2	4	6	7	14	18	30
TOTAL SINGLE DX	48	3.6	5	2	2	3	4	8	8	10
MULTIPLE DX	320	6.5	36	2	3	5	7	12	17	32
TOTAL										
0–19 Years	3	12.5	62	8	8	8	16	27	27	27
20–34	3	5.2	8	1	3	3	8	8	8	8
35–49	23	4.7	20	2	2	3	6	7	8	32
50–64	68	4.5	35	2	2	3	5	7	10	41
65+	271	6.6	33	2	3	6	7	13	17	30
GRAND TOTAL	368	6.1	33	2	3	5	7	12	15	31

42.4: EXCISION OF ESOPHAGUS. Formerly included in operation group(s) 597.

Type of Patients	Observed Patients	Avg. Stay	Vari-ance	10th	25th	50th	75th	90th	95th	99th
1. SINGLE DX										
0–19 Years	2	8.3	<1	8	8	8	8	10	10	10
20–34	2	8.6	6	8	5	10	10	10	10	10
35–49	0									
50–64	4	7.3	<1	7	7	7	7	7	10	11
65+	2	9.8	<1	9	10	10	10	10	10	10
2. MULTIPLE DX										
0–19 Years	24	18.4	243	8	10	12	24	57	>99	>99
20–34	18	9.4	8	8	8	9	10	15	15	3
35–49	90	12.1	35	8	9	10	14	17	20	51
50–64	309	14.6	85	8	9	11	17	27	36	54
65+	375	16.0	134	8	10	12	17	29	44	64
TOTAL SINGLE DX	10	7.9	2	7	7	7	10	10	10	11
MULTIPLE DX	816	15.1	111	8	9	12	17	29	40	64
TOTAL										
0–19 Years	26	17.7	232	8	9	12	20	57	>99	>99
20–34	20	9.3	8	7	8	9	10	15	15	20
35–49	90	12.1	35	8	9	10	14	17	20	51
50–64	313	14.3	84	7	8	11	17	27	36	54
65+	377	16.0	134	8	10	12	17	29	44	64
GRAND TOTAL	826	14.9	110	8	9	11	16	29	39	64

Length of Stay by Diagnosis and Operation, United States, 1997

United States, October 1995–September 1996 Data, by Operation

42.41: PARTIAL ESOPHAGECTOMY. Formerly included in operation group(s) 597.

Type of Patients	Observed Patients	Avg. Stay	Variance	10th	25th	50th	75th	90th	95th	99th
1. SINGLE DX										
0–19 Years	1	8.0	0	8	8	8	8	8	8	8
20–34	1	5.0	0	5	5	5	5	5	5	5
35–49	0									
50–64	1	10.0	0	10	10	10	10	10	10	10
65+	1	9.0	0	9	9	9	9	9	9	9
2. MULTIPLE DX										
0–19 Years	11	18.0	284	6	10	15	57	>99	>99	>99
20–34	11	9.2	5	8	8	9	9	11	11	20
35–49	51	12.2	38	8	9	10	14	17	19	51
50–64	173	14.4	88	8	9	11	16	28	38	54
65+	220	15.5	140	7	10	11	17	27	38	65
TOTAL SINGLE DX	4	7.8	3	5	8	8	9	10	10	10
MULTIPLE DX	466	14.6	111	7	9	11	16	27	38	65
TOTAL										
0–19 Years	12	16.2	247	6	8	10	40	>99	>99	>99
20–34	12	9.1	6	8	8	9	9	11	16	20
35–49	51	12.2	38	8	9	10	14	17	19	51
50–64	174	14.4	88	8	9	11	16	28	38	54
65+	221	15.5	140	7	10	11	17	27	38	65
GRAND TOTAL	470	14.5	111	7	9	11	16	27	38	65

42.42: TOTAL ESOPHAGECTOMY. Formerly included in operation group(s) 597.

Type of Patients	Observed Patients	Avg. Stay	Variance	10th	25th	50th	75th	90th	95th	99th
1. SINGLE DX										
0–19 Years	0									
20–34	1	10.0	0	10	10	10	10	10	10	10
35–49	0									
50–64	3	7.2	<1	7	7	7	7	7	9	9
65+	1	10.0	0	10	10	10	10	10	10	10
2. MULTIPLE DX										
0–19 Years	10	17.1	158	8	9	11	20	44	44	44
20–34	7	9.9	17	5	5	10	15	15	15	15
35–49	34	12.9	36	8	10	13	14	17	24	>99
50–64	116	15.0	87	8	9	13	17	26	31	57
65+	141	17.0	131	9	10	13	18	29	46	64
TOTAL SINGLE DX	5	7.9	2	7	7	7	10	10	10	11
MULTIPLE DX	308	16.0	113	8	10	13	17	29	44	61
TOTAL										
0–19 Years	10	17.1	158	8	9	11	20	44	44	44
20–34	8	9.9	13	5	5	10	14	15	15	15
35–49	34	12.9	36	8	10	13	14	17	24	>99
50–64	119	14.2	84	7	8	12	17	24	31	57
65+	142	16.9	130	9	10	13	18	29	46	64
GRAND TOTAL	313	15.7	111	8	10	12	17	29	44	59

42.5: INTRATHOR ESOPH ANAST. Formerly included in operation group(s) 597.

Type of Patients	Observed Patients	Avg. Stay	Variance	10th	25th	50th	75th	90th	95th	99th
1. SINGLE DX										
0–19 Years	3	11.7	5	10	10	10	14	14	14	14
20–34	0									
35–49	1	6.0	0	6	6	6	6	6	6	6
50–64	1	7.0	0	7	7	7	7	7	7	7
65+	0									
2. MULTIPLE DX										
0–19 Years	38	18.4	103	9	13	16	28	38	>99	>99
20–34	5	24.2	50	8	25	26	26	26	26	49
35–49	18	15.9	90	4	10	14	23	31	35	39
50–64	21	11.0	14	8	8	10	12	15	19	28
65+	44	16.2	188	8	9	10	18	25	50	75
TOTAL SINGLE DX	5	8.4	10	6	6	7	10	14	14	14
MULTIPLE DX	126	17.6	121	8	10	16	26	31	39	>99
TOTAL										
0–19 Years	41	18.2	100	10	13	16	28	38	>99	>99
20–34	5	24.2	50	8	25	26	26	26	26	49
35–49	19	14.5	89	4	6	13	23	23	35	39
50–64	22	10.9	14	8	8	10	12	15	19	28
65+	44	16.2	188	8	9	10	18	25	50	75
GRAND TOTAL	131	17.3	120	8	10	15	26	31	39	>99

42.6: ANTESTERNAL ESOPH ANAST. Formerly included in operation group(s) 597.

Type of Patients	Observed Patients	Avg. Stay	Variance	10th	25th	50th	75th	90th	95th	99th
1. SINGLE DX										
0–19 Years	0									
20–34	0									
35–49	0									
50–64	0									
65+	0									
2. MULTIPLE DX										
0–19 Years	3	45.5	100	28	42	42	55	>99	>99	>99
20–34	1	26.0	0	26	26	26	26	26	26	26
35–49	1	42.0	0	42	42	42	42	42	42	42
50–64	0									
65+	5	9.2	9	4	9	10	11	12	12	12
TOTAL SINGLE DX	0									
MULTIPLE DX	10	26.2	321	9	11	26	42	55	55	>99
TOTAL										
0–19 Years	3	45.5	100	28	42	42	55	>99	>99	>99
20–34	1	26.0	0	26	26	26	26	26	26	26
35–49	1	42.0	0	42	42	42	42	42	42	42
50–64	0									
65+	5	9.2	9	4	9	10	11	12	12	12
GRAND TOTAL	10	26.2	321	9	11	26	42	55	55	>99

Length of Stay by Diagnosis and Operation, United States, 1997

United States, October 1995–September 1996 Data, by Operation

42.7: ESOPHAGOMYOTOMY. Formerly included in operation group(s) 597.

Type of Patients	Observed Patients	Avg. Stay	Variance	10th	25th	50th	75th	90th	95th	99th
1. SINGLE DX										
0–19 Years	18	3.4	2	2	2	3	5	5	6	6
20–34	19	3.3	3	2	2	3	5	6	6	6
35–49	8	3.1	3	1	1	4	5	5	5	5
50–64	9	4.2	7	1	2	4	6	9	9	9
65+	0									
2. MULTIPLE DX										
0–19 Years	30	5.9	11	3	4	5	7	10	16	16
20–34	26	6.9	24	3	4	6	7	12	17	25
35–49	57	5.3	8	2	4	5	7	7	9	16
50–64	38	12.9	299	2	4	6	12	33	60	60
65+	50	10.3	132	2	3	7	11	29	34	74
TOTAL SINGLE DX	54	3.5	3	2	2	3	5	6	6	9
MULTIPLE DX	201	7.8	92	2	4	5	7	14	25	60
TOTAL										
0–19 Years	48	4.7	8	2	3	4	6	7	10	16
20–34	45	5.6	19	2	3	5	6	7	17	25
35–49	65	5.2	8	2	4	5	7	7	9	16
50–64	47	11.8	269	2	3	5	10	33	60	60
65+	50	10.3	132	2	3	7	11	29	34	74
GRAND TOTAL	255	7.1	80	2	3	5	7	12	20	60

42.8: OTHER ESOPHAGEAL REPAIR. Formerly included in operation group(s) 597.

Type of Patients	Observed Patients	Avg. Stay	Variance	10th	25th	50th	75th	90th	95th	99th
1. SINGLE DX										
0–19 Years	20	9.5	171	2	2	3	7	28	50	50
20–34	1	2.0	0	2	2	2	2	2	2	2
35–49	2	1.2	<1	1	1	1	1	1	3	3
50–64	1	1.0	0	1	1	1	1	1	1	1
65+	3	4.8	21	1	1	1	10	10	10	10
2. MULTIPLE DX										
0–19 Years	76	15.1	187	2	5	11	21	40	51	>99
20–34	21	9.3	14	6	7	8	10	17	17	21
35–49	44	13.2	69	5	8	12	16	27	28	49
50–64	87	11.3	128	1	3	7	19	25	33	62
65+	170	13.2	158	3	7	10	14	25	48	60
TOTAL SINGLE DX	27	7.5	134	1	2	3	6	19	28	50
MULTIPLE DX	398	12.9	145	2	6	10	16	27	40	62
TOTAL										
0–19 Years	96	13.8	188	2	4	9	19	40	50	>99
20–34	22	9.2	15	6	7	8	9	17	17	21
35–49	46	12.2	74	2	8	12	15	27	28	49
50–64	88	11.2	128	1	3	7	17	23	33	62
65+	173	13.0	157	2	7	10	14	25	48	60
GRAND TOTAL	425	12.6	146	2	5	10	16	27	40	60

42.9: OTHER ESOPHAGEAL OPS. Formerly included in operation group(s) 597.

Type of Patients	Observed Patients	Avg. Stay	Variance	10th	25th	50th	75th	90th	95th	99th
1. SINGLE DX										
0–19 Years	44	1.3	<1	1	1	1	1	2	3	4
20–34	12	1.1	<1	1	1	1	1	1	1	2
35–49	14	1.7	<1	1	1	2	2	2	2	5
50–64	3	1.2	<1	1	1	1	1	2	2	2
65+	19	3.9	29	1	1	1	5	10	17	27
2. MULTIPLE DX										
0–19 Years	198	5.7	72	1	1	2	6	16	24	42
20–34	85	3.8	26	1	1	2	4	6	16	31
35–49	243	5.4	28	1	2	4	6	12	14	33
50–64	516	7.5	63	1	3	4	9	19	24	45
65+	2164	7.4	44	2	3	5	9	15	20	32
TOTAL SINGLE DX	92	1.5	3	1	1	1	1	2	4	10
MULTIPLE DX	3206	7.0	47	1	3	5	9	15	21	32
TOTAL										
0–19 Years	242	4.9	62	1	1	2	5	14	23	42
20–34	97	2.8	19	1	1	1	3	6	6	29
35–49	257	5.2	27	1	2	4	6	12	13	33
50–64	519	7.4	62	1	3	4	9	19	24	45
65+	2183	7.4	44	2	3	5	9	15	20	32
GRAND TOTAL	3298	6.7	46	1	2	5	8	15	20	32

42.92: ESOPHAGEAL DILATION. Formerly included in operation group(s) 597.

Type of Patients	Observed Patients	Avg. Stay	Variance	10th	25th	50th	75th	90th	95th	99th
1. SINGLE DX										
0–19 Years	42	1.3	<1	1	1	1	1	2	3	4
20–34	12	1.1	<1	1	1	1	1	1	1	2
35–49	14	1.7	<1	1	1	2	2	2	2	5
50–64	3	1.2	<1	1	1	1	1	2	2	2
65+	18	3.9	30	1	1	1	5	10	17	27
2. MULTIPLE DX										
0–19 Years	190	5.2	56	1	1	2	6	14	19	36
20–34	85	3.8	26	1	1	2	4	6	16	31
35–49	233	5.3	28	1	2	4	6	12	13	33
50–64	504	7.5	64	1	3	4	9	22	24	45
65+	2151	7.4	44	2	3	5	9	15	20	32
TOTAL SINGLE DX	89	1.5	3	1	1	1	1	2	3	10
MULTIPLE DX	3163	6.9	46	1	3	5	9	15	21	32
TOTAL										
0–19 Years	232	4.5	48	1	1	2	5	14	18	36
20–34	97	2.8	19	1	1	1	3	6	6	29
35–49	247	5.1	27	1	2	4	6	12	12	33
50–64	507	7.4	64	1	3	4	9	22	24	45
65+	2169	7.3	44	2	3	5	9	15	20	32
GRAND TOTAL	3252	6.7	46	1	2	5	8	15	20	32

United States, October 1995–September 1996 Data, by Operation

43.0: GASTROTOMY. Formerly included in operation group(s) 599.

Type of Patients	Observed Patients	Avg. Stay	Variance	10th	25th	50th	75th	90th	95th	99th
1. SINGLE DX										
0–19 Years	14	3.3	1	2	3	4	4	4	5	7
20–34	2	4.3	<1	4	4	4	4	7	7	7
35–49	1	2.0	0	2	2	2	2	2	2	2
50–64	0									
65+	0									
2. MULTIPLE DX										
0–19 Years	22	6.2	21	3	3	5	7	13	17	19
20–34	31	7.2	114	2	3	5	7	11	13	66
35–49	38	9.6	63	4	6	7	8	30	30	30
50–64	34	8.4	143	3	4	6	11	12	13	92
65+	76	10.4	33	5	6	8	15	15	24	30
TOTAL SINGLE DX	17	3.5	1	2	3	4	4	4	5	7
MULTIPLE DX	201	9.0	70	3	5	7	10	15	24	30
TOTAL										
0–19 Years	36	4.7	13	2	3	4	5	7	13	19
20–34	33	6.8	99	2	2	5	7	10	13	66
35–49	39	9.5	63	3	6	7	8	30	30	30
50–64	34	8.4	143	3	4	6	11	12	13	92
65+	76	10.4	33	5	6	8	15	15	24	30
GRAND TOTAL	218	8.4	66	3	4	7	9	15	24	30

43.11: PERC (ENDO) GASTROSTOMY. Formerly included in operation group(s) 600.

Type of Patients	Observed Patients	Avg. Stay	Variance	10th	25th	50th	75th	90th	95th	99th
1. SINGLE DX										
0–19 Years	49	2.6	3	1	2	2	3	6	6	11
20–34	5	7.7	16	2	6	6	12	12	12	12
35–49	13	4.3	16	1	1	2	2	13	13	13
50–64	19	7.0	58	2	2	2	9	23	23	23
65+	70	6.5	79	1	3	3	9	16	33	52
2. MULTIPLE DX										
0–19 Years	1078	8.2	164	1	2	3	9	21	31	85
20–34	234	14.2	156	3	6	14	16	29	37	60
35–49	652	14.7	208	3	6	10	17	33	50	97
50–64	1735	14.1	181	4	7	10	17	32	56	>99
65+	16830	12.8	99	4	7	10	16	24	32	56
TOTAL SINGLE DX	156	5.4	51	1	2	2	6	14	20	43
MULTIPLE DX	20529	12.7	119	3	6	10	16	25	33	66
TOTAL										
0–19 Years	1127	8.1	160	1	2	3	9	20	31	85
20–34	239	14.1	155	3	6	14	16	29	37	60
35–49	665	14.6	208	3	6	10	17	33	50	97
50–64	1754	14.0	180	2	6	10	17	31	56	>99
65+	16900	12.7	99	4	7	10	16	24	32	56
GRAND TOTAL	20685	12.6	119	3	6	10	16	24	33	66

43.1: GASTROSTOMY. Formerly included in operation group(s) 600.

Type of Patients	Observed Patients	Avg. Stay	Variance	10th	25th	50th	75th	90th	95th	99th
1. SINGLE DX										
0–19 Years	83	3.2	8	1	2	2	4	6	8	14
20–34	8	7.9	26	3	5	6	12	19	19	19
35–49	18	4.7	12	1	2	4	6	11	13	13
50–64	23	6.8	54	2	2	4	9	23	23	23
65+	83	6.3	70	1	1	3	8	16	20	52
2. MULTIPLE DX										
0–19 Years	1536	9.0	174	1	2	4	11	23	39	95
20–34	281	13.8	155	3	5	13	15	29	37	60
35–49	763	14.5	196	3	6	10	17	32	47	97
50–64	1999	13.8	173	3	6	10	17	30	47	>99
65+	18252	12.7	99	4	7	10	16	24	32	55
TOTAL SINGLE DX	215	5.1	41	1	2	3	6	13	17	33
MULTIPLE DX	22831	12.6	120	3	6	10	16	25	34	68
TOTAL										
0–19 Years	1619	8.8	169	1	2	4	11	23	35	95
20–34	289	13.7	153	3	5	12	15	29	37	60
35–49	781	14.4	195	3	6	10	17	31	47	>99
50–64	2022	13.8	173	3	6	10	17	30	46	>99
65+	18335	12.7	99	4	7	10	16	24	32	55
GRAND TOTAL	23046	12.5	119	3	6	10	16	24	34	67

43.19: GASTROSTOMY NEC. Formerly included in operation group(s) 600.

Type of Patients	Observed Patients	Avg. Stay	Variance	10th	25th	50th	75th	90th	95th	99th
1. SINGLE DX										
0–19 Years	34	3.9	13	1	2	3	4	8	14	16
20–34	3	8.3	48	3	5	5	19	19	19	19
35–49	5	5.6	1	4	4	6	6	7	7	7
50–64	4	4.1	<1	3	3	4	6	5	5	5
65+	13	4.8	15	1	2	4	6	9	9	18
2. MULTIPLE DX										
0–19 Years	458	10.7	195	2	3	6	12	29	50	95
20–34	47	12.1	146	2	4	10	14	31	32	63
35–49	111	13.4	110	3	5	11	17	30	31	47
50–64	264	12.3	115	3	6	10	15	21	30	59
65+	1422	12.4	97	3	6	10	16	24	32	54
TOTAL SINGLE DX	59	4.4	14	1	2	3	6	8	14	19
MULTIPLE DX	2302	12.0	126	3	5	9	15	25	35	75
TOTAL										
0–19 Years	492	10.3	186	2	3	5	12	29	48	>99
20–34	50	12.0	142	2	4	10	14	31	32	63
35–49	116	13.2	109	3	6	10	17	30	31	47
50–64	268	12.3	114	4	6	10	15	21	30	59
65+	1435	12.3	97	3	6	10	16	24	32	54
GRAND TOTAL	2361	11.8	125	2	5	9	15	25	35	71

Length of Stay by Diagnosis and Operation, United States, 1997

United States, October 1995–September 1996 Data, by Operation

43.3: PYLOROMYOTOMY. Formerly included in operation group(s) 599.

Type of Patients	Observed Patients	Variance	Avg. Stay	Percentiles						
				10th	25th	50th	75th	90th	95th	99th
1. SINGLE DX										
0–19 Years	2246	2	2.5	1	2	2	3	4	4	7
20–34	1	0	1.0	1	1	1	1	1	1	1
35–49	0									
50–64	0									
65+	1		3.0	3	3	3	3	3	3	3
2. MULTIPLE DX										
0–19 Years	1416	24	3.9	2	2	3	4	6	8	23
20–34	1	0	5.0	5	5	5	5	5	5	5
35–49	3	126	7.7	1	1	2	24	24	24	24
50–64	6	21	7.2	2	2	8	10	10	17	17
65+	7	137	15.3	9	9	10	12	45	45	45
TOTAL SINGLE DX	2248	2	2.5	1	2	2	3	4	4	7
MULTIPLE DX	1433	24	4.0	2	2	3	4	6	9	23
TOTAL										
0–19 Years	3662	11	3.1	1	2	3	3	5	6	15
20–34	2	7	2.7	1	1	1	5	5	5	5
35–49	3	126	7.7	1	1	2	24	24	24	24
50–64	6	21	7.2	2	2	8	10	10	17	17
65+	8	131	12.1	3	3	9	12	24	45	45
GRAND TOTAL	3681	11	3.1	1	2	3	3	5	6	15

43.4: LOC EXC GASTRIC LES. Formerly included in operation group(s) 601.

Type of Patients	Observed Patients	Variance	Avg. Stay	Percentiles						
				10th	25th	50th	75th	90th	95th	99th
1. SINGLE DX										
0–19 Years	9	4	4.2	2	2	4	5	7	7	7
20–34	4	37	11.2	1	3	15	15	15	15	15
35–49	8	6	4.2	1	2	4	7	7	7	7
50–64	11	3	6.0	3	5	7	7	8	8	8
65+	8	8	4.7	3	3	4	6	6	13	13
2. MULTIPLE DX										
0–19 Years	21	267	14.2	2	4	5	13	45	49	49
20–34	54	17	6.2	3	5	5	6	9	11	22
35–49	162	69	8.2	2	4	6	9	16	29	29
50–64	350	34	6.1	1	2	4	7	13	17	25
65+	1255	38	7.6	2	4	6	9	15	18	33
TOTAL SINGLE DX	40	15	5.8	2	3	5	7	15	15	15
MULTIPLE DX	1842	41	7.2	2	3	6	9	14	18	32
TOTAL										
0–19 Years	30	223	11.9	2	3	5	12	43	45	49
20–34	58	19	6.4	3	5	6	6	11	15	22
35–49	170	66	8.0	2	4	6	9	16	29	29
50–64	361	33	6.1	1	2	4	7	13	16	25
65+	1263	37	7.6	2	4	6	9	15	18	33
GRAND TOTAL	1882	41	7.2	2	3	6	9	14	18	32

43.41: ENDO EXC GASTRIC LES. Formerly included in operation group(s) 601.

Type of Patients	Observed Patients	Variance	Avg. Stay	Percentiles						
				10th	25th	50th	75th	90th	95th	99th
1. SINGLE DX										
0–19 Years	1	0	2.0	2	2	2	2	2	2	2
20–34	2	26	13.0	1	15	15	15	15	15	15
35–49	2	<1	1.5	1	2	2	2	2	2	2
50–64	2	1	4.3	3	3	5	5	5	5	5
65+	2	<1	3.7	3	3	4	4	4	4	4
2. MULTIPLE DX										
0–19 Years	5	302	10.7	2	2	2	7	45	45	45
20–34	36	46	5.0	1	2	3	5	6	15	43
35–49	96	8	4.8	2	3	4	6	9	10	14
50–64	218	15	4.4	1	2	3	6	11	12	17
65+	906	27	6.4	2	3	5	8	13	16	27
TOTAL SINGLE DX	9	39	6.4	1	1	3	15	15	15	15
MULTIPLE DX	1261	24	5.7	2	3	4	7	12	15	24
TOTAL										
0–19 Years	6	275	9.8	2	2	2	7	45	45	45
20–34	38	50	5.9	1	2	4	6	15	15	43
35–49	98	8	4.7	2	3	4	6	8	10	14
50–64	220	15	4.4	1	2	3	6	11	12	17
65+	908	27	6.4	2	3	5	8	13	16	27
GRAND TOTAL	1270	24	5.7	1	3	4	7	12	15	24

43.42: LOC GASTRIC LES EXC NEC. Formerly included in operation group(s) 601.

Type of Patients	Observed Patients	Variance	Avg. Stay	Percentiles						
				10th	25th	50th	75th	90th	95th	99th
1. SINGLE DX										
0–19 Years	8	3	4.5	2	3	5	5	7	7	7
20–34	2	0	3.0	3	3	3	3	3	3	3
35–49	6	2	5.9	4	5	6	7	7	7	7
50–64	8	2	6.6	4	6	7	7	8	8	8
65+	6	11	5.0	3	3	4	6	13	13	13
2. MULTIPLE DX										
0–19 Years	13	283	16.0	4	5	5	39	43	49	49
20–34	18	4	6.7	6	6	6	6	10	11	13
35–49	59	96	10.8	5	6	7	12	16	17	75
50–64	115	58	11.2	4	7	8	14	22	24	38
65+	318	51	11.1	6	7	9	13	18	27	39
TOTAL SINGLE DX	30	4	5.7	3	4	6	7	7	8	13
MULTIPLE DX	523	57	10.5	6	6	8	12	17	24	40
TOTAL										
0–19 Years	21	227	12.6	3	4	5	12	43	49	49
20–34	20	4	6.6	6	6	6	6	10	11	13
35–49	65	88	10.2	5	6	7	12	16	17	75
50–64	123	55	10.8	5	7	8	13	22	24	38
65+	324	51	11.1	6	7	9	13	18	27	39
GRAND TOTAL	553	56	10.3	5	6	8	12	17	23	40

Length of Stay by Diagnosis and Operation, United States, 1997

United States, October 1995–September 1996 Data, by Operation

43.7: PART GASTRECTOMY W ANAST. Formerly included in operation group(s) 602.

Type of Patients	Observed Patients	Avg. Stay	Variance	10th	25th	50th	75th	90th	95th	99th
1. SINGLE DX										
0–19 Years	0									
20–34	5	7.4	10	5	5	6	9	13	13	13
35–49	26	9.9	6	6	8	11	11	11	11	11
50–64	21	6.8	6	4	5	6	8	9	10	20
65+	8	7.5	5	4	7	8	8	9	14	14
2. MULTIPLE DX										
0–19 Years	7	15.5	55	7	7	12	22	24	27	27
20–34	55	16.4	45	7	11	16	24	24	24	25
35–49	345	12.7	116	6	8	10	14	18	28	58
50–64	563	13.0	89	6	8	10	15	25	30	57
65+	1344	15.4	107	7	9	12	18	29	38	61
TOTAL SINGLE DX	60	9.6	7	6	7	11	11	11	11	13
MULTIPLE DX	2314	14.3	103	7	8	11	16	26	35	58
TOTAL										
0–19 Years	7	15.5	55	7	7	12	22	24	27	27
20–34	60	16.2	46	7	10	15	24	24	24	25
35–49	371	11.9	85	6	8	11	12	16	22	58
50–64	584	12.8	87	6	8	9	15	25	30	55
65+	1352	15.3	107	7	9	12	18	29	38	61
GRAND TOTAL	2374	13.9	97	6	8	11	16	25	35	57

43.8: OTH PARTIAL GASTRECTOMY. Formerly included in operation group(s) 602.

Type of Patients	Observed Patients	Avg. Stay	Variance	10th	25th	50th	75th	90th	95th	99th
1. SINGLE DX										
0–19 Years	0									
20–34	4	5.4	2	4	4	6	6	6	8	8
35–49	10	7.4	4	5	6	8	10	10	10	10
50–64	11	8.9	22	5	5	6	15	15	15	15
65+	8	6.6	24	2	3	4	9	18	18	18
2. MULTIPLE DX										
0–19 Years	6	17.3	152	6	7	20	39	>99	>99	>99
20–34	32	10.5	60	3	6	8	13	17	38	38
35–49	122	12.4	139	6	7	8	14	22	52	57
50–64	167	10.8	89	5	6	8	11	19	30	55
65+	397	13.1	78	6	7	10	17	23	30	55
TOTAL SINGLE DX	33	7.4	16	3	5	6	9	15	15	18
MULTIPLE DX	724	12.3	95	5	7	8	15	23	33	57
TOTAL										
0–19 Years	6	17.3	152	6	7	20	39	>99	>99	>99
20–34	36	9.9	56	3	6	8	13	16	21	38
35–49	132	12.3	135	6	7	8	13	22	52	57
50–64	178	10.7	87	5	6	8	11	18	33	55
65+	405	13.0	77	6	7	10	17	23	29	55
GRAND TOTAL	757	12.1	93	7	7	8	15	22	31	57

43.5: PROXIMAL GASTRECTOMY. Formerly included in operation group(s) 602.

Type of Patients	Observed Patients	Avg. Stay	Variance	10th	25th	50th	75th	90th	95th	99th
1. SINGLE DX										
0–19 Years	0									
20–34	0									
35–49	2	8.0	0	8	8	8	8	8	8	8
50–64	4	9.9	8	6	8	8	12	14	14	14
65+	1	9.0	0	9	9	9	9	9	9	9
2. MULTIPLE DX										
0–19 Years	0									
20–34	5	25.5	342	9	13	15	49	49	49	49
35–49	30	12.4	84	7	7	9	16	18	29	69
50–64	87	13.1	55	8	10	11	14	20	26	50
65+	189	17.4	157	8	9	13	21	35	37	94
TOTAL SINGLE DX	7	8.9	4	8	8	8	9	12	12	14
MULTIPLE DX	311	15.7	128	7	9	12	18	27	37	59
TOTAL										
0–19 Years	0									
20–34	5	25.5	342	9	13	15	49	49	49	49
35–49	32	11.9	77	7	7	8	15	18	25	69
50–64	91	13.0	54	8	10	11	14	20	26	50
65+	190	17.4	157	8	9	13	21	35	37	59
GRAND TOTAL	318	15.6	126	7	9	12	18	27	37	59

43.6: DISTAL GASTRECTOMY. Formerly included in operation group(s) 602.

Type of Patients	Observed Patients	Avg. Stay	Variance	10th	25th	50th	75th	90th	95th	99th
1. SINGLE DX										
0–19 Years	3	5.8	2	3	6	6	6	6	9	9
20–34	13	4.6	5	2	2	5	7	7	7	7
35–49	19	5.0	3	4	4	4	6	7	8	13
50–64	9	6.5	1	5	6	6	8	8	8	8
65+	5	7.0	3	4	6	7	8	9	9	9
2. MULTIPLE DX										
0–19 Years	7	17.9	172	2	6	24	26	35	35	35
20–34	38	10.3	26	6	6	9	13	20	22	23
35–49	141	10.4	39	6	7	9	12	17	23	35
50–64	229	12.1	68	6	7	10	14	20	26	49
65+	398	14.7	94	7	9	11	18	28	39	50
TOTAL SINGLE DX	49	5.3	3	4	4	5	6	8	8	10
MULTIPLE DX	813	13.1	79	6	8	10	15	24	29	48
TOTAL										
0–19 Years	10	11.5	117	2	6	6	15	35	35	35
20–34	51	8.9	27	4	6	7	11	18	20	23
35–49	160	9.2	36	4	6	8	10	15	19	32
50–64	238	11.8	67	6	7	10	14	19	26	49
65+	403	14.7	94	7	9	11	18	28	39	50
GRAND TOTAL	862	12.5	78	7	8	10	15	23	29	41

Length of Stay by Diagnosis and Operation, United States, 1997

United States, October 1995–September 1996 Data, by Operation

43.89: PARTIAL GASTRECTOMY NEC. Formerly included in operation group(s) 602.

Type of Patients	Observed Patients	Avg. Stay	Vari-ance	10th	25th	50th	75th	90th	95th	99th
1. SINGLE DX										
0–19 Years	0									
20–34	4	5.4	2	4	4	6	6	6	8	8
35–49	10	7.4	4	5	6	8	10	10	10	10
50–64	11	8.9	22	5	5	6	15	15	15	15
65+	8	6.6	24	2	3	4	9	18	18	18
2. MULTIPLE DX										
0–19 Years	6	17.3	152	6	7	20	39	>99	>99	>99
20–34	32	10.5	60	3	6	8	13	17	38	38
35–49	120	12.5	140	6	7	8	14	22	52	57
50–64	164	10.8	90	5	6	8	11	19	34	55
65+	392	13.1	76	6	7	10	17	23	29	55
TOTAL SINGLE DX	33	7.4	16	3	5	6	9	15	15	18
MULTIPLE DX	714	12.3	94	5	7	8	15	23	33	57
TOTAL										
0–19 Years	6	17.3	152	6	7	20	39	>99	>99	>99
20–34	36	9.9	56	3	6	8	13	16	21	38
35–49	130	12.3	136	6	7	8	13	22	52	57
50–64	175	10.8	88	5	6	8	11	18	33	55
65+	400	13.0	76	6	7	10	17	23	29	55
GRAND TOTAL	747	12.1	93	5	7	8	15	23	32	57

43.99: TOTAL GASTRECTOMY NEC. Formerly included in operation group(s) 603.

Type of Patients	Observed Patients	Avg. Stay	Vari-ance	10th	25th	50th	75th	90th	95th	99th
1. SINGLE DX										
0–19 Years	0									
20–34	1	4.0	0	4	4	4	4	4	4	4
35–49	6	9.2	4	8	9	9	9	9	16	16
50–64	9	8.8	4	8	8	8	8	11	15	16
65+	3	10.8	<1	10	10	11	11	12	12	12
2. MULTIPLE DX										
0–19 Years	4	17.7	449	3	3	13	16	56	56	56
20–34	15	17.7	64	9	13	15	23	28	35	42
35–49	149	13.8	101	7	9	9	14	35	35	55
50–64	384	13.1	53	8	9	11	14	21	27	43
65+	572	14.7	72	8	9	12	17	24	30	48
TOTAL SINGLE DX	19	8.9	5	8	8	9	9	11	15	16
MULTIPLE DX	1124	14.0	71	8	9	11	15	24	32	48
TOTAL										
0–19 Years	4	17.7	449	3	3	13	16	56	56	56
20–34	16	16.8	72	7	13	15	23	28	30	42
35–49	155	13.5	95	7	9	9	14	35	35	55
50–64	393	12.9	51	8	9	11	14	21	26	43
65+	575	14.7	72	8	9	12	17	23	30	48
GRAND TOTAL	1143	13.8	70	8	9	11	15	24	32	48

43.9: TOTAL GASTRECTOMY. Formerly included in operation group(s) 603.

Type of Patients	Observed Patients	Avg. Stay	Vari-ance	10th	25th	50th	75th	90th	95th	99th
1. SINGLE DX										
0–19 Years	0									
20–34	1	4.0	0	4	4	4	4	4	4	4
35–49	6	9.2	4	8	8	8	8	11	15	16
50–64	9	8.8	4	8	8	8	8	11	15	16
65+	3	10.8	<1	10	10	11	11	12	12	12
2. MULTIPLE DX										
0–19 Years	5	23.1	472	3	3	13	44	56	56	56
20–34	15	17.7	64	9	13	15	23	28	35	42
35–49	154	13.7	100	7	9	9	14	35	35	55
50–64	394	13.0	52	8	9	11	14	21	27	43
65+	595	14.7	71	8	9	12	18	24	30	48
TOTAL SINGLE DX	19	8.9	5	8	8	9	9	11	15	16
MULTIPLE DX	1163	14.0	71	8	9	11	16	24	32	48
TOTAL										
0–19 Years	5	23.1	472	3	3	13	44	56	56	56
20–34	16	16.8	72	7	13	15	23	28	30	42
35–49	160	13.4	94	7	9	9	14	35	35	55
50–64	403	12.9	51	8	9	11	14	21	26	43
65+	598	14.7	71	8	9	12	18	24	30	48
GRAND TOTAL	1182	13.8	70	8	9	11	15	24	32	48

44.0: VAGOTOMY. Formerly included in operation group(s) 604.

Type of Patients	Observed Patients	Avg. Stay	Vari-ance	10th	25th	50th	75th	90th	95th	99th
1. SINGLE DX										
0–19 Years	1	4.0	0	4	4	4	4	4	4	4
20–34	9	6.0	3	4	4	6	8	8	9	9
35–49	23	6.0	9	4	5	5	7	7	10	18
50–64	21	7.5	7	5	6	7	8	11	13	17
65+	2	9.3	7	7	7	11	11	11	11	11
2. MULTIPLE DX										
0–19 Years	9	14.6	192	3	7	10	19	31	54	54
20–34	79	7.7	57	3	5	6	7	14	19	48
35–49	219	9.8	46	4	5	7	13	18	21	37
50–64	200	11.4	76	5	6	9	13	21	30	44
65+	314	13.7	77	7	8	10	16	24	35	50
TOTAL SINGLE DX	56	6.5	8	4	5	6	7	9	13	18
MULTIPLE DX	821	10.9	69	4	6	8	14	20	30	44
TOTAL										
0–19 Years	10	13.8	185	3	4	10	14	31	54	54
20–34	88	7.6	55	3	5	6	7	14	19	42
35–49	242	9.4	44	4	5	7	12	18	21	37
50–64	221	11.1	71	5	6	8	12	20	30	42
65+	316	13.7	77	7	8	10	16	24	35	50
GRAND TOTAL	877	10.7	67	4	6	8	13	20	29	43

United States, October 1995–September 1996 Data, by Operation

44.01: TRUNCAL VAGOTOMY. Formerly included in operation group(s) 604.

Type of Patients	Observed Patients	Avg. Stay	Variance	10th	25th	50th	75th	90th	95th	99th
1. SINGLE DX										
0–19 Years	0									
20–34	4	4.7	<1	4	4	4	5	6	6	6
35–49	11	6.4	13	5	5	5	6	10	18	18
50–64	8	7.6	6	5	7	7	7	11	14	17
65+	2	9.3	7	7	7	11	11	11	11	11
2. MULTIPLE DX										
0–19 Years	6	8.0	12	3	4	10	10	10	14	14
20–34	32	12.9	188	4	5	8	18	19	42	77
35–49	130	10.0	41	4	6	8	13	18	19	38
50–64	121	12.4	94	5	7	9	16	30	30	44
65+	194	12.5	51	7	8	10	15	21	27	45
TOTAL SINGLE DX	25	6.7	10	4	5	6	7	10	17	18
MULTIPLE DX	483	11.8	70	5	7	9	15	20	30	44
TOTAL										
0–19 Years	6	8.0	12	3	4	10	10	10	14	14
20–34	36	12.0	175	4	5	7	18	19	42	77
35–49	141	9.6	40	4	5	8	12	18	19	34
50–64	129	12.1	90	5	7	9	15	30	30	44
65+	196	12.5	51	7	8	10	15	21	27	45
GRAND TOTAL	508	11.5	68	5	7	9	14	20	30	43

44.13: GASTROSCOPY NEC. Formerly included in operation group(s) 598.

Type of Patients	Observed Patients	Avg. Stay	Variance	10th	25th	50th	75th	90th	95th	99th
1. SINGLE DX										
0–19 Years	20	1.3	<1	1	1	1	2	2	3	3
20–34	6	2.7	3	1	1	2	3	6	6	6
35–49	11	2.4		1	1	2	3	4	4	4
50–64	6	13.7	507	1	1	2	15	56	56	56
65+	9	13.8	217	3	3	3	23	47	47	47
2. MULTIPLE DX										
0–19 Years	53	5.5	29	1	2	4	7	9	16	33
20–34	86	4.9	17	1	2	4	7	9	14	22
35–49	187	5.4	11	2	3	5	6	10	14	18
50–64	253	4.9	20	2	3	4	6	10	11	21
65+	669	7.5	56	2	3	5	9	15	18	36
TOTAL SINGLE DX	52	4.5	88	1	1	2	3	6	23	56
MULTIPLE DX	1248	6.2	37	1	3	5	7	12	17	28
TOTAL										
0–19 Years	73	4.7	26	1	1	4	6	7	15	33
20–34	92	4.7	16	1	2	5	6	9	14	22
35–49	198	5.3	11	2	3	5	6	10	14	18
50–64	259	5.0	24	2	3	5	6	10	13	21
65+	678	7.6	58	2	3	5	9	15	19	40
GRAND TOTAL	1300	6.2	39	1	3	5	7	12	18	31

44.1: GASTRIC DXTIC PX. Formerly included in operation group(s) 598, 601, 606, 631.

Type of Patients	Observed Patients	Avg. Stay	Variance	10th	25th	50th	75th	90th	95th	99th
1. SINGLE DX										
0–19 Years	29	1.7	<1	1	1	1	2	3	4	5
20–34	10	2.5	2	1	2	2	3	5	6	6
35–49	13	2.1	1	1	1	2	4	5	4	4
50–64	12	8.1	176	1	1	4	10	15	56	56
65+	13	9.8	169	1	1	3	20	23	47	47
2. MULTIPLE DX										
0–19 Years	89	4.8	22	1	2	4	6	9	15	26
20–34	142	4.8	24	1	1	3	7	11	12	22
35–49	368	5.7	20	2	3	5	7	14	14	22
50–64	506	5.3	18	2	3	5	7	11	14	21
65+	1339	7.3	46	2	3	5	9	15	18	32
TOTAL SINGLE DX	77	4.0	59	1	1	2	3	6	20	47
MULTIPLE DX	2444	6.2	33	2	3	5	8	13	17	27
TOTAL										
0–19 Years	118	4.2	20	1	1	3	6	8	15	26
20–34	152	4.7	23	1	1	3	6	11	12	22
35–49	381	5.7	20	2	3	5	7	14	14	22
50–64	518	5.3	19	2	3	4	7	11	14	21
65+	1352	7.3	47	2	3	5	9	15	19	32
GRAND TOTAL	2521	6.2	33	2	3	5	8	12	17	27

44.14: CLSD (ENDO) GASTRIC BX. Formerly included in operation group(s) 601.

Type of Patients	Observed Patients	Avg. Stay	Variance	10th	25th	50th	75th	90th	95th	99th
1. SINGLE DX										
0–19 Years	6	2.7	1	1	2	2	4	4	4	4
20–34	4	2.2	1	1	1	2	4	4	4	4
35–49	5	1.0	0	1	1	1	1	1	1	1
50–64	5	5.3	15	2	2	4	10	10	10	10
65+	4	2.3	2	1	1	3	3	4	4	4
2. MULTIPLE DX										
0–19 Years	19	2.3	2	1	1	2	3	4	4	7
20–34	51	4.0	11	1	1	3	6	11	11	11
35–49	159	5.7	23	2	3	4	7	14	14	22
50–64	213	5.6	15	2	3	4	7	11	14	23
65+	590	6.6	32	2	3	5	8	13	18	28
TOTAL SINGLE DX	21	3.2	7	1	1	2	4	10	10	10
MULTIPLE DX	1032	5.8	24	2	3	4	7	12	14	25
TOTAL										
0–19 Years	25	2.4	2	1	1	2	3	4	4	7
20–34	55	3.9	11	1	1	3	6	11	11	11
35–49	161	5.6	23	2	3	4	7	14	14	22
50–64	218	5.6	15	2	3	4	7	11	14	23
65+	594	6.5	32	2	3	5	8	12	18	28
GRAND TOTAL	1053	5.8	24	2	3	4	7	12	14	25

Length of Stay by Diagnosis and Operation, United States, 1997

United States, October 1995–September 1996 Data, by Operation

44.2: PYLOROPLASTY. Formerly included in operation group(s) 604.

Type of Patients	Observed Patients	Avg. Stay	Vari-ance	10th	25th	50th	75th	90th	95th	99th
1. SINGLE DX										
0–19 Years	19	2.4	3	1	2	2	5	5	5	9
20–34	6	4.6	5	1	4	5	7	7	7	7
35–49	11	5.3	2	4	5	5	5	8	8	8
50–64	8	3.8	3	3	3	3	4	7	7	8
65+	6	9.8	56	4	6	7	12	27	27	27
2. MULTIPLE DX										
0–19 Years	68	9.5	84	4	4	5	12	22	32	42
20–34	54	7.4	29	3	4	7	9	11	16	38
35–49	136	10.5	63	3	6	8	18	18	21	34
50–64	190	9.2	61	2	5	7	12	15	22	51
65+	407	10.0	49	3	6	8	13	19	25	35
TOTAL SINGLE DX	50	4.1	9	1	2	3	5	7	8	12
MULTIPLE DX	855	9.7	56	3	5	8	12	18	24	39
TOTAL										
0–19 Years	87	8.3	77	2	4	4	9	20	31	42
20–34	60	7.2	28	3	4	7	8	11	16	38
35–49	147	10.2	61	3	6	8	18	18	20	28
50–64	198	8.9	59	2	5	7	11	15	21	51
65+	413	10.0	49	3	6	8	13	19	25	35
GRAND TOTAL	905	9.4	55	3	5	7	12	18	24	39

44.29: OTHER PYLOROPLASTY. Formerly included in operation group(s) 604.

Type of Patients	Observed Patients	Avg. Stay	Vari-ance	10th	25th	50th	75th	90th	95th	99th
1. SINGLE DX										
0–19 Years	17	2.4	3	1	2	2	3	5	5	9
20–34	4	6.1	1	5	5	7	7	7	7	7
35–49	9	5.4	1	5	5	5	5	8	8	8
50–64	6	4.0	3	3	3	3	5	7	7	8
65+	5	10.6	59	6	6	7	12	27	27	27
2. MULTIPLE DX										
0–19 Years	63	9.8	85	4	4	5	12	22	32	42
20–34	38	8.2	29	4	6	7	9	13	16	38
35–49	81	12.4	69	6	7	9	18	18	23	34
50–64	119	11.6	69	6	6	9	13	21	26	51
65+	230	12.4	48	6	8	11	14	22	28	36
TOTAL SINGLE DX	41	4.2	9	2	2	3	5	7	8	12
MULTIPLE DX	531	11.6	62	5	7	9	14	20	26	43
TOTAL										
0–19 Years	80	8.5	79	2	4	4	11	22	31	42
20–34	42	8.1	28	4	6	7	9	13	16	38
35–49	90	11.9	68	5	7	9	18	18	22	34
50–64	125	10.8	68	5	6	9	13	20	26	51
65+	235	12.4	49	6	8	11	14	22	28	36
GRAND TOTAL	572	11.1	61	4	6	9	14	20	26	43

44.3: GASTROENTEROSTOMY. Formerly included in operation group(s) 606.

Type of Patients	Observed Patients	Avg. Stay	Vari-ance	10th	25th	50th	75th	90th	95th	99th
1. SINGLE DX										
0–19 Years	7	4.8	<1	4	5	5	5	5	5	6
20–34	56	4.6	1	3	4	5	5	5	7	8
35–49	46	4.4	2	3	4	4	5	5	7	10
50–64	15	6.7	5	5	5	6	8	8	11	13
65+	6	7.0	21	4	4	4	8	9	21	21
2. MULTIPLE DX										
0–19 Years	54	10.3	278	4	4	4	8	19	47	96
20–34	567	5.6	27	4	4	5	5	7	9	23
35–49	968	6.6	33	4	4	5	6	10	19	31
50–64	581	9.0	70	4	5	6	10	17	24	43
65+	787	17.5	115	7	9	14	22	32	36	57
TOTAL SINGLE DX	130	5.2	4	3	4	5	6	8	8	13
MULTIPLE DX	2957	9.3	84	4	5	5	10	20	28	47
TOTAL										
0–19 Years	61	9.8	252	4	4	5	6	19	39	83
20–34	623	5.5	24	4	4	5	5	7	9	23
35–49	1014	6.5	31	4	4	5	6	10	19	31
50–64	596	8.9	66	4	5	6	9	16	23	43
65+	793	17.3	116	7	9	14	22	32	36	57
GRAND TOTAL	3087	9.0	80	4	4	5	9	20	27	45

44.31: HIGH GASTRIC BYPASS. Formerly included in operation group(s) 606.

Type of Patients	Observed Patients	Avg. Stay	Vari-ance	10th	25th	50th	75th	90th	95th	99th
1. SINGLE DX										
0–19 Years	4	4.0	0	4	4	4	4	4	4	4
20–34	23	4.5	<1	3	4	5	5	5	5	7
35–49	20	4.0	<1	3	4	4	4	5	5	5
50–64	6	5.5	<1	5	5	5	6	6	6	6
65+	0									
2. MULTIPLE DX										
0–19 Years	12	4.5	2	4	4	4	5	5	5	11
20–34	258	4.9	4	4	4	5	5	6	7	13
35–49	429	5.4	14	4	4	5	5	7	9	16
50–64	148	5.8	12	4	4	5	6	8	9	16
65+	14	6.3	22	3	4	5	6	11	21	21
TOTAL SINGLE DX	53	4.6	<1	3	4	5	5	6	6	7
MULTIPLE DX	861	5.3	10	4	4	5	5	7	8	14
TOTAL										
0–19 Years	16	4.5	2	4	4	5	5	5	5	11
20–34	281	4.9	4	4	4	5	5	6	7	10
35–49	449	5.3	14	4	5	5	5	7	9	16
50–64	154	5.8	10	4	5	5	6	8	9	13
65+	14	6.3	22	3	4	5	6	11	21	21
GRAND TOTAL	914	5.2	9	4	4	5	5	7	8	14

Length of Stay by Diagnosis and Operation, United States, 1997

United States, October 1995–September 1996 Data, by Operation

44.39: GASTROENTEROSTOMY NEC. Formerly included in operation group(s) 606.

Type of Patients	Observed Patients	Avg. Stay	Vari-ance	10th	25th	50th	75th	90th	95th	99th
1. SINGLE DX										
0–19 Years	3	5.0	<1	5	5	5	5	5	5	6
20–34	33	4.7	1	3	4	4	5	7	7	8
35–49	26	5.1	3	3	4	5	5	7	7	10
50–64	9	8.0	7	4	8	8	8	11	13	16
65+	6	7.0	21	4	4	4	8	9	21	21
2. MULTIPLE DX										
0–19 Years	42	16.2	488	3	4	7	15	47	82	96
20–34	309	6.5	53	3	4	5	6	9	23	33
35–49	539	7.8	48	4	5	5	8	19	21	34
50–64	433	10.0	84	4	5	7	12	20	26	50
65+	773	17.6	115	7	9	15	22	32	36	57
TOTAL SINGLE DX	77	5.8	6	4	4	5	8	8	10	16
MULTIPLE DX	2096	11.5	112	4	5	7	14	24	32	54
TOTAL										
0–19 Years	45	14.5	428	4	4	6	12	28	68	96
20–34	342	6.3	47	3	4	5	6	8	18	31
35–49	565	7.7	47	4	5	5	7	19	21	34
50–64	442	9.9	80	4	5	7	11	20	26	50
65+	779	17.4	115	7	9	14	22	32	36	57
GRAND TOTAL	2173	11.2	108	4	5	7	14	24	31	53

44.41: SUT GASTRIC ULCER SITE. Formerly included in operation group(s) 606.

Type of Patients	Observed Patients	Avg. Stay	Vari-ance	10th	25th	50th	75th	90th	95th	99th
1. SINGLE DX										
0–19 Years	2	4.6	1	4	4	4	6	6	6	6
20–34	20	5.8	1	4	6	6	6	6	6	6
35–49	30	6.6	4	4	6	6	8	8	8	9
50–64	15	6.2	3	4	5	6	7	9	9	15
65+	4	5.5	3	4	4	5	8	8	8	8
2. MULTIPLE DX										
0–19 Years	17	16.5	633	7	8	8	8	77	92	92
20–34	54	9.0	36	4	8	7	8	19	26	26
35–49	168	9.7	65	5	6	7	9	16	25	41
50–64	199	9.7	63	4	6	7	12	17	22	45
65+	468	12.7	75	6	7	10	15	22	28	43
TOTAL SINGLE DX	71	6.2	3	4	5	6	7	8	9	11
MULTIPLE DX	906	11.1	86	5	6	8	13	21	26	49
TOTAL										
0–19 Years	19	15.9	609	6	8	8	8	15	92	92
20–34	74	8.5	32	4	6	7	9	17	26	26
35–49	198	9.2	56	5	6	7	9	15	25	41
50–64	214	9.5	61	4	6	7	12	17	22	45
65+	472	12.6	75	6	7	10	15	22	28	43
GRAND TOTAL	977	10.8	82	5	6	8	12	20	26	45

44.4: CNTRL PEPTIC ULCER HEMOR. Formerly included in operation group(s) 605, 606.

Type of Patients	Observed Patients	Avg. Stay	Vari-ance	10th	25th	50th	75th	90th	95th	99th
1. SINGLE DX										
0–19 Years	10	6.6	5	4	6	6	7	12	12	12
20–34	78	6.6	10	2	5	6	10	10	10	10
35–49	116	5.0	5	2	3	5	6	8	8	8
50–64	80	4.4	5	2	3	4	6	8	8	9
65+	43	5.2	16	2	2	5	6	8	14	21
2. MULTIPLE DX										
0–19 Years	72	11.1	309	3	4	7	8	21	49	92
20–34	468	6.5	34	2	3	5	7	12	17	28
35–49	1519	5.9	38	2	3	4	7	10	13	40
50–64	2253	7.1	81	3	3	5	7	13	22	54
65+	7006	7.5	54	2	3	5	9	15	21	41
TOTAL SINGLE DX	327	5.5	8	2	3	6	7	10	10	12
MULTIPLE DX	11318	7.1	59	2	3	5	8	14	20	47
TOTAL										
0–19 Years	82	10.8	286	3	4	7	8	15	49	92
20–34	546	6.5	28	3	3	5	9	10	17	28
35–49	1635	5.8	36	2	3	4	7	10	13	40
50–64	2333	7.0	79	3	3	5	7	13	22	54
65+	7049	7.5	54	2	3	5	9	15	21	41
GRAND TOTAL	11645	7.1	58	2	3	5	8	13	20	47

44.42: SUT DUODENAL ULCER SITE. Formerly included in operation group(s) 606.

Type of Patients	Observed Patients	Avg. Stay	Vari-ance	10th	25th	50th	75th	90th	95th	99th
1. SINGLE DX										
0–19 Years	6	7.4	4	6	6	7	7	12	12	12
20–34	40	8.1	6	5	6	10	10	10	10	10
35–49	60	5.5	2	3	4	6	6	7	8	10
50–64	31	5.2	5	3	3	5	7	8	8	12
65+	9	8.1	26	5	5	6	7	19	21	21
2. MULTIPLE DX										
0–19 Years	26	11.1	142	4	5	7	11	21	49	56
20–34	124	9.5	50	4	6	7	10	17	17	48
35–49	354	9.1	54	5	6	9	9	13	24	45
50–64	337	17.8	279	5	7	10	19	54	54	54
65+	991	14.8	136	6	8	10	17	30	47	56
TOTAL SINGLE DX	146	6.8	7	3	5	6	10	10	10	12
MULTIPLE DX	1832	13.7	154	5	7	9	15	29	47	54
TOTAL										
0–19 Years	32	10.5	123	5	5	7	11	21	49	56
20–34	164	8.9	32	5	6	7	10	12	17	48
35–49	414	8.6	48	6	6	9	9	13	20	45
50–64	368	16.9	269	5	8	9	18	54	54	54
65+	1000	14.8	136	6	8	10	17	30	47	56
GRAND TOTAL	1978	13.0	143	5	6	9	14	27	47	54

Length of Stay by Diagnosis and Operation, United States, 1997

United States, October 1995–September 1996 Data, by Operation

44.43: ENDO CNTRL GASTRIC BLEED. Formerly included in operation group(s) 605.

Type of Patients	Observed Patients	Avg. Stay	Variance	Percentiles						
				10th	25th	50th	75th	90th	95th	99th
1. SINGLE DX										
0–19 Years	2	6.1	9	3	3	8	8	8	8	8
20–34	17	2.3	1	2	2	2	3	5	5	7
35–49	26	2.5	2	1	1	2	3	5	5	5
50–64	33	2.7	1	2	2	2	3	4	5	6
65+	30	3.8	7	2	2	3	5	6	9	14
2. MULTIPLE DX										
0–19 Years	27	4.4	22	2	3	3	4	6	23	23
20–34	282	3.9	11	2	2	3	4	6	10	15
35–49	977	4.4	23	2	2	3	5	7	10	28
50–64	1695	4.6	17	2	3	4	6	8	10	26
65+	5480	5.9	26	2	3	4	7	11	15	26
TOTAL SINGLE DX	108	2.7	3	1	2	2	3	5	6	9
MULTIPLE DX	8461	5.3	24	2	3	4	6	10	14	26
TOTAL										
0–19 Years	29	4.5	21	2	3	3	4	8	11	23
20–34	299	3.7	10	2	2	3	4	6	10	15
35–49	1003	4.3	23	2	2	3	5	7	10	28
50–64	1728	4.6	17	2	3	4	5	7	10	26
65+	5510	5.9	26	2	3	4	7	11	15	26
GRAND TOTAL	8569	5.3	23	2	3	4	6	10	13	26

44.6: OTHER GASTRIC REPAIR. Formerly included in operation group(s) 606.

Type of Patients	Observed Patients	Avg. Stay	Variance	Percentiles						
				10th	25th	50th	75th	90th	95th	99th
1. SINGLE DX										
0–19 Years	296	3.4	5	1	2	3	4	6	8	12
20–34	277	2.4	2	1	1	2	3	4	5	7
35–49	447	2.4	2	1	1	2	3	4	5	7
50–64	178	2.7	2	1	2	2	3	5	6	7
65+	44	2.5	3	1	1	2	4	5	6	8
2. MULTIPLE DX										
0–19 Years	2412	12.1	199	2	4	7	15	30	48	>99
20–34	1060	4.5	25	2	2	3	5	8	12	30
35–49	2349	4.2	22	1	2	3	5	7	10	26
50–64	1780	4.7	38	2	2	3	5	8	11	39
65+	1411	8.2	72	2	3	5	10	18	26	43
TOTAL SINGLE DX	1242	2.7	3	1	2	2	3	5	6	8
MULTIPLE DX	9012	6.9	89	2	2	4	7	15	26	57
TOTAL										
0–19 Years	2708	11.1	185	2	4	6	13	28	45	>99
20–34	1337	4.0	20	1	2	3	4	7	10	28
35–49	2796	3.9	19	1	2	3	4	7	10	26
50–64	1958	4.5	36	1	2	3	5	8	10	38
65+	1455	7.9	70	2	3	5	9	17	25	43
GRAND TOTAL	10254	6.3	79	1	2	4	6	14	23	55

44.5: REVISION GASTRIC ANAST. Formerly included in operation group(s) 606.

Type of Patients	Observed Patients	Avg. Stay	Variance	Percentiles						
				10th	25th	50th	75th	90th	95th	99th
1. SINGLE DX										
0–19 Years	0									
20–34	5	7.0	4	6	6	6	9	9	9	9
35–49	4	4.6	1	4	4	4	4	7	7	7
50–64	8	11.4	37	5	8	9	15	15	26	26
65+	1	8.0	0	8	8	8	8	8	8	8
2. MULTIPLE DX										
0–19 Years	16	13.7	118	7	8	8	14	42	42	42
20–34	39	8.9	94	3	4	6	8	16	37	39
35–49	204	9.3	48	4	5	7	11	18	23	37
50–64	169	9.9	50	5	6	7	11	17	25	39
65+	92	19.3	157	8	12	15	24	34	44	69
TOTAL SINGLE DX	18	7.4	16	4	4	6	9	10	15	26
MULTIPLE DX	520	10.8	78	4	6	8	13	21	29	44
TOTAL										
0–19 Years	16	13.7	118	7	8	8	14	42	42	42
20–34	44	8.5	76	3	4	6	9	12	37	39
35–49	208	9.2	48	4	5	7	11	17	23	37
50–64	177	9.9	49	5	6	7	11	17	25	39
65+	93	19.3	157	8	12	15	24	34	44	69
GRAND TOTAL	538	10.7	76	4	6	8	13	20	29	43

44.63: CLOSE STOM FISTULA NEC. Formerly included in operation group(s) 606.

Type of Patients	Observed Patients	Avg. Stay	Variance	Percentiles						
				10th	25th	50th	75th	90th	95th	99th
1. SINGLE DX										
0–19 Years	30	1.3	<1	1	1	1	1	2	3	4
20–34	0									
35–49	3	8.0	14	5	5	5	12	12	12	12
50–64	2	6.4	26	2	2	2	11	11	11	11
65+	1	10.0	0	10	10	10	10	10	10	10
2. MULTIPLE DX										
0–19 Years	107	4.3	81	1	1	2	3	10	14	48
20–34	8	6.0	24	1	1	5	9	16	16	16
35–49	25	13.1	105	4	4	7	26	26	26	37
50–64	28	26.5	262	5	10	35	39	39	39	72
65+	108	14.2	148	3	6	10	19	36	43	47
TOTAL SINGLE DX	36	2.1	7	1	1	1	2	5	10	12
MULTIPLE DX	276	11.4	166	1	2	7	16	32	39	48
TOTAL										
0–19 Years	137	3.6	64	1	1	2	2	6	13	48
20–34	8	6.0	24	1	1	5	9	16	16	16
35–49	28	12.9	103	4	4	7	26	26	26	37
50–64	30	25.6	269	4	9	32	39	39	39	72
65+	109	14.1	147	3	6	10	19	36	43	47
GRAND TOTAL	312	10.5	157	1	2	5	13	26	39	48

Length of Stay by Diagnosis and Operation, United States, 1997

United States, October 1995–September 1996 Data, by Operation

44.66: CREAT EG SPHINCT COMPET. Formerly included in operation group(s) 606.

Type of Patients	Observed Patients	Avg. Stay	Variance	Percentiles						
				10th	25th	50th	75th	90th	95th	99th
1. SINGLE DX										
0–19 Years	237	3.7	5	1	2	3	5	7	8	12
20–34	246	2.3	1	1	2	3	5	7	8	6
35–49	406	2.2	2	1	2	3	5	7	8	7
50–64	167	2.5	2	1	2	2	3	4	5	6
65+	41	2.4	3	1	2	2	3	5	5	8
2. MULTIPLE DX										
0–19 Years	2062	12.9	211	3	5	7	16	33	50	>99
20–34	732	3.7	17	1	2	2	4	6	8	27
35–49	1926	3.6	15	1	2	3	4	6	8	25
50–64	1561	3.9	19	1	2	3	5	7	9	23
65+	1037	5.9	37	2	3	4	7	11	18	34
TOTAL SINGLE DX	1097	2.6	3	1	2	2	3	4	6	8
MULTIPLE DX	7318	6.5	88	2	2	3	6	14	24	59
TOTAL										
0–19 Years	2299	11.9	197	3	4	7	14	29	47	>99
20–34	978	3.3	13	1	2	2	3	6	7	25
35–49	2332	3.3	13	1	2	3	4	6	7	20
50–64	1728	3.8	18	1	2	3	5	7	9	22
65+	1078	5.6	35	2	2	4	6	11	17	27
GRAND TOTAL	8415	5.9	77	1	2	3	6	12	22	56

44.69: GASTRIC REPAIR NEC. Formerly included in operation group(s) 606.

Type of Patients	Observed Patients	Avg. Stay	Variance	Percentiles						
				10th	25th	50th	75th	90th	95th	99th
1. SINGLE DX										
0–19 Years	10	2.9	2	1	2	3	3	3	6	8
20–34	26	4.4	1	3	4	5	5	6	6	8
35–49	31	4.3	<1	3	4	4	5	5	7	7
50–64	7	5.2	2	3	4	6	6	7	7	7
65+	2	5.5	4	4	4	4	7	7	7	7
2. MULTIPLE DX										
0–19 Years	100	7.6	80	1	2	4	9	20	31	>99
20–34	193	5.2	23	3	4	4	5	8	11	42
35–49	292	6.0	17	3	4	5	7	10	12	21
50–64	119	7.2	61	3	4	5	8	13	20	87
65+	104	13.2	139	4	6	10	14	27	34	83
TOTAL SINGLE DX	76	4.3	2	3	3	4	5	6	6	8
MULTIPLE DX	808	7.3	58	3	4	5	8	13	20	42
TOTAL										
0–19 Years	110	7.2	75	1	2	4	9	20	31	>99
20–34	219	5.1	20	3	4	4	5	7	10	42
35–49	323	5.9	15	3	4	5	8	10	12	20
50–64	126	7.1	57	3	4	5	8	12	18	56
65+	106	13.1	138	4	6	10	14	27	34	83
GRAND TOTAL	884	7.1	53	3	4	5	8	13	20	42

44.9: OTHER STOMACH OPERATIONS. Formerly included in operation group(s) 606.

Type of Patients	Observed Patients	Avg. Stay	Variance	Percentiles						
				10th	25th	50th	75th	90th	95th	99th
1. SINGLE DX										
0–19 Years	2	3.2	<1	3	3	3	3	3	5	5
20–34	3	4.3	<1	4	4	4	5	5	5	5
35–49	3	6.4	2	6	5	7	7	7	7	7
50–64	1	5.0	0	5	5	5	5	5	5	5
65+	0									
2. MULTIPLE DX										
0–19 Years	12	15.6	140	7	12	12	12	29	54	54
20–34	5	4.0	4	1	3	4	4	7	7	7
35–49	31	15.8	247	3	5	11	20	59	59	>99
50–64	15	10.1	29	7	7	8	9	17	17	28
65+	38	12.9	56	5	8	11	18	19	25	37
TOTAL SINGLE DX	8	4.8	3	3	3	5	7	7	7	7
MULTIPLE DX	101	13.7	140	4	7	11	18	23	37	59
TOTAL										
0–19 Years	14	11.6	129	3	3	12	12	29	29	54
20–34	7	4.2	2	3	4	4	5	5	7	7
35–49	34	14.9	231	3	5	11	20	25	59	>99
50–64	16	9.8	29	6	7	7	9	17	17	28
65+	38	12.9	56	5	8	11	18	19	25	37
GRAND TOTAL	109	12.7	133	3	5	9	16	22	37	59

45.0: ENTEROTOMY. Formerly included in operation group(s) 610.

Type of Patients	Observed Patients	Avg. Stay	Variance	Percentiles						
				10th	25th	50th	75th	90th	95th	99th
1. SINGLE DX										
0–19 Years	9	10.3	26	3	5	13	14	16	16	16
20–34	4	7.1	13	2	6	6	11	11	11	11
35–49	5	2.4	<1	2	2	2	3	4	4	4
50–64	7	4.3	2	2	2	5	5	5	5	9
65+	7	2.9	3	2	2	2	3	4	8	8
2. MULTIPLE DX										
0–19 Years	37	19.1	310	5	7	12	22	52	58	73
20–34	47	8.4	44	5	5	7	8	12	25	46
35–49	71	9.2	42	4	5	7	11	17	18	38
50–64	113	9.6	66	3	5	7	12	15	19	58
65+	257	11.1	49	4	7	10	14	18	24	39
TOTAL SINGLE DX	32	4.7	10	2	2	5	5	8	13	16
MULTIPLE DX	525	10.8	75	4	6	9	13	18	25	53
TOTAL										
0–19 Years	46	17.7	274	5	6	12	19	50	58	73
20–34	51	8.3	42	4	5	7	9	12	25	46
35–49	76	8.4	42	3	5	7	10	16	18	38
50–64	120	8.6	58	3	5	6	11	15	19	58
65+	264	10.8	49	4	6	10	13	18	24	39
GRAND TOTAL	557	10.2	72	4	5	8	12	17	24	52

Length of Stay by Diagnosis and Operation, United States, 1997

United States, October 1995–September 1996 Data, by Operation

45.1: SMALL BOWEL DXTIC PX. Formerly included in operation group(s) 607, 618, 631.

Type of Patients	Observed Patients	Avg. Stay	Vari-ance	10th	25th	50th	75th	90th	95th	99th
1. SINGLE DX										
0–19 Years	762	2.3	7	1	1	1	3	5	6	12
20–34	700	3.3	5	1	2	3	5	6	7	10
35–49	804	2.8	4	1	2	2	4	5	7	11
50–64	475	2.8	5	1	2	2	3	5	7	11
65+	439	4.5	15	2	2	3	5	9	14	17
2. MULTIPLE DX										
0–19 Years	4308	5.6	52	1	2	3	6	11	18	37
20–34	10209	4.7	22	1	2	3	6	10	13	23
35–49	23945	4.9	23	2	2	3	6	9	13	25
50–64	29768	5.8	36	2	3	4	7	11	15	40
65+	84428	6.4	32	2	3	5	8	12	16	28
TOTAL SINGLE DX	3180	3.0	7	1	1	2	4	6	7	13
MULTIPLE DX	152658	5.9	31	2	3	4	7	11	15	29
TOTAL										
0–19 Years	5070	5.1	47	1	2	3	6	10	16	35
20–34	10909	4.6	21	1	2	3	5	9	13	23
35–49	24749	4.8	22	2	2	3	6	9	13	25
50–64	30243	5.7	36	2	3	4	7	11	15	40
65+	84867	6.4	31	2	3	5	8	12	16	28
GRAND TOTAL	155838	5.8	31	2	3	4	7	11	15	29

45.14: CLSD (ENDO) SM INTEST BX. Formerly included in operation group(s) 607.

Type of Patients	Observed Patients	Avg. Stay	Vari-ance	10th	25th	50th	75th	90th	95th	99th
1. SINGLE DX										
0–19 Years	3	1.4	<1	1	1	1	1	3	3	3
20–34	8	4.7	7	2	3	4	6	6	13	13
35–49	7	4.9	5	1	6	6	6	6	7	7
50–64	2	2.9	2	2	2	2	4	4	4	4
65+	5	6.3	10	2	3	8	10	10	10	10
2. MULTIPLE DX										
0–19 Years	47	8.4	89	2	3	6	13	19	26	>99
20–34	55	6.1	57	1	2	4	8	15	17	51
35–49	92	5.5	17	2	3	4	7	10	15	23
50–64	110	6.4	29	2	3	5	8	13	14	29
65+	199	7.1	28	3	4	5	9	14	18	27
TOTAL SINGLE DX	25	4.8	8	1	2	5	6	8	10	13
MULTIPLE DX	503	6.6	36	2	3	5	8	14	18	27
TOTAL										
0–19 Years	50	8.1	87	2	3	5	13	19	26	>99
20–34	63	5.9	51	1	2	4	8	10	17	51
35–49	99	5.5	16	2	3	5	8	10	15	23
50–64	112	6.3	29	2	3	5	8	13	14	29
65+	204	7.0	28	3	4	5	9	14	18	27
GRAND TOTAL	528	6.6	35	2	3	5	8	13	18	27

45.13: SM BOWEL ENDOSCOPY NEC. Formerly included in operation group(s) 618.

Type of Patients	Observed Patients	Avg. Stay	Vari-ance	10th	25th	50th	75th	90th	95th	99th
1. SINGLE DX										
0–19 Years	228	1.9	3	1	1	1	3	3	5	6
20–34	366	3.8	5	1	2	3	5	6	8	9
35–49	415	2.8	3	1	2	2	4	5	7	9
50–64	244	2.5	4	1	1	2	3	4	6	9
65+	226	4.1	12	1	2	3	5	9	11	20
2. MULTIPLE DX										
0–19 Years	1098	4.5	39	1	2	3	5	9	15	30
20–34	4082	4.6	22	1	2	3	6	9	12	24
35–49	9961	4.9	23	2	2	4	6	9	13	23
50–64	12165	5.6	28	2	3	4	7	11	14	26
65+	34911	6.6	34	2	3	5	8	13	17	30
TOTAL SINGLE DX	1479	3.1	6	1	1	2	4	6	7	11
MULTIPLE DX	62217	5.9	31	2	3	4	7	12	15	28
TOTAL										
0–19 Years	1326	4.1	34	1	1	2	5	8	13	29
20–34	4448	4.5	20	1	2	3	6	9	11	23
35–49	10376	4.9	22	1	2	3	6	9	13	22
50–64	12409	5.5	27	2	3	4	6	11	14	26
65+	35137	6.5	34	2	3	5	8	13	17	30
GRAND TOTAL	63696	5.8	30	2	3	4	7	12	15	28

45.16: EGD WITH CLOSED BIOPSY. Formerly included in operation group(s) 607.

Type of Patients	Observed Patients	Avg. Stay	Vari-ance	10th	25th	50th	75th	90th	95th	99th
1. SINGLE DX										
0–19 Years	527	2.4	8	1	1	2	3	5	7	12
20–34	323	2.6	3	1	2	2	3	4	6	10
35–49	378	2.9	5	1	2	2	4	5	6	13
50–64	221	3.1	7	1	2	2	4	5	7	20
65+	206	4.9	17	2	2	3	5	12	16	17
2. MULTIPLE DX										
0–19 Years	3136	5.9	56	1	2	4	7	12	19	40
20–34	6045	4.8	23	1	2	3	5	10	14	23
35–49	13829	4.8	22	2	2	3	6	9	13	26
50–64	17443	5.9	42	2	3	4	7	11	17	40
65+	49204	6.3	30	2	3	5	8	12	16	27
TOTAL SINGLE DX	1655	2.9	7	1	1	2	3	5	7	15
MULTIPLE DX	89657	5.8	32	2	3	4	7	11	16	30
TOTAL										
0–19 Years	3663	5.4	50	1	2	3	6	11	17	36
20–34	6368	4.7	22	1	2	3	5	10	14	23
35–49	14207	4.8	22	2	2	3	6	9	13	26
50–64	17664	5.9	42	2	3	4	7	11	17	40
65+	49410	6.3	30	2	3	5	8	12	16	27
GRAND TOTAL	91312	5.8	32	2	3	4	7	11	15	30

United States, October 1995–September 1996 Data, by Operation

45.2: LG INTESTINE DXTIC PX. Formerly included in operation group(s) 607, 618, 631.

Type of Patients	Observed Patients	Avg. Stay	Variance	10th	25th	50th	75th	90th	95th	99th
1. SINGLE DX										
0–19 Years	362	4.1	16	1	1	3	6	9	12	18
20–34	546	3.6	8	1	1	3	5	7	9	13
35–49	610	4.8	31	1	2	3	5	8	13	29
50–64	469	3.6	7	1	2	3	5	7	7	12
65+	460	3.4	24	1	1	3	4	6	8	15
2. MULTIPLE DX										
0–19 Years	1224	5.7	49	1	2	4	7	11	16	29
20–34	3728	5.2	18	2	2	4	6	10	13	23
35–49	7095	5.4	29	2	3	4	6	10	14	27
50–64	10181	5.7	27	2	3	4	7	11	14	28
65+	37076	6.6	32	2	3	5	8	12	17	29
TOTAL SINGLE DX	2447	4.0	19	1	2	3	5	7	9	29
MULTIPLE DX	59304	6.2	31	2	3	5	8	12	16	28
TOTAL										
0–19 Years	1586	5.3	42	1	2	4	6	10	15	28
20–34	4274	5.0	20	1	2	4	6	10	13	22
35–49	7705	5.4	29	2	2	4	6	10	14	29
50–64	10650	5.6	26	2	3	4	7	10	14	28
65+	37536	6.6	32	2	3	5	8	12	17	29
GRAND TOTAL	61751	6.1	30	2	3	5	7	11	16	28

45.22: ENDO LG BOWEL THRU STOMA. Formerly included in operation group(s) 631.

Type of Patients	Observed Patients	Avg. Stay	Variance	10th	25th	50th	75th	90th	95th	99th
1. SINGLE DX										
0–19 Years	1	2.0	0	2	2	2	2	2	2	2
20–34	2	6.7	24	1	1	10	10	10	10	10
35–49	0									
50–64	1	3.0	0	3	3	3	3	3	3	3
65+	2	6.4	53	2	2	2	14	14	14	14
2. MULTIPLE DX										
0–19 Years	3	7.4	14	4	4	9	9	11	11	11
20–34	11	6.9	18	3	4	5	8	13	13	20
35–49	34	5.5	12	2	4	4	6	11	14	16
50–64	39	5.0	20	2	4	4	6	11	15	20
65+	236	6.0	26	2	3	5	8	12	14	28
TOTAL SINGLE DX	6	3.5	12	2	2	2	3	10	10	14
MULTIPLE DX	323	5.7	22	2	3	4	7	12	14	22
TOTAL										
0–19 Years	4	2.8	5	2	2	2	2	4	9	11
20–34	13	6.9	18	2	4	5	8	13	13	20
35–49	34	5.5	12	2	4	4	6	11	14	16
50–64	40	5.0	19	2	4	4	5	11	15	20
65+	238	6.0	26	2	3	5	8	12	14	28
GRAND TOTAL	329	5.7	22	2	3	4	7	12	14	22

45.23: COLONOSCOPY. Formerly included in operation group(s) 618.

Type of Patients	Observed Patients	Avg. Stay	Variance	10th	25th	50th	75th	90th	95th	99th
1. SINGLE DX										
0–19 Years	44	2.9	7	1	1	2	4	6	8	12
20–34	114	3.3	4	1	2	3	4	6	6	9
35–49	181	3.5	7	1	2	3	5	7	9	13
50–64	178	2.9	3	1	2	3	3	5	6	10
65+	227	2.9	34	1	1	2	3	5	7	14
2. MULTIPLE DX										
0–19 Years	178	4.6	17	2	3	3	5	9	12	20
20–34	831	5.1	19	2	2	3	5	9	14	22
35–49	2268	5.1	25	2	3	4	6	9	13	32
50–64	4114	5.5	27	2	3	4	7	10	13	28
65+	17391	6.1	26	2	3	5	7	11	15	27
TOTAL SINGLE DX	744	3.2	14	1	1	3	4	6	7	13
MULTIPLE DX	24782	5.8	26	2	3	4	7	11	15	27
TOTAL										
0–19 Years	222	4.4	16	1	2	3	5	8	12	19
20–34	945	4.8	17	1	2	4	6	10	14	21
35–49	2449	4.9	23	2	2	4	6	9	13	30
50–64	4292	5.4	27	2	3	4	7	10	13	28
65+	17618	6.0	26	2	3	5	7	11	15	27
GRAND TOTAL	25526	5.7	26	2	3	4	7	11	15	27

45.24: FLEXIBLE SIGMOIDOSCOPY. Formerly included in operation group(s) 631.

Type of Patients	Observed Patients	Avg. Stay	Variance	10th	25th	50th	75th	90th	95th	99th
1. SINGLE DX										
0–19 Years	46	3.1	9	1	1	2	4	9	9	12
20–34	122	3.9	11	1	2	3	4	7	9	16
35–49	114	7.0	72	1	2	4	6	29	29	29
50–64	90	3.4	17	1	1	3	4	7	7	7
65+	93	3.3	8	1	1	3	4	7	7	15
2. MULTIPLE DX										
0–19 Years	135	5.0	23	1	2	4	7	9	15	23
20–34	702	5.0	22	1	2	4	7	9	11	22
35–49	1234	5.0	29	1	2	4	6	9	12	23
50–64	1697	5.6	31	1	2	4	7	11	13	33
65+	6582	7.0	38	2	3	5	9	13	17	33
TOTAL SINGLE DX	465	4.7	34	1	2	3	5	8	16	29
MULTIPLE DX	10350	6.3	35	2	3	5	8	12	16	30
TOTAL										
0–19 Years	181	4.5	20	1	2	3	6	9	12	19
20–34	824	4.9	20	1	2	4	7	9	11	21
35–49	1348	5.2	35	1	2	4	6	11	13	29
50–64	1787	5.4	30	1	2	4	7	11	13	29
65+	6675	7.0	38	2	3	5	8	13	17	32
GRAND TOTAL	10815	6.2	35	2	3	5	8	12	16	29

Length of Stay by Diagnosis and Operation, United States, 1997

United States, October 1995–September 1996 Data, by Operation

45.25: CLSD (ENDO) LG INTEST BX. Formerly included in operation group(s) 607.

Type of Patients	Observed Patients	Avg. Stay	Vari-ance	Percentiles						
				10th	25th	50th	75th	90th	95th	99th
1. SINGLE DX										
0–19 Years	263	4.5	18	1	1	4	6	9	13	21
20–34	305	3.7	9	1	2	3	5	7	11	13
35–49	312	4.7	23	2	2	4	4	8	11	29
50–64	196	4.1	6	2	2	4	5	7	8	13
65+	137	4.3	15	1	2	3	6	8	9	27
2. MULTIPLE DX										
0–19 Years	882	6.0	59	1	2	4	7	12	18	41
20–34	2177	5.2	22	2	2	4	6	10	12	24
35–49	3541	5.8	32	2	3	4	7	10	12	26
50–64	4304	5.9	25	2	3	5	7	11	15	27
65+	12831	7.1	36	2	3	6	9	13	18	33
TOTAL SINGLE DX	1213	4.2	14	1	2	3	5	8	11	21
MULTIPLE DX	23735	6.4	33	2	3	5	8	12	17	29
TOTAL										
0–19 Years	1145	5.7	50	1	2	4	7	11	16	29
20–34	2482	5.0	20	2	2	4	6	10	12	22
35–49	3853	5.7	31	2	3	4	6	10	16	28
50–64	4500	5.8	24	2	3	5	7	11	14	27
65+	12968	7.1	36	2	3	6	9	13	18	33
GRAND TOTAL	24948	6.3	32	2	3	5	8	12	16	29

45.30: ENDO EXC/DESTR DUOD LES. Formerly included in operation group(s) 607.

Type of Patients	Observed Patients	Avg. Stay	Vari-ance	Percentiles						
				10th	25th	50th	75th	90th	95th	99th
1. SINGLE DX										
0–19 Years	0									
20–34	0									
35–49	3	1.4	1	1	1	1	1	4	4	4
50–64	3	1.4	1	1	1	1	1	4	4	4
65+	0									
2. MULTIPLE DX										
0–19 Years	2	8.1	1	7	7	9	9	9	9	9
20–34	18	3.9	3	2	2	3	6	6	7	7
35–49	46	3.5	12	1	1	2	4	7	9	18
50–64	85	4.3	10	2	2	4	5	8	8	16
65+	270	6.6	30	3	3	5	8	12	18	32
TOTAL SINGLE DX	6	1.4	1	1	1	1	1	4	4	4
MULTIPLE DX	421	5.5	23	2	3	4	7	9	15	32
TOTAL										
0–19 Years	2	8.1	1	7	7	9	9	9	9	9
20–34	18	3.9	3	2	2	3	6	6	7	7
35–49	49	3.4	12	1	1	2	4	6	9	18
50–64	88	4.3	10	2	3	4	5	8	8	16
65+	270	6.6	30	3	3	5	8	12	18	32
GRAND TOTAL	427	5.4	23	2	3	4	7	9	15	32

45.3: LOC EXC/DESTR SMB LES. Formerly included in operation group(s) 607.

Type of Patients	Observed Patients	Avg. Stay	Vari-ance	Percentiles						
				10th	25th	50th	75th	90th	95th	99th
1. SINGLE DX										
0–19 Years	49	3.8	15	1	2	3	5	6	7	21
20–34	19	2.8	2	2	2	2	3	5	6	8
35–49	12	3.5	4	1	2	2	5	6	6	9
50–64	10	5.6	19	2	2	4	8	12	12	12
65+	2	8.7	<1	7	9	9	9	9	9	9
2. MULTIPLE DX										
0–19 Years	151	6.8	63	3	4	5	7	10	18	82
20–34	100	5.9	11	2	4	6	7	9	12	19
35–49	147	6.0	26	2	3	5	7	11	15	29
50–64	204	7.4	41	2	4	5	8	13	27	28
65+	501	8.2	60	3	4	6	9	16	21	46
TOTAL SINGLE DX	92	3.8	12	1	2	3	5	7	9	21
MULTIPLE DX	1103	7.2	47	2	4	5	8	13	20	34
TOTAL										
0–19 Years	200	5.9	51	2	3	5	7	9	17	80
20–34	119	5.3	11	2	3	5	7	8	10	19
35–49	159	5.8	24	2	3	5	7	11	15	29
50–64	214	7.3	41	2	4	5	8	13	27	28
65+	503	8.2	59	3	4	6	9	16	21	46
GRAND TOTAL	1195	6.9	44	2	3	5	8	12	19	33

45.33: LOC EXC SM BOWEL LES NEC. Formerly included in operation group(s) 607.

Type of Patients	Observed Patients	Avg. Stay	Vari-ance	Percentiles						
				10th	25th	50th	75th	90th	95th	99th
1. SINGLE DX										
0–19 Years	42	2.9	2	1	2	3	4	5	5	7
20–34	18	2.7	2	2	2	3	3	4	6	8
35–49	7	3.4	4	2	2	3	4	6	9	9
50–64	1	2.0	0	2	2	2	2	2	2	2
65+	0									
2. MULTIPLE DX										
0–19 Years	125	5.8	35	3	4	5	7	9	11	>99
20–34	69	6.4	13	3	4	6	8	10	12	19
35–49	60	5.9	11	3	3	5	7	11	14	16
50–64	58	7.0	25	4	5	5	7	12	14	28
65+	86	10.4	59	4	7	8	11	20	24	35
TOTAL SINGLE DX	68	2.9	2	1	2	2	4	5	6	8
MULTIPLE DX	398	6.9	31	3	4	6	8	11	16	33
TOTAL										
0–19 Years	167	4.9	27	2	3	4	6	8	9	63
20–34	87	5.5	13	2	3	5	7	9	12	19
35–49	67	5.6	10	2	5	5	7	10	13	16
50–64	59	7.0	25	4	5	5	7	12	14	28
65+	86	10.4	59	4	7	8	11	20	24	35
GRAND TOTAL	466	6.2	29	2	3	5	7	11	14	28

Length of Stay by Diagnosis and Operation, United States, 1997

United States, October 1995–September 1996 Data, by Operation

45.4: LOC DESTR LG BOWEL LES. Formerly included in operation group(s) 607.

Type of Patients	Observed Patients	Avg. Stay	Variance	10th	25th	50th	75th	90th	95th	99th
1. SINGLE DX										
0–19 Years	29	1.5	<1	1	1	1	2	3	3	4
20–34	13	2.3	3	1	2	2	2	4	4	7
35–49	23	2.7	12	1	2	2	2	4	5	30
50–64	41	2.5	6	1	1	1	3	6	6	13
65+	76	4.5	15	1	2	4	6	8	11	24
2. MULTIPLE DX										
0–19 Years	57	5.6	255	1	3	5	5	5	17	80
20–34	140	4.6	17	1	3	3	6	8	11	17
35–49	766	4.6	19	2	2	4	6	8	12	21
50–64	2177	5.2	17	2	3	4	7	9	12	21
65+	9383	6.0	26	2	3	5	7	12	15	26
TOTAL SINGLE DX	182	2.9	9	1	1	2	3	6	7	13
MULTIPLE DX	12523	5.7	25	2	3	4	7	11	14	24
TOTAL										
0–19 Years	86	4.9	212	1	1	1	3	5	15	80
20–34	153	4.3	16	1	2	3	5	7	10	17
35–49	789	4.6	19	2	2	4	6	8	12	21
50–64	2218	5.1	17	2	3	4	7	9	12	21
65+	9459	6.0	26	2	3	5	7	12	15	26
GRAND TOTAL	12705	5.7	25	2	3	4	7	11	14	24

45.41: LOC EXC LG BOWEL LES. Formerly included in operation group(s) 607.

Type of Patients	Observed Patients	Avg. Stay	Variance	10th	25th	50th	75th	90th	95th	99th
1. SINGLE DX										
0–19 Years	3	2.5	3	1	1	1	2	4	4	4
20–34	8	2.4	1	2	2	2	2	4	4	7
35–49	10	2.6	<1	1	2	3	3	4	4	4
50–64	11	1.7	2	1	1	1	1	4	5	6
65+	20	4.9	6	2	3	5	6	8	9	9
2. MULTIPLE DX										
0–19 Years	15	22.5	999	1	3	5	17	80	80	80
20–34	26	4.6	5	2	3	4	6	7	10	10
35–49	55	4.7	12	2	3	4	5	8	13	19
50–64	87	7.1	18	2	5	7	9	10	14	22
65+	205	8.8	65	3	5	6	9	15	32	40
TOTAL SINGLE DX	52	2.6	4	1	1	2	4	6	6	9
MULTIPLE DX	388	8.0	93	3	4	5	8	14	21	40
TOTAL										
0–19 Years	18	21.1	954	1	3	5	17	80	80	80
20–34	34	3.5	4	2	2	3	4	7	7	10
35–49	65	4.4	11	2	3	3	5	7	13	19
50–64	98	5.8	19	1	2	5	8	9	14	21
65+	225	8.5	62	3	5	6	8	15	32	40
GRAND TOTAL	440	7.2	83	2	3	5	7	13	19	40

45.42: ENDO COLON POLYPECTOMY. Formerly included in operation group(s) 607.

Type of Patients	Observed Patients	Avg. Stay	Variance	10th	25th	50th	75th	90th	95th	99th
1. SINGLE DX										
0–19 Years	24	1.5	<1	1	1	1	2	3	3	3
20–34	1	1.0	0	1	1	1	1	1	1	1
35–49	4	9.9	127	2	2	8	8	30	30	30
50–64	21	3.8	12	1	1	2	6	11	11	13
65+	44	4.8	25	1	1	3	6	11	18	24
2. MULTIPLE DX										
0–19 Years	35	1.6	<1	1	1	1	3	3	4	5
20–34	92	4.7	23	1	2	3	6	9	14	34
35–49	603	4.8	22	1	2	4	6	9	12	23
50–64	1788	5.3	19	2	3	4	7	9	12	21
65+	7708	6.1	25	2	3	5	8	12	15	25
TOTAL SINGLE DX	94	3.7	22	1	1	2	5	8	12	30
MULTIPLE DX	10226	5.8	24	2	3	5	7	11	15	23
TOTAL										
0–19 Years	59	1.5	<1	1	1	1	2	3	3	5
20–34	93	4.6	23	1	2	3	5	9	12	34
35–49	607	4.8	23	2	2	4	6	9	13	25
50–64	1809	5.3	19	2	3	4	7	9	12	21
65+	7752	6.1	25	2	3	5	8	12	15	25
GRAND TOTAL	10320	5.8	24	2	3	4	7	11	15	24

45.43: ENDO DESTR COLON LES NEC. Formerly included in operation group(s) 607.

Type of Patients	Observed Patients	Avg. Stay	Variance	10th	25th	50th	75th	90th	95th	99th
1. SINGLE DX										
0–19 Years	2	1.6	<1	1	1	2	2	2	2	2
20–34	4	3.6	1	1	3	4	4	5	5	5
35–49	9	2.1	<1	2	2	2	2	4	4	4
50–64	9	2.5	1	1	1	3	3	4	4	4
65+	12	2.4	2	1	2	3	3	6	6	6
2. MULTIPLE DX										
0–19 Years	7	2.3	2	1	1	3	3	3	3	6
20–34	21	4.4	9	1	3	4	5	7	14	14
35–49	104	3.9	7	2	2	3	5	7	7	15
50–64	296	4.0	7	2	3	4	5	6	8	18
65+	1458	5.4	21	2	3	4	6	10	13	22
TOTAL SINGLE DX	36	2.2	<1	1	2	2	2	4	5	6
MULTIPLE DX	1886	5.0	17	2	3	4	6	9	12	22
TOTAL										
0–19 Years	9	2.2	1	1	1	3	3	3	3	6
20–34	25	4.3	9	1	3	4	5	7	14	14
35–49	113	3.6	6	2	2	3	5	7	8	15
50–64	305	4.0	7	2	3	4	5	6	8	18
65+	1470	5.4	21	2	3	4	6	10	13	22
GRAND TOTAL	1922	5.0	17	2	3	4	6	9	12	22

Length of Stay by Diagnosis and Operation, United States, 1997

United States, October 1995–September 1996 Data, by Operation

45.61: MULT SEG SM BOWEL RESECT. Formerly included in operation group(s) 608.

Type of Patients	Observed Patients	Avg. Stay	Vari-ance	Percentiles						
				10th	25th	50th	75th	90th	95th	99th
1. SINGLE DX										
0–19 Years	2	9.1	1	8	8	10	10	10	10	10
20–34	4	10.7	35	6	7	7	18	18	18	18
35–49	2	7.0	0	7	7	7	7	7	7	7
50–64	5	7.9	9	5	6	6	9	9	15	15
65+	0									
2. MULTIPLE DX										
0–19 Years	34	11.8	70	8	8	8	14	30	>99	>99
20–34	66	9.9	71	5	6	7	8	26	31	39
35–49	88	18.1	224	6	9	16	22	27	40	87
50–64	117	13.5	130	5	7	9	18	28	36	60
65+	254	17.3	103	8	10	15	22	31	37	65
TOTAL SINGLE DX	13	8.7	14	6	6	7	9	15	18	18
MULTIPLE DX	559	15.0	130	6	7	11	20	29	37	87
TOTAL										
0–19 Years	36	11.7	69	8	8	8	14	30	>99	>99
20–34	70	9.9	70	5	6	7	8	23	31	39
35–49	90	17.9	222	6	8	16	22	27	40	87
50–64	122	13.3	128	5	7	9	17	26	36	60
65+	254	17.3	103	8	10	15	22	31	37	65
GRAND TOTAL	572	14.9	129	6	7	11	20	29	37	87

45.62: PART SM BOWEL RESECT NEC. Formerly included in operation group(s) 608.

Type of Patients	Observed Patients	Avg. Stay	Vari-ance	Percentiles						
				10th	25th	50th	75th	90th	95th	99th
1. SINGLE DX										
0–19 Years	102	8.4	32	4	5	6	13	13	15	31
20–34	85	5.7	6	3	4	5	7	8	10	15
35–49	77	6.4	5	3	5	6	7	9	9	13
50–64	71	7.6	17	4	5	6	10	14	14	24
65+	42	8.5	32	4	5	7	11	12	14	37
2. MULTIPLE DX										
0–19 Years	782	16.2	402	5	6	8	22	75	>99	>99
20–34	912	10.2	75	4	6	8	11	18	25	49
35–49	1685	10.6	61	5	6	8	12	18	26	46
50–64	1961	12.6	115	5	6	10	15	24	35	62
65+	4784	14.0	95	6	8	11	16	24	33	59
TOTAL SINGLE DX	377	7.1	18	3	5	6	8	13	14	24
MULTIPLE DX	10124	12.8	119	5	7	10	15	24	35	85
TOTAL										
0–19 Years	884	15.1	356	5	5	8	17	66	>99	>99
20–34	997	9.7	70	4	5	8	11	17	24	43
35–49	1762	10.3	59	5	6	8	12	18	25	45
50–64	2032	12.4	112	5	6	9	15	24	34	59
65+	4826	13.9	95	6	8	11	16	24	33	59
GRAND TOTAL	10501	12.6	116	5	7	9	15	24	34	84

45.5: INTESTINAL SEG ISOLATION. Formerly included in operation group(s) 610.

Type of Patients	Observed Patients	Avg. Stay	Vari-ance	Percentiles						
				10th	25th	50th	75th	90th	95th	99th
1. SINGLE DX										
0–19 Years	3	4.8	2	4	4	4	5	7	7	7
20–34	1	6.0	0	6	6	6	6	6	6	6
35–49	2	8.1	3	5	9	9	9	9	9	9
50–64	2	3.7	3	3	3	3	3	7	7	7
65+	0									
2. MULTIPLE DX										
0–19 Years	13	10.8	100	4	6	9	>99	>99	>99	>99
20–34	6	12.9	121	5	6	7	18	39	39	39
35–49	14	9.6	29	6	6	6	11	20	20	20
50–64	15	11.6	40	6	6	8	18	23	23	23
65+	25	13.6	179	7	8	9	16	16	31	85
TOTAL SINGLE DX	8	5.6	4	3	4	6	7	9	9	9
MULTIPLE DX	73	12.3	122	6	7	8	16	23	85	>99
TOTAL										
0–19 Years	16	9.5	84	4	4	9	>99	>99	>99	>99
20–34	7	10.4	86	6	6	6	7	20	39	39
35–49	16	9.4	26	5	6	6	11	18	20	20
50–64	17	10.5	42	3	6	8	13	23	23	23
65+	25	13.6	179	7	8	9	16	16	31	85
GRAND TOTAL	81	11.7	115	5	6	8	16	23	85	>99

45.6: OTHER SM BOWEL EXCISION. Formerly included in operation group(s) 608.

Type of Patients	Observed Patients	Avg. Stay	Vari-ance	Percentiles						
				10th	25th	50th	75th	90th	95th	99th
1. SINGLE DX										
0–19 Years	104	8.4	32	4	5	6	13	13	15	31
20–34	91	5.8	7	3	4	5	7	8	10	15
35–49	80	6.4	5	3	5	6	7	9	9	12
50–64	77	7.6	16	4	5	6	9	14	14	24
65+	43	8.5	31	4	5	7	11	12	14	37
2. MULTIPLE DX										
0–19 Years	824	16.1	390	5	6	8	21	70	>99	>99
20–34	984	10.2	75	4	6	8	11	18	26	45
35–49	1789	10.9	71	5	6	8	12	20	27	46
50–64	2098	12.7	116	5	6	9	15	24	35	60
65+	5069	14.1	96	6	8	11	17	25	33	59
TOTAL SINGLE DX	395	7.2	18	3	5	6	8	13	14	24
MULTIPLE DX	10764	13.0	120	5	7	10	15	24	35	86
TOTAL										
0–19 Years	928	15.0	348	5	5	8	17	66	>99	>99
20–34	1075	9.8	70	4	5	8	11	17	24	42
35–49	1869	10.6	68	5	6	8	12	19	26	46
50–64	2175	12.5	113	5	6	9	15	24	34	60
65+	5112	14.1	96	6	8	11	17	25	33	59
GRAND TOTAL	11159	12.7	117	5	7	8	15	24	35	84

Length of Stay by Diagnosis and Operation, United States, 1997

United States, October 1995–September 1996 Data, by Operation

45.7: PART LG BOWEL EXCISION. Formerly included in operation group(s) 609.

Type of Patients	Observed Patients	Avg. Stay	Variance	10th	25th	50th	75th	90th	95th	99th
1. SINGLE DX										
0–19 Years	132	6.4	17	4	4	5	7	9	12	24
20–34	250	6.3	6	4	5	6	7	9	11	15
35–49	571	6.0	6	4	5	6	7	8	10	13
50–64	769	6.1	7	4	5	6	7	8	9	13
65+	586	7.0	8	4	6	7	8	9	10	15
2. MULTIPLE DX										
0–19 Years	710	12.6	178	5	6	8	15	31	52	>99
20–34	1855	9.3	47	5	6	7	10	16	22	42
35–49	5619	9.2	41	5	6	7	10	15	21	36
50–64	11201	9.8	45	5	6	8	11	17	23	37
65+	31607	11.5	61	6	7	9	13	20	26	44
TOTAL SINGLE DX	2308	6.3	7	4	5	6	7	9	10	15
MULTIPLE DX	50992	10.7	56	5	6	8	12	19	24	42
TOTAL										
0–19 Years	842	11.5	154	4	6	7	13	25	40	>99
20–34	2105	8.9	44	4	6	7	10	15	21	42
35–49	6190	8.9	39	5	6	8	10	14	20	36
50–64	11970	9.5	43	6	6	8	11	17	23	36
65+	32193	11.4	60	6	7	9	13	20	26	44
GRAND TOTAL	53300	10.4	55	5	6	8	12	18	24	42

45.72: CECECTOMY. Formerly included in operation group(s) 609.

Type of Patients	Observed Patients	Avg. Stay	Variance	10th	25th	50th	75th	90th	95th	99th
1. SINGLE DX										
0–19 Years	46	6.2	21	4	4	5	7	9	14	40
20–34	64	5.5	3	3	4	5	7	7	8	11
35–49	48	5.6	3	3	5	5	7	8	8	10
50–64	30	4.9	4	3	3	5	6	8	8	10
65+	20	7.4	3	5	7	8	8	10	10	10
2. MULTIPLE DX										
0–19 Years	163	12.7	274	5	6	8	14	32	93	>99
20–34	357	8.6	30	4	5	7	10	15	20	29
35–49	462	10.1	91	5	5	7	10	18	34	50
50–64	423	9.3	46	5	6	8	10	17	21	37
65+	938	13.1	88	6	7	10	17	23	37	42
TOTAL SINGLE DX	208	5.8	7	3	4	5	7	8	10	11
MULTIPLE DX	2343	11.0	86	5	6	8	12	20	31	50
TOTAL										
0–19 Years	209	11.2	221	4	5	7	12	21	84	>99
20–34	421	8.2	27	4	5	7	9	14	20	29
35–49	510	9.2	77	4	5	7	9	15	31	50
50–64	453	9.1	44	5	6	7	10	16	21	37
65+	958	12.8	86	6	7	10	16	22	36	42
GRAND TOTAL	2551	10.4	80	5	6	8	11	20	27	50

45.71: MULT SEG LG BOWEL RESECT. Formerly included in operation group(s) 609.

Type of Patients	Observed Patients	Avg. Stay	Variance	10th	25th	50th	75th	90th	95th	99th
1. SINGLE DX										
0–19 Years	0									
20–34	0									
35–49	1	7.0	0	7	7	7	7	7	7	7
50–64	1	5.0	0	5	5	5	5	5	5	5
65+	3	7.5	2	6	8	8	9	9	9	9
2. MULTIPLE DX										
0–19 Years	12	17.8	130	5	7	20	23	40	40	40
20–34	13	9.3	85	5	5	5	6	29	34	34
35–49	34	7.6	13	5	5	8	9	10	15	26
50–64	71	11.8	52	6	7	9	14	21	25	38
65+	213	15.7	96	6	9	14	19	27	37	99
TOTAL SINGLE DX	5	6.3	2	5	5	6	8	9	9	9
MULTIPLE DX	343	13.1	83	5	7	9	16	23	36	44
TOTAL										
0–19 Years	12	17.8	130	5	7	20	23	40	40	40
20–34	13	9.3	85	5	5	5	6	29	34	34
35–49	35	7.6	13	5	5	8	10	10	15	26
50–64	72	11.6	52	6	7	9	14	21	25	38
65+	216	15.7	96	6	9	14	19	27	37	99
GRAND TOTAL	348	13.0	83	5	7	9	16	23	36	44

45.73: RIGHT HEMICOLECTOMY. Formerly included in operation group(s) 609.

Type of Patients	Observed Patients	Avg. Stay	Variance	10th	25th	50th	75th	90th	95th	99th
1. SINGLE DX										
0–19 Years	36	6.3	20	4	4	6	6	7	24	24
20–34	77	5.8	4	4	5	6	6	8	9	11
35–49	125	5.8	4	4	4	6	7	8	9	13
50–64	208	5.8	7	4	4	6	7	8	9	16
65+	230	6.5	10	4	5	6	7	9	10	20
2. MULTIPLE DX										
0–19 Years	229	10.8	94	5	6	7	12	24	42	>99
20–34	579	9.0	44	5	6	7	10	16	21	41
35–49	1384	9.2	34	5	6	7	11	15	20	36
50–64	3289	10.2	50	5	7	8	11	23	23	35
65+	12392	10.9	50	7	7	9	13	19	25	40
TOTAL SINGLE DX	676	6.0	8	4	4	6	7	8	10	20
MULTIPLE DX	17873	10.5	49	5	6	8	12	19	23	39
TOTAL										
0–19 Years	265	9.8	81	4	6	7	10	21	35	>99
20–34	656	8.6	40	4	6	7	10	15	18	38
35–49	1509	9.0	33	5	6	7	10	14	19	36
50–64	3497	10.0	49	6	6	8	11	22	23	35
65+	12622	10.8	50	7	7	9	13	19	25	39
GRAND TOTAL	18549	10.3	48	5	6	8	12	18	23	38

Length of Stay by Diagnosis and Operation, United States, 1997

United States, October 1995–September 1996 Data, by Operation

45.74: TRANSVERSE COLON RESECT. Formerly included in operation group(s) 609.

Type of Patients	Observed Patients	Avg. Stay	Vari-ance	Percentiles						
				10th	25th	50th	75th	90th	95th	99th
1. SINGLE DX										
0–19 Years	2	5.5	<1	5	5	5	5	7	7	7
20–34	6	5.2	2	5	5	5	5	6	7	9
35–49	11	5.4	2	4	4	5	6	8	8	8
50–64	22	6.1	3	4	5	6	7	8	10	11
65+	22	6.9	13	4	5	6	7	10	11	23
2. MULTIPLE DX										
0–19 Years	44	14.7	214	4	6	8	17	35	56	62
20–34	67	11.8	78	4	6	8	15	25	28	48
35–49	146	10.5	63	5	6	8	11	19	26	52
50–64	401	9.8	55	5	6	8	11	18	20	56
65+	1303	11.2	51	5	7	9	13	19	25	42
TOTAL SINGLE DX	63	6.0	6	4	5	6	7	8	10	11
MULTIPLE DX	1961	10.8	57	5	7	9	13	18	25	45
TOTAL										
0–19 Years	46	13.3	193	4	5	8	13	35	56	62
20–34	73	11.4	76	4	6	8	14	25	28	45
35–49	157	10.3	61	5	6	8	11	19	26	41
50–64	423	9.7	54	5	6	8	11	17	20	56
65+	1325	11.1	51	5	7	9	13	19	25	42
GRAND TOTAL	2024	10.7	57	5	7	8	12	18	24	45

45.75: LEFT HEMICOLECTOMY. Formerly included in operation group(s) 609.

Type of Patients	Observed Patients	Avg. Stay	Vari-ance	Percentiles						
				10th	25th	50th	75th	90th	95th	99th
1. SINGLE DX										
0–19 Years	3	6.3	<1	6	6	5	6	9	9	9
20–34	19	6.7	1	5	6	7	7	7	9	12
35–49	68	6.4	5	4	5	6	8	9	10	13
50–64	95	6.5	4	4	5	6	8	9	9	10
65+	65	7.1	5	5	5	6	8	9	11	15
2. MULTIPLE DX										
0–19 Years	55	13.5	213	5	6	8	13	32	45	>99
20–34	185	11.2	95	4	6	8	13	22	29	42
35–49	712	10.0	39	5	6	8	12	17	21	38
50–64	1672	10.4	48	6	7	8	11	18	23	37
65+	4449	12.4	71	6	7	10	14	21	28	46
TOTAL SINGLE DX	250	6.6	4	4	5	6	8	9	9	13
MULTIPLE DX	7073	11.5	64	6	7	9	13	20	26	43
TOTAL										
0–19 Years	58	13.2	205	5	6	8	13	32	44	>99
20–34	204	10.6	84	5	6	8	12	22	26	42
35–49	780	9.7	38	5	6	8	12	16	21	37
50–64	1767	10.1	46	5	6	8	11	17	23	35
65+	4514	12.3	71	6	7	10	14	21	28	46
GRAND TOTAL	7323	11.3	63	6	7	9	13	20	25	43

45.76: SIGMOIDECTOMY. Formerly included in operation group(s) 609.

Type of Patients	Observed Patients	Avg. Stay	Vari-ance	Percentiles						
				10th	25th	50th	75th	90th	95th	99th
1. SINGLE DX										
0–19 Years	16	9.0	33	4	5	8	11	22	22	22
20–34	64	7.4	10	4	5	7	9	13	13	15
35–49	261	6.2	7	4	5	6	7	8	8	19
50–64	362	6.1	3	4	5	6	7	8	9	11
65+	213	7.2	4	5	6	7	8	9	11	13
2. MULTIPLE DX										
0–19 Years	67	10.4	77	4	6	8	13	19	29	>99
20–34	451	8.5	30	4	6	7	9	14	18	36
35–49	2419	8.8	33	5	6	7	10	14	18	31
50–64	4410	9.3	37	5	6	8	10	16	20	34
65+	10138	11.4	62	6	7	9	13	20	25	47
TOTAL SINGLE DX	916	6.4	5	4	5	6	7	9	10	14
MULTIPLE DX	17485	10.2	50	5	6	8	12	17	23	38
TOTAL										
0–19 Years	83	10.3	72	4	6	8	12	19	29	>99
20–34	515	8.4	28	5	6	7	9	13	18	30
35–49	2680	8.5	31	5	6	7	10	14	18	31
50–64	4772	9.0	35	5	6	7	10	15	20	32
65+	10351	11.3	61	6	7	9	13	19	25	47
GRAND TOTAL	18401	10.0	48	5	6	8	11	17	22	38

45.79: PART LG BOWEL EXC NEC. Formerly included in operation group(s) 609.

Type of Patients	Observed Patients	Avg. Stay	Vari-ance	Percentiles						
				10th	25th	50th	75th	90th	95th	99th
1. SINGLE DX										
0–19 Years	29	6.4	4	5	5	6	7	8	12	15
20–34	20	6.6	15	3	4	5	8	11	14	19
35–49	57	6.6	5	4	5	7	8	10	10	13
50–64	51	7.3	58	3	5	6	7	10	12	52
65+	33	7.4	18	6	6	7	7	8	9	25
2. MULTIPLE DX										
0–19 Years	140	14.7	212	5	6	8	20	33	40	>99
20–34	203	9.9	68	4	6	8	10	16	23	57
35–49	462	9.1	58	3	6	7	10	16	24	42
50–64	935	9.7	53	5	6	8	11	16	22	45
65+	2174	12.4	79	5	7	10	14	23	32	47
TOTAL SINGLE DX	190	6.9	19	4	5	6	7	9	10	25
MULTIPLE DX	3914	11.1	76	5	6	8	12	20	29	47
TOTAL										
0–19 Years	169	13.4	188	5	6	7	19	33	38	96
20–34	223	9.7	65	4	5	8	10	15	22	57
35–49	519	8.8	52	3	6	7	10	15	21	41
50–64	986	9.7	53	5	6	8	11	16	22	45
65+	2207	12.3	78	5	7	9	14	23	32	47
GRAND TOTAL	4104	10.9	74	5	6	8	12	20	28	47

Length of Stay by Diagnosis and Operation, United States, 1997

United States, October 1995–September 1996 Data, by Operation

45.8: TOT INTRA-ABD COLECTOMY. Formerly included in operation group(s) 609.

Type of Patients	Observed Patients	Avg. Stay	Variance	10th	25th	50th	75th	90th	95th	99th
1. SINGLE DX										
0–19 Years	51	7.6	8	5	6	7	9	10	11	24
20–34	56	6.7	9	4	5	6	7	9	10	23
35–49	55	9.8	19	6	7	8	11	16	19	21
50–64	22	7.8	11	5	6	7	8	11	13	21
65+	9	8.7	8	6	6	8	10	10	17	17
2. MULTIPLE DX										
0–19 Years	129	16.9	165	7	8	13	23	30	46	57
20–34	345	12.3	61	6	7	9	16	23	25	39
35–49	463	13.0	85	6	7	9	15	23	33	51
50–64	446	12.2	82	6	7	10	14	21	28	63
65+	769	18.1	174	8	9	14	22	31	45	76
TOTAL SINGLE DX	193	8.2	14	5	6	7	9	16	16	21
MULTIPLE DX	2152	14.7	123	6	8	11	18	28	35	65
TOTAL										
0–19 Years	180	14.9	147	6	7	10	21	24	46	57
20–34	401	11.5	57	5	6	8	15	23	25	39
35–49	518	12.7	79	6	7	9	15	22	30	51
50–64	468	12.0	81	6	7	10	14	21	28	57
65+	778	18.1	174	8	9	14	22	31	45	76
GRAND TOTAL	2345	14.2	117	6	7	10	17	27	33	63

45.91: SM-TO-SM BOWEL ANAST. Formerly included in operation group(s) 611.

Type of Patients	Observed Patients	Avg. Stay	Variance	10th	25th	50th	75th	90th	95th	99th
1. SINGLE DX										
0–19 Years	12	10.8	38	5	7	10	15	17	17	32
20–34	2	7.9	3	6	6	6	8	9	9	9
35–49	3	5.6	5	3	3	6	8	8	8	8
50–64	0									
65+	1	5.0	0	5	5	5	5	5	5	5
2. MULTIPLE DX										
0–19 Years	125	26.5	309	8	13	20	43	48	59	82
20–34	23	10.6	30	5	6	10	14	20	20	23
35–49	75	14.1	118	6	8	9	18	27	33	59
50–64	109	14.5	132	6	9	11	16	32	45	57
65+	255	14.4	66	7	9	12	17	26	33	41
TOTAL SINGLE DX	18	9.9	34	3	6	9	15	15	17	32
MULTIPLE DX	587	17.2	173	6	9	13	20	37	48	60
TOTAL										
0–19 Years	137	25.3	306	8	11	19	37	48	59	82
20–34	25	10.5	30	5	6	10	14	20	20	23
35–49	78	13.9	117	6	8	9	18	27	33	59
50–64	109	14.5	132	6	9	11	16	32	45	57
65+	256	14.4	66	7	9	12	17	26	33	41
GRAND TOTAL	605	17.0	170	6	9	13	20	37	48	60

45.9: INTESTINAL ANASTOMOSIS. Formerly included in operation group(s) 611.

Type of Patients	Observed Patients	Avg. Stay	Variance	10th	25th	50th	75th	90th	95th	99th
1. SINGLE DX										
0–19 Years	31	7.7	19	4	5	6	8	15	15	32
20–34	24	5.9	3	4	5	6	7	8	8	9
35–49	18	6.0	2	5	5	6	7	8	9	10
50–64	24	6.2	2	4	6	6	7	8	10	10
65+	16	8.2	13	5	5	7	13	13	13	14
2. MULTIPLE DX										
0–19 Years	208	20.9	300	5	8	15	29	48	48	82
20–34	157	8.8	27	5	6	7	9	16	20	30
35–49	347	10.6	65	5	7	8	12	19	26	56
50–64	529	11.0	69	5	7	8	13	20	25	45
65+	1083	12.2	51	6	8	11	13	21	27	41
TOTAL SINGLE DX	113	6.8	9	4	5	6	7	10	13	17
MULTIPLE DX	2324	12.3	90	5	7	9	14	22	31	48
TOTAL										
0–19 Years	239	19.1	282	5	7	13	25	48	48	82
20–34	181	8.4	25	4	6	7	9	15	20	30
35–49	365	10.2	61	5	6	8	12	18	26	46
50–64	553	10.8	68	5	6	8	13	19	25	45
65+	1099	12.1	51	6	8	11	13	21	27	41
GRAND TOTAL	2437	12.0	88	5	7	9	13	22	30	48

45.93: SMALL-TO-LARGE BOWEL NEC. Formerly included in operation group(s) 611.

Type of Patients	Observed Patients	Avg. Stay	Variance	10th	25th	50th	75th	90th	95th	99th
1. SINGLE DX										
0–19 Years	8	6.0	6	4	5	5	5	12	12	12
20–34	4	6.4	2	5	5	6	8	8	8	8
35–49	2	6.6	<1	6	6	7	10	10	10	10
50–64	4	7.8	4	6	6	7	10	10	10	10
65+	2	12.0	12	8	8	14	14	14	14	14
2. MULTIPLE DX										
0–19 Years	27	14.4	268	5	6	9	15	19	64	79
20–34	44	10.2	51	5	6	7	10	24	30	32
35–49	105	11.8	77	4	7	10	14	21	30	58
50–64	169	12.6	59	5	7	10	17	24	26	39
65+	357	13.5	53	7	9	11	16	23	29	40
TOTAL SINGLE DX	20	6.7	5	5	5	6	8	10	12	14
MULTIPLE DX	702	12.8	67	6	7	11	15	23	29	42
TOTAL										
0–19 Years	35	11.8	203	5	5	7	14	18	19	79
20–34	48	10.0	49	5	6	7	10	24	30	32
35–49	107	11.5	75	5	7	9	13	21	30	58
50–64	173	12.5	59	5	7	10	17	24	25	39
65+	359	13.5	53	7	9	11	16	23	29	40
GRAND TOTAL	722	12.6	67	5	7	11	15	23	29	42

Length of Stay by Diagnosis and Operation, United States, 1997

United States, October 1995–September 1996 Data, by Operation

46.01: SM BOWEL EXTERIORIZATION. Formerly included in operation group(s) 610.

Type of Patients	Observed Patients	Avg. Stay	Variance	10th	25th	50th	75th	90th	95th	99th
1. SINGLE DX										
0–19 Years	8	11.6	106	3	8	8	9	34	34	34
20–34	7	7.3	3	5	6	7	9	9	9	9
35–49	3	5.7	1	4	5	5	7	7	7	7
50–64	3	5.2	2	2	5	6	6	6	6	6
65+	1	8.0	0	8	8	8	8	8	8	8
2. MULTIPLE DX										
0–19 Years	34	18.1	376	4	7	11	20	64	72	>99
20–34	38	9.4	82	5	5	5	9	17	30	46
35–49	64	9.5	22	5	6	9	12	14	19	26
50–64	72	18.3	402	6	6	10	21	45	74	74
65+	160	18.2	133	6	8	17	26	42	42	>99
TOTAL SINGLE DX	22	8.7	54	4	5	8	8	9	34	34
MULTIPLE DX	368	16.3	206	5	7	11	22	42	45	>99
TOTAL										
0–19	42	17.3	348	4	7	11	18	43	72	>99
20–34	45	9.1	74	5	5	6	9	17	23	46
35–49	67	9.4	22	5	6	9	11	14	19	26
50–64	75	17.9	394	6	8	10	21	45	74	74
65+	161	18.1	133	6	8	17	26	42	42	>99
GRAND TOTAL	390	15.9	202	5	6	11	21	42	43	>99

45.94: LG-TO-LG BOWEL ANAST. Formerly included in operation group(s) 611.

Type of Patients	Observed Patients	Avg. Stay	Variance	10th	25th	50th	75th	90th	95th	99th
1. SINGLE DX										
0–19 Years	2	5.2	<1	5	5	5	5	6	6	6
20–34	12	5.7	2	4	5	6	7	7	7	8
35–49	6	5.5	1	5	5	5	5	7	9	9
50–64	11	6.0	2	5	6	6	7	8	8	8
65+	11	6.7	4	4	5	7	7	9	12	12
2. MULTIPLE DX										
0–19 Years	25	9.3	41	5	6	7	8	24	25	25
20–34	36	7.3	14	4	6	7	8	10	10	31
35–49	107	8.3	22	5	5	7	10	13	15	31
50–64	184	7.8	18	4	6	7	8	14	16	21
65+	390	9.7	18	6	7	9	11	13	18	24
TOTAL SINGLE DX	42	5.8	2	5	5	6	7	7	8	9
MULTIPLE DX	742	8.9	20	5	6	8	10	13	17	24
TOTAL										
0–19	27	8.9	38	5	5	7	8	24	25	25
20–34	48	6.9	11	4	5	7	7	9	10	20
35–49	113	7.9	20	5	5	7	10	12	15	31
50–64	195	7.7	17	4	6	7	8	11	16	21
65+	401	9.7	18	6	7	9	11	13	17	24
GRAND TOTAL	784	8.7	19	5	6	8	10	13	17	24

46.03: LG BOWEL EXTERIORIZATION. Formerly included in operation group(s) 610.

Type of Patients	Observed Patients	Avg. Stay	Variance	10th	25th	50th	75th	90th	95th	99th
1. SINGLE DX										
0–19 Years	30	5.8	7	2	4	5	8	10	10	12
20–34	6	4.6	2	3	3	5	6	6	6	6
35–49	9	3.5	3	2	2	4	5	5	7	7
50–64	9	5.7	3	3	4	6	6	8	8	8
65+	8	9.1	5	7	7	10	11	11	11	11
2. MULTIPLE DX										
0–19 Years	120	10.0	97	4	5	8	11	15	22	53
20–34	73	10.0	44	4	4	8	14	20	23	28
35–49	155	11.0	98	5	7	8	13	21	24	81
50–64	309	12.1	73	5	6	9	15	25	27	41
65+	944	13.1	70	5	7	11	16	24	28	43
TOTAL SINGLE DX	62	5.9	7	3	4	6	8	10	11	12
MULTIPLE DX	1601	12.4	75	5	7	10	15	24	27	43
TOTAL										
0–19	150	9.3	85	3	5	8	11	14	19	53
20–34	79	9.6	43	4	4	8	13	20	23	28
35–49	164	10.7	96	5	6	7	13	21	24	55
50–64	318	11.9	72	5	6	9	15	25	27	41
65+	952	13.1	69	5	7	11	16	24	28	43
GRAND TOTAL	1663	12.1	74	4	7	10	15	24	27	43

46.0: EXTERIORIZATION OF BOWEL. Formerly included in operation group(s) 610.

Type of Patients	Observed Patients	Avg. Stay	Variance	10th	25th	50th	75th	90th	95th	99th
1. SINGLE DX										
0–19 Years	39	7.6	40	3	4	6	9	10	18	34
20–34	14	5.8	4	3	5	6	7	9	9	9
35–49	12	4.3	3	2	2	5	5	7	7	7
50–64	12	5.6	3	3	5	6	6	8	8	8
65+	12	8.3	8	4	7	8	11	11	11	11
2. MULTIPLE DX										
0–19 Years	159	12.6	200	4	6	9	12	29	53	>99
20–34	117	11.8	99	4	5	8	14	28	36	36
35–49	230	10.2	72	4	6	8	12	19	23	38
50–64	395	13.0	135	5	6	9	15	25	32	74
65+	1135	14.0	84	5	8	12	18	26	30	55
TOTAL SINGLE DX	89	6.8	22	3	4	6	8	10	11	34
MULTIPLE DX	2036	13.1	106	5	7	10	16	25	33	72
TOTAL										
0–19	198	11.8	179	4	5	8	12	25	43	97
20–34	131	11.3	94	4	5	8	14	27	36	36
35–49	242	9.9	71	4	6	7	12	18	23	38
50–64	407	12.8	132	5	6	9	15	25	31	74
65+	1147	13.9	83	5	8	12	17	26	30	54
GRAND TOTAL	2125	12.9	104	5	7	10	16	25	32	70

Length of Stay by Diagnosis and Operation, United States, 1997

United States, October 1995–September 1996 Data, by Operation

46.1: COLOSTOMY. Formerly included in operation group(s) 612.

Type of Patients	Observed Patients	Avg. Stay	Variance	10th	25th	50th	75th	90th	95th	99th
1. SINGLE DX										
0–19 Years	46	6.3	10	3	4	6	8	10	10	23
20–34	6	3.9	8	2	2	2	6	10	11	11
35–49	10	5.3	7	4	4	4	5	11	11	13
50–64	17	8.6	12	3	6	9	12	13	13	14
65+	9	8.2	13	4	5	7	12	12	13	13
2. MULTIPLE DX										
0–19 Years	230	12.1	221	3	5	8	12	21	36	96
20–34	105	11.5	82	3	5	9	13	27	34	40
35–49	260	14.2	118	5	6	11	18	33	38	58
50–64	564	14.0	136	5	7	10	17	31	34	64
65+	1517	13.6	97	6	8	11	16	24	33	53
TOTAL SINGLE DX	88	6.5	11	3	4	6	9	11	12	14
MULTIPLE DX	2676	13.5	121	5	7	11	16	26	34	59
TOTAL										
0–19 Years	276	11.2	194	3	5	8	12	21	35	96
20–34	111	11.1	81	3	5	8	13	26	34	40
35–49	270	13.7	116	4	6	10	17	31	38	47
50–64	581	13.9	134	5	7	10	16	31	34	64
65+	1526	13.6	97	6	8	11	16	24	33	53
GRAND TOTAL	2764	13.3	119	5	7	10	15	26	34	59

46.11: TEMPORARY COLOSTOMY. Formerly included in operation group(s) 612.

Type of Patients	Observed Patients	Avg. Stay	Variance	10th	25th	50th	75th	90th	95th	99th
1. SINGLE DX										
0–19 Years	15	6.0	18	3	3	6	6	8	12	23
20–34	5	3.7	9	2	2	2	4	7	11	11
35–49	2	4.0	0	4	4	4	4	4	4	4
50–64	5	8.0	20	2	2	10	10	14	14	14
65+	2	10.8	9	8	8	13	13	13	13	13
2. MULTIPLE DX										
0–19 Years	90	14.1	351	4	6	9	13	27	40	96
20–34	39	9.8	46	2	4	9	13	16	22	37
35–49	73	19.2	149	6	8	14	26	38	38	41
50–64	157	17.0	214	5	7	12	21	40	53	64
65+	343	14.1	90	6	8	12	17	24	29	48
TOTAL SINGLE DX	29	5.4	13	2	3	4	6	10	13	23
MULTIPLE DX	702	15.1	170	5	7	11	18	28	38	80
TOTAL										
0–19 Years	105	13.4	326	3	6	8	12	25	36	94
20–34	44	9.2	46	2	3	8	13	16	22	37
35–49	75	17.6	155	4	7	13	26	38	38	41
50–64	162	16.8	211	5	7	12	21	40	53	64
65+	345	14.1	90	6	8	12	17	24	29	48
GRAND TOTAL	731	14.7	167	5	7	11	18	27	38	68

46.10: COLOSTOMY NOS. Formerly included in operation group(s) 612.

Type of Patients	Observed Patients	Avg. Stay	Variance	10th	25th	50th	75th	90th	95th	99th
1. SINGLE DX										
0–19 Years	24	6.7	7	4	4	7	10	10	10	13
20–34	0									
35–49	3	7.2	13	5	5	5	13	13	13	13
50–64	11	8.7	10	5	6	9	12	13	13	13
65+	5	8.3	12	4	5	7	12	12	12	12
2. MULTIPLE DX										
0–19 Years	98	9.6	58	4	5	8	12	21	26	>99
20–34	38	12.1	107	5	5	8	12	34	34	40
35–49	83	12.5	96	4	6	12	15	28	43	>99
50–64	183	14.8	141	6	7	11	16	33	33	89
65+	519	13.9	132	5	8	11	16	26	34	75
TOTAL SINGLE DX	43	7.3	9	4	5	7	10	12	13	13
MULTIPLE DX	921	13.4	123	5	7	11	15	27	34	86
TOTAL										
0–19 Years	122	9.1	49	4	5	7	12	16	26	>99
20–34	38	12.1	107	5	5	8	12	34	34	40
35–49	86	12.3	94	4	6	11	15	28	40	>99
50–64	194	14.5	136	6	8	11	15	33	33	73
65+	524	13.9	131	5	8	11	16	26	34	75
GRAND TOTAL	964	13.1	119	5	7	10	15	26	34	78

46.13: PERMANENT COLOSTOMY. Formerly included in operation group(s) 612.

Type of Patients	Observed Patients	Avg. Stay	Variance	10th	25th	50th	75th	90th	95th	99th
1. SINGLE DX										
0–19 Years	7	5.7	7	2	3	7	7	7	7	12
20–34	1	6.0	0	6	6	6	6	6	6	6
35–49	5	7.9	8	4	6	7	11	11	11	11
50–64	1	11.0	0	11	11	11	11	11	11	11
65+	2	4.5	6	3	3	3	7	7	7	7
2. MULTIPLE DX										
0–19 Years	42	12.1	215	3	3	7	15	24	57	57
20–34	28	13.5	97	4	7	9	17	30	30	55
35–49	104	11.9	88	5	6	8	15	22	31	45
50–64	224	11.6	74	5	7	9	11	25	34	38
65+	654	13.1	69	5	8	11	15	22	29	43
TOTAL SINGLE DX	16	6.5	9	2	4	7	7	11	11	12
MULTIPLE DX	1052	12.5	79	5	7	10	15	23	33	45
TOTAL										
0–19 Years	49	11.1	186	3	3	7	12	21	57	57
20–34	29	13.3	96	4	6	9	17	30	30	55
35–49	109	11.8	86	5	6	9	15	22	31	45
50–64	225	11.6	74	5	7	9	11	24	34	38
65+	656	13.1	69	5	8	11	15	22	29	43
GRAND TOTAL	1068	12.4	78	5	7	10	15	23	33	43

Length of Stay by Diagnosis and Operation, United States, 1997

United States, October 1995–September 1996 Data, by Operation

46.2: ILEOSTOMY. Formerly included in operation group(s) 612.

Type of Patients	Observed Patients	Vari-ance	Avg. Stay	Percentiles						
				10th	25th	50th	75th	90th	95th	99th
1. SINGLE DX										
0–19 Years	3	0	8.0	8	8	8	>99	>99	>99	>99
20–34	8	50	14.3	5	7	20	20	20	20	20
35–49	5	31	10.4	3	5	9	16	16	16	16
50–64	1	0	5.0	5	5	5	5	5	5	5
65+	2	13	8.6	5	5	11	11	11	11	11
2. MULTIPLE DX										
0–19 Years	63	659	21.7	4	7	11	30	90	>99	>99
20–34	36	59	11.8	5	7	10	14	23	25	46
35–49	90	70	11.3	4	6	9	16	21	26	46
50–64	60	79	13.1	7	8	12	17	>99	>99	>99
65+	96	140	15.9	4	7	12	19	38	39	59
TOTAL SINGLE DX	19	39	11.1	5	7	9	20	20	>99	>99
MULTIPLE DX	345	227	15.3	5	7	11	18	39	76	>99
TOTAL										
0–19 Years	66	632	20.9	4	7	10	30	98	>99	>99
20–34	44	58	12.3	5	7	10	16	21	25	46
35–49	95	68	11.3	4	6	9	16	20	26	46
50–64	61	78	12.9	7	8	12	17	>99	>99	>99
65+	98	139	15.9	4	7	12	19	38	39	59
GRAND TOTAL	364	218	15.1	5	7	11	19	39	76	>99

46.32: PERC (ENDO) JEJUNOSTOMY. Formerly included in operation group(s) 612.

Type of Patients	Observed Patients	Avg. Stay	Vari-ance	Percentiles						
				10th	25th	50th	75th	90th	95th	99th
1. SINGLE DX										
0–19 Years	0									
20–34	0									
35–49	0									
50–64	1	5.0	0	5	5	5	5	5	5	5
65+	0									
2. MULTIPLE DX										
0–19 Years	45	10.2	85	4	7	8	11	15	24	53
20–34	21	14.5	69	4	8	14	21	21	35	35
35–49	37	17.4	306	3	6	14	19	43	70	70
50–64	73	19.3	247	3	7	12	40	40	40	52
65+	290	13.4	105	4	6	10	19	25	30	52
TOTAL SINGLE DX	1	5.0	0	5	5	5	5	5	5	5
MULTIPLE DX	466	14.4	145	4	6	10	20	33	40	53
TOTAL										
0–19 Years	45	10.2	85	4	7	8	11	15	24	53
20–34	21	14.5	69	4	8	14	21	21	35	35
35–49	37	17.4	306	3	6	14	19	43	70	70
50–64	74	19.3	247	3	7	12	40	40	40	52
65+	290	13.4	105	4	6	10	19	25	30	52
GRAND TOTAL	467	14.4	145	4	6	10	20	33	40	53

46.3: OTHER ENTEROSTOMY. Formerly included in operation group(s) 612.

Type of Patients	Observed Patients	Vari-ance	Avg. Stay	Percentiles						
				10th	25th	50th	75th	90th	95th	99th
1. SINGLE DX										
0–19 Years	4	21	7.0	3	3	3	12	12	12	12
20–34	2	2	1.6	1	1	1	1	5	5	5
35–49	5	1	3.2	1	2	4	4	4	4	4
50–64	2	<1	6.0	6	6	6	6	6	6	6
65+	7	18	3.5	1	1	3	4	5	16	16
2. MULTIPLE DX										
0–19 Years	128	138	12.9	2	6	8	17	30	37	>99
20–34	53	276	19.9	4	5	12	45	45	45	45
35–49	119	178	14.9	4	7	13	19	34	70	>99
50–64	185	221	15.6	3	5	9	22	40	40	57
65+	695	158	15.4	4	7	11	22	36	41	65
TOTAL SINGLE DX	20	10	4.8	1	3	4	6	11	12	16
MULTIPLE DX	1180	177	15.4	3	6	11	22	39	45	88
TOTAL										
0–19 Years	132	136	12.7	2	6	8	17	30	37	>99
20–34	55	278	19.4	4	5	12	45	45	45	45
35–49	124	177	14.5	4	6	11	18	34	70	>99
50–64	187	214	15.1	3	5	9	21	40	40	57
65+	702	158	15.3	4	7	11	22	36	41	65
GRAND TOTAL	1200	176	15.2	3	6	11	21	38	44	88

46.39: ENTEROSTOMY NEC. Formerly included in operation group(s) 612.

Type of Patients	Observed Patients	Avg. Stay	Vari-ance	Percentiles						
				10th	25th	50th	75th	90th	95th	99th
1. SINGLE DX										
0–19 Years	4	7.0	21	3	3	3	12	12	12	12
20–34	2	1.6	2	1	1	1	1	5	5	5
35–49	5	3.2	1	1	2	4	4	4	4	4
50–64	1	6.0	0	6	6	6	6	6	6	6
65+	7	3.5	18	1	1	3	4	5	16	16
2. MULTIPLE DX										
0–19 Years	83	13.9	155	2	5	9	25	31	41	>99
20–34	32	21.3	319	4	5	12	45	45	45	45
35–49	82	14.2	144	4	8	13	18	32	88	>99
50–64	112	12.5	179	3	5	9	17	27	33	98
65+	404	16.8	190	3	7	12	22	41	41	65
TOTAL SINGLE DX	19	4.8	11	1	3	4	6	11	12	16
MULTIPLE DX	713	15.9	194	3	6	12	22	41	45	>99
TOTAL										
0–19 Years	87	13.7	152	2	5	9	24	30	38	>99
20–34	34	20.6	321	4	5	12	45	45	45	45
35–49	87	13.8	143	4	7	11	17	32	81	>99
50–64	113	12.0	168	3	5	8	16	25	32	98
65+	411	16.7	190	3	7	12	22	41	41	65
GRAND TOTAL	732	15.6	192	3	6	11	22	41	45	>99

United States, October 1995–September 1996 Data, by Operation

46.4: INTESTINAL STOMA REV. Formerly included in operation group(s) 611.

Type of Patients	Observed Patients	Avg. Stay	Variance	10th	25th	50th	75th	90th	95th	99th
1. SINGLE DX										
0-19 Years	14	2.0	3	1	1	1	2	4	7	7
20-34	7	2.4	2	1	2	2	2	5	5	5
35-49	18	3.5	12	1	1	2	4	7	14	14
50-64	15	4.1	8	1	2	3	6	9	9	9
65+	26	5.0	12	2	3	5	6	7	9	21
2. MULTIPLE DX										
0-19 Years	75	6.2	27	2	2	5	10	11	16	38
20-34	90	8.6	88	2	4	6	8	21	24	46
35-49	206	8.0	55	2	3	6	9	20	20	47
50-64	276	5.9	33	1	2	4	8	11	15	30
65+	699	7.3	51	2	3	6	8	13	19	41
TOTAL SINGLE DX	80	3.4	9	1	1	2	5	7	9	14
MULTIPLE DX	1346	7.1	49	2	3	6	8	13	20	41
TOTAL										
0-19 Years	89	5.5	25	1	2	4	9	11	15	38
20-34	97	7.8	82	2	3	5	8	17	23	46
35-49	224	7.7	54	2	3	6	9	20	20	47
50-64	291	5.8	33	1	2	4	8	11	15	30
65+	725	7.2	50	2	3	6	8	13	19	41
GRAND TOTAL	1426	6.9	47	1	3	5	8	13	20	41

46.42: PERICOLOSTOMY HERNIA REP. Formerly included in operation group(s) 611.

Type of Patients	Observed Patients	Avg. Stay	Variance	10th	25th	50th	75th	90th	95th	99th
1. SINGLE DX										
0-19 Years	0									
20-34	2	2.3	<1	2	2	2	3	3	3	3
35-49	3	2.3	2	1	2	2	4	4	4	4
50-64	6	6.3	8	2	4	6	9	9	9	9
65+	11	4.4	13	1	2	4	5	6	16	16
2. MULTIPLE DX										
0-19 Years	3	2.8	7	1	1	1	6	7	7	7
20-34	12	5.7	26	1	2	5	6	9	13	31
35-49	40	4.4	19	1	2	3	5	8	13	18
50-64	90	4.1	13	1	1	2	7	10	10	15
65+	322	7.1	28	3	4	6	8	12	19	31
TOTAL SINGLE DX	22	4.6	10	2	2	4	6	9	9	16
MULTIPLE DX	467	6.0	25	2	3	5	8	11	15	31
TOTAL										
0-19 Years	3	2.8	7	1	1	1	6	7	7	7
20-34	14	5.1	24	1	2	5	6	8	13	31
35-49	43	4.4	19	2	2	3	5	8	11	18
50-64	96	4.2	13	1	1	2	7	10	10	15
65+	333	7.1	28	3	4	6	8	12	19	31
GRAND TOTAL	489	6.0	25	2	3	5	8	11	15	27

46.41: SM BOWEL STOMA REVISION. Formerly included in operation group(s) 611.

Type of Patients	Observed Patients	Avg. Stay	Variance	10th	25th	50th	75th	90th	95th	99th
1. SINGLE DX										
0-19 Years	4	1.5	<1	1	1	1	2	2	2	2
20-34	3	1.9	<1	1	2	2	2	2	2	2
35-49	7	5.5	9	2	4	4	6	12	12	12
50-64	5	2.4	<1	1	2	3	3	3	3	3
65+	5	5.3	5	1	3	7	7	7	7	7
2. MULTIPLE DX										
0-19 Years	39	7.2	24	2	3	7	10	12	16	>99
20-34	51	9.2	93	2	4	7	8	21	24	61
35-49	106	9.4	66	3	5	6	13	20	23	47
50-64	95	7.8	46	3	4	6	9	15	28	31
65+	122	7.3	93	1	2	5	8	15	28	36
TOTAL SINGLE DX	24	3.2	6	1	2	2	4	7	7	12
MULTIPLE DX	413	8.2	68	2	3	6	10	20	26	47
TOTAL										
0-19 Years	43	6.6	24	1	2	6	10	11	16	>99
20-34	54	8.5	89	2	5	6	8	21	23	61
35-49	113	9.3	65	2	5	6	13	20	23	47
50-64	100	7.6	46	2	3	5	9	15	28	31
65+	127	7.2	90	1	2	5	8	15	27	36
GRAND TOTAL	437	8.0	67	2	3	6	9	20	24	47

46.43: LG BOWEL STOMA REV NEC. Formerly included in operation group(s) 611.

Type of Patients	Observed Patients	Avg. Stay	Variance	10th	25th	50th	75th	90th	95th	99th
1. SINGLE DX										
0-19 Years	10	2.3	4	1	1	1	3	7	7	7
20-34	2	3.1	4	1	1	5	5	5	5	5
35-49	7	2.9	13	1	1	1	3	6	14	14
50-64	3	2.6	2	1	1	2	4	4	4	4
65+	10	5.1	16	2	3	4	6	9	9	21
2. MULTIPLE DX										
0-19 Years	33	5.2	30	2	2	4	5	9	16	38
20-34	27	8.7	104	2	4	6	8	13	46	46
35-49	58	6.9	35	2	3	6	9	12	13	45
50-64	81	7.0	46	2	3	6	9	13	19	42
65+	242	7.3	60	1	3	5	8	13	17	41
TOTAL SINGLE DX	32	3.2	10	1	1	2	4	6	9	14
MULTIPLE DX	441	7.1	54	2	3	5	9	13	17	41
TOTAL										
0-19 Years	43	4.5	25	1	2	4	5	7	14	38
20-34	29	8.0	95	1	4	5	7	13	46	46
35-49	65	6.3	34	1	2	5	9	12	13	25
50-64	84	6.9	45	2	3	5	9	13	19	42
65+	252	7.2	58	1	3	5	8	13	17	41
GRAND TOTAL	473	6.8	52	1	3	5	8	13	16	41

Percentiles apply to the 10th–99th columns.

Length of Stay by Diagnosis and Operation, United States, 1997

United States, October 1995–September 1996 Data, by Operation

46.5: CLOSURE INTESTINAL STOMA. Formerly included in operation group(s) 611.

Type of Patients	Observed Patients	Avg. Stay	Vari-ance	10th	25th	50th	75th	90th	95th	99th
1. SINGLE DX										
0–19 Years	245	5.6	3	4	4	6	6	8	9	10
20–34	212	5.1	3	3	4	5	6	7	9	9
35–49	247	4.9	4	3	4	4	6	7	8	10
50–64	162	5.8	3	4	5	6	6	9	9	11
65+	99	5.9	4	3	4	6	7	8	9	10
2. MULTIPLE DX										
0–19 Years	761	7.6	61	4	4	6	8	12	24	56
20–34	662	6.4	16	3	4	5	8	10	13	22
35–49	1226	7.1	34	4	5	6	8	10	13	28
50–64	1397	7.4	18	4	5	7	8	11	14	21
65+	2265	8.5	34	4	6	7	10	14	18	29
TOTAL SINGLE DX	965	5.4	3	3	4	5	6	8	9	10
MULTIPLE DX	6311	7.6	32	4	5	6	8	12	16	28
TOTAL										
0–19 Years	1006	7.1	47	4	4	6	7	10	19	44
20–34	874	6.1	13	3	4	5	7	10	11	21
35–49	1473	6.7	31	4	4	6	8	10	12	26
50–64	1559	7.2	16	4	5	6	8	11	14	19
65+	2364	8.4	33	4	6	7	10	14	17	29
GRAND TOTAL	7276	7.3	29	4	5	6	8	11	15	26

46.51: SM BOWEL STOMA CLOSURE. Formerly included in operation group(s) 611.

Type of Patients	Observed Patients	Avg. Stay	Vari-ance	10th	25th	50th	75th	90th	95th	99th
1. SINGLE DX										
0–19 Years	89	6.0	5	3	4	6	8	9	9	10
20–34	60	4.3	4	3	3	4	5	6	7	13
35–49	49	4.0	6	1	3	4	6	7	8	11
50–64	22	7.0	6	3	5	9	9	9	9	9
65+	9	4.1	3	3	3	3	6	7	8	8
2. MULTIPLE DX										
0–19 Years	334	9.6	116	4	5	6	9	20	27	64
20–34	344	6.8	21	3	4	6	9	10	13	26
35–49	373	6.1	27	3	4	5	7	10	12	29
50–64	301	8.2	34	3	4	6	11	16	16	28
65+	312	8.4	42	3	5	7	10	14	18	38
TOTAL SINGLE DX	229	5.3	6	3	4	5	8	9	9	11
MULTIPLE DX	1664	7.7	48	3	4	6	9	14	18	43
TOTAL										
0–19 Years	423	8.8	93	3	4	6	9	19	26	56
20–34	404	6.5	19	3	4	5	8	10	13	25
35–49	422	5.9	25	3	4	5	7	9	12	29
50–64	323	8.1	32	3	4	7	10	16	16	28
65+	321	8.3	42	3	5	7	10	14	17	38
GRAND TOTAL	1893	7.4	44	3	4	6	9	13	17	41

46.52: LG BOWEL STOMA CLOSURE. Formerly included in operation group(s) 611.

Type of Patients	Observed Patients	Avg. Stay	Vari-ance	10th	25th	50th	75th	90th	95th	99th
1. SINGLE DX										
0–19 Years	155	5.3	2	4	5	6	6	6	7	9
20–34	152	5.4	2	4	5	5	6	7	8	9
35–49	198	5.0	3	3	4	5	6	7	8	9
50–64	140	5.6	2	4	5	5	6	7	8	11
65+	90	6.2	3	4	5	6	7	8	9	11
2. MULTIPLE DX										
0–19 Years	424	6.3	20	3	4	6	7	9	11	24
20–34	315	6.1	13	3	5	5	7	9	11	19
35–49	853	7.5	37	4	5	6	8	10	13	28
50–64	1093	7.2	14	4	5	7	8	10	13	19
65+	1951	8.5	33	5	6	7	10	13	18	26
TOTAL SINGLE DX	735	5.4	3	3	4	5	6	7	8	10
MULTIPLE DX	4636	7.5	26	4	5	7	8	11	15	24
TOTAL										
0–19 Years	579	6.0	15	4	5	6	6	8	10	24
20–34	467	5.9	10	3	5	5	7	9	10	17
35–49	1051	7.0	32	4	5	6	8	10	12	22
50–64	1233	7.0	13	4	5	6	8	10	13	19
65+	2041	8.5	32	4	6	7	9	13	17	24
GRAND TOTAL	5371	7.2	24	4	5	6	8	11	14	23

46.6: FIXATION OF INTESTINE. Formerly included in operation group(s) 611.

Type of Patients	Observed Patients	Avg. Stay	Vari-ance	10th	25th	50th	75th	90th	95th	99th
1. SINGLE DX										
0–19 Years	4	5.8	19	3	3	4	4	13	13	13
20–34	2	5.1	<1	5	5	5	5	6	6	6
35–49	1	6.0	0	6	6	6	6	6	6	6
50–64	2	7.3	20	5	5	5	5	15	15	15
65+	0									
2. MULTIPLE DX										
0–19 Years	11	15.2	597	2	5	5	11	74	74	>99
20–34	10	2.9	5	1	1	1	5	6	7	7
35–49	20	7.9	22	5	6	6	7	19	20	20
50–64	15	10.8	29	3	5	12	15	18	18	18
65+	48	9.7	23	3	6	10	12	16	18	23
TOTAL SINGLE DX	9	6.1	13	3	4	5	6	13	15	15
MULTIPLE DX	104	8.8	68	2	5	6	12	18	19	74
TOTAL										
0–19 Years	15	12.5	445	2	3	5	11	74	74	>99
20–34	12	3.1	5	1	1	1	5	6	6	7
35–49	21	7.9	21	5	6	6	7	19	20	20
50–64	17	10.5	29	3	5	12	15	18	18	18
65+	48	9.7	23	3	6	10	12	16	18	23
GRAND TOTAL	113	8.7	65	2	4	6	12	16	18	74

Length of Stay by Diagnosis and Operation, United States, 1997

United States, October 1995–September 1996 Data, by Operation

46.7: OTHER INTESTINAL REPAIR. Formerly included in operation group(s) 611.

Type of Patients	Observed Patients	Avg. Stay	Vari-ance	10th	25th	50th	75th	90th	95th	99th
1. SINGLE DX										
0–19 Years	58	5.6	4	4	5	5	6	9	10	13
20–34	54	5.6	7	3	5	5	6	7	10	25
35–49	29	5.8	7	3	4	5	8	11	11	11
50–64	11	6.9	4	5	6	7	7	10	10	10
65+	3	7.3	4	5	8	8	8	8	8	8
2. MULTIPLE DX										
0–19 Years	324	10.9	189	1	5	7	11	23	44	>99
20–34	588	8.6	48	4	5	7	10	17	22	39
35–49	586	10.1	90	3	5	7	12	17	26	62
50–64	504	13.5	156	5	7	9	16	28	44	72
65+	951	14.9	169	5	7	11	19	26	37	71
TOTAL SINGLE DX	155	5.9	6	3	5	6	6	8	10	13
MULTIPLE DX	2953	12.0	137	4	6	8	13	24	35	71
TOTAL										
0–19 Years	382	10.2	168	1	5	7	10	20	37	92
20–34	642	8.3	44	3	5	6	9	16	21	37
35–49	615	10.0	88	4	5	7	12	17	25	62
50–64	515	13.3	151	5	7	9	15	28	42	72
65+	954	14.9	169	5	7	11	18	26	37	71
GRAND TOTAL	3108	11.6	132	4	5	8	13	24	34	71

46.74: CLOSURE SMB FISTULA NEC. Formerly included in operation group(s) 611.

Type of Patients	Observed Patients	Avg. Stay	Vari-ance	10th	25th	50th	75th	90th	95th	99th
1. SINGLE DX										
0–19 Years	4	2.6	3	1	1	3	4	6	6	6
20–34	1	3.0	0	3	3	3	3	3	3	6
35–49	1	8.0	0	8	8	8	8	8	8	8
50–64	2	6.8	<1	7	7	7	7	7	7	7
65+	0									
2. MULTIPLE DX										
0–19 Years	14	11.9	313	4	5	6	18	28	>99	>99
20–34	37	12.7	94	5	6	9	20	28	39	>99
35–49	85	10.4	109	5	7	7	9	18	32	76
50–64	97	20.5	371	5	7	13	28	58	58	76
65+	130	19.2	109	7	11	21	25	29	31	94
TOTAL SINGLE DX	8	5.4	5	1	3	7	7	7	7	8
MULTIPLE DX	363	16.6	203	5	7	12	24	32	58	94
TOTAL										
0–19 Years	18	9.2	240	1	4	5	11	18	94	>99
20–34	38	12.1	93	3	5	9	20	27	39	>99
35–49	86	10.4	108	5	7	7	9	18	32	76
50–64	99	19.4	355	5	7	12	25	58	58	76
65+	130	19.2	109	7	11	21	25	29	31	94
GRAND TOTAL	371	16.1	200	5	7	11	24	31	58	94

46.73: SMALL BOWEL SUTURE NEC. Formerly included in operation group(s) 611.

Type of Patients	Observed Patients	Avg. Stay	Vari-ance	10th	25th	50th	75th	90th	95th	99th
1. SINGLE DX										
0–19 Years	32	5.3	<1	4	5	5	6	6	6	10
20–34	32	5.9	15	3	4	5	7	8	9	25
35–49	12	4.7	1	3	4	5	6	8	9	6
50–64	4	5.7	7	2	2	7	8	8	8	8
65+	1	8.0	0	8	8	8	8	8	8	8
2. MULTIPLE DX										
0–19 Years	160	7.7	94	1	2	6	8	16	25	65
20–34	276	7.7	38	3	5	6	9	15	17	36
35–49	222	9.1	49	4	5	7	11	16	22	39
50–64	201	11.9	87	5	8	9	13	23	33	76
65+	343	12.9	82	4	7	11	17	23	27	55
TOTAL SINGLE DX	81	5.6	6	4	5	5	6	8	8	10
MULTIPLE DX	1202	10.0	74	3	5	8	12	19	25	50
TOTAL										
0–19 Years	192	7.3	80	1	4	6	8	13	25	65
20–34	308	7.6	36	3	5	6	8	14	17	29
35–49	234	9.0	48	3	5	7	10	15	22	39
50–64	205	11.9	87	5	8	9	13	23	33	76
65+	344	12.8	81	4	7	11	16	23	26	55
GRAND TOTAL	1283	9.7	71	3	5	8	12	19	25	50

46.75: SUTURE LG BOWEL LAC. Formerly included in operation group(s) 611.

Type of Patients	Observed Patients	Avg. Stay	Vari-ance	10th	25th	50th	75th	90th	95th	99th
1. SINGLE DX										
0–19 Years	8	5.4	6	3	3	5	7	9	9	9
20–34	13	4.7	4	2	2	5	6	7	8	8
35–49	10	4.9	7	3	4	4	5	11	11	11
50–64	3	8.2	6	5	5	10	10	10	10	11
65+	1	5.0	0	5	5	5	5	5	5	5
2. MULTIPLE DX										
0–19 Years	66	14.8	306	5	6	7	13	60	60	60
20–34	171	8.5	42	4	5	6	10	14	24	37
35–49	140	7.2	60	3	4	6	8	11	17	43
50–64	86	9.1	56	4	5	6	8	18	22	47
65+	232	14.7	269	5	6	9	14	31	71	71
TOTAL SINGLE DX	35	5.8	7	2	4	5	8	10	10	11
MULTIPLE DX	695	11.0	159	4	5	7	11	19	34	71
TOTAL										
0–19 Years	74	14.1	292	4	6	7	13	60	60	60
20–34	184	8.3	41	3	5	6	10	14	22	37
35–49	150	7.1	57	3	4	5	8	11	15	43
50–64	89	9.0	53	4	5	6	9	18	20	44
65+	233	14.7	268	5	6	9	14	31	71	71
GRAND TOTAL	730	10.8	154	4	5	7	11	19	32	71

Length of Stay by Diagnosis and Operation, United States, 1997

United States, October 1995–September 1996 Data, by Operation

46.79: REPAIR OF INTESTINE NEC. Formerly included in operation group(s) 611.

Type of Patients	Observed Patients	Avg. Stay	Vari-ance	10th	25th	50th	75th	90th	95th	99th
1. SINGLE DX										
0–19 Years	9	7.6	11	4	6	6	9	13	13	13
20–34	5	6.0	<1	6	6	6	6	6	7	7
35–49	4	9.3	0	8	9	9	11	11	11	11
50–64	1	6.0	0	6	6	6	6	6	6	6
65+	1	1.0	0	1	1	1	1	1	1	1
2. MULTIPLE DX										
0–19 Years	47	17.5	432	5	6	12	17	47	92	>99
20–34	50	8.7	17	5	6	7	10	14	23	>99
35–49	89	11.1	51	4	7	12	12	15	22	49
50–64	78	14.4	141	4	7	11	19	32	49	49
65+	156	13.1	92	5	7	10	18	23	33	65
TOTAL SINGLE DX	20	6.5	4	5	6	6	6	9	11	13
MULTIPLE DX	420	13.0	129	5	7	11	15	22	36	92
TOTAL										
0–19 Years	56	16.2	388	5	6	11	16	43	92	>99
20–34	55	7.6	12	5	6	6	8	12	15	23
35–49	93	11.1	49	5	7	12	12	15	22	49
50–64	79	14.1	139	4	7	11	19	31	49	49
65+	157	13.0	92	5	7	10	18	23	33	65
GRAND TOTAL	440	12.5	122	5	6	9	14	21	34	92

46.8: BOWEL DILATION & MANIP. Formerly included in operation group(s) 611.

Type of Patients	Observed Patients	Avg. Stay	Vari-ance	10th	25th	50th	75th	90th	95th	99th
1. SINGLE DX										
0–19 Years	225	3.3	3	1	2	3	4	6	6	9
20–34	11	3.3	3	1	2	3	5	6	6	7
35–49	15	8.3	99	1	2	5	7	30	30	30
50–64	13	2.6	4	1	1	2	4	6	6	6
65+	10	2.5	3	1	1	2	3	5	5	7
2. MULTIPLE DX										
0–19 Years	357	6.9	54	2	3	5	9	12	18	35
20–34	81	6.5	39	2	4	6	7	10	13	38
35–49	152	7.3	21	2	4	7	9	15	15	21
50–64	221	7.9	41	1	5	6	12	16	19	29
65+	854	10.7	61	3	5	9	15	20	24	36
TOTAL SINGLE DX	274	3.4	7	1	2	3	4	6	6	9
MULTIPLE DX	1665	8.7	54	2	4	7	11	17	21	35
TOTAL										
0–19 Years	582	5.7	39	2	3	4	7	10	15	28
20–34	92	6.2	36	2	3	5	7	10	12	38
35–49	167	7.4	25	2	4	7	9	15	15	25
50–64	234	7.8	41	1	2	6	12	16	19	29
65+	864	10.7	61	3	5	9	15	20	24	36
GRAND TOTAL	1939	7.9	50	2	3	6	10	16	20	35

46.81: INTRA-ABD SM BOWEL MANIP. Formerly included in operation group(s) 611.

Type of Patients	Observed Patients	Avg. Stay	Vari-ance	10th	25th	50th	75th	90th	95th	99th
1. SINGLE DX										
0–19 Years	90	4.0	4	2	2	4	6	6	7	10
20–34	7	3.8	4	1	3	4	6	6	7	7
35–49	8	13.5	130	5	5	7	30	30	30	30
50–64	4	2.5	5	1	1	1	5	6	6	6
65+	1	1.0	0	1	1	1	1	1	1	1
2. MULTIPLE DX										
0–19 Years	174	7.2	75	3	4	5	7	12	19	81
20–34	41	6.9	33	4	5	6	7	10	10	53
35–49	69	9.1	17	4	6	8	13	15	15	18
50–64	105	9.6	29	4	5	8	12	16	21	29
65+	252	12.4	38	6	8	11	16	19	21	35
TOTAL SINGLE DX	110	4.3	12	1	2	4	6	6	7	30
MULTIPLE DX	641	9.4	50	4	5	8	12	18	20	34
TOTAL										
0–19 Years	264	6.1	53	2	3	5	6	10	16	42
20–34	48	6.6	31	3	5	6	7	10	10	53
35–49	77	9.4	25	4	6	8	14	15	18	30
50–64	109	9.5	30	4	5	8	12	15	21	29
65+	253	12.3	38	6	8	11	16	19	21	35
GRAND TOTAL	751	8.6	47	3	4	7	11	17	19	31

46.82: INTRA-ABD LG BOWEL MANIP. Formerly included in operation group(s) 611.

Type of Patients	Observed Patients	Avg. Stay	Vari-ance	10th	25th	50th	75th	90th	95th	99th
1. SINGLE DX										
0–19 Years	80	3.0	2	2	2	3	3	4	5	8
20–34	1	2.0	0	2	2	2	2	2	2	2
35–49	3	3.0	2	1	1	4	4	4	4	4
50–64	4	2.8	2	2	2	2	4	5	5	5
65+	1	1.0	0	1	1	1	1	1	1	1
2. MULTIPLE DX										
0–19 Years	136	6.0	16	2	3	5	10	10	11	19
20–34	19	3.6	7	1	2	3	4	6	12	13
35–49	18	7.2	6	4	7	7	8	11	12	15
50–64	27	7.4	15	2	4	6	10	13	14	19
65+	88	10.0	82	2	5	8	12	21	23	45
TOTAL SINGLE DX	89	3.0	2	2	2	3	3	4	5	8
MULTIPLE DX	288	6.8	31	2	3	5	10	12	16	23
TOTAL										
0–19 Years	216	5.1	13	2	3	3	7	10	10	18
20–34	20	3.6	7	1	2	3	4	6	9	13
35–49	21	6.8	7	4	5	7	7	11	12	15
50–64	31	7.0	16	2	4	6	10	13	14	19
65+	89	9.9	82	2	5	8	12	20	23	45
GRAND TOTAL	377	6.0	27	2	3	4	9	10	14	23

Length of Stay by Diagnosis and Operation, United States, 1997

United States, October 1995–September 1996 Data, by Operation

46.85: DILATION OF INTESTINE. Formerly included in operation group(s) 611.

Type of Patients	Observed Patients	Avg. Stay	Vari-ance	Percentiles						
				10th	25th	50th	75th	90th	95th	99th
1. SINGLE DX										
0–19 Years	17	1.2	<1	1	1	1	1	2	2	2
20–34	2	2.8	<1	2	3	3	3	3	3	3
35–49	4	1.9	<1	1	2	2	2	3	3	3
50–64	5	2.3	4	1	1	1	3	6	6	6
65+	6	2.6	3	1	2	2	3	5	7	7
2. MULTIPLE DX										
0–19 Years	16	4.1	18	1	1	3	5	6	8	20
20–34	20	8.4	83	2	3	6	8	18	38	38
35–49	64	5.0	22	2	2	3	7	11	14	23
50–64	85	6.7	48	1	3	3	15	16	16	29
65+	499	10.0	68	3	4	8	14	23	24	38
TOTAL SINGLE DX	34	1.7	1	1	1	1	2	3	3	7
MULTIPLE DX	684	8.6	62	1	3	6	13	18	24	35
TOTAL										
0–19 Years	33	2.3	9	1	1	1	2	5	6	20
20–34	22	7.9	78	2	2	5	8	14	38	38
35–49	68	4.9	21	1	2	3	5	11	14	23
50–64	90	6.7	48	1	4	8	15	16	16	29
65+	505	9.9	68	2	4	8	13	23	24	38
GRAND TOTAL	718	8.3	62	1	3	5	12	18	24	35

47.0: APPENDECTOMY. Formerly included in operation group(s) 613.

Type of Patients	Observed Patients	Avg. Stay	Vari-ance	Percentiles						
				10th	25th	50th	75th	90th	95th	99th
1. SINGLE DX										
0–19 Years	14164	2.6	3	1	1	2	3	5	6	8
20–34	10921	2.2	2	1	1	2	3	4	5	7
35–49	4860	2.5	3	1	2	2	3	4	5	9
50–64	1472	3.0	4	1	2	3	4	5	7	8
65+	286	4.0	6	2	2	3	5	7	11	11
2. MULTIPLE DX										
0–19 Years	8903	4.6	15	1	2	3	6	9	11	19
20–34	7968	3.7	11	1	2	3	5	7	9	16
35–49	6071	4.6	12	1	2	4	6	9	11	16
50–64	3520	5.4	16	2	3	5	7	10	13	18
65+	2877	7.0	26	2	4	6	9	12	15	26
TOTAL SINGLE DX	31703	2.5	3	1	1	2	3	4	6	8
MULTIPLE DX	29339	4.6	15	1	2	4	6	9	11	19
TOTAL										
0–19 Years	23067	3.3	9	1	2	2	4	7	8	14
20–34	18889	2.9	6	1	2	2	3	5	7	12
35–49	10931	3.6	9	1	2	3	5	7	9	15
50–64	4992	4.6	13	2	3	4	6	9	11	17
65+	3163	6.7	25	2	4	6	8	12	14	26
GRAND TOTAL	61042	3.5	9	1	2	3	4	7	9	15

46.9: OTHER INTESTINAL OPS. Formerly included in operation group(s) 611.

Type of Patients	Observed Patients	Avg. Stay	Vari-ance	Percentiles						
				10th	25th	50th	75th	90th	95th	99th
1. SINGLE DX										
0–19 Years	2	2.7	2	2	2	2	4	4	4	4
20–34	1	8.0	0	8	8	8	8	8	8	8
35–49	3	5.0	0	5	5	5	5	5	5	5
50–64	3	5.3	2	4	4	5	7	7	7	7
65+	0									
2. MULTIPLE DX										
0–19 Years	23	16.0	329	6	6	9	19	33	63	>99
20–34	39	17.1	324	4	6	9	20	61	61	68
35–49	80	9.4	34	4	5	7	14	18	20	25
50–64	79	10.0	30	5	6	9	11	16	22	25
65+	77	14.0	93	7	7	11	18	35	38	46
TOTAL SINGLE DX	7	5.3	4	2	4	5	7	8	8	8
MULTIPLE DX	298	12.7	116	5	7	10	15	24	38	61
TOTAL										
0–19 Years	25	15.6	324	6	6	9	19	33	63	>99
20–34	40	16.9	320	4	6	9	20	39	61	68
35–49	81	9.4	34	4	5	7	14	18	20	25
50–64	82	9.9	30	5	6	9	11	16	22	25
65+	77	14.0	93	7	7	11	18	35	38	46
GRAND TOTAL	305	12.6	116	5	7	10	15	23	38	61

47.1: INCIDENTAL APPENDECTOMY. Formerly included in operation group(s) 613.

Type of Patients	Observed Patients	Avg. Stay	Vari-ance	Percentiles						
				10th	25th	50th	75th	90th	95th	99th
1. SINGLE DX										
0–19 Years	44	2.4	1	1	1	2	3	4	5	5
20–34	52	2.8	1	1	2	3	4	4	5	5
35–49	25	3.7	4	2	2	4	4	6	8	11
50–64	6	2.3	1	2	2	2	2	3	6	6
65+	0									
2. MULTIPLE DX										
0–19 Years	86	5.8	60	2	2	4	6	10	22	22
20–34	107	3.6	7	1	2	3	4	6	7	19
35–49	78	4.7	22	1	2	3	6	13	15	23
50–64	32	7.7	32	2	5	5	9	13	14	34
65+	30	12.1	206	5	5	7	11	28	31	82
TOTAL SINGLE DX	127	2.8	2	1	2	3	4	4	5	8
MULTIPLE DX	333	5.3	43	1	2	4	6	10	15	28
TOTAL										
0–19 Years	130	4.6	42	1	2	3	4	8	12	22
20–34	159	3.3	5	1	2	3	3	5	6	14
35–49	103	4.4	17	2	2	4	5	9	15	23
50–64	38	5.4	26	2	5	4	7	12	13	34
65+	30	12.1	206	5	5	7	11	28	31	82
GRAND TOTAL	460	4.5	31	1	2	3	5	8	12	23

Length of Stay by Diagnosis and Operation, United States, 1997

United States, October 1995–September 1996 Data, by Operation

47.2: DRAIN APPENDICEAL ABSC. Formerly included in operation group(s) 614.

Type of Patients	Observed Patients	Avg. Stay	Variance	Percentiles						
				10th	25th	50th	75th	90th	95th	99th
1. SINGLE DX										
0–19 Years	37	5.7	13	2	2	6	8	10	11	17
20–34	17	5.0	4	4	4	4	6	8	10	10
35–49	13	6.3	5	2	5	7	8	8	8	8
50–64	3	4.2	<1	4	4	4	4	6	6	6
65+	1	7.0	0	7	7	7	7	7	7	7
2. MULTIPLE DX										
0–19 Years	41	6.3	9	4	5	5	7	9	12	17
20–34	32	7.9	44	4	5	6	8	14	16	40
35–49	44	7.4	9	4	5	8	8	10	14	17
50–64	25	10.6	31	4	5	11	14	16	26	26
65+	26	8.7	74	3	3	6	10	23	23	46
TOTAL SINGLE DX	71	5.2	6	2	4	4	7	8	10	15
MULTIPLE DX	168	7.8	28	3	5	6	9	14	16	26
TOTAL										
0–19 Years	78	6.1	10	2	5	5	7	10	12	17
20–34	49	6.5	28	4	4	5	7	10	14	33
35–49	57	7.1	8	3	5	7	9	9	14	17
50–64	28	7.2	25	4	4	4	11	14	14	26
65+	27	8.7	72	3	3	6	10	20	23	46
GRAND TOTAL	239	6.8	21	3	4	5	8	12	14	26

47.9: OTHER APPENDICEAL OPS. Formerly included in operation group(s) 614.

Type of Patients	Observed Patients	Avg. Stay	Variance	Percentiles						
				10th	25th	50th	75th	90th	95th	99th
1. SINGLE DX										
0–19 Years	2	5.3	3	4	4	4	7	7	7	7
20–34	2	5.1	1	4	4	6	6	6	6	6
35–49	1	12.0	0	12	12	12	12	12	12	12
50–64	0									
65+	0									
2. MULTIPLE DX										
0–19 Years	51	6.0	29	3	3	4	7	9	14	28
20–34	6	3.8	3	3	3	3	4	5	9	9
35–49	3	4.9	9	2	2	5	8	8	8	8
50–64	1	9.0	0	9	9	9	9	9	9	9
65+	2	8.1	8	6	6	10	10	10	10	10
TOTAL SINGLE DX	5	5.8	6	4	4	6	7	7	12	12
MULTIPLE DX	63	5.6	24	3	3	4	7	9	11	28
TOTAL										
0–19 Years	53	5.9	28	3	4	4	7	9	14	28
20–34	8	4.0	3	3	3	3	4	6	8	9
35–49	4	6.3	17	2	2	5	8	12	12	12
50–64	1	9.0	0	9	9	9	9	9	9	9
65+	2	8.1	8	6	6	10	10	10	10	10
GRAND TOTAL	68	5.6	23	3	3	4	7	9	11	28

48.0: PROCTOTOMY. Formerly included in operation group(s) 616.

Type of Patients	Observed Patients	Avg. Stay	Variance	Percentiles						
				10th	25th	50th	75th	90th	95th	99th
1. SINGLE DX										
0–19 Years	5	3.1	6	1	1	1	6	6	6	6
20–34	24	2.0	3	1	1	1	2	3	6	7
35–49	25	2.1	4	1	1	1	2	4	7	8
50–64	9	1.1	<1	1	1	1	1	2	2	2
65+	2	1.0	0	1	1	1	1	1	1	1
2. MULTIPLE DX										
0–19 Years	22	5.4	13	2	3	4	8	12	12	18
20–34	47	3.8	11	1	3	4	4	5	10	19
35–49	63	3.3	11	1	1	3	4	8	8	21
50–64	48	4.1	11	2	2	3	4	9	13	13
65+	58	5.7	49	1	2	3	7	9	20	54
TOTAL SINGLE DX	65	2.0	3	1	1	1	2	5	7	8
MULTIPLE DX	238	4.2	17	1	2	3	4	8	13	21
TOTAL										
0–19 Years	27	5.0	13	1	3	4	7	10	12	17
20–34	71	3.5	10	1	2	3	4	5	7	19
35–49	88	3.0	9	1	1	2	4	7	8	21
50–64	57	3.7	11	1	2	2	4	8	13	13
65+	60	5.7	48	1	2	3	7	9	20	54
GRAND TOTAL	303	3.8	15	1	2	3	4	8	12	20

48.1: PROCTOSTOMY. Formerly included in operation group(s) 618.

Type of Patients	Observed Patients	Avg. Stay	Variance	Percentiles						
				10th	25th	50th	75th	90th	95th	99th
1. SINGLE DX										
0–19 Years	0									
20–34	0									
35–49	0									
65+	0									
2. MULTIPLE DX										
0–19 Years	0									
20–34	0									
35–49	0									
50–64	1	5.0	0	5	5	5	5	5	5	5
65+	2	9.0	3	8	8	8	11	11	11	11
TOTAL SINGLE DX	0									
MULTIPLE DX	3	7.4	6	5	5	8	8	11	11	11
TOTAL										
0–19 Years	0									
20–34	0									
35–49	0									
50–64	1	5.0	0	5	5	5	5	5	5	5
65+	2	9.0	3	8	8	8	11	11	11	11
GRAND TOTAL	3	7.4	6	5	5	8	8	11	11	11

Length of Stay by Diagnosis and Operation, United States, 1997

United States, October 1995–September 1996 Data, by Operation

48.2: RECTAL/PERIRECT DXTIC PX. Formerly included in operation group(s) 615, 618, 631.

Type of Patients	Observed Patients	Avg. Stay	Variance	10th	25th	50th	75th	90th	95th	99th
1. SINGLE DX										
0–19 Years	181	2.7	5	1	1	2	3	5	6	16
20–34	66	1.9	4	1	1	1	2	4	6	11
35–49	60	2.1	4	1	1	1	2	4	7	8
50–64	21	2.2	4	1	1	2	2	5	7	9
65+	27	3.6	18	1	1	2	4	10	15	15
2. MULTIPLE DX										
0–19 Years	463	7.4	85	1	2	5	9	14	24	52
20–34	390	4.3	22	1	1	3	6	9	10	19
35–49	508	4.9	25	1	2	3	6	10	14	26
50–64	582	5.6	23	2	2	4	6	11	16	26
65+	1954	6.5	36	2	3	5	8	13	17	31
TOTAL SINGLE DX	355	2.4	5	1	1	1	3	5	7	11
MULTIPLE DX	3897	5.9	37	1	2	4	7	12	16	31
TOTAL										
0–19 Years	644	5.9	64	1	2	3	7	12	19	44
20–34	456	3.9	19	1	1	3	5	9	10	17
35–49	568	4.6	23	1	2	3	6	10	13	25
50–64	603	5.4	23	1	2	4	6	11	15	26
65+	1981	6.5	36	2	3	5	8	13	17	31
GRAND TOTAL	4252	5.6	35	2	2	4	7	11	15	28

48.24: CLSD (ENDO) RECTAL BX. Formerly included in operation group(s) 615.

Type of Patients	Observed Patients	Avg. Stay	Variance	10th	25th	50th	75th	90th	95th	99th
1. SINGLE DX										
0–19 Years	134	3.0	6	1	1	2	4	5	7	16
20–34	27	3.5	5	1	2	3	4	6	7	11
35–49	21	3.4	7	1	2	2	4	7	8	12
50–64	8	1.7	2	1	1	1	2	3	6	10
65+	12	3.9	20	1	2	2	4	14	14	14
2. MULTIPLE DX										
0–19 Years	368	7.7	93	1	3	5	9	15	28	66
20–34	239	5.4	26	2	3	4	7	10	11	23
35–49	306	5.5	26	2	2	4	7	12	15	25
50–64	355	5.2	16	1	3	5	6	10	12	25
65+	1146	6.9	37	2	4	6	8	13	17	27
TOTAL SINGLE DX	202	3.0	6	1	1	2	4	6	8	16
MULTIPLE DX	2414	6.3	39	2	3	5	8	12	16	33
TOTAL										
0–19 Years	502	6.2	71	1	2	4	7	12	21	47
20–34	266	5.3	25	1	3	4	7	10	11	23
35–49	327	5.4	25	1	2	4	7	11	14	25
50–64	363	5.0	16	1	2	4	6	10	12	25
65+	1158	6.9	37	2	4	6	8	13	17	27
GRAND TOTAL	2616	6.1	37	1	3	5	7	11	16	29

48.23: RIGID PROCTSIGMOIDOSCOPY. Formerly included in operation group(s) 631.

Type of Patients	Observed Patients	Avg. Stay	Variance	10th	25th	50th	75th	90th	95th	99th
1. SINGLE DX										
0–19 Years	30	1.8	3	1	1	1	2	4	6	11
20–34	39	1.4	2	1	1	1	1	2	3	9
35–49	37	1.8	2	1	1	1	2	4	4	8
50–64	11	2.9	4	1	1	2	5	7	7	7
65+	15	3.4	17	1	1	2	4	10	15	15
2. MULTIPLE DX										
0–19 Years	52	6.7	36	1	2	4	11	19	19	26
20–34	146	2.9	13	1	1	1	4	7	9	13
35–49	190	3.8	20	1	2	3	4	7	10	27
50–64	207	6.1	34	2	3	4	7	13	20	26
65+	765	5.9	35	1	3	4	7	12	15	31
TOTAL SINGLE DX	132	1.8	3	1	1	1	2	4	6	10
MULTIPLE DX	1360	5.2	31	1	2	4	6	11	15	28
TOTAL										
0–19 Years	82	4.6	28	1	1	2	6	11	19	21
20–34	185	2.5	10	1	1	1	3	6	8	12
35–49	227	3.5	18	1	1	2	4	7	10	27
50–64	218	5.9	33	2	3	4	7	13	20	26
65+	780	5.9	34	1	3	4	7	12	15	31
GRAND TOTAL	1492	4.8	29	1	1	3	6	10	14	27

48.3: LOC DESTR RECTAL LESION. Formerly included in operation group(s) 615.

Type of Patients	Observed Patients	Avg. Stay	Variance	10th	25th	50th	75th	90th	95th	99th
1. SINGLE DX										
0–19 Years	14	1.3	<1	1	1	1	2	2	2	3
20–34	9	4.7	11	2	2	4	9	9	9	9
35–49	24	2.1	1	1	1	2	3	4	5	6
50–64	47	1.9	3	1	1	1	2	3	6	8
65+	72	1.4	<1	1	1	1	2	2	3	4
2. MULTIPLE DX										
0–19 Years	20	4.0	22	1	1	1	5	12	12	19
20–34	43	3.7	9	1	2	2	4	8	13	13
35–49	152	4.0	13	1	2	3	5	10	15	15
50–64	326	4.2	27	1	2	3	5	10	15	30
65+	1405	5.4	42	2	2	3	7	13	17	25
TOTAL SINGLE DX	166	1.7	2	1	1	1	2	3	4	9
MULTIPLE DX	1946	5.0	36	1	2	3	6	11	16	25
TOTAL										
0–19 Years	34	2.8	14	1	1	1	2	7	12	19
20–34	52	3.8	10	1	2	3	4	8	13	13
35–49	176	3.8	12	1	2	3	4	9	13	15
50–64	373	3.9	24	1	2	3	5	9	12	30
65+	1477	5.1	40	1	2	3	6	12	17	23
GRAND TOTAL	2112	4.7	34	1	2	3	5	11	15	23

Length of Stay by Diagnosis and Operation, United States, 1997

United States, October 1995–September 1996 Data, by Operation

48.35: LOC EXC RECTAL LES/TISS. Formerly included in operation group(s) 615.

Type of Patients	Observed Patients	Avg. Stay	Vari-ance	Percentiles						
				10th	25th	50th	75th	90th	95th	99th
1. SINGLE DX										
0–19 Years	3	1.4	<1	1	1	1	2	2	2	2
20–34	4	6.4	10	2	3	9	9	9	9	9
35–49	21	2.2	2	1	1	2	2	5	5	6
50–64	41	1.9	3	1	1	1	3	3	6	8
65+	58	1.6	<1	1	1	1	2	3	3	4
2. MULTIPLE DX										
0–19 Years	8	4.8	19	1	2	3	6	12	12	12
20–34	11	2.3	4	1	1	2	4	7	12	9
35–49	65	3.5	14	1	2	2	4	7	7	9
50–64	145	4.1	46	1	1	2	4	8	19	30
65+	615	5.0	57	1	1	3	6	11	15	22
TOTAL SINGLE DX	127	1.9	2	1	1	1	2	3	5	9
MULTIPLE DX	844	4.7	51	1	1	3	5	10	15	28
TOTAL										
0–19 Years	11	4.0	17	1	1	2	5	12	12	12
20–34	15	3.7	10	3	3	3	7	7	9	9
35–49	86	3.2	11	1	1	2	3	6	10	15
50–64	186	3.6	37	1	2	2	3	6	15	30
65+	673	4.7	53	1	1	3	5	10	14	22
GRAND TOTAL	971	4.3	46	1	1	2	4	9	14	25

48.4: PULL-THRU RECT RESECTION. Formerly included in operation group(s) 617.

Type of Patients	Observed Patients	Avg. Stay	Vari-ance	Percentiles						
				10th	25th	50th	75th	90th	95th	99th
1. SINGLE DX										
0–19 Years	101	7.0	16	4	5	7	8	9	14	28
20–34	2	7.5	5	6	6	6	10	10	10	10
35–49	3	5.0	8	1	1	6	6	8	8	8
50–64	2	3.3	10	2	2	2	2	10	10	10
65+	4	3.7	7	1	1	4	5	8	8	8
2. MULTIPLE DX										
0–19 Years	237	8.0	31	4	5	7	9	12	20	33
20–34	21	8.7	21	3	6	8	11	13	16	22
35–49	24	8.8	27	3	3	8	12	17	18	18
50–64	23	11.5	19	4	7	14	14	14	17	19
65+	116	6.5	16	3	4	6	8	10	15	23
TOTAL SINGLE DX	112	6.8	16	4	5	7	8	9	12	28
MULTIPLE DX	421	7.8	27	3	5	7	9	14	17	33
TOTAL										
0–19 Years	338	7.7	27	4	5	7	9	11	17	33
20–34	23	8.6	20	3	6	8	10	13	16	22
35–49	27	8.5	27	2	3	8	12	17	18	18
50–64	25	10.7	23	3	7	14	14	14	17	19
65+	120	6.5	16	2	4	6	8	10	15	23
GRAND TOTAL	533	7.7	25	3	5	7	9	14	17	31

48.36: ENDO RECTAL POLYPECTOMY. Formerly included in operation group(s) 615.

Type of Patients	Observed Patients	Avg. Stay	Vari-ance	Percentiles						
				10th	25th	50th	75th	90th	95th	99th
1. SINGLE DX										
0–19 Years	11	1.3	<1	1	1	1	2	2	2	3
20–34	2	3.0	0	3	3	3	3	3	3	3
35–49	2	2.3	<1	1	1	1	2	2	2	2
50–64	4	1.7	<1	1	1	2	2	2	2	2
65+	7	1.8	1	1	1	1	2	4	4	4
2. MULTIPLE DX										
0–19 Years	10	2.3	9	1	2	2	4	6	12	12
20–34	26	3.7	11	2	2	2	4	8	13	13
35–49	81	4.5	13	2	2	3	4	11	14	14
50–64	155	4.5	14	2	2	3	5	11	13	17
65+	632	5.8	26	2	3	4	7	13	17	21
TOTAL SINGLE DX	26	1.5	<1	1	1	1	2	2	3	4
MULTIPLE DX	904	5.3	22	2	2	3	6	12	17	19
TOTAL										
0–19 Years	21	1.8	4	1	1	1	1	3	6	12
20–34	28	3.7	10	2	2	3	4	8	13	13
35–49	83	4.4	13	2	2	3	4	11	14	14
50–64	159	4.4	14	2	2	3	5	11	13	17
65+	639	5.8	26	2	3	4	7	13	17	21
GRAND TOTAL	930	5.2	22	1	2	3	6	12	17	19

48.5: ABD-PERINEAL RECT RESECT. Formerly included in operation group(s) 617.

Type of Patients	Observed Patients	Avg. Stay	Vari-ance	Percentiles						
				10th	25th	50th	75th	90th	95th	99th
1. SINGLE DX										
0–19 Years	5	7.3	1	6	7	7	8	8	8	11
20–34	9	7.0	3	5	6	7	8	9	8	9
35–49	28	6.9	5	5	5	6	8	9	10	18
50–64	66	8.3	10	4	6	8	10	12	12	20
65+	23	7.9	9	4	7	8	10	11	13	15
2. MULTIPLE DX										
0–19 Years	3	8.5	7	6	6	10	10	11	11	11
20–34	69	9.9	48	5	6	8	12	16	27	36
35–49	270	10.1	34	5	7	8	12	18	20	28
50–64	682	10.3	26	6	7	9	12	18	20	28
65+	1459	11.7	41	7	8	9	13	19	25	36
TOTAL SINGLE DX	131	7.9	8	5	6	8	9	12	12	18
MULTIPLE DX	2483	11.0	36	6	7	9	13	18	22	34
TOTAL										
0–19 Years	8	7.5	2	6	7	7	8	10	11	11
20–34	78	9.7	45	5	6	8	10	15	23	36
35–49	298	9.9	33	5	7	8	12	18	20	26
50–64	748	10.1	25	6	7	9	12	17	20	28
65+	1482	11.6	41	7	8	9	13	19	25	36
GRAND TOTAL	2614	10.8	35	6	7	9	12	18	22	34

Length of Stay by Diagnosis and Operation, United States, 1997

United States, October 1995–September 1996 Data, by Operation

48.6: OTHER RECTAL RESECTION. Formerly included in operation group(s) 617.

Type of Patients	Observed Patients	Avg. Stay	Vari-ance	10th	25th	50th	75th	90th	95th	99th
1. SINGLE DX										
0–19 Years	42	5.8	3	4	5	5	6	8	11	13
20–34	14	5.2	2	4	4	5	6	8	8	8
35–49	62	6.3	4	4	5	6	7	9	9	11
50–64	121	6.2	3	4	5	6	7	8	8	10
65+	98	6.0	13	1	4	7	7	9	11	14
2. MULTIPLE DX										
0–19 Years	105	9.0	101	4	5	7	9	14	22	80
20–34	94	8.0	28	4	5	7	9	13	20	25
35–49	499	8.7	47	5	6	7	9	13	17	62
50–64	1319	8.1	19	5	6	7	9	12	15	24
65+	3125	10.0	43	5	7	8	11	16	21	35
TOTAL SINGLE DX	337	6.1	7	4	5	6	7	9	10	13
MULTIPLE DX	5142	9.2	38	5	6	8	10	15	20	33
TOTAL										
0–19 Years	147	7.9	70	4	5	6	8	13	18	36
20–34	108	7.6	25	4	5	7	9	11	19	25
35–49	561	8.5	43	5	6	7	9	13	15	62
50–64	1440	8.0	18	6	6	7	9	11	15	24
65+	3223	9.8	42	5	7	8	11	16	21	35
GRAND TOTAL	5479	9.0	36	5	6	8	10	14	19	33

48.62: ANT RECT RESECT W COLOST. Formerly included in operation group(s) 617.

Type of Patients	Observed Patients	Avg. Stay	Vari-ance	10th	25th	50th	75th	90th	95th	99th
1. SINGLE DX										
0–19 Years	0									
20–34	0									
35–49	7	6.8	1	5	6	7	8	8	8	8
50–64	7	5.9	3	4	4	6	7	8	8	8
65+	6	11.0	13	8	11	11	11	12	22	22
2. MULTIPLE DX										
0–19 Years	5	9.5	38	2	7	8	19	19	19	19
20–34	7	10.5	29	6	6	9	13	20	20	20
35–49	64	8.6	11	6	6	8	11	14	15	23
50–64	168	9.7	21	6	8	8	11	15	17	28
65+	378	12.6	60	7	7	10	15	20	25	48
TOTAL SINGLE DX	19	8.5	12	4	6	8	11	11	12	22
MULTIPLE DX	622	11.2	44	6	7	9	13	20	24	42
TOTAL										
0–19 Years	5	9.5	38	2	7	8	19	19	19	19
20–34	7	10.5	29	6	6	9	13	20	20	20
35–49	70	8.5	10	6	7	8	11	13	15	23
50–64	175	9.7	20	6	7	8	11	15	17	28
65+	384	12.6	59	7	7	10	15	20	25	48
GRAND TOTAL	641	11.1	43	6	7	9	13	20	24	41

48.63: ANTERIOR RECT RESECT NEC. Formerly included in operation group(s) 617.

Type of Patients	Observed Patients	Avg. Stay	Vari-ance	10th	25th	50th	75th	90th	95th	99th
1. SINGLE DX										
0–19 Years	0									
20–34	9	6.1	2	4	5	6	6	8	8	8
35–49	38	6.8	3	4	5	7	8	9	10	11
50–64	94	6.2	3	4	5	6	7	8	8	10
65+	62	6.9	13	1	6	7	9	9	10	14
2. MULTIPLE DX										
0–19 Years	1	18.0	0	18	18	18	18	18	18	18
20–34	36	6.6	4	4	5	7	9	9	10	11
35–49	295	7.7	12	5	6	7	9	10	13	28
50–64	878	7.8	11	5	6	7	9	11	13	22
65+	2078	9.6	32	6	7	8	10	15	20	32
TOTAL SINGLE DX	203	6.6	6	4	5	7	7	9	9	13
MULTIPLE DX	3288	8.8	25	5	6	8	10	13	17	30
TOTAL										
0–19 Years	1	18.0	0	18	18	18	18	18	18	18
20–34	45	6.5	3	4	5	7	7	9	9	11
35–49	333	7.6	11	5	6	7	9	10	12	28
50–64	972	7.7	11	5	6	7	9	11	13	21
65+	2140	9.5	32	6	7	8	10	15	19	32
GRAND TOTAL	3491	8.7	24	5	6	8	10	13	16	30

48.69: RECTAL RESECTION NEC. Formerly included in operation group(s) 617.

Type of Patients	Observed Patients	Avg. Stay	Vari-ance	10th	25th	50th	75th	90th	95th	99th
1. SINGLE DX										
0–19 Years	3	5.3	2	5	5	5	5	5	10	10
20–34	5	4.5	2	4	4	4	4	8	8	8
35–49	17	5.0	3	4	4	4	6	7	8	9
50–64	20	6.1	2	1	1	6	7	7	7	10
65+	28	4.7	8	3	4	7	7	7	7	10
2. MULTIPLE DX										
0–19 Years	17	17.5	673	3	4	5	25	80	80	80
20–34	48	8.5	40	3	5	7	9	18	20	40
35–49	135	10.4	123	5	6	7	10	15	24	62
50–64	262	8.2	50	2	6	7	10	13	22	29
65+	645	9.6	68	3	6	8	12	16	21	40
TOTAL SINGLE DX	73	4.9	6	1	3	6	7	7	8	10
MULTIPLE DX	1107	9.4	79	3	6	7	11	16	22	62
TOTAL										
0–19 Years	20	14.5	532	4	5	5	8	80	80	80
20–34	53	7.8	36	4	4	6	9	14	19	40
35–49	152	9.9	116	4	6	7	10	15	23	62
50–64	282	8.1	48	2	5	7	10	13	20	27
65+	673	9.0	63	2	5	7	11	16	21	40
GRAND TOTAL	1180	9.0	74	2	5	7	10	15	21	54

Length of Stay by Diagnosis and Operation, United States, 1997

United States, October 1995–September 1996 Data, by Operation

48.7: REPAIR OF RECTUM. Formerly included in operation group(s) 618.

Type of Patients	Observed Patients	Avg. Stay	Vari-ance	10th	25th	50th	75th	90th	95th	99th
1. SINGLE DX										
0–19 Years	17	4.7	2	3	4	5	5	5	8	8
20–34	17	3.8	3	2	2	4	5	6	7	7
35–49	17	3.2	2	1	2	4	5	6	5	7
50–64	11	3.9	3	2	2	5	5	6	6	6
65+	10	2.8	2	1	1	3	4	5	5	5
2. MULTIPLE DX										
0–19 Years	90	6.4	19	2	3	5	8	14	15	20
20–34	62	5.9	14	1	2	5	9	9	12	22
35–49	102	6.5	57	2	3	4	7	11	28	35
50–64	115	6.0	14	2	4	5	8	10	11	18
65+	421	6.4	22	1	3	6	8	11	13	25
TOTAL SINGLE DX	72	4.2	2	2	3	5	5	5	7	8
MULTIPLE DX	790	6.3	24	2	3	5	8	11	14	28
TOTAL										
0–19 Years	107	5.7	13	2	4	5	7	11	14	16
20–34	79	5.5	13	1	2	5	8	9	12	15
35–49	119	6.2	54	2	3	4	7	10	24	35
50–64	126	5.9	14	2	4	5	8	10	11	18
65+	431	6.4	22	1	3	6	8	11	13	25
GRAND TOTAL	862	6.1	23	2	3	5	8	11	13	27

48.8: PERIRECT TISS INC/EXC. Formerly included in operation group(s) 616.

Type of Patients	Observed Patients	Avg. Stay	Vari-ance	10th	25th	50th	75th	90th	95th	99th
1. SINGLE DX										
0–19 Years	94	2.1	2	1	1	2	3	3	4	7
20–34	268	2.0	2	1	1	2	3	3	6	8
35–49	270	2.1	2	1	1	2	3	4	5	6
50–64	115	2.0	2	1	1	1	3	4	6	8
65+	25	2.5	3	1	1	2	3	5	7	7
2. MULTIPLE DX										
0–19 Years	146	4.7	16	1	2	4	6	9	12	23
20–34	404	3.2	14	1	1	4	4	6	9	16
35–49	710	3.8	19	1	1	3	5	8	11	16
50–64	598	7.5	158	1	2	3	7	16	29	75
65+	450	6.8	47	1	3	5	8	15	18	41
TOTAL SINGLE DX	772	2.1	2	1	1	2	3	4	5	8
MULTIPLE DX	2308	5.2	64	1	2	3	6	10	15	41
TOTAL										
0–19 Years	240	3.8	12	1	2	3	4	8	9	19
20–34	672	2.7	9	1	1	3	3	5	8	12
35–49	980	3.4	15	1	1	2	4	7	10	14
50–64	713	6.6	136	1	2	3	6	14	29	75
65+	475	6.6	46	1	3	4	7	15	18	41
GRAND TOTAL	3080	4.4	49	1	1	3	5	9	13	29

48.76: PROCTOPEXY NEC. Formerly included in operation group(s) 618.

Type of Patients	Observed Patients	Avg. Stay	Vari-ance	10th	25th	50th	75th	90th	95th	99th
1. SINGLE DX										
0–19 Years	1	5.0	0	5	5	5	5	5	5	5
20–34	4	3.9	2	3	3	3	5	6	6	6
35–49	3	3.3	2	1	2	3	4	4	4	4
50–64	4	2.4	2	1	2	2	4	6	6	6
65+	6	3.1	2	1	2	2	4	5	5	5
2. MULTIPLE DX										
0–19 Years	11	7.5	36	1	2	7	14	15	15	15
20–34	6	2.8	5	1	1	1	6	6	6	6
35–49	36	5.2	24	1	2	3	8	9	15	28
50–64	54	4.6	6	2	3	4	6	8	10	14
65+	223	5.8	21	1	3	5	8	9	13	25
TOTAL SINGLE DX	18	4.4	1	2	4	5	5	5	5	6
MULTIPLE DX	330	5.5	19	1	3	5	7	9	13	25
TOTAL										
0–19 Years	12	6.0	16	2	5	5	5	14	14	15
20–34	10	3.2	4	1	1	3	6	6	6	6
35–49	39	5.0	22	1	2	4	7	9	15	28
50–64	58	4.5	6	2	3	4	5	8	10	14
65+	229	5.8	21	1	3	5	8	9	13	25
GRAND TOTAL	348	5.5	18	1	3	5	7	9	13	25

48.81: PERIRECTAL INCISION. Formerly included in operation group(s) 616.

Type of Patients	Observed Patients	Avg. Stay	Vari-ance	10th	25th	50th	75th	90th	95th	99th
1. SINGLE DX										
0–19 Years	92	2.1	2	1	1	2	3	3	4	7
20–34	267	2.0	2	1	1	2	3	3	6	8
35–49	264	2.1	2	1	1	2	3	4	5	6
50–64	108	2.4	2	1	1	2	3	4	6	8
65+	22	2.3	2	1	1	2	3	5	5	5
2. MULTIPLE DX										
0–19 Years	141	4.8	16	1	2	4	6	9	12	23
20–34	390	3.2	9	1	1	4	4	6	9	16
35–49	678	3.7	14	1	1	3	5	7	10	15
50–64	572	7.4	159	1	2	3	7	14	29	75
65+	417	6.8	45	1	3	4	8	15	18	41
TOTAL SINGLE DX	753	2.1	2	1	1	2	3	4	5	8
MULTIPLE DX	2198	5.1	62	1	2	3	6	10	15	32
TOTAL										
0–19 Years	233	3.8	13	1	2	3	4	9	10	19
20–34	657	2.7	7	1	1	2	3	5	7	12
35–49	942	3.2	11	1	1	3	4	6	8	14
50–64	680	6.7	141	1	2	3	6	13	29	75
65+	439	6.6	44	1	3	4	7	15	18	30
GRAND TOTAL	2951	4.3	48	1	1	3	5	8	13	29

Length of Stay by Diagnosis and Operation, United States, 1997

United States, October 1995–September 1996 Data, by Operation

48.9: OTH RECTAL/PERIRECT OP. Formerly included in operation group(s) 618.

Type of Patients	Observed Patients	Avg. Stay	Vari-ance	10th	25th	50th	75th	90th	95th	99th
1. SINGLE DX										
0–19 Years	10	3.0	4	1	1	2	4	7	7	7
20–34	0									
35–49	3	2.0	<1	2	2	2	2	2	2	2
50–64	3	1.7	2	1	1	1	1	2	2	2
65+	1	2.0	0	2	2	2	2	2	2	2
2. MULTIPLE DX										
0–19 Years	19	3.7	24	1	1	2	3	10	13	27
20–34	12	8.4	33	2	3	10	13	17	17	17
35–49	12	3.1	6	1	1	3	4	4	6	14
50–64	14	3.6	10	1	2	3	5	8	12	12
65+	11	12.6	162	2	5	10	17	28	49	49
TOTAL SINGLE DX	17	2.3	2	1	2	2	2	4	6	7
MULTIPLE DX	68	4.9	38	1	1	3	5	13	17	28
TOTAL										
0–19 Years	29	3.5	18	1	1	2	4	7	10	27
20–34	12	8.4	33	2	3	10	13	17	17	17
35–49	15	2.6	4	1	1	2	4	4	4	14
50–64	17	3.2	9	1	2	2	5	7	8	12
65+	12	12.1	159	2	5	6	17	28	49	49
GRAND TOTAL	85	4.2	29	1	2	2	4	11	14	27

49.0: PERIANAL TISS INC/EXC. Formerly included in operation group(s) 622.

Type of Patients	Observed Patients	Avg. Stay	Vari-ance	10th	25th	50th	75th	90th	95th	99th
1. SINGLE DX										
0–19 Years	64	2.0	1	1	1	2	3	3	4	5
20–34	142	1.9	2	1	1	1	2	3	4	7
35–49	162	2.1	2	1	1	2	2	3	5	7
50–64	53	2.3	4	1	1	2	3	4	6	12
65+	11	5.8	55	1	1	3	5	21	21	21
2. MULTIPLE DX										
0–19 Years	82	3.7	16	1	1	3	4	9	10	25
20–34	247	3.6	14	1	2	3	4	7	9	23
35–49	430	4.3	10	1	2	4	6	6	9	16
50–64	316	5.2	41	1	2	4	7	10	12	25
65+	241	5.9	40	2	2	4	8	12	16	29
TOTAL SINGLE DX	432	2.1	3	1	1	2	3	4	5	8
MULTIPLE DX	1316	4.6	23	1	2	3	6	9	11	25
TOTAL										
0–19 Years	146	2.8	9	1	1	2	3	4	8	14
20–34	389	3.0	10	1	1	3	4	5	8	23
35–49	592	3.9	9	1	2	3	6	6	8	16
50–64	369	4.6	35	2	2	3	6	9	12	24
65+	252	5.9	40	1	2	4	8	12	16	29
GRAND TOTAL	1748	4.0	19	1	2	3	5	7	11	23

49.01: INC PERIANAL ABSCESS. Formerly included in operation group(s) 622.

Type of Patients	Observed Patients	Avg. Stay	Vari-ance	10th	25th	50th	75th	90th	95th	99th
1. SINGLE DX										
0–19 Years	57	2.1	1	1	1	2	3	4	4	5
20–34	136	1.9	2	1	1	1	3	4	4	7
35–49	153	2.1	2	1	2	2	3	4	5	7
50–64	49	2.4	5	1	1	2	3	4	8	12
65+	8	6.6	65	1	3	3	5	21	21	21
2. MULTIPLE DX										
0–19 Years	74	3.7	15	1	1	3	4	9	10	25
20–34	235	3.7	15	1	2	3	5	7	10	27
35–49	402	4.4	11	1	2	4	6	7	9	20
50–64	302	5.4	43	1	2	3	7	10	12	31
65+	224	5.8	41	1	2	4	8	12	16	29
TOTAL SINGLE DX	403	2.1	3	1	1	2	3	4	5	8
MULTIPLE DX	1237	4.7	24	1	2	3	6	9	12	26
TOTAL										
0–19 Years	131	2.9	9	1	1	2	3	5	9	14
20–34	371	3.1	11	1	1	2	4	5	8	23
35–49	555	4.0	10	1	2	3	6	8	8	16
50–64	351	4.8	37	1	2	3	6	10	12	24
65+	232	5.8	42	1	2	4	8	12	16	29
GRAND TOTAL	1640	4.1	20	1	2	3	6	8	11	23

49.1: INC/EXC OF ANAL FISTULA. Formerly included in operation group(s) 619.

Type of Patients	Observed Patients	Avg. Stay	Vari-ance	10th	25th	50th	75th	90th	95th	99th
1. SINGLE DX										
0–19 Years	13	2.1	2	1	1	1	3	4	5	5
20–34	26	2.0	<1	1	2	2	2	3	3	3
35–49	53	1.7	1	1	1	1	3	3	3	6
50–64	24	1.8	<1	1	1	1	2	3	4	4
65+	13	1.7	<1	1	1	1	2	3	3	3
2. MULTIPLE DX										
0–19 Years	27	2.7	4	1	1	2	3	6	6	10
20–34	118	3.1	8	1	1	2	4	5	9	15
35–49	189	3.7	30	1	1	2	4	6	15	23
50–64	132	3.8	20	1	1	2	4	9	16	19
65+	107	7.5	62	2	2	4	11	19	19	46
TOTAL SINGLE DX	129	1.8	1	1	1	1	2	3	3	6
MULTIPLE DX	573	4.0	26	1	1	2	4	9	16	21
TOTAL										
0–19 Years	40	2.4	3	1	1	2	3	5	6	9
20–34	144	3.0	7	1	1	2	3	6	8	13
35–49	242	3.1	22	1	1	2	3	6	11	23
50–64	156	3.4	17	1	1	2	4	8	16	19
65+	120	6.9	58	1	2	4	9	19	19	46
GRAND TOTAL	702	3.5	22	1	1	2	4	8	14	19

Length of Stay by Diagnosis and Operation, United States, 1997

United States, October 1995–September 1996 Data, by Operation

49.11: ANAL FISTULOTOMY. Formerly included in operation group(s) 619.

Type of Patients	Observed Patients	Avg. Stay	Vari-ance	Percentiles						
				10th	25th	50th	75th	90th	95th	99th
1. SINGLE DX										
0–19 Years	9	1.6	1	1	1	1	1	3	4	4
20–34	8	2.0	<1	1	2	2	2	3	3	3
35–49	19	2.4	1	1	1	3	3	3	3	5
50–64	8	1.7	<1	1	1	2	2	2	2	2
65+	5	2.1	<1	1	1	2	3	3	3	3
2. MULTIPLE DX										
0–19 Years	13	3.0	5	1	1	3	5	6	6	10
20–34	55	3.0	5	1	2	3	5	5	5	15
35–49	95	3.9	40	1	1	2	3	9	15	23
50–64	48	5.4	25	1	2	3	7	16	16	17
65+	51	6.1	41	1	1	3	9	14	19	34
TOTAL SINGLE DX	49	2.1	<1	1	1	2	3	3	3	5
MULTIPLE DX	262	3.9	24	1	1	2	5	8	15	23
TOTAL										
0–19 Years	22	2.2	3	1	1	1	3	5	6	10
20–34	63	2.9	5	1	2	2	4	5	5	15
35–49	114	3.5	31	1	1	2	3	6	15	23
50–64	56	4.8	23	1	2	3	7	13	16	17
65+	56	5.7	39	1	1	3	9	13	16	24
GRAND TOTAL	311	3.6	20	1	1	2	4	7	13	23

49.12: ANAL FISTULECTOMY. Formerly included in operation group(s) 619.

Type of Patients	Observed Patients	Avg. Stay	Vari-ance	Percentiles						
				10th	25th	50th	75th	90th	95th	99th
1. SINGLE DX										
0–19 Years	4	3.2	2	2	2	3	5	5	5	5
20–34	18	2.0	<1	1	2	2	2	3	3	3
35–49	34	1.4	1	1	1	1	1	2	3	6
50–64	16	1.8	1	1	1	2	2	4	4	4
65+	8	1.5	<1	1	1	1	2	2	3	3
2. MULTIPLE DX										
0–19 Years	14	2.6	2	1	1	2	3	4	6	9
20–34	63	3.4	12	1	1	2	4	9	11	18
35–49	94	3.6	20	1	1	2	3	9	13	17
50–64	84	2.9	15	1	1	2	2	6	8	21
65+	56	8.4	72	1	3	4	14	19	19	46
TOTAL SINGLE DX	80	1.7	1	1	1	1	2	3	4	6
MULTIPLE DX	311	4.2	29	1	1	2	4	9	18	19
TOTAL										
0–19 Years	18	2.7	2	1	2	2	3	5	5	9
20–34	81	3.0	9	1	1	2	3	8	11	13
35–49	128	2.8	14	1	1	1	2	9	9	17
50–64	100	2.7	13	1	1	2	5	6	8	21
65+	64	7.5	68	1	2	4	13	19	19	46
GRAND TOTAL	391	3.5	23	1	1	2	3	9	16	19

49.2: ANAL & PERIANAL DXTIC PX. Formerly included in operation group(s) 620, 622, 631.

Type of Patients	Observed Patients	Avg. Stay	Vari-ance	Percentiles						
				10th	25th	50th	75th	90th	95th	99th
1. SINGLE DX										
0–19 Years	33	4.4	3	2	3	5	5	6	7	8
20–34	13	1.9	<1	1	1	2	2	3	3	4
35–49	6	2.2	9	1	1	2	2	10	10	10
50–64	5	4.1	4	1	2	4	7	7	7	7
65+	2	2.0	0	2	2	2	2	2	2	2
2. MULTIPLE DX										
0–19 Years	108	5.2	9	3	4	5	6	7	7	12
20–34	39	4.7	48	1	1	3	6	8	12	52
35–49	69	4.4	41	1	1	2	5	11	26	26
50–64	39	4.9	40	1	2	4	5	9	10	43
65+	140	4.0	13	1	2	3	4	7	10	22
TOTAL SINGLE DX	59	3.4	4	1	2	3	5	6	7	8
MULTIPLE DX	395	4.5	24	1	2	4	6	8	12	26
TOTAL										
0–19 Years	141	5.0	8	2	4	5	6	7	7	12
20–34	52	3.7	33	1	1	2	5	8	8	27
35–49	75	4.3	40	1	1	1	5	11	26	26
50–64	44	4.8	35	1	2	4	5	9	10	43
65+	142	4.0	13	1	2	3	4	7	10	22
GRAND TOTAL	454	4.4	22	1	2	4	5	7	10	26

49.21: ANOSCOPY. Formerly included in operation group(s) 631.

Type of Patients	Observed Patients	Avg. Stay	Vari-ance	Percentiles						
				10th	25th	50th	75th	90th	95th	99th
1. SINGLE DX										
0–19 Years	33	4.4	3	2	3	5	5	6	7	8
20–34	13	1.9	<1	1	1	2	2	3	3	4
35–49	2	1.0	0	1	1	1	1	1	1	1
50–64	3	3.4	1	1	4	4	4	4	4	4
65+	2	2.0	0	2	2	2	2	2	2	2
2. MULTIPLE DX										
0–19 Years	104	5.3	10	2	4	5	6	7	7	12
20–34	29	4.4	28	1	1	2	6	8	8	27
35–49	47	4.4	17	1	2	3	6	8	15	23
50–64	32	3.7	6	1	2	3	5	7	9	10
65+	119	3.6	8	1	2	3	4	7	8	16
TOTAL SINGLE DX	53	3.3	3	1	2	3	5	6	6	8
MULTIPLE DX	331	4.3	11	1	2	4	6	7	9	20
TOTAL										
0–19 Years	137	5.1	8	2	4	5	6	7	7	12
20–34	42	3.4	19	1	1	2	4	8	8	27
35–49	49	4.3	16	1	2	3	6	8	15	23
50–64	35	3.7	5	1	2	3	5	7	9	10
65+	121	3.6	8	1	2	3	4	7	8	16
GRAND TOTAL	384	4.1	10	1	2	4	5	7	8	16

Length of Stay by Diagnosis and Operation, United States, 1997

United States, October 1995–September 1996 Data, by Operation

49.3: LOC DESTR ANAL LES NEC. Formerly included in operation group(s) 620.

Type of Patients	Observed Patients	Avg. Stay	Variance	10th	25th	50th	75th	90th	95th	99th
1. SINGLE DX										
0–19 Years	8	1.3	<1	1	1	1	1	2	2	4
20–34	24	1.5	1	1	1	1	2	3	4	6
35–49	15	2.0	1	1	1	2	3	4	4	4
50–64	9	1.4	<1	1	1	1	2	2	2	2
65+	8	2.2	1	1	1	2	4	4	4	4
2. MULTIPLE DX										
0–19 Years	20	7.7	87	1	2	4	7	30	30	30
20–34	69	3.9	23	1	1	2	4	9	15	27
35–49	123	6.5	29	1	2	6	11	14	14	22
50–64	79	3.3	15	1	1	2	7	7	15	18
65+	162	6.5	97	1	1	3	6	13	28	44
TOTAL SINGLE DX	64	1.6	1	1	1	1	2	3	4	6
MULTIPLE DX	453	5.6	50	1	1	3	7	14	15	44
TOTAL										
0–19 Years	28	5.8	70	1	1	2	7	10	30	30
20–34	93	3.3	18	1	1	2	3	9	12	17
35–49	138	6.3	28	1	2	4	11	14	14	22
50–64	88	3.1	14	1	1	2	3	6	14	18
65+	170	6.4	95	1	1	3	6	13	28	44
GRAND TOTAL	517	5.2	47	1	1	3	6	14	14	34

49.4: HEMORRHOID PROCEDURES. Formerly included in operation group(s) 621, 622, 631.

Type of Patients	Observed Patients	Avg. Stay	Variance	10th	25th	50th	75th	90th	95th	99th
1. SINGLE DX										
0–19 Years	5	1.4	<1	1	1	1	1	3	3	3
20–34	100	1.8	1	1	1	1	2	3	4	5
35–49	176	2.2	4	1	2	2	3	4	5	6
50–64	86	1.6	<1	1	1	1	2	3	3	5
65+	28	1.7	1	1	1	1	2	3	4	6
2. MULTIPLE DX										
0–19 Years	15	2.6	3	1	2	2	4	5	5	8
20–34	525	2.6	9	1	1	2	3	4	7	23
35–49	1277	2.2	4	1	1	2	2	4	6	10
50–64	1010	3.0	10	1	1	3	4	6	8	16
65+	1129	4.3	20	1	1	3	6	12	14	19
TOTAL SINGLE DX	395	1.9	2	1	1	2	2	4	4	6
MULTIPLE DX	3956	2.9	10	1	1	2	3	6	9	15
TOTAL										
0–19 Years	20	2.5	3	1	1	2	4	4	5	8
20–34	625	2.4	8	1	1	2	3	4	6	14
35–49	1453	2.2	4	1	1	2	3	5	6	10
50–64	1096	2.9	10	1	1	3	3	5	8	15
65+	1157	4.2	19	1	1	3	5	11	14	19
GRAND TOTAL	4351	2.8	10	1	1	2	3	6	8	15

49.39: OTH LOC DESTR ANAL LES. Formerly included in operation group(s) 620.

Type of Patients	Observed Patients	Avg. Stay	Variance	10th	25th	50th	75th	90th	95th	99th
1. SINGLE DX										
0–19 Years	8	1.3	<1	1	1	1	1	2	2	4
20–34	22	1.4	1	1	1	1	2	3	4	6
35–49	15	2.0	1	1	1	2	3	4	4	4
50–64	8	1.5	<1	1	1	1	2	2	2	2
65+	7	2.2	1	1	1	2	4	4	4	4
2. MULTIPLE DX										
0–19 Years	19	8.1	96	1	2	4	8	30	30	30
20–34	65	4.3	24	1	1	2	7	10	15	27
35–49	116	6.6	27	1	2	6	11	14	14	18
50–64	72	3.3	16	1	1	2	3	7	15	18
65+	141	6.4	89	1	1	3	6	14	28	44
TOTAL SINGLE DX	60	1.6	1	1	1	1	2	3	4	6
MULTIPLE DX	413	5.7	47	1	1	3	7	14	15	34
TOTAL										
0–19 Years	27	6.0	76	1	1	2	7	30	30	30
20–34	87	3.5	20	1	1	2	3	9	12	27
35–49	131	6.3	27	1	2	5	11	14	14	18
50–64	80	3.2	15	1	1	2	3	6	15	18
65+	148	6.3	87	1	1	3	6	13	28	44
GRAND TOTAL	473	5.3	44	1	1	3	6	14	14	34

49.46: EXC OF HEMORRHOIDS. Formerly included in operation group(s) 621.

Type of Patients	Observed Patients	Avg. Stay	Variance	10th	25th	50th	75th	90th	95th	99th
1. SINGLE DX										
0–19 Years	3	2.2	1	3	3	3	3	3	3	3
20–34	89	1.7	<1	1	1	1	2	3	3	5
35–49	162	2.3	4	1	1	2	3	4	5	5
50–64	79	1.6	<1	1	1	1	2	3	3	5
65+	27	1.7	1	1	1	1	2	3	4	6
2. MULTIPLE DX										
0–19 Years	13	2.6	3	1	1	2	4	4	5	8
20–34	484	2.4	7	1	1	2	3	4	6	13
35–49	1185	2.1	3	1	1	2	2	4	5	10
50–64	918	2.8	9	1	1	2	3	5	8	15
65+	961	4.1	19	1	1	2	5	11	14	19
TOTAL SINGLE DX	360	2.0	2	1	1	2	2	4	4	6
MULTIPLE DX	3561	2.7	9	1	1	2	3	6	8	14
TOTAL										
0–19 Years	16	2.6	3	1	1	2	4	4	5	8
20–34	573	2.3	6	1	1	2	3	4	5	12
35–49	1347	2.1	3	1	1	2	3	4	5	10
50–64	997	2.6	8	1	1	2	3	5	8	15
65+	988	4.0	19	1	1	2	5	11	14	19
GRAND TOTAL	3921	2.7	8	1	1	2	3	5	8	14

Length of Stay by Diagnosis and Operation, United States, 1997

United States, October 1995–September 1996 Data, by Operation

49.5: ANAL SPHINCTER DIVISION. Formerly included in operation group(s) 622.

Type of Patients	Observed Patients	Avg. Stay	Variance	10th	25th	50th	75th	90th	95th	99th
1. SINGLE DX										
0–19 Years	2	1.0	0	1	1	1	1	1	1	1
20–34	9	1.9	2	1	1	1	2	4	4	4
35–49	16	2.0	1	1	1	2	2	4	4	5
50–64	5	2.0	<1	1	1	2	2	3	3	3
65+	3	1.3	<1	1	1	1	2	2	2	2
2. MULTIPLE DX										
0–19 Years	10	4.5	8	2	2	5	6	7	7	14
20–34	31	2.7	5	1	1	2	4	4	6	18
35–49	55	2.6	9	1	1	2	3	6	10	12
50–64	49	3.2	5	1	1	2	4	6	6	10
65+	83	6.3	41	1	2	4	7	16	17	38
TOTAL SINGLE DX	35	1.9	1	1	1	1	2	4	4	5
MULTIPLE DX	228	3.8	18	1	1	3	5	7	11	19
TOTAL										
0–19 Years	12	4.1	8	1	2	5	6	7	7	14
20–34	40	2.6	5	1	1	2	4	4	5	9
35–49	71	2.5	8	1	1	2	3	6	10	11
50–64	54	3.1	5	1	1	2	4	6	6	10
65+	86	6.2	40	1	2	4	7	16	17	38
GRAND TOTAL	263	3.6	17	1	1	2	4	7	11	19

49.6: EXCISION OF ANUS. Formerly included in operation group(s) 622.

Type of Patients	Observed Patients	Avg. Stay	Variance	10th	25th	50th	75th	90th	95th	99th
1. SINGLE DX										
0–19 Years	0									
20–34	0									
35–49	0									
50–64	1	5.0	0	5	5	5	5	5	5	5
65+	0									
2. MULTIPLE DX										
0–19 Years	0									
20–34	2	3.0	2	1	1	4	4	4	4	4
35–49	4	1.9	1	1	1	2	2	5	5	5
50–64	1	3.0	0	3	3	3	3	3	3	3
65+	3	2.2	3	1	1	2	2	5	5	5
TOTAL SINGLE DX	1	5.0	0	5	5	5	5	5	5	5
MULTIPLE DX	10	2.4	2	1	1	2	4	4	5	5
TOTAL										
0–19 Years	0									
20–34	2	3.0	2	1	1	4	4	4	4	4
35–49	4	1.9	1	1	1	2	2	5	5	5
50–64	2	4.0	2	3	3	3	5	5	5	5
65+	3	2.2	3	1	1	2	2	5	5	5
GRAND TOTAL	11	2.5	2	1	1	2	4	5	5	5

49.7: REPAIR OF ANUS. Formerly included in operation group(s) 622.

Type of Patients	Observed Patients	Avg. Stay	Variance	10th	25th	50th	75th	90th	95th	99th
1. SINGLE DX										
0–19 Years	123	2.4	3	1	1	2	3	5	6	8
20–34	39	3.2	10	1	2	2	4	5	11	17
35–49	43	3.1	2	1	2	3	5	5	6	6
50–64	24	1.9	1	1	1	3	2	4	4	7
65+	13	2.4	1	1	1	2	3	4	4	4
2. MULTIPLE DX										
0–19 Years	297	4.3	9	1	2	4	5	7	9	16
20–34	115	3.6	5	1	2	3	4	6	8	12
35–49	148	3.2	4	1	2	2	3	5	6	11
50–64	99	2.5	5	1	1	2	3	5	5	10
65+	131	4.9	19	2	3	4	6	10	16	>99
TOTAL SINGLE DX	242	2.6	4	1	1	2	3	5	6	8
MULTIPLE DX	790	3.8	9	1	2	3	5	7	9	17
TOTAL										
0–19 Years	420	3.7	8	1	2	3	5	6	9	16
20–34	154	3.5	7	1	2	3	4	6	8	12
35–49	191	3.2	4	1	2	3	4	5	6	11
50–64	123	2.5	4	1	1	2	3	4	5	8
65+	144	4.7	19	2	3	4	6	10	16	>99
GRAND TOTAL	1032	3.5	8	1	2	3	4	6	8	16

49.79: ANAL SPHINCTER REP NEC. Formerly included in operation group(s) 622.

Type of Patients	Observed Patients	Avg. Stay	Variance	10th	25th	50th	75th	90th	95th	99th
1. SINGLE DX										
0–19 Years	113	2.6	3	1	1	2	3	5	6	8
20–34	30	3.1	10	1	2	2	4	5	6	17
35–49	34	3.2	4	2	2	3	5	5	6	6
50–64	20	1.9	1	1	1	2	2	4	4	7
65+	8	2.4	1	1	2	2	3	4	4	4
2. MULTIPLE DX										
0–19 Years	284	4.2	8	1	2	4	5	7	9	16
20–34	95	3.6	5	1	2	3	4	6	9	12
35–49	116	3.2	4	1	2	3	4	5	7	11
50–64	70	2.4	2	1	1	2	3	5	5	7
65+	105	5.0	22	2	3	4	5	8	11	38
TOTAL SINGLE DX	205	2.7	4	1	1	2	3	5	6	8
MULTIPLE DX	670	3.8	8	1	2	3	5	6	9	16
TOTAL										
0–19 Years	397	3.8	7	1	2	3	5	6	9	14
20–34	125	3.5	7	1	2	3	4	5	8	17
35–49	150	3.2	4	1	2	3	4	6	6	11
50–64	90	2.3	2	1	1	2	3	4	6	7
65+	113	4.8	21	2	3	4	5	8	11	16
GRAND TOTAL	875	3.5	8	1	2	3	4	6	8	14

Length of Stay by Diagnosis and Operation, United States, 1997

United States, October 1995–September 1996 Data, by Operation

49.9: OTH OPERATIONS ON ANUS. Formerly included in operation group(s) 622.

Type of Patients	Observed Patients	Avg. Stay	Variance	Percentiles						
				10th	25th	50th	75th	90th	95th	99th
1. SINGLE DX										
0–19 Years	12	3.0	2	1	2	3	3	6	6	6
20–34	2	1.0	0	1	1	1	1	1	1	1
35–49	5	1.7	<1	1	1	1	3	3	3	3
50–64	5	1.4	<1	1	1	1	2	2	2	2
65+	0									
2. MULTIPLE DX										
0–19 Years	24	6.7	47	3	3	5	6	13	30	30
20–34	19	3.8	6	1	1	3	6	6	8	8
35–49	31	5.0	30	1	1	3	8	16	19	19
50–64	29	3.0	5	1	1	2	4	5	8	11
65+	45	4.3	27	1	1	2	6	12	16	28
TOTAL SINGLE DX	24	2.1	2	1	1	2	3	3	4	6
MULTIPLE DX	148	4.5	24	1	1	3	6	8	14	30
TOTAL										
0–19 Years	36	5.4	34	2	3	3	6	12	13	30
20–34	21	3.7	6	1	1	3	6	6	8	8
35–49	36	3.7	21	1	1	2	4	8	9	19
50–64	34	2.7	4	1	1	2	4	5	7	11
65+	45	4.3	27	1	1	2	6	12	16	28
GRAND TOTAL	172	4.0	20	1	1	3	5	8	13	28

50.0: HEPATOTOMY. Formerly included in operation group(s) 623.

Type of Patients	Observed Patients	Avg. Stay	Variance	Percentiles						
				10th	25th	50th	75th	90th	95th	99th
1. SINGLE DX										
0–19 Years	1	2.0	0	2	2	2	2	2	2	2
20–34	2	9.0	0	9	9	9	9	9	9	9
35–49	4	6.4	58	2	4	5	5	5	31	31
50–64	5	3.0	4	1	1	2	5	5	5	5
65+	0									
2. MULTIPLE DX										
0–19 Years	17	22.4	876	3	4	10	20	86	86	86
20–34	28	10.2	105	4	6	6	12	23	26	66
35–49	40	22.1	276	4	7	16	44	44	44	44
50–64	52	13.4	168	3	5	10	17	34	34	75
65+	109	11.3	62	2	7	10	15	20	23	41
TOTAL SINGLE DX	12	5.9	32	2	2	5	9	9	9	31
MULTIPLE DX	246	14.3	195	3	6	10	17	34	44	75
TOTAL										
0–19 Years	18	22.0	865	3	4	10	20	86	86	86
20–34	30	10.1	97	4	6	7	10	18	26	66
35–49	44	20.8	276	4	5	16	44	44	44	44
50–64	57	12.8	164	3	5	10	15	34	34	75
65+	109	11.3	62	2	7	10	15	20	23	41
GRAND TOTAL	258	14.0	191	3	6	10	16	34	44	75

50.1: HEPATIC DXTIC PX. Formerly included in operation group(s) 624, 631.

Type of Patients	Observed Patients	Avg. Stay	Variance	Percentiles						
				10th	25th	50th	75th	90th	95th	99th
1. SINGLE DX										
0–19 Years	227	2.7	10	1	1	1	3	6	9	12
20–34	75	2.7	6	1	1	1	4	6	6	14
35–49	125	1.7	7	1	1	1	1	3	5	10
50–64	83	2.8	12	1	1	1	3	5	12	18
65+	53	3.5	13	1	1	2	5	9	11	17
2. MULTIPLE DX										
0–19 Years	821	8.5	220	1	1	4	9	19	28	97
20–34	446	7.4	65	1	2	5	9	17	22	42
35–49	1262	7.1	59	1	2	5	9	15	20	44
50–64	1722	7.9	51	1	3	6	10	17	22	33
65+	2849	8.5	46	2	4	7	11	16	20	35
TOTAL SINGLE DX	563	2.5	9	1	1	1	3	5	8	17
MULTIPLE DX	7100	8.0	73	1	3	6	10	16	22	42
TOTAL										
0–19 Years	1048	7.0	172	1	1	3	7	16	25	97
20–34	521	6.2	54	1	1	4	8	15	21	36
35–49	1387	6.5	56	1	3	4	8	14	19	44
50–64	1805	7.5	50	1	3	6	10	16	22	33
65+	2902	8.5	46	2	4	7	11	16	20	35
GRAND TOTAL	7663	7.5	70	1	2	5	10	16	21	39

50.11: CLSD (PERC) LIVER BIOPSY. Formerly included in operation group(s) 624.

Type of Patients	Observed Patients	Avg. Stay	Variance	Percentiles						
				10th	25th	50th	75th	90th	95th	99th
1. SINGLE DX										
0–19 Years	196	2.2	9	1	1	1	2	5	6	15
20–34	63	1.9	5	1	1	1	2	4	5	15
35–49	112	1.3	1	1	1	1	1	2	3	9
50–64	71	2.9	12	1	1	1	3	7	12	18
65+	47	3.5	14	1	1	2	5	9	11	17
2. MULTIPLE DX										
0–19 Years	678	5.8	55	1	1	3	7	16	20	37
20–34	381	7.0	62	1	2	4	9	16	22	36
35–49	1119	6.6	50	1	2	5	8	14	18	35
50–64	1449	7.5	41	2	3	6	9	16	21	32
65+	2468	8.4	43	2	4	7	11	15	19	35
TOTAL SINGLE DX	489	2.1	8	1	1	1	2	4	7	15
MULTIPLE DX	6095	7.4	47	1	3	6	10	16	20	33
TOTAL										
0–19 Years	874	4.9	45	1	1	2	5	14	19	35
20–34	444	5.9	55	1	1	3	8	15	20	36
35–49	1231	5.9	47	1	3	6	8	14	18	33
50–64	1520	7.2	41	2	3	6	9	16	21	32
65+	2515	8.3	43	2	4	7	11	15	19	35
GRAND TOTAL	6584	6.9	46	1	2	5	9	15	19	33

Length of Stay by Diagnosis and Operation, United States, 1997

United States, October 1995–September 1996 Data, by Operation

50.12: OPEN BIOPSY OF LIVER. Formerly included in operation group(s) 624.

Type of Patients	Observed Patients	Avg. Stay	Vari-ance	10th	25th	50th	75th	90th	95th	99th
1. SINGLE DX										
0–19 Years	31	5.1	8	1	3	5	7	9	10	12
20–34	12	4.5	1	3	4	4	6	6	6	7
35–49	13	5.9	50	2	2	5	5	10	10	40
50–64	12	2.6	13	1	1	1	4	5	5	18
65+	6	3.0	2	1	2	2	5	5	5	5
2. MULTIPLE DX										
0–19 Years	143	19.5	761	2	4	8	18	97	97	>99
20–34	64	9.8	75	3	5	6	14	22	25	>99
35–49	140	11.6	120	2	5	9	14	26	43	47
50–64	273	9.7	98	1	4	7	13	23	30	43
65+	381	9.6	61	3	5	8	13	18	23	35
TOTAL SINGLE DX	74	4.2	13	1	1	4	5	7	9	18
MULTIPLE DX	1001	11.6	212	2	4	7	14	23	33	97
TOTAL										
0–19 Years	174	16.5	636	2	4	7	16	49	97	97
20–34	76	7.6	51	3	4	6	7	16	25	71
35–49	153	11.1	116	2	5	8	13	25	40	47
50–64	285	8.7	91	1	2	6	10	19	30	43
65+	387	9.5	61	3	5	8	13	18	23	35
GRAND TOTAL	1075	10.6	192	2	4	7	13	21	30	97

50.22: PARTIAL HEPATECTOMY. Formerly included in operation group(s) 624.

Type of Patients	Observed Patients	Avg. Stay	Vari-ance	10th	25th	50th	75th	90th	95th	99th
1. SINGLE DX										
0–19 Years	4	3.8	3	2	2	5	5	5	6	6
20–34	8	5.5	1	5	5	5	5	5	8	10
35–49	18	6.5	24	3	3	5	7	17	17	17
50–64	4	7.1	7	4	6	6	11	11	11	11
65+	6	8.1	17	2	5	7	12	12	12	12
2. MULTIPLE DX										
0–19 Years	35	11.9	94	5	6	10	12	19	43	49
20–34	67	8.2	67	5	6	6	7	11	20	52
35–49	111	8.9	91	5	5	6	8	14	15	63
50–64	178	7.9	28	4	5	7	8	12	17	34
65+	260	9.5	44	5	6	8	10	16	21	39
TOTAL SINGLE DX	40	6.3	13	3	5	5	7	12	17	17
MULTIPLE DX	651	8.9	56	5	6	7	9	14	19	52
TOTAL										
0–19 Years	39	11.3	91	5	6	9	12	19	23	49
20–34	75	7.9	62	5	6	6	7	9	17	52
35–49	129	8.7	86	4	5	6	8	14	16	63
50–64	182	7.9	28	4	5	7	8	11	17	34
65+	266	9.4	43	5	6	8	10	16	21	39
GRAND TOTAL	691	8.8	55	5	6	7	9	14	18	51

50.2: LOC EXC/DESTR LIVER LES. Formerly included in operation group(s) 624.

Type of Patients	Observed Patients	Avg. Stay	Vari-ance	10th	25th	50th	75th	90th	95th	99th
1. SINGLE DX										
0–19 Years	18	3.5	2	1	3	3	5	5	6	6
20–34	13	5.2	3	4	5	5	5	8	9	10
35–49	31	5.2	15	2	3	4	6	8	17	17
50–64	10	6.0	11	1	4	6	8	11	11	12
65+	11	6.3	16	1	2	6	12	12	12	12
2. MULTIPLE DX										
0–19 Years	51	9.9	64	5	6	7	11	15	20	49
20–34	107	7.4	58	4	5	6	6	9	15	52
35–49	177	8.1	86	1	5	6	8	14	17	63
50–64	289	6.8	26	1	4	6	8	11	15	30
65+	440	8.7	36	4	6	7	10	14	18	34
TOTAL SINGLE DX	83	4.9	10	2	3	4	6	8	12	17
MULTIPLE DX	1064	8.0	47	4	5	6	9	14	17	44
TOTAL										
0–19 Years	69	8.1	55	3	5	6	10	12	19	49
20–34	120	7.3	55	4	5	6	6	9	15	52
35–49	208	7.8	79	2	4	6	8	14	17	61
50–64	299	6.8	26	1	4	6	8	11	15	30
65+	451	8.6	36	4	6	7	10	14	18	34
GRAND TOTAL	1147	7.8	46	3	5	6	9	13	17	43

50.29: DESTR HEPATIC LESION NEC. Formerly included in operation group(s) 624.

Type of Patients	Observed Patients	Avg. Stay	Vari-ance	10th	25th	50th	75th	90th	95th	99th
1. SINGLE DX										
0–19 Years	10	3.5	2	1	3	3	4	5	5	6
20–34	5	4.0	10	1	1	4	4	9	9	9
35–49	13	3.8	1	2	3	4	4	6	6	6
50–64	6	5.4	13	1	2	4	8	8	12	12
65+	5	4.0	6	1	1	4	6	7	7	7
2. MULTIPLE DX										
0–19 Years	16	6.9	4	5	6	7	7	8	11	16
20–34	40	6.2	39	3	4	6	6	7	8	24
35–49	64	6.9	76	1	1	5	9	13	23	29
50–64	102	5.7	20	3	5	6	8	9	14	23
65+	168	7.9	26	3	5	6	10	14	18	26
TOTAL SINGLE DX	39	3.9	4	1	3	4	5	6	8	9
MULTIPLE DX	390	6.8	34	1	4	6	8	12	15	29
TOTAL										
0–19 Years	26	5.5	6	3	4	6	7	7	11	16
20–34	45	6.1	38	3	4	6	6	9	15	24
35–49	77	6.5	67	1	2	5	8	12	18	29
50–64	108	5.7	19	1	1	6	8	9	14	23
65+	173	7.8	26	3	5	6	9	14	18	26
GRAND TOTAL	429	6.6	32	1	4	6	8	12	15	29

Length of Stay by Diagnosis and Operation, United States, 1997

United States, October 1995–September 1996 Data, by Operation

50.5: LIVER TRANSPLANT. Formerly included in operation group(s) 624.

Type of Patients	Observed Patients	Avg. Stay	Variance	10th	25th	50th	75th	90th	95th	99th
1. SINGLE DX										
0–19 Years	3	10.8	28	8	8	10	10	25	25	25
20–34	1	14.0	0	14	14	14	14	14	14	14
35–49	3	12.4	24	7	7	13	17	17	17	17
50–64	5	11.7	2	10	11	11	13	15	15	15
65+	1	11.0	0	11	11	11	11	11	11	11
2. MULTIPLE DX										
0–19 Years	149	29.9	371	11	14	24	50	62	>99	>99
20–34	36	26.7	285	12	15	21	31	58	71	>99
35–49	282	25.5	382	10	12	19	30	67	70	97
50–64	241	24.2	301	10	12	18	32	66	>99	>99
65+	48	27.8	407	9	14	22	33	67	77	>99
TOTAL SINGLE DX	13	12.3	12	8	10	12	14	17	17	25
MULTIPLE DX	756	26.3	355	10	13	21	36	65	85	>99
TOTAL										
0–19 Years	152	29.5	372	11	14	23	47	61	99	>99
20–34	37	25.3	269	13	14	19	31	42	71	>99
35–49	285	25.3	379	10	11	18	29	67	70	97
50–64	246	23.9	297	10	12	18	32	66	>99	>99
65+	49	27.5	405	9	13	22	33	67	77	>99
GRAND TOTAL	769	26.0	351	10	12	20	34	65	85	>99

50.59: LIVER TRANSPLANT NEC. Formerly included in operation group(s) 624.

Type of Patients	Observed Patients	Avg. Stay	Variance	10th	25th	50th	75th	90th	95th	99th
1. SINGLE DX										
0–19 Years	3	10.8	28	8	8	10	10	25	25	25
20–34	1	14.0	0	14	14	14	14	14	14	14
35–49	3	12.4	24	7	7	13	17	17	17	17
50–64	5	11.7	2	10	11	11	13	15	15	15
65+	1	11.0	0	11	11	11	11	11	11	11
2. MULTIPLE DX										
0–19 Years	149	29.9	371	11	14	24	50	62	>99	>99
20–34	36	26.7	285	12	15	21	31	58	71	>99
35–49	281	25.6	382	10	12	19	30	67	70	97
50–64	239	24.2	301	10	12	18	32	66	>99	>99
65+	47	27.2	404	9	14	22	33	67	77	>99
TOTAL SINGLE DX	13	12.3	12	8	10	12	14	17	17	25
MULTIPLE DX	752	26.3	355	10	13	21	36	65	85	>99
TOTAL										
0–19 Years	152	29.5	372	11	14	23	47	61	99	>99
20–34	37	25.3	269	13	14	19	31	42	71	>99
35–49	284	25.4	380	10	11	18	29	67	70	97
50–64	244	23.9	297	10	12	18	32	66	>99	>99
65+	48	26.9	400	9	13	22	33	67	77	>99
GRAND TOTAL	765	26.0	351	10	12	20	34	65	85	>99

50.3: HEPATIC LOBECTOMY. Formerly included in operation group(s) 624.

Type of Patients	Observed Patients	Avg. Stay	Variance	10th	25th	50th	75th	90th	95th	99th
1. SINGLE DX										
0–19 Years	12	7.0	5	5	6	7	8	10	10	15
20–34	5	6.0	3	3	6	6	7	8	8	9
35–49	7	6.3	1	5	6	6	7	7	7	9
50–64	8	5.4	2	4	4	6	6	7	7	7
65+	0									
2. MULTIPLE DX										
0–19 Years	36	11.7	56	6	8	9	13	22	33	39
20–34	29	8.4	14	5	6	7	7	13	19	21
35–49	92	9.3	23	6	6	8	11	13	15	29
50–64	162	9.7	41	6	7	8	10	15	25	35
65+	200	14.2	177	6	9	9	16	24	35	81
TOTAL SINGLE DX	32	6.4	3	4	6	6	7	8	10	10
MULTIPLE DX	519	11.6	97	6	7	8	13	21	28	64
TOTAL										
0–19 Years	48	10.8	50	5	7	8	13	17	33	33
20–34	34	8.1	13	5	6	7	9	13	19	21
35–49	99	9.0	21	6	6	8	10	13	15	29
50–64	170	9.6	40	6	7	8	10	15	25	35
65+	200	14.2	177	6	7	9	16	24	35	81
GRAND TOTAL	551	11.3	93	6	7	8	12	20	26	64

50.4: TOTAL HEPATECTOMY. Formerly included in operation group(s) 624.

Type of Patients	Observed Patients	Avg. Stay	Variance	10th	25th	50th	75th	90th	95th	99th
1. SINGLE DX										
0–19 Years	2	6.1	<1	6	6	6	6	6	7	7
20–34	3	6.7	2	5	5	7	8	8	8	8
35–49	0									
50–64	0									
65+	0									
2. MULTIPLE DX										
0–19 Years	5	47.4	384	14	41	58	65	65	65	65
20–34	3	2.9	4	1	1	1	5	5	5	5
35–49	2	17.1	84	11	11	11	28	28	28	28
50–64	9	12.8	136	1	5	9	21	37	37	37
65+	4	8.5	11	5	5	9	9	13	13	13
TOTAL SINGLE DX	5	6.3	<1	5	5	6	7	8	8	8
MULTIPLE DX	23	17.2	362	1	5	9	21	58	65	65
TOTAL										
0–19 Years	7	32.2	657	6	6	28	58	65	65	65
20–34	6	3.8	4	1	1	5	5	7	5	5
35–49	2	17.1	84	11	11	11	28	28	28	28
50–64	9	12.8	136	1	5	9	21	37	37	37
65+	4	8.5	11	5	5	9	9	13	13	13
GRAND TOTAL	28	15.6	323	1	5	9	14	41	65	65

Length of Stay by Diagnosis and Operation, United States, 1997

United States, October 1995–September 1996 Data, by Operation

50.6: REPAIR OF LIVER. Formerly included in operation group(s) 624.

Type of Patients	Observed Patients	Avg. Stay	Vari-ance	10th	25th	50th	75th	90th	95th	99th
1. SINGLE DX										
0–19 Years	5	2.7	2	1	2	2	3	5	5	7
20–34	18	4.5	12	2	2	4	5	11	15	15
35–49	4	3.0	<1	1	3	3	4	4	4	4
50–64	1	7.0	0	7	7	7	7	7	7	7
65+	0									
2. MULTIPLE DX										
0–19 Years	128	11.7	81	4	6	8	18	21	22	41
20–34	264	9.8	76	4	5	7	10	19	27	50
35–49	143	11.2	129	4	5	7	12	26	35	62
50–64	55	9.7	42	4	7	9	11	12	17	42
65+	62	13.8	100	6	8	10	18	25	31	50
TOTAL SINGLE DX	28	4.0	8	2	2	3	5	7	11	15
MULTIPLE DX	652	10.9	87	4	5	8	12	21	27	47
TOTAL										
0–19 Years	133	11.5	81	4	6	8	15	21	22	41
20–34	282	9.6	74	4	5	7	10	19	27	47
35–49	147	11.0	128	4	5	7	12	25	33	57
50–64	56	9.6	41	4	7	9	11	12	17	42
65+	62	13.8	100	6	8	10	18	25	31	50
GRAND TOTAL	680	10.7	86	4	5	7	12	21	27	47

50.9: OTHER LIVER OPERATIONS. Formerly included in operation group(s) 623, 624.

Type of Patients	Observed Patients	Avg. Stay	Vari-ance	10th	25th	50th	75th	90th	95th	99th
1. SINGLE DX										
0–19 Years	1	5.0	0	5	5	5	5	5	5	5
20–34	10	4.6	8	2	3	3	6	12	12	12
35–49	5	4.9	13	1	1	6	7	10	10	10
50–64	6	2.4	<1	1	2	3	3	3	3	3
65+	11	5.2	35	1	1	1	8	9	20	20
2. MULTIPLE DX										
0–19 Years	16	29.4	349	6	7	28	48	48	48	63
20–34	45	9.4	33	3	4	9	12	16	20	23
35–49	109	17.0	342	4	6	11	20	29	77	77
50–64	177	9.1	42	2	3	7	14	19	21	25
65+	264	11.2	100	3	5	9	13	22	35	41
TOTAL SINGLE DX	33	4.3	13	1	2	3	6	9	12	20
MULTIPLE DX	611	11.8	137	3	5	9	14	23	32	77
TOTAL										
0–19 Years	17	28.2	359	5	7	28	48	48	48	63
20–34	55	8.5	32	3	4	7	12	16	16	23
35–49	114	16.8	339	4	6	11	20	29	77	77
50–64	183	8.9	42	2	3	7	14	19	21	25
65+	275	11.1	99	3	5	8	13	21	34	41
GRAND TOTAL	644	11.5	134	3	4	8	14	23	29	77

50.61: CLOSURE OF LIVER LAC. Formerly included in operation group(s) 624.

Type of Patients	Observed Patients	Avg. Stay	Vari-ance	10th	25th	50th	75th	90th	95th	99th
1. SINGLE DX										
0–19 Years	4	2.5	2	1	2	2	3	5	5	5
20–34	18	4.5	12	2	2	4	5	11	15	15
35–49	4	3.0	<1	1	3	3	4	4	4	4
50–64	1	7.0	0	7	7	7	7	7	7	7
65+	0									
2. MULTIPLE DX										
0–19 Years	115	11.5	75	4	6	8	15	21	22	37
20–34	243	9.1	69	4	5	7	10	18	24	47
35–49	135	11.0	126	4	5	7	12	25	33	62
50–64	47	9.1	23	6	7	9	11	11	12	40
65+	48	14.2	111	6	9	11	19	25	31	50
TOTAL SINGLE DX	27	3.9	8	2	2	3	5	7	11	15
MULTIPLE DX	588	10.5	83	4	5	7	12	21	27	47
TOTAL										
0–19 Years	119	11.3	75	4	5	7	15	21	22	37
20–34	261	8.9	67	3	5	7	10	17	22	47
35–49	139	10.8	124	4	5	7	12	25	33	62
50–64	48	9.0	23	4	7	9	11	11	12	40
65+	48	14.2	111	6	9	11	19	25	31	50
GRAND TOTAL	615	10.3	82	4	5	7	11	21	27	47

50.91: PERC LIVER ASPIRATION. Formerly included in operation group(s) 623.

Type of Patients	Observed Patients	Avg. Stay	Vari-ance	10th	25th	50th	75th	90th	95th	99th
1. SINGLE DX										
0–19 Years	1	5.0	0	5	5	5	5	5	5	5
20–34	9	4.9	8	3	3	3	6	12	12	12
35–49	5	4.9	13	1	1	6	7	10	10	10
50–64	6	2.4	<1	1	2	3	3	3	3	3
65+	10	5.6	37	1	1	1	8	20	20	20
2. MULTIPLE DX										
0–19 Years	14	30.8	332	6	11	28	48	48	48	63
20–34	43	9.4	33	3	4	9	12	16	20	23
35–49	90	18.1	358	5	7	11	22	35	77	77
50–64	148	9.5	43	3	3	8	14	21	21	25
65+	228	12.4	103	4	7	9	14	24	40	41
TOTAL SINGLE DX	31	4.5	13	1	3	3	6	9	12	20
MULTIPLE DX	523	12.6	143	3	5	9	15	24	39	77
TOTAL										
0–19 Years	15	29.4	348	5	7	28	48	48	48	63
20–34	52	8.7	32	3	4	7	12	16	16	23
35–49	95	17.8	355	5	7	11	22	35	77	77
50–64	154	9.3	43	3	3	7	14	20	21	25
65+	238	12.2	102	4	7	9	14	23	40	41
GRAND TOTAL	554	12.2	140	3	5	9	15	24	35	77

Length of Stay by Diagnosis and Operation, United States, 1997

United States, October 1995–September 1996 Data, by Operation

51.0: GB INC & CHOLECYSTOSTOMY. Formerly included in operation group(s) 629.

Type of Patients	Observed Patients	Avg. Stay	Vari-ance	Percentiles						
				10th	25th	50th	75th	90th	95th	99th
1. SINGLE DX										
0–19 Years	2	5.2	4	4	4	4	7	7	7	7
20–34	1	1.0	0	1	1	1	1	1	1	1
35–49	6	3.6	3	2	2	4	4	6	8	8
50–64	5	5.7	59	2	2	2	8	24	24	24
65+	5	10.7	16	4	8	12	14	15	15	15
2. MULTIPLE DX										
0–19 Years	8	14.9	26	15	15	15	15	15	15	17
20–34	17	7.1	33	4	4	5	8	12	24	26
35–49	49	9.3	64	3	5	6	10	19	31	41
50–64	93	8.6	60	3	4	6	11	17	23	35
65+	352	12.2	77	4	6	11	15	24	30	59
TOTAL SINGLE DX	19	6.0	31	2	2	4	8	14	15	24
MULTIPLE DX	519	11.3	69	4	6	10	15	21	27	53
TOTAL										
0–19 Years	10	14.8	26	15	15	15	15	15	15	17
20–34	18	7.0	33	2	4	5	8	12	24	26
35–49	55	8.6	60	2	4	6	10	18	29	41
50–64	98	8.5	60	3	4	6	10	17	23	35
65+	357	12.2	76	4	6	11	15	24	30	59
GRAND TOTAL	538	11.2	69	3	5	10	15	21	26	53

51.10: ERCP. Formerly included in operation group(s) 628.

Type of Patients	Observed Patients	Avg. Stay	Vari-ance	Percentiles						
				10th	25th	50th	75th	90th	95th	99th
1. SINGLE DX										
0–19 Years	36	3.4	12	1	1	3	4	7	15	15
20–34	177	2.9	4	1	1	2	4	6	7	11
35–49	212	3.3	7	1	2	2	4	7	8	13
50–64	173	2.8	6	1	1	2	4	6	8	11
65+	113	3.8	18	1	1	2	5	9	10	24
2. MULTIPLE DX										
0–19 Years	99	5.1	32	1	2	3	6	10	19	33
20–34	908	5.7	31	1	2	4	7	11	15	29
35–49	1650	6.4	36	2	3	5	8	12	17	32
50–64	1937	6.2	34	2	3	5	7	12	16	28
65+	4435	7.0	29	2	4	6	9	13	17	27
TOTAL SINGLE DX	711	3.1	8	1	1	2	4	6	8	13
MULTIPLE DX	9029	6.5	32	2	3	5	8	13	17	28
TOTAL										
0–19 Years	135	4.7	28	1	2	3	5	8	18	33
20–34	1085	5.3	28	1	2	4	6	10	15	27
35–49	1862	6.0	34	2	3	4	7	11	17	29
50–64	2110	5.9	33	1	2	4	7	12	15	27
65+	4548	7.0	29	2	4	6	9	13	17	27
GRAND TOTAL	9740	6.3	31	2	3	5	8	12	17	27

51.1: BILIARY TRACT DXTIC PX. Formerly included in operation group(s) 628, 629, 631.

Type of Patients	Observed Patients	Avg. Stay	Vari-ance	Percentiles						
				10th	25th	50th	75th	90th	95th	99th
1. SINGLE DX										
0–19 Years	39	3.3	12	1	1	2	4	6	15	15
20–34	182	2.8	4	1	1	2	3	6	7	11
35–49	217	3.3	7	2	2	2	4	6	8	13
50–64	186	2.8	5	1	1	2	4	6	8	11
65+	124	3.5	16	1	1	2	4	7	10	24
2. MULTIPLE DX										
0–19 Years	108	5.1	31	1	2	3	6	10	19	33
20–34	944	5.7	31	1	3	4	7	11	15	27
35–49	1722	6.5	40	2	3	5	8	12	17	39
50–64	2075	6.1	34	2	3	5	7	12	15	28
65+	4825	7.0	30	2	4	6	9	14	17	27
TOTAL SINGLE DX	748	3.1	8	1	1	2	4	6	8	13
MULTIPLE DX	9674	6.5	33	2	3	5	8	13	17	29
TOTAL										
0–19 Years	147	4.6	26	1	2	3	5	10	15	28
20–34	1126	5.3	28	1	3	4	6	10	15	27
35–49	1939	6.1	38	2	3	4	7	11	17	38
50–64	2261	5.8	32	1	2	4	7	12	15	27
65+	4949	6.9	30	2	3	6	9	13	17	27
GRAND TOTAL	10422	6.2	32	1	3	5	8	12	16	28

51.14: CLSD BD/SPHINCT ODDI BX. Formerly included in operation group(s) 628.

Type of Patients	Observed Patients	Avg. Stay	Vari-ance	Percentiles						
				10th	25th	50th	75th	90th	95th	99th
1. SINGLE DX										
0–19 Years	0									
20–34	0									
35–49	1	2.0	0	2	2	2	2	2	2	2
50–64	6	1.6	<1	1	1	1	1	1	2	2
65+	5	1.2	<1	1	1	2	1	1	3	4
2. MULTIPLE DX										
0–19 Years	2	2.0	0	2	2	2	2	2	2	2
20–34	14	6.4	31	3	4	4	7	19	19	19
35–49	18	6.3	59	2	3	4	6	10	26	39
50–64	64	3.6	11	1	1	3	6	10	10	15
65+	226	6.4	41	1	3	4	9	13	14	36
TOTAL SINGLE DX	12	1.3	<1	1	1	1	2	2	2	4
MULTIPLE DX	324	5.9	36	1	2	4	8	13	14	36
TOTAL										
0–19 Years	2	2.0	0	2	2	2	2	2	2	2
20–34	14	6.4	31	3	4	4	7	19	19	19
35–49	19	6.2	57	2	3	3	6	10	26	39
50–64	70	3.5	10	1	1	2	5	9	10	15
65+	231	6.2	40	1	3	4	9	13	14	36
GRAND TOTAL	336	5.6	35	1	2	4	7	13	14	26

Length of Stay by Diagnosis and Operation, United States, 1997

United States, October 1995–September 1996 Data, by Operation

51.2: CHOLECYSTECTOMY. Formerly included in operation group(s) 625, 626.

Type of Patients	Observed Patients	Avg. Stay	Vari-ance	10th	25th	50th	75th	90th	95th	99th
1. SINGLE DX										
0–19 Years	689	2.0	2	1	1	2	2	4	4	8
20–34	6762	1.9	2	1	1	1	2	3	4	7
35–49	6269	2.0	2	1	1	1	2	4	5	7
50–64	3968	2.0	2	1	1	1	3	4	5	7
65+	1793	2.7	5	1	1	2	4	6	7	8
2. MULTIPLE DX										
0–19 Years	1156	4.4	16	1	2	3	5	8	13	18
20–34	11418	3.7	17	1	2	3	5	7	9	18
35–49	16641	3.8	16	1	1	3	5	7	10	19
50–64	19791	4.4	19	1	2	3	6	8	11	20
65+	33870	6.5	36	1	3	5	8	13	17	31
TOTAL SINGLE DX	19481	2.0	2	1	1	1	2	4	5	7
MULTIPLE DX	82876	4.8	25	1	2	4	6	10	13	24
TOTAL										
0–19 Years	1845	3.4	12	1	1	2	4	7	10	14
20–34	18180	3.0	12	1	1	2	4	6	7	13
35–49	22910	3.3	12	1	1	2	4	7	9	16
50–64	23759	3.9	16	1	2	3	5	8	10	19
65+	35663	6.3	35	1	3	5	8	12	16	30
GRAND TOTAL	102357	4.2	21	1	1	3	5	9	12	22

51.22: CHOLECYSTECTOMY NOS. Formerly included in operation group(s) 625.

Type of Patients	Observed Patients	Avg. Stay	Vari-ance	10th	25th	50th	75th	90th	95th	99th
1. SINGLE DX										
0–19 Years	65	3.4	7	1	2	3	4	5	9	17
20–34	695	3.7	6	2	2	3	5	6	7	9
35–49	794	3.5	3	1	2	3	4	6	7	10
50–64	666	3.9	4	2	3	4	5	6	7	10
65+	353	4.7	9	2	3	4	6	8	8	14
2. MULTIPLE DX										
0–19 Years	250	6.1	29	2	3	5	7	10	15	25
20–34	2263	5.8	28	3	4	5	7	9	13	24
35–49	3913	6.1	24	2	3	5	7	10	13	27
50–64	5505	6.7	29	3	4	5	8	11	15	28
65+	11984	8.7	41	3	5	7	10	15	20	34
TOTAL SINGLE DX	2573	3.8	5	2	2	3	5	6	8	10
MULTIPLE DX	23915	7.3	34	3	4	6	9	13	17	30
TOTAL										
0–19 Years	315	5.5	25	2	3	5	7	10	13	21
20–34	2958	5.3	24	2	3	4	6	9	11	22
35–49	4707	5.6	22	2	4	5	7	10	12	23
50–64	6171	6.4	27	3	4	5	8	11	14	28
65+	12337	8.5	41	3	5	7	10	15	20	33
GRAND TOTAL	26488	6.9	32	3	4	6	8	12	16	29

51.23: LAPSCP CHOLECYSTECTOMY. Formerly included in operation group(s) 626.

Type of Patients	Observed Patients	Avg. Stay	Vari-ance	10th	25th	50th	75th	90th	95th	99th
1. SINGLE DX										
0–19 Years	624	1.9	2	1	1	2	2	4	4	6
20–34	6067	1.7	1	1	1	1	2	3	4	7
35–49	5475	1.8	2	1	1	1	2	3	4	7
50–64	3302	1.7	2	1	1	1	2	3	4	6
65+	1440	2.1	3	1	1	2	2	4	6	8
2. MULTIPLE DX										
0–19 Years	906	3.9	12	1	2	3	5	8	13	14
20–34	9155	3.2	13	1	1	2	4	6	8	15
35–49	12728	3.1	11	1	1	2	4	6	8	16
50–64	14286	3.5	12	1	1	2	5	7	9	16
65+	21886	5.3	29	1	3	4	7	11	14	29
TOTAL SINGLE DX	16908	1.8	2	1	1	1	2	3	4	7
MULTIPLE DX	58961	3.9	18	1	1	3	5	8	10	20
TOTAL										
0–19 Years	1530	3.0	8	1	1	2	4	6	9	14
20–34	15222	2.5	8	1	1	2	3	5	6	11
35–49	18203	2.7	8	1	1	2	3	5	7	13
50–64	17588	3.1	10	1	2	3	4	6	8	14
65+	23326	5.1	28	1	2	4	7	10	14	27
GRAND TOTAL	75869	3.3	14	1	1	2	4	7	9	18

51.3: BILIARY TRACT ANAST. Formerly included in operation group(s) 629.

Type of Patients	Observed Patients	Avg. Stay	Vari-ance	10th	25th	50th	75th	90th	95th	99th
1. SINGLE DX										
0–19 Years	41	8.7	17	5	6	8	10	13	22	22
20–34	7	5.2	4	4	4	4	6	8	9	12
35–49	7	5.2	<1	4	5	5	6	6	7	7
50–64	10	6.7	1	6	7	7	7	7	7	10
65+	11	8.2	8	4	6	7	11	12	13	13
2. MULTIPLE DX										
0–19 Years	82	14.4	77	6	8	13	20	23	32	51
20–34	83	10.2	22	6	7	8	13	16	19	27
35–49	182	10.9	66	4	6	8	12	20	27	46
50–64	412	12.7	65	6	7	10	15	23	26	45
65+	1055	13.0	55	7	8	11	16	23	27	40
TOTAL SINGLE DX	76	7.4	10	4	6	7	8	12	13	22
MULTIPLE DX	1814	12.6	59	6	7	10	15	22	27	45
TOTAL										
0–19 Years	123	12.4	63	5	7	10	15	22	27	51
20–34	90	9.6	23	5	7	8	13	16	19	27
35–49	189	10.8	65	4	6	8	12	20	25	46
50–64	422	12.2	62	6	7	10	15	22	25	45
65+	1066	13.0	55	7	8	11	16	23	27	40
GRAND TOTAL	1890	12.3	58	6	7	10	15	22	27	44

Length of Stay by Diagnosis and Operation, United States, 1997

United States, October 1995–September 1996 Data, by Operation

51.32: GB-TO-INTESTINE ANAST. Formerly included in operation group(s) 629.

Type of Patients	Observed Patients	Avg. Stay	Vari-ance	10th	25th	50th	75th	90th	95th	99th
1. SINGLE DX										
0–19 Years	1	5.0	0	5	5	5	5	5	5	5
20–34	0									
35–49	1	6.0	0	6	6	6	6	6	6	6
50–64	3	6.9	<1	7	7	7	7	7	7	7
65+	3	7.9	22	4	4	6	13	13	13	13
2. MULTIPLE DX										
0–19 Years	8	12.5	40	9	11	11	14	14	14	38
20–34	8	12.8	54	9	7	9	15	27	27	27
35–49	42	9.0	53	4	4	8	9	20	23	46
50–64	124	12.2	62	6	6	11	14	23	28	39
65+	320	13.5	74	6	7	10	18	23	30	47
TOTAL SINGLE DX	8	6.9	1	6	7	7	7	7	7	13
MULTIPLE DX	502	12.5	70	5	7	10	16	23	28	47
TOTAL										
0–19 Years	9	11.0	41	5	9	11	12	14	14	38
20–34	8	12.8	54	6	7	9	15	27	27	27
35–49	43	9.0	96	4	8	8	9	20	23	46
50–64	127	11.0	53	6	6	11	14	23	28	39
65+	323	13.5	74	6	7	10	18	23	30	47
GRAND TOTAL	510	12.1	67	5	7	9	15	23	27	47

51.4: INC BILE DUCT OBSTR. Formerly included in operation group(s) 629.

Type of Patients	Observed Patients	Avg. Stay	Vari-ance	10th	25th	50th	75th	90th	95th	99th
1. SINGLE DX										
0–19 Years	3	7.2	7	5	5	8	8	11	11	11
20–34	14	4.4	8	2	3	3	6	11	12	12
35–49	7	7.1	12	2	6	8	11	11	12	12
50–64	7	6.7	27	5	5	5	5	8	24	24
65+	7	4.1	10	1	1	4	4	11	11	12
2. MULTIPLE DX										
0–19 Years	12	6.0	9	2	3	7	9	9	11	11
20–34	58	12.1	313	2	3	7	9	9	65	65
35–49	95	14.6	393	2	3	8	12	68	68	68
50–64	153	8.9	51	2	5	8	11	15	19	39
65+	420	11.6	79	2	5	10	16	24	24	44
TOTAL SINGLE DX	38	5.8	19	2	4	5	6	11	12	24
MULTIPLE DX	738	11.3	139	2	5	8	13	24	28	68
TOTAL										
0–19 Years	15	6.1	9	2	3	7	9	10	11	11
20–34	72	11.3	287	2	3	6	9	19	65	65
35–49	102	14.3	377	2	3	8	11	68	68	68
50–64	160	8.7	50	2	5	7	11	14	19	39
65+	427	11.4	79	2	5	10	16	24	24	44
GRAND TOTAL	776	11.0	134	2	5	8	13	24	28	68

51.36: CHOLEDOCHOENTEROSTOMY. Formerly included in operation group(s) 629.

Type of Patients	Observed Patients	Avg. Stay	Vari-ance	10th	25th	50th	75th	90th	95th	99th
1. SINGLE DX										
0–19 Years	11	7.8	6	5	6	7	8	13	13	14
20–34	6	4.9	3	4	4	4	6	6	8	12
35–49	5	5.0	<1	4	3	5	6	6	6	6
50–64	6	4.0	2	3	3	3	6	6	6	6
65+	7	7.5	4	6	7	7	9	11	11	11
2. MULTIPLE DX										
0–19 Years	16	8.9	32	4	6	7	10	17	19	31
20–34	46	9.8	20	6	7	8	13	15	16	32
35–49	96	12.6	96	6	8	10	15	22	37	50
50–64	240	12.9	59	6	8	11	16	23	24	39
65+	647	13.1	50	7	9	11	16	23	27	36
TOTAL SINGLE DX	35	6.1	6	4	4	6	7	9	11	13
MULTIPLE DX	1045	12.7	56	6	8	11	15	23	26	39
TOTAL										
0–19 Years	27	8.4	20	5	6	7	10	13	17	31
20–34	52	8.9	20	4	6	8	12	15	16	32
35–49	101	12.2	94	5	6	9	15	22	37	50
50–64	246	12.8	59	6	7	11	16	23	24	39
65+	654	13.0	50	7	8	11	16	23	27	36
GRAND TOTAL	1080	12.5	56	6	8	10	15	22	26	39

51.43: INSERT CBD-HEP TUBE. Formerly included in operation group(s) 629.

Type of Patients	Observed Patients	Avg. Stay	Vari-ance	10th	25th	50th	75th	90th	95th	99th
1. SINGLE DX										
0–19 Years	1	5.0	0	5	5	5	5	5	5	5
20–34	5	3.5	5	2	2	3	3	6	9	9
35–49	0									
50–64	3	17.0	99	3	9	24	24	24	24	24
65+	2	5.5	18	1	1	8	8	8	8	8
2. MULTIPLE DX										
0–19 Years	6	7.0	5	5	6	7	9	9	9	9
20–34	19	8.6	23	4	5	9	10	19	19	19
35–49	42	7.0	37	1	2	6	9	11	20	27
50–64	91	9.0	78	2	3	6	12	16	27	57
65+	196	12.5	109	2	4	9	22	24	28	52
TOTAL SINGLE DX	11	8.1	71	2	3	3	9	24	24	24
MULTIPLE DX	354	10.6	91	2	4	8	15	24	27	52
TOTAL										
0–19 Years	7	6.8	5	5	5	7	9	9	9	9
20–34	24	7.6	23	3	4	6	9	13	19	19
35–49	42	7.0	37	1	2	6	9	11	20	27
50–64	94	9.2	80	2	3	6	12	18	27	57
65+	198	12.5	109	2	4	9	22	24	28	52
GRAND TOTAL	365	10.6	91	2	4	8	15	24	27	52

Length of Stay by Diagnosis and Operation, United States, 1997

United States, October 1995–September 1996 Data, by Operation

51.5: OTHER BILE DUCT INCISION. Formerly included in operation group(s) 629.

Type of Patients	Observed Patients	Avg. Stay	Vari-ance	Percentiles						
				10th	25th	50th	75th	90th	95th	99th
1. SINGLE DX										
0–19 Years	1	9.0	0	9	9	9	9	9	9	9
20–34	1	1.0	0	1	1	1	1	1	1	1
35–49	4	5.4	3	4	5	5	5	8	11	11
50–64	3	5.8	12	2	2	6	10	10	10	10
65+	2	2.2	1	1	1	3	3	3	3	3
2. MULTIPLE DX										
0–19 Years	7	5.1	10	4	4	4	4	8	14	14
20–34	16	6.8	11	5	5	6	7	7	9	24
35–49	38	8.1	40	3	3	7	10	15	15	40
50–64	50	14.5	139	3	5	9	31	31	31	38
65+	110	12.6	46	5	8	11	17	23	24	36
TOTAL SINGLE DX	11	5.4	6	3	4	5	6	9	10	11
MULTIPLE DX	221	11.6	74	3	5	8	15	24	31	37
TOTAL										
0–19 Years	8	5.7	10	4	4	4	8	9	14	14
20–34	17	6.7	12	5	5	6	7	7	9	24
35–49	42	7.5	33	3	4	6	10	15	15	35
50–64	53	14.3	138	3	5	9	31	31	31	38
65+	112	12.5	47	5	8	11	17	23	24	36
GRAND TOTAL	232	11.3	72	3	5	8	15	24	31	37

51.6: LOC EXC BD & S OF O LES. Formerly included in operation group(s) 628, 629.

Type of Patients	Observed Patients	Avg. Stay	Vari-ance	Percentiles						
				10th	25th	50th	75th	90th	95th	99th
1. SINGLE DX										
0–19 Years	13	8.3	12	5	6	7	10	14	14	14
20–34	3	4.7	1	4	4	4	6	7	7	7
35–49	2	6.3	21	1	1	9	9	9	9	9
50–64	6	6.5	5	6	6	6	8	9	9	9
65+	1	9.0	0	9	9	9	9	9	9	9
2. MULTIPLE DX										
0–19 Years	18	9.7	10	5	8	11	11	13	15	18
20–34	19	7.2	13	4	5	7	8	9	11	23
35–49	27	8.3	21	4	5	8	9	17	18	21
50–64	44	9.5	36	3	7	7	10	20	23	34
65+	73	10.1	46	4	6	9	13	20	23	48
TOTAL SINGLE DX	25	6.9	10	4	4	6	8	14	14	14
MULTIPLE DX	181	9.3	32	4	6	8	11	17	21	34
TOTAL										
0–19 Years	31	9.3	11	5	7	10	11	14	14	18
20–34	22	6.5	11	4	4	6	8	9	11	23
35–49	29	8.2	20	4	5	8	9	15	18	21
50–64	50	9.4	34	5	7	7	10	20	23	34
65+	74	10.0	45	4	6	9	13	20	23	48
GRAND TOTAL	206	9.1	30	4	6	8	11	16	21	34

51.7: REPAIR OF BILE DUCTS. Formerly included in operation group(s) 629.

Type of Patients	Observed Patients	Avg. Stay	Vari-ance	Percentiles						
				10th	25th	50th	75th	90th	95th	99th
1. SINGLE DX										
0–19 Years	1	6.0	0	6	6	6	6	6	6	6
20–34	5	3.1	4	2	2	2	3	8	8	8
35–49	6	4.2	3	3	4	4	4	7	10	10
50–64	3	5.5	3	4	4	4	7	7	7	7
65+	1	3.0	0	3	3	3	3	3	3	3
2. MULTIPLE DX										
0–19 Years	10	12.3	118	3	6	6	12	31	37	37
20–34	33	5.7	13	3	4	5	6	8	14	22
35–49	44	8.5	59	3	4	6	10	18	26	42
50–64	51	10.2	58	4	5	7	15	15	27	39
65+	50	12.8	110	5	6	10	15	18	29	52
TOTAL SINGLE DX	16	3.7	4	2	2	3	4	7	8	10
MULTIPLE DX	188	9.8	70	4	5	6	14	18	27	51
TOTAL										
0–19 Years	11	11.6	109	5	6	6	12	31	37	37
20–34	38	5.0	12	2	3	4	6	8	10	22
35–49	50	7.7	51	3	4	5	10	16	21	42
50–64	54	10.2	58	4	5	7	15	15	27	39
65+	51	12.7	110	5	6	10	15	18	29	52
GRAND TOTAL	204	9.1	67	3	4	6	12	17	26	51

51.8: SPHINCTER OF ODDI OP NEC. Formerly included in operation group(s) 628, 629.

Type of Patients	Observed Patients	Avg. Stay	Vari-ance	Percentiles						
				10th	25th	50th	75th	90th	95th	99th
1. SINGLE DX										
0–19 Years	13	3.1	5	2	2	3	3	4	12	12
20–34	189	2.4	4	1	1	2	3	4	6	7
35–49	196	2.5	5	1	1	2	4	5	6	11
50–64	145	2.2	2	1	1	2	3	4	5	9
65+	144	2.0	3	1	1	1	2	4	6	8
2. MULTIPLE DX										
0–19 Years	83	5.7	29	2	3	5	6	10	17	27
20–34	742	4.8	15	1	2	4	6	9	13	21
35–49	1178	5.4	33	1	2	4	7	10	15	33
50–64	1490	5.5	32	1	3	4	7	11	15	32
65+	4776	6.2	32	1	3	5	8	13	17	30
TOTAL SINGLE DX	687	2.3	4	1	1	2	3	4	6	9
MULTIPLE DX	8269	5.8	31	1	2	4	7	12	16	30
TOTAL										
0–19 Years	96	5.5	27	2	3	4	6	10	17	27
20–34	931	4.3	13	1	2	3	5	8	12	19
35–49	1374	5.0	30	1	2	3	6	9	14	28
50–64	1635	5.1	29	1	3	4	7	10	15	32
65+	4920	6.1	32	1	3	5	8	12	16	30
GRAND TOTAL	8956	5.5	29	1	2	4	7	11	15	30

Length of Stay by Diagnosis and Operation, United States, 1997

United States, October 1995–September 1996 Data, by Operation

51.84: ENDO AMPULLA & BD DILAT. Formerly included in operation group(s) 628.

Type of Patients	Observed Patients	Avg. Stay	Variance	10th	25th	50th	75th	90th	95th	99th
1. SINGLE DX										
0–19 Years	0									
20–34	6	2.3	<1	1	2	3	3	3	3	3
35–49	4	2.9	1	1	2	3	4	4	4	4
50–64	4	5.0	11	1	3	3	9	9	9	9
65+	6	3.8	2	2	2	5	5	5	5	5
2. MULTIPLE DX										
0–19 Years	8	2.8	5	1	2	2	4	4	4	12
20–34	34	4.7	8	2	3	4	5	7	7	16
35–49	64	4.2	11	1	2	3	5	7	13	17
50–64	71	5.8	13	1	3	7	7	9	12	19
65+	150	4.4	12	1	3	3	5	7	10	18
TOTAL SINGLE DX	20	3.7	6	1	2	3	4	9	9	9
MULTIPLE DX	327	4.7	12	1	3	4	6	7	12	17
TOTAL										
0–19 Years	8	2.8	5	1	2	2	4	4	4	12
20–34	40	4.4	8	2	3	4	5	7	7	16
35–49	68	4.1	11	2	2	3	5	7	12	17
50–64	75	5.8	13	1	3	7	7	9	12	19
65+	156	4.4	11	1	3	3	5	7	10	18
GRAND TOTAL	347	4.7	12	1	3	4	6	7	11	17

51.85: ENDO SPHINCTOT/PAPILLOT. Formerly included in operation group(s) 628.

Type of Patients	Observed Patients	Avg. Stay	Variance	10th	25th	50th	75th	90th	95th	99th
1. SINGLE DX										
0–19 Years	7	3.8	9	2	3	3	3	12	12	12
20–34	108	2.1	<1	1	2	2	2	3	4	6
35–49	112	2.4	2	1	1	2	4	4	5	7
50–64	85	2.3	4	1	1	1	3	5	6	10
65+	65	1.5	1	1	1	1	2	3	4	7
2. MULTIPLE DX										
0–19 Years	41	7.6	56	2	3	5	8	27	27	27
20–34	389	5.0	16	1	2	4	6	10	13	22
35–49	650	5.7	31	1	2	4	8	11	16	28
50–64	747	5.9	47	1	2	4	7	12	21	32
65+	2274	5.7	27	1	2	5	7	11	15	28
TOTAL SINGLE DX	377	2.1	2	1	1	2	3	4	5	7
MULTIPLE DX	4101	5.7	31	1	2	4	7	11	15	32
TOTAL										
0–19 Years	48	7.2	52	2	3	5	7	17	27	27
20–34	497	4.1	13	1	2	3	5	8	12	21
35–49	762	5.2	28	1	2	4	7	10	15	28
50–64	832	5.5	44	1	2	4	6	11	21	32
65+	2339	5.5	26	1	2	4	7	11	15	25
GRAND TOTAL	4478	5.3	29	1	2	4	7	11	15	31

51.87: ENDO INSERT BD STENT. Formerly included in operation group(s) 628.

Type of Patients	Observed Patients	Avg. Stay	Variance	10th	25th	50th	75th	90th	95th	99th
1. SINGLE DX										
0–19 Years	3	2.4	<1	2	2	2	2	4	4	4
20–34	8	2.2	2	1	1	2	3	4	5	5
35–49	26	3.4	18	1	1	2	3	8	13	19
50–64	20	1.8	2	1	1	1	2	2	5	9
65+	23	3.5	7	1	1	3	6	7	8	11
2. MULTIPLE DX										
0–19 Years	9	3.5	<1	3	3	3	4	5	5	5
20–34	77	6.1	13	1	3	6	7	11	14	17
35–49	178	4.9	15	2	2	4	7	10	11	20
50–64	310	5.1	19	1	2	4	7	11	13	20
65+	1017	6.4	26	1	3	5	8	14	16	22
TOTAL SINGLE DX	80	2.4	7	1	1	2	2	5	8	13
MULTIPLE DX	1591	5.9	23	1	3	5	8	12	16	20
TOTAL										
0–19 Years	12	3.4	<1	3	3	3	4	5	5	5
20–34	85	5.9	13	2	3	5	7	10	14	17
35–49	204	4.7	15	2	2	4	7	10	11	19
50–64	330	4.4	17	1	2	3	6	10	13	17
65+	1040	6.4	26	1	3	5	8	13	16	22
GRAND TOTAL	1671	5.7	22	1	2	4	8	12	15	20

51.88: ENDO RMVL BILIARY STONE. Formerly included in operation group(s) 628.

Type of Patients	Observed Patients	Avg. Stay	Variance	10th	25th	50th	75th	90th	95th	99th
1. SINGLE DX										
0–19 Years	2	1.5	<1	1	1	2	2	2	2	2
20–34	63	2.6	6	1	1	2	3	6	6	6
35–49	52	2.4	3	1	1	2	3	5	6	6
50–64	33	2.0	1	1	1	1	3	3	3	4
65+	48	2.0	3	1	2	2	2	4	6	9
2. MULTIPLE DX										
0–19 Years	20	5.4	12	1	3	5	8	8	8	24
20–34	184	3.6	8	1	2	3	4	6	9	16
35–49	211	3.7	11	1	2	3	5	7	8	19
50–64	286	4.6	11	1	3	4	6	9	10	15
65+	1155	6.9	45	1	3	5	8	15	19	30
TOTAL SINGLE DX	198	2.2	3	1	1	2	3	5	6	7
MULTIPLE DX	1856	5.8	33	1	2	4	7	11	19	30
TOTAL										
0–19 Years	22	5.2	12	1	3	5	8	8	8	24
20–34	247	3.4	7	1	2	3	4	6	8	16
35–49	263	3.4	10	1	2	3	5	9	8	19
50–64	319	4.3	10	1	2	4	5	8	10	15
65+	1203	6.6	44	1	2	5	8	15	19	30
GRAND TOTAL	2054	5.4	31	1	2	4	6	10	17	30

Length of Stay by Diagnosis and Operation, United States, 1997

United States, October 1995–September 1996 Data, by Operation

51.9: OTHER BILIARY TRACT OPS. Formerly included in operation group(s) 627, 629.

Type of Patients	Observed Patients	Avg. Stay	Vari-ance	Percentiles						
				10th	25th	50th	75th	90th	95th	99th
1. SINGLE DX										
0–19 Years	1	3.0	0	3	3	3	3	3	3	3
20–34	6	1.9	3	1	1	1	2	6	6	6
35–49	12	3.5	14	1	2	2	2	9	13	13
50–64	6	1.9	1	1	1	2	2	4	4	4
65+	14	3.5	19	1	1	1	4	11	17	17
2. MULTIPLE DX										
0–19 Years	34	6.8	48	1	2	6	8	14	16	46
20–34	59	4.6	19	1	2	3	6	7	7	25
35–49	127	7.4	38	2	3	6	11	12	15	34
50–64	227	6.0	30	2	3	4	7	11	15	32
65+	584	8.9	60	2	4	7	12	19	20	34
TOTAL SINGLE DX	39	3.0	13	1	1	2	3	9	13	17
MULTIPLE DX	1031	7.6	48	2	3	6	10	16	19	34
TOTAL										
0–19 Years	35	6.7	48	1	2	6	8	14	16	46
20–34	65	4.5	18	1	2	3	6	7	10	25
35–49	139	7.2	38	1	3	6	10	12	15	34
50–64	233	5.9	29	2	3	4	7	10	15	32
65+	598	8.8	59	2	4	7	12	19	20	34
GRAND TOTAL	1070	7.5	48	2	3	6	10	16	19	34

52.0: PANCREATOTOMY. Formerly included in operation group(s) 630.

Type of Patients	Observed Patients	Avg. Stay	Vari-ance	Percentiles						
				10th	25th	50th	75th	90th	95th	99th
1. SINGLE DX										
0–19 Years	3	2.6	1	1	1	3	3	4	4	4
20–34	4	10.4	52	2	7	10	20	20	20	20
35–49	3	5.3	11	2	2	8	8	8	8	8
50–64	4	5.2	16	2	2	3	11	11	11	11
65+	0									
2. MULTIPLE DX										
0–19 Years	14	16.1	61	5	10	18	21	21	21	39
20–34	73	15.9	257	5	6	11	20	42	73	>99
35–49	150	23.1	348	4	9	17	31	64	64	>99
50–64	127	16.8	206	4	7	13	24	41	61	>99
65+	143	21.5	244	5	10	20	26	48	54	73
TOTAL SINGLE DX	14	5.7	24	2	2	3	8	11	20	20
MULTIPLE DX	507	20.2	278	5	8	15	28	48	64	>99
TOTAL										
0–19 Years	17	14.7	72	3	7	18	21	21	21	39
20–34	77	15.8	252	5	6	10	20	38	73	>99
35–49	153	22.9	348	4	9	17	31	64	64	>99
50–64	131	16.5	204	4	7	13	22	41	61	>99
65+	143	21.5	244	5	10	20	26	48	54	73
GRAND TOTAL	521	20.0	277	4	8	15	27	48	64	>99

51.98: PERC OP ON BIL TRACT NEC. Formerly included in operation group(s) 627.

Type of Patients	Observed Patients	Avg. Stay	Vari-ance	Percentiles						
				10th	25th	50th	75th	90th	95th	99th
1. SINGLE DX										
0–19 Years	1	3.0	0	3	3	3	3	3	3	3
20–34	5	2.0	3	1	1	1	2	6	6	6
35–49	9	4.1	18	1	2	2	6	13	13	13
50–64	3	1.5	<1	1	1	1	2	2	2	2
65+	10	3.6	22	1	1	1	3	10	17	17
2. MULTIPLE DX										
0–19 Years	22	6.2	43	1	2	6	7	14	16	35
20–34	31	5.6	23	1	1	6	7	10	13	27
35–49	82	6.7	22	2	3	6	11	11	15	25
50–64	175	5.3	16	2	3	4	7	10	12	23
65+	368	8.4	50	2	3	6	11	19	20	34
TOTAL SINGLE DX	28	3.2	15	1	1	2	3	9	13	17
MULTIPLE DX	678	7.1	37	2	3	6	9	15	19	34
TOTAL										
0–19 Years	23	6.1	42	2	2	6	7	14	16	35
20–34	36	5.4	22	1	1	6	7	9	13	27
35–49	91	6.5	22	1	3	6	11	11	15	25
50–64	178	5.3	16	1	3	4	7	10	12	23
65+	378	8.4	50	2	3	6	11	19	20	34
GRAND TOTAL	706	7.0	37	1	3	6	9	15	19	34

52.1: PANCREATIC DXTIC PX. Formerly included in operation group(s) 628, 630, 631.

Type of Patients	Observed Patients	Avg. Stay	Vari-ance	Percentiles						
				10th	25th	50th	75th	90th	95th	99th
1. SINGLE DX										
0–19 Years	1	1.0	0	1	1	1	1	1	1	1
20–34	4	3.0	6	1	1	2	4	7	7	7
35–49	14	3.5	5	1	2	3	4	8	8	8
50–64	13	8.3	30	2	3	7	15	15	15	15
65+	13	4.4	28	1	1	1	7	11	18	18
2. MULTIPLE DX										
0–19 Years	4	6.6	9	5	5	5	6	12	12	12
20–34	50	21.2	301	1	4	13	41	41	41	41
35–49	149	7.8	47	3	3	6	10	16	21	38
50–64	243	7.2	51	2	3	5	9	15	17	39
65+	609	8.7	55	2	4	7	11	19	22	39
TOTAL SINGLE DX	45	4.9	22	1	1	3	7	15	15	18
MULTIPLE DX	1055	8.9	77	2	3	6	11	19	28	41
TOTAL										
0–19 Years	5	3.9	13	1	1	5	5	6	12	12
20–34	54	20.8	302	1	4	13	41	41	41	41
35–49	163	7.5	45	2	3	5	10	15	20	38
50–64	256	7.3	50	2	3	5	9	15	17	39
65+	622	8.6	55	2	3	7	11	19	22	39
GRAND TOTAL	1100	8.8	76	2	3	6	11	19	27	41

United States, October 1995–September 1996 Data, by Operation

52.11: PANC ASP (NEEDLE) BX. Formerly included in operation group(s) 630.

Type of Patients	Observed Patients	Avg. Stay	Variance	10th	25th	50th	75th	90th	95th	99th
1. SINGLE DX										
0–19 Years	1	1.0	0	1	1	1	1	1	1	1
20–34	1	1.0	0	1	1	1	1	1	1	1
35–49	9	2.5	2	1	1	2	4	4	5	5
50–64	5	11.1	35	1	4	15	15	15	15	15
65+	9	4.2	14	1	1	2	7	11	11	11
2. MULTIPLE DX										
0–19 Years	0									
20–34	28	26.3	274	4	6	41	41	41	41	41
35–49	81	7.4	49	1	3	4	10	16	21	38
50–64	136	6.7	45	2	2	4	8	15	17	39
65+	395	8.9	48	2	4	7	12	19	21	31
TOTAL SINGLE DX	25	5.0	27	1	1	2	7	15	15	15
MULTIPLE DX	640	9.3	86	2	3	7	11	19	34	41
TOTAL										
0–19 Years	1	1.0	0	1	1	1	1	1	1	1
20–34	29	26.0	278	4	6	34	41	41	41	41
35–49	90	7.0	47	1	3	4	10	16	21	38
50–64	141	6.8	45	2	2	4	9	15	17	39
65+	404	8.9	47	2	4	7	12	19	21	31
GRAND TOTAL	665	9.2	85	2	3	6	11	19	34	41

52.2: PANC/PANC DUCT LES DESTR. Formerly included in operation group(s) 628, 630.

Type of Patients	Observed Patients	Avg. Stay	Variance	10th	25th	50th	75th	90th	95th	99th
1. SINGLE DX										
0–19 Years	3	7.9	25	4	4	4	9	16	16	16
20–34	1	6.0	0	6	6	6	6	6	6	6
35–49	3	6.9	1	6	6	6	8	8	8	8
50–64	3	3.9	2	2	2	5	5	5	5	5
65+	0									
2. MULTIPLE DX										
0–19 Years	3	11.3	128	5	5	5	10	34	34	34
20–34	26	32.3	926	5	6	16	60	97	>99	>99
35–49	71	38.5	684	7	11	35	71	71	80	83
50–64	75	20.6	477	5	6	13	58	>99	>99	>99
65+	54	26.2	358	7	11	20	42	55	61	>99
TOTAL SINGLE DX	10	6.4	10	4	5	6	8	9	16	16
MULTIPLE DX	229	29.0	614	5	8	22	55	71	>99	>99
TOTAL										
0–19 Years	6	9.7	78	4	5	5	10	16	34	34
20–34	27	32.0	923	5	6	16	60	97	>99	>99
35–49	74	37.2	695	7	11	30	71	71	80	83
50–64	78	20.2	472	5	6	12	46	>99	>99	>99
65+	54	26.2	358	7	11	20	42	55	61	>99
GRAND TOTAL	239	28.2	611	5	8	20	55	71	>99	>99

52.3: PANCREATIC CYST MARSUP. Formerly included in operation group(s) 630.

Type of Patients	Observed Patients	Avg. Stay	Variance	10th	25th	50th	75th	90th	95th	99th
1. SINGLE DX										
0–19 Years	0									
20–34	1	13.0	0	13	13	13	13	13	13	13
35–49	2	2.2	1	1	1	3	3	3	3	3
50–64	2	4.3	<1	4	4	4	4	6	6	6
65+	0									
2. MULTIPLE DX										
0–19 Years	3	9.7	17	4	10	10	10	16	16	16
20–34	9	16.1	300	6	7	12	16	29	71	71
35–49	27	29.2	858	5	8	17	50	89	89	89
50–64	12	16.3	211	6	7	10	23	34	56	56
65+	13	20.7	510	7	7	8	24	42	61	97
TOTAL SINGLE DX	5	4.1	6	1	3	4	4	6	6	13
MULTIPLE DX	64	22.2	580	6	7	10	25	56	89	97
TOTAL										
0–19 Years	3	9.7	17	4	10	10	10	16	16	16
20–34	10	16.0	288	6	7	12	16	29	71	71
35–49	29	27.1	844	3	7	14	34	89	89	89
50–64	14	12.6	176	4	7	9	10	34	56	56
65+	13	20.7	510	7	7	8	24	42	61	97
GRAND TOTAL	69	20.3	550	4	7	10	23	56	89	89

52.4: INT DRAIN PANC CYST. Formerly included in operation group(s) 630.

Type of Patients	Observed Patients	Avg. Stay	Variance	10th	25th	50th	75th	90th	95th	99th
1. SINGLE DX										
0–19 Years	0									
20–34	4	5.4	<1	5	5	5	6	6	6	6
35–49	8	6.5	21	2	3	5	8	9	20	20
50–64	2	6.5	<1	6	6	6	7	7	7	7
65+	1	9.0	0	9	9	9	9	9	9	9
2. MULTIPLE DX										
0–19 Years	6	10.1	2	10	10	10	10	10	13	14
20–34	21	17.4	272	7	9	12	19	39	69	69
35–49	59	11.4	150	5	5	8	11	20	36	74
50–64	64	14.2	123	5	9	9	15	27	43	59
65+	45	12.1	43	6	8	11	14	19	29	>99
TOTAL SINGLE DX	15	6.4	12	2	5	5	8	9	9	14
MULTIPLE DX	195	12.9	114	5	8	10	13	24	36	69
TOTAL										
0–19 Years	6	10.1	2	10	10	10	10	10	13	14
20–34	25	16.0	255	5	7	11	17	39	61	69
35–49	67	11.1	143	5	5	7	11	19	35	74
50–64	66	14.1	122	5	9	9	15	27	43	59
65+	46	12.1	43	6	8	11	14	19	29	>99
GRAND TOTAL	210	12.7	113	5	7	10	13	24	35	69

United States, October 1995–September 1996 Data, by Operation

52.5: PARTIAL PANCREATECTOMY. Formerly included in operation group(s) 630.

Type of Patients	Observed Patients	Avg. Stay	Vari-ance	10th	25th	50th	75th	90th	95th	99th
1. SINGLE DX										
0–19 Years	6	8.0	1	7	7	8	9	9	11	11
20–34	6	6.0	2	4	5	6	7	8	8	8
35–49	9	7.3	10	4	5	7	8	15	15	15
50–64	6	10.4	18	5	6	10	15	15	15	15
65+	5	7.9	6	5	7	7	8	12	12	12
2. MULTIPLE DX										
0–19 Years	42	24.2	852	7	8	12	21	92	92	>99
20–34	72	13.2	124	6	7	9	16	22	30	64
35–49	174	18.7	236	6	8	10	32	42	44	71
50–64	164	18.2	323	6	8	13	18	62	69	69
65+	244	12.9	111	6	7	9	14	26	34	58
TOTAL SINGLE DX	32	7.9	8	5	6	7	9	12	15	15
MULTIPLE DX	696	16.1	245	6	7	10	17	40	50	92
TOTAL										
0–19 Years	48	21.6	754	7	8	10	17	92	92	>99
20–34	78	12.5	117	5	7	9	15	22	30	64
35–49	183	18.5	233	6	7	10	32	42	44	71
50–64	170	18.0	316	6	8	13	18	44	69	69
65+	249	12.8	110	6	7	9	13	26	34	58
GRAND TOTAL	728	15.9	239	6	7	10	17	38	50	92

52.52: DISTAL PANCREATECTOMY. Formerly included in operation group(s) 630.

Type of Patients	Observed Patients	Avg. Stay	Vari-ance	10th	25th	50th	75th	90th	95th	99th
1. SINGLE DX										
0–19 Years	6	8.0	1	7	7	8	9	9	11	11
20–34	6	6.0	2	4	5	6	7	8	8	8
35–49	8	7.9	9	5	7	7	8	15	15	15
50–64	6	10.4	18	5	6	10	15	15	15	15
65+	5	7.9	6	5	7	7	8	12	12	12
2. MULTIPLE DX										
0–19 Years	34	14.8	220	7	8	9	12	33	44	85
20–34	64	12.7	107	6	7	9	15	19	30	69
35–49	142	15.8	192	6	7	9	19	40	40	71
50–64	130	11.6	56	5	7	10	14	18	27	62
65+	179	11.7	82	6	7	9	12	20	34	50
TOTAL SINGLE DX	31	8.0	8	5	6	7	9	12	15	15
MULTIPLE DX	549	12.9	114	6	7	9	13	25	37	62
TOTAL										
0–19 Years	40	13.3	181	7	8	9	12	21	44	85
20–34	70	12.0	100	5	7	9	12	18	28	64
35–49	150	15.6	189	6	7	9	19	40	40	71
50–64	136	11.5	54	5	7	10	14	18	24	62
65+	184	11.7	82	6	7	9	12	20	34	50
GRAND TOTAL	580	12.7	110	6	7	9	13	24	35	55

52.6: TOTAL PANCREATECTOMY. Formerly included in operation group(s) 630.

Type of Patients	Observed Patients	Avg. Stay	Vari-ance	10th	25th	50th	75th	90th	95th	99th
1. SINGLE DX										
0–19 Years	0									
20–34	0									
35–49	0									
50–64	1	12.0	0	12	12	12	12	12	12	12
65+	0									
2. MULTIPLE DX										
0–19 Years	2	44.9	>999	9	9	9	81	81	81	81
20–34	12	21.3	177	8	11	15	31	44	44	52
35–49	24	14.2	164	7	11	11	11	25	55	74
50–64	35	18.3	448	6	7	10	21	71	88	>99
65+	38	22.1	168	10	14	16	26	37	37	93
TOTAL SINGLE DX	1	12.0	0	12	12	12	12	12	12	12
MULTIPLE DX	111	17.6	255	7	11	11	20	37	57	88
TOTAL										
0–19 Years	2	44.9	>999	9	9	9	81	81	81	81
20–34	12	21.3	177	8	11	15	31	44	44	52
35–49	24	14.2	164	7	11	11	11	25	55	74
50–64	36	18.2	444	6	7	11	21	71	88	>99
65+	38	22.1	168	10	14	16	26	37	37	93
GRAND TOTAL	112	17.6	255	7	11	11	20	37	57	88

52.7: RAD PANC/DUODENECTOMY. Formerly included in operation group(s) 630.

Type of Patients	Observed Patients	Avg. Stay	Vari-ance	10th	25th	50th	75th	90th	95th	99th
1. SINGLE DX										
0–19 Years	0									
20–34	1	11.0	0	11	11	11	11	11	11	11
35–49	1	9.0	0	9	9	9	9	9	9	9
50–64	9	12.1	14	7	8	11	15	15	19	19
65+	3	13.2	27	7	7	15	18	18	18	18
2. MULTIPLE DX										
0–19 Years	1	20.0	0	20	20	20	20	20	20	20
20–34	26	22.9	322	11	11	13	36	49	59	77
35–49	151	16.2	60	10	11	13	20	25	30	49
50–64	369	17.7	150	9	11	14	19	32	41	68
65+	569	18.7	104	9	11	15	27	33	36	52
TOTAL SINGLE DX	14	12.0	14	7	8	11	15	17	18	19
MULTIPLE DX	1116	18.1	118	9	11	14	23	33	37	66
TOTAL										
0–19 Years	1	20.0	0	20	20	20	20	20	20	20
20–34	27	22.7	318	9	11	13	36	49	59	77
35–49	152	16.1	60	10	11	13	20	25	30	49
50–64	378	17.6	148	9	11	14	19	32	40	68
65+	572	18.7	103	9	11	15	27	33	36	52
GRAND TOTAL	1130	18.0	117	9	11	14	23	33	37	66

Length of Stay by Diagnosis and Operation, United States, 1997

United States, October 1995–September 1996 Data, by Operation

52.93: ENDO INSERT PANC STENT. Formerly included in operation group(s) 628.

Type of Patients	Observed Patients	Avg. Stay	Variance	10th	25th	50th	75th	90th	95th	99th
1. SINGLE DX										
0–19 Years	2	11.3	115			18	18	18	18	18
20–34	10	2.3	6	1	1	3	5	4	4	5
35–49	11	3.6	6	1	2	3	5	8	9	9
50–64	7	1.8	<1	1	1	2	2	3	3	3
65+	12	2.4	3	1	1	3	3	3	6	9
2. MULTIPLE DX										
0–19 Years	9	4.3	7	1	1	6	6	7	9	9
20–34	53	4.5	16	2	3	5	5	9	10	25
35–49	146	5.6	24	1	3	5	7	10	13	30
50–64	143	5.0	20	1	2	4	6	10	14	24
65+	307	6.7	23	2	4	5	8	12	18	25
TOTAL SINGLE DX	42	2.6	5	1	1	2	3	5	8	9
MULTIPLE DX	658	5.7	22	1	3	5	7	11	14	24
TOTAL										
0–19 Years	11	5.2	22	1	1	6	6	9	18	18
20–34	63	4.2	15	1	2	3	5	9	10	25
35–49	157	5.5	23	1	3	4	6	10	13	30
50–64	150	4.9	20	1	2	4	6	10	14	24
65+	319	6.2	23	1	3	5	8	12	16	22
GRAND TOTAL	700	5.5	22	1	3	4	7	11	14	24

52.96: PANCREATIC ANASTOMOSIS. Formerly included in operation group(s) 630.

Type of Patients	Observed Patients	Avg. Stay	Variance	10th	25th	50th	75th	90th	95th	99th
1. SINGLE DX										
0–19 Years	3	9.1	5	6	6	10	10	11	11	11
20–34	3	6.2	<1	5	5	6	7	7	7	7
35–49	2	11.0	7	5	12	12	12	12	12	12
50–64	2	8.0	0	8	8	8	8	8	8	8
65+	0									
2. MULTIPLE DX										
0–19 Years	5	9.8	16	5	5	12	12	12	17	17
20–34	41	16.2	181	6	6	12	23	41	48	57
35–49	129	15.9	188	6	8	11	17	32	43	80
50–64	93	14.1	101	6	8	10	18	25	29	62
65+	50	12.2	52	6	7	11	16	17	30	41
TOTAL SINGLE DX	10	9.2	7	5	7	10	12	12	12	12
MULTIPLE DX	318	14.7	139	6	7	11	17	29	43	64
TOTAL										
0–19 Years	8	9.6	13	5	5	11	12	12	17	17
20–34	44	15.7	177	6	6	10	21	33	48	57
35–49	131	15.8	183	6	8	11	16	32	43	80
50–64	95	14.0	100	6	8	10	17	25	29	62
65+	50	12.2	52	6	7	11	16	17	30	41
GRAND TOTAL	328	14.6	136	6	7	11	17	28	41	62

52.8: TRANSPLANT OF PANCREAS. Formerly included in operation group(s) 630.

Type of Patients	Observed Patients	Avg. Stay	Variance	10th	25th	50th	75th	90th	95th	99th
1. SINGLE DX										
0–19 Years	0									
20–34	0									
35–49	0									
50–64	0									
65+	0									
2. MULTIPLE DX										
0–19 Years	0									
20–34	16	12.2	163	2	2	11	24	>99	>99	>99
35–49	41	15.1	171	6	8	11	15	45	56	>99
50–64	4	14.2	26	5	10	18	18	18	18	18
65+	0									
TOTAL SINGLE DX	0									
MULTIPLE DX	61	14.4	165	6	7	11	16	45	56	>99
TOTAL										
0–19 Years	0									
20–34	16	12.2	163	2	2	11	24	>99	>99	>99
35–49	41	15.1	171	6	8	11	15	45	56	>99
50–64	4	14.2	26	5	10	18	18	18	18	18
65+	0									
GRAND TOTAL	61	14.4	165	6	7	11	16	45	56	>99

52.9: OTHER OPS ON PANCREAS. Formerly included in operation group(s) 628, 630.

Type of Patients	Observed Patients	Avg. Stay	Variance	10th	25th	50th	75th	90th	95th	99th
1. SINGLE DX										
0–19 Years	6	8.8	35	1	6	10	11	18	18	18
20–34	17	3.5	19	1	1	2	4	6	7	24
35–49	17	5.8	19	1	2	5	12	12	12	12
50–64	11	3.4	8	1	1	2	3	3	6	8
65+	14	2.4	3	1	1	3	3	3	6	9
2. MULTIPLE DX										
0–19 Years	24	6.7	26	1	4	6	8	12	17	23
20–34	127	7.4	79	2	3	5	8	14	26	48
35–49	333	10.1	126	2	4	7	12	24	31	51
50–64	278	8.4	68	1	3	6	10	18	23	46
65+	420	7.4	31	2	4	6	9	13	18	30
TOTAL SINGLE DX	65	3.7	14	1	1	3	4	9	12	18
MULTIPLE DX	1182	8.4	75	2	3	6	10	17	25	47
TOTAL										
0–19 Years	30	7.0	27	1	4	6	10	12	18	23
20–34	144	7.1	75	2	3	5	7	14	25	48
35–49	350	9.9	122	2	4	7	12	24	30	51
50–64	289	8.3	67	1	3	6	10	18	23	46
65+	434	7.0	31	1	3	5	9	13	18	30
GRAND TOTAL	1247	8.1	72	1	3	6	10	17	24	46

Length of Stay by Diagnosis and Operation, United States, 1997

United States, October 1995–September 1996 Data, by Operation

53.0: UNILAT IH REPAIR. Formerly included in operation group(s) 632.

Type of Patients	Observed Patients	Avg. Stay	Vari-ance	Percentiles						
				10th	25th	50th	75th	90th	95th	99th
1. SINGLE DX										
0–19 Years	559	1.3	<1	1	1	1	1	2	2	4
20–34	339	1.6	<1	1	1	1	2	2	3	4
35–49	391	1.6	<1	1	1	1	2	2	3	5
50–64	354	2.0	3	1	1	1	2	4	5	8
65+	428	1.6	1	1	1	1	2	3	4	6
2. MULTIPLE DX										
0–19 Years	736	5.3	212	1	1	1	3	8	62	>99
20–34	325	2.1	4	1	1	1	3	4	5	9
35–49	695	2.5	12	1	1	1	3	6	8	17
50–64	1259	3.3	11	1	1	2	4	6	9	19
65+	5108	4.0	27	1	1	2	5	8	12	24
TOTAL SINGLE DX	2071	1.6	1	1	1	1	2	3	4	6
MULTIPLE DX	8123	3.7	40	1	1	2	4	7	11	36
TOTAL										
0–19 Years	1295	3.7	129	1	1	1	2	5	16	>99
20–34	664	1.9	3	1	1	1	2	3	4	8
35–49	1086	2.2	8	1	1	1	2	4	6	13
50–64	1613	3.0	10	1	1	2	4	6	8	15
65+	5536	3.8	25	1	1	2	5	8	11	22
GRAND TOTAL	10194	3.3	33	1	1	2	4	6	10	26

53.01: UNILAT REP DIRECT IH. Formerly included in operation group(s) 632.

Type of Patients	Observed Patients	Avg. Stay	Vari-ance	Percentiles						
				10th	25th	50th	75th	90th	95th	99th
1. SINGLE DX										
0–19 Years	48	1.5	<1	1	1	1	2	3	3	3
20–34	35	1.6	<1	1	1	1	2	3	3	4
35–49	45	1.8	1	1	1	1	2	3	4	10
50–64	35	3.3	5	1	1	3	4	8	8	8
65+	49	1.7	2	1	1	1	2	4	4	7
2. MULTIPLE DX										
0–19 Years	91	3.7	86	1	1	1	3	8	58	>99
20–34	42	3.0	4	1	2	3	4	6	8	9
35–49	114	2.4	6	1	1	1	3	6	7	10
50–64	212	2.9	11	1	1	2	3	5	8	18
65+	642	3.7	16	1	1	2	5	8	12	20
TOTAL SINGLE DX	212	2.2	3	1	1	1	3	4	6	8
MULTIPLE DX	1101	3.4	20	1	1	2	4	7	11	26
TOTAL										
0–19 Years	139	3.0	63	1	1	1	2	8	36	>99
20–34	77	2.6	3	1	1	2	3	5	7	9
35–49	159	2.2	5	1	1	1	3	5	6	10
50–64	247	3.0	10	1	1	2	4	6	8	16
65+	691	3.6	16	1	1	2	5	8	11	20
GRAND TOTAL	1313	3.2	17	1	1	2	4	7	10	24

53.00: UNILAT IH REPAIR NOS. Formerly included in operation group(s) 632.

Type of Patients	Observed Patients	Avg. Stay	Vari-ance	Percentiles						
				10th	25th	50th	75th	90th	95th	99th
1. SINGLE DX										
0–19 Years	163	1.3	<1	1	1	1	1	2	3	5
20–34	55	1.8	<1	1	1	1	2	3	3	4
35–49	40	1.9	<1	1	1	1	2	4	4	5
50–64	46	2.5	3	1	1	1	5	5	6	6
65+	47	1.5	1	1	1	1	1	3	4	6
2. MULTIPLE DX										
0–19 Years	251	6.9	344	1	1	1	2	17	71	>99
20–34	43	2.9	7	1	1	2	3	6	7	15
35–49	90	3.3	12	1	1	2	4	8	9	17
50–64	124	2.9	7	1	1	2	4	6	8	13
65+	478	4.6	17	1	2	3	6	9	13	19
TOTAL SINGLE DX	351	1.7	1	1	1	1	2	3	5	6
MULTIPLE DX	986	4.8	114	1	1	2	4	8	13	85
TOTAL										
0–19 Years	414	5.1	236	1	1	1	2	5	52	98
20–34	98	2.2	3	1	1	2	2	4	5	9
35–49	130	2.9	10	1	1	2	4	6	7	17
50–64	170	2.8	6	1	1	2	4	6	7	13
65+	525	4.2	16	1	2	3	6	9	12	17
GRAND TOTAL	1337	4.0	86	1	1	2	4	7	11	77

53.02: UNILAT REP INDIRECT IH. Formerly included in operation group(s) 632.

Type of Patients	Observed Patients	Avg. Stay	Vari-ance	Percentiles						
				10th	25th	50th	75th	90th	95th	99th
1. SINGLE DX										
0–19 Years	323	1.3	<1	1	1	1	1	2	2	4
20–34	82	1.5	<1	1	1	1	2	2	3	4
35–49	66	1.6	<1	1	1	1	2	2	3	5
50–64	45	1.9	2	1	1	2	3	3	4	11
65+	70	2.0	1	1	1	2	3	3	4	7
2. MULTIPLE DX										
0–19 Years	372	4.6	151	1	1	1	3	9	47	>99
20–34	74	2.3	7	1	1	1	3	4	7	21
35–49	116	3.0	13	1	1	2	3	6	9	19
50–64	186	3.8	10	1	3	4	4	4	5	13
65+	823	4.4	24	1	1	3	5	9	13	25
TOTAL SINGLE DX	586	1.5	<1	1	1	1	2	2	3	4
MULTIPLE DX	1571	4.1	50	1	1	3	4	8	12	70
TOTAL										
0–19 Years	695	3.1	83	1	1	1	2	5	10	>99
20–34	156	1.9	4	1	1	1	2	3	4	8
35–49	182	2.5	9	1	1	2	4	5	5	18
50–64	231	3.6	10	1	2	4	4	6	7	11
65+	893	4.2	23	1	1	3	5	9	13	25
GRAND TOTAL	2157	3.4	38	1	1	2	4	6	9	47

Length of Stay by Diagnosis and Operation, United States, 1997

United States, October 1995–September 1996 Data, by Operation

53.03: UNILAT REP DIR IH/GRAFT. Formerly included in operation group(s) 632.

Type of Patients	Observed Patients	Avg. Stay	Vari-ance	Percentiles						
				10th	25th	50th	75th	90th	95th	99th
1. SINGLE DX										
0–19 Years	3	1.8	<1	1	2	2	2	2	2	2
20–34	36	1.5	<1	1	1	1	2	2	3	3
35–49	78	1.4	<1	1	1	1	2	2	3	4
50–64	83	1.6	1	1	1	1	2	3	3	4
65+	90	1.3	<1	1	1	1	2	2	2	4
2. MULTIPLE DX										
0–19 Years	5	5.5	8	1	3	6	8	8	8	8
20–34	49	1.8	2	1	1	1	2	3	4	7
35–49	150	2.0	15	1	1	1	2	4	6	13
50–64	300	3.0	8	1	1	2	4	7	8	13
65+	1146	3.5	21	1	1	2	4	8	10	20
TOTAL SINGLE DX	290	1.5	<1	1	1	1	2	2	3	4
MULTIPLE DX	1650	3.2	17	1	1	2	4	7	10	18
TOTAL										
0–19 Years	8	4.3	8	1	2	3	8	8	8	8
20–34	85	1.7	2	1	1	1	2	3	3	7
35–49	228	1.9	11	1	1	1	2	3	6	8
50–64	383	2.6	7	1	1	2	3	7	8	13
65+	1236	3.3	20	1	1	2	4	7	10	20
GRAND TOTAL	1940	2.9	15	1	1	2	3	6	9	16

53.04: UNILAT INDIRECT IH/GRAFT. Formerly included in operation group(s) 632.

Type of Patients	Observed Patients	Avg. Stay	Vari-ance	Percentiles						
				10th	25th	50th	75th	90th	95th	99th
1. SINGLE DX										
0–19 Years	12	1.2	<1	1	1	1	1	2	2	2
20–34	79	1.6	<1	1	1	1	2	2	3	3
35–49	72	1.6	<1	1	1	1	2	3	4	4
50–64	64	1.6	<1	1	1	1	2	3	3	4
65+	78	1.4	<1	1	1	1	1	2	2	4
2. MULTIPLE DX										
0–19 Years	10	1.4	<1	1	1	1	2	2	2	3
20–34	69	1.7	3	1	1	1	2	3	4	6
35–49	105	2.5	10	1	1	1	2	3	4	12
50–64	209	3.3	15	1	1	2	3	7	12	19
65+	1074	4.3	50	1	1	2	5	8	12	51
TOTAL SINGLE DX	305	1.5	<1	1	1	1	2	2	4	5
MULTIPLE DX	1467	3.8	37	1	1	2	4	7	11	51
TOTAL										
0–19 Years	22	1.3	<1	1	1	1	2	2	2	3
20–34	148	1.7	2	1	1	1	2	3	3	5
35–49	177	2.1	6	1	1	1	2	4	7	10
50–64	273	3.0	13	1	1	2	3	7	10	19
65+	1152	4.0	46	1	1	2	4	8	12	51
GRAND TOTAL	1772	3.3	30	1	1	2	3	7	9	24

53.05: UNILAT REP IH/GRAFT NOS. Formerly included in operation group(s) 632.

Type of Patients	Observed Patients	Avg. Stay	Vari-ance	Percentiles						
				10th	25th	50th	75th	90th	95th	99th
1. SINGLE DX										
0–19 Years	10	1.2	<1	1	1	1	1	1	3	3
20–34	52	1.4	<1	1	1	1	2	2	3	4
35–49	90	1.5	<1	1	1	1	2	2	3	3
50–64	81	1.6	2	1	1	1	2	2	3	10
65+	94	1.8	1	2	2	2	2	3	4	6
2. MULTIPLE DX										
0–19 Years	7	4.1	5	1	1	5	5	7	7	7
20–34	48	1.7	2	1	1	1	2	3	4	7
35–49	120	2.6	11	1	1	1	2	4	9	22
50–64	228	3.4	16	1	1	2	4	10	10	25
65+	945	3.8	22	1	2	3	5	7	11	20
TOTAL SINGLE DX	327	1.6	<1	1	1	1	2	2	3	6
MULTIPLE DX	1348	3.4	18	1	2	2	4	7	10	20
TOTAL										
0–19 Years	17	2.2	4	1	1	1	3	5	7	7
20–34	100	1.7	2	1	1	1	2	3	4	6
35–49	210	2.1	6	1	1	2	2	3	5	15
50–64	309	3.0	13	1	1	2	4	8	10	17
65+	1039	3.6	20	1	2	3	5	7	11	19
GRAND TOTAL	1675	3.0	15	1	1	2	3	6	10	19

53.1: BILAT IH REPAIR. Formerly included in operation group(s) 633.

Type of Patients	Observed Patients	Avg. Stay	Vari-ance	Percentiles						
				10th	25th	50th	75th	90th	95th	99th
1. SINGLE DX										
0–19 Years	523	1.2	<1	1	1	1	1	2	2	3
20–34	30	1.1	<1	1	1	1	1	1	2	4
35–49	74	1.4	<1	1	1	1	2	2	3	3
50–64	89	1.3	<1	1	1	1	1	2	3	5
65+	84	2.0	4	1	1	1	2	4	6	8
2. MULTIPLE DX										
0–19 Years	1151	17.4	832	1	1	2	53	91	>99	>99
20–34	61	2.1	2	1	1	2	2	3	4	6
35–49	143	2.0	3	1	1	2	2	3	4	11
50–64	277	2.7	9	1	1	2	3	6	6	17
65+	942	3.4	21	1	2	2	4	7	11	23
TOTAL SINGLE DX	800	1.3	<1	1	1	1	1	2	3	6
MULTIPLE DX	2574	10.5	490	1	1	2	5	73	94	>99
TOTAL										
0–19 Years	1674	12.9	653	1	1	1	9	84	>99	>99
20–34	91	1.7	1	1	1	1	2	3	4	6
35–49	217	1.8	3	1	1	2	2	4	4	8
50–64	366	2.3	7	1	1	2	2	4	9	14
65+	1026	3.3	20	1	2	2	4	6	11	22
GRAND TOTAL	3374	8.3	390	1	1	1	4	57	85	>99

Length of Stay by Diagnosis and Operation, United States, 1997

United States, October 1995–September 1996 Data, by Operation

53.10: BILAT IH REPAIR NOS. Formerly included in operation group(s) 633.

Type of Patients	Observed Patients	Avg. Stay	Vari-ance	10th	25th	50th	75th	90th	95th	99th
1. SINGLE DX										
0–19 Years	182	1.2	<1	1	1	1	1	2	2	3
20–34	1	1.0	0	1	1	1	1	2	2	1
35–49	3	1.4	<1	1	1	1	2	2	2	2
50–64	4	1.7	6	1	1	1	1	1	9	9
65+	5	2.9	3	1	1	4	4	4	5	5
2. MULTIPLE DX										
0–19 Years	445	20.6	945	1	1	3	60	91	>99	>99
20–34	3	1.3	<1	1	1	1	1	2	2	2
35–49	4	1.1	<1	1	1	1	1	2	2	2
50–64	20	2.6	4	1	1	2	3	6	8	8
65+	65	5.6	44	1	1	3	5	22	22	23
TOTAL SINGLE DX	195	1.2	<1	1	1	1	1	2	2	4
MULTIPLE DX	537	18.7	865	1	1	3	53	85	>99	>99
TOTAL										
0–19 Years	627	15.7	777	1	1	2	35	85	>99	>99
20–34	4	1.3	<1	1	1	1	2	2	2	2
35–49	7	1.1	<1	1	1	1	1	2	2	2
50–64	24	2.4	5	1	1	2	3	6	8	9
65+	70	5.4	41	1	1	3	5	22	22	23
GRAND TOTAL	732	14.5	714	1	1	2	9	85	>99	>99

53.12: BILAT INDIRECT IH REPAIR. Formerly included in operation group(s) 633.

Type of Patients	Observed Patients	Avg. Stay	Vari-ance	10th	25th	50th	75th	90th	95th	99th
1. SINGLE DX										
0–19 Years	287	1.2	<1	1	1	1	1	2	2	4
20–34	2	1.4	<1	1	1	1	2	2	2	2
35–49	4	1.6	<1	1	1	2	2	2	2	2
50–64	3	1.2	<1	1	1	1	1	1	2	2
65+	7	2.4	1	1	1	4	4	4	4	4
2. MULTIPLE DX										
0–19 Years	586	15.0	728	1	1	3	23	86	>99	>99
20–34	9	1.3	<1	1	1	1	2	2	2	2
35–49	7	1.7	<1	1	1	2	2	3	3	3
50–64	7	7.5	50	1	2	2	14	17	17	17
65+	69	3.4	19	1	1	3	5	10	13	27
TOTAL SINGLE DX	303	1.3	<1	1	1	1	1	2	2	4
MULTIPLE DX	678	14.0	681	1	1	2	16	84	>99	>99
TOTAL										
0–19 Years	873	10.9	551	1	1	1	4	73	>99	>99
20–34	11	1.3	<1	1	1	1	2	2	2	3
35–49	11	1.7	<1	1	1	2	2	3	3	3
50–64	10	6.4	47	1	2	2	14	17	17	17
65+	76	3.3	18	1	1	3	3	10	13	16
GRAND TOTAL	981	10.4	519	1	1	1	4	73	>99	>99

53.14: BILAT DIRECT IH REP-GRFT. Formerly included in operation group(s) 633.

Type of Patients	Observed Patients	Avg. Stay	Vari-ance	10th	25th	50th	75th	90th	95th	99th
1. SINGLE DX										
0–19 Years	0									
20–34	5	1.1	<1	1	1	1	1	1	1	4
35–49	20	1.2	<1	1	1	1	1	2	2	3
50–64	36	1.2	<1	1	1	1	1	1	3	5
65+	18	1.3	2	1	1	1	1	2	2	15
2. MULTIPLE DX										
0–19 Years	1	1.0	0	1	1	1	1	1	1	1
20–34	16	2.3	1	1	2	2	3	3	3	6
35–49	51	1.7	3	1	1	2	2	2	3	8
50–64	88	2.1	3	1	1	2	3	3	4	11
65+	240	3.4	19	1	1	2	3	7	14	16
TOTAL SINGLE DX	79	1.2	<1	1	1	1	1	1	2	4
MULTIPLE DX	396	2.7	12	1	1	2	3	5	9	15
TOTAL										
0–19 Years	1	1.0	0	1	1	1	1	1	1	1
20–34	21	1.6	<1	1	1	1	2	3	3	6
35–49	71	1.6	2	1	1	1	2	2	3	8
50–64	124	1.8	2	1	1	2	3	3	4	11
65+	258	3.1	17	1	1	2	3	5	14	16
GRAND TOTAL	475	2.3	10	1	1	1	2	4	7	14

53.17: BILAT IH REP-GRAFT NOS. Formerly included in operation group(s) 633.

Type of Patients	Observed Patients	Avg. Stay	Vari-ance	10th	25th	50th	75th	90th	95th	99th
1. SINGLE DX										
0–19 Years	5	1.4	<1	1	1	1	2	2	2	2
20–34	8	1.1	<1	1	1	1	1	2	2	2
35–49	16	1.6	<1	1	2	2	2	2	3	3
50–64	14	1.9	2	1	1	2	2	3	4	11
65+	17	2.2	12	1	1	1	2	3	4	20
2. MULTIPLE DX										
0–19 Years	4	15.3	198	2	11	11	17	48	48	48
20–34	13	2.0	<1	1	2	1	2	4	4	4
35–49	18	2.3	5	1	1	2	4	4	5	11
50–64	50	2.5	8	1	1	2	3	5	6	19
65+	164	3.7	24	1	1	2	5	7	10	30
TOTAL SINGLE DX	60	1.7	3	1	1	1	2	2	3	11
MULTIPLE DX	249	3.4	22	1	1	2	4	7	10	30
TOTAL										
0–19 Years	9	8.9	153	1	1	2	11	17	48	48
20–34	21	1.8	<1	1	1	2	2	3	3	4
35–49	34	1.9	3	1	1	1	2	4	5	11
50–64	64	2.3	6	1	1	2	2	4	5	19
65+	181	3.6	23	1	1	2	5	7	10	30
GRAND TOTAL	309	3.1	19	1	1	2	3	7	9	30

United States, October 1995–September 1996 Data, by Operation

53.2: UNILAT FH REPAIR. Formerly included in operation group(s) 634.

Type of Patients	Observed Patients	Avg. Stay	Variance	Percentiles						
				10th	25th	50th	75th	90th	95th	99th
1. SINGLE DX										
0–19 Years	7	1.3	<1	1	1	1	2	2	2	2
20–34	13	1.4	<1	1	1	1	1	3	3	4
35–49	51	1.6	<1	1	1	1	2	2	3	4
50–64	44	1.5	<1	1	1	1	1	3	4	7
65+	77	3.4	3	1	2	3	5	5	5	8
2. MULTIPLE DX										
0–19 Years	3	1.4	<1	1	1	1	1	3	3	3
20–34	18	2.6	8	1	1	2	3	5	5	16
35–49	65	2.2	4	1	1	1	3	6	6	8
50–64	107	3.8	17	1	2	2	5	8	9	16
65+	806	5.8	43	1	2	4	7	12	18	28
TOTAL SINGLE DX	192	2.2	2	1	1	2	3	5	5	5
MULTIPLE DX	999	5.2	38	1	2	3	6	10	16	26
TOTAL										
0–19 Years	10	1.3	<1	1	1	1	2	2	2	3
20–34	31	1.8	4	1	1	1	2	3	4	16
35–49	116	1.8	2	1	1	1	2	3	5	8
50–64	151	3.1	14	1	2	2	4	7	9	16
65+	883	5.5	39	1	2	4	6	11	16	26
GRAND TOTAL	1191	4.5	31	1	1	3	5	9	13	25

53.21: UNILAT FH REP W GRAFT. Formerly included in operation group(s) 634.

Type of Patients	Observed Patients	Avg. Stay	Variance	Percentiles						
				10th	25th	50th	75th	90th	95th	99th
1. SINGLE DX										
0–19 Years	3	1.1	<1	1	1	1	1	1	2	2
20–34	2	1.6	<1	1	1	1	3	3	3	3
35–49	20	1.7	<1	1	1	1	2	2	3	3
50–64	21	1.3	<1	1	1	1	2	2	3	3
65+	43	3.7	2	2	2	4	5	5	5	5
2. MULTIPLE DX										
0–19 Years	0									
20–34	7	1.3	<1	1	1	1	2	2	2	2
35–49	24	1.8	3	1	1	1	2	2	2	8
50–64	43	3.6	24	1	2	2	5	6	7	40
65+	342	5.0	41	1	2	4	6	10	14	24
TOTAL SINGLE DX	89	2.6	2	1	1	2	4	5	5	5
MULTIPLE DX	416	4.6	37	1	2	3	6	9	13	24
TOTAL										
0–19 Years	3	1.1	<1	1	1	1	1	1	2	2
20–34	9	1.5	<1	1	1	1	2	2	3	3
35–49	44	1.8	1	1	1	1	2	2	3	6
50–64	64	2.9	18	1	1	2	3	6	7	9
65+	385	4.8	34	1	2	4	5	8	13	24
GRAND TOTAL	505	4.0	27	1	1	3	5	7	10	22

53.29: UNILAT FH REP NEC. Formerly included in operation group(s) 634.

Type of Patients	Observed Patients	Avg. Stay	Variance	Percentiles						
				10th	25th	50th	75th	90th	95th	99th
1. SINGLE DX										
0–19 Years	4	1.4	<1	1	1	1	2	2	2	2
20–34	11	1.2	<1	1	1	1	1	1	4	4
35–49	31	1.4	<1	1	1	1	1	3	3	4
50–64	23	1.5	2	1	1	1	1	3	4	7
65+	34	2.5	3	1	1	2	3	4	4	8
2. MULTIPLE DX										
0–19 Years	3	1.4	<1	1	1	1	1	3	3	3
20–34	11	3.2	11	1	1	2	4	5	9	16
35–49	41	2.4	4	1	1	1	3	5	7	9
50–64	64	3.9	13	1	2	2	5	9	12	16
65+	464	6.4	44	1	2	5	8	12	21	29
TOTAL SINGLE DX	103	1.6	1	1	1	1	2	3	4	8
MULTIPLE DX	583	5.7	38	1	2	4	7	12	18	28
TOTAL										
0–19 Years	7	1.4	<1	1	1	1	2	2	2	3
20–34	22	2.0	5	1	1	1	2	4	5	16
35–49	72	1.8	2	1	1	1	2	3	5	8
50–64	87	3.2	11	1	1	2	5	8	9	16
65+	498	6.2	42	1	2	4	8	12	20	29
GRAND TOTAL	686	4.9	33	1	1	3	6	10	16	26

53.3: BILAT FH REPAIR. Formerly included in operation group(s) 634.

Type of Patients	Observed Patients	Avg. Stay	Variance	Percentiles						
				10th	25th	50th	75th	90th	95th	99th
1. SINGLE DX										
0–19 Years	0									
20–34	0									
35–49	1	2.0	0	2	2	2	2	2	2	2
50–64	0									
65+	1	1.0	0	1	1	1	1	1	1	1
2. MULTIPLE DX										
0–19 Years	0									
20–34	2	1.3	<1	1	1	1	2	2	2	2
35–49	0									
50–64	2	1.4	<1	1	1	1	1	3	3	3
65+	17	8.5	59	2	4	5	9	16	29	29
TOTAL SINGLE DX	2	1.5	<1	1	1	1	2	2	2	2
MULTIPLE DX	21	7.2	56	1	2	5	9	16	28	29
TOTAL										
0–19 Years	0									
20–34	2	1.3	<1	1	1	1	2	2	2	2
35–49	1	2.0	0	2	2	2	2	2	2	2
50–64	2	1.4	<1	1	1	1	1	3	3	3
65+	18	8.2	59	2	4	5	9	16	29	29
GRAND TOTAL	23	6.8	54	1	2	5	7	16	28	29

Length of Stay by Diagnosis and Operation, United States, 1997

United States, October 1995–September 1996 Data, by Operation

53.4: UMBILICAL HERNIA REPAIR. Formerly included in operation group(s) 635.

Type of Patients	Observed Patients	Avg. Stay	Vari-ance	10th	25th	50th	75th	90th	95th	99th
1. SINGLE DX										
0–19 Years	92	1.9	2	1	1	1	3	3	5	6
20–34	131	1.6	<1	1	1	1	2	3	3	4
35–49	217	1.8	1	1	1	1	2	3	4	8
50–64	132	2.0	2	1	1	2	2	3	5	8
65+	55	2.3	2	1	1	2	3	4	4	9
2. MULTIPLE DX										
0–19 Years	230	8.3	221	1	1	2	8	23	46	90
20–34	200	2.7	8	1	1	2	3	4	6	10
35–49	661	3.1	9	1	1	2	4	6	8	18
50–64	803	3.9	16	1	1	3	4	8	12	16
65+	1130	4.7	22	1	2	3	6	10	13	23
TOTAL SINGLE DX	627	1.9	2	1	1	1	2	3	4	8
MULTIPLE DX	3024	4.2	33	1	1	3	5	8	12	28
TOTAL										
0–19 Years	322	6.7	173	1	1	2	5	18	35	84
20–34	331	2.2	5	1	1	2	3	4	5	10
35–49	878	2.8	7	1	1	2	4	6	7	15
50–64	935	3.5	13	1	1	3	4	7	11	16
65+	1185	4.6	21	1	2	3	6	9	12	23
GRAND TOTAL	3651	3.7	28	1	1	2	4	7	11	24

53.41: UMB HERNIA REPAIR-GRAFT. Formerly included in operation group(s) 635.

Type of Patients	Observed Patients	Avg. Stay	Vari-ance	10th	25th	50th	75th	90th	95th	99th
1. SINGLE DX										
0–19 Years	2	2.5	<1	2	2	3	3	3	3	3
20–34	18	1.9	1	1	1	1	3	4	4	5
35–49	49	1.6	1	1	1	1	2	3	3	8
50–64	44	2.2	3	1	1	2	2	4	8	8
65+	16	2.3	<1	1	2	2	3	4	4	4
2. MULTIPLE DX										
0–19 Years	11	30.2	418	7	10	46	54	>99	>99	>99
20–34	31	2.5	3	1	1	2	3	6	6	8
35–49	154	2.6	5	1	1	2	4	5	6	10
50–64	215	4.0	18	1	1	2	4	12	16	16
65+	285	4.5	17	1	2	4	5	9	11	18
TOTAL SINGLE DX	129	2.0	2	1	1	2	2	3	5	8
MULTIPLE DX	696	4.0	25	1	1	3	5	8	12	37
TOTAL										
0–19 Years	13	27.0	449	3	7	40	53	>99	>99	>99
20–34	49	2.3	3	1	1	2	3	4	6	8
35–49	203	2.4	4	1	1	2	4	5	7	10
50–64	259	3.5	15	1	2	2	4	8	13	16
65+	301	4.4	16	1	2	3	5	9	11	18
GRAND TOTAL	825	3.6	21	1	1	2	4	7	12	19

53.49: UMB HERNIA REPAIR NEC. Formerly included in operation group(s) 635.

Type of Patients	Observed Patients	Avg. Stay	Vari-ance	10th	25th	50th	75th	90th	95th	99th
1. SINGLE DX										
0–19 Years	90	1.9	2	1	1	1	3	3	5	6
20–34	113	1.6	<1	1	1	1	2	3	3	4
35–49	168	1.8	1	1	1	1	2	4	4	7
50–64	88	1.9	2	1	1	2	3	3	4	5
65+	39	2.3	3	1	1	2	3	4	6	9
2. MULTIPLE DX										
0–19 Years	219	7.5	197	1	1	2	7	23	34	84
20–34	169	2.7	9	1	1	2	3	4	6	11
35–49	507	3.3	10	1	1	2	4	7	9	18
50–64	588	3.8	14	1	1	3	5	8	11	17
65+	845	4.8	24	1	2	3	6	10	14	25
TOTAL SINGLE DX	498	1.8	1	1	1	1	2	3	4	6
MULTIPLE DX	2328	4.3	36	1	1	3	5	9	12	28
TOTAL										
0–19 Years	309	6.1	153	1	1	2	5	14	26	84
20–34	282	2.2	5	1	1	2	3	3	4	10
35–49	675	3.0	9	1	1	2	4	6	8	17
50–64	676	3.5	13	1	1	3	4	7	11	15
65+	884	4.7	23	1	2	3	6	10	13	23
GRAND TOTAL	2826	3.8	30	1	1	2	4	8	11	25

53.5: REP OTH ABD WALL HERNIA. Formerly included in operation group(s) 636.

Type of Patients	Observed Patients	Avg. Stay	Vari-ance	10th	25th	50th	75th	90th	95th	99th
1. SINGLE DX										
0–19 Years	39	2.1	2	1	1	1	3	5	6	6
20–34	146	1.8	<1	1	1	2	3	5	3	5
35–49	308	2.6	3	1	1	2	3	6	6	8
50–64	216	2.3	3	1	1	2	3	4	6	11
65+	160	2.3	3	1	1	2	3	5	6	9
2. MULTIPLE DX										
0–19 Years	95	3.8	15	1	1	2	5	10	13	>99
20–34	313	3.6	8	1	2	4	4	5	11	14
35–49	1173	3.8	16	1	2	3	5	7	10	18
50–64	1312	4.4	19	1	2	3	6	9	10	21
65+	2152	5.2	29	1	2	4	7	11	14	27
TOTAL SINGLE DX	869	2.3	3	1	1	2	3	5	6	8
MULTIPLE DX	5045	4.5	21	1	2	3	6	9	12	21
TOTAL										
0–19 Years	134	3.1	11	1	1	2	4	6	11	20
20–34	459	3.1	7	1	1	3	4	4	8	14
35–49	1481	3.5	14	1	2	3	4	7	9	15
50–64	1528	4.1	17	1	2	3	6	8	10	19
65+	2312	5.0	27	2	2	3	6	10	13	26
GRAND TOTAL	5914	4.1	19	1	2	3	5	8	11	20

Length of Stay by Diagnosis and Operation, United States, 1997

United States, October 1995–September 1996 Data, by Operation

53.51: INCISIONAL HERNIA REPAIR. Formerly included in operation group(s) 636.

Type of Patients	Observed Patients	Avg. Stay	Vari-ance	Percentiles						
				10th	25th	50th	75th	90th	95th	99th
1. SINGLE DX										
0–19 Years	15	3.0	3	1	2	3	4	6	6	6
20–34	70	1.5	<1	1	1	2	4	6	6	5
35–49	185	2.8	4	1	1	2	4	6	6	8
50–64	129	2.2	2	1	1	2	3	4	5	7
65+	114	2.0	2	1	1	1	2	4	5	7
2. MULTIPLE DX										
0–19 Years	54	3.8	14	1	1	3	5	12	15	>99
20–34	184	3.8	16	1	2	3	4	13	14	14
35–49	722	3.9	21	1	2	3	5	8	10	20
50–64	833	4.3	19	1	2	3	6	9	11	21
65+	1435	5.0	29	1	2	4	6	11	14	26
TOTAL SINGLE DX	513	2.3	3	1	1	2	3	5	6	8
MULTIPLE DX	3228	4.5	23	1	2	3	6	9	13	22
TOTAL										
0–19 Years	69	3.6	11	1	1	3	5	8	12	>99
20–34	254	3.1	12	1	1	2	3	6	14	14
35–49	907	3.7	17	1	2	3	4	8	10	16
50–64	962	4.0	17	1	2	3	5	8	10	21
65+	1549	4.8	27	1	2	4	6	10	13	25
GRAND TOTAL	3741	4.1	21	1	2	3	5	8	11	21

53.6: REP OTH ABD HERNIA-GRAFT. Formerly included in operation group(s) 636.

Type of Patients	Observed Patients	Avg. Stay	Vari-ance	Percentiles						
				10th	25th	50th	75th	90th	95th	99th
1. SINGLE DX										
0–19 Years	4	3.3	3	1	2	4	5	5	5	5
20–34	195	2.2	1	1	1	2	5	5	4	5
35–49	629	2.6	3	1	1	2	3	5	6	7
50–64	593	2.3	2	1	1	2	3	4	5	8
65+	352	2.6	3	1	1	2	3	5	8	8
2. MULTIPLE DX										
0–19 Years	11	4.3	4	2	3	4	6	6	8	8
20–34	336	3.8	10	1	2	3	4	8	13	13
35–49	2029	4.1	16	1	2	3	5	7	11	29
50–64	2945	3.8	9	1	2	3	5	7	10	15
65+	4533	4.5	20	1	2	3	6	8	11	21
TOTAL SINGLE DX	1773	2.5	3	1	1	2	3	4	5	8
MULTIPLE DX	9854	4.2	15	1	2	3	5	8	10	17
TOTAL										
0–19 Years	15	4.2	4	2	2	4	6	8	8	8
20–34	531	3.1	7	1	2	2	4	6	9	13
35–49	2658	3.8	14	1	2	3	4	7	9	18
50–64	3538	3.6	8	1	2	3	5	7	9	15
65+	4885	4.4	19	1	2	3	5	8	10	19
GRAND TOTAL	11627	3.9	14	1	2	3	5	7	10	16

53.59: ABD WALL HERNIA REP NEC. Formerly included in operation group(s) 636.

Type of Patients	Observed Patients	Avg. Stay	Vari-ance	Percentiles						
				10th	25th	50th	75th	90th	95th	99th
1. SINGLE DX										
0–19 Years	24	1.6	2	1	1	1	1	4	4	6
20–34	76	2.2	<1	1	2	2	3	3	3	4
35–49	123	2.2	2	1	1	1	3	4	4	6
50–64	87	2.3	5	1	1	1	3	6	7	11
65+	46	3.4	4	1	2	3	4	5	9	9
2. MULTIPLE DX										
0–19 Years	41	3.7	17	1	1	2	5	10	11	20
20–34	129	3.5	3	2	2	4	4	4	5	9
35–49	451	3.7	10	1	2	3	4	7	7	16
50–64	479	4.6	19	1	2	3	6	8	10	17
65+	717	5.5	27	1	2	4	7	11	14	29
TOTAL SINGLE DX	356	2.3	3	1	1	2	3	4	5	9
MULTIPLE DX	1817	4.5	18	1	2	4	6	9	11	20
TOTAL										
0–19 Years	65	2.7	11	1	1	1	3	6	10	20
20–34	205	3.2	3	1	2	3	4	5	5	9
35–49	574	3.3	8	1	2	3	4	7	9	15
50–64	566	4.2	18	1	2	3	6	8	9	15
65+	763	5.4	27	1	2	4	7	11	14	28
GRAND TOTAL	2173	4.1	16	1	2	3	5	8	10	20

53.61: INC HERNIA REPAIR-GRAFT. Formerly included in operation group(s) 636.

Type of Patients	Observed Patients	Avg. Stay	Vari-ance	Percentiles						
				10th	25th	50th	75th	90th	95th	99th
1. SINGLE DX										
0–19 Years	3	3.1	4	1	2	2	5	5	5	5
20–34	144	2.3	1	1	1	2	3	4	4	6
35–49	482	2.7	3	1	1	2	3	6	6	7
50–64	447	2.3	2	1	1	2	3	4	5	8
65+	268	2.7	4	1	2	2	3	5	8	8
2. MULTIPLE DX										
0–19 Years	6	3.6	3	2	2	3	6	6	6	6
20–34	256	3.9	11	2	2	3	4	9	13	13
35–49	1541	3.9	11	1	2	3	5	7	11	14
50–64	2279	3.7	9	1	2	3	5	7	8	14
65+	3566	4.5	20	1	2	3	6	8	10	22
TOTAL SINGLE DX	1344	2.5	3	1	1	2	3	4	5	8
MULTIPLE DX	7648	4.1	14	1	2	3	5	7	10	16
TOTAL										
0–19 Years	9	3.5	3	2	2	3	5	6	6	6
20–34	400	3.2	8	1	2	2	4	7	9	13
35–49	2023	3.6	10	1	2	3	5	7	8	14
50–64	2726	3.5	8	1	2	3	5	8	9	14
65+	3834	4.4	19	1	2	3	6	8	10	19
GRAND TOTAL	8992	3.8	13	1	2	3	5	7	9	15

Length of Stay by Diagnosis and Operation, United States, 1997

United States, October 1995–September 1996 Data, by Operation

53.69: ABD HERNIA REP-GRFT NEC. Formerly included in operation group(s) 636.

Type of Patients	Observed Patients	Avg. Stay	Vari-ance	Percentiles						
				10th	25th	50th	75th	90th	95th	99th
1. SINGLE DX										
0–19 Years	1	4.0	0	4	4	4	4	4	4	4
20–34	51	1.8	1	1	1	1	3	3	3	6
35–49	147	2.4	4	1	1	2	3	5	6	8
50–64	146	2.3	2	1	1	2	3	4	5	7
65+	84	2.5	2	1	2	2	3	4	5	7
2. MULTIPLE DX										
0–19 Years	5	5.5	4	3	3	6	6	8	8	8
20–34	80	3.5	7	1	2	3	4	7	9	14
35–49	488	4.7	32	1	2	3	5	8	12	29
50–64	666	4.3	11	1	2	3	5	9	11	16
65+	967	4.5	22	1	2	3	6	9	12	20
TOTAL SINGLE DX	429	2.3	3	1	1	2	3	4	5	7
MULTIPLE DX	2206	4.5	20	1	2	3	5	9	11	29
TOTAL										
0–19 Years	6	5.4	3	3	4	6	6	8	8	8
20–34	131	2.8	5	1	1	2	4	5	7	12
35–49	635	4.2	26	1	2	3	5	7	9	29
50–64	812	3.9	10	1	2	3	5	8	10	15
65+	1051	4.3	20	1	2	3	6	8	11	19
GRAND TOTAL	2635	4.1	18	1	2	3	5	8	10	25

53.8: REPAIR DH, THOR APPR. Formerly included in operation group(s) 637.

Type of Patients	Observed Patients	Avg. Stay	Vari-ance	Percentiles						
				10th	25th	50th	75th	90th	95th	99th
1. SINGLE DX										
0–19 Years	21	5.8	64	2	3	5	6	6	8	49
20–34	2	5.6	<1	5	5	6	6	6	6	6
35–49	9	5.4	11	2	2	5	10	10	10	10
50–64	6	3.1	5	1	1	3	5	6	7	7
65+	2	8.8	3	7	7	10	10	10	10	10
2. MULTIPLE DX										
0–19 Years	78	15.0	242	3	4	9	18	42	49	63
20–34	22	6.2	8	4	4	6	7	10	10	15
35–49	69	6.6	21	4	5	5	7	11	12	16
50–64	80	7.6	54	1	4	6	8	16	23	38
65+	105	10.8	84	5	5	8	13	17	30	52
TOTAL SINGLE DX	40	5.5	43	2	3	5	6	8	10	49
MULTIPLE DX	354	9.9	104	4	5	6	10	17	30	57
TOTAL										
0–19 Years	99	13.1	219	3	4	7	14	40	49	63
20–34	24	6.2	8	4	4	6	7	10	15	15
35–49	78	6.5	20	4	4	5	7	11	12	16
50–64	86	7.3	52	1	4	6	8	16	20	38
65+	107	10.8	83	5	6	8	13	17	30	52
GRAND TOTAL	394	9.5	100	3	5	6	10	17	30	57

53.7: ABD REP-DIAPH HERNIA. Formerly included in operation group(s) 637.

Type of Patients	Observed Patients	Avg. Stay	Vari-ance	Percentiles						
				10th	25th	50th	75th	90th	95th	99th
1. SINGLE DX										
0–19 Years	37	4.5	11	3	3	4	5	7	8	23
20–34	8	6.2	11	3	3	6	9	10	12	12
35–49	18	4.0	11	1	1	6	6	11	13	14
50–64	28	5.7	1	5	6	6	6	6	6	7
65+	20	4.9	5	2	3	5	7	8	9	10
2. MULTIPLE DX										
0–19 Years	165	18.1	422	4	6	10	24	50	97	>99
20–34	51	8.3	88	3	5	6	8	12	19	59
35–49	156	6.0	26	2	3	5	7	11	13	26
50–64	264	6.4	31	2	3	5	7	13	17	28
65+	599	9.4	51	3	5	8	12	16	22	41
TOTAL SINGLE DX	111	5.0	7	2	3	6	6	6	8	14
MULTIPLE DX	1235	9.2	108	2	4	6	11	17	28	87
TOTAL										
0–19 Years	202	14.5	350	3	4	7	17	50	87	>99
20–34	59	8.1	84	3	5	6	8	12	19	59
35–49	174	5.9	25	2	3	5	7	11	12	26
50–64	292	6.3	26	2	3	5	6	12	17	28
65+	619	9.3	50	3	5	8	11	16	22	41
GRAND TOTAL	1346	8.7	98	2	4	6	10	17	27	77

53.9: OTHER HERNIA REPAIR. Formerly included in operation group(s) 637.

Type of Patients	Observed Patients	Avg. Stay	Vari-ance	Percentiles						
				10th	25th	50th	75th	90th	95th	99th
1. SINGLE DX										
0–19 Years	4	7.2	20	2	4	6	12	12	12	12
20–34	5	3.8	2	1	4	4	4	6	6	7
35–49	17	3.3	4	1	1	4	4	6	7	11
50–64	14	4.1	5	2	3	4	4	6	10	13
65+	8	4.7	1	3	5	5	5	5	5	7
2. MULTIPLE DX										
0–19 Years	19	15.8	644	3	5	6	9	41	96	96
20–34	22	6.7	15	1	3	5	10	12	13	13
35–49	47	6.1	38	2	2	5	7	12	15	32
50–64	81	8.8	31	4	5	8	11	14	17	36
65+	168	12.0	133	3	5	9	14	28	42	50
TOTAL SINGLE DX	48	4.2	4	2	3	4	5	5	7	12
MULTIPLE DX	337	9.9	119	2	5	7	12	17	36	50
TOTAL										
0–19 Years	23	14.8	577	3	5	6	9	41	96	96
20–34	27	5.8	13	1	4	5	9	12	13	13
35–49	64	5.6	33	2	2	4	6	11	14	32
50–64	95	7.9	29	3	4	8	9	13	17	36
65+	176	10.8	119	3	5	7	13	20	42	50
GRAND TOTAL	385	8.9	103	2	4	6	10	16	28	50

Length of Stay by Diagnosis and Operation, United States, 1997

United States, October 1995–September 1996 Data, by Operation

54.0: ABDOMINAL WALL INCISION. Formerly included in operation group(s) 638.

Type of Patients	Observed Patients	Avg. Stay	Variance	Percentiles						
				10th	25th	50th	75th	90th	95th	99th
1. SINGLE DX										
0–19 Years	73	2.9	4	1	2	2	4	5	6	10
20–34	90	2.7	3	1	2	2	4	5	6	11
35–49	87	2.8	4	1	2	2	4	4	6	13
50–64	58	5.4	30	1	2	3	8	13	13	34
65+	39	2.5	6	1	1	1	3	5	8	15
2. MULTIPLE DX										
0–19 Years	258	4.8	19	1	2	3	6	11	13	19
20–34	364	5.8	40	1	3	4	6	11	13	47
35–49	700	5.9	42	1	2	4	7	12	17	32
50–64	636	6.5	70	1	2	4	7	13	19	52
65+	900	12.5	244	2	4	7	14	26	52	67
TOTAL SINGLE DX	347	3.1	8	1	2	2	4	5	9	13
MULTIPLE DX	2858	7.7	108	1	3	5	8	15	23	67
TOTAL										
0–19 Years	331	4.4	16	1	2	3	5	10	12	19
20–34	454	5.2	34	1	2	4	6	10	13	41
35–49	787	5.5	38	1	2	4	7	11	16	32
50–64	694	6.4	67	1	2	4	7	13	19	52
65+	939	11.8	235	2	3	7	13	24	52	67
GRAND TOTAL	3205	7.1	98	1	2	4	8	14	21	67

54.1: LAPAROTOMY. Formerly included in operation group(s) 639.

Type of Patients	Observed Patients	Avg. Stay	Variance	Percentiles						
				10th	25th	50th	75th	90th	95th	99th
1. SINGLE DX										
0–19 Years	231	3.5	7	2	2	3	4	6	10	14
20–34	319	3.4	4	1	2	3	4	6	7	12
35–49	204	3.4	4	1	2	3	4	5	7	11
50–64	101	4.7	25	2	2	3	6	8	10	32
65+	50	4.2	8	3	3	3	5	7	7	10
2. MULTIPLE DX										
0–19 Years	687	9.1	144	2	4	6	9	21	36	>99
20–34	1464	6.1	55	2	3	4	7	11	18	36
35–49	1569	8.0	61	2	4	6	7	15	22	41
50–64	1297	9.8	82	2	4	7	12	19	25	52
65+	1929	11.8	100	4	6	9	15	24	31	59
TOTAL SINGLE DX	905	3.6	7	1	2	3	4	6	8	13
MULTIPLE DX	6946	8.9	84	2	4	6	11	19	25	56
TOTAL										
0–19 Years	918	7.6	114	2	3	5	8	17	29	>99
20–34	1783	5.6	47	2	3	4	6	10	17	36
35–49	1773	7.2	55	2	3	5	8	14	21	40
50–64	1398	9.5	79	3	4	7	12	19	25	50
65+	1979	11.5	98	3	6	8	14	24	30	58
GRAND TOTAL	7851	8.2	77	2	3	5	10	18	24	52

54.11: EXPLORATORY LAPAROTOMY. Formerly included in operation group(s) 639.

Type of Patients	Observed Patients	Avg. Stay	Variance	Percentiles						
				10th	25th	50th	75th	90th	95th	99th
1. SINGLE DX										
0–19 Years	181	3.2	6	2	2	2	4	5	8	13
20–34	267	3.4	4	1	2	3	4	6	7	12
35–49	157	3.3	3	1	2	3	4	5	6	10
50–64	75	5.1	29	1	3	4	6	8	14	32
65+	30	3.7	2	3	3	3	4	6	7	8
2. MULTIPLE DX										
0–19 Years	481	9.0	148	2	3	5	9	22	35	>99
20–34	1059	5.9	53	2	3	5	8	10	17	31
35–49	1085	7.3	50	2	4	5	8	14	19	40
50–64	919	9.6	73	3	4	7	12	19	22	40
65+	1434	11.7	92	4	6	9	14	23	29	55
TOTAL SINGLE DX	710	3.5	7	1	2	3	4	6	7	14
MULTIPLE DX	4978	8.7	79	2	4	6	10	18	24	50
TOTAL										
0–19 Years	662	7.2	111	2	2	4	7	16	28	>99
20–34	1326	5.3	42	2	3	4	6	10	14	28
35–49	1242	6.6	44	2	3	5	7	13	17	35
50–64	994	9.2	71	3	4	7	12	19	22	40
65+	1464	11.4	90	3	6	8	14	23	29	55
GRAND TOTAL	5688	7.8	71	2	3	5	9	17	22	43

54.12: REOPEN RECENT LAP SITE. Formerly included in operation group(s) 639.

Type of Patients	Observed Patients	Avg. Stay	Variance	Percentiles						
				10th	25th	50th	75th	90th	95th	99th
1. SINGLE DX										
0–19 Years	8	4.2	2	2	4	4	5	5	7	7
20–34	10	2.9	1	1	2	3	4	4	4	4
35–49	13	3.3	2	1	1	3	4	3	5	8
50–64	9	2.2	1	1	1	3	4	3	4	4
65+	2	4.0	3	3	5	5	5	5	5	5
2. MULTIPLE DX										
0–19 Years	33	7.1	23	2	4	6	8	15	18	22
20–34	81	8.0	91	2	3	5	9	18	18	41
35–49	101	10.3	118	2	4	6	12	27	33	44
50–64	67	9.5	86	2	4	7	15	15	21	66
65+	93	11.6	74	3	6	8	17	29	29	29
TOTAL SINGLE DX	42	3.2	2	1	2	3	4	5	5	8
MULTIPLE DX	375	9.7	91	2	3	6	13	21	29	44
TOTAL										
0–19 Years	41	6.6	21	2	4	6	7	11	18	22
20–34	91	7.1	79	2	3	4	7	18	18	41
35–49	114	9.6	111	2	3	6	11	27	33	44
50–64	76	9.0	83	2	4	6	12	15	21	60
65+	95	11.5	74	3	6	8	17	29	29	29
GRAND TOTAL	417	9.1	86	2	3	6	12	21	29	43

Length of Stay by Diagnosis and Operation, United States, 1997

United States, October 1995–September 1996 Data, by Operation

54.19: LAPAROTOMY NEC. Formerly included in operation group(s) 639.

Type of Patients	Observed Patients	Avg. Stay	Vari-ance	10th	25th	50th	75th	90th	95th	99th
1. SINGLE DX										
0–19 Years	42	5.0	12	1	2	5	7	9	10	18
20–34	42	3.8	5	1	2	4	5	7	7	11
35–49	34	4.1	5	2	3	3	5	7	10	11
50–64	17	3.3	6	1	1	3	5	6	6	10
65+	18	6.4	30	2	3	6	7	10	10	32
2. MULTIPLE DX										
0–19 Years	173	9.7	150	3	4	6	10	19	52	>99
20–34	324	6.3	55	2	3	4	7	13	20	36
35–49	383	9.5	76	2	4	7	11	19	28	56
50–64	311	10.3	100	3	4	7	13	22	27	64
65+	402	12.3	132	4	5	9	15	27	43	>99
TOTAL SINGLE DX	153	4.3	9	1	3	3	6	8	10	11
MULTIPLE DX	1593	9.4	98	2	4	6	11	21	30	69
TOTAL										
0–19 Years	215	9.0	133	3	4	6	9	19	40	>99
20–34	366	6.1	51	2	3	4	7	11	17	36
35–49	417	8.8	70	2	3	7	11	17	25	52
50–64	328	10.0	98	3	4	7	13	22	27	60
65+	420	12.2	130	4	5	9	15	26	43	>99
GRAND TOTAL	1746	9.0	93	2	4	6	11	20	28	67

54.2: ABD REGION DXTIC PX. Formerly included in operation group(s) 631, 638, 640.

Type of Patients	Observed Patients	Avg. Stay	Vari-ance	10th	25th	50th	75th	90th	95th	99th
1. SINGLE DX										
0–19 Years	283	2.8	6	1	1	2	3	5	8	13
20–34	745	2.3	3	1	1	2	3	5	6	8
35–49	308	2.5	4	1	1	2	3	5	7	9
50–64	77	2.7	7	1	1	2	3	5	7	9
65+	48	4.4	16	1	1	3	6	12	12	15
2. MULTIPLE DX										
0–19 Years	601	3.9	26	1	1	3	5	8	12	21
20–34	2155	3.2	11	1	1	2	4	6	8	15
35–49	1546	4.3	16	1	2	3	6	9	12	20
50–64	904	5.8	38	1	2	4	7	13	16	31
65+	1658	8.4	49	1	3	7	12	17	22	32
TOTAL SINGLE DX	1461	2.5	4	1	1	2	3	5	6	12
MULTIPLE DX	6864	4.9	29	1	2	3	6	11	15	26
TOTAL										
0–19 Years	884	3.6	20	1	1	2	4	7	11	17
20–34	2900	2.9	9	1	1	2	4	6	7	13
35–49	1854	4.0	15	1	2	3	5	8	11	17
50–64	981	5.6	37	1	3	3	7	12	16	31
65+	1706	8.3	49	1	3	7	12	17	22	32
GRAND TOTAL	8325	4.4	25	1	1	3	5	10	14	24

54.21: LAPAROSCOPY. Formerly included in operation group(s) 640.

Type of Patients	Observed Patients	Avg. Stay	Vari-ance	10th	25th	50th	75th	90th	95th	99th
1. SINGLE DX										
0–19 Years	248	2.3	2	1	1	2	3	4	4	8
20–34	702	2.3	3	1	1	2	3	5	6	8
35–49	271	2.4	4	1	1	2	3	5	7	9
50–64	49	2.4	3	1	1	2	3	4	6	7
65+	26	2.2	4	1	1	1	2	4	7	12
2. MULTIPLE DX										
0–19 Years	459	3.4	19	1	1	2	4	6	10	17
20–34	1860	3.1	9	1	1	3	4	6	8	13
35–49	1155	3.9	12	1	2	3	5	8	10	15
50–64	387	4.4	22	1	2	3	5	10	14	24
65+	468	6.2	39	1	1	4	9	14	20	32
TOTAL SINGLE DX	1296	2.3	3	1	1	2	3	4	6	8
MULTIPLE DX	4329	3.7	16	1	1	3	5	7	10	19
TOTAL										
0–19 Years	707	3.0	13	1	1	2	3	5	7	17
20–34	2562	2.8	7	1	1	2	3	5	7	12
35–49	1426	3.6	11	1	1	3	5	8	10	15
50–64	436	4.2	20	1	1	3	5	9	13	22
65+	494	6.1	38	1	1	4	9	14	20	32
GRAND TOTAL	5625	3.4	13	1	1	2	4	7	9	17

54.23: PERITONEAL BIOPSY. Formerly included in operation group(s) 638.

Type of Patients	Observed Patients	Avg. Stay	Vari-ance	10th	25th	50th	75th	90th	95th	99th
1. SINGLE DX										
0–19 Years	13	8.8	21	1	5	12	13	13	13	13
20–34	11	3.2	5	1	1	6	6	6	6	6
35–49	17	4.7	7	2	3	4	8	8	8	12
50–64	12	2.9	5	1	2	2	2	6	7	12
65+	16	6.1	19	1	2	4	12	12	12	15
2. MULTIPLE DX										
0–19 Years	57	7.1	57	2	3	5	8	14	16	48
20–34	69	5.9	26	2	3	5	7	9	10	39
35–49	183	6.4	29	2	3	5	7	13	19	25
50–64	310	7.0	56	2	3	5	8	15	17	48
65+	699	9.9	47	3	5	8	13	21	24	31
TOTAL SINGLE DX	69	5.7	18	1	2	4	8	12	13	13
MULTIPLE DX	1318	8.2	48	2	3	6	12	16	22	37
TOTAL										
0–19 Years	70	7.5	48	1	3	5	12	13	15	44
20–34	80	5.6	25	1	3	5	7	9	10	39
35–49	200	6.3	28	2	3	5	7	12	18	25
50–64	322	6.8	54	2	3	4	8	15	17	48
65+	715	9.8	46	3	5	8	13	20	24	31
GRAND TOTAL	1387	8.1	47	2	3	6	11	16	22	33

54.24: CLSD BX INTRA-ABD MASS. Formerly included in operation group(s) 638.

Type of Patients	Observed Patients	Avg. Stay	Vari-ance	10th	25th	50th	75th	90th	95th	99th
1. SINGLE DX										
0–19 Years	2	6.3	10	2	2	8	8	8	8	8
20–34	3	3.8	<1	3	4	4	4	4	4	4
35–49	6	3.3	<1	1	2	4	4	4	4	4
50–64	6	4.5	11	1	2	4	9	9	9	9
65+	5	3.8	14	1	2	3	4	10	10	10
2. MULTIPLE DX										
0–19 Years	19	7.8	13	3	6	8	10	11	11	20
20–34	16	4.7	3	2	3	5	6	7	7	9
35–49	63	6.7	41	1	3	5	8	13	21	34
50–64	107	6.6	29	2	3	6	9	14	19	27
65+	310	8.8	60	3	4	7	10	16	21	41
TOTAL SINGLE DX	22	4.0	6	1	2	4	4	9	9	10
MULTIPLE DX	515	7.9	48	2	4	6	10	14	20	34
TOTAL										
0–19 Years	21	7.7	13	3	5	8	10	11	11	20
20–34	19	4.6	3	2	3	5	6	7	7	9
35–49	69	6.2	37	1	3	4	8	11	21	34
50–64	113	6.5	29	2	3	6	9	14	17	27
65+	315	8.8	60	3	4	7	10	16	21	41
GRAND TOTAL	537	7.8	47	2	4	6	9	14	19	32

54.3: EXC/DESTR ABD WALL LES. Formerly included in operation group(s) 638.

Type of Patients	Observed Patients	Avg. Stay	Vari-ance	10th	25th	50th	75th	90th	95th	99th
1. SINGLE DX										
0–19 Years	32	3.1	6	1	1	2	5	8	8	9
20–34	42	2.1	2	1	1	1	2	5	6	6
35–49	45	4.1	8	1	2	3	8	8	8	8
50–64	29	2.1	4	1	1	2	2	3	5	8
65+	14	2.1	<1	2	2	2	2	3	3	6
2. MULTIPLE DX										
0–19 Years	81	5.7	35	1	2	4	7	12	15	29
20–34	135	6.0	50	1	3	4	7	11	16	35
35–49	269	7.3	106	1	3	4	8	12	18	56
50–64	300	9.1	115	1	3	6	9	23	32	54
65+	466	8.6	70	2	4	6	11	16	22	42
TOTAL SINGLE DX	162	2.7	5	1	1	2	3	6	8	8
MULTIPLE DX	1251	7.9	87	1	3	5	9	15	24	56
TOTAL										
0–19 Years	113	5.1	30	1	1	3	7	10	15	29
20–34	177	4.9	40	1	2	3	6	10	15	35
35–49	314	6.9	95	1	2	4	8	11	18	56
50–64	329	8.2	106	1	3	4	8	22	32	54
65+	480	7.9	67	2	4	5	10	16	21	38
GRAND TOTAL	1413	7.1	78	1	2	4	8	14	22	47

54.25: PERITONEAL LAVAGE. Formerly included in operation group(s) 631.

Type of Patients	Observed Patients	Avg. Stay	Vari-ance	10th	25th	50th	75th	90th	95th	99th
1. SINGLE DX										
0–19 Years	17	3.4	3	1	2	3	5	5	6	8
20–34	26	1.9	3	1	1	1	2	4	5	9
35–49	13	2.0	1	1	1	2	2	4	5	6
50–64	0	2.4	2	1	2	2	4	4	4	4
2. MULTIPLE DX										
0–19 Years	51	3.6	51	1	1	2	4	7	10	65
20–34	200	3.2	30	1	1	2	3	5	12	19
35–49	116	4.0	19	1	1	3	5	8	16	26
50–64	43	6.6	76	2	2	5	8	10	14	73
65+	33	9.3	72	1	2	6	14	19	26	34
TOTAL SINGLE DX	60	2.5	3	1	1	2	3	5	5	8
MULTIPLE DX	443	4.3	41	1	1	2	5	10	16	26
TOTAL										
0–19 Years	68	3.6	39	1	2	2	5	6	8	13
20–34	226	3.0	27	1	1	2	3	6	12	16
35–49	129	3.8	18	1	1	2	4	8	16	26
50–64	47	6.4	72	2	2	4	8	10	14	73
65+	33	9.3	72	1	2	6	14	19	26	34
GRAND TOTAL	503	4.1	37	1	1	2	4	10	15	26

54.4: EXC/DESTR PERITON TISS. Formerly included in operation group(s) 638.

Type of Patients	Observed Patients	Avg. Stay	Vari-ance	10th	25th	50th	75th	90th	95th	99th
1. SINGLE DX										
0–19 Years	85	3.8	5	1	2	4	5	6	6	7
20–34	79	3.0	3	1	2	3	3	5	6	10
35–49	88	3.3	4	2	2	3	4	6	9	12
50–64	54	3.7	4	2	2	3	5	6	9	10
65+	26	3.9	6	2	2	3	6	7	7	16
2. MULTIPLE DX										
0–19 Years	191	8.4	139	2	3	5	8	13	31	70
20–34	290	5.2	26	2	3	4	6	9	13	31
35–49	482	5.6	23	2	3	4	6	10	16	25
50–64	552	8.3	102	3	4	6	8	14	23	58
65+	782	9.8	43	4	6	9	12	17	21	32
TOTAL SINGLE DX	332	3.5	4	2	2	3	5	6	6	10
MULTIPLE DX	2297	7.7	62	2	4	6	9	14	20	50
TOTAL										
0–19 Years	276	6.9	99	2	3	5	6	11	22	70
20–34	369	4.7	22	2	3	3	6	9	11	29
35–49	570	5.2	21	2	3	4	6	9	14	25
50–64	606	7.7	91	2	4	5	8	13	19	58
65+	808	9.6	43	4	6	8	12	16	21	32
GRAND TOTAL	2629	7.1	56	2	3	5	8	14	18	43

Length of Stay by Diagnosis and Operation, United States, 1997

United States, October 1995–September 1996 Data, by Operation

54.5: PERITONEAL ADHESIOLYSIS. Formerly included in operation group(s) 642.

Type of Patients	Observed Patients	Avg. Stay	Vari-ance	Percentiles						
				10th	25th	50th	75th	90th	95th	99th
1. SINGLE DX										
0–19 Years	208	6.6	13	3	5	7	7	10	14	14
20–34	351	4.5	10	2	2	4	6	8	10	17
35–49	463	5.0	10	2	3	4	7	10	11	15
50–64	209	6.0	12	2	4	6	8	9	11	18
65+	117	6.8	8	4	5	6	8	11	11	15
2. MULTIPLE DX										
0–19 Years	869	9.8	82	3	5	8	12	18	27	56
20–34	2430	5.1	23	1	2	4	7	10	13	25
35–49	4139	6.8	36	2	3	5	8	13	17	31
50–64	3373	9.0	58	3	5	7	11	17	22	37
65+	6686	11.3	56	4	7	10	14	20	24	40
TOTAL SINGLE DX	1348	5.5	11	2	3	5	7	10	11	15
MULTIPLE DX	17497	8.6	53	2	4	7	11	17	21	38
TOTAL										
0–19 Years	1077	9.1	68	3	5	7	10	15	24	52
20–34	2781	5.0	22	1	2	4	6	10	13	23
35–49	4602	6.6	34	2	3	5	8	13	17	30
50–64	3582	8.8	55	3	5	7	10	17	21	35
65+	6803	11.2	56	4	7	9	14	19	24	40
GRAND TOTAL	18845	8.3	50	2	4	7	10	16	21	35

54.61: RECLOSE POSTOP DISRUPT. Formerly included in operation group(s) 642.

Type of Patients	Observed Patients	Avg. Stay	Vari-ance	Percentiles						
				10th	25th	50th	75th	90th	95th	99th
1. SINGLE DX										
0–19 Years	6	2.3	3	1	1	2	2	6	6	6
20–34	20	3.0	2	1	2	3	4	6	5	6
35–49	21	3.0	4	1	1	3	4	7	7	10
50–64	10	2.3	1	1	2	2	4	4	4	4
65+	6	3.6	2	1	3	3	5	5	5	5
2. MULTIPLE DX										
0–19 Years	15	6.1	49	2	2	3	8	23	23	27
20–34	48	10.3	289	2	3	3	7	39	61	61
35–49	90	7.7	94	2	2	5	9	12	31	45
50–64	110	6.6	35	1	3	4	9	16	16	29
65+	211	12.3	208	3	5	7	11	36	54	54
TOTAL SINGLE DX	63	2.9	3	1	1	3	4	5	6	7
MULTIPLE DX	474	9.4	145	2	3	6	9	19	45	54
TOTAL										
0–19 Years	21	4.7	36	1	2	3	5	8	23	27
20–34	68	8.6	232	1	3	3	6	14	61	61
35–49	111	7.0	84	1	2	4	8	12	31	45
50–64	120	6.4	34	1	3	4	9	15	16	29
65+	217	12.1	205	3	5	7	11	33	54	54
GRAND TOTAL	537	8.8	136	2	3	6	9	18	43	54

54.6: ABD WALL/PERITON SUTURE. Formerly included in operation group(s) 642.

Type of Patients	Observed Patients	Avg. Stay	Vari-ance	Percentiles						
				10th	25th	50th	75th	90th	95th	99th
1. SINGLE DX										
0–19 Years	17	1.7	1	1	1	1	2	3	4	6
20–34	41	1.5	1	1	1	1	1	3	4	5
35–49	31	2.6	4	1	1	2	4	5	7	10
50–64	15	2.2	1	1	1	2	3	4	4	4
65+	8	3.2	2	2	2	3	5	5	5	5
2. MULTIPLE DX										
0–19 Years	51	9.1	120	1	2	4	8	24	24	58
20–34	120	6.7	126	1	3	4	6	9	18	61
35–49	145	6.5	71	1	2	4	7	11	20	45
50–64	130	6.5	33	1	3	5	9	14	16	29
65+	235	11.8	194	3	5	7	11	24	54	54
TOTAL SINGLE DX	112	1.9	2	1	1	1	2	4	5	7
MULTIPLE DX	681	8.4	119	1	3	5	8	17	30	54
TOTAL										
0–19 Years	68	6.6	92	1	2	3	6	24	24	58
20–34	161	4.6	81	1	1	3	5	8	10	61
35–49	176	5.9	62	1	3	4	7	11	15	45
50–64	145	6.2	32	1	3	4	8	14	16	26
65+	243	11.6	192	3	5	7	10	21	54	54
GRAND TOTAL	793	7.2	105	1	2	4	7	15	24	54

54.7: OTH ABD WALL PERITON REP. Formerly included in operation group(s) 642.

Type of Patients	Observed Patients	Avg. Stay	Vari-ance	Percentiles						
				10th	25th	50th	75th	90th	95th	99th
1. SINGLE DX										
0–19 Years	22	16.2	223	3	7	15	22	35	98	>99
20–34	9	5.1	6	1	3	6	7	7	7	9
35–49	9	4.4	5	2	2	4	6	7	9	9
50–64	7	3.3	5	1	1	3	5	5	8	8
65+	5	1.9	2	1	1	1	2	5	5	5
2. MULTIPLE DX										
0–19 Years	251	28.2	475	5	13	23	41	70	89	>99
20–34	51	6.0	29	1	3	5	6	11	16	30
35–49	67	5.6	32	1	1	4	8	11	19	26
50–64	51	6.3	32	2	3	4	9	10	14	34
65+	47	10.4	48	3	6	8	14	21	22	36
TOTAL SINGLE DX	52	9.4	136	1	3	6	15	22	24	>99
MULTIPLE DX	467	18.3	388	3	5	10	26	53	72	>99
TOTAL										
0–19 Years	273	27.5	468	5	13	23	40	70	90	>99
20–34	60	5.9	26	1	3	5	7	10	16	30
35–49	76	5.5	30	2	2	4	8	11	19	22
50–64	58	6.2	31	2	3	8	9	10	13	34
65+	52	9.9	50	2	6	8	14	21	22	36
GRAND TOTAL	519	17.7	376	2	5	10	25	51	72	>99

Length of Stay by Diagnosis and Operation, United States, 1997

United States, October 1995–September 1996 Data, by Operation

54.9: OTHER ABD REGION OPS. Formerly included in operation group(s) 638, 641, 642.

Type of Patients	Observed Patients	Avg. Stay	Variance	10th	25th	50th	75th	90th	95th	99th
1. SINGLE DX										
0–19 Years	224	4.2	10	1	2	3	5	7	10	15
20–34	116	4.4	16	1	2	3	6	8	9	22
35–49	126	4.8	9	1	2	5	7	7	8	14
50–64	72	4.1	5	1	2	4	5	7	8	13
65+	62	2.9	9	1	1	2	4	6	6	20
2. MULTIPLE DX										
0–19 Years	1799	7.9	104	1	2	5	10	17	27	57
20–34	2157	6.9	63	1	3	5	8	13	22	39
35–49	5880	6.8	41	2	3	5	8	13	17	34
50–64	7241	7.4	57	2	3	6	9	14	20	43
65+	8376	8.1	50	2	4	6	10	16	21	35
TOTAL SINGLE DX	600	4.2	11	1	2	4	6	7	9	15
MULTIPLE DX	25453	7.4	55	2	3	5	9	14	20	39
TOTAL										
0–19 Years	2023	7.4	93	1	2	4	8	15	24	54
20–34	2273	6.8	61	1	3	5	8	13	21	39
35–49	6006	6.7	40	2	3	5	8	13	17	34
50–64	7313	7.3	57	2	3	5	9	13	20	42
65+	8438	8.0	50	2	4	6	10	16	21	35
GRAND TOTAL	26053	7.3	54	2	3	5	9	14	20	39

54.91: PERC ABD DRAINAGE. Formerly included in operation group(s) 638.

Type of Patients	Observed Patients	Avg. Stay	Variance	10th	25th	50th	75th	90th	95th	99th
1. SINGLE DX										
0–19 Years	50	6.2	14	3	4	5	7	15	15	15
20–34	68	5.3	11	2	3	5	7	9	9	17
35–49	80	5.8	10	2	4	7	7	9	9	24
50–64	39	4.3	5	1	2	4	4	7	10	13
65+	31	5.4	13	2	3	6	6	6	10	22
2. MULTIPLE DX										
0–19 Years	295	7.9	53	2	3	6	10	14	20	35
20–34	776	7.2	46	2	4	6	8	14	19	38
35–49	3172	7.2	37	2	4	6	9	13	18	30
50–64	3981	7.5	35	2	4	7	9	13	19	31
65+	5155	8.0	37	2	4	7	10	15	19	30
TOTAL SINGLE DX	268	5.5	11	2	4	5	7	8	12	17
MULTIPLE DX	13379	7.6	38	2	4	6	9	14	19	31
TOTAL										
0–19 Years	345	7.5	45	2	3	6	9	15	17	34
20–34	844	7.0	44	2	3	6	8	13	19	33
35–49	3252	7.1	37	2	4	6	9	13	18	30
50–64	4020	7.4	35	2	4	6	9	13	19	31
65+	5186	8.0	37	2	4	7	10	15	19	30
GRAND TOTAL	13647	7.5	37	2	4	6	9	14	19	31

54.92: RMVL FB PERITON CAVITY. Formerly included in operation group(s) 642.

Type of Patients	Observed Patients	Avg. Stay	Variance	10th	25th	50th	75th	90th	95th	99th
1. SINGLE DX										
0–19 Years	5	2.5	3	1	1	2	3	5	6	6
20–34	5	1.9	4	1	1	2	3	5	8	8
35–49	7	5.2	3	2	6	6	6	6	6	6
50–64	4	3.4	4	1	1	5	5	5	5	5
65+	4	1.1	<1	1	1	1	1	1	1	4
2. MULTIPLE DX										
0–19 Years	24	6.9	61	1	2	4	11	12	27	36
20–34	56	5.3	23	1	2	4	6	13	18	18
35–49	75	9.6	135	2	2	7	9	28	37	37
50–64	67	9.6	105	2	5	7	11	18	27	37
65+	65	9.0	95	3	4	6	11	16	25	30
TOTAL SINGLE DX	25	2.5	5	1	1	1	5	6	6	6
MULTIPLE DX	287	8.4	94	2	3	6	10	17	28	37
TOTAL										
0–19 Years	29	6.2	55	1	2	4	6	11	27	36
20–34	61	5.2	23	1	2	4	6	13	18	18
35–49	82	9.1	121	2	3	6	9	18	37	37
50–64	71	9.2	100	2	5	6	10	18	22	37
65+	69	6.6	79	1	1	4	8	14	18	30
GRAND TOTAL	312	7.5	86	1	2	5	9	15	25	37

54.93: CREATE CUTANEOPERIT FIST. Formerly included in operation group(s) 642.

Type of Patients	Observed Patients	Avg. Stay	Variance	10th	25th	50th	75th	90th	95th	99th
1. SINGLE DX										
0–19 Years	14	6.2	39	1	2	3	14	17	17	17
20–34	16	3.8	5	1	2	3	6	6	8	9
35–49	24	2.0	2	1	1	3	5	7	5	8
50–64	15	3.5	4	1	1	3	5	7	7	7
65+	17	2.3	3	1	1	2	2	4	8	8
2. MULTIPLE DX										
0–19 Years	292	14.7	268	2	4	9	19	37	53	87
20–34	274	12.4	187	2	3	6	14	39	39	41
35–49	620	7.1	53	1	2	5	9	15	21	34
50–64	801	8.0	128	1	3	5	9	16	26	78
65+	857	10.6	105	1	3	8	14	25	29	51
TOTAL SINGLE DX	86	3.3	10	1	2	2	4	7	9	17
MULTIPLE DX	2844	9.7	131	1	2	6	12	24	35	59
TOTAL										
0–19 Years	306	14.3	261	2	3	9	18	35	52	87
20–34	290	11.9	180	2	3	6	13	39	39	40
35–49	644	7.0	52	1	2	5	9	14	20	34
50–64	816	7.9	126	1	2	5	9	16	25	78
65+	874	10.4	104	1	3	7	14	24	29	51
GRAND TOTAL	2930	9.5	128	1	2	6	11	23	35	59

United States, October 1995–September 1996 Data, by Operation

54.94: CREAT PERITONEOVAS SHUNT. Formerly included in operation group(s) 642.

Type of Patients	Observed Patients	Avg. Stay	Variance	Percentiles						
				10th	25th	50th	75th	90th	95th	99th
1. SINGLE DX										
0–19 Years	5	2.6	4	1	1	2	3	6	6	6
20–34	1	2.0	0	2	2	2	3	6	6	6
35–49	2	2.7	<1	2	2	3	3	3	3	3
50–64	3	3.9	10	2	2	2	8	8	8	8
65+	2	2.5	6	1	1	1	5	5	5	5
2. MULTIPLE DX										
0–19 Years	18	14.8	656	2	4	7	9	93	>99	>99
20–34	12	8.6	82	2	3	5	11	28	32	32
35–49	95	11.1	71	2	4	10	15	21	27	35
50–64	176	10.5	100	2	4	8	13	25	29	44
65+	246	10.0	89	2	4	7	13	19	36	36
TOTAL SINGLE DX	13	2.7	4	1	1	2	3	6	6	8
MULTIPLE DX	547	10.5	104	2	4	8	14	21	31	44
TOTAL										
0–19 Years	23	10.5	458	1	2	5	8	51	93	>99
20–34	13	7.8	76	2	3	5	7	28	32	32
35–49	97	11.0	71	2	4	10	15	21	27	35
50–64	179	10.5	100	2	4	8	13	25	29	44
65+	248	9.9	89	2	4	7	13	19	36	36
GRAND TOTAL	560	10.3	103	2	4	8	13	21	31	44

54.95: PERITONEAL INCISION. Formerly included in operation group(s) 642.

Type of Patients	Observed Patients	Avg. Stay	Variance	Percentiles						
				10th	25th	50th	75th	90th	95th	99th
1. SINGLE DX										
0–19 Years	130	3.2	3	1	2	3	4	5	6	10
20–34	14	2.4	2	2	2	2	2	5	5	9
35–49	6	3.3	4	2	2	2	6	6	6	6
50–64	1	8.0	0	8	8	8	8	8	8	8
65+	4	2.3	1	1	1	3	3	3	3	3
2. MULTIPLE DX										
0–19 Years	602	7.3	81	1	2	4	9	15	24	54
20–34	235	6.0	63	1	2	3	7	13	19	50
35–49	347	9.2	102	2	3	6	11	18	28	48
50–64	356	8.6	79	2	3	6	10	19	28	44
65+	309	10.5	117	2	5	7	13	21	29	44
TOTAL SINGLE DX	155	3.1	3	1	2	3	4	5	6	10
MULTIPLE DX	1849	8.1	88	1	3	5	10	17	26	50
TOTAL										
0–19 Years	732	6.6	70	1	2	4	7	14	21	54
20–34	249	5.7	59	1	2	3	6	12	19	50
35–49	353	9.0	101	2	3	6	11	18	28	48
50–64	357	8.6	79	2	3	6	10	19	28	44
65+	313	10.4	117	2	5	7	12	21	29	44
GRAND TOTAL	2004	7.6	82	2	4	5	9	16	24	48

54.98: PERITONEAL DIALYSIS. Formerly included in operation group(s) 641.

Type of Patients	Observed Patients	Avg. Stay	Variance	Percentiles						
				10th	25th	50th	75th	90th	95th	99th
1. SINGLE DX										
0–19 Years	13	2.2	<1	1	1	2	3	3	3	4
20–34	10	5.5	106	1	1	1	2	34	34	34
35–49	7	1.7	<1	1	1	2	2	2	2	2
50–64	9	2.9	5	1	2	2	5	7	7	7
65+	1	2.0	0	2	2	2	2	2	2	2
2. MULTIPLE DX										
0–19 Years	536	4.7	26	1	2	3	6	10	14	25
20–34	782	5.1	21	2	2	4	6	11	11	27
35–49	1520	5.1	18	2	3	4	6	9	12	26
50–64	1804	6.1	68	2	3	4	7	11	16	49
65+	1674	6.5	35	2	3	5	8	14	17	29
TOTAL SINGLE DX	40	3.1	34	1	1	2	3	4	10	34
MULTIPLE DX	6316	5.7	37	2	3	4	7	11	15	29
TOTAL										
0–19 Years	549	4.7	25	1	2	3	6	10	14	25
20–34	792	5.2	22	2	2	4	6	11	11	28
35–49	1527	5.1	18	2	3	4	6	9	12	26
50–64	1813	6.1	67	2	3	4	7	11	16	49
65+	1675	6.5	35	2	3	5	8	14	17	29
GRAND TOTAL	6356	5.7	37	2	3	4	7	11	15	29

55.0: NEPHROTOMY & NEPHROSTOMY. Formerly included in operation group(s) 644, 646.

Type of Patients	Observed Patients	Avg. Stay	Variance	Percentiles						
				10th	25th	50th	75th	90th	95th	99th
1. SINGLE DX										
0–19 Years	58	2.9	4	1	2	3	4	4	7	9
20–34	156	2.9	3	1	2	3	4	5	5	9
35–49	237	3.3	11	1	2	3	4	5	7	27
50–64	166	3.3	4	1	2	3	4	6	6	10
65+	61	3.9	9	1	2	3	4	10	10	10
2. MULTIPLE DX										
0–19 Years	226	7.2	44	1	2	6	10	15	17	40
20–34	605	6.2	52	2	3	4	7	11	16	39
35–49	1019	5.6	32	1	2	4	7	11	16	31
50–64	1256	7.1	41	2	3	5	10	15	18	32
65+	2177	9.2	59	2	4	7	12	18	23	38
TOTAL SINGLE DX	678	3.2	7	1	2	3	4	6	7	12
MULTIPLE DX	5283	7.6	50	2	3	5	10	15	20	36
TOTAL										
0–19 Years	284	6.3	38	1	2	4	8	14	15	35
20–34	761	5.6	45	1	2	4	6	10	14	28
35–49	1256	5.2	30	1	2	4	6	11	15	31
50–64	1422	6.6	37	2	3	5	8	14	17	29
65+	2238	9.1	58	2	4	7	12	18	23	38
GRAND TOTAL	5961	7.1	47	2	3	5	9	15	19	34

United States, October 1995–September 1996 Data, by Operation

55.01: NEPHROTOMY. Formerly included in operation group(s) 646.

Type of Patients	Observed Patients	Avg. Stay	Vari-ance	10th	25th	50th	75th	90th	95th	99th
1. SINGLE DX										
0–19 Years	9	3.2	<1	2	2	4	4	4	4	4
20–34	23	3.2	5	1	2	3	4	5	5	8
35–49	36	6.0	39	2	3	4	6	7	28	28
50–64	35	4.0	4	2	3	4	5	6	8	11
65+	11	7.3	13	1	3	10	10	10	10	10
2. MULTIPLE DX										
0–19 Years	31	9.3	52	1	3	9	12	18	20	35
20–34	64	7.2	36	2	4	6	7	13	13	39
35–49	124	7.1	51	2	3	5	7	13	29	31
50–64	128	6.5	20	2	4	5	8	12	14	27
65+	141	9.8	52	3	5	9	11	17	25	37
TOTAL SINGLE DX	114	4.6	14	2	3	4	5	10	10	28
MULTIPLE DX	488	7.9	45	2	4	6	11	14	21	37
TOTAL										
0–19 Years	40	7.2	43	2	3	4	10	18	18	35
20–34	87	6.2	31	2	3	5	6	13	17	39
35–49	160	7.0	50	2	3	5	7	13	28	31
50–64	163	5.9	18	2	3	5	8	10	13	24
65+	152	9.6	50	3	5	9	11	16	24	37
GRAND TOTAL	602	7.4	41	2	3	5	10	13	18	37

55.02: NEPHROSTOMY. Formerly included in operation group(s) 646.

Type of Patients	Observed Patients	Avg. Stay	Vari-ance	10th	25th	50th	75th	90th	95th	99th
1. SINGLE DX										
0–19 Years	8	2.4	5	1	1	1	2	7	8	8
20–34	14	2.9	6	1	1	2	4	4	9	9
35–49	8	2.7	6	1	2	2	3	4	6	6
50–64	5	2.2	<1	1	2	2	3	5	6	6
65+	2	2.3	1	1	1	3	3	3	3	3
2. MULTIPLE DX										
0–19 Years	35	7.8	63	1	2	5	9	17	26	40
20–34	63	7.0	19	2	3	7	10	13	13	28
35–49	117	8.5	80	2	4	5	11	15	25	48
50–64	162	9.0	60	2	4	7	13	15	17	38
65+	331	10.2	61	3	4	8	15	20	25	33
TOTAL SINGLE DX	37	2.6	4	1	1	2	4	5	8	9
MULTIPLE DX	708	9.2	59	2	4	7	13	18	21	43
TOTAL										
0–19 Years	43	6.6	55	1	2	5	8	14	26	40
20–34	77	6.5	19	2	3	6	10	13	13	14
35–49	125	8.1	77	2	3	5	11	14	21	48
50–64	167	8.9	59	2	4	7	13	15	17	38
65+	333	10.1	61	3	4	8	15	20	25	33
GRAND TOTAL	745	9.0	59	2	4	7	13	18	21	40

55.03: PERC NEPHROSTOMY-NO FRAG. Formerly included in operation group(s) 644.

Type of Patients	Observed Patients	Avg. Stay	Vari-ance	10th	25th	50th	75th	90th	95th	99th
1. SINGLE DX										
0–19 Years	35	3.0	4	1	2	3	3	5	9	9
20–34	81	2.7	2	1	2	2	3	5	5	6
35–49	122	2.8	7	1	2	2	3	5	6	18
50–64	72	3.3	5	1	2	3	4	6	6	10
65+	29	2.9	5	1	2	2	4	5	5	15
2. MULTIPLE DX										
0–19 Years	137	6.4	25	1	2	5	9	14	15	16
20–34	373	6.3	77	1	2	5	7	11	17	66
35–49	606	5.2	25	1	2	4	7	10	15	22
50–64	755	7.4	42	1	3	6	10	16	19	32
65+	1501	9.5	64	2	4	8	12	18	24	40
TOTAL SINGLE DX	339	2.9	5	1	2	2	4	5	6	10
MULTIPLE DX	3372	7.7	54	2	3	6	10	16	21	36
TOTAL										
0–19 Years	172	5.7	22	1	2	4	8	13	15	16
20–34	454	5.6	65	1	2	3	6	11	17	66
35–49	728	4.9	23	1	2	3	6	9	15	22
50–64	827	7.1	40	2	3	5	10	16	18	32
65+	1530	9.4	64	2	4	8	12	18	24	40
GRAND TOTAL	3711	7.3	52	1	3	5	10	15	20	34

55.04: PERC NEPHROSTOMY W FRAG. Formerly included in operation group(s) 644.

Type of Patients	Observed Patients	Avg. Stay	Vari-ance	10th	25th	50th	75th	90th	95th	99th
1. SINGLE DX										
0–19 Years	6	2.4	4	1	1	1	3	6	6	6
20–34	38	3.3	6	1	2	3	4	7	8	14
35–49	71	3.2	6	1	2	3	3	5	6	15
50–64	54	3.0	2	2	2	3	3	5	6	8
65+	19	3.1	2	1	3	3	3	4	8	8
2. MULTIPLE DX										
0–19 Years	23	8.6	99	2	3	7	10	15	46	46
20–34	105	5.1	15	3	4	4	6	9	10	18
35–49	172	4.0	9	1	2	3	5	8	10	15
50–64	211	4.4	19	1	2	3	5	8	10	22
65+	204	5.9	16	2	3	4	7	11	16	19
TOTAL SINGLE DX	188	3.1	4	1	2	3	3	5	7	14
MULTIPLE DX	715	5.1	19	2	3	4	6	9	13	20
TOTAL										
0–19 Years	29	7.7	90	2	2	6	8	15	20	46
20–34	143	4.8	14	2	3	4	6	7	10	18
35–49	243	3.7	9	2	2	3	5	7	8	15
50–64	265	4.1	15	2	3	3	5	7	10	22
65+	223	5.7	16	2	3	4	7	11	16	19
GRAND TOTAL	903	4.7	17	2	2	4	6	9	11	18

Length of Stay by Diagnosis and Operation, United States, 1997

Length of Stay by Diagnosis and Operation, United States, October 1995–September 1996 Data, by Operation

55.1: PYELOTOMY & PYELOSTOMY. Formerly included in operation group(s) 646.

Type of Patients	Observed Patients	Avg. Stay	Vari-ance	10th	25th	50th	75th	90th	95th	99th
1. SINGLE DX										
0–19 Years	15	3.4	3	1	2	3	5	5	6	6
20–34	36	3.1	3	1	2	3	4	5	6	11
35–49	37	4.0	2	2	3	4	5	5	6	7
50–64	26	1.8	2	1	1	1	2	4	5	7
65+	11	5.5	5	2	4	6	8	8	8	8
2. MULTIPLE DX										
0–19 Years	44	6.8	48	3	3	4	7	12	32	32
20–34	79	4.7	9	1	3	5	6	7	7	15
35–49	101	5.5	13	2	3	5	7	9	10	14
50–64	124	5.6	18	1	3	4	7	11	13	21
65+	134	5.2	27	1	2	4	7	10	15	24
TOTAL SINGLE DX	125	3.0	3	1	1	3	4	5	6	8
MULTIPLE DX	482	5.4	20	1	3	5	7	10	13	28
TOTAL										
0–19 Years	59	6.1	41	2	3	4	6	11	14	32
20–34	115	4.2	7	1	2	4	5	7	7	11
35–49	138	5.2	11	2	3	5	7	8	10	14
50–64	150	4.5	16	1	1	4	6	10	13	18
65+	145	5.2	26	1	2	4	7	9	15	24
GRAND TOTAL	607	4.9	18	1	2	4	6	9	12	23

55.2: RENAL DIAGNOSTIC PX. Formerly included in operation group(s) 646, 651, 664.

Type of Patients	Observed Patients	Avg. Stay	Vari-ance	10th	25th	50th	75th	90th	95th	99th
1. SINGLE DX										
0–19 Years	362	2.1	6	1	1	1	2	5	7	12
20–34	111	2.5	7	1	1	1	3	5	8	15
35–49	108	1.5	3	1	1	1	1	2	5	10
50–64	59	1.3	1	1	1	1	1	2	3	7
65+	25	1.7	5	1	1	1	1	3	4	18
2. MULTIPLE DX										
0–19 Years	853	5.5	40	1	1	4	8	12	17	29
20–34	982	5.3	30	1	2	4	7	11	15	26
35–49	1324	5.6	31	1	2	5	6	11	15	27
50–64	975	7.4	56	1	2	6	11	16	18	35
65+	924	8.0	51	1	3	7	10	17	22	33
TOTAL SINGLE DX	665	1.9	5	1	1	1	1	5	6	12
MULTIPLE DX	5058	6.2	41	1	2	5	8	13	18	30
TOTAL										
0–19 Years	1215	4.6	33	1	1	2	6	10	15	29
20–34	1093	5.0	28	1	1	4	6	10	14	24
35–49	1432	5.0	29	1	1	4	6	10	14	26
50–64	1034	6.9	55	1	2	5	10	15	18	35
65+	949	7.8	50	1	3	7	10	17	22	33
GRAND TOTAL	5723	5.6	39	1	1	4	7	13	17	29

55.11: PYELOTOMY. Formerly included in operation group(s) 646.

Type of Patients	Observed Patients	Avg. Stay	Vari-ance	10th	25th	50th	75th	90th	95th	99th
1. SINGLE DX										
0–19 Years	12	3.8	3	1	2	5	5	5	6	6
20–34	35	3.1	3	1	2	3	4	5	6	11
35–49	37	4.0	2	2	3	4	5	5	6	7
50–64	24	2.0	2	1	1	1	3	5	5	7
65+	10	5.3	7	1	4	5	8	8	8	8
2. MULTIPLE DX										
0–19 Years	28	4.4	6	2	3	4	5	7	10	14
20–34	72	4.6	9	1	3	5	6	7	7	9
35–49	84	5.5	8	3	3	5	7	9	10	14
50–64	109	5.5	19	1	3	4	7	13	13	28
65+	113	4.7	28	1	2	4	5	9	14	27
TOTAL SINGLE DX	118	3.1	3	1	1	3	5	5	6	8
MULTIPLE DX	406	5.0	16	1	3	4	7	8	13	20
TOTAL										
0–19 Years	40	4.2	5	2	3	4	5	6	7	14
20–34	107	4.1	7	1	2	4	5	7	7	11
35–49	121	5.0	6	2	3	5	7	8	10	13
50–64	133	4.5	17	1	1	4	6	9	13	21
65+	123	4.7	27	1	2	4	5	9	14	27
GRAND TOTAL	524	4.6	14	1	2	4	6	8	11	18

55.23: CLSD (PERC) RENAL BIOPSY. Formerly included in operation group(s) 646.

Type of Patients	Observed Patients	Avg. Stay	Vari-ance	10th	25th	50th	75th	90th	95th	99th
1. SINGLE DX										
0–19 Years	342	2.0	6	1	1	1	2	5	7	12
20–34	104	2.5	7	1	1	1	3	5	8	15
35–49	95	1.9	5	1	1	1	1	4	7	12
50–64	54	1.3	1	1	1	1	1	2	3	7
65+	23	1.6	5	1	1	1	1	3	4	18
2. MULTIPLE DX										
0–19 Years	777	5.3	36	1	1	4	7	11	17	29
20–34	934	5.2	28	1	2	4	7	11	15	24
35–49	1221	5.5	35	1	2	4	7	11	15	28
50–64	907	7.1	40	1	3	6	11	15	18	26
65+	847	7.9	48	1	3	7	10	17	21	33
TOTAL SINGLE DX	618	2.0	5	1	1	1	2	5	7	12
MULTIPLE DX	4686	6.1	38	1	2	4	8	13	18	29
TOTAL										
0–19 Years	1119	4.4	30	1	1	2	6	9	14	29
20–34	1038	4.9	27	1	1	4	6	10	14	23
35–49	1316	5.2	34	1	1	4	7	11	15	27
50–64	961	6.7	39	1	2	5	10	15	18	25
65+	870	7.7	48	1	3	7	10	17	21	33
GRAND TOTAL	5304	5.6	36	1	1	4	8	13	17	29

Length of Stay by Diagnosis and Operation, United States, 1997

United States, October 1995–September 1996 Data, by Operation

55.24: OPEN BIOPSY OF KIDNEY. Formerly included in operation group(s) 646.

Type of Patients	Observed Patients	Avg. Stay	Variance	Percentiles						
				10th	25th	50th	75th	90th	95th	99th
1. SINGLE DX										
0–19 Years	20	4.7	15	1	1	2	9	9	10	12
20–34	7	3.2	5	1	1	3	3	8	3	8
35–49	11	1.1	<1	1	1	1	1	1	1	3
50–64	2	2.6	<1	2	2	3	4	3	3	3
65+	1	4.0	0	4	4	4	4	4	4	4
2. MULTIPLE DX										
0–19 Years	71	9.3	97	1	4	8	11	18	27	58
20–34	43	8.9	69	2	3	7	13	17	30	39
35–49	94	5.9	46	2	3	3	6	12	20	27
50–64	63	12.9	328	2	6	6	13	36	56	83
65+	61	10.3	94	2	4	7	12	24	31	49
TOTAL SINGLE DX	41	1.4	3	1	1	1	1	2	3	9
MULTIPLE DX	332	9.0	135	2	3	5	11	19	27	57
TOTAL										
0–19 Years	91	8.4	85	1	2	7	9	16	21	54
20–34	50	8.3	64	1	2	7	10	17	30	32
35–49	105	3.0	24	1	1	1	6	6	12	26
50–64	65	12.8	326	2	2	6	13	36	56	83
65+	62	10.2	93	2	4	7	12	24	31	49
GRAND TOTAL	373	6.3	100	1	1	3	8	14	24	56

55.39: LOC DESTR RENAL LES NEC. Formerly included in operation group(s) 646.

Type of Patients	Observed Patients	Avg. Stay	Variance	Percentiles						
				10th	25th	50th	75th	90th	95th	99th
1. SINGLE DX										
0–19 Years	9	4.6	3	3	4	4	5	8	8	8
20–34	5	4.0	2	2	4	4	4	6	6	6
35–49	9	4.2	1	3	4	4	5	5	5	5
50–64	16	3.7	1	3	3	3	4	6	6	6
65+	4	2.5	1	1	2	2	4	4	4	4
2. MULTIPLE DX										
0–19 Years	29	8.3	45	3	5	6	11	14	28	28
20–34	14	4.1	1	3	3	4	5	5	7	8
35–49	49	5.0	5	3	4	5	5	8	11	12
50–64	56	5.4	4	3	5	5	7	8	8	13
65+	113	6.2	39	2	2	5	7	11	15	44
TOTAL SINGLE DX	43	3.8	2	3	3	4	4	5	6	8
MULTIPLE DX	261	5.8	23	2	4	5	6	9	13	28
TOTAL										
0–19 Years	38	7.7	39	3	4	6	8	14	28	28
20–34	19	4.1	1	3	3	4	5	5	7	8
35–49	58	4.9	4	3	4	4	5	7	11	12
50–64	72	4.6	3	3	3	5	5	7	8	9
65+	117	6.0	38	2	2	5	7	11	15	44
GRAND TOTAL	304	5.4	19	2	3	5	6	8	12	28

55.3: LOC EXC/DESTR RENAL LES. Formerly included in operation group(s) 646.

Type of Patients	Observed Patients	Avg. Stay	Variance	Percentiles						
				10th	25th	50th	75th	90th	95th	99th
1. SINGLE DX										
0–19 Years	13	3.9	4	1	3	4	4	8	8	8
20–34	9	4.2	3	3	3	4	6	7	7	7
35–49	9	4.2	1	3	4	4	4	5	5	5
50–64	18	3.6	1	3	3	3	4	6	6	9
65+	6	2.7	1	2	2	2	4	4	4	4
2. MULTIPLE DX										
0–19 Years	31	8.0	43	3	4	6	8	14	28	28
20–34	17	7.4	29	3	4	4	15	16	16	16
35–49	59	4.8	5	3	4	4	6	8	11	12
50–64	69	5.2	4	3	4	5	6	8	8	15
65+	118	6.4	44	2	2	5	7	12	19	44
TOTAL SINGLE DX	55	3.7	2	2	3	4	4	6	6	8
MULTIPLE DX	294	6.0	26	2	4	5	7	11	16	28
TOTAL										
0–19 Years	44	7.1	37	2	4	6	8	13	28	28
20–34	26	6.9	26	3	3	4	6	16	16	16
35–49	68	4.7	4	3	4	4	5	7	10	12
50–64	87	4.6	4	3	3	5	6	7	8	13
65+	124	6.2	43	2	2	5	7	12	19	44
GRAND TOTAL	349	5.6	22	2	3	5	6	9	14	28

55.4: PARTIAL NEPHRECTOMY. Formerly included in operation group(s) 646.

Type of Patients	Observed Patients	Avg. Stay	Variance	Percentiles						
				10th	25th	50th	75th	90th	95th	99th
1. SINGLE DX										
0–19 Years	35	3.8	6	2	3	3	4	6	9	11
20–34	9	6.5	4	3	4	8	8	8	8	8
35–49	19	5.2	<1	3	4	6	8	8	8	8
50–64	31	4.3	<1	3	4	5	5	6	6	6
65+	14	5.3	1	4	5	5	6	7	7	7
2. MULTIPLE DX										
0–19 Years	231	4.6	16	2	3	4	5	8	10	20
20–34	66	6.6	13	3	4	5	7	10	15	19
35–49	126	6.7	44	4	4	6	7	9	12	31
50–64	215	6.9	49	4	4	6	7	9	12	55
65+	297	8.0	28	4	5	7	9	13	19	30
TOTAL SINGLE DX	108	4.8	4	3	3	4	6	8	8	9
MULTIPLE DX	935	6.7	33	3	4	6	7	10	14	30
TOTAL										
0–19 Years	266	4.5	14	2	3	4	5	8	9	20
20–34	75	6.6	11	4	4	6	8	10	13	19
35–49	145	6.3	33	4	4	6	7	9	10	25
50–64	246	6.7	45	4	4	6	7	9	12	55
65+	311	7.9	28	4	5	7	9	12	19	30
GRAND TOTAL	1043	6.5	30	3	4	5	7	10	13	28

Length of Stay by Diagnosis and Operation, United States, 1997

United States, October 1995–September 1996 Data, by Operation

55.5: COMPLETE NEPHRECTOMY. Formerly included in operation group(s) 643.

Type of Patients	Observed Patients	Avg. Stay	Vari-ance	Percentiles						
				10th	25th	50th	75th	90th	95th	99th
1. SINGLE DX										
0–19 Years	213	4.2	8	1	2	4	6	8	8	13
20–34	280	4.5	2	3	4	4	5	6	7	8
35–49	488	4.8	2	3	4	5	6	7	7	9
50–64	309	4.8	2	3	4	5	6	6	7	9
65+	177	5.9	5	4	4	5	7	9	11	12
2. MULTIPLE DX										
0–19 Years	787	6.7	58	2	3	4	8	12	18	51
20–34	641	6.8	45	3	4	5	7	12	16	40
35–49	1516	7.0	33	4	4	5	7	12	17	31
50–64	2478	6.9	28	4	4	6	7	10	14	34
65+	3962	8.4	38	4	5	7	9	15	20	32
TOTAL SINGLE DX	1467	4.8	3	3	4	5	6	7	8	11
MULTIPLE DX	9384	7.5	37	3	4	6	8	13	18	35
TOTAL										
0–19 Years	1000	6.1	47	2	4	4	8	11	15	50
20–34	921	6.1	32	3	4	5	6	9	14	35
35–49	2004	6.5	27	3	4	5	7	10	15	29
50–64	2787	6.6	25	3	4	6	7	10	13	29
65+	4139	8.3	37	4	5	7	9	15	20	31
GRAND TOTAL	10851	7.1	33	3	4	6	8	12	16	31

55.51: NEPHROURETERECTOMY. Formerly included in operation group(s) 643.

Type of Patients	Observed Patients	Avg. Stay	Vari-ance	Percentiles						
				10th	25th	50th	75th	90th	95th	99th
1. SINGLE DX										
0–19 Years	209	4.1	7	1	2	4	6	8	8	10
20–34	279	4.5	2	3	4	4	5	6	7	8
35–49	486	4.8	2	3	4	5	6	7	7	9
50–64	306	4.8	2	3	4	5	6	6	7	8
65+	176	5.9	5	4	4	5	7	9	11	12
2. MULTIPLE DX										
0–19 Years	711	6.0	40	2	3	4	8	11	15	32
20–34	503	6.9	47	3	4	5	7	12	16	41
35–49	1295	6.6	23	4	4	5	7	10	15	26
50–64	2369	6.8	26	4	4	6	7	10	13	31
65+	3908	8.4	37	4	5	7	9	15	20	31
TOTAL SINGLE DX	1456	4.8	3	3	4	5	6	7	8	11
MULTIPLE DX	8786	7.3	33	3	4	6	8	12	17	31
TOTAL										
0–19 Years	920	5.5	32	2	4	4	7	10	13	26
20–34	782	6.0	32	3	4	5	6	8	14	35
35–49	1781	6.2	18	3	4	5	7	9	14	23
50–64	2675	6.6	24	4	4	6	7	9	13	28
65+	4084	8.3	35	4	5	7	9	15	20	31
GRAND TOTAL	10242	6.9	29	3	4	6	8	11	16	29

55.53: REJECTED KID NEPHRECTOMY. Formerly included in operation group(s) 643.

Type of Patients	Observed Patients	Avg. Stay	Vari-ance	Percentiles						
				10th	25th	50th	75th	90th	95th	99th
1. SINGLE DX										
0–19 Years	1	2.0	0	2	2	2	2	2	2	2
20–34	0									
35–49	0									
50–64	1	5.0	0	5	5	5	5	5	5	5
65+	0									
2. MULTIPLE DX										
0–19 Years	30	6.2	12	3	4	6	9	13	13	>99
20–34	110	6.8	47	1	2	6	10	12	20	40
35–49	151	8.4	48	2	4	6	11	17	24	33
50–64	51	8.3	38	3	5	8	9	14	19	39
65+	7	13.9	321	4	4	4	25	26	77	77
TOTAL SINGLE DX	2	3.4	3	2	2	2	5	5	5	5
MULTIPLE DX	349	7.8	53	2	4	6	10	17	24	40
TOTAL										
0–19 Years	31	6.1	12	3	4	6	8	13	13	>99
20–34	110	6.8	47	1	2	6	10	12	20	40
35–49	151	8.4	48	2	4	6	11	17	24	33
50–64	52	8.3	38	3	5	7	9	14	19	39
65+	7	13.9	321	4	4	4	25	26	77	77
GRAND TOTAL	351	7.8	53	2	4	6	10	17	24	40

55.6: KIDNEY TRANSPLANT. Formerly included in operation group(s) 645.

Type of Patients	Observed Patients	Avg. Stay	Vari-ance	Percentiles						
				10th	25th	50th	75th	90th	95th	99th
1. SINGLE DX										
0–19 Years	15	11.4	33	7	7	10	12	25	25	25
20–34	41	6.9	11	4	6	6	7	10	13	19
35–49	70	6.9	10	4	5	6	8	10	12	18
50–64	32	7.1	3	5	6	7	8	9	9	12
65+	3	12.4	16	6	8	15	15	15	15	15
2. MULTIPLE DX										
0–19 Years	310	13.4	68	6	8	11	16	24	34	44
20–34	685	11.2	57	5	7	9	14	19	24	43
35–49	1201	11.0	49	5	7	9	13	19	25	43
50–64	866	11.5	72	5	7	9	13	20	26	48
65+	181	12.6	68	6	7	12	14	23	30	57
TOTAL SINGLE DX	161	7.3	12	4	5	6	8	10	15	20
MULTIPLE DX	3243	11.5	60	5	7	9	14	20	26	44
TOTAL										
0–19 Years	325	13.3	67	6	8	11	16	24	34	44
20–34	726	11.0	55	5	7	9	14	19	23	41
35–49	1271	10.6	47	5	6	9	13	18	24	43
50–64	898	11.3	70	5	7	9	13	19	25	48
65+	184	12.6	67	6	7	12	14	23	30	57
GRAND TOTAL	3404	11.2	58	5	7	9	13	19	25	44

Length of Stay by Diagnosis and Operation, United States, 1997

United States, October 1995–September 1996 Data, by Operation

55.69: KIDNEY TRANSPLANT NEC. Formerly included in operation group(s) 645.

Type of Patients	Observed Patients	Avg. Stay	Vari-ance	10th	25th	50th	75th	90th	95th	99th
1. SINGLE DX										
0–19 Years	15	11.4	33	7	7	10	12	25	25	25
20–34	41	6.9	11	4	6	6	7	10	13	19
35–49	70	6.9	10	4	6	6	8	10	12	18
50–64	32	7.1	3	5	6	7	8	9	9	12
65+	3	12.4	16	6	8	15	15	15	15	15
2. MULTIPLE DX										
0–19 Years	308	13.4	69	6	8	11	16	24	34	44
20–34	681	11.2	57	5	7	9	14	19	24	43
35–49	1198	11.0	49	5	7	9	13	19	25	43
50–64	865	11.5	72	5	7	9	13	20	26	48
65+	180	12.5	69	6	7	12	14	23	30	57
TOTAL SINGLE DX	161	7.3	12	4	5	6	8	10	15	20
MULTIPLE DX	3232	11.5	60	5	7	9	14	20	26	44
TOTAL										
0–19 Years	323	13.4	67	6	8	11	16	24	34	44
20–34	722	11.0	55	5	7	9	14	19	23	41
35–49	1268	10.7	47	5	6	9	13	18	24	43
50–64	897	11.3	70	5	7	9	13	19	25	48
65+	183	12.5	68	6	7	12	14	23	30	57
GRAND TOTAL	3393	11.2	58	5	7	9	13	19	25	44

55.8: OTHER KIDNEY REPAIR. Formerly included in operation group(s) 646.

Type of Patients	Observed Patients	Avg. Stay	Vari-ance	10th	25th	50th	75th	90th	95th	99th
1. SINGLE DX										
0–19 Years	618	3.1	2	1	2	3	4	5	5	7
20–34	83	3.8	4	3	3	3	4	5	6	8
35–49	52	3.1	2	3	2	3	4	5	6	8
50–64	22	4.3	1	3	4	4	5	5	7	9
65+	5	3.6	1	3	3	3	4	4	7	7
2. MULTIPLE DX										
0–19 Years	680	4.1	13	2	3	3	5	7	8	17
20–34	229	4.6	5	3	3	3	5	7	8	16
35–49	164	4.8	6	3	3	4	6	7	7	11
50–64	106	5.4	12	3	3	4	7	10	15	15
65+	107	6.1	9	4	5	6	6	8	10	17
TOTAL SINGLE DX	780	3.2	2	2	2	3	4	5	5	7
MULTIPLE DX	1286	4.6	10	2	3	4	5	7	9	16
TOTAL										
0–19 Years	1298	3.6	8	2	2	3	4	6	7	11
20–34	312	4.4	5	3	3	4	5	6	7	16
35–49	216	4.2	5	3	3	4	6	8	8	10
50–64	128	5.2	10	3	4	4	6	8	13	15
65+	112	6.0	9	4	5	6	6	8	10	17
GRAND TOTAL	2066	4.0	7	2	3	4	5	6	8	15

55.7: NEPHROPEXY. Formerly included in operation group(s) 646.

Type of Patients	Observed Patients	Avg. Stay	Vari-ance	10th	25th	50th	75th	90th	95th	99th
1. SINGLE DX										
0–19 Years	1	2.0	0	2	2	2	2	2	2	2
20–34	2	2.1	<1	2	2	2	2	2	2	2
35–49	2	3.0	0	3	3	3	3	3	3	3
50–64	0									
65+	0									
2. MULTIPLE DX										
0–19 Years	0									
20–34	8	3.3	3	2	2	2	6	6	6	6
35–49	3	4.2	3	2	2	4	6	6	6	6
50–64	1	11.0	0	11	11	11	11	11	11	11
65+	2	4.3	<1	4	4	4	5	5	5	5
TOTAL SINGLE DX	5	2.4	<1	2	2	2	3	3	3	3
MULTIPLE DX	14	4.0	5	2	2	3	6	6	6	11
TOTAL										
0–19 Years	1	2.0	0	2	2	2	2	2	2	2
20–34	10	3.0	2	2	2	2	3	6	6	6
35–49	5	3.4	1	2	3	3	4	6	6	6
50–64	1	11.0	0	11	11	11	11	11	11	11
65+	2	4.3	<1	4	4	4	5	5	5	5
GRAND TOTAL	19	3.5	4	2	2	3	4	6	6	11

55.87: CORRECTION OF UPJ. Formerly included in operation group(s) 646.

Type of Patients	Observed Patients	Avg. Stay	Vari-ance	10th	25th	50th	75th	90th	95th	99th
1. SINGLE DX										
0–19 Years	612	3.1	2	1	2	3	4	5	5	7
20–34	82	3.7	4	3	3	3	4	5	6	8
35–49	51	3.1	2	2	2	3	4	5	6	7
50–64	22	4.3	1	3	4	4	5	5	7	9
65+	5	3.6	1	3	3	3	4	4	7	7
2. MULTIPLE DX										
0–19 Years	649	4.1	13	2	3	3	5	7	8	16
20–34	200	4.4	3	3	3	4	5	6	7	10
35–49	146	4.5	10	3	3	4	6	7	7	10
50–64	97	5.4	10	3	3	4	6	7	15	15
65+	104	6.1	8	4	5	6	6	8	10	15
TOTAL SINGLE DX	772	3.2	2	2	2	3	4	5	5	7
MULTIPLE DX	1196	4.5	10	2	3	4	5	7	8	15
TOTAL										
0–19 Years	1261	3.6	8	2	2	3	4	6	7	11
20–34	282	4.2	3	3	3	4	5	6	6	10
35–49	197	4.0	3	3	3	4	6	6	6	10
50–64	119	5.2	9	3	5	6	6	8	13	15
65+	109	5.9	8	4	5	6	8	8	10	15
GRAND TOTAL	1968	4.0	7	2	3	3	5	6	7	13

Length of Stay by Diagnosis and Operation, United States, 1997

United States, October 1995–September 1996 Data, by Operation

55.9: OTHER RENAL OPERATIONS. Formerly included in operation group(s) 646.

Type of Patients	Observed Patients	Avg. Stay	Vari-ance	10th	25th	50th	75th	90th	95th	99th
1. SINGLE DX										
0–19 Years	3	2.0	<1	1	2	2	2	3	3	3
20–34	5	3.5	11	1	1	2	5	9	9	9
35–49	8	1.9	<1	1	1	1	3	3	3	3
50–64	9	3.0	3	1	1	3	5	5	5	5
65+	1	1.0	0	1	1	1	1	1	1	1
2. MULTIPLE DX										
0–19 Years	45	7.6	40	1	3	7	9	17	23	25
20–34	51	8.7	58	1	3	8	9	25	25	25
35–49	124	5.6	19	1	2	5	7	11	12	20
50–64	167	5.6	23	1	3	5	7	10	14	28
65+	366	6.7	32	1	3	5	9	15	17	24
TOTAL SINGLE DX	26	2.3	3	1	1	2	3	5	5	9
MULTIPLE DX	753	6.5	31	1	3	5	8	14	17	25
TOTAL										
0–19 Years	48	7.2	39	1	2	6	9	17	17	25
20–34	56	8.5	57	1	3	8	8	25	25	25
35–49	132	5.3	18	1	2	5	7	11	12	20
50–64	176	5.5	22	1	2	5	7	10	14	28
65+	367	6.7	32	1	3	5	9	15	17	24
GRAND TOTAL	779	6.4	31	1	2	5	8	13	17	25

56.0: TU RMVL URETERAL OBSTR. Formerly included in operation group(s) 649.

Type of Patients	Observed Patients	Avg. Stay	Vari-ance	10th	25th	50th	75th	90th	95th	99th
1. SINGLE DX										
0–19 Years	129	2.1	1	1	1	2	2	3	4	6
20–34	1115	1.8	1	1	1	2	2	3	4	5
35–49	1309	1.9	1	1	1	2	2	3	4	5
50–64	678	1.7	<1	1	1	1	2	3	3	5
65+	172	1.8	1	1	1	1	2	3	4	5
2. MULTIPLE DX										
0–19 Years	197	3.3	20	1	1	2	3	7	12	12
20–34	1376	2.4	2	1	1	2	3	4	6	8
35–49	2245	2.6	4	1	1	2	3	4	6	10
50–64	1894	2.8	7	1	1	2	3	5	7	13
65+	1852	4.2	16	1	2	3	5	9	11	19
TOTAL SINGLE DX	3403	1.8	1	1	1	2	2	3	4	5
MULTIPLE DX	7564	2.9	7	1	1	2	3	5	8	13
TOTAL										
0–19 Years	326	2.9	13	1	1	2	3	5	8	12
20–34	2491	2.1	2	1	1	2	3	4	5	7
35–49	3554	2.3	3	1	1	2	3	4	5	8
50–64	2572	2.5	5	1	1	2	3	4	6	11
65+	2024	3.9	15	1	2	3	5	8	11	18
GRAND TOTAL	10967	2.5	5	1	1	2	3	5	6	11

55.93: REPL NEPHROSTOMY TUBE. Formerly included in operation group(s) 646.

Type of Patients	Observed Patients	Avg. Stay	Vari-ance	10th	25th	50th	75th	90th	95th	99th
1. SINGLE DX										
0–19 Years	1	2.0	0	2	2	2	2	2	2	2
20–34	1	1.0	0	1	1	1	1	1	1	1
35–49	4	1.0	0	1	1	1	1	1	1	1
50–64	3	2.1	1	1	1	3	3	3	3	3
65+	1	1.0	0	1	1	1	1	1	1	1
2. MULTIPLE DX										
0–19 Years	25	6.5	46	1	1	4	8	23	25	25
20–34	28	6.2	46	1	1	3	8	17	19	32
35–49	65	5.4	19	1	2	5	8	12	12	20
50–64	113	5.1	23	1	2	3	6	9	14	28
65+	255	6.2	30	1	3	5	8	13	15	24
TOTAL SINGLE DX	10	1.4	<1	1	1	1	2	3	3	3
MULTIPLE DX	486	5.9	29	1	2	5	8	13	16	25
TOTAL										
0–19 Years	26	6.0	44	1	1	4	8	15	23	25
20–34	29	6.0	45	1	1	3	8	17	19	32
35–49	69	5.1	19	1	2	4	8	12	12	20
50–64	116	5.0	23	1	2	3	6	9	14	28
65+	256	6.2	30	1	3	5	8	13	15	24
GRAND TOTAL	496	5.8	28	1	2	5	8	13	15	25

56.1: URETERAL MEATOTOMY. Formerly included in operation group(s) 650.

Type of Patients	Observed Patients	Avg. Stay	Vari-ance	10th	25th	50th	75th	90th	95th	99th
1. SINGLE DX										
0–19 Years	1	1.0	0	1	1	1	1	1	1	1
20–34	6	1.5	<1	1	2	2	3	3	3	5
35–49	14	2.4	<1	2	1	2	3	3	3	5
50–64	9	2.0	<1	1	2	2	2	3	4	4
65+	1	6.0	0	6	6	6	6	6	6	6
2. MULTIPLE DX										
0–19 Years	2	3.2	1	2	2	4	4	4	4	4
20–34	18	3.7	9	1	1	3	5	8	8	13
35–49	27	3.8	13	1	1	3	4	10	15	15
50–64	47	3.8	7	1	2	3	6	8	8	11
65+	64	4.8	16	1	2	3	6	13	13	14
TOTAL SINGLE DX	31	2.3	<1	1	2	2	3	3	3	6
MULTIPLE DX	158	4.1	11	1	2	3	5	8	13	15
TOTAL										
0–19 Years	3	2.8	2	2	2	4	4	4	4	4
20–34	24	3.4	8	1	1	2	5	8	8	13
35–49	41	3.1	7	2	2	3	3	6	7	15
50–64	56	3.5	6	1	2	3	4	8	8	11
65+	65	4.8	15	1	2	3	6	13	13	14
GRAND TOTAL	189	3.7	9	1	2	3	4	8	11	14

United States, October 1995–September 1996 Data, by Operation

56.2: URETEROTOMY. Formerly included in operation group(s) 647.

Type of Patients	Observed Patients	Avg. Stay	Vari-ance	Percentiles						
				10th	25th	50th	75th	90th	95th	99th
1. SINGLE DX										
0–19 Years	23	2.9	4	1	1	3	4	5	8	8
20–34	43	2.9	2	1	1	3	4	5	8	6
35–49	55	3.6	11	1	1	3	4	7	13	13
50–64	31	4.7	5	3	3	5	7	7	7	7
65+	17	3.6	<1	3	3	3	4	5	5	7
2. MULTIPLE DX										
0–19 Years	39	3.7	10	1	2	3	6	7	11	16
20–34	82	4.1	9	1	2	3	4	8	10	15
35–49	146	3.8	11	1	2	3	5	7	9	13
50–64	190	4.5	7	2	3	4	5	7	8	15
65+	238	6.4	32	2	3	5	8	13	14	23
TOTAL SINGLE DX	169	3.6	6	1	2	3	4	7	7	13
MULTIPLE DX	695	4.7	16	1	2	4	6	8	12	16
TOTAL										
0–19 Years	62	3.4	8	1	1	3	5	7	8	14
20–34	125	3.7	7	1	2	3	4	8	8	14
35–49	201	3.8	11	1	2	3	5	7	9	13
50–64	221	4.5	6	2	3	4	5	7	8	15
65+	255	6.1	30	2	3	5	8	11	14	21
GRAND TOTAL	864	4.5	14	1	2	4	6	8	11	16

56.31: URETEROSCOPY. Formerly included in operation group(s) 651.

Type of Patients	Observed Patients	Avg. Stay	Vari-ance	Percentiles						
				10th	25th	50th	75th	90th	95th	99th
1. SINGLE DX										
0–19 Years	17	2.0	1	1	1	2	2	4	4	4
20–34	52	2.0	2	1	1	2	2	4	5	5
35–49	64	2.2	2	1	1	2	2	3	4	5
50–64	40	1.9	1	1	1	2	2	3	4	6
65+	10	3.0	3	1	1	3	4	6	6	6
2. MULTIPLE DX										
0–19 Years	17	3.4	2	1	2	4	4	5	5	8
20–34	88	2.6	3	1	2	3	4	5	6	9
35–49	135	3.9	12	1	2	3	4	7	13	18
50–64	130	2.4	5	1	1	1	3	5	6	11
65+	148	3.9	21	1	1	2	4	10	13	23
TOTAL SINGLE DX	183	2.1	2	1	1	2	2	4	5	6
MULTIPLE DX	518	3.3	11	1	1	2	4	7	10	17
TOTAL										
0–19 Years	34	2.7	2	1	1	2	4	4	4	5
20–34	140	2.3	3	1	1	2	3	5	5	7
35–49	199	3.4	9	1	2	2	4	6	13	13
50–64	170	2.3	5	1	1	1	3	5	6	10
65+	158	3.9	20	1	1	2	4	8	13	23
GRAND TOTAL	701	3.0	9	1	1	2	4	6	8	16

56.3: URETERAL DIAGNOSTIC PX. Formerly included in operation group(s) 650, 651, 664.

Type of Patients	Observed Patients	Avg. Stay	Vari-ance	Percentiles						
				10th	25th	50th	75th	90th	95th	99th
1. SINGLE DX										
0–19 Years	18	2.0	1	1	1	2	2	4	4	4
20–34	57	1.9	2	1	1	2	2	3	5	6
35–49	69	2.1	1	1	1	2	2	3	4	5
50–64	44	1.8	1	1	1	2	2	3	4	7
65+	11	2.3	3	1	1	1	4	4	6	6
2. MULTIPLE DX										
0–19 Years	19	3.4	2	1	2	4	4	4	5	8
20–34	98	3.0	3	1	2	3	4	5	6	7
35–49	158	4.0	12	1	2	3	5	7	13	18
50–64	165	2.8	7	1	1	3	4	6	7	14
65+	250	4.1	19	1	1	3	5	10	13	23
TOTAL SINGLE DX	199	2.0	2	1	1	2	2	4	4	6
MULTIPLE DX	690	3.5	11	1	1	3	4	7	11	17
TOTAL										
0–19 Years	37	2.7	2	1	1	2	4	4	4	5
20–34	155	2.6	3	1	1	2	3	4	6	7
35–49	227	3.4	9	1	2	2	5	6	13	15
50–64	209	2.7	6	1	1	2	4	6	6	14
65+	261	4.0	19	1	1	2	5	10	13	21
GRAND TOTAL	889	3.2	10	1	1	2	4	6	9	16

56.4: URETERECTOMY. Formerly included in operation group(s) 650.

Type of Patients	Observed Patients	Avg. Stay	Vari-ance	Percentiles						
				10th	25th	50th	75th	90th	95th	99th
1. SINGLE DX										
0–19 Years	26	4.0	11	1	2	3	4	11	11	11
20–34	5	4.9	<1	4	5	5	5	5	5	5
35–49	7	4.3	3	2	2	5	6	6	6	6
50–64	15	5.4	3	4	4	5	7	7	7	8
65+	15	4.5	4	1	3	5	5	8	8	8
2. MULTIPLE DX										
0–19 Years	188	5.6	41	2	2	4	6	9	13	35
20–34	25	3.9	5	3	3	3	5	5	7	10
35–49	58	4.6	10	1	1	4	5	9	11	16
50–64	86	7.8	16	3	5	7	12	13	15	15
65+	239	6.6	37	2	2	5	9	11	18	31
TOTAL SINGLE DX	68	4.6	6	1	3	4	5	7	11	11
MULTIPLE DX	596	6.0	30	2	3	5	7	11	13	35
TOTAL										
0–19 Years	214	5.5	38	2	2	4	6	10	12	35
20–34	30	4.1	5	3	3	3	5	5	6	10
35–49	65	4.6	10	1	2	5	5	8	11	16
50–64	101	7.5	15	3	4	7	12	13	13	15
65+	254	6.5	36	2	2	5	9	11	17	30
GRAND TOTAL	664	5.9	28	2	3	5	7	11	13	35

Length of Stay by Diagnosis and Operation, United States, 1997

United States, October 1995–September 1996 Data, by Operation

56.41: PARTIAL URETERECTOMY. Formerly included in operation group(s) 650.

Type of Patients	Observed Patients	Avg. Stay	Vari-ance	10th	25th	50th	75th	90th	95th	99th
1. SINGLE DX										
0–19 Years	24	4.1	12	1	2	3	4	11	11	11
20–34	5	4.9	<1	4	5	5	5	5	5	5
35–49	5	3.4	3	2	2	3	5	5	5	5
50–64	13	5.4	3	4	4	5	7	7	7	8
65+	10	4.3	4	1	3	5	5	7	8	8
2. MULTIPLE DX										
0–19 Years	171	5.7	43	2	2	4	6	9	13	35
20–34	23	3.8	2	3	3	3	5	5	7	8
35–49	52	4.6	11	1	2	4	6	5	11	16
50–64	70	7.7	18	3	4	6	13	13	13	15
65+	207	7.2	42	2	3	5	10	12	19	31
TOTAL SINGLE DX	57	4.5	6	1	3	5	5	7	11	11
MULTIPLE DX	523	6.1	32	2	3	5	7	12	13	35
TOTAL										
0–19 Years	195	5.5	40	2	2	4	6	10	11	35
20–34	28	4.0	2	3	3	3	5	5	6	8
35–49	57	4.6	11	1	2	4	6	9	11	16
50–64	83	7.4	17	3	4	6	12	13	13	15
65+	217	7.1	40	2	3	5	10	12	19	31
GRAND TOTAL	580	5.9	30	2	3	5	7	11	13	35

56.51: FORM CUTAN ILEOURETEROST. Formerly included in operation group(s) 648.

Type of Patients	Observed Patients	Avg. Stay	Vari-ance	10th	25th	50th	75th	90th	95th	99th
1. SINGLE DX										
0–19 Years	2	2.5	<1	2	2	3	3	3	3	3
20–34	0									
35–49	0									
50–64	3	9.2	2	6	9	10	10	10	10	10
65+	4	9.7	<1	9	10	10	10	10	10	10
2. MULTIPLE DX										
0–19 Years	17	10.5	8	8	9	10	12	14	17	17
20–34	40	18.9	383	8	9	15	17	30	83	83
35–49	57	15.1	182	6	10	12	16	19	27	85
50–64	112	12.3	47	7	8	12	12	17	27	37
65+	249	14.1	115	7	8	10	14	28	44	52
TOTAL SINGLE DX	9	7.8	10	2	6	10	10	10	10	10
MULTIPLE DX	475	14.0	123	7	8	11	14	23	35	77
TOTAL										
0–19 Years	19	9.5	14	3	9	10	11	14	14	17
20–34	40	18.9	383	8	9	15	17	30	83	83
35–49	57	15.1	182	6	10	12	16	19	27	85
50–64	115	12.3	46	7	9	12	12	17	27	37
65+	253	14.0	112	7	8	10	14	26	44	52
GRAND TOTAL	484	13.8	121	7	8	11	14	23	34	77

56.5: CUTAN URETERO-ILEOSTOMY. Formerly included in operation group(s) 648.

Type of Patients	Observed Patients	Avg. Stay	Vari-ance	10th	25th	50th	75th	90th	95th	99th
1. SINGLE DX										
0–19 Years	2	2.5	<1	2	2	3	3	3	3	3
20–34	2	3.4	3	2	2	2	5	5	5	5
35–49	0									
50–64	4	5.1	19	1	1	1	10	10	10	10
65+	5	9.2	4	8	9	10	10	10	10	10
2. MULTIPLE DX										
0–19 Years	26	10.6	29	5	8	10	14	17	24	24
20–34	60	13.9	292	1	7	10	16	17	79	83
35–49	93	12.9	123	6	7	11	15	18	27	77
50–64	155	11.9	50	7	8	11	12	20	27	42
65+	318	13.4	108	7	8	10	14	24	38	52
TOTAL SINGLE DX	13	6.2	15	1	2	9	10	10	10	10
MULTIPLE DX	652	12.9	110	6	8	10	14	22	30	58
TOTAL										
0–19 Years	28	9.8	32	2	5	10	12	17	24	24
20–34	62	13.7	290	1	7	9	16	17	79	83
35–49	93	12.9	123	6	7	11	15	18	27	77
50–64	159	11.7	51	6	8	11	12	18	27	41
65+	323	13.3	106	7	8	10	14	23	37	52
GRAND TOTAL	665	12.7	109	6	8	10	14	22	29	58

56.6: EXT URIN DIVERSION NEC. Formerly included in operation group(s) 648.

Type of Patients	Observed Patients	Avg. Stay	Vari-ance	10th	25th	50th	75th	90th	95th	99th
1. SINGLE DX										
0–19 Years	8	2.1	1	1	1	2	2	3	5	5
20–34	0									
35–49	0									
50–64	0									
65+	0									
2. MULTIPLE DX										
0–19 Years	36	8.9	110	1	2	6	10	31	31	35
20–34	7	14.0	51	6	9	12	23	23	23	23
35–49	5	8.3	6	3	9	9	10	10	10	10
50–64	8	16.6	46	8	10	23	23	23	23	23
65+	20	9.6	60	1	5	10	11	17	20	40
TOTAL SINGLE DX	8	2.1	1	1	1	2	2	3	5	5
MULTIPLE DX	76	10.9	83	1	5	9	14	23	31	40
TOTAL										
0–19 Years	44	7.8	99	1	2	4	9	21	31	35
20–34	7	14.0	51	6	9	12	23	23	23	23
35–49	5	8.3	6	3	9	9	10	10	10	10
50–64	8	16.6	46	8	10	23	23	23	23	23
65+	20	9.6	60	1	5	10	11	17	20	40
GRAND TOTAL	84	10.2	83	1	3	9	12	23	31	40

Length of Stay by Diagnosis and Operation, United States, 1997

United States, October 1995–September 1996 Data, by Operation

56.7: OTHER URETERAL ANAST. Formerly included in operation group(s) 648.

Type of Patients	Observed Patients	Avg. Stay	Vari-ance	Percentiles						
				10th	25th	50th	75th	90th	95th	99th
1. SINGLE DX										
0–19 Years	1405	3.2	2	2	2	3	4	5	6	7
20–34	28	4.5	2	3	4	4	5	7	7	7
35–49	17	4.2	9	2	2	3	4	10	10	14
50–64	10	5.8	6	5	5	5	6	6	8	19
65+	4	7.3	60	3	4	4	4	22	22	22
2. MULTIPLE DX										
0–19 Years	1994	4.7	14	2	3	4	5	8	10	19
20–34	124	5.5	13	3	4	5	5	10	11	21
35–49	173	7.0	20	3	4	6	8	11	16	24
50–64	109	9.5	29	4	6	8	11	17	20	31
65+	139	9.3	58	4	5	8	10	15	16	60
TOTAL SINGLE DX	1464	3.2	2	2	2	3	4	5	6	7
MULTIPLE DX	2539	5.3	18	2	3	4	6	9	12	20
TOTAL										
0–19 Years	3399	4.1	9	2	3	3	5	6	9	19
20–34	152	5.3	11	3	4	5	5	8	11	21
35–49	190	6.8	20	3	4	6	8	11	16	24
50–64	119	9.2	28	4	5	8	11	17	20	31
65+	143	9.2	58	4	5	8	10	15	16	60
GRAND TOTAL	4003	4.5	13	2	3	4	5	8	10	19

56.8: REPAIR OF URETER. Formerly included in operation group(s) 650.

Type of Patients	Observed Patients	Avg. Stay	Vari-ance	Percentiles						
				10th	25th	50th	75th	90th	95th	99th
1. SINGLE DX										
0–19 Years	16	3.3	3	1	1	4	4	5	7	7
20–34	5	1.2	<1	1	1	1	1	1	3	3
35–49	2	1.1	<1	1	1	1	1	1	2	2
50–64	2	1.0	0	1	1	1	1	1	1	1
65+	1	1.0	0	1	1	1	1	1	1	1
2. MULTIPLE DX										
0–19 Years	56	5.4	17	1	3	4	7	12	14	17
20–34	16	6.0	3	4	5	6	7	9	9	10
35–49	23	4.1	8	2	2	3	5	7	11	15
50–64	22	7.8	33	2	4	7	11	21	21	21
65+	10	4.5	42	1	1	2	5	8	15	39
TOTAL SINGLE DX	26	2.6	3	1	1	2	4	4	7	7
MULTIPLE DX	127	5.4	18	1	3	5	7	11	14	21
TOTAL										
0–19 Years	72	4.8	14	1	2	4	6	11	14	17
20–34	21	5.1	6	1	4	5	7	8	9	10
35–49	25	3.7	8	1	2	3	5	7	11	15
50–64	24	7.3	34	1	3	5	11	16	21	21
65+	11	4.4	42	1	1	2	5	8	15	39
GRAND TOTAL	153	4.9	16	1	2	4	6	10	13	21

56.74: URETERONEOCYSTOSTOMY. Formerly included in operation group(s) 648.

Type of Patients	Observed Patients	Avg. Stay	Vari-ance	Percentiles						
				10th	25th	50th	75th	90th	95th	99th
1. SINGLE DX										
0–19 Years	1392	3.2	2	2	2	3	4	5	6	7
20–34	28	4.5	2	3	4	4	5	7	7	7
35–49	16	4.1	7	2	2	3	4	10	10	10
50–64	8	5.5	<1	5	5	5	6	6	6	8
65+	3	8.0	67	4	4	4	4	22	22	22
2. MULTIPLE DX										
0–19 Years	1946	4.6	11	2	3	4	5	8	10	19
20–34	108	5.2	10	2	4	4	5	9	11	21
35–49	138	6.6	18	3	4	6	8	11	13	24
50–64	77	9.1	27	5	5	7	10	20	20	24
65+	90	7.7	43	4	5	6	8	14	16	60
TOTAL SINGLE DX	1447	3.2	2	2	2	3	4	5	6	7
MULTIPLE DX	2359	5.0	13	2	3	4	6	9	11	20
TOTAL										
0–19 Years	3338	4.0	7	2	3	3	5	6	9	19
20–34	136	5.1	8	3	4	5	5	8	11	21
35–49	154	6.4	17	3	4	5	8	11	13	24
50–64	85	8.8	26	4	5	7	10	20	20	24
65+	93	7.7	43	4	5	6	8	14	16	60
GRAND TOTAL	3806	4.3	10	2	3	3	5	7	9	19

56.9: OTHER URETERAL OPERATION. Formerly included in operation group(s) 650.

Type of Patients	Observed Patients	Avg. Stay	Vari-ance	Percentiles						
				10th	25th	50th	75th	90th	95th	99th
1. SINGLE DX										
0–19 Years	0									
20–34	3	3.5	5	2	2	2	7	7	7	7
35–49	1	1.0	0	1	1	1	1	1	1	1
50–64	0									
65+	1	1.0	0	1	1	1	1	1	1	1
2. MULTIPLE DX										
0–19 Years	3	2.5	<1	2	2	3	3	3	3	3
20–34	5	5.0	36	2	2	3	5	5	24	24
35–49	6	1.7	3	1	1	1	1	6	6	6
50–64	10	3.8	21	1	3	4	6	6	13	29
65+	22	5.8	15	1	3	4	10	10	10	20
TOTAL SINGLE DX	5	2.0	3	1	1	1	2	7	7	7
MULTIPLE DX	46	4.6	19	1	1	3	6	10	10	24
TOTAL										
0–19 Years	3	2.5	<1	2	2	3	3	3	3	3
20–34	8	4.3	22	2	2	3	5	7	7	24
35–49	7	1.6	2	1	1	1	1	6	6	6
50–64	10	3.8	21	1	3	4	6	6	13	29
65+	23	5.0	16	1	3	4	9	10	10	20
GRAND TOTAL	51	4.2	17	1	1	3	6	10	10	24

Length of Stay by Diagnosis and Operation, United States, 1997

United States, October 1995–September 1996 Data, by Operation

57.0: TU BLADDER CLEARANCE. Formerly included in operation group(s) 653.

Type of Patients	Observed Patients	Avg. Stay	Vari-ance	Percentiles						
				10th	25th	50th	75th	90th	95th	99th
1. SINGLE DX										
0–19 Years	4	1.2	<1	1	1	1	1	2	2	2
20–34	12	1.8	1	1	1	1	3	3	2	5
35–49	17	2.2	1	1	1	2	3	3	3	4
50–64	19	1.8	<1	1	1	2	2	2	3	4
65+	26	1.4	2	1	1	1	1	2	3	9
2. MULTIPLE DX										
0–19 Years	32	6.4	148	1	2	2	5	8	36	58
20–34	72	3.1	10	1	1	2	4	7	9	16
35–49	123	3.8	9	1	2	2	5	8	9	14
50–64	226	3.4	11	1	1	2	4	8	9	17
65+	1017	4.9	26	1	2	3	5	11	15	26
TOTAL SINGLE DX	78	1.8	<1	1	1	2	2	3	3	5
MULTIPLE DX	1470	4.5	25	1	2	3	5	9	14	25
TOTAL										
0–19 Years	36	6.2	142	1	2	2	5	8	36	58
20–34	84	2.9	9	1	1	2	3	7	9	16
35–49	140	3.6	9	1	2	2	4	8	9	14
50–64	245	3.3	10	1	1	2	4	7	9	17
65+	1043	4.8	26	1	2	3	5	11	15	26
GRAND TOTAL	1548	4.3	24	1	2	3	5	9	13	25

57.17: PERCUTANEOUS CYSTOSTOMY. Formerly included in operation group(s) 654.

Type of Patients	Observed Patients	Avg. Stay	Vari-ance	Percentiles						
				10th	25th	50th	75th	90th	95th	99th
1. SINGLE DX										
0–19 Years	4	2.4	1	2	2	2	2	3	6	6
20–34	2	4.9	4	2	2	6	6	6	6	6
35–49	3	1.9	<1	2	2	2	2	2	2	2
50–64	0									
65+	3	3.7	4	2	3	3	3	7	7	7
2. MULTIPLE DX										
0–19 Years	68	4.9	21	1	2	3	7	11	17	>99
20–34	26	5.1	9	2	5	5	5	8	10	17
35–49	53	7.5	29	2	6	7	8	10	21	26
50–64	59	6.7	43	2	2	4	9	18	22	27
65+	317	6.9	40	1	2	5	10	15	21	25
TOTAL SINGLE DX	12	2.9	3	2	2	2	3	6	6	7
MULTIPLE DX	523	6.6	36	1	2	5	8	15	21	28
TOTAL										
0–19 Years	72	4.8	20	1	2	3	7	11	17	>99
20–34	28	5.1	9	2	5	5	6	6	10	17
35–49	56	7.2	29	2	5	6	8	10	21	26
50–64	59	6.7	43	2	2	4	9	18	22	27
65+	320	6.9	40	1	2	5	10	15	21	25
GRAND TOTAL	535	6.5	35	1	2	5	8	15	21	27

57.1: CYSTOTOMY & CYSTOSTOMY. Formerly included in operation group(s) 654.

Type of Patients	Observed Patients	Avg. Stay	Vari-ance	Percentiles						
				10th	25th	50th	75th	90th	95th	99th
1. SINGLE DX										
0–19 Years	66	2.9	2	1	2	3	4	5	5	9
20–34	26	3.3	6	1	1	2	4	8	8	8
35–49	56	2.0	2	1	1	2	2	4	4	7
50–64	43	2.1	<1	1	1	2	3	3	4	5
65+	56	3.0	3	1	2	3	3	5	6	10
2. MULTIPLE DX										
0–19 Years	360	5.4	38	1	2	4	7	10	17	45
20–34	146	6.6	27	2	4	5	9	10	14	30
35–49	335	4.9	57	1	2	2	5	10	15	29
50–64	491	5.1	31	1	3	3	6	13	17	23
65+	1494	7.1	48	2	3	5	9	15	20	35
TOTAL SINGLE DX	247	2.5	3	1	1	2	3	4	5	8
MULTIPLE DX	2826	6.1	45	2	2	4	8	14	18	33
TOTAL										
0–19 Years	426	5.1	34	1	2	3	6	10	15	45
20–34	172	6.3	26	2	3	5	9	9	14	30
35–49	391	4.5	51	1	2	3	5	10	15	28
50–64	534	4.9	29	1	2	3	5	12	17	23
65+	1550	6.9	47	2	3	5	9	15	20	35
GRAND TOTAL	3073	5.8	42	2	3	4	7	14	17	33

57.18: S/P CYSTOSTOMY NEC. Formerly included in operation group(s) 654.

Type of Patients	Observed Patients	Avg. Stay	Vari-ance	Percentiles						
				10th	25th	50th	75th	90th	95th	99th
1. SINGLE DX										
0–19 Years	14	2.7	3	1	1	3	3	5	5	9
20–34	10	2.5	2	1	1	2	3	5	5	8
35–49	45	2.6	3	1	2	2	3	4	4	7
50–64	35	2.0	<1	1	2	2	2	3	3	5
65+	44	3.1	3	2	2	3	3	5	6	10
2. MULTIPLE DX										
0–19 Years	62	6.1	68	1	1	3	9	15	26	45
20–34	92	6.3	34	2	3	4	8	13	14	41
35–49	235	4.4	65	2	3	2	4	8	14	63
50–64	358	4.6	27	1	2	3	5	11	17	21
65+	897	7.1	52	2	3	4	9	15	19	37
TOTAL SINGLE DX	148	2.6	3	1	2	2	3	4	5	9
MULTIPLE DX	1644	5.8	50	2	2	3	7	14	17	37
TOTAL										
0–19 Years	76	5.4	57	1	2	3	5	11	15	45
20–34	102	6.1	34	2	3	4	8	12	14	41
35–49	280	4.2	59	2	2	2	4	7	13	29
50–64	393	4.3	25	1	2	3	4	10	17	21
65+	941	6.8	50	2	3	4	8	15	19	37
GRAND TOTAL	1792	5.6	47	2	2	3	6	13	17	35

Length of Stay by Diagnosis and Operation

United States, 1997

United States, October 1995–September 1996 Data, by Operation

57.19: CYSTOTOMY NEC. Formerly included in operation group(s) 654.

Type of Patients	Observed Patients	Avg. Stay	Variance	10th	25th	50th	75th	90th	95th	99th
1. SINGLE DX										
0–19 Years	8	2.7	2	1	1	3	4	4	4	4
20–34	14	3.4	7	1	1	3	4	8	8	8
35–49	8	1.2	<1	1	1	1	1	2	2	5
50–64	8	2.7	1	2	2	2	3	5	5	5
65+	9	2.5	2	1	1	2	4	4	4	6
2. MULTIPLE DX										
0–19 Years	54	4.1	26	2	2	2	3	9	19	27
20–34	26	8.6	15	4	9	9	9	9	15	30
35–49	45	4.9	39	1	1	2	7	15	15	28
50–64	70	6.7	32	1	2	4	9	16	18	22
65+	276	7.2	47	2	3	5	9	15	25	37
TOTAL SINGLE DX	47	2.2	3	1	1	1	3	4	5	8
MULTIPLE DX	471	6.6	40	1	2	5	9	15	21	30
TOTAL										
0–19 Years	62	3.9	23	1	2	2	4	7	16	27
20–34	40	7.5	18	2	4	9	9	9	14	30
35–49	53	3.9	31	1	1	1	5	15	15	28
50–64	78	6.3	30	2	2	4	9	16	18	22
65+	285	7.1	46	2	3	5	9	15	25	37
GRAND TOTAL	518	6.1	37	1	2	4	9	14	19	28

57.3: BLADDER DIAGNOSTIC PX. Formerly included in operation group(s) 651, 652, 654, 664.

Type of Patients	Observed Patients	Avg. Stay	Variance	10th	25th	50th	75th	90th	95th	99th
1. SINGLE DX										
0–19 Years	105	2.8	7	1	1	2	3	4	6	14
20–34	308	2.2	2	1	1	2	3	4	5	7
35–49	361	2.2	3	1	1	2	3	4	5	7
50–64	224	2.3	4	1	1	2	3	4	5	8
65+	142	3.1	6	1	1	2	4	7	8	9
2. MULTIPLE DX										
0–19 Years	364	4.6	22	1	2	3	5	10	16	24
20–34	1058	4.2	22	1	2	3	5	9	11	24
35–49	1857	6.0	87	1	2	4	6	11	16	49
50–64	2477	5.8	39	1	2	4	7	11	18	30
65+	8671	7.5	51	2	3	6	9	15	20	34
TOTAL SINGLE DX	1140	2.3	3	1	1	2	3	4	5	8
MULTIPLE DX	14427	6.6	52	1	2	5	8	13	18	35
TOTAL										
0–19 Years	469	4.2	19	1	2	3	4	9	15	22
20–34	1366	3.7	18	1	2	3	4	7	9	24
35–49	2218	5.3	74	1	2	3	6	10	14	49
50–64	2701	5.5	37	1	2	4	7	11	17	28
65+	8813	7.4	51	2	3	6	9	15	20	34
GRAND TOTAL	15567	6.2	50	1	2	4	8	13	18	34

57.2: VESICOSTOMY. Formerly included in operation group(s) 654.

Type of Patients	Observed Patients	Avg. Stay	Variance	10th	25th	50th	75th	90th	95th	99th
1. SINGLE DX										
0–19 Years	14	2.3	<1	1	2	3	3	4	4	4
20–34	1	3.0	0	3	3	3	3	3	3	3
35–49	1	5.0	0	5	5	5	5	5	5	5
50–64	1	2.0	0	2	2	2	2	2	2	2
65+	0									
2. MULTIPLE DX										
0–19 Years	212	7.3	89	1	1	5	8	17	23	52
20–34	18	8.5	7	5	7	9	10	10	10	20
35–49	45	9.0	5	4	9	10	14	14	10	13
50–64	6	10.0	29	3	5	14	14	14	14	15
65+	18	8.7	31	2	4	6	15	16	16	16
TOTAL SINGLE DX	17	2.4	<1	1	2	3	3	3	4	5
MULTIPLE DX	263	7.8	69	1	2	7	10	15	23	52
TOTAL										
0–19 Years	226	6.9	84	1	1	5	8	17	23	52
20–34	19	8.4	8	5	7	9	10	10	10	20
35–49	10	8.9	5	4	9	10	14	14	10	13
50–64	7	9.3	32	2	3	14	14	14	14	15
65+	18	8.7	31	2	4	6	15	16	16	16
GRAND TOTAL	280	7.4	66	1	2	6	10	15	23	52

57.32: CYSTOSCOPY NEC. Formerly included in operation group(s) 651.

Type of Patients	Observed Patients	Avg. Stay	Variance	10th	25th	50th	75th	90th	95th	99th
1. SINGLE DX										
0–19 Years	98	2.7	6	1	1	2	3	4	5	22
20–34	304	2.2	2	1	1	2	3	4	5	7
35–49	344	2.2	2	1	1	2	3	4	5	7
50–64	209	2.3	4	1	1	2	3	4	5	8
65+	114	3.2	6	1	1	2	4	8	8	11
2. MULTIPLE DX										
0–19 Years	336	4.2	15	1	2	3	5	8	15	18
20–34	980	4.0	20	1	2	3	5	7	10	24
35–49	1654	6.1	92	1	2	4	6	11	17	49
50–64	2102	5.9	39	1	2	4	7	12	18	28
65+	7123	7.5	48	2	3	6	9	14	18	34
TOTAL SINGLE DX	1069	2.3	3	1	1	2	3	4	5	8
MULTIPLE DX	12195	6.5	51	1	3	5	8	13	18	35
TOTAL										
0–19 Years	434	3.8	13	1	2	3	4	7	12	18
20–34	1284	3.6	17	1	2	3	4	7	9	22
35–49	1998	5.4	78	1	2	4	6	10	14	49
50–64	2311	5.5	37	1	2	4	7	11	18	27
65+	7237	7.4	48	2	3	6	9	14	18	34
GRAND TOTAL	13264	6.1	48	1	2	4	8	12	17	33

Length of Stay by Diagnosis and Operation, United States, 1997

57.33: CLSD (TU) BLADDER BIOPSY. Formerly included in operation group(s) 652.

Type of Patients	Observed Patients	Avg. Stay	Vari-ance	10th	25th	50th	75th	90th	95th	99th
1. SINGLE DX										
0–19 Years	5	4.1	20	1	1	3	3	14	14	14
20–34	4	1.7	<1	1	1	2	3	2	2	2
35–49	16	1.8	13	1	1	1	1	2	3	21
50–64	15	1.9	2	1	1	1	2	4	4	7
65+	28	2.8	4	1	1	2	4	6	7	7
2. MULTIPLE DX										
0–19 Years	23	7.1	65	1	2	3	10	15	24	32
20–34	73	6.3	35	1	3	5	9	11	14	38
35–49	188	4.9	28	2	2	3	6	10	12	27
50–64	356	5.3	37	1	2	3	7	11	14	30
65+	1503	7.5	70	1	2	5	10	20	22	39
TOTAL SINGLE DX	68	2.3	10	1	1	1	2	4	7	21
MULTIPLE DX	2143	6.7	59	1	2	4	9	15	20	35
TOTAL										
0–19 Years	28	6.5	57	1	1	3	10	15	24	32
20–34	77	6.2	34	1	2	4	9	11	14	38
35–49	204	4.5	27	2	1	3	6	10	12	26
50–64	371	5.2	36	1	2	3	7	11	14	30
65+	1531	7.4	69	1	2	5	10	20	22	39
GRAND TOTAL	2211	6.6	58	1	2	4	9	15	20	34

57.49: TU DESTR BLADDER LES NEC. Formerly included in operation group(s) 652.

Type of Patients	Observed Patients	Avg. Stay	Vari-ance	10th	25th	50th	75th	90th	95th	99th
1. SINGLE DX										
0–19 Years	5	2.3	1	1	1	3	3	3	3	4
20–34	10	1.4	<1	1	1	1	2	3	3	4
35–49	77	1.7	<1	1	1	1	2	2	3	4
50–64	203	1.7	1	1	1	1	2	3	3	6
65+	419	1.5	1	1	1	1	2	3	3	5
2. MULTIPLE DX										
0–19 Years	41	6.4	96	1	2	3	7	11	27	48
20–34	76	4.3	20	1	1	3	4	11	11	22
35–49	348	3.0	9	1	1	2	3	6	9	18
50–64	1402	3.3	19	1	1	2	4	6	9	21
65+	8301	3.9	22	1	1	2	5	9	12	22
TOTAL SINGLE DX	714	1.6	1	1	1	1	2	3	3	5
MULTIPLE DX	10168	3.8	22	1	1	2	4	8	12	22
TOTAL										
0–19 Years	46	5.9	87	1	2	3	6	11	13	48
20–34	86	3.9	18	1	1	2	4	11	11	22
35–49	425	2.7	8	1	1	2	3	5	9	16
50–64	1605	3.2	18	1	1	2	4	6	8	20
65+	8720	3.8	21	1	1	2	5	8	12	22
GRAND TOTAL	10882	3.6	20	1	1	2	4	8	11	22

57.4: TU EXC/DESTR BLADDER LES. Formerly included in operation group(s) 652.

Type of Patients	Observed Patients	Avg. Stay	Vari-ance	10th	25th	50th	75th	90th	95th	99th
1. SINGLE DX										
0–19 Years	5	2.3	1	1	1	3	3	3	3	4
20–34	10	1.4	<1	1	1	2	2	2	2	2
35–49	77	1.7	<1	1	1	1	2	3	3	4
50–64	203	1.7	1	1	1	1	2	3	3	4
65+	419	1.5	1	1	1	2	2	3	3	5
2. MULTIPLE DX										
0–19 Years	41	6.4	96	1	2	3	7	11	27	48
20–34	77	4.3	19	1	1	2	4	11	11	22
35–49	349	3.0	9	1	1	2	3	6	9	18
50–64	1402	3.3	19	1	1	2	4	6	9	21
65+	8305	3.9	22	1	1	2	5	9	12	22
TOTAL SINGLE DX	714	1.6	1	1	1	1	2	3	3	5
MULTIPLE DX	10174	3.8	22	1	1	2	4	8	12	22
TOTAL										
0–19 Years	46	5.9	87	1	2	3	6	11	13	48
20–34	87	3.9	18	1	1	2	4	11	11	22
35–49	426	2.7	8	1	1	2	3	5	9	16
50–64	1605	3.2	18	1	1	2	4	6	8	20
65+	8724	3.8	21	1	1	2	5	8	12	22
GRAND TOTAL	10888	3.6	20	1	1	2	4	8	11	22

57.5: BLADDER LES DESTR NEC. Formerly included in operation group(s) 654.

Type of Patients	Observed Patients	Avg. Stay	Vari-ance	10th	25th	50th	75th	90th	95th	99th
1. SINGLE DX										
0–19 Years	37	2.6	4	1	1	2	3	5	7	8
20–34	6	4.1	3	2	3	4	5	5	7	7
35–49	9	4.0	2	2	4	4	4	6	6	6
50–64	10	2.9	2	1	3	3	3	5	5	5
65+	4	7.1	13	1	7	7	10	10	10	10
2. MULTIPLE DX										
0–19 Years	54	4.8	25	1	3	4	5	7	15	33
20–34	21	6.9	34	3	4	5	7	11	26	26
35–49	31	5.0	3	3	4	5	6	8	9	10
50–64	72	6.1	13	2	4	5	7	10	14	19
65+	167	6.6	30	2	4	6	8	10	13	33
TOTAL SINGLE DX	66	3.0	5	1	1	3	4	7	7	10
MULTIPLE DX	345	5.9	22	2	3	5	7	9	12	28
TOTAL										
0–19 Years	91	3.9	17	1	1	3	5	6	7	33
20–34	27	6.5	31	3	4	5	7	11	26	26
35–49	40	4.9	3	3	4	4	6	8	9	10
50–64	82	5.8	13	3	4	5	7	10	10	19
65+	171	6.6	29	2	4	6	8	10	13	28
GRAND TOTAL	411	5.4	20	1	3	5	7	8	11	26

Length of Stay by Diagnosis and Operation, United States, 1997

57.59: OTH BLADDER LESION DESTR. Formerly included in operation group(s) 654.

Type of Patients	Observed Patients	Avg. Stay	Vari-ance	Percentiles						
				10th	25th	50th	75th	90th	95th	99th
1. SINGLE DX										
0–19 Years	6	3.0	1	2	2	3	3	5	5	6
20–34	0									
35–49	9	4.0	2	2	4	4	4	6	6	6
50–64	8	2.8	1	1	3	3	3	4	5	5
65+	4	7.1	13	1	7	7	10	10	10	10
2. MULTIPLE DX										
0–19 Years	27	4.8	9	3	3	4	6	7	7	18
20–34	11	9.8	67	2	7	7	8	26	26	26
35–49	27	5.0	3	3	4	5	6	8	9	9
50–64	66	6.0	14	3	4	5	7	11	14	19
65+	164	6.6	30	2	4	6	8	10	13	33
TOTAL SINGLE DX	**27**	**3.9**	**5**	**2**	**2**	**3**	**5**	**7**	**10**	**10**
MULTIPLE DX	**295**	**6.1**	**21**	**3**	**4**	**6**	**7**	**9**	**13**	**26**
TOTAL										
0–19 Years	33	4.4	8	2	3	3	6	7	7	18
20–34	11	9.8	67	2	7	7	8	26	26	26
35–49	36	4.9	3	3	4	5	6	6	8	9
50–64	74	5.8	14	3	3	5	7	11	14	19
65+	168	6.6	30	2	4	6	8	10	13	28
GRAND TOTAL	**322**	**5.9**	**20**	**2**	**3**	**5**	**7**	**9**	**12**	**19**

57.6: PARTIAL CYSTECTOMY. Formerly included in operation group(s) 654.

Type of Patients	Observed Patients	Avg. Stay	Vari-ance	Percentiles						
				10th	25th	50th	75th	90th	95th	99th
1. SINGLE DX										
0–19 Years	3	2.3	2	1	1	3	3	4	4	4
20–34	3	6.0	1	5	5	5	7	7	7	7
35–49	10	5.4	3	3	4	5	7	7	8	8
50–64	15	4.4	4	2	3	5	5	7	8	8
65+	12	4.5	2	3	3	5	5	6	7	7
2. MULTIPLE DX										
0–19 Years	11	8.6	10	6	6	9	10	10	18	18
20–34	15	5.6	11	4	5	5	5	7	9	34
35–49	29	6.2	13	4	5	5	6	11	15	18
50–64	59	6.3	19	3	3	5	8	11	13	30
65+	295	8.7	40	3	5	8	10	15	19	35
TOTAL SINGLE DX	**43**	**4.5**	**3**	**3**	**3**	**5**	**5**	**7**	**7**	**8**
MULTIPLE DX	**409**	**7.6**	**30**	**3**	**5**	**6**	**9**	**14**	**18**	**33**
TOTAL										
0–19 Years	14	6.9	16	1	3	8	9	10	10	18
20–34	18	5.6	11	5	5	5	5	7	9	34
35–49	39	6.1	12	4	5	5	6	11	15	18
50–64	74	6.0	17	3	3	5	7	11	13	17
65+	307	8.5	39	3	5	7	10	15	19	35
GRAND TOTAL	**452**	**7.3**	**29**	**3**	**4**	**6**	**8**	**13**	**18**	**32**

57.7: TOTAL CYSTECTOMY. Formerly included in operation group(s) 654.

Type of Patients	Observed Patients	Avg. Stay	Vari-ance	Percentiles						
				10th	25th	50th	75th	90th	95th	99th
1. SINGLE DX										
0–19 Years	1	7.0	0	7	7	7	7	7	7	7
20–34	0									
35–49	6	7.9	3	7	8	8	8	9	9	12
50–64	29	7.5	4	6	6	7	9	11	11	11
65+	26	8.8	10	6	6	9	10	12	13	20
2. MULTIPLE DX										
0–19 Years	3	10.2	20	6	6	9	15	15	15	15
20–34	11	11.6	32	6	6	14	14	14	21	31
35–49	120	12.0	50	7	9	9	13	18	24	46
50–64	507	11.0	31	7	8	9	12	18	22	30
65+	1285	12.6	52	7	8	10	14	22	24	42
TOTAL SINGLE DX	**62**	**8.0**	**6**	**6**	**6**	**8**	**9**	**11**	**11**	**16**
MULTIPLE DX	**1926**	**12.1**	**47**	**7**	**8**	**10**	**14**	**21**	**23**	**42**
TOTAL										
0–19 Years	4	8.8	14	6	6	7	9	15	15	15
20–34	11	11.6	32	6	6	14	14	14	21	31
35–49	126	11.7	47	7	8	9	13	17	21	46
50–64	536	10.8	30	7	8	9	12	17	22	27
65+	1311	12.5	52	7	8	10	14	22	23	42
GRAND TOTAL	**1988**	**12.0**	**46**	**7**	**8**	**10**	**14**	**21**	**23**	**42**

57.71: RADICAL CYSTECTOMY. Formerly included in operation group(s) 654.

Type of Patients	Observed Patients	Avg. Stay	Vari-ance	Percentiles						
				10th	25th	50th	75th	90th	95th	99th
1. SINGLE DX										
0–19 Years	1	7.0	0	7	7	7	7	7	7	7
20–34	0									
35–49	5	8.2	<1	8	8	8	8	9	9	12
50–64	26	7.7	4	6	6	7	10	11	11	11
65+	23	8.8	10	6	6	9	10	13	16	20
2. MULTIPLE DX										
0–19 Years	2	13.9	7	9	15	15	15	15	15	15
20–34	5	13.9	2	14	14	14	14	14	14	21
35–49	97	13.0	70	7	8	10	16	21	31	47
50–64	472	11.0	31	7	8	9	12	18	22	30
65+	1175	12.5	51	7	8	10	14	22	23	38
TOTAL SINGLE DX	**55**	**8.1**	**6**	**6**	**7**	**8**	**9**	**11**	**11**	**16**
MULTIPLE DX	**1751**	**12.1**	**46**	**7**	**8**	**10**	**14**	**21**	**23**	**38**
TOTAL										
0–19 Years	3	9.8	15	7	7	7	15	15	15	15
20–34	5	13.9	2	14	14	14	14	14	14	21
35–49	102	12.4	64	7	8	9	15	20	29	47
50–64	498	10.8	30	7	8	9	12	17	21	30
65+	1198	12.5	50	7	8	10	14	22	23	38
GRAND TOTAL	**1806**	**12.0**	**45**	**7**	**8**	**10**	**14**	**21**	**22**	**38**

United States, October 1995–September 1996 Data, by Operation

57.8: OTH URIN BLADDER REPAIR. Formerly included in operation group(s) 654.

Type of Patients	Observed Patients	Avg. Stay	Vari-ance	10th	25th	50th	75th	90th	95th	99th
1. SINGLE DX										
0–19 Years	19	6.6	24	2	2	4	11	13	16	21
20–34	41	3.0	4	1	2	3	4	6	4	11
35–49	149	2.1	2	1	1	2	3	4	4	8
50–64	88	2.4	1	1	2	2	2	4	5	6
65+	45	1.9	3	1	1	2	2	3	4	10
2. MULTIPLE DX										
0–19 Years	403	9.2	74	4	5	8	10	14	24	44
20–34	190	7.2	48	2	2	5	9	14	22	31
35–49	436	5.0	32	1	2	3	6	11	15	20
50–64	360	5.8	71	1	1	3	7	11	21	44
65+	511	6.3	50	1	2	4	8	12	18	32
TOTAL SINGLE DX	342	2.5	4	1	1	2	3	4	6	11
MULTIPLE DX	1900	6.7	58	1	2	5	9	12	18	39
TOTAL										
0–19	422	9.1	72	3	5	7	10	14	23	44
20–34	231	6.4	43	1	2	5	8	13	18	30
35–49	585	4.1	24	1	1	2	5	9	12	17
50–64	448	5.0	55	1	2	2	5	10	18	44
65+	556	5.9	47	1	2	3	8	12	17	32
GRAND TOTAL	2242	5.9	50	1	2	4	8	12	17	37

57.87: URINARY BLADDER RECONST. Formerly included in operation group(s) 654.

Type of Patients	Observed Patients	Avg. Stay	Vari-ance	10th	25th	50th	75th	90th	95th	99th
1. SINGLE DX										
0–19 Years	9	8.8	12	2	7	11	11	13	13	13
20–34	4	6.8	4	4	7	7	7	7	11	11
35–49	0									
50–64	1	6.0	0	6	6	6	6	6	6	6
65+	0									
2. MULTIPLE DX										
0–19 Years	227	9.3	75	5	6	8	10	13	16	35
20–34	28	9.7	11	5	7	10	13	13	14	15
35–49	41	9.6	8	6	8	10	12	12	14	17
50–64	16	9.4	13	3	7	9	11	14	18	18
65+	11	8.5	14	2	7	10	12	12	12	12
TOTAL SINGLE DX	14	8.3	11	2	7	8	11	13	13	13
MULTIPLE DX	323	9.3	60	5	6	8	11	13	16	28
TOTAL										
0–19	236	9.3	72	5	6	8	10	13	16	35
20–34	32	9.3	11	5	7	10	13	13	14	15
35–49	41	9.6	8	6	8	10	12	12	14	17
50–64	17	9.2	13	3	7	9	11	14	18	18
65+	11	8.5	14	2	7	10	12	12	12	12
GRAND TOTAL	337	9.3	58	5	6	8	11	13	15	28

57.84: REP OTH FISTULA BLADDER. Formerly included in operation group(s) 654.

Type of Patients	Observed Patients	Avg. Stay	Vari-ance	10th	25th	50th	75th	90th	95th	99th
1. SINGLE DX										
0–19 Years	1	3.0	0	3	3	3	3	3	3	3
20–34	19	3.4	3	2	2	3	4	5	7	11
35–49	54	2.8	2	1	2	2	4	4	5	7
50–64	8	3.6	<1	2	4	4	4	4	5	5
65+	1	10.0	0	10	10	10	10	10	10	10
2. MULTIPLE DX										
0–19 Years	17	5.6	21	2	4	5	6	7	7	24
20–34	39	4.1	13	1	1	4	5	7	8	18
35–49	123	4.6	8	1	3	4	5	8	9	17
50–64	43	5.2	50	1	2	3	5	10	11	51
65+	27	10.6	105	2	3	8	15	25	27	59
TOTAL SINGLE DX	83	3.1	2	1	2	3	4	5	6	10
MULTIPLE DX	249	5.1	25	1	2	4	6	9	14	27
TOTAL										
0–19	18	5.2	18	2	3	5	6	7	7	24
20–34	58	3.8	10	1	2	3	5	7	8	18
35–49	177	4.0	7	1	2	4	5	7	7	17
50–64	51	4.7	36	1	3	4	5	8	11	51
65+	28	10.6	99	2	3	8	14	25	27	59
GRAND TOTAL	332	4.5	19	1	2	4	5	8	11	24

57.89: BLADDER REPAIR NEC. Formerly included in operation group(s) 654.

Type of Patients	Observed Patients	Avg. Stay	Vari-ance	10th	25th	50th	75th	90th	95th	99th
1. SINGLE DX										
0–19 Years	0									
20–34	12	2.0	1	1	1	1	3	4	4	4
35–49	86	1.7	2	1	1	1	2	3	3	10
50–64	74	2.1	<1	1	2	2	2	4	4	5
65+	42	1.7	<1	1	1	2	2	3	3	4
2. MULTIPLE DX										
0–19 Years	37	6.3	14	2	4	6	7	12	12	22
20–34	38	4.9	28	2	2	6	7	9	14	31
35–49	155	3.4	23	1	1	2	3	5	17	20
50–64	196	4.3	62	1	1	2	4	10	10	44
65+	259	3.4	24	1	1	2	3	6	14	21
TOTAL SINGLE DX	214	1.8	1	1	1	2	2	3	4	5
MULTIPLE DX	685	4.0	36	1	1	2	4	9	14	44
TOTAL										
0–19	37	6.3	14	2	4	6	7	12	12	22
20–34	50	4.3	24	1	2	2	6	9	9	31
35–49	241	2.7	15	1	1	2	3	4	8	17
50–64	270	3.7	44	1	1	2	3	6	10	44
65+	301	3.1	21	1	1	2	3	5	14	21
GRAND TOTAL	899	3.4	27	1	1	2	3	6	10	29

United States, October 1995–September 1996 Data, by Operation

57.9: OTHER BLADDER OPERATIONS. Formerly included in operation group(s) 664.

Type of Patients	Observed Patients	Avg. Stay	Vari-ance	Percentiles						
				10th	25th	50th	75th	90th	95th	99th
1. SINGLE DX										
0–19 Years	22	1.7	<1	1	1	2	2	3	3	3
20–34	14	2.4	<1	1	1	3	3	3	3	4
35–49	15	1.8	4	1	1	1	2	3	6	13
50–64	23	3.4	3	1	1	5	5	5	5	5
65+	53	1.8	1	1	1	1	2	3	4	6
2. MULTIPLE DX										
0–19 Years	160	4.8	25	1	2	3	7	11	13	34
20–34	194	3.8	45	1	1	2	4	7	13	21
35–49	302	4.8	50	1	1	2	5	10	15	51
50–64	574	5.2	28	2	2	4	6	11	16	24
65+	3542	5.8	26	2	3	4	7	11	14	23
TOTAL SINGLE DX	127	2.2	2	1	1	2	3	5	5	6
MULTIPLE DX	4772	5.5	30	1	2	4	7	11	15	24
TOTAL										
0–19 Years	182	4.5	24	1	1	2	6	11	13	34
20–34	208	3.7	42	1	1	2	3	7	12	21
35–49	317	4.8	50	1	1	2	5	10	15	51
50–64	597	5.1	28	2	2	4	6	11	16	24
65+	3595	5.7	25	2	3	4	7	11	14	23
GRAND TOTAL	4899	5.4	29	1	2	4	7	11	15	24

57.93: CONTROL BLADDER HEMOR. Formerly included in operation group(s) 654.

Type of Patients	Observed Patients	Avg. Stay	Vari-ance	Percentiles						
				10th	25th	50th	75th	90th	95th	99th
1. SINGLE DX										
0–19 Years	0									
20–34	1	1.0	0	1	1	1	1	1	1	1
35–49	0									
50–64	1	1.0	0	1	1	1	1	1	1	1
65+	5	2.6	<1	2	2	2	4	4	4	4
2. MULTIPLE DX										
0–19 Years	8	9.8	81	1	2	3	21	21	21	21
20–34	17	5.2	46	1	2	2	4	21	21	21
35–49	31	9.9	230	2	3	5	5	51	51	51
50–64	71	3.4	27	1	1	2	3	5	9	32
65+	361	5.5	21	2	2	4	7	12	13	21
TOTAL SINGLE DX	7	2.2	1	1	2	2	3	4	4	4
MULTIPLE DX	488	5.7	56	1	2	4	7	12	17	51
TOTAL										
0–19 Years	8	9.8	81	1	2	3	21	21	21	21
20–34	18	5.0	45	1	1	2	3	21	21	21
35–49	31	9.9	230	2	3	5	5	51	51	51
50–64	72	3.4	27	1	1	2	3	5	9	32
65+	366	5.4	21	2	2	4	7	11	13	21
GRAND TOTAL	495	5.7	56	1	2	4	7	11	17	51

57.91: BLADDER SPHINCTEROTOMY. Formerly included in operation group(s) 654.

Type of Patients	Observed Patients	Avg. Stay	Vari-ance	Percentiles						
				10th	25th	50th	75th	90th	95th	99th
1. SINGLE DX										
0–19 Years	2	1.6	<1	1	1	2	2	2	2	2
20–34	1	2.0	0	2	2	2	2	2	2	2
35–49	7	1.3	<1	1	1	1	1	2	2	2
50–64	11	1.3	<1	1	1	1	1	3	3	3
65+	21	1.2	<1	1	1	1	1	2	2	2
2. MULTIPLE DX										
0–19 Years	4	6.4	54	1	3	3	17	17	17	17
20–34	18	6.2	36	1	2	3	13	19	19	19
35–49	57	5.2	33	1	1	2	12	15	15	15
50–64	114	3.5	18	1	1	2	7	11	11	21
65+	522	4.2	32	1	1	2	5	10	12	29
TOTAL SINGLE DX	42	1.3	<1	1	1	1	1	2	2	3
MULTIPLE DX	715	4.3	30	1	2	2	5	11	15	24
TOTAL										
0–19 Years	6	4.4	35	1	1	2	3	17	17	17
20–34	19	6.1	35	2	2	3	13	13	19	19
35–49	64	5.0	32	1	1	2	7	15	15	15
50–64	125	3.4	17	1	1	2	5	11	11	21
65+	543	4.0	30	1	1	2	5	9	11	28
GRAND TOTAL	757	4.1	29	1	1	2	4	11	15	22

57.94: INSERT INDWELL URIN CATH. Formerly included in operation group(s) 664.

Type of Patients	Observed Patients	Avg. Stay	Vari-ance	Percentiles						
				10th	25th	50th	75th	90th	95th	99th
1. SINGLE DX										
0–19 Years	19	1.8	<1	1	1	2	2	3	3	3
20–34	12	2.5	<1	1	2	3	3	3	3	4
35–49	8	2.3	9	1	1	1	5	6	13	13
50–64	9	4.3	2	1	4	5	5	5	5	5
65+	22	2.8	1	2	2	3	3	4	5	6
2. MULTIPLE DX										
0–19 Years	137	4.8	24	1	2	3	7	11	13	34
20–34	145	3.4	47	1	1	2	3	6	9	16
35–49	197	3.6	13	1	1	2	5	8	9	21
50–64	360	6.1	30	2	3	5	7	15	17	23
65+	2424	6.1	24	2	3	5	7	12	15	21
TOTAL SINGLE DX	70	2.7	2	1	2	3	3	5	5	6
MULTIPLE DX	3263	5.7	26	1	3	4	7	11	15	21
TOTAL										
0–19 Years	156	4.4	22	1	1	2	6	11	13	34
20–34	157	3.3	43	1	1	2	3	6	8	16
35–49	205	3.6	13	1	1	2	5	8	9	21
50–64	369	6.0	29	2	3	5	7	15	16	23
65+	2446	6.1	24	2	3	5	7	12	15	21
GRAND TOTAL	3333	5.6	26	1	3	4	7	11	15	21

Length of Stay by Diagnosis and Operation, United States, 1997

United States, October 1995–September 1996 Data, by Operation

58.0: URETHROTOMY. Formerly included in operation group(s) 658.

Type of Patients	Observed Patients	Avg. Stay	Variance	10th	25th	50th	75th	90th	95th	99th
1. SINGLE DX										
0–19 Years	7	1.9	2	1	1	1	3	5	5	5
20–34	4	2.1	<1	2	2	2	2	3	3	3
35–49	1	2.0	0	2	2	2	2	2	2	2
50–64	4	2.4	2	1	1	3	3	4	4	4
65+	1	2.0	0	2	2	2	2	2	2	2
2. MULTIPLE DX										
0–19 Years	9	2.8	6	1	1	2	3	8	8	8
20–34	13	5.2	13	1	3	5	5	12	12	14
35–49	10	4.4	42	1	1	3	7	7	10	35
50–64	12	7.6	89	2	2	3	14	20	35	35
65+	63	7.2	89	1	1	3	8	28	28	34
TOTAL SINGLE DX	17	2.0	<1	1	1	2	2	3	4	5
MULTIPLE DX	107	6.5	74	1	1	3	7	27	28	35
TOTAL										
0–19 Years	16	2.4	4	1	1	1	3	5	7	8
20–34	17	4.2	11	1	2	3	5	10	12	14
35–49	11	4.3	40	1	1	2	7	7	10	35
50–64	16	6.6	76	1	2	3	5	20	35	35
65+	64	7.1	87	1	1	2	8	28	28	34
GRAND TOTAL	124	6.0	67	1	1	2	6	20	28	35

58.1: URETHRAL MEATOTOMY. Formerly included in operation group(s) 655.

Type of Patients	Observed Patients	Avg. Stay	Variance	10th	25th	50th	75th	90th	95th	99th
1. SINGLE DX										
0–19 Years	4	1.0	0	1	1	1	1	1	1	1
20–34	1	1.0	0	1	1	1	1	1	1	1
35–49	0									
50–64	0									
65+	0									
2. MULTIPLE DX										
0–19 Years	9	3.0	5	1	2	3	3	4	10	10
20–34	3	1.5	<1	1	1	2	2	2	2	2
35–49	11	3.0	10	1	1	1	4	8	8	15
50–64	15	2.9	14	1	2	1	2	12	13	13
65+	30	4.7	11	1	1	4	7	8	10	17
TOTAL SINGLE DX	5	1.0	0	1	1	1	1	1	1	1
MULTIPLE DX	68	3.6	10	1	1	3	5	8	10	15
TOTAL										
0–19 Years	13	2.8	4	1	1	3	3	4	10	10
20–34	4	1.4	<1	1	1	1	2	2	2	2
35–49	11	3.0	10	1	1	1	4	8	8	15
50–64	15	2.9	14	1	1	1	2	12	13	13
65+	30	4.7	11	1	1	4	7	8	10	17
GRAND TOTAL	73	3.6	10	1	1	3	5	8	10	15

58.2: URETHRAL DIAGNOSTIC PX. Formerly included in operation group(s) 651, 656, 658, 664.

Type of Patients	Observed Patients	Avg. Stay	Variance	10th	25th	50th	75th	90th	95th	99th
1. SINGLE DX										
0–19 Years	2	2.0	1	1	1	3	3	3	3	3
20–34	6	1.5	1	1	1	1	1	4	4	4
35–49	7	1.3	<1	1	1	1	1	1	3	4
50–64	3	1.0	0	1	1	1	1	1	1	1
65+	3	1.7	<1	1	1	2	2	2	2	2
2. MULTIPLE DX										
0–19 Years	8	4.6	18	1	1	4	7	8	14	14
20–34	11	3.1	4	1	1	2	5	6	6	6
35–49	28	6.0	21	2	3	3	13	13	13	13
50–64	25	6.0	11	1	3	6	7	11	11	12
65+	69	8.9	90	2	3	5	15	17	37	37
TOTAL SINGLE DX	21	1.3	<1	1	1	1	1	2	3	4
MULTIPLE DX	141	7.0	49	1	3	5	10	15	17	37
TOTAL										
0–19 Years	10	4.2	16	1	1	3	7	8	14	14
20–34	17	2.6	3	1	1	2	4	6	6	6
35–49	35	4.6	19	1	1	3	5	13	13	13
50–64	28	5.1	13	1	1	6	6	11	11	12
65+	72	8.8	89	2	2	5	13	17	37	37
GRAND TOTAL	162	6.1	46	1	2	4	7	13	17	37

58.3: EXC/DESTR URETHRAL LES. Formerly included in operation group(s) 656.

Type of Patients	Observed Patients	Avg. Stay	Variance	10th	25th	50th	75th	90th	95th	99th
1. SINGLE DX										
0–19 Years	32	2.1	2	1	1	1	3	4	6	7
20–34	48	1.5	<1	1	1	1	2	2	3	4
35–49	41	1.5	<1	1	1	1	2	2	3	4
50–64	13	1.4	<1	1	1	1	2	2	3	3
65+	7	1.9	<1	1	1	2	3	3	3	3
2. MULTIPLE DX										
0–19 Years	94	5.3	44	1	1	3	7	13	25	36
20–34	40	1.9	5	1	1	1	3	3	5	15
35–49	72	2.4	18	1	1	1	2	4	4	27
50–64	63	2.4	4	1	2	2	3	5	6	9
65+	171	4.1	19	1	2	2	5	8	14	22
TOTAL SINGLE DX	141	1.7	1	1	1	1	2	3	4	6
MULTIPLE DX	440	3.5	23	1	1	2	3	8	13	25
TOTAL										
0–19 Years	126	4.5	36	1	1	3	5	9	15	36
20–34	88	1.8	3	1	1	1	2	3	3	15
35–49	113	2.2	14	1	1	1	2	4	4	27
50–64	76	2.3	4	1	1	2	3	5	6	9
65+	178	4.0	19	1	2	2	5	8	14	22
GRAND TOTAL	581	3.1	19	1	1	2	3	6	10	25

Length of Stay by Diagnosis and Operation, United States, 1997

United States, October 1995–September 1996 Data, by Operation

58.31: ENDO URETHRAL LES DESTR. Formerly included in operation group(s) 656.

Type of Patients	Observed Patients	Avg. Stay	Vari-ance	Percentiles						
				10th	25th	50th	75th	90th	95th	99th
1. SINGLE DX										
0–19 Years	18	2.6	2	1	1	2	3	6	6	6
20–34	16	1.4	<1	1	1	1	1	2	2	2
35–49	13	1.3	<1	1	1	1	2	2	2	2
50–64	1	1.0	0	1	1	1	1	1	1	1
65+	6	1.6	<1	1	1	1	1	3	3	3
2. MULTIPLE DX										
0–19 Years	58	5.5	52	1	1	3	8	14	25	36
20–34	17	2.7	14	1	1	1	3	7	15	15
35–49	31	2.4	26	1	1	1	2	3	4	32
50–64	23	2.5	7	1	1	1	3	6	9	13
65+	89	4.5	16	1	2	3	5	10	14	18
TOTAL SINGLE DX	54	1.8	1	1	1	1	2	3	4	6
MULTIPLE DX	218	4.0	30	1	1	2	4	9	14	32
TOTAL										
0–19 Years	76	5.0	43	1	1	3	6	10	15	36
20–34	33	2.1	8	1	1	1	2	3	7	15
35–49	44	2.2	20	1	1	1	2	3	4	32
50–64	24	2.4	7	1	1	1	3	6	9	13
65+	95	4.4	16	1	2	3	5	10	14	18
GRAND TOTAL	272	3.6	26	1	1	2	3	8	14	27

58.4: REPAIR OF URETHRA. Formerly included in operation group(s) 656.

Type of Patients	Observed Patients	Avg. Stay	Vari-ance	Percentiles						
				10th	25th	50th	75th	90th	95th	99th
1. SINGLE DX										
0–19 Years	475	2.0	3	1	1	1	2	4	6	9
20–34	49	2.5	2	1	2	2	3	5	6	9
35–49	60	1.8	1	1	1	2	3	3	4	7
50–64	34	2.5	1	1	2	2	3	4	5	5
65+	23	2.2	3	1	1	2	3	4	4	11
2. MULTIPLE DX										
0–19 Years	502	3.5	10	1	1	2	5	8	9	17
20–34	123	3.1	11	1	1	2	4	7	8	20
35–49	151	3.9	13	2	2	3	4	7	10	17
50–64	155	3.4	17	1	2	3	4	5	6	17
65+	142	4.2	16	1	1	3	8	8	8	21
TOTAL SINGLE DX	641	2.1	3	1	1	1	2	4	6	8
MULTIPLE DX	1073	3.6	12	1	1	3	5	8	9	18
TOTAL										
0–19 Years	977	2.7	7	1	1	2	3	7	8	12
20–34	172	2.9	9	1	1	2	3	7	7	17
35–49	211	3.2	10	1	2	3	4	5	6	15
50–64	189	3.2	14	1	1	2	4	5	6	17
65+	165	3.9	14	1	1	3	7	8	8	19
GRAND TOTAL	1714	3.0	9	1	1	2	4	7	8	14

58.39: URETHRA LES DESTR NEC. Formerly included in operation group(s) 656.

Type of Patients	Observed Patients	Avg. Stay	Vari-ance	Percentiles						
				10th	25th	50th	75th	90th	95th	99th
1. SINGLE DX										
0–19 Years	14	1.6	2	1	1	1	1	3	3	7
20–34	32	1.6	<1	1	1	1	2	2	3	4
35–49	28	1.5	<1	1	1	1	2	2	3	4
50–64	12	1.5	<1	1	1	1	2	2	3	3
65+	1	3.0	0	3	3	3	3	3	3	3
2. MULTIPLE DX										
0–19 Years	36	5.0	30	1	2	3	5	8	18	25
20–34	23	1.6	1	1	1	1	2	3	4	5
35–49	41	2.4	10	1	1	2	2	4	4	27
50–64	40	2.4	10	1	1	2	3	5	5	7
65+	82	3.6	22	1	2	2	3	7	18	23
TOTAL SINGLE DX	87	1.6	1	1	1	1	2	3	3	7
MULTIPLE DX	222	3.0	15	1	1	2	3	5	7	25
TOTAL										
0–19 Years	50	3.8	23	1	1	2	5	7	16	25
20–34	55	1.6	<1	1	1	1	2	3	4	5
35–49	69	2.2	8	1	1	2	2	4	4	13
50–64	52	2.3	2	1	1	2	3	4	5	7
65+	83	3.6	21	1	2	2	3	7	18	23
GRAND TOTAL	309	2.7	12	1	1	2	3	5	7	23

58.45: HYPOSPAD/EPISPADIAS REP. Formerly included in operation group(s) 656.

Type of Patients	Observed Patients	Avg. Stay	Vari-ance	Percentiles						
				10th	25th	50th	75th	90th	95th	99th
1. SINGLE DX										
0–19 Years	418	2.0	3	1	1	1	2	4	6	9
20–34	5	1.0	0	1	1	1	1	1	1	1
35–49	0	1.0	0	1	1	1	1	1	1	1
50–64	0									
65+										
2. MULTIPLE DX										
0–19 Years	339	3.1	9	1	1	2	4	7	8	20
20–34	11	2.1	2	1	1	2	2	3	3	8
35–49	6	3.0	3	3	3	3	3	5	5	8
50–64	4	1.2	<1	1	1	1	1	2	2	2
65+	1	7.0	0	7	7	7	7	7	7	7
TOTAL SINGLE DX	424	2.0	3	1	1	1	2	4	6	9
MULTIPLE DX	361	3.1	9	1	1	2	4	7	8	18
TOTAL										
0–19 Years	757	2.5	6	1	1	2	3	6	7	10
20–34	16	1.8	2	1	1	1	2	3	3	8
35–49	7	2.7	<1	1	1	1	3	3	3	8
50–64	4	1.2	<1	1	1	1	1	2	2	2
65+	1	7.0	0	7	7	7	7	7	7	7
GRAND TOTAL	785	2.5	6	1	1	2	3	5	7	10

Length of Stay by Diagnosis and Operation, United States, 1997

United States, October 1995–September 1996 Data, by Operation

58.49: URETHRAL REPAIR NEC. Formerly included in operation group(s) 656.

Type of Patients	Observed Patients	Avg. Stay	Vari-ance	10th	25th	50th	75th	90th	95th	99th
1. SINGLE DX										
0–19 Years	24	1.9	2	1	1	2	2	4	6	6
20–34	30	2.4	1	2	2	2	2	4	5	8
35–49	50	1.8	1	1	1	1	3	3	3	5
50–64	27	2.4	1	1	2	2	3	3	5	6
65+	20	2.0	1	1	1	2	3	4	4	4
2. MULTIPLE DX										
0–19 Years	53	4.2	7	1	2	4	6	7	8	11
20–34	64	2.7	10	1	1	1	3	6	7	20
35–49	92	3.7	10	2	2	3	4	6	10	11
50–64	104	2.8	3	1	2	3	4	5	5	6
65+	94	3.0	15	1	1	2	3	6	10	22
TOTAL SINGLE DX	151	2.0	1	1	1	2	3	3	4	6
MULTIPLE DX	407	3.2	9	1	1	3	4	6	7	18
TOTAL										
0–19 Years	77	3.5	6	1	1	2	6	7	7	11
20–34	94	2.6	8	1	1	2	3	5	7	20
35–49	142	2.9	7	1	1	3	3	4	7	10
50–64	131	2.7	2	1	2	2	3	5	5	6
65+	114	2.7	12	1	1	2	3	4	7	21
GRAND TOTAL	558	2.9	7	1	1	2	3	5	7	14

58.6: URETHRAL DILATION. Formerly included in operation group(s) 657.

Type of Patients	Observed Patients	Avg. Stay	Vari-ance	10th	25th	50th	75th	90th	95th	99th
1. SINGLE DX										
0–19 Years	7	2.1	5	1	1	1	2	7	7	7
20–34	17	1.2	<1	1	1	1	1	2	2	3
35–49	20	2.7	5	1	1	2	3	5	7	12
50–64	6	1.2	<1	1	1	1	1	2	2	2
65+	8	1.2	<1	1	1	1	1	1	4	4
2. MULTIPLE DX										
0–19 Years	41	3.3	6	1	1	3	4	7	7	13
20–34	94	3.5	15	1	2	3	4	6	9	12
35–49	174	7.3	174	1	2	3	7	10	62	62
50–64	232	4.8	25	1	2	4	5	10	12	31
65+	1129	6.9	35	2	3	5	9	14	17	28
TOTAL SINGLE DX	58	1.9	3	1	1	1	2	3	5	12
MULTIPLE DX	1670	6.3	49	1	2	5	8	13	16	34
TOTAL										
0–19 Years	48	3.2	6	1	1	2	4	7	7	13
20–34	111	3.3	14	1	2	2	4	6	9	12
35–49	194	6.8	158	1	2	3	6	10	22	62
50–64	238	4.6	24	1	2	3	5	10	12	28
65+	1137	6.9	35	2	3	5	9	14	17	28
GRAND TOTAL	1728	6.1	48	1	2	4	7	12	16	34

58.5: URETHRAL STRICTURE REL. Formerly included in operation group(s) 658.

Type of Patients	Observed Patients	Avg. Stay	Vari-ance	10th	25th	50th	75th	90th	95th	99th
1. SINGLE DX										
0–19 Years	10	1.6	1	1	1	1	2	4	4	4
20–34	16	1.8	3	1	1	1	2	3	9	9
35–49	18	3.0	14	1	1	1	3	12	12	12
50–64	13	1.5	1	1	1	1	1	4	4	4
65+	25	1.9	4	1	1	1	2	3	7	10
2. MULTIPLE DX										
0–19 Years	31	2.8	5	1	1	2	4	4	6	16
20–34	73	4.9	19	1	1	4	8	10	12	21
35–49	146	7.8	50	1	2	5	18	18	18	19
50–64	265	3.8	38	1	1	2	4	8	12	38
65+	956	4.6	29	1	2	3	6	10	14	25
TOTAL SINGLE DX	82	1.9	4	1	1	1	2	4	6	12
MULTIPLE DX	1471	4.9	34	1	1	3	6	11	18	25
TOTAL										
0–19 Years	41	2.6	5	1	1	2	4	4	5	16
20–34	89	4.4	18	1	1	3	6	10	11	21
35–49	164	7.6	49	1	2	4	18	18	18	19
50–64	278	3.7	36	1	1	2	4	8	11	34
65+	981	4.6	28	1	2	3	6	10	14	25
GRAND TOTAL	1553	4.7	33	1	1	3	6	11	18	23

58.9: OTHER URETHRAL OPS. Formerly included in operation group(s) 658.

Type of Patients	Observed Patients	Avg. Stay	Vari-ance	10th	25th	50th	75th	90th	95th	99th
1. SINGLE DX										
0–19 Years	7	3.0	3	1	1	4	4	4	6	6
20–34	2	1.0	0	1	1	1	1	1	1	1
35–49	4	1.1	<1	1	1	1	1	1	2	2
50–64	9	1.3	<1	1	1	1	2	2	2	2
65+	23	1.2	<1	1	1	1	1	2	2	3
2. MULTIPLE DX										
0–19 Years	40	4.4	6	1	2	5	6	8	8	10
20–34	26	4.2	22	1	2	3	4	8	11	30
35–49	34	7.1	78	1	2	4	6	29	29	29
50–64	158	2.8	9	1	1	2	3	7	9	11
65+	599	2.6	6	1	1	2	3	4	7	12
TOTAL SINGLE DX	45	1.4	<1	1	1	1	1	2	4	4
MULTIPLE DX	857	2.9	11	1	1	2	3	5	9	16
TOTAL										
0–19 Years	47	4.0	6	1	2	4	6	8	8	10
20–34	28	4.0	22	1	2	3	4	8	11	30
35–49	38	3.9	46	1	1	1	4	7	29	29
50–64	167	2.8	8	1	1	2	3	6	9	11
65+	622	2.5	6	1	1	2	3	4	6	12
GRAND TOTAL	902	2.8	10	1	1	2	3	5	8	14

Length of Stay by Diagnosis and Operation, United States, 1997

United States, October 1995–September 1996 Data, by Operation

58.93: IMPLANTATION OF AUS. Formerly included in operation group(s) 658.

Type of Patients	Observed Patients	Avg. Stay	Vari-ance	Percentiles						
				10th	25th	50th	75th	90th	95th	99th
1. SINGLE DX										
0–19 Years	2	4.0	0	4	4	4	4	4	4	4
20–34	0									
35–49	2	1.0	0	1	1	1	1	1	1	1
50–64	8	1.3	<1	1	1	1	1	2	2	2
65+	19	1.2	<1	1	1	1	1	2	2	3
2. MULTIPLE DX										
0–19 Years	31	5.1	5	2	3	5	7	8	8	10
20–34	15	3.4	3	1	3	4	4	4	6	8
35–49	14	3.3	3	1	1	4	4	5	5	7
50–64	126	2.3	4	1	1	2	3	6	7	11
65+	482	2.1	2	1	1	2	3	4	4	5
TOTAL SINGLE DX	31	1.3	<1	1	1	1	1	2	4	4
MULTIPLE DX	668	2.3	3	1	1	2	3	4	5	8
TOTAL										
0–19 Years	33	5.0	4	2	4	5	6	8	8	10
20–34	15	3.4	3	1	3	4	4	4	4	8
35–49	16	1.6	2	1	1	4	4	4	4	7
50–64	134	2.2	4	1	1	2	3	3	5	11
65+	501	2.0	2	1	1	2	3	4	4	5
GRAND TOTAL	699	2.2	2	1	1	2	3	4	4	8

59.1: PERIVESICAL INCISION. Formerly included in operation group(s) 663.

Type of Patients	Observed Patients	Avg. Stay	Vari-ance	Percentiles						
				10th	25th	50th	75th	90th	95th	99th
1. SINGLE DX										
0–19 Years	0									
20–34	0									
35–49	2	3.0	0	3	3	3	3	3	3	3
50–64	0									
65+	1	4.0	0	4	4	4	4	4	4	4
2. MULTIPLE DX										
0–19 Years	0									
20–34	4	4.3	2	2	5	5	5	5	5	5
35–49	7	1.3	<1	1	1	1	1	2	3	4
50–64	3	11.6	55	4	5	18	18	18	18	18
65+	5	4.3	13	1	1	1	4	10	10	10
TOTAL SINGLE DX	3	3.3	<1	3	3	3	4	4	4	4
MULTIPLE DX	19	2.4	10	1	1	1	3	5	5	18
TOTAL										
0–19 Years	0									
20–34	4	4.3	2	2	5	5	5	5	5	5
35–49	9	1.3	<1	1	1	1	1	3	3	4
50–64	3	11.6	55	4	5	18	18	18	18	18
65+	6	4.3	11	1	1	4	4	10	10	10
GRAND TOTAL	22	2.4	10	1	1	1	3	5	5	18

59.0: RETROPERITON DISSECTION. Formerly included in operation group(s) 663.

Type of Patients	Observed Patients	Avg. Stay	Vari-ance	Percentiles						
				10th	25th	50th	75th	90th	95th	99th
1. SINGLE DX										
0–19 Years	5	3.4	2	2	2	3	5	5	5	5
20–34	3	2.4	3	1	1	1	3	5	5	5
35–49	5	4.9	13	3	3	6	6	6	15	15
50–64	3	4.3	4	2	2	6	6	6	6	6
65+	1	7.0	0	7	7	7	7	7	7	7
2. MULTIPLE DX										
0–19 Years	14	6.2	26	2	3	4	8	15	20	20
20–34	37	4.6	10	3	4	4	4	6	8	27
35–49	69	6.8	28	3	4	5	7	14	15	27
50–64	85	9.4	45	3	5	7	14	18	18	33
65+	84	9.8	82	3	5	7	10	16	34	40
TOTAL SINGLE DX	17	4.0	7	2	3	3	5	6	7	15
MULTIPLE DX	289	7.4	41	3	4	5	8	14	18	34
TOTAL										
0–19 Years	19	5.0	17	2	3	4	6	8	15	20
20–34	40	4.6	10	3	4	4	4	6	8	27
35–49	74	6.6	27	3	4	4	7	14	15	27
50–64	88	9.3	45	3	5	7	14	18	18	33
65+	85	9.8	81	3	5	7	10	16	34	40
GRAND TOTAL	306	7.3	40	3	4	5	8	14	18	34

59.2: PERIRENAL DXTIC PX. Formerly included in operation group(s) 663, 664.

Type of Patients	Observed Patients	Avg. Stay	Vari-ance	Percentiles						
				10th	25th	50th	75th	90th	95th	99th
1. SINGLE DX										
0–19 Years	1	11.0	0	11	11	11	11	11	11	11
20–34	0									
35–49	1	2.0	0	2	2	2	2	2	2	2
50–64	0									
65+	0									
2. MULTIPLE DX										
0–19 Years	1	1.0	0	1	1	1	1	1	1	1
20–34	3	6.2	2	5	5	5	8	8	8	8
35–49	1	6.0	0	6	6	6	6	6	6	6
50–64	2	6.1	21	4	4	6	6	14	14	14
65+	2	8.2	7	6	6	10	10	10	10	10
TOTAL SINGLE DX	2	6.7	24	2	2	11	11	11	11	11
MULTIPLE DX	9	5.7	8	1	4	5	6	8	10	14
TOTAL										
0–19 Years	2	6.8	29	1	1	11	11	11	11	11
20–34	3	6.2	2	5	5	5	8	8	8	8
35–49	2	4.4	4	2	2	6	4	6	6	6
50–64	2	6.1	21	4	4	6	4	14	14	14
65+	2	8.2	7	6	6	10	10	10	10	10
GRAND TOTAL	11	6.0	11	2	4	6	8	11	11	14

Length of Stay by Diagnosis and Operation, United States, 1997

United States, October 1995–September 1996 Data, by Operation

59.3: URETHROVES JUNCT PLICAT. Formerly included in operation group(s) 660.

Type of Patients	Observed Patients	Avg. Stay	Vari-ance	Percentiles						
				10th	25th	50th	75th	90th	95th	99th
1. SINGLE DX										
0–19 Years	0									
20–34	0									
35–49	2	2.9	<1	3	3	3	3	3	3	3
50–64	1	3.0	0	3	3	3	3	3	3	3
65+	1	1.0	0	1	1	1	1	1	1	1
2. MULTIPLE DX										
0–19 Years	0									
20–34	4	2.6	<1	2	2	3	3	3	3	3
35–49	12	2.5	<1	2	2	3	3	3	3	3
50–64	15	2.6	1	1	2	3	4	4	4	4
65+	19	2.8	2	1	2	2	4	5	5	8
TOTAL SINGLE DX	4	2.6	<1	1	3	3	3	3	3	3
MULTIPLE DX	50	2.7	1	1	2	2	3	4	5	5
TOTAL										
0–19 Years	0									
20–34	4	2.6	<1	2	2	3	3	3	3	3
35–49	14	2.7	<1	2	2	3	3	3	3	3
50–64	16	2.6	1	1	2	3	3	4	4	4
65+	20	2.6	2	1	2	2	4	5	5	8
GRAND TOTAL	54	2.6	1	1	2	3	3	4	5	5

59.4: SUPRAPUBIC SLING OP. Formerly included in operation group(s) 660.

Type of Patients	Observed Patients	Avg. Stay	Vari-ance	Percentiles						
				10th	25th	50th	75th	90th	95th	99th
1. SINGLE DX										
0–19 Years	1	2.0	0	2	2	2	2	2	2	2
20–34	8	1.7	<1	1	1	2	2	2	3	3
35–49	44	2.1	<1	1	2	2	3	3	4	4
50–64	89	1.8	<1	1	1	2	2	3	4	4
65+	61	2.0	1	1	1	2	3	3	4	5
2. MULTIPLE DX										
0–19 Years	12	3.4	1	2	3	3	3	6	6	6
20–34	24	2.4	<1	1	2	3	3	3	3	7
35–49	212	2.6	2	1	2	2	3	4	5	7
50–64	307	3.1	10	1	2	3	3	4	6	20
65+	354	2.9	5	1	2	3	4	5	5	9
TOTAL SINGLE DX	203	1.9	<1	1	1	2	2	3	4	5
MULTIPLE DX	909	2.9	6	1	2	3	3	4	5	20
TOTAL										
0–19 Years	13	3.3	1	2	3	3	3	6	6	6
20–34	32	2.3	<1	1	1	3	3	3	3	3
35–49	256	2.5	2	1	2	2	3	4	5	7
50–64	396	2.8	8	1	2	2	3	4	5	20
65+	415	2.7	4	1	2	2	4	4	5	8
GRAND TOTAL	1112	2.7	5	1	2	2	3	4	5	13

59.5: RETROPUBIC URETHRAL SUSP. Formerly included in operation group(s) 659.

Type of Patients	Observed Patients	Avg. Stay	Vari-ance	Percentiles						
				10th	25th	50th	75th	90th	95th	99th
1. SINGLE DX										
0–19 Years	3	3.7	1	1	4	4	4	4	4	4
20–34	61	3.0	1	2	2	3	4	4	4	8
35–49	341	2.5	<1	2	2	2	3	4	4	6
50–64	311	2.9	<1	1	2	3	3	4	5	5
65+	137	2.6	<1	1	2	3	3	4	4	5
2. MULTIPLE DX										
0–19 Years	2	3.0	0	3	3	3	3	3	3	3
20–34	97	2.9	<1	2	2	3	3	3	3	5
35–49	824	2.9	2	2	2	3	4	4	5	8
50–64	1085	3.1	3	2	2	3	4	5	6	9
65+	932	3.6	3	2	2	3	4	6	6	10
TOTAL SINGLE DX	853	2.7	1	2	2	3	3	4	5	6
MULTIPLE DX	2940	3.1	2	2	2	3	4	5	6	9
TOTAL										
0–19 Years	5	3.6	<1	3	4	4	4	4	4	4
20–34	158	2.9	1	2	2	3	4	4	4	5
35–49	1165	2.8	1	2	2	3	3	4	5	7
50–64	1396	3.1	2	2	2	3	4	5	6	9
65+	1069	3.5	3	2	2	3	4	5	6	9
GRAND TOTAL	3793	3.0	2	2	2	3	4	5	6	8

59.6: PARAURETHRAL SUSPENSION. Formerly included in operation group(s) 660.

Type of Patients	Observed Patients	Avg. Stay	Vari-ance	Percentiles						
				10th	25th	50th	75th	90th	95th	99th
1. SINGLE DX										
0–19 Years	0									
20–34	5	1.9	<1	2	2	2	2	3	3	3
35–49	25	2.0	<1	2	2	2	2	3	3	3
50–64	18	1.9	<1	2	2	2	2	2	3	3
65+	15	2.2	<1	2	2	2	3	3	3	4
2. MULTIPLE DX										
0–19 Years	1	1.0	0	1	1	1	1	1	1	1
20–34	7	1.9	1	1	1	2	3	3	3	6
35–49	98	2.3	2	1	2	2	3	3	6	7
50–64	128	2.3	1	1	2	2	3	3	4	5
65+	136	2.5	3	1	1	2	3	4	5	10
TOTAL SINGLE DX	63	2.0	<1	1	2	2	2	3	3	3
MULTIPLE DX	370	2.3	2	1	2	2	3	4	5	7
TOTAL										
0–19 Years	1	1.0	0	1	1	1	1	1	1	1
20–34	12	1.9	<1	1	1	2	2	3	3	6
35–49	123	2.2	2	1	2	2	3	3	4	7
50–64	146	2.2	<1	1	1	2	3	3	4	5
65+	151	2.5	3	1	1	2	3	4	5	10
GRAND TOTAL	433	2.3	2	1	2	2	3	3	5	7

Length of Stay by Diagnosis and Operation, United States, 1997

United States, October 1995–September 1996 Data, by Operation

59.7: OTH URINARY INCONT REP. Formerly included in operation group(s) 660.

Type of Patients	Observed Patients	Avg. Stay	Variance	10th	25th	50th	75th	90th	95th	99th
1. SINGLE DX										
0–19 Years	2	1.7	<1	1	1	2	2	2	2	2
20–34	91	2.0	<1	1	1	2	3	3	3	8
35–49	661	1.9	<1	1	1	2	2	3	4	6
50–64	663	2.1	<1	1	1	2	3	3	4	5
65+	318	1.6	<1	1	1	1	2	3	3	5
2. MULTIPLE DX										
0–19 Years	9	3.2	5	2	2	2	4	7	7	7
20–34	166	2.6	1	1	2	2	4	4	4	5
35–49	1619	2.3	1	1	2	2	3	3	4	6
50–64	2307	2.4	1	1	2	2	3	4	5	7
65+	2367	2.6	3	1	2	2	3	4	6	10
TOTAL SINGLE DX	1735	1.9	<1	1	1	2	2	3	3	5
MULTIPLE DX	6468	2.4	2	1	2	2	3	4	5	7
TOTAL										
0–19 Years	11	3.0	4	2	2	2	2	7	7	7
20–34	257	2.4	1	1	2	2	3	3	4	5
35–49	2280	2.2	1	1	2	2	3	3	4	6
50–64	2970	2.3	1	1	1	2	3	4	4	6
65+	2685	2.4	3	1	2	2	3	4	5	8
GRAND TOTAL	8203	2.3	2	1	1	2	3	4	4	7

59.71: LEVATOR MUSC SUSPENSION. Formerly included in operation group(s) 660.

Type of Patients	Observed Patients	Avg. Stay	Variance	10th	25th	50th	75th	90th	95th	99th
1. SINGLE DX										
0–19 Years	0									
20–34	0									
35–49	21	2.0	<1	1	1	2	2	4	4	6
50–64	22	2.4	<1	2	2	2	3	3	3	5
65+	4	2.2		2	2	2	2	2	5	5
2. MULTIPLE DX										
0–19 Years	2	2.0	0	2	2	2	2	2	2	2
20–34	1	1.0	0	1	1	1	1	1	1	1
35–49	43	2.0	1	1	1	2	2	3	4	5
50–64	79	2.8	2	1	2	2	3	5	6	7
65+	93	2.8	3	1	2	2	4	5	6	11
TOTAL SINGLE DX	47	2.1	<1	1	1	2	2	3	4	5
MULTIPLE DX	218	2.6	2	1	2	2	3	4	6	7
TOTAL										
0–19 Years	2	2.0	0	2	2	2	2	2	2	2
20–34	1	1.0	0	1	1	1	1	1	1	1
35–49	64	2.0	1	1	1	2	3	4	4	5
50–64	101	2.7	2	2	2	2	3	5	6	7
65+	97	2.8	3	1	2	2	4	5	6	6
GRAND TOTAL	265	2.5	2	1	2	2	3	4	5	7

59.79: URIN INCONT REPAIR NEC. Formerly included in operation group(s) 660.

Type of Patients	Observed Patients	Avg. Stay	Variance	10th	25th	50th	75th	90th	95th	99th
1. SINGLE DX										
0–19 Years	0									
20–34	91	2.0	1	1	1	2	3	3	3	8
35–49	638	1.9	<1	1	1	2	2	3	4	6
50–64	639	2.1	<1	1	1	2	3	3	4	5
65+	306	1.6	<1	1	1	1	2	3	3	5
2. MULTIPLE DX										
0–19 Years	5	5.4	5	1	4	7	7	7	7	7
20–34	164	2.7	1	1	2	3	4	4	4	5
35–49	1568	2.3	1	1	2	2	3	3	4	6
50–64	2214	2.4	2	1	2	2	3	4	5	7
65+	2222	2.6	3	1	2	2	3	4	5	10
TOTAL SINGLE DX	1674	1.9	<1	1	1	2	2	3	3	5
MULTIPLE DX	6173	2.4	2	1	2	2	3	4	5	7
TOTAL										
0–19 Years	5	5.4	5	1	4	7	7	7	7	7
20–34	255	2.4	1	1	2	2	3	4	4	5
35–49	2206	2.2	1	1	2	2	3	3	4	6
50–64	2853	2.3	1	1	2	2	3	4	4	6
65+	2528	2.4	3	1	2	2	3	4	5	9
GRAND TOTAL	7847	2.3	2	1	1	2	3	4	4	7

59.8: URETERAL CATHETERIZATION. Formerly included in operation group(s) 661.

Type of Patients	Observed Patients	Avg. Stay	Variance	10th	25th	50th	75th	90th	95th	99th
1. SINGLE DX										
0–19 Years	53	2.0	3	1	1	1	3	4	5	10
20–34	378	1.7	<1	1	1	1	2	3	4	4
35–49	523	1.8	2	1	1	1	2	3	4	7
50–64	270	2.0	4	1	1	1	2	3	4	13
65+	88	2.0	2	2	1	2	3	4	4	9
2. MULTIPLE DX										
0–19 Years	210	3.7	16	1	1	3	4	7	12	28
20–34	1079	2.9	6	1	1	2	4	5	7	11
35–49	1694	3.1	8	1	2	2	4	5	9	13
50–64	1668	4.1	16	1	2	3	5	8	11	22
65+	2281	5.7	30	2	2	4	7	12	17	25
TOTAL SINGLE DX	1312	1.8	2	1	1	1	2	3	4	9
MULTIPLE DX	6932	4.0	17	1	2	3	5	8	12	21
TOTAL										
0–19 Years	263	3.4	14	1	1	3	4	6	10	28
20–34	1457	2.5	5	1	1	2	3	3	8	10
35–49	2217	2.8	7	1	1	2	3	5	8	13
50–64	1938	3.7	14	1	2	3	5	8	10	19
65+	2369	5.6	29	2	2	4	7	12	16	25
GRAND TOTAL	8244	3.6	15	1	1	2	4	8	10	19

Length of Stay by Diagnosis and Operation, United States, 1997

United States, October 1995–September 1996 Data, by Operation

59.9: OTHER URINARY SYSTEM OPS. Formerly included in operation group(s) 662, 663.

Type of Patients	Observed Patients	Avg. Stay	Vari-ance	10th	25th	50th	75th	90th	95th	99th
1. SINGLE DX										
0–19 Years	0									
20–34	6	2.6	4	1	1	2	2	6	6	6
35–49	7	1.7	<1	1	1	2	2	3	4	4
50–64	6	1.6	<1	1	1	1	2	3	3	3
65+	1	2.0	0	2	2	2	2	2	2	2
2. MULTIPLE DX										
0–19 Years	9	3.6	14	1	1	2	6	6	13	13
20–34	22	4.1	3	2	4	4	4	7	7	10
35–49	49	3.8	18	1	1	3	5	6	8	10
50–64	52	7.6	24	2	3	8	11	12	18	26
65+	132	6.5	43	2	2	5	8	13	17	24
TOTAL SINGLE DX	20	2.0	2	1	1	2	2	4	6	6
MULTIPLE DX	264	5.9	30	1	2	5	8	11	14	26
TOTAL										
0–19 Years	9	3.6	14	1	1	2	6	6	13	13
20–34	28	3.9	4	1	2	4	4	7	7	10
35–49	56	3.7	17	1	1	3	5	6	8	26
50–64	58	7.3	25	1	3	6	11	12	18	18
65+	133	6.5	43	2	2	5	8	13	17	24
GRAND TOTAL	284	5.7	29	1	2	4	7	11	14	24

60.1: PROS/SEM VESICL DXTIC PX. Formerly included in operation group(s) 667, 677.

Type of Patients	Observed Patients	Avg. Stay	Vari-ance	10th	25th	50th	75th	90th	95th	99th
1. SINGLE DX										
0–19 Years	2	4.6	20	1	1	1	9	9	9	9
20–34	1	1.0	0	1	1	1	1	1	1	1
35–49	1	3.0	0	3	3	3	3	3	3	3
50–64	6	3.2	2	1	3	3	3	6	6	6
65+	13	2.2	1	2	2	2	2	4	5	5
2. MULTIPLE DX										
0–19 Years	1	9.0	0	9	9	9	9	9	9	9
20–34	2	5.8	11	4	4	4	10	10	10	10
35–49	15	4.3	17	1	1	3	5	14	14	14
50–64	174	6.6	31	2	3	5	9	12	19	36
65+	797	12.9	321	2	4	7	12	26	71	71
TOTAL SINGLE DX	23	2.2	2	1	1	2	3	4	5	9
MULTIPLE DX	989	11.6	269	2	4	7	12	21	71	71
TOTAL										
0–19 Years	3	7.7	9	1	1	9	9	9	9	9
20–34	3	1.4	3	1	1	1	1	1	4	10
35–49	16	4.2	16	1	1	3	5	14	14	14
50–64	180	6.4	30	1	3	5	8	12	17	36
65+	810	12.7	317	2	4	7	12	25	71	71
GRAND TOTAL	1012	11.2	262	1	3	6	11	20	71	71

60.0: INCISION OF PROSTATE. Formerly included in operation group(s) 667.

Type of Patients	Observed Patients	Avg. Stay	Vari-ance	10th	25th	50th	75th	90th	95th	99th
1. SINGLE DX										
0–19 Years	0									
20–34	2	1.0	0	1	1	1	1	1	1	1
35–49	7	1.4	<1	1	1	1	2	2	2	2
50–64	14	1.4	<1	1	1	1	2	2	2	3
65+	26	1.7	1	1	2	2	2	3	4	6
2. MULTIPLE DX										
0–19 Years	0									
20–34	3	1.9	<1	1	1	2	2	2	2	2
35–49	32	2.3	12	1	1	2	4	4	5	22
50–64	79	5.6	34	1	3	3	8	18	18	18
65+	173	4.0	20	1	2	2	6	8	10	22
TOTAL SINGLE DX	49	1.5	<1	1	1	1	2	2	3	6
MULTIPLE DX	287	4.1	23	1	1	2	5	9	15	22
TOTAL										
0–19 Years	0									
20–34	5	1.5	<1	1	1	1	2	2	2	2
35–49	39	2.2	11	1	1	2	2	4	5	22
50–64	93	5.0	32	1	1	2	5	15	18	18
65+	199	3.8	19	1	1	2	5	8	9	22
GRAND TOTAL	336	3.8	22	1	1	2	4	9	15	21

60.11: CLSD (PERC) PROSTATIC BX. Formerly included in operation group(s) 667.

Type of Patients	Observed Patients	Avg. Stay	Vari-ance	10th	25th	50th	75th	90th	95th	99th
1. SINGLE DX										
0–19 Years	1	1.0	0	1	1	1	1	1	1	1
20–34	1	1.0	0	1	1	1	1	1	1	1
35–49	1	3.0	0	3	3	3	3	3	3	3
50–64	6	3.2	2	1	3	3	3	6	6	6
65+	12	2.2	1	2	2	2	2	4	5	5
2. MULTIPLE DX										
0–19 Years	1	9.0	0	9	9	9	9	9	9	9
20–34	2	5.8	11	4	4	4	10	10	10	10
35–49	15	4.3	17	1	1	3	5	14	14	14
50–64	174	6.6	31	2	3	5	9	12	19	36
65+	784	12.9	323	2	4	7	12	25	71	71
TOTAL SINGLE DX	21	2.0	2	1	1	2	3	3	5	6
MULTIPLE DX	976	11.6	270	2	4	7	12	21	71	71
TOTAL										
0–19 Years	2	7.5	11	1	1	9	9	9	9	9
20–34	3	1.4	3	1	1	1	1	1	4	10
35–49	16	4.2	16	1	1	3	5	14	14	14
50–64	180	6.4	30	1	3	5	8	12	17	36
65+	796	12.8	319	2	4	7	12	25	71	71
GRAND TOTAL	997	11.3	264	1	3	6	11	20	71	71

Length of Stay by Diagnosis and Operation, United States, 1997

United States, October 1995–September 1996 Data, by Operation

60.2: TU PROSTATECTOMY. Formerly included in operation group(s) 667.

Type of Patients	Observed Patients	Avg. Stay	Variance	10th	25th	50th	75th	90th	95th	99th
1. SINGLE DX										
0–19 Years	0									
20–34	3	2.6	<1	1	3	3	3	3	3	3
35–49	64	1.6	<1	1	1	2	2	2	2	3
50–64	668	1.9	<1	1	1	2	2	3	3	5
65+	1239	2.0	1	1	1	2	2	3	4	6
2. MULTIPLE DX										
0–19 Years	3	1.6	<1	1	1	2	2	2	2	2
20–34	10	2.4	10	1	1	1	2	7	7	16
35–49	289	3.9	20	1	2	2	4	10	17	17
50–64	6146	2.9	9	1	2	2	3	5	7	16
65+	32597	4.0	22	1	2	3	4	8	12	24
TOTAL SINGLE DX	1974	1.9	1	1	1	2	2	3	3	6
MULTIPLE DX	39045	3.7	19	1	2	3	4	7	11	22
TOTAL										
0–19 Years	3	1.6	<1	1	1	2	2	2	2	2
20–34	13	2.4	7	1	1	1	3	5	7	16
35–49	353	3.3	15	1	1	2	3	6	17	17
50–64	6814	2.8	8	1	1	2	3	5	7	15
65+	33836	3.9	21	1	2	3	4	8	11	23
GRAND TOTAL	41019	3.6	18	1	1	2	4	7	11	21

60.29: TU PROSTATECTOMY NEC. Formerly included in operation group(s) 667.

Type of Patients	Observed Patients	Avg. Stay	Variance	10th	25th	50th	75th	90th	95th	99th
1. SINGLE DX										
0–19 Years	0									
20–34	3	2.8	<1	1	3	3	3	3	3	3
35–49	56	1.6	<1	1	1	2	2	2	2	3
50–64	599	2.0	<1	1	1	2	3	3	3	5
65+	1081	2.0	1	1	1	2	2	3	4	6
2. MULTIPLE DX										
0–19 Years	2	2.0	0	2	2	2	2	2	2	2
20–34	9	2.5	11	1	1	1	2	7	7	16
35–49	261	4.1	21	1	2	2	4	11	17	17
50–64	5614	2.9	9	1	2	2	3	5	7	16
65+	29576	4.0	21	1	2	3	4	8	12	23
TOTAL SINGLE DX	1738	2.0	1	1	1	2	2	3	3	6
MULTIPLE DX	35462	3.7	19	1	2	3	4	7	11	21
TOTAL										
0–19 Years	2	2.0	0	2	2	2	2	2	2	2
20–34	11	2.6	7	1	1	2	3	5	7	16
35–49	317	3.4	16	1	1	2	3	7	17	17
50–64	6213	2.8	8	1	2	2	3	5	7	15
65+	30657	3.9	20	1	2	3	4	8	11	22
GRAND TOTAL	37200	3.6	18	1	2	2	4	7	10	21

60.21: TULIP PROCEDURE. Formerly included in operation group(s) 666.

Type of Patients	Observed Patients	Avg. Stay	Variance	10th	25th	50th	75th	90th	95th	99th
1. SINGLE DX										
0–19 Years	0									
20–34	1	1.0	0	1	1	1	1	1	1	1
35–49	8	1.0	<1	1	1	1	1	1	1	2
50–64	69	1.3	1	1	1	1	1	2	3	3
65+	158	1.7	<1	1	1	1	2	3	3	4
2. MULTIPLE DX										
0–19 Years	1	1.0	0	1	1	1	1	1	1	1
20–34	1	1.0	0	1	1	1	1	1	1	1
35–49	28	2.0	4	1	1	2	2	3	7	7
50–64	532	2.0	4	1	1	2	2	3	5	12
65+	3021	4.0	29	1	2	2	4	9	13	29
TOTAL SINGLE DX	236	1.5	<1	1	1	1	2	3	3	4
MULTIPLE DX	3583	3.6	25	1	1	2	4	8	12	29
TOTAL										
0–19 Years	1	1.0	0	1	1	1	1	1	1	1
20–34	2	1.0	0	1	1	1	1	1	1	1
35–49	36	1.8	3	1	1	1	1	2	4	10
50–64	601	2.0	4	1	1	1	2	3	5	10
65+	3179	3.9	28	1	2	2	4	9	13	29
GRAND TOTAL	3819	3.5	24	1	1	2	4	8	11	28

60.3: SUPRAPUBIC PROSTATECTOMY. Formerly included in operation group(s) 666.

Type of Patients	Observed Patients	Avg. Stay	Variance	10th	25th	50th	75th	90th	95th	99th
1. SINGLE DX										
0–19 Years	0									
20–34	0									
35–49										
50–64	4	6.4	6	3	3	7	9	9	9	9
65+	3	9.5	26	4	8	8	16	16	16	16
2. MULTIPLE DX										
0–19 Years	0									
20–34	0									
35–49	1	5.0	0	5	5	5	5	5	5	5
50–64	151	6.2	7	5	5	6	7	8	12	>99
65+	708	7.9	28	4	5	7	9	13	15	33
TOTAL SINGLE DX	7	7.4	13	3	4	7	9	9	16	16
MULTIPLE DX	860	7.5	23	4	5	6	8	13	15	35
TOTAL										
0–19 Years	0									
20–34	0									
35–49	1	5.0	0	5	5	5	5	5	5	5
50–64	155	6.2	7	5	5	6	7	8	12	>99
65+	711	7.9	28	4	5	7	9	13	15	33
GRAND TOTAL	867	7.5	23	5	5	6	8	13	15	35

Length of Stay by Diagnosis and Operation, United States, 1997

United States, October 1995–September 1996 Data, by Operation

60.4: RETROPUBIC PROSTATECTOMY. Formerly included in operation group(s) 666.

Type of Patients	Observed Patients	Avg. Stay	Vari- ance	Percentiles						
				10th	25th	50th	75th	90th	95th	99th
1. SINGLE DX										
0–19 Years	0									
20–34	0									
35–49	3	3.6	1	2	2	4	4	5	5	5
50–64	59	4.6	2	3	3	5	6	6	6	7
65+	30	2.8	2	2	2	2	3	5	6	7
2. MULTIPLE DX										
0–19 Years	7	3.7	31	1	1	1	1	17	17	17
20–34	0									
35–49	13	4.3	2	3	4	4	5	7	7	7
50–64	309	4.7	7	3	3	4	5	7	7	15
65+	640	5.9	13	3	4	5	7	10	12	20
TOTAL SINGLE DX	92	3.9	3	2	2	4	6	6	6	7
MULTIPLE DX	969	5.4	11	3	3	5	6	8	12	18
TOTAL										
0–19 Years	7	3.7	31	1	1	1	1	17	17	17
20–34	0									
35–49	16	4.1	2	2	4	4	5	7	7	7
50–64	368	4.7	6	3	3	4	6	7	7	12
65+	670	5.7	12	3	4	5	6	9	12	20
GRAND TOTAL	1061	5.2	10	3	3	5	6	8	11	17

60.5: RADICAL PROSTATECTOMY. Formerly included in operation group(s) 666.

Type of Patients	Observed Patients	Avg. Stay	Vari- ance	Percentiles						
				10th	25th	50th	75th	90th	95th	99th
1. SINGLE DX										
0–19 Years	0									
20–34	0									
35–49	140	3.3	1	2	2	3	4	4	5	8
50–64	1773	3.8	1	3	3	4	5	5	6	7
65+	945	3.8	2	3	3	4	4	5	6	8
2. MULTIPLE DX										
0–19 Years	1	2.0	0	2	2	2	2	2	2	2
20–34	0									
35–49	410	4.2	3	3	3	4	5	6	7	9
50–64	6868	4.4	4	3	3	4	5	6	7	13
65+	7010	4.7	6	3	3	4	5	7	9	14
TOTAL SINGLE DX	2858	3.8	1	3	3	4	4	5	6	8
MULTIPLE DX	14289	4.6	5	3	3	4	5	7	8	13
TOTAL										
0–19 Years	1	2.0	0	2	2	2	2	2	2	2
20–34	0									
35–49	550	3.9	2	2	3	4	4	6	7	8
50–64	8641	4.3	4	3	3	4	5	6	7	12
65+	7955	4.6	5	3	3	4	5	7	8	13
GRAND TOTAL	17147	4.4	4	3	3	4	5	6	7	12

60.6: OTHER PROSTATECTOMY. Formerly included in operation group(s) 666.

Type of Patients	Observed Patients	Avg. Stay	Vari- ance	Percentiles						
				10th	25th	50th	75th	90th	95th	99th
1. SINGLE DX										
0–19 Years	0									
20–34	0									
35–49	2	1.0	0	1	1	1	1	1	1	1
50–64	38	1.9	2	1	1	1	3	3	4	9
65+	43	2.0	1	1	1	2	2	4	4	6
2. MULTIPLE DX										
0–19 Years	0									
20–34	2	5.5	9	1	7	7	7	7	7	7
35–49	4	7.8	47	2	3	6	18	18	18	18
50–64	111	3.4	5	1	2	3	4	6	7	13
65+	267	3.0	11	1	2	2	3	6	7	15
TOTAL SINGLE DX	83	1.9	1	1	1	2	2	3	4	8
MULTIPLE DX	384	3.2	10	1	2	2	4	6	7	16
TOTAL										
0–19 Years	0									
20–34	2	5.5	9	1	7	7	7	7	7	7
35–49	6	6.2	44	1	2	3	6	18	18	18
50–64	149	3.0	5	1	1	2	4	5	6	11
65+	310	2.8	9	1	2	2	3	5	6	13
GRAND TOTAL	467	2.9	8	1	1	2	3	5	7	13

60.7: SEMINAL VESICLE OPS. Formerly included in operation group(s) 667.

Type of Patients	Observed Patients	Avg. Stay	Vari- ance	Percentiles						
				10th	25th	50th	75th	90th	95th	99th
1. SINGLE DX										
0–19 Years	0									
20–34	2	1.0	0	1	1	1	1	1	1	1
35–49	2	2.1	2	1	1	1	4	4	4	4
50–64	1	1.0	0	1	1	1	1	1	1	1
65+	1	1.0	0	1	1	1	1	1	1	1
2. MULTIPLE DX										
0–19 Years	2	3.0	0	3	3	3	3	3	3	3
20–34	2	1.6	<1	1	1	1	2	2	2	2
35–49	2	3.3	5	1	1	5	5	5	5	5
50–64	3	4.7	10	2	2	2	8	8	8	8
65+	0									
TOTAL SINGLE DX	6	1.4	1	1	1	1	1	4	4	4
MULTIPLE DX	9	3.2	4	1	2	3	3	8	8	8
TOTAL										
0–19 Years	2	3.0	0	3	3	3	3	3	3	3
20–34	4	1.3	<1	1	1	1	2	2	2	2
35–49	4	2.6	3	1	1	2	4	5	5	5
50–64	4	3.8	10	1	1	1	8	8	8	8
65+	1	1.0	0	1	1	1	1	1	1	1
GRAND TOTAL	15	2.5	4	1	1	2	3	5	8	8

Length of Stay by Diagnosis and Operation, United States, 1997

United States, October 1995–September 1996 Data, by Operation

60.94: CNTRL POSTOP PROS HEMOR. Formerly included in operation group(s) 667.

Type of Patients	Observed Patients	Avg. Stay	Vari-ance	10th	25th	50th	75th	90th	95th	99th
1. SINGLE DX										
0–19 Years	0									
20–34	0									
35–49	1	2.0	0	2	2	2	2	2	2	2
50–64	1	1.0	0	1	1	1	1	1	1	1
65+	5	2.5	7	1	1	2	2	9	9	9
2. MULTIPLE DX										
0–19 Years	2	2.0	0	2	2	2	2	2	2	2
20–34	1	4.0	0	4	4	4	4	4	4	4
35–49	2	3.1	<1	3	3	3	3	4	4	4
50–64	32	3.7	19	1	2	3	4	6	14	25
65+	286	7.7	66	1	2	4	11	20	20	30
TOTAL SINGLE DX	7	2.1	5	1	1	2	2	2	9	9
MULTIPLE DX	323	7.2	61	1	2	4	8	20	20	30
TOTAL										
0–19 Years	2	2.0	0	2	2	2	2	2	2	2
20–34	1	4.0	0	4	4	4	4	4	4	4
35–49	3	3.0	<1	2	3	3	3	4	4	4
50–64	33	3.7	19	1	2	3	4	6	14	25
65+	291	7.7	65	1	2	4	11	20	20	30
GRAND TOTAL	330	7.2	61	1	2	4	8	20	20	30

61.0: SCROTUM & TUNICA VAG I&D. Formerly included in operation group(s) 668.

Type of Patients	Observed Patients	Avg. Stay	Vari-ance	10th	25th	50th	75th	90th	95th	99th
1. SINGLE DX										
0–19 Years	52	2.0	2	1	1	1	3	3	5	8
20–34	51	1.6	2	1	1	1	3	3	4	11
35–49	36	2.8	5	1	2	2	3	5	9	11
50–64	19	3.7	4	1	2	5	5	5	5	11
65+	3	2.2	1	1	2	2	2	5	5	5
2. MULTIPLE DX										
0–19 Years	47	3.0	8	1	1	2	4	6	9	11
20–34	80	3.9	6	1	2	4	5	6	7	13
35–49	195	5.4	39	1	2	3	6	12	14	50
50–64	134	4.9	15	2	3	3	7	10	11	16
65+	142	5.7	21	2	3	5	6	11	15	24
TOTAL SINGLE DX	161	2.1	3	1	1	2	3	5	5	11
MULTIPLE DX	598	4.9	22	1	2	4	6	10	12	22
TOTAL										
0–19 Years	99	2.5	5	1	1	2	3	5	8	11
20–34	131	3.1	6	1	2	3	5	5	6	11
35–49	231	5.1	36	1	2	3	6	11	13	37
50–64	153	4.8	14	2	3	3	6	10	11	16
65+	145	5.6	21	2	3	5	7	10	14	24
GRAND TOTAL	759	4.3	19	1	2	3	5	9	11	21

60.8: PERIPROSTATIC INC OR EXC. Formerly included in operation group(s) 667.

Type of Patients	Observed Patients	Avg. Stay	Vari-ance	10th	25th	50th	75th	90th	95th	99th
1. SINGLE DX										
0–19 Years	0									
20–34	0									
35–49	0									
50–64	2	2.4	<1	2	2	2	3	3	3	3
65+	0									
2. MULTIPLE DX										
0–19 Years	0									
20–34	0									
35–49	1	1.0	0	1	1	1	1	1	1	1
50–64	8	3.0	5	2	2	2	3	6	6	11
65+	31	3.1	5	1	1	2	6	6	7	8
TOTAL SINGLE DX	2	2.4	<1	2	2	2	3	3	3	3
MULTIPLE DX	40	3.1	5	1	1	2	6	6	7	10
TOTAL										
0–19 Years	0									
20–34	0									
35–49	1	1.0	0	1	1	1	1	1	1	1
50–64	10	2.9	5	2	2	2	3	6	6	11
65+	31	3.1	5	1	1	2	6	6	7	8
GRAND TOTAL	42	3.1	5	1	1	2	6	6	7	10

60.9: OTHER PROSTATIC OPS. Formerly included in operation group(s) 667.

Type of Patients	Observed Patients	Avg. Stay	Vari-ance	10th	25th	50th	75th	90th	95th	99th
1. SINGLE DX										
0–19 Years	0									
20–34	0									
35–49	1	2.0	0	2	2	2	2	2	2	2
50–64	12	1.4	<1	1	1	1	1	3	3	4
65+	27	1.7	2	1	1	1	2	3	4	9
2. MULTIPLE DX										
0–19 Years	2	2.0	0	2	2	2	2	2	2	2
20–34	3	1.1	<1	1	1	1	1	1	1	4
35–49	5	4.1	9	3	3	3	4	12	12	12
50–64	54	3.5	18	1	1	3	4	6	12	25
65+	368	6.8	58	1	2	3	8	20	20	30
TOTAL SINGLE DX	40	1.5	1	1	1	1	2	3	3	4
MULTIPLE DX	432	6.2	53	1	2	3	6	20	20	30
TOTAL										
0–19 Years	2	2.0	0	2	2	2	2	2	2	2
20–34	3	1.1	<1	1	1	1	1	1	1	4
35–49	6	3.9	8	3	3	3	4	12	12	12
50–64	66	2.9	14	1	1	2	3	5	11	25
65+	395	6.6	57	1	2	3	7	20	20	30
GRAND TOTAL	472	5.8	50	1	1	3	5	20	20	30

United States, October 1995–September 1996 Data, by Operation

61.1: SCROTUM/TUNICA DXTIC PX. Formerly included in operation group(s) 668, 677.

Type of Patients	Observed Patients	Avg. Stay	Vari-ance	Percentiles						
				10th	25th	50th	75th	90th	95th	99th
1. SINGLE DX										
0–19 Years	2	1.2	<1	1	1	1	1		2	2
20–34	0									
35–49	0									
50–64	0									
65+	0									
2. MULTIPLE DX										
0–19 Years	0									
20–34	1	6.0	0	6	6	6	6	6	6	6
35–49	0									
50–64	1	23.0	0	23	23	23	23	23	23	23
65+	6	15.5	15	10	15	15	16	17	24	24
TOTAL SINGLE DX	**2**	**1.2**	**<1**	**1**	**1**	**1**	**1**		**2**	**2**
MULTIPLE DX	**8**	**15.4**	**20**	**10**	**15**	**15**	**16**	**23**	**24**	**24**
TOTAL										
0–19 Years	2	1.2	<1	1	1	1	1		2	2
20–34	1	6.0	0	6	6	6	6	6	6	6
35–49	0									
50–64	1	23.0	0	23	23	23	23	23	23	23
65+	6	15.5	15	10	15	15	16	17	24	24
GRAND TOTAL	**10**	**12.2**	**51**	**1**	**6**	**15**	**15**	**23**	**24**	**24**

61.2: EXCISION OF HYDROCELE. Formerly included in operation group(s) 668.

Type of Patients	Observed Patients	Avg. Stay	Vari-ance	Percentiles						
				10th	25th	50th	75th	90th	95th	99th
1. SINGLE DX										
0–19 Years	1	1.0	0	1	1	1	1	1	1	1
20–34	3	1.0	0	1	1	1	1	1	1	1
35–49	4	1.6	1	1	1	1	2	2	4	4
50–64	8	1.9	2	1	1	1	2	4	6	6
65+	5	1.0	0	1	1	1	1	1	1	1
2. MULTIPLE DX										
0–19 Years	22	2.5	3	1	1	2	4	4	4	5
20–34	8	2.4	2	1	1	2	4	4	6	6
35–49	20	6.1	27	1	2	3	11	13	18	18
50–64	27	2.7	5	1	1	2	7	9	9	9
65+	61	3.3	10	1	1	2	4	6	10	18
TOTAL SINGLE DX	**21**	**1.3**	**<1**	**1**	**1**	**1**	**1**	**2**	**2**	**6**
MULTIPLE DX	**138**	**3.4**	**11**	**1**	**1**	**2**	**4**	**7**	**11**	**18**
TOTAL										
0–19 Years	23	2.5	3	1	1	2	4	4	4	5
20–34	11	2.1	2	1	1	1	3	4	4	6
35–49	24	4.8	24	1	1	2	7	13	13	18
50–64	35	2.5	4	1	1	1	3	6	8	9
65+	66	2.6	8	1	1	1	3	6	7	15
GRAND TOTAL	**159**	**2.9**	**9**	**1**	**1**	**2**	**4**	**6**	**10**	**18**

61.3: SCROTAL LES EXC/DESTR. Formerly included in operation group(s) 668.

Type of Patients	Observed Patients	Avg. Stay	Vari-ance	Percentiles						
				10th	25th	50th	75th	90th	95th	99th
1. SINGLE DX										
0–19 Years	5	1.4	<1	1	1		1	3	3	3
20–34	7	2.6	<1	1	2	3	3	4	4	4
35–49	5	3.4	1	2	2	3	5	5	5	5
50–64	2	7.0	0	7	7	7	7	7	7	7
65+	4	4.1	27	1	1	1	12	12	12	12
2. MULTIPLE DX										
0–19 Years	9	2.5	5	2	2	3	3	3	11	11
20–34	16	7.1	54	1	3	4	8	19	22	27
35–49	37	5.8	39	1	2	3	8	12	22	28
50–64	45	10.2	164	1	4	6	14	22	59	>99
65+	44	9.6	95	2	4	6	11	22	31	49
TOTAL SINGLE DX	**23**	**3.2**	**7**	**1**	**1**	**3**	**4**	**7**	**7**	**12**
MULTIPLE DX	**151**	**7.0**	**84**	**1**	**2**	**4**	**8**	**15**	**27**	**59**
TOTAL										
0–19 Years	14	2.4	4	1	2	2	2	3	9	11
20–34	23	5.2	36	3	3	3	7	9	19	27
35–49	42	5.6	37	1	2	3	8	12	18	28
50–64	47	10.0	153	1	4	7	11	22	59	>99
65+	48	9.2	91	2	4	6	11	22	29	49
GRAND TOTAL	**174**	**6.5**	**76**	**1**	**2**	**4**	**8**	**14**	**22**	**59**

61.4: SCROTUM & TUNICA VAG REP. Formerly included in operation group(s) 668.

Type of Patients	Observed Patients	Avg. Stay	Vari-ance	Percentiles						
				10th	25th	50th	75th	90th	95th	99th
1. SINGLE DX										
0–19 Years	18	1.1	<1	1	1	1	1	1	2	2
20–34	7	2.1	2	1	1	1	4	4	4	4
35–49	3	2.6	3	3	3	2	5	5	5	5
50–64	1	3.0	0	3	3	3	3	3	3	3
65+	2	1.5	<1	1	1	1	2	2	2	2
2. MULTIPLE DX										
0–19 Years	13	4.8	162	1	1	3	3	4	5	71
20–34	14	3.9	76	1	1	2	2	3	38	38
35–49	16	3.2	13	1	2	2	3	13	13	13
50–64	20	4.2	35	1	1	3	5	6	10	36
65+	26	7.5	129	1	2	3	7	17	43	43
TOTAL SINGLE DX	**31**	**1.4**	**<1**	**1**	**1**	**1**	**1**	**2**	**4**	**5**
MULTIPLE DX	**89**	**4.5**	**66**	**1**	**1**	**2**	**4**	**10**	**13**	**43**
TOTAL										
0–19 Years	31	2.2	51	1	1	1	1	3	4	71
20–34	21	3.2	48	1	1	1	2	4	9	38
35–49	19	3.1	13	1	1	3	5	13	13	13
50–64	21	4.2	35	1	1	3	6	6	10	36
65+	28	7.1	123	1	2	2	7	17	43	43
GRAND TOTAL	**120**	**3.6**	**50**	**1**	**1**	**2**	**3**	**6**	**13**	**43**

Length of Stay by Diagnosis and Operation, United States, 1997

United States, October 1995–September 1996 Data, by Operation

61.9: OTH SCROT/TUNICA VAG OPS. Formerly included in operation group(s) 668.

Type of Patients	Observed Patients	Avg. Stay	Variance	10th	25th	50th	75th	90th	95th	99th
1. SINGLE DX										
0–19 Years	0									
20–34	0									
35–49	0									
50–64	0									
65+	0									
2. MULTIPLE DX										
0–19 Years	0									
20–34	1	4.0	0	4	4	4	4	4	4	4
35–49	5	4.4	9	1	1	5	7	9	9	9
50–64	7	12.7	138	2	2	7	26	28	28	28
65+	19	7.8	7	5	7	7	8	12	13	15
TOTAL SINGLE DX	0									
MULTIPLE DX	32	8.1	42	2	5	7	9	15	26	28
TOTAL										
0–19 Years	0									
20–34	1	4.0	0	4	4	4	4	4	4	4
35–49	5	4.4	9	1	1	5	7	9	9	9
50–64	7	12.7	138	2	2	7	26	28	28	28
65+	19	7.8	7	5	7	7	8	12	13	15
GRAND TOTAL	32	8.1	42	2	5	7	9	15	26	28

62.1: TESTES DXTIC PX. Formerly included in operation group(s) 671, 677.

Type of Patients	Observed Patients	Avg. Stay	Variance	10th	25th	50th	75th	90th	95th	99th
1. SINGLE DX										
0–19 Years	11	3.3	17	2	2	2	3	7	7	26
20–34	4	1.1	<1	1	1	1	1	2	2	2
35–49	1	1.0	0	1	1	1	1	1	1	1
50–64	0									
65+	0									
2. MULTIPLE DX										
0–19 Years	17	12.1	96	2	2	6	21	21	21	32
20–34	11	2.5	23	1	1	1	1	5	18	18
35–49	3	5.3	7	1	6	6	6	8	8	8
50–64	4	1.7	3	1	1	3	6	6	6	6
65+	6	6.3	87	3	3	3	6	15	35	35
TOTAL SINGLE DX	16	2.7	14	1	1	2	2	7	7	26
MULTIPLE DX	41	5.2	61	1	1	1	5	21	21	32
TOTAL										
0–19 Years	28	8.0	78	2	2	3	18	21	21	32
20–34	15	2.4	22	1	1	1	1	5	18	18
35–49	4	3.9	9	1	6	6	6	8	8	8
50–64	4	1.7	3	1	1	3	6	6	6	6
65+	6	6.3	87	3	3	3	6	15	35	35
GRAND TOTAL	57	4.7	52	1	1	2	4	18	21	32

62.0: INCISION OF TESTIS. Formerly included in operation group(s) 671.

Type of Patients	Observed Patients	Avg. Stay	Variance	10th	25th	50th	75th	90th	95th	99th
1. SINGLE DX										
0–19 Years	21	1.8	1	1	1	1	2	4	4	4
20–34	6	1.3	<1	1	1	1	2	2	2	2
35–49	2	1.3	<1	1	1	1	1	1	1	1
50–64	1	1.0	0	1	1	1	1	1	1	1
65+	0									
2. MULTIPLE DX										
0–19 Years	11	1.8	<1	1	1	2	3	3	3	4
20–34	12	4.0	11	1	1	3	6	7	13	13
35–49	10	2.7	14	1	2	1	2	6	14	14
50–64	8	4.9	15	1	2	3	9	11	11	11
65+	6	4.5	8	1	2	3	8	8	8	8
TOTAL SINGLE DX	30	1.7	1	1	1	1	2	4	4	4
MULTIPLE DX	47	3.0	9	1	2	2	3	7	9	14
TOTAL										
0–19 Years	32	1.8	1	1	1	2	2	4	4	4
20–34	18	3.2	9	1	1	1	5	7	13	13
35–49	12	2.5	13	1	2	2	2	6	14	14
50–64	9	4.7	15	1	2	2	9	11	11	11
65+	6	4.5	8	1	2	3	8	8	8	8
GRAND TOTAL	77	2.5	6	1	1	2	3	6	8	13

62.2: TESTICULAR LES DESTR/EXC. Formerly included in operation group(s) 671.

Type of Patients	Observed Patients	Avg. Stay	Variance	10th	25th	50th	75th	90th	95th	99th
1. SINGLE DX										
0–19 Years	55	1.0	<1	1	1	1	1	1	1	2
20–34	10	1.1	<1	1	1	1	1	1	1	2
35–49	2	1.0	0	1	1	1	1	1	1	1
50–64	0									
65+	0									
2. MULTIPLE DX										
0–19 Years	37	1.4	<1	1	1	1	1	3	4	4
20–34	6	2.7	7	1	1	2	2	8	8	8
35–49	3	6.5	25	2	2	11	11	11	11	11
50–64	2	1.0	0	1	1	1	1	1	1	1
65+	2	5.3	7	2	2	7	7	7	7	7
TOTAL SINGLE DX	67	1.0	<1	1	1	1	1	1	1	2
MULTIPLE DX	50	1.7	3	1	1	1	1	4	7	11
TOTAL										
0–19 Years	92	1.2	<1	1	1	1	1	2	2	4
20–34	16	1.3	1	1	1	1	2	2	2	8
35–49	5	3.7	20	2	2	7	7	11	11	11
50–64	2	1.0	0	1	1	1	1	1	1	1
65+	2	5.3	7	2	2	7	7	7	7	7
GRAND TOTAL	117	1.3	1	1	1	1	1	2	3	8

Length of Stay by Diagnosis and Operation, United States, 1997

United States, October 1995–September 1996 Data, by Operation

62.3: UNILATERAL ORCHIECTOMY. Formerly included in operation group(s) 669.

Type of Patients	Observed Patients	Avg. Stay	Vari-ance	Percentiles						
				10th	25th	50th	75th	90th	95th	99th
1. SINGLE DX										
0–19 Years	194	1.2	<1	1	1	1	1	2	2	5
20–34	136	1.8	4	1	1	1	2	2	3	9
35–49	66	1.4	1	1	1	1	1	2	4	7
50–64	20	2.8	8	1	1	1	3	8	9	10
65+	18	2.6	4	1	1	2	4	6	6	8
2. MULTIPLE DX										
0–19 Years	206	2.8	20	1	1	2	3	4	6	22
20–34	162	4.1	43	1	1	2	5	9	13	17
35–49	156	3.8	14	1	1	3	5	9	12	15
50–64	99	7.8	47	1	2	5	14	17	19	22
65+	280	6.9	65	1	2	5	9	14	16	73
TOTAL SINGLE DX	434	1.5	2	1	1	1	1	2	5	8
MULTIPLE DX	903	4.8	40	1	1	3	6	11	15	26
TOTAL										
0–19 Years	400	2.1	11	1	1	1	2	4	5	12
20–34	298	3.0	25	1	1	1	3	7	9	17
35–49	222	3.0	11	1	1	1	4	7	10	15
50–64	119	7.2	45	1	2	4	11	17	17	22
65+	298	6.7	63	1	2	5	9	14	16	73
GRAND TOTAL	1337	3.7	30	1	1	2	4	9	13	21

62.41: RMVL BOTH TESTES. Formerly included in operation group(s) 669.

Type of Patients	Observed Patients	Avg. Stay	Vari-ance	Percentiles						
				10th	25th	50th	75th	90th	95th	99th
1. SINGLE DX										
0–19 Years	4	1.0	0	1	1	1	1	1	1	1
20–34	2	1.2	<1	1	1	1	1	2	2	2
35–49	2	1.4	<1	1	1	1	2	2	2	2
50–64	3	1.0	0	1	1	1	1	1	1	1
65+	59	1.6	<1	1	1	1	2	2	3	5
2. MULTIPLE DX										
0–19 Years	8	2.8	3	2	2	2	3	6	6	6
20–34	3	6.6	18	3	3	4	5	9	11	11
35–49	8	7.1	14	2	3	8	10	12	12	12
50–64	99	4.7	28	2	2	2	5	12	17	25
65+	950	7.0	49	1	2	4	10	17	18	31
TOTAL SINGLE DX	70	1.5	<1	1	1	1	2	2	3	5
MULTIPLE DX	1068	6.7	47	1	2	4	9	17	18	31
TOTAL										
0–19 Years	12	2.5	3	1	2	2	2	6	6	6
20–34	5	4.3	17	1	1	3	4	11	11	11
35–49	10	5.6	17	1	2	5	10	10	12	12
50–64	102	4.7	27	2	2	2	5	12	17	25
65+	1009	6.6	48	1	2	3	9	17	18	31
GRAND TOTAL	1138	6.4	45	1	2	3	9	17	18	30

62.4: BILATERAL ORCHIECTOMY. Formerly included in operation group(s) 669.

Type of Patients	Observed Patients	Avg. Stay	Vari-ance	Percentiles						
				10th	25th	50th	75th	90th	95th	99th
1. SINGLE DX										
0–19 Years	4	1.0	0	1	1	1	1	1	1	1
20–34	3	1.8	<1	1	1	1	3	3	3	3
35–49	3	1.2	<1	1	2	2	2	2	2	2
50–64	3	1.0	0	1	1	1	1	1	1	1
65+	59	1.6	<1	1	1	2	2	2	3	5
2. MULTIPLE DX										
0–19 Years	10	2.8	3	1	2	2	4	6	6	6
20–34	9	2.6	9	1	1	1	3	8	11	11
35–49	10	8.2	11	2	8	10	10	10	12	12
50–64	99	4.7	28	2	2	2	5	12	12	25
65+	961	6.9	48	1	2	4	10	17	18	31
TOTAL SINGLE DX	72	1.6	<1	1	1	1	2	2	3	5
MULTIPLE DX	1089	6.6	46	1	2	3	9	17	18	30
TOTAL										
0–19 Years	14	2.5	3	1	1	2	2	6	6	6
20–34	12	2.5	8	1	1	1	3	8	11	11
35–49	13	6.2	16	2	2	8	10	10	12	12
50–64	102	4.7	27	2	2	2	5	12	12	25
65+	1020	6.5	47	1	2	3	9	17	18	31
GRAND TOTAL	1161	6.3	44	1	2	3	9	17	17	30

62.5: ORCHIOPEXY. Formerly included in operation group(s) 670.

Type of Patients	Observed Patients	Avg. Stay	Vari-ance	Percentiles						
				10th	25th	50th	75th	90th	95th	99th
1. SINGLE DX										
0–19 Years	410	1.2	<1	1	1	1	1	2	2	4
20–34	109	1.1	<1	1	1	1	1	2	2	3
35–49	15	1.2	<1	1	1	1	1	2	2	2
50–64	1	3.0	0	3	3	3	3	3	3	3
65+	1	2.0	0	2	2	2	2	2	2	2
2. MULTIPLE DX										
0–19 Years	339	2.1	32	1	1	1	1	3	5	21
20–34	46	1.5	<1	1	1	1	2	3	3	3
35–49	17	1.6	1	1	1	1	1	4	4	4
50–64	6	2.5	8	2	2	1	5	6	7	15
65+	6	9.7	85	2	2	6	12	30	30	30
TOTAL SINGLE DX	536	1.2	<1	1	1	1	1	2	2	4
MULTIPLE DX	414	2.0	27	1	1	1	1	3	5	15
TOTAL										
0–19 Years	749	1.6	15	1	1	1	1	2	4	9
20–34	155	1.2	<1	1	1	1	1	3	4	3
35–49	32	1.5	<1	1	1	1	1	3	4	4
50–64	7	2.6	7	1	2	1	3	6	7	15
65+	7	8.8	81	2	2	6	12	30	30	31
GRAND TOTAL	950	1.5	11	1	1	1	1	2	4	7

Length of Stay by Diagnosis and Operation, United States, 1997

United States, October 1995–September 1996 Data, by Operation

62.6: REPAIR OF TESTES. Formerly included in operation group(s) 671.

Type of Patients	Observed Patients	Avg. Stay	Vari-ance	Percentiles						
				10th	25th	50th	75th	90th	95th	99th
1. SINGLE DX										
0–19 Years	3	1.0	0	1	1	1	1	1	1	1
20–34	6	1.4	1	1	1	1	1	4	4	4
35–49	0									
50–64	0									
65+	0									
2. MULTIPLE DX										
0–19 Years	6	1.2	<1	1	1	1	1	2	2	4
20–34	8	1.3	<1	1	1	1	1	2	3	3
35–49	2	15.8	233	2	2	29	29	29	29	29
50–64	1	1.0	0	1	1	1	1	1	1	1
65+	0									
TOTAL SINGLE DX	9	1.3	<1	1	1	1	1	1	4	4
MULTIPLE DX	17	1.9	18	1	1	1	1	2	3	29
TOTAL										
0–19 Years	9	1.2	<1	1	1	1	1	1	2	4
20–34	14	1.3	<1	1	1	1	1	3	3	4
35–49	2	15.8	233	2	2	29	29	29	29	29
50–64	1	1.0	0	1	1	1	1	1	1	1
65+	0									
GRAND TOTAL	26	1.8	14	1	1	1	1	2	3	29

62.9: OTHER TESTICULAR OPS. Formerly included in operation group(s) 671.

Type of Patients	Observed Patients	Avg. Stay	Vari-ance	Percentiles						
				10th	25th	50th	75th	90th	95th	99th
1. SINGLE DX										
0–19 Years	1	4.0	0	4	4	4	4	4	4	4
20–34	1	2.0	0	2	2	2	2	2	2	2
35–49	0									
50–64	0									
65+	0									
2. MULTIPLE DX										
0–19 Years	1	1.0	0	1	1	1	1	1	1	1
20–34	0									
35–49	8	5.3	4	2	4	6	7	7	7	7
50–64	3	6.2	1	4	6	6	7	7	7	7
65+	2	10.5	59	2	2	15	15	15	15	15
TOTAL SINGLE DX	2	2.2	<1	2	2	2	2	2	4	4
MULTIPLE DX	14	3.8	10	1	1	2	6	7	7	15
TOTAL										
0–19 Years	2	1.1	<1	1	1	1	1	1	1	4
20–34	1	2.0	0	2	2	2	2	2	2	2
35–49	8	5.3	4	2	4	6	7	7	7	7
50–64	3	6.2	1	4	6	6	7	7	7	7
65+	2	10.5	59	2	2	15	15	15	15	15
GRAND TOTAL	16	3.5	9	1	1	2	6	7	7	15

62.7: INSERT TESTICULAR PROSTH. Formerly included in operation group(s) 671.

Type of Patients	Observed Patients	Avg. Stay	Vari-ance	Percentiles						
				10th	25th	50th	75th	90th	95th	99th
1. SINGLE DX										
0–19 Years	1	1.0	0	1	1	1	1	1	1	1
20–34	1	1.0	0	1	1	1	1	1	1	1
35–49	0									
50–64	0									
65+	0									
2. MULTIPLE DX										
0–19 Years	1	1.0	0	1	1	1	1	1	1	1
20–34	0									
35–49	1	2.0	0	2	2	2	2	2	2	2
50–64	0									
65+	0									
TOTAL SINGLE DX	2	1.0	0	1	1	1	1	1	1	1
MULTIPLE DX	2	1.4	<1	1	1	1	2	2	2	2
TOTAL										
0–19 Years	2	1.0	0	1	1	1	1	1	1	1
20–34	1	1.0	0	1	1	1	1	1	1	1
35–49	1	2.0	0	2	2	2	2	2	2	2
50–64	0									
65+	0									
GRAND TOTAL	4	1.2	<1	1	1	1	1	2	2	2

63.0: SPERMATIC CORD DXTIC PX. Formerly included in operation group(s) 673, 677.

Type of Patients	Observed Patients	Avg. Stay	Vari-ance	Percentiles						
				10th	25th	50th	75th	90th	95th	99th
1. SINGLE DX										
0–19 Years	0									
20–34	0									
35–49	0									
50–64	0									
65+	0									
2. MULTIPLE DX										
0–19 Years	0									
20–34	1	1.0	0	1	1	1	1	1	1	1
35–49	0									
50–64	0									
65+	0									
TOTAL SINGLE DX	0									
MULTIPLE DX	1	1.0	0	1	1	1	1	1	1	1
TOTAL										
0–19 Years	0									
20–34	1	1.0	0	1	1	1	1	1	1	1
35–49	0									
50–64	0									
65+	0									
GRAND TOTAL	1	1.0	0	1	1	1	1	1	1	1

Length of Stay by Diagnosis and Operation, United States, 1997

United States, October 1995–September 1996 Data, by Operation

63.1: EXC SPERMATIC VARICOCELE. Formerly included in operation group(s) 673.

Type of Patients	Observed Patients	Avg. Stay	Variance	10th	25th	50th	75th	90th	95th	99th
1. SINGLE DX										
0–19 Years	41	1.2	<1	1	1	1	1	2	3	3
20–34	14	2.5	7	1	1	1	1	8	8	8
35–49	9	1.7	<1	1	1	1	3	3	3	3
50–64	12	1.1	<1	1	1	1	1	1	2	2
65+	6	1.2	<1	1	1	1	1	2	2	2
2. MULTIPLE DX										
0–19 Years	69	2.2	26	1	1	1	3	2	11	26
20–34	28	2.6	7	1	1	1	3	8	9	9
35–49	43	3.2	41	1	1	2	2	4	13	44
50–64	36	4.4	55	1	1	2	3	6	31	31
65+	103	5.0	35	1	1	2	7	12	18	35
TOTAL SINGLE DX	82	1.4	1	1	1	1	1	3	3	8
MULTIPLE DX	279	3.5	34	1	1	1	3	9	13	31
TOTAL										
0–19 Years	110	2.0	19	1	1	1	1	2	3	23
20–34	42	2.5	7	1	1	1	3	8	9	9
35–49	52	3.1	37	1	1	2	2	4	6	44
50–64	48	3.1	35	1	1	2	3	6	31	31
65+	109	4.9	34	1	1	2	7	11	18	35
GRAND TOTAL	361	3.0	28	1	1	1	2	8	11	31

63.2: EXC EPIDIDYMIS CYST. Formerly included in operation group(s) 673.

Type of Patients	Observed Patients	Avg. Stay	Variance	10th	25th	50th	75th	90th	95th	99th
1. SINGLE DX										
0–19 Years	1	1.0	0	1	1	1	1	1	1	1
20–34	3	1.2	<1	1	1	1	1	2	2	2
35–49	4	1.4	<1	1	1	2	2	2	2	2
50–64	1	1.0	0	1	1	1	1	1	1	1
65+	3	1.0	0	1	1	1	1	1	1	1
2. MULTIPLE DX										
0–19 Years	1	3.0	0	3	3	3	3	3	3	3
20–34	2	1.0	0	1	1	1	1	1	1	1
35–49	5	2.1	<1	2	2	2	2	4	5	6
50–64	17	2.0	3	1	1	2	2	5	5	7
65+	22	3.3	5	2	2	2	4	6	9	11
TOTAL SINGLE DX	12	1.2	<1	1	1	1	1	2	2	2
MULTIPLE DX	47	2.2	3	1	1	2	2	6	6	9
TOTAL										
0–19 Years	2	1.9	1	1	1	1	3	3	3	3
20–34	5	1.0	<1	1	1	1	1	1	1	2
35–49	9	1.9	<1	1	1	2	2	2	2	6
50–64	18	2.0	3	1	2	2	2	5	5	7
65+	25	3.1	5	2	2	2	4	6	6	11
GRAND TOTAL	59	2.1	3	1	1	1	2	5	6	9

63.3: EXC SPERM CORD LES NEC. Formerly included in operation group(s) 673.

Type of Patients	Observed Patients	Avg. Stay	Variance	10th	25th	50th	75th	90th	95th	99th
1. SINGLE DX										
0–19 Years	11	1.0	<1	1	1	1	1	1	1	2
20–34	5	2.3	3	1	1	1	5	5	5	5
35–49	0									
50–64	0									
65+	1	1.0	0	1	1	1	1	1	1	1
2. MULTIPLE DX										
0–19 Years	10	2.0	2	1	1	1	3	3	6	6
20–34	3	4.1	3	1	2	5	5	5	5	5
35–49	9	9.3	55	1	2	10	17	21	21	21
50–64	7	2.0	5	1	1	1	2	4	9	9
65+	14	3.3	3	2	3	3	4	4	8	8
TOTAL SINGLE DX	17	1.1	<1	1	1	1	1	1	1	5
MULTIPLE DX	43	3.3	12	1	1	3	4	6	10	21
TOTAL										
0–19 Years	21	1.4	1	1	1	1	1	3	3	6
20–34	8	3.4	4	1	1	5	5	5	5	9
35–49	9	9.3	55	1	2	10	17	21	21	21
50–64	7	2.0	5	1	1	1	2	4	9	9
65+	15	2.4	3	1	1	2	3	4	4	8
GRAND TOTAL	60	2.3	8	1	1	1	3	5	6	17

63.4: EPIDIDYMECTOMY. Formerly included in operation group(s) 673.

Type of Patients	Observed Patients	Avg. Stay	Variance	10th	25th	50th	75th	90th	95th	99th
1. SINGLE DX										
0–19 Years	3	1.7	3	1	1	1	1	6	6	6
20–34	1	2.0	0	2	2	2	2	2	2	2
35–49	6	3.0	2	1	1	4	4	4	4	4
50–64	0									
65+	1	1.0	0	1	1	1	1	1	1	1
2. MULTIPLE DX										
0–19 Years	3	3.3	2	2	2	3	5	5	5	5
20–34	3	4.5	8	1	3	3	7	7	7	7
35–49	18	6.0	25	1	1	5	11	11	13	17
50–64	12	2.9	7	1	1	1	5	8	8	8
65+	9	4.8	7	1	3	5	7	8	8	8
TOTAL SINGLE DX	11	2.5	2	1	1	2	4	4	4	6
MULTIPLE DX	45	4.1	14	1	1	2	7	11	11	13
TOTAL										
0–19 Years	6	2.5	3	1	1	2	5	5	6	6
20–34	4	3.4	6	2	2	2	7	7	7	7
35–49	24	4.9	18	1	1	4	8	11	11	17
50–64	12	2.9	7	1	1	1	5	8	8	8
65+	10	4.2	8	1	3	4	7	8	8	8
GRAND TOTAL	56	3.8	12	1	1	2	6	8	11	13

Length of Stay by Diagnosis and Operation, United States, 1997

United States, October 1995–September 1996 Data, by Operation

63.5: SPERM CORD/EPID REPAIR. Formerly included in operation group(s) 673.

Type of Patients	Observed Patients	Avg. Stay	Vari-ance	Percentiles						
				10th	25th	50th	75th	90th	95th	99th
1. SINGLE DX										
0–19 Years	19	1.1	<1	1	1	1	1	1	2	4
20–34	6	1.6	2	1	1	1	1	4	4	4
35–49	0									
50–64	0									
65+	0									
2. MULTIPLE DX										
0–19 Years	7	1.1	<1	1	1	1	1	1	2	2
20–34	5	1.2	<1	1	1	1	1	2	2	2
35–49	1	2.0	0	2	2	2	2	2	2	2
50–64	1	1.0	0	1	1	1	1	1	1	1
65+	1	5.0	0	5	5	5	5	5	5	5
TOTAL SINGLE DX	25	1.2	<1	1	1	1	1	2	2	4
MULTIPLE DX	15	1.4	<1	1	1	1	2	2	5	5
TOTAL										
0–19 Years	26	1.1	<1	1	1	1	1	1	2	2
20–34	11	1.4	<1	1	1	1	1	2	4	4
35–49	1	2.0	0	2	2	2	2	2	2	2
50–64	1	1.0	0	1	1	1	1	1	1	1
65+	1	5.0	0	5	5	5	5	5	5	5
GRAND TOTAL	40	1.3	<1	1	1	1	1	2	2	5

63.6: VASOTOMY. Formerly included in operation group(s) 672.

Type of Patients	Observed Patients	Avg. Stay	Vari-ance	Percentiles						
				10th	25th	50th	75th	90th	95th	99th
1. SINGLE DX										
0–19 Years	0									
20–34	0									
35–49	0									
50–64	0									
65+	0									
2. MULTIPLE DX										
0–19 Years	0									
20–34	0									
35–49	1	1.0	0	1	1	1	1	1	1	1
50–64	0									
65+	0									
TOTAL SINGLE DX	0									
MULTIPLE DX	1	1.0	0	1	1	1	1	1	1	1
TOTAL										
0–19 Years	0									
20–34	0									
35–49	1	1.0	0	1	1	1	1	1	1	1
50–64	0									
65+	0									
GRAND TOTAL	1	1.0	0	1	1	1	1	1	1	1

63.7: VASECTOMY & VAS DEF LIG. Formerly included in operation group(s) 672.

Type of Patients	Observed Patients	Avg. Stay	Vari-ance	Percentiles						
				10th	25th	50th	75th	90th	95th	99th
1. SINGLE DX										
0–19 Years	0									
20–34	2	1.0	0	1	1	1	1	1	1	1
35–49	0									
50–64	1	1.0	0	1	1	1	1	1	1	1
65+	0									
2. MULTIPLE DX										
0–19 Years	0									
20–34	1	1.0	0	1	1	1	1	1	1	1
35–49	5	2.5	2	1	1	3	3	5	5	5
50–64	3	9.5	19	2	11	11	12	12	12	12
65+	1	4.0	0	4	4	4	4	4	4	4
TOTAL SINGLE DX	3	1.0	0	1	1	1	1	1	1	1
MULTIPLE DX	10	3.9	12	1	1	3	4	11	12	12
TOTAL										
0–19 Years	0									
20–34	3	1.0	0	1	1	1	1	1	1	1
35–49	5	2.5	2	1	1	3	3	5	5	5
50–64	4	6.7	30	1	11	11	11	12	12	12
65+	1	4.0	0	4	4	4	4	4	4	4
GRAND TOTAL	13	3.1	10	1	1	2	4	11	11	12

63.8: VAS DEF & EPID REPAIR. Formerly included in operation group(s) 673.

Type of Patients	Observed Patients	Avg. Stay	Vari-ance	Percentiles						
				10th	25th	50th	75th	90th	95th	99th
1. SINGLE DX										
0–19 Years	0									
20–34	3	1.6	<1	1	1	2	2	2	2	2
35–49	1	1.0	0	1	1	1	1	1	1	1
50–64	1	1.0	0	1	1	1	1	1	1	1
65+	0									
2. MULTIPLE DX										
0–19 Years	0									
20–34	5	1.1	<1	1	1	1	1	1	2	2
35–49	5	2.4	3	1	1	1	5	5	5	5
50–64	0									
65+	0									
TOTAL SINGLE DX	5	1.3	<1	1	1	1	2	2	2	2
MULTIPLE DX	10	1.6	2	1	1	1	1	5	5	5
TOTAL										
0–19 Years	0									
20–34	8	1.2	<1	1	1	1	1	2	2	2
35–49	6	2.2	3	1	1	1	5	5	5	5
50–64	1	1.0	0	1	1	1	1	1	1	1
65+	0									
GRAND TOTAL	15	1.5	1	1	1	1	1	2	5	5

Length of Stay by Diagnosis and Operation, United States, 1997

United States, October 1995–September 1996 Data, by Operation

64.1: PENILE DIAGNOSTIC PX. Formerly included in operation group(s) 676, 677.

Type of Patients	Observed Patients	Avg. Stay	Variance	10th	25th	50th	75th	90th	95th	99th
1. SINGLE DX										
0–19 Years	1	1.0	0	1	1	1	1	1	1	1
20–34	0									
35–49	2	2.5	<1	2	2	2	3	3	3	3
50–64	1	3.0	0	3	3	3	3	3	3	3
65+	2	3.5	<1	3	3	3	4	4	4	4
2. MULTIPLE DX										
0–19 Years	4	4.0	13	2	2	2	5	5	14	14
20–34	4	3.4	15	1	1	1	9	9	9	9
35–49	5	6.6	24	3	3	5	10	10	19	19
50–64	7	7.8	24	1	4	6	9	17	17	17
65+	28	8.4	75	1	3	5	10	27	27	36
TOTAL SINGLE DX	6	2.8	<1	1	2	3	3	4	4	4
MULTIPLE DX	48	7.2	53	1	2	5	9	19	27	28
TOTAL										
0–19 Years	5	3.7	12	1	1	2	5	5	14	14
20–34	4	3.4	15	1	1	1	9	9	9	9
35–49	7	5.9	23	3	3	3	7	10	19	19
50–64	8	7.2	23	3	4	6	9	17	17	17
65+	30	8.1	72	1	3	5	10	23	27	36
GRAND TOTAL	54	6.9	51	1	2	5	9	19	27	28

64.2: LOC EXC/DESTR PENILE LES. Formerly included in operation group(s) 676.

Type of Patients	Observed Patients	Avg. Stay	Variance	10th	25th	50th	75th	90th	95th	99th
1. SINGLE DX										
0–19 Years	6	1.6	<1	1	1	2	2	2	2	2
20–34	2	1.3	<1	1	1	2	2	2	2	2
35–49	16	1.7	<1	1	1	1	2	2	2	3
50–64	31	1.5	<1	1	1	1	2	2	3	3
65+	7	3.6	19	1	1	2	2	13	13	13
2. MULTIPLE DX										
0–19 Years	16	2.1	1	1	1	2	3	3	3	6
20–34	25	4.9	10	2	3	4	7	10	10	14
35–49	23	4.2	8	1	2	5	5	10	10	13
50–64	53	5.9	41	1	2	3	9	15	19	>99
65+	43	6.0	40	3	3	5	5	9	17	34
TOTAL SINGLE DX	62	1.8	3	1	1	2	2	2	3	13
MULTIPLE DX	160	5.1	27	1	2	4	5	10	13	34
TOTAL										
0–19 Years	22	2.0	<1	1	1	2	2	3	3	6
20–34	27	4.7	10	2	2	4	7	10	10	14
35–49	39	3.4	7	1	2	2	5	5	10	11
50–64	84	4.2	30	1	1	2	4	11	18	38
65+	50	5.8	38	2	3	5	5	9	17	34
GRAND TOTAL	222	4.3	24	1	2	3	5	10	12	27

63.9: OTH SPERM CORD/EPID OPS. Formerly included in operation group(s) 673.

Type of Patients	Observed Patients	Avg. Stay	Variance	10th	25th	50th	75th	90th	95th	99th
1. SINGLE DX										
0–19 Years	2	1.6	<1	1	1	2	2	2	2	2
20–34	1	1.0	0	1	1	1	1	1	1	1
35–49	1	2.0	0	2	2	2	2	2	2	2
50–64	0									
65+	0									
2. MULTIPLE DX										
0–19 Years	2	2.2	1	1	1	3	3	3	3	3
20–34	6	2.9	8	2	2	2	3	4	10	15
35–49	3	7.1	94	1	1	1	21	21	21	21
50–64	1	5.0	0	5	5	5	5	5	5	5
65+	3	3.7	2	1	3	5	5	5	5	5
TOTAL SINGLE DX	4	1.6	<1	1	1	2	2	2	2	2
MULTIPLE DX	15	3.6	17	1	2	2	3	5	15	21
TOTAL										
0–19 Years	4	1.8	<1	1	1	2	2	3	3	3
20–34	7	2.8	8	2	2	2	2	4	10	15
35–49	4	6.4	84	1	1	1	21	21	21	21
50–64	1	5.0	0	5	5	5	5	5	5	5
65+	3	3.7	2	1	3	5	5	5	5	5
GRAND TOTAL	19	3.3	16	1	2	2	3	5	15	21

64.0: CIRCUMCISION. Formerly included in operation group(s) 677.

Type of Patients	Observed Patients	Avg. Stay	Variance	10th	25th	50th	75th	90th	95th	99th
1. SINGLE DX										
0–19 Years	149248	1.7	<1	1	1	2	2	3	3	4
20–34	8	1.8	<1	1	1	2	2	3	3	3
35–49	3	1.2	<1	1	1	1	1	3	3	3
50–64	0									
65+	3	3.9	10	1	1	1	7	7	7	7
2. MULTIPLE DX										
0–19 Years	160519	2.7	17	1	1	2	3	4	6	19
20–34	20	3.2	9	1	2	2	3	6	9	16
35–49	54	5.0	19	1	2	5	6	8	16	22
50–64	59	6.9	78	1	1	4	11	14	22	64
65+	121	5.8	39	1	2	3	7	12	17	39
TOTAL SINGLE DX	149262	1.7	<1	1	1	2	2	3	3	4
MULTIPLE DX	160773	2.7	17	1	1	2	3	4	6	19
TOTAL										
0–19 Years	309767	2.2	9	1	1	2	2	3	4	12
20–34	28	2.9	8	1	2	2	3	6	9	16
35–49	57	4.6	18	1	1	3	6	8	12	22
50–64	59	6.9	78	1	1	4	11	14	22	64
65+	124	5.7	38	1	2	3	7	12	17	39
GRAND TOTAL	310035	2.2	9	1	1	2	2	3	4	12

Length of Stay by Diagnosis and Operation, United States, 1997

United States, October 1995–September 1996 Data, by Operation

64.3: AMPUTATION OF PENIS. Formerly included in operation group(s) 676.

Type of Patients	Observed Patients	Avg. Stay	Vari- ance	10th	25th	50th	75th	90th	95th	99th
1. SINGLE DX										
0–19 Years	1	2.0	0	2	2	2	2	2	2	2
20–34	0									
35–49	4	1.9	2	1	1	1	2	4	4	4
50–64	13	2.5	4	1	1	2	2	4	6	10
65+	8	5.4	4	1	6	6	6	6	7	9
2. MULTIPLE DX										
0–19 Years	2	10.2	80	1	1	17	17	17	17	17
20–34	3	4.6	8	1	1	6	7	7	7	7
35–49	8	12.0	287	1	2	3	21	21	57	57
50–64	43	10.2	135	2	2	5	11	37	37	38
65+	79	4.8	40	1	2	3	5	9	13	29
TOTAL SINGLE DX	26	3.8	6	1	2	4	6	6	7	10
MULTIPLE DX	135	7.2	92	1	2	4	8	17	37	38
TOTAL										
0–19 Years	3	7.2	64	1	1	2	17	17	17	17
20–34	3	4.6	8	1	1	6	7	7	7	7
35–49	12	9.0	222	1	2	2	10	21	57	57
50–64	56	8.8	119	1	2	4	11	37	37	38
65+	87	4.9	34	1	2	4	6	9	13	29
GRAND TOTAL	161	6.6	79	1	2	4	6	13	26	38

64.4: PENILE REP/PLASTIC OPS. Formerly included in operation group(s) 676.

Type of Patients	Observed Patients	Avg. Stay	Vari- ance	10th	25th	50th	75th	90th	95th	99th
1. SINGLE DX										
0–19 Years	43	1.5	2	1	1	1	1	2	4	9
20–34	40	1.8	<1	1	1	2	3	3	3	3
35–49	23	1.5	<1	1	1	1	1	2	3	4
50–64	21	1.2	<1	1	1	1	1	2	3	3
65+	2	2.0	0	2	2	2	2	2	2	2
2. MULTIPLE DX										
0–19 Years	84	3.2	23	1	1	2	3	7	11	35
20–34	35	2.6	6	1	1	2	2	8	9	9
35–49	40	8.6	245	1	2	3	6	23	64	65
50–64	45	2.8	4	1	2	3	4	4	5	11
65+	24	4.3	53	1	2	3	3	8	9	45
TOTAL SINGLE DX	129	1.6	<1	1	1	1	2	3	3	6
MULTIPLE DX	228	3.8	51	1	1	2	3	7	11	45
TOTAL										
0–19 Years	127	2.6	17	1	1	1	2	4	9	19
20–34	75	2.1	3	1	1	2	3	7	9	9
35–49	63	4.6	119	1	1	2	3	6	22	64
50–64	66	2.4	3	1	1	2	4	4	5	11
65+	26	4.2	51	1	2	3	3	8	9	45
GRAND TOTAL	357	2.9	32	1	1	2	3	4	8	23

64.5: SEX TRANSFORMATION NEC. Formerly included in operation group(s) 676.

Type of Patients	Observed Patients	Avg. Stay	Vari- ance	10th	25th	50th	75th	90th	95th	99th
1. SINGLE DX										
0–19 Years	0									
20–34	0									
35–49	0									
50–64	0									
65+	0									
2. MULTIPLE DX										
0–19 Years	0									
20–34	0									
35–49	0									
50–64	0									
65+	0									
TOTAL SINGLE DX	0									
MULTIPLE DX	0									
TOTAL										
0–19 Years	0									
20–34	0									
35–49	0									
50–64	0									
65+	0									
GRAND TOTAL	0									

64.9: OTHER MALE GENITAL OPS. Formerly included in operation group(s) 675, 676, 677.

Type of Patients	Observed Patients	Avg. Stay	Vari- ance	10th	25th	50th	75th	90th	95th	99th
1. SINGLE DX										
0–19 Years	25	1.4	<1	1	1	1	1	3	4	4
20–34	42	1.7	<1	1	1	2	2	3	3	4
35–49	114	1.8	1	1	1	1	2	3	4	7
50–64	200	1.7	1	1	1	1	2	3	3	8
65+	150	1.6	<1	1	1	1	2	2	3	5
2. MULTIPLE DX										
0–19 Years	134	3.0	10	1	1	2	3	5	11	19
20–34	131	3.4	18	1	1	2	4	7	11	24
35–49	481	2.3	5	1	1	1	2	4	6	12
50–64	1287	2.2	9	1	1	2	2	4	6	14
65+	1125	2.7	12	1	1	2	3	6	9	13
TOTAL SINGLE DX	531	1.7	1	1	1	1	2	3	4	7
MULTIPLE DX	3158	2.4	10	1	1	2	3	5	7	14
TOTAL										
0–19 Years	159	2.6	8	1	1	2	3	5	7	15
20–34	173	3.0	14	1	1	2	3	7	9	18
35–49	595	2.2	4	1	1	2	3	4	5	11
50–64	1487	2.1	8	1	1	1	2	4	6	13
65+	1275	2.5	11	1	1	2	3	5	8	13
GRAND TOTAL	3689	2.3	8	1	1	2	2	4	7	13

Length of Stay by Diagnosis and Operation

United States, October 1995–September 1996 Data, by Operation

64.95: INSERT/REPL NON-IPP NOS. Formerly included in operation group(s) 675.

Type of Patients	Observed Patients	Avg. Stay	Vari-ance	Percentiles						
				10th	25th	50th	75th	90th	95th	99th
1. SINGLE DX										
0–19 Years	0									
20–34	0									
35–49	9	1.6	<1	1	1	2	2	2	3	3
50–64	21	1.5	2	1	1	1	2	2	3	6
65+	27	1.7	<1	1	1	1	2	3	3	4
2. MULTIPLE DX										
0–19 Years	0									
20–34	8	1.3	<1	1	1	1	1	2	3	5
35–49	56	2.0	4	1	1	2	2	3	4	5
50–64	147	1.6	1	1	1	1	2	3	3	6
65+	108	1.6	1	1	1	1	2	3	4	7
TOTAL SINGLE DX	57	1.5	1	1	1	1	2	3	3	6
MULTIPLE DX	319	1.7	2	1	1	1	2	3	3	6
TOTAL										
0–19 Years	0									
20–34	8	1.3	<1	1	1	1	1	2	3	5
35–49	65	2.0	3	1	1	2	2	3	4	5
50–64	168	1.6	1	1	1	1	2	3	3	6
65+	135	1.7	1	1	1	1	2	3	4	7
GRAND TOTAL	376	1.7	2	1	1	1	2	3	3	6

64.97: INSERT OR REPL IPP. Formerly included in operation group(s) 675.

Type of Patients	Observed Patients	Avg. Stay	Vari-ance	Percentiles						
				10th	25th	50th	75th	90th	95th	99th
1. SINGLE DX										
0–19 Years	0									
20–34	6	1.6	<1	1	1	2	2	2	2	2
35–49	66	1.6	<1	1	1	1	2	2	3	4
50–64	144	1.4	<1	1	1	1	2	2	3	4
65+	104	1.5	<1	1	1	1	2	2	3	5
2. MULTIPLE DX										
0–19 Years	0									
20–34	39	2.7	3	1	1	2	4	5	6	8
35–49	285	1.9	2	1	1	2	2	3	3	9
50–64	913	1.7	1	1	1	1	2	3	4	6
65+	744	1.9	2	1	1	1	2	3	4	8
TOTAL SINGLE DX	320	1.5	<1	1	1	1	2	3	3	4
MULTIPLE DX	1981	1.8	2	1	1	1	2	3	4	7
TOTAL										
0–19 Years	0									
20–34	45	2.6	3	1	1	2	3	5	6	7
35–49	351	1.8	1	1	1	2	2	3	3	8
50–64	1057	1.7	1	1	1	1	2	3	4	6
65+	848	1.8	2	1	1	1	2	3	4	8
GRAND TOTAL	2301	1.7	1	1	1	1	2	3	4	7

64.96: RMVL INT PENILE PROSTH. Formerly included in operation group(s) 676.

Type of Patients	Observed Patients	Avg. Stay	Vari-ance	Percentiles						
				10th	25th	50th	75th	90th	95th	99th
1. SINGLE DX										
0–19 Years	0									
20–34	1	1.0	0	1	1	1	1	1	1	1
35–49	5	4.5	7	2	2	4	8	8	8	8
50–64	17	3.1	2	1	3	3	3	5	8	8
65+	14	1.7	1	1	1	2	2	2	2	10
2. MULTIPLE DX										
0–19 Years	0									
20–34	11	7.4	75	2	3	3	7	24	31	31
35–49	39	3.8	15	1	1	3	5	7	13	20
50–64	144	5.1	50	1	2	3	6	11	13	65
65+	152	3.9	39	1	1	2	4	8	12	21
TOTAL SINGLE DX	37	2.3	2	1	1	2	3	3	5	8
MULTIPLE DX	346	4.5	43	1	2	3	5	9	12	24
TOTAL										
0–19 Years	0									
20–34	12	6.8	72	1	3	3	7	24	24	31
35–49	44	3.8	15	1	2	3	5	8	12	20
50–64	161	4.8	42	1	2	3	5	10	13	23
65+	166	3.3	30	1	1	2	3	7	8	18
GRAND TOTAL	383	4.1	35	1	2	2	4	8	12	23

65.0: OOPHOROTOMY. Formerly included in operation group(s) 681.

Type of Patients	Observed Patients	Avg. Stay	Vari-ance	Percentiles						
				10th	25th	50th	75th	90th	95th	99th
1. SINGLE DX										
0–19 Years	22	1.4	<1	1	1	1	2	2	3	6
20–34	25	2.2	2	1	1	2	3	3	4	9
35–49	6	2.5	3	1	2	2	2	7	7	7
50–64	0									
65+	0									
2. MULTIPLE DX										
0–19 Years	29	3.8	3	2	3	3	5	7	7	7
20–34	135	3.0	6	1	1	3	4	6	8	12
35–49	61	2.2	5	1	1	1	3	5	6	16
50–64	3	10.9	26	1	5	14	14	14	14	14
65+	3	5.3	17	2	2	6	6	13	13	13
TOTAL SINGLE DX	53	2.0	2	1	1	2	2	3	4	9
MULTIPLE DX	231	3.0	7	1	1	2	4	6	8	14
TOTAL										
0–19 Years	51	3.1	4	1	1	3	5	7	7	7
20–34	160	2.8	5	1	1	2	3	6	8	12
35–49	67	2.2	5	1	1	1	3	5	6	16
50–64	3	10.9	26	1	5	14	14	14	14	14
65+	3	5.3	17	2	2	6	6	13	13	13
GRAND TOTAL	284	2.8	7	1	1	2	3	6	7	14

Length of Stay by Diagnosis and Operation, United States, 1997

United States, October 1995–September 1996 Data, by Operation

65.1: DXTIC PX ON OVARIES. Formerly included in operation group(s) 678, 681, 704.

Type of Patients	Observed Patients	Avg. Stay	Vari-ance	10th	25th	50th	75th	90th	95th	99th
1. SINGLE DX										
0–19 Years	6	2.3	<1	1	2	3	3	3	3	3
20–34	17	2.6	1	1	2	3	3	3	5	6
35–49	5	1.9	3	1	1	1	1	6	6	6
50–64	1	2.0	0	2	2	2	2	2	2	2
65+	3	2.5	<1	2	2	2	3	3	3	3
2. MULTIPLE DX										
0–19 Years	24	3.0	7	1	1	2	4	5	8	13
20–34	79	2.2	3	1	1	2	3	4	5	8
35–49	61	2.3	7	1	1	2	3	3	5	11
50–64	26	5.2	12	2	2	5	6	9	13	17
65+	27	12.0	55	5	7	9	18	23	27	32
TOTAL SINGLE DX	32	2.4	1	1	1	3	3	3	4	6
MULTIPLE DX	217	3.2	13	1	1	2	3	6	9	20
TOTAL										
0–19 Years	30	2.8	6	1	1	2	3	5	8	12
20–34	96	2.3	2	1	1	2	3	4	5	6
35–49	66	2.3	3	1	1	2	3	3	5	11
50–64	27	5.0	12	2	2	5	6	9	13	17
65+	30	10.9	58	5	5	9	17	20	27	32
GRAND TOTAL	249	3.1	12	1	1	2	3	5	9	19

65.22: OVARIAN WEDGE RESECTION. Formerly included in operation group(s) 678.

Type of Patients	Observed Patients	Avg. Stay	Vari-ance	10th	25th	50th	75th	90th	95th	99th
1. SINGLE DX										
0–19 Years	11	2.6	<1	2	2	3	3	3	3	3
20–34	39	1.8	2	1	2	1	3	3	3	9
35–49	9	2.0	<1	1	2	2	2	3	3	3
50–64	1	2.0	0	2	2	2	2	2	2	2
65+	1	6.0	0	6	6	6	6	6	6	6
2. MULTIPLE DX										
0–19 Years	30	2.5	<1	2	2	2	3	4	4	4
20–34	192	2.7	2	1	2	2	3	4	6	8
35–49	59	2.9	1	2	2	3	4	4	5	6
50–64	2	6.4	9	5	5	5	5	11	11	11
65+	2	4.2	3	3	3	3	6	6	6	6
TOTAL SINGLE DX	61	2.0	2	1	1	2	3	3	4	9
MULTIPLE DX	285	2.7	2	1	2	2	3	4	6	8
TOTAL										
0–19 Years	41	2.5	<1	2	2	3	3	3	4	4
20–34	231	2.5	3	1	1	2	3	4	6	9
35–49	68	2.8	1	1	2	3	4	5	5	6
50–64	3	5.5	10	2	5	5	6	11	11	11
65+	3	4.9	2	3	3	6	6	6	6	6
GRAND TOTAL	346	2.6	2	1	2	2	3	4	6	8

65.2: LOC EXC/DESTR OVARY LES. Formerly included in operation group(s) 678.

Type of Patients	Observed Patients	Avg. Stay	Vari-ance	10th	25th	50th	75th	90th	95th	99th
1. SINGLE DX										
0–19 Years	317	3.0	2	1	2	3	4	4	4	6
20–34	975	2.3	1	1	2	2	3	3	4	6
35–49	256	2.3	1	1	2	2	3	4	5	6
50–64	25	3.2	1	2	3	3	4	4	5	5
65+	12	4.3	5	1	2	4	6	8	8	9
2. MULTIPLE DX										
0–19 Years	553	2.6	3	1	1	2	3	4	5	8
20–34	3185	2.7	3	1	2	2	3	4	5	8
35–49	1499	3.1	7	1	2	2	3	5	7	12
50–64	165	5.3	19	2	2	4	7	10	13	18
65+	179	8.3	49	3	4	6	11	23	27	32
TOTAL SINGLE DX	1585	2.5	1	1	2	2	3	4	4	6
MULTIPLE DX	5581	3.0	6	1	2	3	3	5	7	13
TOTAL										
0–19 Years	870	2.7	2	1	2	2	4	4	5	7
20–34	4160	2.6	3	1	2	2	3	4	5	8
35–49	1755	3.0	6	1	2	3	3	5	7	10
50–64	190	5.0	18	2	2	4	6	10	13	18
65+	191	8.1	48	2	4	6	11	17	19	36
GRAND TOTAL	7166	2.9	5	1	2	2	3	5	6	19

65.29: LOC EXC/DESTR OV LES NEC. Formerly included in operation group(s) 678.

Type of Patients	Observed Patients	Avg. Stay	Vari-ance	10th	25th	50th	75th	90th	95th	99th
1. SINGLE DX										
0–19 Years	304	3.0	2	1	2	3	4	4	4	6
20–34	926	2.3	<1	1	2	2	3	3	4	5
35–49	245	2.4	1	1	2	2	4	4	5	5
50–64	24	3.2	1	2	3	3	4	4	5	5
65+	11	4.1	5	1	2	4	6	8	8	9
2. MULTIPLE DX										
0–19 Years	513	2.5	3	1	2	2	3	4	5	7
20–34	2973	2.7	3	2	2	2	3	4	5	8
35–49	1437	3.1	7	1	2	2	5	5	7	12
50–64	163	5.2	20	2	2	4	7	10	13	18
65+	177	8.4	50	3	4	6	11	17	19	36
TOTAL SINGLE DX	1510	2.5	1	1	2	2	3	4	4	5
MULTIPLE DX	5263	3.0	6	1	2	3	3	5	7	13
TOTAL										
0–19 Years	817	2.7	2	1	2	2	4	4	5	7
20–34	3899	2.6	3	1	2	3	3	4	5	8
35–49	1682	3.0	6	1	2	3	5	5	7	10
50–64	187	5.0	18	2	2	4	6	10	13	18
65+	188	8.2	48	2	4	6	11	17	19	36
GRAND TOTAL	6773	2.9	5	1	2	2	3	4	6	11

Length of Stay by Diagnosis and Operation, United States, 1997

United States, October 1995–September 1996 Data, by Operation

65.3: UNILATERAL OOPHORECTOMY. Formerly included in operation group(s) 679.

Type of Patients	Observed Patients	Avg. Stay	Vari-ance	10th	25th	50th	75th	90th	95th	99th
1. SINGLE DX										
0–19 Years	97	3.5	14	1	2	2	3	5	15	15
20–34	301	2.4	<1	1	2	2	3	3	4	5
35–49	169	2.4	<1	1	2	2	3	3	4	5
50–64	22	2.8	<1	2	3	3	3	3	4	5
65+	8	4.2	8	2	2	4	4	11	11	11
2. MULTIPLE DX										
0–19 Years	124	3.3	4	2	2	3	3	5	7	11
20–34	816	2.9	3	1	2	3	3	5	6	8
35–49	820	3.3	5	2	2	3	3	5	7	14
50–64	180	4.9	44	2	2	3	5	8	13	42
65+	185	6.1	21	2	3	4	8	13	15	21
TOTAL SINGLE DX	597	2.6	3	1	2	2	3	4	4	15
MULTIPLE DX	2125	3.4	8	2	2	3	3	6	8	14
TOTAL										
0–19 Years	221	3.4	8	1	2	3	3	5	11	15
20–34	1117	2.8	2	1	2	2	3	4	6	7
35–49	989	3.2	5	2	2	3	4	5	6	14
50–64	202	4.5	37	2	2	3	5	7	13	42
65+	193	6.1	21	2	3	4	8	12	15	21
GRAND TOTAL	2722	3.3	8	2	2	3	3	5	7	15

65.5: BILATERAL OOPHORECTOMY. Formerly included in operation group(s) 680.

Type of Patients	Observed Patients	Avg. Stay	Vari-ance	10th	25th	50th	75th	90th	95th	99th
1. SINGLE DX										
0–19 Years	4	1.7	6	1	1	1	1	1	10	10
20–34	12	2.6	1	1	2	2	3	4	5	5
35–49	21	1.9	1	1	1	2	3	4	4	5
50–64	11	3.2	3	1	2	3	3	7	7	7
65+	8	2.8	<1	2	2	3	4	4	4	4
2. MULTIPLE DX										
0–19 Years	9	4.2	6	2	2	4	8	8	8	8
20–34	85	2.5	1	2	2	2	3	4	5	6
35–49	280	3.7	7	2	2	3	4	6	9	14
50–64	131	4.1	11	2	3	3	4	7	8	21
65+	149	6.6	54	3	3	5	8	12	17	27
TOTAL SINGLE DX	56	2.3	2	1	1	2	3	4	5	7
MULTIPLE DX	654	3.9	15	2	2	3	4	7	10	17
TOTAL										
0–19 Years	13	3.6	7	1	1	2	5	8	8	10
20–34	97	2.5	1	2	2	2	3	4	5	6
35–49	301	3.5	6	2	2	3	4	6	9	14
50–64	142	4.0	11	2	3	3	4	7	8	21
65+	157	6.5	53	3	3	4	8	12	17	27
GRAND TOTAL	710	3.8	14	2	2	3	4	7	9	17

65.4: UNILATERAL S-O. Formerly included in operation group(s) 679.

Type of Patients	Observed Patients	Avg. Stay	Vari-ance	10th	25th	50th	75th	90th	95th	99th
1. SINGLE DX										
0–19 Years	152	3.2	2	2	2	3	4	5	5	11
20–34	498	2.4	1	1	2	2	3	4	4	6
35–49	411	2.4	2	1	2	2	3	4	4	7
50–64	87	2.8	2	1	2	2	3	4	4	7
65+	23	2.6	3	1	1	2	3	6	8	8
2. MULTIPLE DX										
0–19 Years	345	4.2	13	2	2	3	5	7	9	19
20–34	2498	3.2	3	2	2	3	4	5	7	10
35–49	3198	3.2	6	1	2	3	4	5	7	12
50–64	647	3.8	10	1	2	3	4	7	10	17
65+	546	5.7	26	2	3	4	7	10	13	25
TOTAL SINGLE DX	1171	2.6	2	1	2	2	3	4	5	7
MULTIPLE DX	7234	3.4	7	2	2	3	4	6	8	13
TOTAL										
0–19 Years	497	3.9	10	2	2	3	4	7	9	13
20–34	2996	3.0	3	2	2	3	3	5	6	9
35–49	3609	3.1	5	1	2	3	4	5	7	12
50–64	734	3.7	9	1	2	3	4	6	10	15
65+	569	5.5	26	2	3	4	7	10	12	25
GRAND TOTAL	8405	3.3	7	1	2	3	4	5	8	12

65.51: RMVL BOTH OV-SAME OP. Formerly included in operation group(s) 680.

Type of Patients	Observed Patients	Avg. Stay	Vari-ance	10th	25th	50th	75th	90th	95th	99th
1. SINGLE DX										
0–19 Years	4	1.7	6	1	1	1	1	1	10	10
20–34	8	2.0	<1	1	1	2	2	4	4	4
35–49	12	1.5	<1	1	1	1	2	2	4	4
50–64	11	3.2	3	1	2	3	3	7	7	7
65+	7	3.1	<1	2	2	3	4	4	4	4
2. MULTIPLE DX										
0–19 Years	9	4.2	6	2	2	4	8	8	8	8
20–34	47	2.8	1	2	2	3	3	4	5	7
35–49	181	3.8	7	2	2	3	4	7	12	14
50–64	108	3.9	10	1	3	3	4	7	8	14
65+	123	7.2	66	3	3	5	8	14	19	27
TOTAL SINGLE DX	42	2.1	2	1	1	2	3	4	4	7
MULTIPLE DX	468	4.3	20	2	2	3	4	8	12	19
TOTAL										
0–19 Years	13	3.6	7	1	1	2	5	8	8	10
20–34	55	2.6	1	2	2	3	3	4	5	7
35–49	193	3.6	7	1	2	3	4	6	12	14
50–64	119	3.9	9	1	3	3	4	7	8	13
65+	130	7.1	65	2	3	5	8	14	19	27
GRAND TOTAL	510	4.2	19	2	2	3	4	8	12	19

Length of Stay by Diagnosis and Operation, United States, 1997

United States, October 1995–September 1996 Data, by Operation

65.52: RMVL REMAINING OVARY. Formerly included in operation group(s) 680.

Type of Patients	Observed Patients	Avg. Stay	Variance	10th	25th	50th	75th	90th	95th	99th
1. SINGLE DX										
0–19 Years	0									
20–34	4	3.4	<1	3	3	3	3	5	5	5
35–49	9	2.6	<1	2	2	2	3	4	5	5
50–64	0									
65+	1	2.0	0	2	2	2	2	2	2	2
2. MULTIPLE DX										
0–19 Years	0									
20–34	38	2.4	1	2	2	2	2	5	5	6
35–49	99	3.5	5	1	2	3	4	6	9	9
50–64	23	5.2	22	2	3	3	5	8	21	21
65+	26	4.5	7	3	3	3	6	8	10	15
TOTAL SINGLE DX	14	2.8	<1	2	2	3	3	5	5	5
MULTIPLE DX	186	3.2	5	2	2	2	4	5	8	10
TOTAL										
0–19 Years	0									
20–34	42	2.5	1	2	2	2	3	5	5	6
35–49	108	3.4	5	2	2	3	4	6	9	9
50–64	23	5.2	22	3	3	3	5	8	21	21
65+	27	4.5	7	3	3	3	6	8	10	15
GRAND TOTAL	200	3.2	5	2	2	2	4	5	8	10

65.61: RMVL BOTH OV & FALL-1 OP. Formerly included in operation group(s) 680.

Type of Patients	Observed Patients	Avg. Stay	Variance	10th	25th	50th	75th	90th	95th	99th
1. SINGLE DX										
0–19 Years	4	3.2	2	2	2	4	4	5	5	5
20–34	40	2.6	<1	2	2	3	3	3	4	4
35–49	124	2.7	1	2	2	3	3	4	5	7
50–64	159	2.7	1	2	3	3	3	3	5	7
65+	68	3.5	2	2	3	3	4	5	6	7
2. MULTIPLE DX										
0–19 Years	7	4.2	5	1	3	4	6	6	9	9
20–34	558	3.4	6	2	2	3	4	6	10	12
35–49	2774	3.5	9	2	2	3	4	5	8	14
50–64	1876	4.3	17	2	3	3	5	8	11	26
65+	1540	6.1	33	2	3	4	7	11	15	39
TOTAL SINGLE DX	395	2.8	1	2	2	3	3	4	5	7
MULTIPLE DX	6755	4.2	16	2	2	3	4	8	10	22
TOTAL										
0–19 Years	11	3.6	3	2	2	4	4	6	6	9
20–34	598	3.3	5	2	2	3	4	6	9	12
35–49	2898	3.4	9	2	2	3	4	5	8	14
50–64	2035	4.2	16	2	3	3	5	7	10	26
65+	1608	6.0	32	2	3	4	7	11	15	39
GRAND TOTAL	7150	4.1	16	2	2	3	4	8	10	22

65.6: BILAT SALPINGO-OOPHORECT. Formerly included in operation group(s) 680.

Type of Patients	Observed Patients	Avg. Stay	Variance	10th	25th	50th	75th	90th	95th	99th
1. SINGLE DX										
0–19 Years	4	3.2	2	2	2	4	4	5	5	5
20–34	50	2.7	<1	2	2	3	3	4	5	5
35–49	150	2.7	1	2	2	3	3	4	4	5
50–64	168	2.7	1	2	2	3	3	4	4	7
65+	69	3.5	2	3	3	3	4	5	6	7
2. MULTIPLE DX										
0–19 Years	8	4.1	5	1	3	4	6	6	9	9
20–34	766	3.2	5	2	2	3	4	5	9	11
35–49	3248	3.5	9	2	2	3	4	6	8	14
50–64	1998	4.3	17	2	3	3	4	7	11	26
65+	1641	5.9	31	2	3	4	7	11	15	39
TOTAL SINGLE DX	441	2.8	1	2	2	3	3	4	5	7
MULTIPLE DX	7661	4.1	15	2	2	3	4	7	10	21
TOTAL										
0–19 Years	12	3.6	5	2	2	4	4	6	6	9
20–34	816	3.2	5	2	2	3	4	5	8	11
35–49	3398	3.4	8	2	2	3	4	5	8	14
50–64	2166	4.1	15	2	2	3	4	7	10	26
65+	1710	5.9	31	3	3	4	7	11	15	39
GRAND TOTAL	8102	4.0	14	2	2	3	4	7	10	20

65.62: RMVL REM OVARY & TUBE. Formerly included in operation group(s) 680.

Type of Patients	Observed Patients	Avg. Stay	Variance	10th	25th	50th	75th	90th	95th	99th
1. SINGLE DX										
0–19 Years	0									
20–34	10	3.2	1	2	2	4	4	5	5	5
35–49	26	2.5	<1	2	2	2	3	4	5	5
50–64	9	2.4	<1	2	2	2	3	3	3	5
65+	1	2.0	0	2	2	2	2	2	2	2
2. MULTIPLE DX										
0–19 Years	1	3.0	0	3	3	3	3	3	3	3
20–34	208	2.7	3	1	2	2	3	4	5	10
35–49	474	3.3	7	1	2	3	4	5	7	21
50–64	122	3.4	9	2	3	4	4	5	7	14
65+	101	4.4	9	2	3	4	4	7	11	20
TOTAL SINGLE DX	46	2.8	1	2	2	2	3	4	5	5
MULTIPLE DX	906	3.2	6	1	2	3	4	5	7	13
TOTAL										
0–19 Years	1	3.0	0	3	3	3	3	3	3	3
20–34	218	2.8	2	2	2	2	3	4	5	10
35–49	500	3.3	7	1	2	3	4	5	7	21
50–64	131	3.3	8	2	2	3	3	5	7	14
65+	102	4.4	9	2	3	4	4	7	11	20
GRAND TOTAL	952	3.2	6	1	2	3	4	5	7	12

Length of Stay by Diagnosis and Operation, United States, 1997

United States, October 1995–September 1996 Data, by Operation

65.7: REPAIR OF OVARY. Formerly included in operation group(s) 681.

Type of Patients	Observed Patients	Avg. Stay	Vari-ance	10th	25th	50th	75th	90th	95th	99th
1. SINGLE DX										
0–19 Years	11	5.4	28	1	1	3	14	14	14	14
20–34	17	2.3	<1	2	2	2	3	3	3	5
35–49	5	2.1	<1	2	2	2	2	3	3	3
50–64	0									
65+	0									
2. MULTIPLE DX										
0–19 Years	18	2.0	2	1	1	1	3	4	5	7
20–34	61	3.4	19	1	2	3	4	5	5	36
35–49	21	2.9	<1	2	2	3	3	4	4	4
50–64	0									
65+	0									
TOTAL SINGLE DX	33	4.1	19	1	2	2	3	14	14	14
MULTIPLE DX	100	3.0	12	1	2	3	4	5	5	7
TOTAL										
0–19 Years	29	4.0	20	1	1	2	4	14	14	14
20–34	78	3.2	15	1	2	3	4	5	5	36
35–49	26	2.8	<1	2	2	3	3	4	4	4
50–64	0									
65+	0									
GRAND TOTAL	133	3.4	15	1	2	3	4	5	14	14

65.9: OTHER OVARIAN OPERATIONS. Formerly included in operation group(s) 681.

Type of Patients	Observed Patients	Avg. Stay	Vari-ance	10th	25th	50th	75th	90th	95th	99th
1. SINGLE DX										
0–19 Years	62	1.9	2	1	1	1	3	3	3	5
20–34	90	2.0	2	1	1	2	3	4	5	5
35–49	22	2.1	2	1	1	2	3	4	5	8
50–64	2	7.0	7	1	8	8	8	8	8	8
65+	0									
2. MULTIPLE DX										
0–19 Years	83	2.5	6	1	1	2	3	4	5	8
20–34	348	3.4	13	1	1	2	4	7	9	21
35–49	175	3.7	13	1	2	3	5	7	11	23
50–64	7	3.3	3	1	2	3	5	5	5	5
65+	8	4.3	12	3	3	3	4	8	9	19
TOTAL SINGLE DX	176	2.0	2	1	1	2	3	3	5	8
MULTIPLE DX	621	3.3	12	1	1	2	4	7	9	21
TOTAL										
0–19 Years	145	2.2	4	1	1	2	3	4	4	7
20–34	438	3.0	10	1	1	2	3	6	8	21
35–49	197	3.5	12	1	2	3	4	7	11	23
50–64	9	4.8	7	1	2	5	8	8	8	8
65+	8	4.3	12	3	3	3	4	8	9	19
GRAND TOTAL	797	3.0	9	1	1	2	3	6	8	21

65.8: TUBO-OVARIAN ADHESIO. Formerly included in operation group(s) 681.

Type of Patients	Observed Patients	Avg. Stay	Vari-ance	10th	25th	50th	75th	90th	95th	99th
1. SINGLE DX										
0–19 Years	3	2.4	<1	1	2	3	3	3	3	3
20–34	17	2.1	3	1	2	2	2	3	3	8
35–49	16	2.5	<1	1	2	3	3	3	3	3
50–64	2	3.0	0	3	3	3	3	3	3	3
65+	1	5.0	0	5	5	5	5	5	5	5
2. MULTIPLE DX										
0–19 Years	33	3.5	3	1	2	3	5	5	7	8
20–34	417	2.6	2	1	2	3	3	4	5	9
35–49	290	2.8	3	1	2	3	3	4	5	8
50–64	49	3.7	4	2	3	4	4	6	7	11
65+	17	6.7	74	2	3	4	7	9	13	42
TOTAL SINGLE DX	39	2.3	<1	1	2	2	3	3	3	5
MULTIPLE DX	806	2.8	4	1	2	3	3	4	5	9
TOTAL										
0–19 Years	36	3.4	3	1	2	3	5	5	7	8
20–34	434	2.6	2	1	2	3	3	4	5	9
35–49	306	2.8	3	1	2	3	3	4	5	8
50–64	51	3.7	4	2	3	4	4	6	7	11
65+	18	6.7	72	2	3	4	7	9	13	42
GRAND TOTAL	845	2.8	4	1	2	3	3	4	5	9

65.91: ASPIRATION OF OVARY. Formerly included in operation group(s) 681.

Type of Patients	Observed Patients	Avg. Stay	Vari-ance	10th	25th	50th	75th	90th	95th	99th
1. SINGLE DX										
0–19 Years	56	2.3	2	1	1	2	3	3	3	5
20–34	78	2.1	2	1	1	1	3	4	5	5
35–49	18	2.2	2	1	1	2	2	4	5	5
50–64	2	7.0	7	8	8	8	8	8	8	8
65+	0									
2. MULTIPLE DX										
0–19 Years	70	2.5	6	1	1	2	3	4	5	8
20–34	308	3.1	7	1	1	2	4	7	8	11
35–49	164	3.8	14	1	2	3	4	8	11	23
50–64	7	3.3	3	1	3	3	5	5	5	5
65+	7	4.2	12	3	3	3	6	9	8	19
TOTAL SINGLE DX	154	2.2	2	1	1	2	3	4	5	8
MULTIPLE DX	556	3.2	9	1	1	2	4	6	8	12
TOTAL										
0–19 Years	126	2.4	5	1	1	2	3	4	4	7
20–34	386	2.8	6	1	1	2	3	6	7	11
35–49	182	3.6	13	2	2	3	4	7	11	23
50–64	9	4.8	7	1	2	5	8	8	8	8
65+	7	4.2	12	3	3	3	6	9	8	19
GRAND TOTAL	710	2.9	7	1	1	2	3	6	8	12

Length of Stay by Diagnosis and Operation, United States, 1997

United States, October 1995–September 1996 Data, by Operation

66.0: SALPINGOSTOMY/SALPINGOT. Formerly included in operation group(s) 684.

Type of Patients	Observed Patients	Avg. Stay	Vari-ance	Percentiles						
				10th	25th	50th	75th	90th	95th	99th
1. SINGLE DX										
0–19 Years	58	1.7	<1	1	1	1	2	3	3	4
20–34	643	1.6	<1	1	1	1	2	3	3	4
35–49	106	2.1	<1	1	1	2	3	3	3	5
50–64	0									
65+	0									
2. MULTIPLE DX										
0–19 Years	88	2.1	3	1	1	1	2	5	7	7
20–34	903	2.2	2	1	1	2	3	4	4	9
35–49	200	2.3	2	1	1	2	3	5	5	7
50–64	2	5.8	4	4	4	7	7	7	7	7
65+	1	1.0	0	1	1	1	1	1	1	1
TOTAL SINGLE DX	807	1.7	<1	1	1	1	2	3	3	4
MULTIPLE DX	1194	2.2	2	1	1	2	3	4	5	9
TOTAL										
0–19 Years	146	1.9	2	1	1	1	2	3	5	7
20–34	1546	1.9	2	1	1	2	2	3	4	7
35–49	306	2.2	2	1	1	2	3	5	5	6
50–64	2	5.8	4	4	4	7	7	7	7	7
65+	1	1.0	0	1	1	1	1	1	1	1
GRAND TOTAL	2001	2.0	2	1	1	2	2	3	4	7

66.01: SALPINGOTOMY. Formerly included in operation group(s) 684.

Type of Patients	Observed Patients	Avg. Stay	Vari-ance	Percentiles						
				10th	25th	50th	75th	90th	95th	99th
1. SINGLE DX										
0–19 Years	5	1.4	<1	1	1	1	1	3	3	3
20–34	58	1.7	1	1	1	1	2	3	3	5
35–49	17	1.7	<1	1	1	2	2	2	3	4
50–64	0									
65+	0									
2. MULTIPLE DX										
0–19 Years	15	3.2	7	1	1	2	6	7	7	9
20–34	130	2.9	4	1	2	2	3	6	8	9
35–49	34	2.1	2	1	1	2	2	4	4	8
50–64	1	4.0	0	4	4	4	4	4	4	4
65+	0									
TOTAL SINGLE DX	80	1.7	1	1	1	1	2	3	4	5
MULTIPLE DX	180	2.8	4	1	1	2	3	5	7	9
TOTAL										
0–19 Years	20	2.5	5	1	1	1	3	7	7	9
20–34	188	2.6	3	1	1	2	3	5	7	9
35–49	51	2.0	1	1	1	2	2	4	4	8
50–64	1	4.0	0	4	4	4	4	4	4	4
65+	0									
GRAND TOTAL	260	2.5	3	1	1	2	3	4	7	9

66.02: SALPINGOSTOMY. Formerly included in operation group(s) 684.

Type of Patients	Observed Patients	Avg. Stay	Vari-ance	Percentiles						
				10th	25th	50th	75th	90th	95th	99th
1. SINGLE DX										
0–19 Years	53	1.7	<1	1	1	1	2	3	3	4
20–34	585	1.6	<1	1	1	1	2	3	3	4
35–49	89	2.1	<1	1	1	2	3	3	3	5
50–64	0									
65+	0									
2. MULTIPLE DX										
0–19 Years	73	1.9	2	1	1	1	2	4	5	7
20–34	773	2.0	2	1	1	2	2	4	4	7
35–49	166	2.3	2	1	1	2	3	5	5	6
50–64	1	7.0	0	7	7	7	7	7	7	7
65+	1	1.0	0	1	1	1	1	1	1	1
TOTAL SINGLE DX	727	1.7	<1	1	1	1	2	3	3	4
MULTIPLE DX	1014	2.0	2	1	1	2	2	4	4	7
TOTAL										
0–19 Years	126	1.8	1	1	1	1	2	3	4	7
20–34	1358	1.8	1	1	1	2	2	3	4	5
35–49	255	2.2	2	1	1	2	3	4	5	6
50–64	1	7.0	0	7	7	7	7	7	7	7
65+	1	1.0	0	1	1	1	1	1	1	1
GRAND TOTAL	1741	1.9	1	1	1	2	2	3	4	5

66.1: FALLOPIAN TUBE DXTIC PX. Formerly included in operation group(s) 684, 704.

Type of Patients	Observed Patients	Avg. Stay	Vari-ance	Percentiles						
				10th	25th	50th	75th	90th	95th	99th
1. SINGLE DX										
0–19 Years	0									
20–34	1	3.0	0	3	3	3	3	3	3	3
35–49	0									
50–64	0									
65+	0									
2. MULTIPLE DX										
0–19 Years	1	2.0	0	2	2	2	2	2	2	2
20–34	6	2.4	3	2	2	2	2	2	8	8
35–49	5	3.8	2	2	3	4	5	5	5	5
50–64	3	3.2	1	2	3	3	3	4	4	5
65+	1	10.0	0	10	10	10	10	10	10	10
TOTAL SINGLE DX	1	3.0	0	3	3	3	3	3	3	3
MULTIPLE DX	16	3.0	5	2	2	2	3	5	8	10
TOTAL										
0–19 Years	1	2.0	0	2	2	2	2	2	2	2
20–34	7	2.5	3	2	2	2	2	3	8	8
35–49	5	3.8	2	2	3	4	5	5	5	5
50–64	3	3.2	1	2	3	3	3	4	5	5
65+	1	10.0	0	10	10	10	10	10	10	10
GRAND TOTAL	17	3.0	5	2	2	2	3	5	8	10

Length of Stay by Diagnosis and Operation, United States, 1997

United States, October 1995–September 1996 Data, by Operation

66.2: BILAT ENDO OCCL FALL. Formerly included in operation group(s) 682.

Type of Patients	Observed Patients	Avg. Stay	Vari-ance	10th	25th	50th	75th	90th	95th	99th
1. SINGLE DX										
0–19 Years	0									
20–34	43	1.6	<1	1	1	1	2	3	3	5
35–49	12	1.4	<1	1	1	1	2	2	2	2
50–64	0									
65+	0									
2. MULTIPLE DX										
0–19 Years	4	2.9	1	2	2	2	4	4	4	4
20–34	1041	1.9	<1	1	1	2	2	3	3	5
35–49	262	1.8	2	1	1	1	2	3	4	10
50–64	1	1.0	0	1	1	1	1	1	1	1
65+	0									
TOTAL SINGLE DX	55	1.6	<1	1	1	1	2	2	3	5
MULTIPLE DX	1308	1.9	1	1	1	2	2	3	3	5
TOTAL										
0–19 Years	4	2.9	1	2	2	2	4	4	4	4
20–34	1084	1.9	<1	1	1	2	2	3	3	5
35–49	274	1.8	2	1	1	1	2	3	4	10
50–64	1	1.0	0	1	1	1	1	1	1	1
65+	0									
GRAND TOTAL	1363	1.9	1	1	1	2	2	3	3	5

66.22: BILAT ENDO LIG/DIV FALL. Formerly included in operation group(s) 682.

Type of Patients	Observed Patients	Avg. Stay	Vari-ance	10th	25th	50th	75th	90th	95th	99th
1. SINGLE DX										
0–19 Years	0									
20–34	10	2.3	1	1	2	2	2	5	5	5
35–49	4	1.6	<1	1	1	2	2	2	2	2
50–64	0									
65+	0									
2. MULTIPLE DX										
0–19 Years	0									
20–34	277	2.0	<1	1	1	2	2	3	3	5
35–49	71	1.7	<1	1	1	2	2	3	3	3
50–64	0									
65+	0									
TOTAL SINGLE DX	14	2.3	1	1	2	2	2	3	5	5
MULTIPLE DX	348	2.0	<1	1	1	2	2	3	3	4
TOTAL										
0–19 Years	0									
20–34	287	2.0	<1	1	1	2	2	3	3	5
35–49	75	1.7	<1	1	1	2	2	3	3	3
50–64	0									
65+	0									
GRAND TOTAL	362	2.0	<1	1	1	2	2	3	3	5

66.29: BILAT ENDO OCCL FALL NEC. Formerly included in operation group(s) 682.

Type of Patients	Observed Patients	Avg. Stay	Vari-ance	10th	25th	50th	75th	90th	95th	99th
1. SINGLE DX										
0–19 Years	0									
20–34	32	1.4	<1	1	1	1	2	2	3	4
35–49	8	1.3	<1	1	1	1	2	2	2	2
50–64	0									
65+	0									
2. MULTIPLE DX										
0–19 Years	4	2.9	1	2	2	2	4	4	4	4
20–34	749	1.8	<1	1	1	2	2	3	3	6
35–49	190	1.9	3	1	1	1	2	3	5	11
50–64	1	1.0	0	1	1	1	1	1	1	1
65+	0									
TOTAL SINGLE DX	40	1.4	<1	1	1	1	2	2	3	4
MULTIPLE DX	944	1.8	1	1	1	2	2	3	3	7
TOTAL										
0–19 Years	4	2.9	1	2	2	2	4	4	4	4
20–34	781	1.8	<1	1	1	2	2	3	3	6
35–49	198	1.9	3	1	1	1	2	3	5	10
50–64	1	1.0	0	1	1	1	1	1	1	1
65+	0									
GRAND TOTAL	984	1.8	1	1	1	2	2	3	3	7

66.3: OTH BILAT FALL DESTR/EXC. Formerly included in operation group(s) 683.

Type of Patients	Observed Patients	Avg. Stay	Vari-ance	10th	25th	50th	75th	90th	95th	99th
1. SINGLE DX										
0–19 Years	1	2.0	0	2	2	2	2	2	2	2
20–34	328	2.0	<1	1	1	2	2	3	4	5
35–49	70	2.2	<1	1	2	2	3	3	3	4
50–64	1	1.0	0	1	1	1	1	1	1	1
65+	0									
2. MULTIPLE DX										
0–19 Years	44	3.3	26	1	2	2	3	3	7	29
20–34	16091	1.8	<1	1	1	2	2	3	3	3
35–49	3783	2.0	1	1	2	2	2	3	3	5
50–64	4	1.6	<1	1	1	2	2	2	2	2
65+	0									
TOTAL SINGLE DX	400	2.0	<1	1	1	2	2	3	4	5
MULTIPLE DX	19922	1.9	1	1	1	2	2	3	3	4
TOTAL										
0–19 Years	45	3.2	26	1	2	2	3	3	7	29
20–34	16419	1.8	<1	1	1	2	2	3	3	4
35–49	3853	2.0	1	1	2	2	2	3	3	5
50–64	5	1.5	<1	1	1	1	2	2	2	2
65+	0									
GRAND TOTAL	20322	1.9	1	1	1	2	2	3	3	4

United States, October 1995–September 1996 Data, by Operation

66.32: BILAT FALL LIG & DIV NEC. Formerly included in operation group(s) 683.

Type of Patients	Observed Patients	Avg. Stay	Variance	Percentiles 10th	25th	50th	75th	90th	95th	99th
1. SINGLE DX										
0–19 Years	1	2.0	0	2	2	2	2	2	2	2
20–34	168	1.8	<1	1	1	2	2	3	4	5
35–49	38	2.4	<1	1	2	2	3	3	3	3
50–64	0									
65+	0									
2. MULTIPLE DX										
0–19 Years	32	2.4	1	1	1	2	3	3	3	7
20–34	10088	1.8	<1	1	1	2	2	3	3	4
35–49	2439	2.0	2	1	2	2	2	3	3	5
50–64	4	1.6	<1	1	1	2	2	2	2	2
65+	0									
TOTAL SINGLE DX	207	1.9	<1	1	1	2	2	3	4	5
MULTIPLE DX	12563	1.8	1	1	1	2	2	3	3	4
TOTAL										
0–19 Years	33	2.4	1	2	2	2	3	3	3	7
20–34	10256	1.8	<1	1	1	2	2	3	3	4
35–49	2477	2.0	1	1	2	2	2	3	3	5
50–64	4	1.6	<1	1	1	2	2	2	2	2
65+	0									
GRAND TOTAL	12770	1.8	1	1	1	2	2	3	3	4

66.4: TOT UNILAT SALPINGECTOMY. Formerly included in operation group(s) 684.

Type of Patients	Observed Patients	Avg. Stay	Variance	Percentiles 10th	25th	50th	75th	90th	95th	99th
1. SINGLE DX										
0–19 Years	12	2.9	4	1	1	2	4	8	8	8
20–34	61	2.2	1	1	1	2	3	4	4	8
35–49	39	2.4	2	1	2	2	3	3	6	6
50–64	3	2.2	<1	2	2	2	2	2	4	4
65+	0									
2. MULTIPLE DX										
0–19 Years	41	2.4	1	2	2	2	3	5	5	6
20–34	292	2.8	2	2	2	3	3	5	6	8
35–49	192	3.9	7	1	2	3	6	8	8	11
50–64	20	3.9	5	2	3	3	5	8	9	8
65+	11	3.4	12	2	2	2	4	5	9	23
TOTAL SINGLE DX	115	2.3	2	1	1	2	3	4	5	8
MULTIPLE DX	556	3.2	4	1	2	3	4	6	8	9
TOTAL										
0–19 Years	53	2.5	2	1	2	2	3	4	5	8
20–34	353	2.7	2	1	2	2	3	4	6	8
35–49	231	3.8	6	1	2	3	5	8	8	11
50–64	23	3.6	4	2	3	3	4	8	9	8
65+	11	3.4	12	2	2	2	4	5	9	23
GRAND TOTAL	671	3.1	4	1	2	3	4	6	8	8

66.39: BILAT FALL DESTR NEC. Formerly included in operation group(s) 683.

Type of Patients	Observed Patients	Avg. Stay	Variance	Percentiles 10th	25th	50th	75th	90th	95th	99th
1. SINGLE DX										
0–19 Years	0									
20–34	159	2.2	<1	2	2	2	2	3	3	6
35–49	32	2.0	<1	1	1	2	2	3	4	4
50–64	1	1.0	0	1	1	1	1	1	1	1
65+	0									
2. MULTIPLE DX										
0–19 Years	12	6.4	107	1	1	2	4	29	29	29
20–34	5964	1.9	<1	1	1	2	2	3	3	4
35–49	1337	2.1	1	1	2	2	2	3	4	5
50–64	0									
65+	0									
TOTAL SINGLE DX	192	2.2	<1	1	2	2	3	3	4	4
MULTIPLE DX	7313	1.9	1	1	1	2	2	3	3	4
TOTAL										
0–19 Years	12	6.4	107	1	1	2	4	29	29	29
20–34	6123	1.9	<1	1	1	2	2	3	3	4
35–49	1369	2.1	1	1	1	2	2	3	4	5
50–64	1	1.0	0	1	1	1	1	1	1	1
65+	0									
GRAND TOTAL	7505	1.9	1	1	1	2	2	3	3	4

66.5: TOT BILAT SALPINGECTOMY. Formerly included in operation group(s) 683.

Type of Patients	Observed Patients	Avg. Stay	Variance	Percentiles 10th	25th	50th	75th	90th	95th	99th
1. SINGLE DX										
0–19 Years	3	1.5	1	1	1	1	1	4	4	4
20–34	19	1.8	2	1	1	1	3	3	3	7
35–49	14	2.6	2	1	1	3	3	4	4	7
50–64	0									
65+	0									
2. MULTIPLE DX										
0–19 Years	4	4.3	2	4	4	4	6	6	6	6
20–34	134	2.8	4	1	2	2	3	4	6	14
35–49	100	3.0	3	1	2	3	4	5	6	8
50–64	11	2.3	2	2	2	3	4	4	5	5
65+	11	4.2	6	3	3	4	4	10	10	10
TOTAL SINGLE DX	36	2.1	1	1	1	1	3	4	4	7
MULTIPLE DX	260	2.9	4	1	2	3	4	5	6	14
TOTAL										
0–19 Years	7	3.2	4	1	1	4	4	6	6	6
20–34	153	2.7	4	1	2	2	3	5	6	14
35–49	114	2.9	3	1	2	3	3	5	6	8
50–64	11	2.3	2	2	2	3	4	4	5	5
65+	11	4.2	6	3	3	4	4	10	10	10
GRAND TOTAL	296	2.8	4	1	2	3	3	4	6	10

Length of Stay by Diagnosis and Operation, United States, 1997

United States, October 1995–September 1996 Data, by Operation

66.6: OTHER SALPINGECTOMY. Formerly included in operation group(s) 683, 684.

Type of Patients	Observed Patients	Avg. Stay	Variance	Percentiles						
				10th	25th	50th	75th	90th	95th	99th
1. SINGLE DX										
0–19 Years	127	1.9	<1	1	1	2	2	3	4	4
20–34	1691	1.9	<1	1	1	2	2	3	4	5
35–49	469	2.0	<1	1	1	2	3	3	4	4
50–64	6	1.1	<1	1	1	1	1	1	2	3
65+	0									
2. MULTIPLE DX										
0–19 Years	253	2.6	2	1	2	3	3	4	4	8
20–34	3590	2.5	2	1	2	3	3	4	4	6
35–49	1314	2.7	4	1	1	2	3	5	6	11
50–64	30	4.1	4	2	3	3	6	8	8	9
65+	16	5.3	27	2	3	4	5	9	12	30
TOTAL SINGLE DX	2293	1.9	<1	1	1	2	3	3	4	5
MULTIPLE DX	5203	2.5	2	1	2	2	3	4	5	8
TOTAL										
0–19 Years	380	2.3	2	1	1	2	3	4	4	8
20–34	5281	2.3	2	1	1	2	3	4	4	6
35–49	1783	2.5	3	1	1	2	3	5	6	8
50–64	36	2.9	5	1	1	2	3	7	8	8
65+	16	5.3	27	2	3	4	5	9	12	30
GRAND TOTAL	7496	2.4	2	1	1	2	3	4	4	7

66.62: RMVL FALL & TUBAL PREG. Formerly included in operation group(s) 684.

Type of Patients	Observed Patients	Avg. Stay	Variance	Percentiles						
				10th	25th	50th	75th	90th	95th	99th
1. SINGLE DX										
0–19 Years	91	1.8	<1	1	1	2	2	3	4	5
20–34	1565	1.9	<1	1	1	2	3	3	4	5
35–49	415	2.0	<1	1	1	2	3	3	4	4
50–64	0									
65+	0									
2. MULTIPLE DX										
0–19 Years	181	2.6	2	1	2	3	3	4	4	8
20–34	3094	2.5	2	1	2	3	3	4	4	6
35–49	1047	2.5	3	1	1	2	3	4	6	8
50–64	1	1.0	0	1	1	1	1	1	1	1
65+	0									
TOTAL SINGLE DX	2071	2.0	<1	1	1	2	3	3	4	5
MULTIPLE DX	4323	2.5	2	1	1	2	3	4	5	7
TOTAL										
0–19 Years	272	2.3	2	1	1	2	3	4	4	8
20–34	4659	2.3	1	1	1	2	3	4	4	6
35–49	1462	2.4	2	1	1	2	3	4	5	8
50–64	1	1.0	0	1	1	1	1	1	1	1
65+	0									
GRAND TOTAL	6394	2.3	2	1	1	2	3	4	4	7

66.61: EXC/DESTR FALL LES. Formerly included in operation group(s) 684.

Type of Patients	Observed Patients	Avg. Stay	Variance	Percentiles						
				10th	25th	50th	75th	90th	95th	99th
1. SINGLE DX										
0–19 Years	24	2.3	<1	1	2	2	3	3	4	4
20–34	19	1.7	<1	1	1	1	2	3	3	3
35–49	15	2.0	<1	2	2	2	2	3	3	3
50–64	3	1.6	<1	1	1	1	2	3	3	3
65+	0									
2. MULTIPLE DX										
0–19 Years	47	2.6	1	1	2	3	3	4	4	6
20–34	126	2.5	4	1	1	2	3	4	5	14
35–49	74	2.7	3	1	2	3	3	5	5	8
50–64	22	4.5	5	2	3	4	6	8	8	9
65+	10	5.7	42	2	4	4	5	12	30	30
TOTAL SINGLE DX	61	2.0	<1	1	2	2	2	3	3	4
MULTIPLE DX	279	2.8	4	1	2	2	3	4	6	12
TOTAL										
0–19 Years	71	2.6	1	1	2	2	3	4	4	6
20–34	145	2.4	4	1	1	2	3	4	4	14
35–49	89	2.5	2	1	2	3	3	5	5	8
50–64	25	4.3	5	2	3	3	6	8	8	9
65+	10	5.7	42	2	4	4	5	12	30	30
GRAND TOTAL	340	2.6	4	1	2	2	3	4	5	10

66.69: PARTIAL FALL RMVL NEC. Formerly included in operation group(s) 684.

Type of Patients	Observed Patients	Avg. Stay	Variance	Percentiles						
				10th	25th	50th	75th	90th	95th	99th
1. SINGLE DX										
0–19 Years	12	2.3	<1	2	2	2	3	3	3	3
20–34	99	2.0	<1	1	1	2	3	3	3	3
35–49	36	2.1	1	1	1	2	3	3	4	6
50–64	3	1.0	<1	1	1	1	1	1	1	2
65+	0									
2. MULTIPLE DX										
0–19 Years	24	2.8	6	1	2	2	3	4	5	23
20–34	274	2.8	2	1	2	3	3	5	5	9
35–49	156	3.5	8	1	2	3	4	6	13	13
50–64	6	3.6	2	3	3	3	3	7	7	7
65+	6	4.7	8	2	3	4	9	9	9	9
TOTAL SINGLE DX	150	1.9	<1	1	1	2	2	3	3	4
MULTIPLE DX	466	3.1	5	1	2	3	4	5	7	13
TOTAL										
0–19 Years	36	2.5	4	1	2	2	3	4	4	5
20–34	373	2.5	2	1	2	2	3	4	5	8
35–49	192	3.3	7	1	2	3	4	6	9	13
50–64	9	1.9	2	1	1	1	4	8	7	9
65+	6	4.7	8	2	3	4	9	9	9	9
GRAND TOTAL	616	2.7	4	1	2	2	3	4	6	13

Length of Stay by Diagnosis and Operation, United States, 1997

United States, October 1995–September 1996 Data, by Operation

66.7: REPAIR OF FALLOPIAN TUBE. Formerly included in operation group(s) 684.

Type of Patients	Observed Patients	Avg. Stay	Variance	10th	25th	50th	75th	90th	95th	99th
1. SINGLE DX										
0–19 Years	1	2.0	0	2	2	2	2	2	2	2
20–34	233	1.7	<1	1	1	2	2	3	3	4
35–49	167	1.8	<1	1	1	2	2	3	3	5
50–64	0									
65+	0									
2. MULTIPLE DX										
0–19 Years	6	2.8	2	1	2	2	5	5	5	5
20–34	428	2.3	<1	1	1	2	3	3	4	5
35–49	234	2.1	1	1	1	2	3	3	4	7
50–64	0									
65+	0									
TOTAL SINGLE DX	401	1.7	<1	1	1	2	2	3	3	4
MULTIPLE DX	668	2.2	1	1	2	2	3	3	4	5
TOTAL										
0–19 Years	7	2.7	2	1	2	2	3	5	5	5
20–34	661	2.0	<1	1	1	2	3	3	4	4
35–49	401	1.9	1	1	1	2	2	3	4	5
50–64	0									
65+	0									
GRAND TOTAL	1069	2.0	<1	1	1	2	2	3	4	5

66.8: FALL TUBE INSUFFLATION. Formerly included in operation group(s) 684.

Type of Patients	Observed Patients	Avg. Stay	Variance	10th	25th	50th	75th	90th	95th	99th
1. SINGLE DX										
0–19 Years	1	6.0	0	6	6	6	6	6	6	6
20–34	5	1.4	<1	1	1	1	2	2	3	3
35–49	0									
50–64	0									
65+	0									
2. MULTIPLE DX										
0–19 Years	0									
20–34	10	1.5	<1	1	1	1	2	2	2	2
35–49	6	1.7	<1	1	1	1	3	3	3	3
50–64	0									
65+	0									
TOTAL SINGLE DX	6	2.0	3	1	1	1	2	6	6	6
MULTIPLE DX	16	1.6	<1	1	1	1	2	3	3	3
TOTAL										
0–19 Years	1	6.0	0	6	6	6	6	6	6	6
20–34	15	1.4	<1	1	1	1	2	2	2	3
35–49	6	1.7	<1	1	1	1	3	3	3	3
50–64	0									
65+	0									
GRAND TOTAL	22	1.7	1	1	1	1	2	3	3	6

66.79: FALL TUBE REPAIR NEC. Formerly included in operation group(s) 684.

Type of Patients	Observed Patients	Avg. Stay	Variance	10th	25th	50th	75th	90th	95th	99th
1. SINGLE DX										
0–19 Years	1	2.0	0	2	2	2	2	2	2	2
20–34	167	1.6	<1	1	1	1	2	2	3	4
35–49	126	1.7	<1	1	1	2	2	3	3	4
50–64	0									
65+	0									
2. MULTIPLE DX										
0–19 Years	5	3.0	2	1	2	2	2	5	5	5
20–34	328	2.2	<1	1	2	2	3	3	4	5
35–49	189	2.0	1	1	1	2	2	3	3	7
50–64	0									
65+	0									
TOTAL SINGLE DX	294	1.7	<1	1	1	2	2	3	3	4
MULTIPLE DX	522	2.1	1	1	1	2	3	3	4	5
TOTAL										
0–19 Years	6	2.8	2	1	2	2	5	5	5	5
20–34	495	1.9	<1	1	1	2	2	3	3	5
35–49	315	1.9	1	1	1	2	2	3	3	5
50–64	0									
65+	0									
GRAND TOTAL	816	1.9	<1	1	1	2	2	3	3	5

66.9: OTHER FALLOPIAN TUBE OPS. Formerly included in operation group(s) 684.

Type of Patients	Observed Patients	Avg. Stay	Variance	10th	25th	50th	75th	90th	95th	99th
1. SINGLE DX										
0–19 Years	4	1.2	<1	1	1	1	1	2	3	3
20–34	17	1.4	<1	1	1	1	2	2	2	3
35–49	26	1.1	<1	1	1	1	1	1	2	2
50–64	0									
65+	0									
2. MULTIPLE DX										
0–19 Years	8	3.5	5	1	2	3	7	7	7	7
20–34	88	1.9	1	1	1	2	2	3	4	4
35–49	46	2.0	1	1	1	2	3	3	4	5
50–64	0									
65+	0									
TOTAL SINGLE DX	47	1.2	<1	1	1	1	1	2	2	3
MULTIPLE DX	142	2.0	2	1	1	2	2	3	4	7
TOTAL										
0–19 Years	12	2.4	4	1	1	2	3	7	7	7
20–34	105	1.9	1	1	1	2	2	3	4	4
35–49	72	1.7	1	1	1	1	2	3	3	5
50–64	0									
65+	0									
GRAND TOTAL	189	1.8	1	1	1	2	2	3	4	7

Length of Stay by Diagnosis and Operation, United States, 1997

United States, October 1995–September 1996 Data, by Operation

67.0: CERVICAL CANAL DILATION. Formerly included in operation group(s) 697.

Type of Patients	Observed Patients	Avg. Stay	Vari-ance	10th	25th	50th	75th	90th	95th	99th
1. SINGLE DX										
0–19 Years	0									
20–34	3	1.8	<1	1	2	2	2	2	2	2
35–49	3	3.1	1	2	2	2	4	4	4	4
50–64	3	1.6	<1	1	1	2	2	2	2	2
65+	4	2.8	<1	2	3	3	3	3	3	3
2. MULTIPLE DX										
0–19 Years	2	1.0	0	1	1	1	1	1	1	1
20–34	7	2.3	<1	1	1	2	3	3	4	4
35–49	11	2.5	2	2	2	2	3	4	6	6
50–64	8	2.6	2	2	2	3	3	5	5	5
65+	7	5.4	30	2	2	2	4	15	15	15
TOTAL SINGLE DX	13	2.3	<1	1	2	2	3	3	4	4
MULTIPLE DX	35	2.8	8	1	2	2	3	5	6	15
TOTAL										
0–19 Years	2	1.0	0	1	1	1	1	1	1	1
20–34	10	2.2	<1	1	2	2	3	3	4	4
35–49	14	2.6	2	2	2	2	3	4	6	6
50–64	11	2.3	2	2	2	3	3	5	5	5
65+	11	4.4	20	2	2	3	3	15	15	15
GRAND TOTAL	48	2.7	6	1	2	2	3	4	5	15

67.1: CERVICAL DIAGNOSTIC PX. Formerly included in operation group(s) 686, 704.

Type of Patients	Observed Patients	Avg. Stay	Vari-ance	10th	25th	50th	75th	90th	95th	99th
1. SINGLE DX										
0–19 Years	0									
20–34	7	2.4	4	1	1	2	3	7	7	7
35–49	6	1.2	<1	1	1	1	1	2	2	3
50–64	12	1.4	<1	1	1	1	1	3	4	4
65+	4	2.3	10	1	1	1	1	9	9	9
2. MULTIPLE DX										
0–19 Years	4	3.3	16	2	2	2	2	2	15	15
20–34	61	6.4	63	1	1	3	9	19	26	38
35–49	136	7.1	43	1	2	4	12	17	17	22
50–64	85	7.8	47	2	2	6	13	20	20	23
65+	171	7.8	44	2	3	7	10	14	18	39
TOTAL SINGLE DX	29	1.6	2	1	1	1	1	3	4	9
MULTIPLE DX	457	7.3	48	1	2	5	10	17	20	32
TOTAL										
0–19 Years	4	3.3	16	2	2	2	2	2	15	15
20–34	68	6.2	60	1	1	3	9	16	26	38
35–49	142	6.5	42	1	1	4	10	17	17	22
50–64	97	7.3	47	1	2	5	12	20	20	23
65+	175	7.7	44	2	3	7	9	14	18	39
GRAND TOTAL	486	6.9	47	1	2	4	9	17	20	31

67.12: CERVICAL BIOPSY NEC. Formerly included in operation group(s) 686.

Type of Patients	Observed Patients	Avg. Stay	Vari-ance	10th	25th	50th	75th	90th	95th	99th
1. SINGLE DX										
0–19 Years	0									
20–34	5	3.0	7	1	1	2	7	7	7	7
35–49	5	1.8	<1	1	1	2	2	3	3	3
50–64	9	1.6	<1	1	1	1	2	4	4	4
65+	3	2.8	13	1	1	1	1	9	9	9
2. MULTIPLE DX										
0–19 Years	4	3.3	16	2	2	2	2	2	15	15
20–34	48	6.6	54	1	1	3	9	19	26	26
35–49	116	7.7	46	1	2	5	17	17	17	22
50–64	74	6.1	30	2	2	4	7	15	18	23
65+	140	7.9	45	2	4	7	10	16	19	36
TOTAL SINGLE DX	22	2.1	4	1	1	1	2	4	7	9
MULTIPLE DX	382	7.2	45	1	2	5	9	17	19	28
TOTAL										
0–19 Years	4	3.3	16	2	2	2	2	2	15	15
20–34	53	6.5	53	1	1	3	9	19	26	26
35–49	121	7.5	46	1	2	4	17	17	17	22
50–64	83	5.8	30	2	3	4	7	15	18	23
65+	143	7.8	45	2	4	7	9	15	19	36
GRAND TOTAL	404	7.1	45	1	2	5	9	17	18	27

67.2: CONIZATION OF CERVIX. Formerly included in operation group(s) 685.

Type of Patients	Observed Patients	Avg. Stay	Vari-ance	10th	25th	50th	75th	90th	95th	99th
1. SINGLE DX										
0–19 Years	0									
20–34	13	1.5	<1	1	1	1	2	2	3	3
35–49	13	2.2	2	1	1	1	3	5	5	5
50–64	3	1.7	<1	1	1	1	3	3	3	3
65+	0									
2. MULTIPLE DX										
0–19 Years	1	3.0	0	3	3	3	3	3	3	3
20–34	42	2.1	2	1	1	2	3	4	5	9
35–49	54	3.7	27	1	1	2	3	10	10	27
50–64	28	2.0	4	1	1	1	2	3	6	10
65+	23	3.0	5	1	1	2	4	5	7	13
TOTAL SINGLE DX	29	1.9	1	1	1	1	3	3	5	5
MULTIPLE DX	148	2.7	12	1	1	2	3	6	10	13
TOTAL										
0–19 Years	1	3.0	0	3	3	3	3	3	3	3
20–34	55	2.0	2	1	1	2	2	3	5	7
35–49	67	3.4	23	1	1	2	3	10	10	27
50–64	31	2.0	4	1	1	2	3	6	6	10
65+	23	3.0	5	1	2	2	4	5	7	13
GRAND TOTAL	177	2.6	10	1	1	2	3	5	9	13

United States, October 1995–September 1996 Data, by Operation

67.3: EXC/DESTR CERV LES NEC. Formerly included in operation group(s) 686.

Type of Patients	Observed Patients	Avg. Stay	Variance	10th	25th	50th	75th	90th	95th	99th
1. SINGLE DX										
0–19 Years	2	2.2	1	1	1	3	3	3	3	3
20–34	21	1.2	<1	1	1	1	3	2	2	2
35–49	11	1.5	<1	1	1	1	2	3	3	3
50–64	6	1.5	<1	1	1	1	2	3	3	3
65+	0									
2. MULTIPLE DX										
0–19 Years	12	2.4	7	1	1	1	3	5	10	10
20–34	99	1.6	2	1	1	1	2	4	4	6
35–49	107	2.8	7	1	1	2	3	7	9	14
50–64	67	5.0	19	1	3	4	7	8	10	27
65+	76	5.5	33	2	2	3	7	10	15	30
TOTAL SINGLE DX	40	1.3	<1	1	1	1	1	2	3	3
MULTIPLE DX	361	2.7	11	1	1	1	3	6	8	15
TOTAL										
0–19 Years	14	2.3	6	1	1	1	3	5	10	10
20–34	120	1.5	2	1	1	1	2	3	4	6
35–49	118	2.7	7	1	1	2	3	7	9	14
50–64	73	4.9	19	1	2	3	7	8	10	27
65+	76	5.5	33	2	2	3	7	10	15	30
GRAND TOTAL	401	2.6	10	1	1	1	3	6	8	15

67.39: CERV LES EXC/DESTR NEC. Formerly included in operation group(s) 686.

Type of Patients	Observed Patients	Avg. Stay	Variance	10th	25th	50th	75th	90th	95th	99th
1. SINGLE DX										
0–19 Years	2	2.2	1	1	1	3	3	3	3	3
20–34	9	1.5	<1	1	1	1	1	2	2	2
35–49	8	1.6	<1	1	1	1	3	3	3	3
50–64	3	2.1	<1	1	1	2	3	3	3	3
65+	0									
2. MULTIPLE DX										
0–19 Years	7	4.0	10	1	1	4	5	10	10	10
20–34	71	1.5	1	1	1	1	1	4	4	6
35–49	82	2.7	8	1	1	2	3	7	9	14
50–64	58	4.5	22	1	2	3	6	7	17	27
65+	66	6.3	39	2	3	4	8	11	15	30
TOTAL SINGLE DX	22	1.6	<1	1	1	1	2	3	3	3
MULTIPLE DX	284	2.5	11	1	1	1	3	6	9	16
TOTAL										
0–19 Years	9	3.5	9	1	1	3	5	10	10	10
20–34	80	1.5	1	1	1	1	1	4	4	6
35–49	90	2.6	7	1	1	2	3	7	9	14
50–64	61	4.5	22	1	2	3	5	7	17	27
65+	66	6.3	39	2	3	4	8	11	15	30
GRAND TOTAL	306	2.5	11	1	1	1	3	6	9	15

67.4: AMPUTATION OF CERVIX. Formerly included in operation group(s) 686.

Type of Patients	Observed Patients	Avg. Stay	Variance	10th	25th	50th	75th	90th	95th	99th
1. SINGLE DX										
0–19 Years	0									
20–34	0									
35–49	5	2.0	<1	2	2	2	2	2	3	3
50–64	5	2.5	<1	1	2	3	3	3	3	3
65+	14	1.7	1	1	1	1	3	3	4	4
2. MULTIPLE DX										
0–19 Years	0									
20–34	9	3.9	5	2	2	3	5	8	9	9
35–49	34	3.0	6	1	1	2	5	7	7	8
50–64	26	2.7	2	1	2	3	3	4	4	8
65+	127	3.8	11	1	2	3	5	6	9	20
TOTAL SINGLE DX	24	2.0	<1	1	1	2	3	3	3	4
MULTIPLE DX	196	3.5	9	1	2	3	4	6	8	19
TOTAL										
0–19 Years	0									
20–34	9	3.9	5	2	2	3	5	8	9	9
35–49	39	2.9	5	1	1	2	4	7	7	8
50–64	31	2.7	2	1	2	3	3	4	4	8
65+	141	3.7	11	1	2	3	4	6	9	20
GRAND TOTAL	220	3.4	8	1	2	3	4	6	7	19

67.5: INT CERVICAL OS REPAIR. Formerly included in operation group(s) 687.

Type of Patients	Observed Patients	Avg. Stay	Variance	10th	25th	50th	75th	90th	95th	99th
1. SINGLE DX										
0–19 Years	51	3.4	34	1	1	1	3	6	18	45
20–34	627	2.2	5	1	1	1	2	5	6	10
35–49	119	2.2	5	1	1	1	2	7	9	9
50–64	0									
65+	0									
2. MULTIPLE DX										
0–19 Years	48	6.8	76	1	3	5	8	11	13	58
20–34	711	4.8	57	1	1	3	5	10	16	40
35–49	167	3.7	45	1	1	2	4	6	8	49
50–64	3	1.0	0	2	2	3	4	4	4	4
65+	2	3.0	1	2	2	3	4	4	4	4
TOTAL SINGLE DX	797	2.3	7	1	1	1	2	5	7	11
MULTIPLE DX	931	4.7	56	1	1	3	5	10	13	40
TOTAL										
0–19 Years	99	4.9	56	1	1	3	6	11	13	58
20–34	1338	3.7	36	1	1	2	4	7	10	33
35–49	286	3.2	32	1	1	1	4	6	8	18
50–64	3	1.0	0	2	2	3	4	4	4	4
65+	2	3.0	1	2	2	3	4	4	4	4
GRAND TOTAL	1728	3.6	36	1	1	2	4	7	10	33

Length of Stay by Diagnosis and Operation, United States, 1997

67.6: OTHER REPAIR OF CERVIX. Formerly included in operation group(s) 687.

Type of Patients	Observed Patients	Avg. Stay	Vari-ance	Percentiles						
				10th	25th	50th	75th	90th	95th	99th
1. SINGLE DX										
0–19 Years	0									
20–34	11	1.2	<1	1	1	1	1	2	2	2
35–49	13	1.2	<1	1	1	1	1	3	3	3
50–64	1	1.0	0	1	1	1	1	1	1	1
65+	0									
2. MULTIPLE DX										
0–19 Years	1	1.0	0	1	1	1	1	1	1	1
20–34	34	4.1	16	1	1	3	4	12	12	12
35–49	17	4.0	23	1	1	2	4	12	16	16
50–64	5	1.8	<1	1	1	1	3	3	3	3
65+	1	6.0	0	6	6	6	6	6	6	6
TOTAL SINGLE DX	25	1.2	<1	1	1	1	1	2	2	3
MULTIPLE DX	58	3.7	16	1	1	2	3	12	12	16
TOTAL										
0–19 Years	1	1.0	0	1	1	1	1	1	1	1
20–34	45	3.5	15	1	1	2	3	12	12	12
35–49	30	2.7	14	1	1	1	2	10	12	16
50–64	6	1.7	<1	1	1	1	3	3	3	3
65+	1	6.0	0	6	6	6	6	6	6	6
GRAND TOTAL	83	3.1	13	1	1	2	3	12	12	12

68.1: UTER/ADNEXA DXTIC PX. Formerly included in operation group(s) 688, 697, 704.

Type of Patients	Observed Patients	Avg. Stay	Vari-ance	Percentiles						
				10th	25th	50th	75th	90th	95th	99th
1. SINGLE DX										
0–19 Years	2	1.2	<1	1	1	1	1	1	3	3
20–34	18	1.8	1	1	1	1	4	4	4	4
35–49	15	3.0	5	1	1	2	4	7	7	7
50–64	6	2.3	2	1	1	2	4	4	4	4
65+	6	2.6	6	1	1	1	3	5	9	9
2. MULTIPLE DX										
0–19 Years	12	5.8	12	1	3	9	9	9	9	9
20–34	137	3.5	16	1	2	2	4	6	9	26
35–49	357	4.0	18	1	1	3	5	13	30	>99
50–64	195	6.1	41	1	2	5	9	11	14	27
65+	315	9.5	79	2	3	6	13	23	24	37
TOTAL SINGLE DX	47	2.3	3	1	1	1	3	4	7	9
MULTIPLE DX	1016	6.3	50	1	2	4	8	18	23	>99
TOTAL										
0–19 Years	14	4.9	13	1	1	3	9	9	9	9
20–34	155	3.3	15	1	2	2	4	6	9	26
35–49	372	3.9	17	1	2	3	5	12	24	>99
50–64	201	6.0	40	1	2	4	9	11	14	27
65+	321	9.3	79	2	3	6	13	23	24	37
GRAND TOTAL	1063	6.0	48	1	2	4	7	16	23	>99

68.0: HYSTEROTOMY. Formerly included in operation group(s) 688.

Type of Patients	Observed Patients	Avg. Stay	Vari-ance	Percentiles						
				10th	25th	50th	75th	90th	95th	99th
1. SINGLE DX										
0–19 Years	1	1.0	0	1	1	1	1	1	1	1
20–34	7	2.1	<1	2	2	2	2	3	3	3
35–49	0									
50–64	0									
65+	0									
2. MULTIPLE DX										
0–19 Years	2	4.6	1	2	5	5	5	5	5	5
20–34	21	3.8	4	1	3	3	5	7	7	8
35–49	13	2.7	9	2	2	2	2	8	8	16
50–64	5	4.1	9	2	2	3	5	11	11	11
65+	4	3.3	1	1	3	4	4	4	4	4
TOTAL SINGLE DX	8	2.0	<1	1	2	2	2	3	3	3
MULTIPLE DX	45	3.2	7	2	2	2	3	5	7	16
TOTAL										
0–19 Years	3	3.1	4	1	1	2	5	5	5	5
20–34	28	3.4	4	1	2	3	5	7	7	8
35–49	13	2.7	9	2	2	2	2	8	8	16
50–64	5	4.1	9	2	2	3	5	11	11	11
65+	4	3.3	1	1	3	4	4	4	4	4
GRAND TOTAL	53	3.1	7	2	2	2	3	5	7	16

68.16: CLSD UTERINE BX. Formerly included in operation group(s) 688.

Type of Patients	Observed Patients	Avg. Stay	Vari-ance	Percentiles						
				10th	25th	50th	75th	90th	95th	99th
1. SINGLE DX										
0–19 Years	2	1.2	<1	1	1	1	1	1	3	3
20–34	9	1.7	1	1	1	1	2	4	4	4
35–49	6	1.9	<1	1	1	1	3	3	3	4
50–64	4	2.8	2	1	2	4	4	5	5	5
65+	4	3.1	2	2	2	3	5	5	5	5
2. MULTIPLE DX										
0–19 Years	8	2.7	<1	1	2	3	3	4	4	4
20–34	84	3.8	20	1	2	2	4	8	10	30
35–49	280	4.3	20	1	2	3	6	18	>99	>99
50–64	163	6.5	24	3	3	5	9	11	14	24
65+	284	9.7	83	2	3	6	13	23	26	37
TOTAL SINGLE DX	25	1.9	2	1	1	1	3	4	4	5
MULTIPLE DX	819	6.8	53	1	2	4	9	20	24	>99
TOTAL										
0–19 Years	10	2.2	1	1	1	3	3	3	4	4
20–34	93	3.4	18	1	2	3	4	8	8	26
35–49	286	4.2	20	1	2	3	6	18	>99	>99
50–64	167	6.4	24	1	3	5	9	11	14	24
65+	288	9.7	82	2	3	6	13	23	25	37
GRAND TOTAL	844	6.6	52	1	2	4	9	19	24	>99

Length of Stay by Diagnosis and Operation, United States, 1997

United States, October 1995–September 1996 Data, by Operation

68.2: UTERINE LES EXC/DESTR. Formerly included in operation group(s) 688.

Type of Patients	Observed Patients	Avg. Stay	Variance	10th	25th	50th	75th	90th	95th	99th
1. SINGLE DX										
0–19 Years	7	2.0	<1	1	2	2	2	2	3	3
20–34	685	2.6	<1	2	2	2	3	4	4	5
35–49	682	2.5	<1	2	2	2	3	3	4	4
50–64	22	1.3	<1	1	1	1	1	3	3	3
65+	2	2.5	1	1	1	3	3	3	3	3
2. MULTIPLE DX										
0–19 Years	23	3.5	3	1	2	3	5	7	7	7
20–34	2826	2.8	2	2	2	3	3	4	5	7
35–49	3683	3.1	2	2	2	3	4	5	5	8
50–64	159	3.2	10	2	2	3	3	5	8	17
65+	84	5.3	27	1	2	3	8	11	13	29
TOTAL SINGLE DX	1398	2.5	<1	1	2	2	3	3	4	5
MULTIPLE DX	6775	3.0	3	2	2	3	3	4	5	8
TOTAL										
0–19 Years	30	3.0	3	1	2	2	3	5	7	7
20–34	3511	2.8	2	2	2	3	3	4	5	7
35–49	4365	3.0	2	2	2	3	3	5	5	8
50–64	181	3.2	8	1	2	3	3	4	7	17
65+	86	5.2	26	1	2	3	8	11	13	29
GRAND TOTAL	8173	2.9	2	2	2	3	3	4	5	8

68.29: UTER LES EXC/DESTR NEC. Formerly included in operation group(s) 688.

Type of Patients	Observed Patients	Avg. Stay	Variance	10th	25th	50th	75th	90th	95th	99th
1. SINGLE DX										
0–19 Years	7	2.0	<1	1	2	2	2	2	3	3
20–34	682	2.6	<1	2	2	2	3	4	4	5
35–49	682	2.5	<1	2	2	2	3	3	4	4
50–64	22	1.3	<1	1	1	1	1	3	3	3
65+	2	2.5	1	1	1	3	3	3	3	3
2. MULTIPLE DX										
0–19 Years	22	3.6	3	2	2	3	5	7	7	7
20–34	2824	2.8	2	2	2	3	3	4	5	7
35–49	3679	3.1	2	2	2	3	4	5	5	8
50–64	159	3.2	10	2	2	3	3	5	8	17
65+	84	5.3	27	2	2	3	8	11	13	29
TOTAL SINGLE DX	1395	2.5	<1	1	2	2	3	3	4	5
MULTIPLE DX	6768	3.0	3	2	2	3	3	4	5	8
TOTAL										
0–19 Years	29	3.0	3	2	2	2	3	5	7	7
20–34	3506	2.8	2	2	2	3	3	4	5	7
35–49	4361	3.0	2	2	2	3	3	5	5	8
50–64	181	3.2	8	1	1	2	3	4	7	17
65+	86	5.2	26	2	2	3	8	11	13	29
GRAND TOTAL	8163	2.9	2	2	2	3	3	4	5	8

68.3: SUBTOT ABD HYSTERECTOMY. Formerly included in operation group(s) 689.

Type of Patients	Observed Patients	Avg. Stay	Variance	10th	25th	50th	75th	90th	95th	99th
1. SINGLE DX										
0–19 Years	1	3.0	0	3	3	3	3	3	3	3
20–34	16	3.6	<1	3	3	4	4	4	4	4
35–49	66	2.9	2	2	2	3	3	4	7	7
50–64	13	4.2	2	2	3	5	5	6	6	6
65+	0									
2. MULTIPLE DX										
0–19 Years	4	2.6	<1	2	2	3	3	3	3	3
20–34	226	3.9	9	2	3	3	4	6	9	14
35–49	1431	3.5	6	2	2	3	4	5	7	14
50–64	363	4.9	23	3	3	4	5	8	14	26
65+	178	8.9	37	4	5	7	10	17	23	29
TOTAL SINGLE DX	96	3.2	2	2	2	3	4	5	7	7
MULTIPLE DX	2202	4.1	12	2	3	3	4	7	10	21
TOTAL										
0–19 Years	5	2.6	<1	2	2	3	3	3	3	3
20–34	242	3.9	8	2	3	3	4	6	9	14
35–49	1497	3.5	5	2	2	3	4	5	7	14
50–64	376	4.9	23	3	3	4	5	8	13	26
65+	178	8.9	37	4	5	7	10	17	23	29
GRAND TOTAL	2298	4.1	12	2	3	3	4	7	10	18

68.4: TOTAL ABD HYSTERECTOMY. Formerly included in operation group(s) 689.

Type of Patients	Observed Patients	Avg. Stay	Variance	10th	25th	50th	75th	90th	95th	99th
1. SINGLE DX										
0–19 Years	4	4.2	3	3	3	3	6	7	7	7
20–34	739	2.9	<1	2	2	3	3	4	4	7
35–49	2538	2.9	<1	2	2	3	3	4	5	7
50–64	923	3.2	<1	2	3	3	4	4	5	6
65+	388	3.7	9	3	3	3	4	5	6	12
2. MULTIPLE DX										
0–19 Years	56	4.2	28	2	2	3	4	6	13	32
20–34	11959	3.1	2	2	2	3	3	4	5	9
35–49	57446	3.3	3	2	3	3	4	5	7	10
50–64	17601	3.7	6	3	3	4	5	7	9	13
65+	9605	5.4	17	3	3	4	6	9	12	23
TOTAL SINGLE DX	4592	3.0	1	2	2	3	3	4	4	7
MULTIPLE DX	96667	3.5	5	2	3	3	4	5	7	12
TOTAL										
0–19 Years	60	4.2	27	2	2	3	4	6	13	32
20–34	12698	3.1	2	2	2	3	3	4	5	9
35–49	59984	3.2	3	2	2	3	3	5	5	10
50–64	18524	3.7	5	2	3	4	4	5	7	13
65+	9993	5.3	17	3	3	4	6	9	12	22
GRAND TOTAL	101259	3.5	4	2	3	3	4	5	6	12

Length of Stay by Diagnosis and Operation, United States, 1997

United States, October 1995–September 1996 Data, by Operation

68.5: VAGINAL HYSTERECTOMY. Formerly included in operation group(s) 690.

Type of Patients	Observed Patients	Avg. Stay	Vari-ance	Percentiles						
				10th	25th	50th	75th	90th	95th	99th
1. SINGLE DX										
0–19 Years	2	1.8	<1	1	2	2	2	2	2	2
20–34	963	1.8	<1	1	1	2	2	2	3	4
35–49	1692	1.9	<1	1	1	2	2	3	3	4
50–64	776	2.4	2	1	2	2	3	3	4	6
65+	602	2.9	1	2	2	3	3	4	5	6
2. MULTIPLE DX										
0–19 Years	13	2.6	3	1	2	2	2	5	5	10
20–34	8059	2.0	<1	1	1	2	2	3	3	5
35–49	26330	2.2	1	1	2	2	3	3	4	6
50–64	9263	2.5	1	1	2	2	3	4	4	6
65+	7674	3.2	3	2	2	3	4	5	6	10
TOTAL SINGLE DX	4035	2.1	1	1	1	2	2	3	4	5
MULTIPLE DX	51339	2.3	1	1	2	2	3	3	4	6
TOTAL										
0–19 Years	15	2.5	3	1	2	2	2	5	5	10
20–34	9022	2.0	<1	1	1	2	2	3	3	5
35–49	28022	2.1	1	1	2	2	3	3	4	5
50–64	10039	2.5	1	1	2	2	3	4	4	6
65+	8276	3.2	3	2	2	3	4	5	6	9
GRAND TOTAL	55374	2.3	1	2	2	2	3	3	4	6

68.6: RADICAL ABD HYSTERECTOMY. Formerly included in operation group(s) 691.

Type of Patients	Observed Patients	Avg. Stay	Vari-ance	Percentiles						
				10th	25th	50th	75th	90th	95th	99th
1. SINGLE DX										
0–19 Years	1	4.0	0	4	4	4	4	4	4	4
20–34	64	4.4	2	3	3	4	5	6	7	8
35–49	112	5.2	2	3	4	5	6	8	8	8
50–64	33	4.8	5	3	4	4	6	8	8	14
65+	14	4.1	4	2	3	4	5	6	9	9
2. MULTIPLE DX										
0–19 Years	2	4.0	8	3	3	3	3	11	11	11
20–34	229	5.4	5	3	4	5	6	7	10	14
35–49	588	5.5	4	4	4	5	6	8	8	11
50–64	324	6.3	10	3	4	6	7	10	13	16
65+	265	7.7	30	4	5	6	8	13	20	36
TOTAL SINGLE DX	224	4.9	3	3	4	5	6	8	8	8
MULTIPLE DX	1408	6.0	11	4	4	5	7	9	11	21
TOTAL										
0–19 Years	3	4.0	6	3	3	3	4	4	11	11
20–34	293	5.2	5	3	4	5	6	7	9	14
35–49	700	5.4	3	4	4	5	7	8	8	11
50–64	357	6.2	10	4	4	6	7	9	13	16
65+	279	7.5	30	4	5	6	8	13	20	36
GRAND TOTAL	1632	5.9	10	3	4	5	7	8	11	20

68.7: RADICAL VAG HYSTERECTOMY. Formerly included in operation group(s) 691.

Type of Patients	Observed Patients	Avg. Stay	Vari-ance	Percentiles						
				10th	25th	50th	75th	90th	95th	99th
1. SINGLE DX										
0–19 Years	0									
20–34	6	2.9	3	2	2	2	3	7	7	7
35–49	6	2.3	<1	1	2	2	3	4	4	4
50–64	4	2.6	<1	2	2	2	3	4	4	4
65+	1	5.0	0	5	5	5	5	5	5	5
2. MULTIPLE DX										
0–19 Years	0									
20–34	22	2.9	6	2	2	2	3	4	6	14
35–49	62	2.2	<1	1	2	2	2	3	3	5
50–64	31	3.0	2	2	3	3	3	5	5	10
65+	20	4.5	12	2	2	4	5	7	15	15
TOTAL SINGLE DX	17	2.7	2	2	2	2	3	5	5	7
MULTIPLE DX	135	2.7	3	1	2	2	3	4	5	14
TOTAL										
0–19 Years	0									
20–34	28	2.9	6	2	2	2	3	5	6	14
35–49	68	2.2	<1	1	2	2	3	3	4	5
50–64	35	3.0	2	2	2	3	3	5	5	10
65+	21	4.5	11	2	2	4	5	7	15	15
GRAND TOTAL	152	2.7	3	2	2	2	3	4	5	14

68.8: PELVIC EVISCERATION. Formerly included in operation group(s) 691.

Type of Patients	Observed Patients	Avg. Stay	Vari-ance	Percentiles						
				10th	25th	50th	75th	90th	95th	99th
1. SINGLE DX										
0–19 Years	0									
20–34	3	5.4	41	1	1	3	3	15	15	15
35–49	0									
50–64	3	8.2	68	3	3	4	18	18	18	18
65+	2	15.0	36	8	8	19	19	19	19	19
2. MULTIPLE DX										
0–19 Years	0									
20–34	8	14.4	28	5	13	15	16	23	23	23
35–49	35	13.6	155	3	5	9	17	28	30	66
50–64	80	15.7	126	8	9	13	15	27	35	66
65+	124	17.5	176	8	10	12	20	32	39	86
TOTAL SINGLE DX	8	9.8	57	1	3	8	18	19	19	19
MULTIPLE DX	247	16.5	160	7	10	13	20	32	39	74
TOTAL										
0–19 Years	0									
20–34	11	12.0	46	3	5	13	16	18	23	23
35–49	35	13.6	155	3	5	9	17	28	30	66
50–64	83	15.6	126	8	9	13	15	27	35	66
65+	126	17.5	174	8	10	12	20	32	39	86
GRAND TOTAL	255	16.4	159	7	10	13	20	32	39	74

Length of Stay by Diagnosis and Operation, United States, 1997

United States, October 1995–September 1996 Data, by Operation

68.9: HYSTERECTOMY NEC & NOS. Formerly included in operation group(s) 689.

Type of Patients	Observed Patients	Avg. Stay	Vari-ance	Percentiles						
				10th	25th	50th	75th	90th	95th	99th
1. SINGLE DX										
0–19 Years	0									
20–34	8	2.5	1	1	2	3	3	3	3	6
35–49	10	3.0	1	2	2	3	4	5	5	5
50–64	6	2.8	<1	2	3	3	3	3	3	4
65+	1	3.0	0	3	3	3	3	3	3	3
2. MULTIPLE DX										
0–19 Years	2	2.3	5	1	1	1	5	5	5	5
20–34	47	3.1	5	2	2	3	4	5	6	8
35–49	229	2.6	4	1	2	2	3	3	4	9
50–64	62	3.2	5	1	2	3	3	6	9	11
65+	41	6.2	32	2	3	4	7	18	18	18
TOTAL SINGLE DX	25	2.8	<1	2	2	3	3	4	5	6
MULTIPLE DX	381	3.1	8	1	2	3	3	5	7	18
TOTAL										
0–19 Years	2	2.3	5	1	1	1	5	5	5	5
20–34	55	3.0	5	2	2	3	3	5	6	6
35–49	239	2.6	4	1	2	2	3	3	4	8
50–64	68	3.1	4	1	2	3	3	6	9	11
65+	42	6.1	32	2	3	4	7	18	18	18
GRAND TOTAL	406	3.1	7	1	2	3	3	5	6	18

69.0: UTERINE D&C. Formerly included in operation group(s) 692, 693.

Type of Patients	Observed Patients	Avg. Stay	Vari-ance	Percentiles						
				10th	25th	50th	75th	90th	95th	99th
1. SINGLE DX										
0–19 Years	573	1.3	<1	1	1	1	1	2	3	4
20–34	2734	1.3	<1	1	1	1	1	2	2	4
35–49	825	1.3	<1	1	1	1	1	2	3	6
50–64	49	1.6	<1	1	1	1	2	3	3	4
65+	26	1.6	<1	1	1	1	2	3	3	5
2. MULTIPLE DX										
0–19 Years	522	2.2	5	1	1	1	3	4	5	13
20–34	3742	2.4	6	1	1	2	3	4	6	12
35–49	2038	2.6	8	1	1	2	3	5	7	12
50–64	518	5.3	93	1	2	2	4	11	18	65
65+	826	5.7	37	2	2	4	8	12	15	35
TOTAL SINGLE DX	4207	1.3	<1	1	1	1	1	2	3	4
MULTIPLE DX	7646	2.9	16	1	1	2	3	6	8	18
TOTAL										
0–19 Years	1095	1.6	3	1	1	1	2	3	4	8
20–34	6476	1.9	4	1	1	1	2	3	5	10
35–49	2863	2.2	6	1	1	1	3	5	7	11
50–64	567	5.1	89	1	1	2	5	10	17	65
65+	852	5.6	37	2	2	4	7	12	15	35
GRAND TOTAL	11853	2.3	11	1	1	1	2	4	6	18

69.01: D&C FOR TERM OF PREG. Formerly included in operation group(s) 692.

Type of Patients	Observed Patients	Avg. Stay	Vari-ance	Percentiles						
				10th	25th	50th	75th	90th	95th	99th
1. SINGLE DX										
0–19 Years	18	1.5	<1	1	1	1	2	3	3	3
20–34	63	1.3	<1	1	1	1	2	3	3	3
35–49	14	2.6	3	1	1	2	5	5	5	8
50–64	1	1.0	0	1	1	1	1	1	1	1
65+	0									
2. MULTIPLE DX										
0–19 Years	26	4.9	61	1	1	2	4	19	19	38
20–34	166	2.6	10	1	1	1	3	6	8	15
35–49	57	2.2	6	1	1	1	3	4	7	14
50–64	0									
65+	0									
TOTAL SINGLE DX	96	1.6	1	1	1	1	2	3	4	5
MULTIPLE DX	249	2.6	12	1	1	1	3	6	8	19
TOTAL										
0–19 Years	44	3.0	31	1	1	1	2	4	15	38
20–34	229	2.4	9	1	1	1	2	5	8	15
35–49	71	2.2	6	1	1	1	3	5	7	14
50–64	1	1.0	0	1	1	1	1	1	1	1
65+	0									
GRAND TOTAL	345	2.4	10	1	1	1	2	5	8	19

69.02: D&C POST DEL OR AB. Formerly included in operation group(s) 693.

Type of Patients	Observed Patients	Avg. Stay	Vari-ance	Percentiles						
				10th	25th	50th	75th	90th	95th	99th
1. SINGLE DX										
0–19 Years	514	1.2	<1	1	1	1	1	2	2	4
20–34	2423	1.2	<1	1	1	1	1	2	2	4
35–49	695	1.2	<1	1	1	1	1	2	2	5
50–64	1	1.0	0	1	1	1	1	1	1	1
65+	0									
2. MULTIPLE DX										
0–19 Years	401	2.1	4	1	1	1	3	4	5	11
20–34	2803	2.4	6	1	1	2	3	4	6	12
35–49	794	2.3	5	1	1	2	3	5	7	12
50–64	2	2.6	4	4	4	4	4	4	4	4
65+	0									
TOTAL SINGLE DX	3633	1.2	<1	1	1	1	1	2	2	4
MULTIPLE DX	4000	2.3	5	1	1	2	3	4	6	12
TOTAL										
0–19 Years	915	1.5	2	1	1	1	2	3	4	8
20–34	5226	1.9	4	1	1	1	2	3	5	10
35–49	1489	1.8	3	1	1	1	1	3	4	8
50–64	3	1.4	1	1	1	1	1	4	4	4
65+	0									
GRAND TOTAL	7633	1.8	3	1	1	1	2	3	4	9

Length of Stay by Diagnosis and Operation, United States, 1997

United States, October 1995–September 1996 Data, by Operation

69.09: D&C NEC. Formerly included in operation group(s) 693.

Type of Patients	Observed Patients	Avg. Stay	Variance	10th	25th	50th	75th	90th	95th	99th
1. SINGLE DX										
0–19 Years	41	2.3	3	1	1	2	3	4	5	7
20–34	248	1.5	<1	1	1	1	2	3	5	5
35–49	116	1.5	1	1	1	1	2	3	3	7
50–64	47	1.6	<1	1	1	1	2	3	4	4
65+	26	1.6	<1	1	1	1	2	3	3	5
2. MULTIPLE DX										
0–19 Years	95	2.2	2	1	1	2	3	4	5	7
20–34	773	2.5	5	1	1	2	3	4	6	11
35–49	1187	2.8	11	1	1	2	3	5	8	12
50–64	516	5.3	93	1	1	2	6	11	18	65
65+	826	5.7	37	1	2	4	8	12	15	35
TOTAL SINGLE DX	478	1.6	1	1	1	1	2	3	4	7
MULTIPLE DX	3397	3.7	30	1	1	2	4	8	11	25
TOTAL										
0–19 Years	136	2.2	2	1	1	2	3	4	5	7
20–34	1021	2.2	4	1	1	2	3	4	5	10
35–49	1303	2.7	10	1	1	2	3	5	8	12
50–64	563	5.1	89	1	1	2	5	10	17	65
65+	852	5.6	37	2	2	4	7	12	15	35
GRAND TOTAL	3875	3.5	27	1	1	2	4	7	11	22

69.19: EXC UTER/SUPP STRUCT NEC. Formerly included in operation group(s) 697.

Type of Patients	Observed Patients	Avg. Stay	Variance	10th	25th	50th	75th	90th	95th	99th
1. SINGLE DX										
0–19 Years	13	2.6	<1	2	2	3	3	3	3	3
20–34	30	3.2	1	2	2	4	4	4	4	5
35–49	19	2.7	1	1	2	3	4	4	4	4
50–64	1	1.0	0	1	1	1	1	1	1	1
65+	1	4.0	0	4	4	4	4	4	4	4
2. MULTIPLE DX										
0–19 Years	26	2.8	2	1	2	3	3	6	6	6
20–34	154	2.7	2	1	2	3	3	4	6	9
35–49	118	3.0	3	1	2	3	3	5	6	8
50–64	33	5.7	8	3	3	6	6	7	9	16
65+	13	5.4	8	1	3	7	7	9	10	11
TOTAL SINGLE DX	64	3.1	1	2	2	3	4	4	4	5
MULTIPLE DX	344	3.1	4	1	2	3	3	6	7	10
TOTAL										
0–19 Years	39	2.7	2	1	2	3	3	4	6	6
20–34	184	2.8	2	1	2	3	3	4	4	9
35–49	137	2.9	3	1	2	3	3	5	6	7
50–64	34	5.6	8	3	3	6	7	7	9	16
65+	14	5.3	7	1	3	7	7	9	10	11
GRAND TOTAL	408	3.1	3	1	2	3	4	5	7	9

69.1: EXC/DESTR UTER/SUPP LES. Formerly included in operation group(s) 697.

Type of Patients	Observed Patients	Avg. Stay	Variance	10th	25th	50th	75th	90th	95th	99th
1. SINGLE DX										
0–19 Years	13	2.6	<1	2	2	3	3	3	3	3
20–34	30	3.2	1	2	2	4	4	4	4	5
35–49	19	2.7	1	1	2	3	4	4	4	4
50–64	1	1.0	0	1	1	1	1	1	1	1
65+	1	4.0	0	4	4	4	4	4	4	4
2. MULTIPLE DX										
0–19 Years	26	2.8	2	1	2	3	3	6	6	6
20–34	154	2.7	2	1	2	3	3	4	4	9
35–49	118	3.0	3	1	2	3	3	5	5	8
50–64	33	5.7	8	3	3	6	6	7	9	16
65+	13	5.4	8	1	3	7	7	9	10	11
TOTAL SINGLE DX	64	3.1	1	2	2	3	4	4	4	5
MULTIPLE DX	344	3.1	4	1	2	3	3	6	7	10
TOTAL										
0–19 Years	39	2.7	2	1	2	3	3	4	6	6
20–34	184	2.8	2	1	2	3	3	4	4	9
35–49	137	2.9	3	1	2	3	3	5	6	7
50–64	34	5.6	8	3	3	6	7	7	9	16
65+	14	5.3	7	1	3	7	7	9	10	11
GRAND TOTAL	408	3.1	3	1	2	3	4	5	7	9

69.2: UTERINE SUPP STRUCT REP. Formerly included in operation group(s) 696.

Type of Patients	Observed Patients	Avg. Stay	Variance	10th	25th	50th	75th	90th	95th	99th
1. SINGLE DX										
0–19 Years	1	3.0	0	3	3	3	3	3	3	3
20–34	8	2.3	<1	1	2	2	3	3	3	3
35–49	8	2.0	<1	2	2	2	2	3	3	3
50–64	1	1.0	0	1	1	1	1	1	1	1
65+	6	2.4	<1	1	1	3	3	3	4	4
2. MULTIPLE DX										
0–19 Years	7	4.7	11	1	2	4	10	10	10	10
20–34	63	2.2	2	1	1	2	3	4	4	9
35–49	34	3.0	3	1	2	3	4	5	6	8
50–64	8	2.2	<1	2	2	3	4	3	4	4
65+	25	2.9	4	1	1	3	4	5	6	10
TOTAL SINGLE DX	24	2.2	<1	1	2	2	3	3	3	4
MULTIPLE DX	137	2.6	3	1	2	2	3	4	6	10
TOTAL										
0–19 Years	8	4.4	10	2	2	4	5	10	10	10
20–34	71	2.2	1	1	1	2	3	4	4	5
35–49	42	2.7	2	1	2	2	4	5	6	9
50–64	9	2.1	<1	1	2	2	3	3	4	4
65+	31	2.8	3	1	1	3	4	5	6	10
GRAND TOTAL	161	2.6	3	1	2	2	3	4	5	10

Length of Stay by Diagnosis and Operation, United States, 1997

United States, October 1995–September 1996 Data, by Operation

69.3: PARACERV UTERINE DENERV. Formerly included in operation group(s) 696.

Type of Patients	Observed Patients	Avg. Stay	Vari-ance	10th	25th	50th	75th	90th	95th	99th
1. SINGLE DX										
0–19 Years	0									
20–34	1	3.0	0	3	3	3	3	3	3	3
35–49	0									
50–64	0									
65+	0									
2. MULTIPLE DX										
0–19 Years	2	1.7	1	1	1	1	3	3	3	3
20–34	6	2.0	<1	2	2	2	2	2	2	3
35–49	2	1.4	<1	1	1	1	2	2	2	2
50–64	0									
65+	0									
TOTAL SINGLE DX	1	3.0	0	3	3	3	3	3	3	3
MULTIPLE DX	10	2.0	<1	2	2	2	2	2	3	3
TOTAL										
0–19 Years	2	1.7	1	1	1	1	3	3	3	3
20–34	7	2.1	<1	2	2	2	2	2	3	3
35–49	2	1.4	<1	1	1	1	2	2	2	2
50–64	0									
65+	0									
GRAND TOTAL	11	2.0	<1	2	2	2	2	2	3	3

69.4: UTERINE REPAIR. Formerly included in operation group(s) 697.

Type of Patients	Observed Patients	Avg. Stay	Vari-ance	10th	25th	50th	75th	90th	95th	99th
1. SINGLE DX										
0–19 Years	2	3.0	0	3	3	3	3	3	3	3
20–34	4	5.7	4	3	3	7	7	7	7	7
35–49	1	6.0	0	6	6	6	6	6	6	6
50–64	0									
65+	0									
2. MULTIPLE DX										
0–19 Years	5	3.9	3	3	3	3	4	8	8	8
20–34	36	2.1	3	1	1	1	3	4	5	10
35–49	19	3.7	<1	3	3	4	4	5	5	7
50–64	4	12.5	79	1	20	20	20	20	20	20
65+	3	5.0	14	2	2	2	9	9	9	9
TOTAL SINGLE DX	7	4.7	4	3	3	3	7	7	7	7
MULTIPLE DX	67	3.1	12	1	1	3	4	5	9	20
TOTAL										
0–19 Years	7	3.5	2	3	3	3	3	4	8	8
20–34	40	2.4	4	3	1	1	3	5	7	9
35–49	20	3.8	<1	3	3	4	4	5	6	7
50–64	4	12.5	79	1	20	20	20	20	20	20
65+	3	5.0	14	2	2	2	9	9	9	9
GRAND TOTAL	74	3.2	11	1	1	3	4	6	8	20

69.5: ASP CURETTAGE UTERUS. Formerly included in operation group(s) 694, 695.

Type of Patients	Observed Patients	Avg. Stay	Vari-ance	10th	25th	50th	75th	90th	95th	99th
1. SINGLE DX										
0–19 Years	397	1.2	<1	1	1	1	1	2	2	3
20–34	1904	1.3	<1	1	1	1	1	2	3	5
35–49	520	1.2	<1	1	1	1	1	2	3	5
50–64	1	2.0	0	2	2	2	2	2	2	2
65+	1	1.0	0	1	1	1	1	1	1	1
2. MULTIPLE DX										
0–19 Years	255	2.2	4	1	1	2	2	5	6	9
20–34	1564	2.3	6	1	1	2	2	5	6	11
35–49	531	2.5	10	1	1	1	3	5	9	18
50–64	27	3.7	23	1	1	2	4	9	10	30
65+	38	8.9	39	2	3	8	13	16	17	23
TOTAL SINGLE DX	2823	1.2	<1	1	1	1	1	2	2	4
MULTIPLE DX	2415	2.4	7	1	1	2	3	5	7	14
TOTAL										
0–19 Years	652	1.5	2	1	1	1	2	3	4	7
20–34	3468	1.8	3	1	1	1	2	3	4	9
35–49	1051	1.7	5	1	1	1	2	3	5	10
50–64	28	3.6	22	1	2	2	4	9	10	30
65+	39	8.8	39	2	3	8	13	16	17	23
GRAND TOTAL	5238	1.8	4	1	1	1	2	3	5	10

69.51: ASP CURETTAGE-PREG TERM. Formerly included in operation group(s) 694.

Type of Patients	Observed Patients	Avg. Stay	Vari-ance	10th	25th	50th	75th	90th	95th	99th
1. SINGLE DX										
0–19 Years	20	1.7	1	1	1	1	2	3	3	6
20–34	89	2.1	7	1	1	1	2	3	3	13
35–49	22	1.5	3	1	1	1	1	1	9	9
50–64	0									
65+	0									
2. MULTIPLE DX										
0–19 Years	33	2.4	4	1	1	2	3	5	8	10
20–34	203	3.4	13	1	1	2	4	9	10	17
35–49	55	4.0	15	1	1	2	5	9	9	21
50–64	2	1.0	0	1	1	1	1	1	1	1
65+	0									
TOTAL SINGLE DX	131	2.0	5	1	1	1	2	3	6	13
MULTIPLE DX	293	3.4	12	1	1	2	4	9	10	16
TOTAL										
0–19 Years	53	2.1	3	1	1	2	2	3	6	10
20–34	292	3.0	11	1	1	2	3	8	11	14
35–49	77	3.3	13	1	1	1	5	9	9	21
50–64	2	1.0	0	1	1	1	1	1	1	1
65+	0									
GRAND TOTAL	424	2.9	10	1	1	2	3	8	9	14

Length of Stay by Diagnosis and Operation, United States, 1997

United States, October 1995–September 1996 Data, by Operation

69.52: ASP CURETTE POST DEL/AB. Formerly included in operation group(s) 695.

Type of Patients	Observed Patients	Avg. Stay	Vari-ance	10th	25th	50th	75th	90th	95th	99th
1. SINGLE DX										
0–19 Years	355	1.1	<1	1	1	1	1	1	2	3
20–34	1736	1.2	<1	1	1	1	1	1	2	5
35–49	477	1.2	<1	1	1	1	1	2	2	3
50–64	1	2.0	0	2	2	2	2	2	2	2
65+	0									
2. MULTIPLE DX										
0–19 Years	197	2.2	4	1	1	2	2	5	7	9
20–34	1262	2.1	4	1	1	2	2	4	5	9
35–49	405	2.4	8	1	1	1	3	4	6	18
50–64	1	1.0	0	1	1	1	1	1	1	1
65+	0									
TOTAL SINGLE DX	2569	1.2	<1	1	1	1	1	2	2	4
MULTIPLE DX	1865	2.2	5	1	1	2	2	4	6	10
TOTAL										
0–19 Years	552	1.5	2	1	1	1	1	2	4	7
20–34	2998	1.7	3	1	1	1	2	3	4	7
35–49	882	1.6	3	1	1	1	1	3	4	10
50–64	2	1.8	<1	1	2	2	2	2	2	2
65+	0									
GRAND TOTAL	4434	1.6	3	1	1	1	2	3	4	7

69.59: ASP CURETTAGE UTERUS NEC. Formerly included in operation group(s) 695.

Type of Patients	Observed Patients	Avg. Stay	Vari-ance	10th	25th	50th	75th	90th	95th	99th
1. SINGLE DX										
0–19 Years	22	1.1	<1	1	1	1	1	2	2	2
20–34	79	1.1	<1	1	1	1	1	1	2	4
35–49	21	1.1	<1	1	1	1	1	2	2	2
50–64	0									
65+	1	1.0	0	1	1	1	1	1	1	1
2. MULTIPLE DX										
0–19 Years	25	2.1	1	1	1	2	3	4	4	6
20–34	99	2.3	4	1	1	2	2	4	5	11
35–49	71	2.4	13	1	1	1	2	4	6	14
50–64	24	3.8	24	1	1	2	4	9	10	30
65+	38	8.9	39	2	3	8	13	16	17	23
TOTAL SINGLE DX	123	1.1	<1	1	1	1	1	1	2	4
MULTIPLE DX	257	3.3	18	1	1	2	3	9	12	17
TOTAL										
0–19 Years	47	1.6	<1	1	1	1	2	3	4	4
20–34	178	1.4	1	1	1	1	1	2	2	6
35–49	92	2.2	11	1	1	1	2	4	6	10
50–64	24	3.8	24	1	1	2	4	9	10	30
65+	39	8.8	39	2	3	8	13	16	17	23
GRAND TOTAL	380	2.1	9	1	1	1	2	4	7	16

69.6: MENSTRUAL EXTRACTION. Formerly included in operation group(s) 704.

Type of Patients	Observed Patients	Avg. Stay	Vari-ance	10th	25th	50th	75th	90th	95th	99th
1. SINGLE DX										
0–19 Years	0									
20–34	0									
35–49	1	1.0	0	1	1	1	1	1	1	1
50–64	0									
65+	0									
2. MULTIPLE DX										
0–19 Years	0									
20–34	0									
35–49	1	2.0	0	2	2	2	2	2	2	2
50–64	0									
65+	0									
TOTAL SINGLE DX	1	1.0	0	1	1	1	1	1	1	1
MULTIPLE DX	1	2.0	0	2	2	2	2	2	2	2
TOTAL										
0–19 Years	0									
20–34	0									
35–49	2	1.4	<1	1	1	1	2	2	2	2
50–64	0									
65+	0									
GRAND TOTAL	2	1.4	<1	1	1	1	2	2	2	2

69.7: INSERTION OF IUD. Formerly included in operation group(s) 704.

Type of Patients	Observed Patients	Avg. Stay	Vari-ance	10th	25th	50th	75th	90th	95th	99th
1. SINGLE DX										
0–19 Years	0									
20–34	0									
35–49	0									
50–64	0									
65+	0									
2. MULTIPLE DX										
0–19 Years	0									
20–34	0									
35–49	1	19.0	0	19	19	19	19	19	19	19
50–64	0									
65+	0									
TOTAL SINGLE DX	0									
MULTIPLE DX	1	19.0	0	19	19	19	19	19	19	19
TOTAL										
0–19 Years	0									
20–34	0									
35–49	1	19.0	0	19	19	19	19	19	19	19
50–64	0									
65+	0									
GRAND TOTAL	1	19.0	0	19	19	19	19	19	19	19

Length of Stay by Diagnosis and Operation, United States, 1997

United States, October 1995–September 1996 Data, by Operation

69.9: OTHER OPS UTERUS/ADNEXA. Formerly included in operation group(s) 697, 704.

Type of Patients	Observed Patients	Avg. Stay	Vari-ance	Percentiles						
				10th	25th	50th	75th	90th	95th	99th
1. SINGLE DX										
0–19 Years	18	3.0	12	1	1	1	3	10	10	10
20–34	99	1.4	2	1	1	1	1	2	2	10
35–49	65	1.6	<1	1	1	1	2	3	3	5
50–64	23	2.4	1	2	2	2	3	4	5	5
65+	8	3.7	7	2	2	2	5	9	9	9
2. MULTIPLE DX										
0–19 Years	126	1.4	2	1	1	1	1	1	4	10
20–34	487	1.7	5	1	1	1	1	3	4	10
35–49	139	2.1	6	1	1	1	2	4	5	11
50–64	39	3.2	27	2	2	2	3	4	5	44
65+	32	2.9	1	2	2	3	4	4	4	6
TOTAL SINGLE DX	213	1.8	3	1	1	1	2	3	5	10
MULTIPLE DX	823	1.7	5	1	1	1	2	3	4	10
TOTAL										
0–19 Years	144	1.5	3	1	1	1	1	3	4	10
20–34	586	1.6	5	1	1	1	1	3	4	10
35–49	204	1.9	5	1	1	1	2	4	5	11
50–64	62	2.9	18	2	2	2	3	4	5	44
65+	40	3.0	2	2	2	3	4	4	6	9
GRAND TOTAL	1036	1.7	5	1	1	1	2	3	4	10

69.96: RMVL CERVICAL CERCLAGE. Formerly included in operation group(s) 697.

Type of Patients	Observed Patients	Avg. Stay	Vari-ance	Percentiles						
				10th	25th	50th	75th	90th	95th	99th
1. SINGLE DX										
0–19 Years	5	5.8	19	1	1	10	10	10	10	10
20–34	43	1.3	<1	1	1	1	1	2	2	5
35–49	11	1.3	<1	1	1	1	1	2	2	4
50–64	0									
65+	0									
2. MULTIPLE DX										
0–19 Years	12	4.1	24	1	1	2	5	10	10	26
20–34	218	2.7	13	1	1	2	3	5	7	25
35–49	49	2.8	16	1	1	2	3	6	7	13
50–64	1	5.0	0	5	5	5	5	5	5	5
65+	0									
TOTAL SINGLE DX	59	1.6	4	1	1	1	1	2	4	10
MULTIPLE DX	280	2.7	14	1	1	2	3	5	8	25
TOTAL										
0–19 Years	17	4.8	22	1	1	3	10	10	10	26
20–34	261	2.4	11	1	1	1	3	4	6	17
35–49	60	2.4	12	1	1	1	3	4	6	13
50–64	1	5.0	0	5	5	5	5	5	5	5
65+	0									
GRAND TOTAL	339	2.5	12	1	1	1	3	5	7	17

69.93: INSERTION OF LAMINARIA. Formerly included in operation group(s) 697.

Type of Patients	Observed Patients	Avg. Stay	Vari-ance	Percentiles						
				10th	25th	50th	75th	90th	95th	99th
1. SINGLE DX										
0–19 Years	10	1.2	<1	1	1	1	1	2	3	10
20–34	37	2.1	6	1	1	1	2	4	10	10
35–49	11	1.5	1	1	1	1	2	2	5	5
50–64	0									
65+	0									
2. MULTIPLE DX										
0–19 Years	107	1.2	<1	1	1	1	1	1	4	4
20–34	226	1.1	<1	1	1	1	1	2	2	3
35–49	45	1.5	<1	1	1	1	2	2	3	6
50–64	0									
65+	0									
TOTAL SINGLE DX	58	1.7	3	1	1	1	2	3	5	10
MULTIPLE DX	378	1.2	<1	1	1	1	1	2	2	4
TOTAL										
0–19 Years	117	1.2	<1	1	1	1	1	1	4	4
20–34	263	1.2	<1	1	1	1	1	2	2	4
35–49	56	1.5	<1	1	1	1	2	2	3	5
50–64	0									
65+	0									
GRAND TOTAL	436	1.2	<1	1	1	1	1	2	2	4

70.0: CULDOCENTESIS. Formerly included in operation group(s) 700.

Type of Patients	Observed Patients	Avg. Stay	Vari-ance	Percentiles						
				10th	25th	50th	75th	90th	95th	99th
1. SINGLE DX										
0–19 Years	3	2.1	<1	2	2	2	2	3	3	3
20–34	31	1.9	1	1	1	1	2	4	4	5
35–49	6	1.9	1	1	1	2	2	3	5	5
50–64	0									
65+	0									
2. MULTIPLE DX										
0–19 Years	22	2.2	4	1	1	1	3	6	7	8
20–34	83	2.9	4	1	1	2	4	6	7	10
35–49	39	4.8	15	2	2	3	6	10	13	19
50–64	5	5.0	5	3	4	5	5	12	12	12
65+	10	13.2	33	5	8	18	18	18	20	20
TOTAL SINGLE DX	40	1.9	1	1	1	2	2	4	4	5
MULTIPLE DX	159	3.9	15	1	2	3	5	8	12	19
TOTAL										
0–19 Years	25	2.2	3	1	1	1	3	4	6	8
20–34	114	2.6	3	1	2	2	3	5	6	8
35–49	45	4.4	14	2	2	3	5	9	11	19
50–64	5	5.0	5	3	4	5	5	12	12	12
65+	10	13.2	33	5	8	18	18	18	20	20
GRAND TOTAL	199	3.4	12	1	1	2	4	7	10	18

Length of Stay by Diagnosis and Operation, United States, 1997

United States, October 1995–September 1996 Data, by Operation

70.1: INC VAGINA & CUL-DE-SAC. Formerly included in operation group(s) 700.

Type of Patients	Observed Patients	Avg. Stay	Vari-ance	Percentiles						
				10th	25th	50th	75th	90th	95th	99th
1. SINGLE DX										
0–19 Years	9	2.5	2	1	2	2	2	5	7	7
20–34	37	4.9	11	1	2	4	6	12	12	13
35–49	28	3.5	4	1	2	3	5	6	8	8
50–64	10	3.4	8	1	2	2	4	9	9	9
65+	3	1.2	<1	1	1	1	1	2	2	2
2. MULTIPLE DX										
0–19 Years	55	4.4	7	2	2	4	7	7	10	15
20–34	157	6.4	19	2	3	5	11	12	12	20
35–49	203	6.3	13	2	4	6	7	10	13	20
50–64	53	6.6	19	2	3	6	9	10	15	25
65+	78	9.5	72	1	3	7	15	23	24	34
TOTAL SINGLE DX	87	3.9	9	1	2	3	6	8	12	12
MULTIPLE DX	546	6.4	22	2	3	5	8	12	15	24
TOTAL										
0–19 Years	64	4.2	7	2	2	4	7	7	9	15
20–34	194	6.1	18	2	3	5	10	12	12	18
35–49	231	6.1	13	2	4	6	7	10	12	19
50–64	63	6.1	18	2	3	5	9	10	15	25
65+	81	8.8	71	1	2	6	15	23	24	34
GRAND TOTAL	633	6.1	21	2	3	5	8	12	14	24

70.2: VAG/CUL-DE-SAC DXTIC PX. Formerly included in operation group(s) 700, 704.

Type of Patients	Observed Patients	Avg. Stay	Vari-ance	Percentiles						
				10th	25th	50th	75th	90th	95th	99th
1. SINGLE DX										
0–19 Years	48	3.6	4	1	1	4	5	6	6	7
20–34	12	2.0	<1	1	2	2	2	3	6	5
35–49	3	2.3		1	2	2	2	4	4	4
50–64	4	2.9	4	1	1	3	3	8	8	8
65+	3	6.3	15	1	5	5	10	10	10	10
2. MULTIPLE DX										
0–19 Years	188	5.2	8	3	4	5	6	7	7	21
20–34	43	4.1	21	1	2	4	4	14	14	18
35–49	51	5.5	30	1	2	4	7	13	13	31
50–64	45	6.6	59	1	2	3	7	22	25	31
65+	142	7.4	35	2	3	6	10	15	18	36
TOTAL SINGLE DX	70	3.3	4	1	2	3	5	6	7	10
MULTIPLE DX	469	5.9	26	2	3	5	7	12	15	27
TOTAL										
0–19 Years	236	4.8	8	2	4	5	6	7	7	19
20–34	55	3.6	18	1	2	2	3	12	14	15
35–49	54	5.4	29	1	2	4	7	13	13	31
50–64	49	6.3	55	1	2	3	7	22	25	25
65+	145	7.4	35	2	3	6	10	15	18	36
GRAND TOTAL	539	5.6	24	1	2	4	6	11	15	25

70.12: CULDOTOMY. Formerly included in operation group(s) 700.

Type of Patients	Observed Patients	Avg. Stay	Vari-ance	Percentiles						
				10th	25th	50th	75th	90th	95th	99th
1. SINGLE DX										
0–19 Years	6	2.6	2	2	2	2	2	5	7	7
20–34	24	5.9	11	1	3	6	7	12	12	13
35–49	12	4.0	5	2	2	3	5	8	8	8
50–64	1	4.0	0	4	4	4	4	4	4	4
65+	0									
2. MULTIPLE DX										
0–19 Years	19	5.3	8	3	4	4	6	10	12	>99
20–34	90	6.4	16	2	3	5	8	11	14	21
35–49	118	7.0	13	3	5	7	8	11	14	24
50–64	27	7.2	12	3	4	7	9	10	15	17
65+	31	14.2	84	3	7	15	19	24	31	49
TOTAL SINGLE DX	43	5.0	10	2	2	5	6	12	12	13
MULTIPLE DX	285	7.4	25	3	4	7	9	13	18	27
TOTAL										
0–19 Years	25	4.7	8	2	3	4	5	10	12	>99
20–34	114	6.2	15	2	3	6	8	12	12	20
35–49	130	6.8	13	2	5	7	7	10	14	24
50–64	28	7.2	12	3	4	7	9	10	15	17
65+	31	14.2	84	3	7	15	19	24	31	49
GRAND TOTAL	328	7.1	24	2	4	6	8	12	16	25

70.3: LOC EXC/DESTR VAG/CUL. Formerly included in operation group(s) 700.

Type of Patients	Observed Patients	Avg. Stay	Vari-ance	Percentiles						
				10th	25th	50th	75th	90th	95th	99th
1. SINGLE DX										
0–19 Years	11	1.3	<1	1	1	1	1	2	3	3
20–34	27	1.9	1	1	1	2	2	4	4	7
35–49	12	2.1	2	1	1	2	3	5	5	5
50–64	10	2.3	<1	1	1	3	3	3	3	3
65+	8	2.0	2	1	1	1	2	5	5	5
2. MULTIPLE DX										
0–19 Years	65	2.0	2	1	1	1	2	4	5	8
20–34	234	2.6	5	1	1	2	3	7	7	7
35–49	113	2.7	7	1	1	2	3	4	5	18
50–64	66	3.5	6	1	2	3	4	6	7	12
65+	104	4.0	11	1	2	3	5	8	11	18
TOTAL SINGLE DX	68	1.9	1	1	1	2	2	4	5	7
MULTIPLE DX	582	2.9	7	1	1	2	3	7	7	12
TOTAL										
0–19 Years	76	1.9	2	1	1	2	2	4	5	8
20–34	261	2.6	5	1	1	2	3	7	7	7
35–49	125	2.6	6	1	1	2	3	4	5	18
50–64	76	3.4	6	1	2	3	4	6	7	12
65+	112	3.9	11	1	2	3	5	8	11	18
GRAND TOTAL	650	2.8	6	1	1	2	3	6	7	12

Length of Stay by Diagnosis and Operation, United States, 1997

United States, October 1995–September 1996 Data, by Operation

70.33: EXC/DESTR VAG LESION. Formerly included in operation group(s) 700.

Type of Patients	Observed Patients	Avg. Stay	Variance	10th	25th	50th	75th	90th	95th	99th
1. SINGLE DX										
0–19 Years	5	1.5	<1	1	1	1	2	3	3	3
20–34	23	1.8	1	1	1	1	2	3	3	3
35–49	12	2.1	2	1	1	2	3	5	5	5
50–64	4	1.0	0	1	1	1	1	1	1	1
65+	6	1.3	<1	1	1	1	1	2	2	2
2. MULTIPLE DX										
0–19 Years	33	2.6	4	1	1	2	3	5	6	8
20–34	149	1.6	<1	1	1	2	3	5	6	5
35–49	80	2.8	9	1	1	2	3	4	6	23
50–64	62	3.6	7	1	2	3	4	6	8	12
65+	95	3.7	10	1	2	3	4	7	10	18
TOTAL SINGLE DX	50	1.8	1	1	1	2	2	3	3	7
MULTIPLE DX	419	2.6	6	1	1	2	3	5	7	14
TOTAL										
0–19 Years	38	2.5	4	1	1	2	3	5	6	8
20–34	172	1.6	<1	1	1	2	2	2	2	5
35–49	92	2.7	8	1	1	2	3	4	5	18
50–64	66	3.5	7	1	2	3	4	6	8	12
65+	101	3.6	9	1	2	3	4	7	10	18
GRAND TOTAL	469	2.6	6	1	1	2	3	5	6	12

70.4: VAGINAL OBLITERATION. Formerly included in operation group(s) 700.

Type of Patients	Observed Patients	Avg. Stay	Variance	10th	25th	50th	75th	90th	95th	99th
1. SINGLE DX										
0–19 Years	0									
20–34	0									
35–49	3	1.9	1	1	1	1	3	3	3	3
50–64	4	1.6	<1	1	1	2	2	3	2	2
65+	7	2.0	1	1	1	2	3	3	3	5
2. MULTIPLE DX										
0–19 Years	2	6.0	3	3	7	7	7	7	7	7
20–34	5	3.6	<1	3	3	4	4	4	4	4
35–49	27	5.4	40	1	3	4	4	11	26	26
50–64	24	5.9	21	1	2	7	8	9	15	22
65+	75	3.2	6	1	2	2	4	6	8	18
TOTAL SINGLE DX	14	1.9	1	1	2	2	3	3	3	5
MULTIPLE DX	133	4.2	17	1	2	3	5	8	9	26
TOTAL										
0–19 Years	2	6.0	3	3	7	7	7	7	7	7
20–34	5	3.6	<1	3	3	4	4	4	4	4
35–49	30	5.2	39	1	2	4	4	11	26	26
50–64	28	5.5	21	1	2	4	8	9	15	22
65+	82	3.0	6	1	1	2	4	6	7	11
GRAND TOTAL	147	3.9	16	1	2	3	4	8	9	26

70.5: CYSTOCELE/RECTOCELE REP. Formerly included in operation group(s) 698.

Type of Patients	Observed Patients	Avg. Stay	Variance	10th	25th	50th	75th	90th	95th	99th
1. SINGLE DX										
0–19 Years	1	7.0	0	7	7	7	7	7	7	7
20–34	68	1.6	<1	1	1	1	2	2	2	4
35–49	323	1.9	<1	1	1	2	2	3	3	5
50–64	814	1.9	<1	1	1	2	2	3	3	5
65+	845	2.2	1	1	1	2	3	3	4	5
2. MULTIPLE DX										
0–19 Years	2	1.8	2	1	1	1	4	4	4	4
20–34	228	2.3	1	1	2	2	4	4	4	5
35–49	1492	2.3	1	2	2	2	3	4	4	6
50–64	3342	2.4	2	2	2	3	3	4	4	7
65+	4965	2.8	3	2	2	3	3	4	5	8
TOTAL SINGLE DX	2051	2.0	<1	1	1	2	2	3	4	5
MULTIPLE DX	10029	2.6	2	1	2	2	3	4	5	7
TOTAL										
0–19 Years	3	3.2	8	1	1	1	7	7	7	7
20–34	296	2.1	1	1	1	2	3	4	4	5
35–49	1815	2.3	1	1	2	2	3	3	4	6
50–64	4156	2.3	1	1	2	2	3	4	4	6
65+	5810	2.7	3	2	2	3	3	4	5	8
GRAND TOTAL	12080	2.5	2	1	2	2	4	4	5	7

70.50: REP CYSTOCELE/RECTOCELE. Formerly included in operation group(s) 698.

Type of Patients	Observed Patients	Avg. Stay	Variance	10th	25th	50th	75th	90th	95th	99th
1. SINGLE DX										
0–19 Years	0									
20–34	23	2.1	<1	1	2	2	2	3	4	4
35–49	153	2.1	<1	1	2	2	2	3	4	5
50–64	411	2.2	<1	1	2	2	3	3	4	5
65+	441	2.6	1	1	2	3	3	4	4	5
2. MULTIPLE DX										
0–19 Years	0									
20–34	112	2.6	1	1	2	3	3	4	4	6
35–49	842	2.4	1	1	2	2	3	4	4	6
50–64	1958	2.7	2	2	2	3	3	4	5	8
65+	2829	3.0	3	2	2	3	4	4	5	8
TOTAL SINGLE DX	1028	2.3	<1	1	2	2	3	3	4	5
MULTIPLE DX	5741	2.8	2	2	2	3	3	4	5	7
TOTAL										
0–19 Years	0									
20–34	135	2.5	<1	1	2	3	3	4	4	5
35–49	995	2.4	1	1	2	2	3	4	4	5
50–64	2369	2.6	1	1	2	3	3	4	5	7
65+	3270	2.9	2	2	2	3	4	4	5	8
GRAND TOTAL	6769	2.7	2	1	2	3	3	4	5	7

Length of Stay by Diagnosis and Operation, United States, 1997

United States, October 1995–September 1996 Data, by Operation

70.51: CYSTOCELE REPAIR. Formerly included in operation group(s) 698.

Type of Patients	Observed Patients	Avg. Stay	Variance	10th	25th	50th	75th	90th	95th	99th
1. SINGLE DX										
0–19 Years	0									
20–34	9	1.7	<1	1	1	2	2	2	2	3
35–49	40	1.8	<1	1	1	2	2	3	3	3
50–64	170	1.9	<1	1	1	2	2	3	3	5
65+	206	2.0	1	1	1	2	2	3	4	5
2. MULTIPLE DX										
0–19 Years	0									
20–34	41	2.3	2	1	1	2	3	4	4	5
35–49	324	2.3	1	1	2	2	3	3	4	6
50–64	677	2.1	2	1	1	2	3	3	4	5
65+	1176	2.7	4	1	2	2	3	4	5	10
TOTAL SINGLE DX	425	1.9	<1	1	1	2	2	3	3	5
MULTIPLE DX	2218	2.4	2	1	2	2	3	4	4	7
TOTAL										
0–19 Years	0									
20–34	50	2.3	1	1	1	2	3	4	4	5
35–49	364	2.2	<1	1	2	2	3	3	4	6
50–64	847	2.1	<1	1	1	2	3	3	4	5
65+	1382	2.6	3	1	2	2	3	4	5	9
GRAND TOTAL	2643	2.3	2	1	2	2	3	4	4	7

70.52: RECTOCELE REPAIR. Formerly included in operation group(s) 698.

Type of Patients	Observed Patients	Avg. Stay	Variance	10th	25th	50th	75th	90th	95th	99th
1. SINGLE DX										
0–19 Years	1	7.0	0	7	7	7	7	7	7	7
20–34	36	1.3	<1	1	1	1	2	2	3	3
35–49	130	1.8	<1	1	1	2	2	3	3	5
50–64	233	1.6	<1	1	1	2	2	3	3	5
65+	198	1.7	<1	1	1	2	2	3	3	4
2. MULTIPLE DX										
0–19 Years	2	1.8	2	1	1	1	4	4	4	4
20–34	75	1.9	1	1	1	2	2	4	4	5
35–49	326	2.1	2	1	1	2	3	4	5	6
50–64	707	2.0	2	1	1	2	3	4	5	7
65+	960	2.5	3	1	2	2	3	4	5	9
TOTAL SINGLE DX	598	1.7	<1	1	1	2	2	3	3	4
MULTIPLE DX	2070	2.2	2	1	2	2	3	4	5	7
TOTAL										
0–19 Years	3	3.2	8	1	1	1	7	7	7	7
20–34	111	1.7	1	1	1	2	2	3	4	4
35–49	456	2.0	1	1	1	2	3	3	4	5
50–64	940	1.9	<1	1	2	2	3	3	4	6
65+	1158	2.4	3	1	2	2	3	4	5	8
GRAND TOTAL	2668	2.1	2	1	2	2	3	4	4	7

70.6: VAGINAL CONSTR/RECONST. Formerly included in operation group(s) 699.

Type of Patients	Observed Patients	Avg. Stay	Variance	10th	25th	50th	75th	90th	95th	99th
1. SINGLE DX										
0–19 Years	9	5.5	2	4	5	6	6	6	7	8
20–34	1	9.0	0	9	9	9	9	9	9	9
35–49	0									
50–64	1	8.0	0	8	8	8	8	8	8	8
65+	0									
2. MULTIPLE DX										
0–19 Years	34	7.4	10	3	6	7	9	11	12	20
20–34	7	7.6	13	2	5	9	9	12	12	12
35–49	4	3.7	2	2	2	4	4	6	6	6
50–64	6	7.1	19	2	4	7	7	17	17	17
65+	7	6.9	6	4	4	9	9	9	9	9
TOTAL SINGLE DX	11	5.7	2	4	6	6	6	7	8	9
MULTIPLE DX	58	7.2	10	3	4	7	9	10	12	20
TOTAL										
0–19 Years	43	6.7	8	4	6	6	8	9	11	20
20–34	8	7.7	13	2	5	9	9	12	12	12
35–49	4	3.7	2	2	2	4	4	6	6	6
50–64	7	7.3	15	2	5	7	7	10	17	17
65+	7	6.9	6	4	4	9	9	9	9	9
GRAND TOTAL	69	6.7	8	3	5	6	9	9	12	17

70.7: OTHER VAGINAL REPAIR. Formerly included in operation group(s) 699.

Type of Patients	Observed Patients	Avg. Stay	Variance	10th	25th	50th	75th	90th	95th	99th
1. SINGLE DX										
0–19 Years	62	1.5	1	1	1	1	2	2	3	7
20–34	173	1.8	1	1	1	1	2	3	4	5
35–49	110	1.9	1	1	1	2	2	3	4	5
50–64	106	2.5	2	1	1	2	3	4	5	6
65+	92	2.7	1	1	2	3	3	4	5	6
2. MULTIPLE DX										
0–19 Years	148	3.2	7	1	1	2	4	6	8	13
20–34	300	2.6	4	1	1	2	3	5	6	11
35–49	353	3.6	14	1	2	3	4	6	8	16
50–64	505	3.6	19	1	2	3	4	7	8	14
65+	801	4.4	21	2	2	3	5	8	11	19
TOTAL SINGLE DX	543	2.0	1	1	1	2	3	4	4	6
MULTIPLE DX	2107	3.7	16	1	2	3	4	7	9	15
TOTAL										
0–19 Years	210	2.6	6	1	1	2	3	6	7	11
20–34	473	2.3	3	1	1	2	3	4	5	8
35–49	463	3.1	11	1	1	3	4	6	6	15
50–64	611	3.4	16	1	2	3	4	6	8	12
65+	893	4.2	20	2	2	3	4	8	11	19
GRAND TOTAL	2650	3.3	13	1	2	3	4	6	8	14

Length of Stay by Diagnosis and Operation, United States, 1997

United States, October 1995–September 1996 Data, by Operation

70.71: SUTURE VAGINA LACERATION. Formerly included in operation group(s) 699.

Type of Patients	Observed Patients	Avg. Stay	Vari-ance	Percentiles						
				10th	25th	50th	75th	90th	95th	99th
1. SINGLE DX										
0–19 Years	28	1.3	<1	1	1	1	2	2	2	3
20–34	21	1.3	<1	1	1	1	1	2	3	3
35–49	12	1.5	<1	1	1	1	2	3	4	4
50–64	7	2.4	<1	1	2	2	3	3	4	4
65+	2	2.9	1	2	2	2	4	4	4	4
2. MULTIPLE DX										
0–19 Years	51	2.3	3	1	1	2	3	4	6	9
20–34	57	1.8	2	1	1	1	2	3	5	7
35–49	46	2.7	8	1	1	2	3	5	6	15
50–64	31	2.3	2	1	2	2	3	3	4	8
65+	49	3.4	3	2	2	3	4	6	7	9
TOTAL SINGLE DX	70	1.4	<1	1	1	1	2	3	3	4
MULTIPLE DX	234	2.4	4	1	1	2	3	5	6	9
TOTAL										
0–19 Years	79	1.8	2	1	1	1	2	3	4	9
20–34	78	1.7	2	1	1	1	2	3	5	7
35–49	58	2.5	7	1	1	2	3	4	5	15
50–64	38	2.3	1	2	2	2	3	3	3	8
65+	51	3.4	3	2	2	3	4	6	7	9
GRAND TOTAL	304	2.2	3	1	1	2	3	4	5	9

70.73: REP RECTOVAGINAL FISTULA. Formerly included in operation group(s) 699.

Type of Patients	Observed Patients	Avg. Stay	Vari-ance	Percentiles						
				10th	25th	50th	75th	90th	95th	99th
1. SINGLE DX										
0–19 Years	10	1.4	<1	1	1	1	2	2	2	2
20–34	137	1.9	1	1	1	2	2	3	4	5
35–49	61	2.0	1	1	2	2	3	3	4	6
50–64	8	3.8	<1	3	4	4	4	4	5	5
65+	5	1.9	4	1	1	1	2	7	7	7
2. MULTIPLE DX										
0–19 Years	23	3.3	9	1	1	2	5	6	13	13
20–34	179	2.9	4	1	2	3	3	4	6	14
35–49	136	3.7	10	1	2	3	5	5	8	16
50–64	45	4.8	9	2	2	6	7	7	8	14
65+	41	7.1	21	2	3	7	12	14	15	18
TOTAL SINGLE DX	221	2.1	1	1	1	2	3	4	4	5
MULTIPLE DX	424	3.7	10	1	1	3	5	7	10	15
TOTAL										
0–19 Years	33	3.0	8	1	1	2	4	6	6	13
20–34	316	2.4	3	1	1	2	3	4	5	8
35–49	197	2.9	7	1	1	2	5	5	7	10
50–64	53	4.4	7	2	2	4	6	7	7	14
65+	46	6.8	22	2	3	6	11	14	15	17
GRAND TOTAL	645	3.0	7	1	1	2	4	6	7	14

70.77: VAGINAL SUSP & FIXATION. Formerly included in operation group(s) 699.

Type of Patients	Observed Patients	Avg. Stay	Vari-ance	Percentiles						
				10th	25th	50th	75th	90th	95th	99th
1. SINGLE DX										
0–19 Years	0									
20–34	1	3.0	0	3	3	3	3	3	3	3
35–49	22	1.6	<1	1	1	1	2	3	3	4
50–64	79	2.3	<1	1	1	2	3	4	4	5
65+	79	2.8	1	2	2	3	3	4	5	6
2. MULTIPLE DX										
0–19 Years	4	5.0	2	5	5	5	5	8	8	8
20–34	9	4.7	3	5	5	6	6	6	6	6
35–49	83	3.0	1	2	2	3	3	4	6	6
50–64	341	3.1	4	1	2	3	3	5	7	10
65+	584	3.5	5	2	2	3	4	6	8	10
TOTAL SINGLE DX	181	2.3	1	1	1	2	3	4	4	5
MULTIPLE DX	1021	3.4	4	2	2	3	4	6	7	10
TOTAL										
0–19 Years	4	5.0	2	5	5	5	5	8	8	8
20–34	10	4.7	3	2	3	6	6	6	6	6
35–49	105	2.6	2	1	2	3	3	4	6	6
50–64	420	2.9	3	1	2	3	3	4	6	9
65+	663	3.5	5	2	2	3	4	5	8	10
GRAND TOTAL	1202	3.2	4	1	2	3	4	5	6	10

70.79: VAGINAL REPAIR NEC. Formerly included in operation group(s) 699.

Type of Patients	Observed Patients	Avg. Stay	Vari-ance	Percentiles						
				10th	25th	50th	75th	90th	95th	99th
1. SINGLE DX										
0–19 Years	20	1.8	3	1	1	1	2	3	7	7
20–34	12	1.3	<1	1	1	1	1	2	2	5
35–49	10	2.3	2	1	1	2	3	5	5	5
50–64	8	1.2	<1	1	1	1	1	2	2	2
65+	5	1.7	<1	1	1	1	2	2	2	2
2. MULTIPLE DX										
0–19 Years	64	3.8	6	1	2	3	6	7	9	11
20–34	37	2.5	6	1	1	2	3	5	5	20
35–49	59	2.7	4	1	2	2	3	5	5	13
50–64	42	2.8	2	1	2	2	3	4	5	8
65+	54	3.1	2	1	2	3	4	5	6	7
TOTAL SINGLE DX	55	1.5	1	1	1	1	2	2	5	7
MULTIPLE DX	256	3.1	4	1	2	3	4	6	7	10
TOTAL										
0–19 Years	84	3.2	6	1	1	2	5	7	8	10
20–34	49	1.9	4	1	1	1	2	4	5	6
35–49	69	2.7	4	1	2	2	3	4	5	13
50–64	50	2.5	2	1	2	3	3	4	5	8
65+	59	3.1	2	1	2	3	4	5	6	7
GRAND TOTAL	311	2.7	4	1	1	2	3	5	7	9

Length of Stay by Diagnosis and Operation, United States, 1997

United States, October 1995–September 1996 Data, by Operation

70.8: VAGINAL VAULT OBLIT. Formerly included in operation group(s) 700.

Type of Patients	Observed Patients	Avg. Stay	Vari-ance	Percentiles						
				10th	25th	50th	75th	90th	95th	99th
1. SINGLE DX										
0–19 Years	0									
20–34	0									
35–49	2	2.0	0	2	2	2	2	2	2	2
50–64	5	1.7	1	1	1	1	2	4	4	4
65+	39	2.2	1	1	2	2	2	4	5	5
2. MULTIPLE DX										
0–19 Years	1	3.0	0	3	3	3	3	3	3	3
20–34	3	2.8	6	1	1	1	6	6	6	6
35–49	10	2.8	3	2	2	1	3	5	7	7
50–64	17	2.2	6	1	1	1	3	3	12	12
65+	239	3.1	13	1	2	2	4	5	7	19
TOTAL SINGLE DX	46	2.1	1	1	1	2	2	4	4	5
MULTIPLE DX	270	3.0	13	1	2	2	3	5	7	14
TOTAL										
0–19 Years	1	3.0	0	3	3	3	3	3	3	3
20–34	3	2.8	6	1	1	1	6	6	6	6
35–49	12	2.7	2	2	2	2	3	5	7	7
50–64	22	2.1	5	1	1	1	2	3	4	12
65+	278	2.9	12	1	2	2	3	5	7	14
GRAND TOTAL	316	2.9	11	1	1	2	3	4	7	14

70.92: CUL-DE-SAC OPERATION NEC. Formerly included in operation group(s) 700.

Type of Patients	Observed Patients	Avg. Stay	Vari-ance	Percentiles						
				10th	25th	50th	75th	90th	95th	99th
1. SINGLE DX										
0–19 Years	0									
20–34	5	2.4	<1	2	2	2	3	3	3	3
35–49	22	2.4	<1	1	2	2	3	4	4	4
50–64	59	2.0	<1	1	1	2	3	3	3	4
65+	92	2.0	1	1	1	2	2	3	4	4
2. MULTIPLE DX										
0–19 Years	1	1.0	0	1	1	1	1	1	1	1
20–34	31	2.5	2	1	2	2	3	3	5	10
35–49	261	2.8	2	1	2	3	3	5	5	8
50–64	874	2.5	1	2	2	2	3	4	5	6
65+	1832	3.0	3	2	2	3	3	5	6	10
TOTAL SINGLE DX	178	2.1	1	1	1	2	3	3	4	4
MULTIPLE DX	2999	2.8	2	1	2	3	3	4	5	9
TOTAL										
0–19 Years	1	1.0	0	1	1	1	1	1	1	1
20–34	36	2.5	2	1	2	2	3	3	4	10
35–49	283	2.8	2	1	2	3	3	5	5	8
50–64	933	2.5	1	2	2	2	3	4	5	6
65+	1924	3.0	3	1	2	3	3	4	6	10
GRAND TOTAL	3177	2.8	2	1	2	2	3	4	5	9

70.9: OTH VAG & CUL-DE-SAC OPS. Formerly included in operation group(s) 700.

Type of Patients	Observed Patients	Avg. Stay	Vari-ance	Percentiles						
				10th	25th	50th	75th	90th	95th	99th
1. SINGLE DX										
0–19 Years	1	1.0	0	1	1	1	1	1	1	1
20–34	7	2.5	<1	2	2	2	3	3	3	4
35–49	38	2.6	3	1	2	2	3	4	7	7
50–64	75	2.0	<1	1	1	2	3	3	4	7
65+	107	2.0	1	1	1	2	2	3	4	4
2. MULTIPLE DX										
0–19 Years	4	7.7	29	1	2	8	14	14	14	14
20–34	34	2.5	2	1	2	2	3	3	5	10
35–49	280	2.9	2	1	2	3	3	5	5	8
50–64	904	2.5	1	1	2	2	3	4	5	6
65+	1907	3.0	3	2	2	3	3	5	6	10
TOTAL SINGLE DX	228	2.1	1	1	1	2	3	3	4	7
MULTIPLE DX	3129	2.8	2	1	2	3	3	4	5	9
TOTAL										
0–19 Years	5	6.3	31	1	1	8	8	14	14	14
20–34	41	2.5	2	2	2	2	3	3	4	10
35–49	318	2.8	2	1	2	3	3	5	5	8
50–64	979	2.5	1	1	2	2	3	4	4	6
65+	2014	2.9	3	1	2	3	3	5	6	10
GRAND TOTAL	3357	2.8	2	1	2	2	3	4	5	9

71.0: INC VULVA & PERINEUM. Formerly included in operation group(s) 701.

Type of Patients	Observed Patients	Avg. Stay	Vari-ance	Percentiles						
				10th	25th	50th	75th	90th	95th	99th
1. SINGLE DX										
0–19 Years	27	2.6	10	1	1	2	2	4	14	14
20–34	34	2.8	9	1	2	3	3	4	6	7
35–49	12	1.9	<1	1	1	2	2	3	3	5
50–64	6	2.6	<1	1	2	3	3	3	3	3
65+	3	2.8	4	1	3	3	5	5	5	5
2. MULTIPLE DX										
0–19 Years	66	4.0	18	1	2	3	5	7	11	27
20–34	120	4.0	9	1	2	3	5	7	11	15
35–49	128	5.3	14	2	3	5	6	9	11	21
50–64	92	7.1	37	3	3	5	9	14	15	37
65+	72	8.8	67	2	5	7	10	18	20	61
TOTAL SINGLE DX	82	2.6	5	1	1	2	3	4	6	14
MULTIPLE DX	478	5.4	25	1	2	4	6	11	14	27
TOTAL										
0–19 Years	93	3.3	14	1	1	2	4	7	11	27
20–34	154	3.7	8	1	2	3	5	6	9	14
35–49	140	5.1	14	1	3	5	6	9	11	21
50–64	98	6.7	36	3	3	5	8	14	14	37
65+	75	8.6	66	1	4	6	10	18	20	61
GRAND TOTAL	560	4.9	23	1	2	3	6	10	14	23

Length of Stay by Diagnosis and Operation, United States, 1997

United States, October 1995–September 1996 Data, by Operation

71.09: INC VULVA/PERINEUM NEC. Formerly included in operation group(s) 701.

Type of Patients	Observed Patients	Avg. Stay	Vari-ance	10th	25th	50th	75th	90th	95th	99th
1. SINGLE DX										
0-19 Years	25	2.7	12	1	1	1	2	9	14	14
20-34	34	2.8	9	1	1	3	3	4	6	7
35-49	12	1.9	<1	1	1	2	2	3	3	5
50-64	6	2.6	<1	1	2	3	3	3	3	5
65+	3	2.8	4	1	1	3	5	5	5	5
2. MULTIPLE DX										
0-19 Years	62	4.1	18	1	2	3	5	7	11	27
20-34	119	4.0	9	1	2	3	5	7	11	15
35-49	128	5.3	14	2	3	5	6	9	11	21
50-64	91	7.1	37	3	5	5	10	14	15	37
65+	68	9.0	68	3	5	7	11	20	20	61
TOTAL SINGLE DX	80	2.7	5	1	1	2	3	4	7	14
MULTIPLE DX	468	5.4	26	1	2	4	6	11	14	27
TOTAL										
0-19 Years	87	3.5	16	1	1	2	4	8	11	27
20-34	153	3.7	8	1	2	3	5	6	9	14
35-49	140	5.1	14	2	3	5	6	9	11	21
50-64	97	6.7	36	3	3	5	8	14	14	37
65+	71	8.8	67	2	5	7	10	20	20	61
GRAND TOTAL	548	4.9	23	1	2	4	6	10	14	23

71.2: BARTHOLIN'S GLAND OPS. Formerly included in operation group(s) 701.

Type of Patients	Observed Patients	Avg. Stay	Vari-ance	10th	25th	50th	75th	90th	95th	99th
1. SINGLE DX										
0-19 Years	20	2.1	2	1	1	2	2	5	5	5
20-34	66	1.7	<1	1	1	1	2	3	4	4
35-49	35	1.3	<1	1	1	1	1	2	3	4
50-64	6	1.3	<1	1	1	1	1	3	3	3
65+	0									
2. MULTIPLE DX										
0-19 Years	37	1.7	4	1	1	1	2	3	3	13
20-34	109	2.0	3	1	1	1	2	3	5	12
35-49	65	2.4	4	1	1	2	3	4	7	>99
50-64	34	4.1	8	1	3	3	5	6	7	23
65+	12	5.4	15	1	2	6	6	9	15	17
TOTAL SINGLE DX	127	1.7	1	1	1	1	2	3	4	5
MULTIPLE DX	257	2.5	5	1	1	2	3	5	6	13
TOTAL										
0-19 Years	57	1.8	3	1	1	1	2	3	5	7
20-34	175	1.9	2	1	1	1	2	3	5	10
35-49	100	2.0	3	1	1	2	3	4	6	12
50-64	40	3.9	8	1	2	3	5	6	7	23
65+	12	5.4	15	1	2	6	6	9	15	17
GRAND TOTAL	384	2.2	4	1	1	2	3	5	6	12

71.1: VULVAR DIAGNOSTIC PX. Formerly included in operation group(s) 701, 704.

Type of Patients	Observed Patients	Avg. Stay	Vari-ance	10th	25th	50th	75th	90th	95th	99th
1. SINGLE DX										
0-19 Years	2	5.0	1	4	4	6	6	6	6	6
20-34	1	1.0	0	1	1	1	1	1	1	1
35-49	2	4.5	<1	3	3	5	5	5	5	5
50-64	3	5.5	34	1	1	1	11	11	11	11
65+	3	5.8	26	3	3	4	4	16	16	16
2. MULTIPLE DX										
0-19 Years	8	7.0	22	1	4	6	10	14	14	14
20-34	21	3.2	5	1	2	3	5	6	6	12
35-49	24	2.8	13	1	1	1	3	5	6	20
50-64	23	4.5	9	2	2	3	6	5	10	14
65+	60	9.4	64	3	3	8	11	28	28	28
TOTAL SINGLE DX	11	4.7	11	1	3	4	6	11	11	16
MULTIPLE DX	136	7.3	52	1	3	5	8	18	28	28
TOTAL										
0-19 Years	10	6.4	16	1	4	6	10	14	14	14
20-34	22	3.1	5	1	2	3	3	5	6	12
35-49	26	2.9	12	1	1	1	1	5	6	20
50-64	26	4.6	10	2	2	3	6	10	11	14
65+	63	9.3	63	3	3	8	11	28	28	28
GRAND TOTAL	147	7.2	50	1	3	5	8	18	28	28

71.3: LOC VULVAR/PERI EXC NEC. Formerly included in operation group(s) 701.

Type of Patients	Observed Patients	Avg. Stay	Vari-ance	10th	25th	50th	75th	90th	95th	99th
1. SINGLE DX										
0-19 Years	13	1.6	<1	1	1	1	2	3	3	4
20-34	13	3.0	5	1	2	2	3	4	10	10
35-49	23	2.7	3	1	2	2	3	6	7	7
50-64	10	1.4	<1	1	1	1	2	2	2	3
65+	9	3.8	7	2	2	4	6	7	9	9
2. MULTIPLE DX										
0-19 Years	67	2.1	4	1	1	2	2	3	4	8
20-34	315	2.9	57	1	1	2	2	3	4	69
35-49	124	2.7	10	1	1	2	3	5	9	23
50-64	71	4.0	45	1	2	2	3	6	14	27
65+	141	5.6	47	1	2	4	7	10	24	50
TOTAL SINGLE DX	68	2.5	4	1	1	2	3	5	7	10
MULTIPLE DX	718	3.5	44	1	1	2	3	6	10	34
TOTAL										
0-19 Years	80	2.0	3	1	1	2	2	3	4	8
20-34	328	2.9	55	1	1	2	3	5	4	69
35-49	147	2.7	9	1	1	2	3	6	9	11
50-64	81	3.8	42	1	2	2	3	6	14	27
65+	150	5.5	46	1	2	4	7	10	16	50
GRAND TOTAL	786	3.4	41	1	1	2	3	6	9	32

Length of Stay by Diagnosis and Operation, United States, 1997

United States, October 1995–September 1996 Data, by Operation

71.4: OPERATIONS ON CLITORIS. Formerly included in operation group(s) 701.

Type of Patients	Observed Patients	Avg. Stay	Vari-ance	Percentiles 10th	25th	50th	75th	90th	95th	99th
1. SINGLE DX										
0–19 Years	16	2.5	6	1	1	1	2	7	7	7
20–34	1	1.0	0	1	1	1	1	7	1	1
35–49	0									
50–64	0									
65+	1	3.0	0	3	3	3	3	3	3	3
2. MULTIPLE DX										
0–19 Years	25	2.4	2	1	1	3	3	4	4	6
20–34	8	2.4	<1	2	2	3	3	3	3	3
35–49	3	3.6	2	2	2	3	5	5	5	5
50–64	0									
65+	0									
TOTAL SINGLE DX	18	2.5	5	1	1	1	3	7	7	7
MULTIPLE DX	36	2.5	1	1	2	2	3	4	4	6
TOTAL										
0–19 Years	41	2.5	4	1	1	2	3	7	7	7
20–34	9	2.4	<1	2	2	2	3	3	3	3
35–49	3	3.6	2	2	2	3	5	5	5	5
50–64	0									
65+	1	3.0	0	3	3	3	3	3	3	3
GRAND TOTAL	54	2.5	3	1	1	2	3	5	7	7

71.5: RADICAL VULVECTOMY. Formerly included in operation group(s) 702.

Type of Patients	Observed Patients	Avg. Stay	Vari-ance	Percentiles 10th	25th	50th	75th	90th	95th	99th
1. SINGLE DX										
0–19 Years	0									
20–34	2	4.0	2	3	3	4	5	5	5	5
35–49	14	3.4	1	2	3	4	4	4	5	5
50–64	17	4.1	3	2	3	4	6	7	7	7
65+	29	5.0	4	3	4	4	7	8	8	8
2. MULTIPLE DX										
0–19 Years	0									
20–34	16	7.4	158	3	4	4	6	9	24	65
35–49	56	6.9	45	2	3	5	8	17	21	34
50–64	77	9.0	189	3	4	5	8	18	55	79
65+	316	7.9	36	3	4	6	10	15	19	29
TOTAL SINGLE DX	62	4.3	3	2	3	4	5	7	8	8
MULTIPLE DX	465	7.9	60	3	4	6	9	15	20	55
TOTAL										
0–19 Years	0									
20–34	18	7.3	154	3	4	4	6	9	24	65
35–49	70	6.0	35	2	3	4	6	12	21	34
50–64	94	8.2	163	2	3	5	7	17	23	79
65+	345	7.7	35	3	4	6	9	15	18	29
GRAND TOTAL	527	7.6	55	2	4	6	8	15	19	38

71.6: OTHER VULVECTOMY. Formerly included in operation group(s) 702.

Type of Patients	Observed Patients	Avg. Stay	Vari-ance	Percentiles 10th	25th	50th	75th	90th	95th	99th
1. SINGLE DX										
0–19 Years	0									
20–34	9	2.1	2	1	1	1	4	4	4	4
35–49	30	2.0	2	1	1	1	2	4	6	6
50–64	24	2.7	12	1	1	1	3	5	15	15
65+	26	2.5	2	1	2	2	3	4	4	7
2. MULTIPLE DX										
0–19 Years	0									
20–34	30	2.6	7	1	2	1	4	6	7	15
35–49	78	3.8	11	1	2	2	5	8	10	14
50–64	88	4.4	44	1	1	2	5	7	11	37
65+	229	4.2	22	1	2	3	5	7	11	17
TOTAL SINGLE DX	89	2.4	4	1	1	2	3	4	6	15
MULTIPLE DX	425	4.1	24	1	2	3	5	7	10	24
TOTAL										
0–19 Years	0									
20–34	39	2.5	6	1	1	1	4	6	7	15
35–49	108	3.2	9	1	1	2	4	7	10	14
50–64	112	4.1	39	1	1	2	5	7	13	37
65+	255	4.0	20	1	2	3	5	6	10	17
GRAND TOTAL	514	3.8	22	1	1	3	5	7	10	22

71.61: UNILATERAL VULVECTOMY. Formerly included in operation group(s) 702.

Type of Patients	Observed Patients	Avg. Stay	Vari-ance	Percentiles 10th	25th	50th	75th	90th	95th	99th
1. SINGLE DX										
0–19 Years	0									
20–34	6	2.2	2	1	1	1	4	4	4	4
35–49	20	2.0	2	1	1	2	3	4	4	6
50–64	16	1.9	2	1	1	1	2	3	5	5
65+	22	2.2	2	1	2	2	2	3	7	7
2. MULTIPLE DX										
0–19 Years	0									
20–34	17	2.5	5	1	1	1	4	7	7	10
35–49	52	3.4	9	1	1	2	5	7	10	14
50–64	59	4.3	52	1	1	2	4	8	30	37
65+	168	3.9	9	1	2	3	5	6	9	17
TOTAL SINGLE DX	64	2.1	2	1	1	2	2	4	5	7
MULTIPLE DX	296	3.8	17	1	1	3	5	6	10	24
TOTAL										
0–19 Years	0									
20–34	23	2.4	5	1	1	1	4	4	7	10
35–49	72	2.9	7	1	1	2	4	6	10	14
50–64	75	3.9	44	1	1	1	4	7	15	37
65+	190	3.7	9	2	2	3	5	6	8	17
GRAND TOTAL	360	3.6	15	1	1	2	5	6	9	24

Length of Stay by Diagnosis and Operation, United States, 1997

United States, October 1995–September 1996 Data, by Operation

71.7: VULVAR & PERINEAL REPAIR. Formerly included in operation group(s) 703.

Type of Patients	Observed Patients	Avg. Stay	Vari-ance	10th	25th	50th	75th	90th	95th	99th
1. SINGLE DX										
0–19 Years	45	1.2	<1	1	1	1	1	2	2	3
20–34	51	1.7	1	1	1	1	2	3	3	4
35–49	22	1.9	1	1	1	2	2	3	3	4
50–64	21	2.2	<1	1	2	2	3	3	5	5
65+	17	2.1	1	1	1	2	3	4	4	4
2. MULTIPLE DX										
0–19 Years	66	1.9	2	1	1	1	2	4	5	9
20–34	148	2.0	6	1	1	1	2	3	4	12
35–49	99	2.4	4	1	1	2	3	5	6	13
50–64	120	2.6	2	1	2	2	3	4	4	6
65+	179	3.7	18	1	2	3	4	6	12	21
TOTAL SINGLE DX	156	1.6	<1	1	1	1	2	3	3	4
MULTIPLE DX	612	2.6	8	1	1	2	3	4	6	21
TOTAL										
0–19 Years	111	1.6	1	1	1	1	2	3	4	6
20–34	199	1.9	5	1	1	1	2	3	4	12
35–49	121	2.3	3	1	2	2	3	4	6	13
50–64	141	2.6	2	1	2	2	3	4	4	6
65+	196	3.6	17	1	2	3	4	5	10	21
GRAND TOTAL	768	2.4	7	1	1	2	3	4	5	16

71.71: SUTURE VULVAR/PERI LAC. Formerly included in operation group(s) 703.

Type of Patients	Observed Patients	Avg. Stay	Vari-ance	10th	25th	50th	75th	90th	95th	99th
1. SINGLE DX										
0–19 Years	39	1.1	<1	1	1	1	1	2	2	2
20–34	22	1.9	<1	1	1	2	2	3	3	3
35–49	12	2.2	<1	1	2	2	3	3	3	3
50–64	9	3.0	2	2	2	3	4	5	5	5
65+	9	1.8	1	1	1	1	3	3	4	4
2. MULTIPLE DX										
0–19 Years	48	1.9	2	1	1	1	2	4	6	9
20–34	72	2.0	3	1	1	2	2	3	3	12
35–49	31	2.7	4	1	2	2	3	5	7	7
50–64	60	2.8	3	2	2	3	3	4	4	6
65+	95	2.9	3	1	2	2	4	5	6	12
TOTAL SINGLE DX	91	1.5	<1	1	1	1	2	3	3	5
MULTIPLE DX	306	2.5	3	1	1	2	3	4	6	12
TOTAL										
0–19 Years	87	1.6	2	1	1	1	2	3	4	6
20–34	94	2.0	2	1	1	2	2	3	3	12
35–49	43	2.7	4	1	2	2	3	5	7	7
50–64	69	2.8	3	2	2	3	3	4	5	6
65+	104	2.8	3	1	2	2	3	4	6	12
GRAND TOTAL	397	2.3	3	1	1	2	3	4	5	10

71.79: VULVAR/PERINEUM REP NEC. Formerly included in operation group(s) 703.

Type of Patients	Observed Patients	Avg. Stay	Vari-ance	10th	25th	50th	75th	90th	95th	99th
1. SINGLE DX										
0–19 Years	6	1.6	<1	1	1	1	2	2	3	3
20–34	24	1.5	<1	1	1	1	2	3	3	4
35–49	9	1.6	<1	1	1	1	2	2	2	4
50–64	12	1.9	<1	2	2	2	2	2	2	3
65+	8	2.5	1	2	2	3	3	4	4	4
2. MULTIPLE DX										
0–19 Years	17	1.7	1	1	1	1	2	4	4	5
20–34	65	1.8	2	1	1	1	3	3	5	5
35–49	62	2.0	2	1	1	2	2	3	5	6
50–64	60	2.4	2	2	2	2	4	4	4	5
65+	78	4.1	23	2	2	3	4	7	21	21
TOTAL SINGLE DX	59	1.6	<1	1	1	1	2	3	3	4
MULTIPLE DX	282	2.6	9	1	1	2	3	4	5	21
TOTAL										
0–19 Years	23	1.7	1	1	1	1	2	3	4	5
20–34	89	1.7	1	1	1	1	2	3	4	5
35–49	71	2.0	2	1	1	2	2	3	5	6
50–64	72	2.3	1	2	2	2	3	4	4	6
65+	86	4.0	22	2	2	3	4	6	21	21
GRAND TOTAL	341	2.4	8	1	1	2	3	4	5	21

71.8: OTHER VULVAR OPERATIONS. Formerly included in operation group(s) 703.

Type of Patients	Observed Patients	Avg. Stay	Vari-ance	10th	25th	50th	75th	90th	95th	99th
1. SINGLE DX										
0–19 Years	1	4.0	0	4	4	4	4	4	4	4
20–34	0									
35–49	0									
50–64	1	5.0	0	5	5	5	5	5	5	5
65+	1	3.0	0	3	3	3	3	3	3	3
2. MULTIPLE DX										
0–19 Years	1	5.0	0	5	5	5	5	5	5	5
20–34	1	1.0	0	1	1	1	1	1	1	1
35–49	1	3.0	0	3	3	3	3	3	3	3
50–64	0									
65+	1	3.0	0	3	3	3	3	3	3	3
TOTAL SINGLE DX	3	3.8	<1	3	3	4	5	5	5	5
MULTIPLE DX	4	3.2	2	1	3	3	5	5	5	5
TOTAL										
0–19 Years	2	4.7	<1	4	4	5	5	5	5	5
20–34	1	1.0	0	1	1	1	1	1	1	1
35–49	1	3.0	0	3	3	3	3	3	3	3
50–64	1	5.0	0	5	5	5	5	5	5	5
65+	2	3.0	0	3	3	3	3	3	3	3
GRAND TOTAL	7	3.4	2	1	3	3	5	5	5	5

Length of Stay by Diagnosis and Operation, United States, 1997

United States, October 1995–September 1996 Data, by Operation

71.9: OTHER FEMALE GENITAL OPS. Formerly included in operation group(s) 703.

Type of Patients	Observed Patients	Avg. Stay	Vari-ance	10th	25th	50th	75th	90th	95th	99th
1. SINGLE DX										
0–19 Years	2	2.5	2	2	2	2	2	6	6	6
20–34	0									
35–49	0									
50–64	0									
65+	0									
2. MULTIPLE DX										
0–19 Years	2	2.6	<1	1	3	3	3	3	3	3
20–34	0									
35–49	1	3.0	0	3	3	3	3	3	3	3
50–64	1	2.0	0	2	2	2	2	2	2	2
65+	1	2.0	0	2	2	2	2	2	2	2
TOTAL SINGLE DX	2	2.5	2	2	2	2	2	6	6	6
MULTIPLE DX	5	2.4	<1	2	2	3	3	3	3	3
TOTAL										
0–19 Years	4	2.6	1	2	2	2	3	3	6	6
20–34	0									
35–49	1	3.0	0	3	3	3	3	3	3	3
50–64	1	2.0	0	2	2	2	2	2	2	2
65+	1	2.0	0	2	2	2	2	2	2	2
GRAND TOTAL	7	2.5	1	2	2	2	3	3	6	6

72.0: LOW FORCEPS OPERATION. Formerly included in operation group(s) 705.

Type of Patients	Observed Patients	Avg. Stay	Vari-ance	10th	25th	50th	75th	90th	95th	99th
1. SINGLE DX										
0–19 Years	83	1.8	<1	1	1	2	2	2	3	4
20–34	397	1.7	<1	1	1	2	2	2	3	3
35–49	47	1.9	<1	1	1	2	2	3	3	3
50–64	0									
65+	0									
2. MULTIPLE DX										
0–19 Years	578	2.4	4	1	1	2	3	3	5	10
20–34	2906	2.1	3	1	1	2	2	3	4	9
35–49	509	2.1	2	2	2	2	2	3	4	8
50–64	0									
65+	0									
TOTAL SINGLE DX	527	1.7	<1	1	1	2	2	2	3	3
MULTIPLE DX	3993	2.1	3	1	1	2	2	3	4	8
TOTAL										
0–19 Years	661	2.3	4	1	1	2	3	3	5	8
20–34	3303	2.0	3	1	1	2	2	3	3	7
35–49	556	2.1	2	1	1	2	2	3	3	8
50–64	0									
65+	0									
GRAND TOTAL	4520	2.1	3	1	1	2	2	3	4	8

72.1: LOW FORCEPS W EPISIOTOMY. Formerly included in operation group(s) 705.

Type of Patients	Observed Patients	Avg. Stay	Vari-ance	10th	25th	50th	75th	90th	95th	99th
1. SINGLE DX										
0–19 Years	1164	1.9	2	1	1	2	2	3	3	4
20–34	5109	1.8	<1	1	1	2	2	3	3	3
35–49	509	1.8	<1	1	1	2	2	3	3	3
50–64	0									
65+	0									
2. MULTIPLE DX										
0–19 Years	2794	2.0	2	1	1	2	2	3	3	6
20–34	16353	2.0	1	1	1	2	2	3	3	5
35–49	2424	2.1	2	1	1	2	3	3	4	6
50–64	0									
65+	0									
TOTAL SINGLE DX	6782	1.8	<1	1	1	2	2	3	3	3
MULTIPLE DX	21571	2.0	2	1	1	2	2	3	3	5
TOTAL										
0–19 Years	3958	2.0	2	1	1	2	2	3	3	6
20–34	21462	2.0	1	1	1	2	2	3	3	5
35–49	2933	2.1	2	1	1	2	2	3	4	6
50–64	0									
65+	0									
GRAND TOTAL	28353	2.0	1	1	1	2	2	3	3	5

72.2: MID FORCEPS OPERATION. Formerly included in operation group(s) 707.

Type of Patients	Observed Patients	Avg. Stay	Vari-ance	10th	25th	50th	75th	90th	95th	99th
1. SINGLE DX										
0–19 Years	55	1.4	<1	1	1	1	2	2	3	4
20–34	216	1.8	<1	1	1	1	2	2	3	3
35–49	24	1.3	<1	1	1	1	1	2	3	3
50–64	1	1.0	0	1	1	1	1	1	1	1
65+	0									
2. MULTIPLE DX										
0–19 Years	175	2.2	2	1	2	2	2	3	4	9
20–34	1040	2.2	2	1	2	2	3	3	4	5
35–49	164	2.2	3	1	2	2	3	3	3	6
50–64	0									
65+	0									
TOTAL SINGLE DX	296	1.6	<1	1	1	2	2	2	3	3
MULTIPLE DX	1379	2.2	2	1	2	2	3	3	4	5
TOTAL										
0–19 Years	230	1.9	1	1	1	2	2	3	4	9
20–34	1256	2.1	2	1	1	2	2	3	4	5
35–49	188	2.1	3	1	1	2	2	3	3	5
50–64	1	1.0	0	1	1	1	1	1	1	1
65+	0									
GRAND TOTAL	1675	2.1	2	1	1	2	2	3	4	5

Length of Stay by Diagnosis and Operation, United States, 1997

United States, October 1995–September 1996 Data, by Operation

72.21: MID FORCEPS W EPISIOTOMY. Formerly included in operation group(s) 707.

Type of Patients	Observed Patients	Avg. Stay	Variance	10th	25th	50th	75th	90th	95th	99th
1. SINGLE DX										
0–19 Years	51	1.4	<1	1	1	1	2	2	3	3
20–34	196	1.8	<1	1	1	2	2	3	3	3
35–49	21	1.2	<1	1	1	1	1	2	2	2
50–64	1	1.0	0	1	1	1	1	1	1	1
65+	0									
2. MULTIPLE DX										
0–19 Years	149	2.1	1	1	2	2	2	3	4	7
20–34	890	2.2	3	1	2	2	3	3	4	5
35–49	135	2.2	3	1	2	2	3	3	3	5
50–64	0									
65+	0									
TOTAL SINGLE DX	269	1.6	<1	1	1	2	2	2	3	3
MULTIPLE DX	1174	2.2	2	1	2	2	3	3	4	5
TOTAL										
0–19 Years	200	1.8	<1	1	1	2	2	3	3	5
20–34	1086	2.1	2	1	2	2	2	3	4	5
35–49	156	2.0	3	1	1	2	2	3	3	4
50–64	1	1.0	0	1	1	1	1	1	1	1
65+	0									
GRAND TOTAL	1443	2.0	2	1	1	2	2	3	3	5

72.3: HIGH FORCEPS OPERATION. Formerly included in operation group(s) 707.

Type of Patients	Observed Patients	Avg. Stay	Variance	10th	25th	50th	75th	90th	95th	99th
1. SINGLE DX										
0–19 Years	1	1.0	0	1	1	1	1	1	1	1
20–34	7	1.7	<1	1	1	2	2	2	3	3
35–49	0									
50–64	0									
65+	0									
2. MULTIPLE DX										
0–19 Years	3	2.0	0	2	2	2	2	2	2	2
20–34	16	2.1	<1	2	2	2	2	3	3	3
35–49	2	2.0	<1	2	2	2	2	3	3	3
50–64	0									
65+	0									
TOTAL SINGLE DX	8	1.6	<1	1	1	2	2	2	3	3
MULTIPLE DX	21	2.0	<1	2	2	2	2	2	3	3
TOTAL										
0–19 Years	4	1.7	<1	1	1	2	2	2	2	2
20–34	23	2.0	<1	2	2	2	2	3	3	3
35–49	2	2.0	<1	2	2	2	2	3	3	2
50–64	0									
65+	0									
GRAND TOTAL	29	1.9	<1	2	2	2	2	2	3	3

72.4: FORCEPS ROT FETAL HEAD. Formerly included in operation group(s) 707.

Type of Patients	Observed Patients	Avg. Stay	Variance	10th	25th	50th	75th	90th	95th	99th
1. SINGLE DX										
0–19 Years	10	1.7	<1	1	1	2	2	2	2	2
20–34	56	1.9	<1	1	2	2	2	3	3	2
35–49	4	2.1	<1	1	1	2	3	3	3	3
50–64	0									
65+	0									
2. MULTIPLE DX										
0–19 Years	42	2.1	<1	1	2	2	2	3	3	5
20–34	216	2.1	<1	1	2	2	3	3	3	4
35–49	33	2.2	1	1	2	2	2	3	3	6
50–64	0									
65+	0									
TOTAL SINGLE DX	70	1.8	<1	1	1	2	2	2	3	3
MULTIPLE DX	291	2.1	<1	1	2	2	3	3	3	5
TOTAL										
0–19 Years	52	1.9	<1	1	2	2	2	2	3	5
20–34	272	2.1	<1	1	2	2	3	3	3	3
35–49	37	2.2	1	1	2	2	3	3	3	6
50–64	0									
65+	0									
GRAND TOTAL	361	2.0	<1	1	2	2	2	3	3	4

72.5: BREECH EXTRACTION. Formerly included in operation group(s) 706.

Type of Patients	Observed Patients	Avg. Stay	Variance	10th	25th	50th	75th	90th	95th	99th
1. SINGLE DX										
0–19 Years	18	1.3	<1	1	1	1	2	2	2	2
20–34	118	1.5	<1	1	1	1	2	2	2	4
35–49	24	1.6	<1	1	1	2	2	2	2	3
50–64	0									
65+	0									
2. MULTIPLE DX										
0–19 Years	144	2.5	16	1	1	2	2	4	6	22
20–34	858	2.7	9	1	1	2	3	5	11	12
35–49	194	3.0	15	1	1	2	3	5	12	15
50–64	1	12.0	0	12	12	12	12	12	12	12
65+	0									
TOTAL SINGLE DX	160	1.5	<1	1	1	1	2	2	2	3
MULTIPLE DX	1197	2.7	11	1	1	2	3	5	11	13
TOTAL										
0–19 Years	162	2.4	15	1	1	2	2	4	6	22
20–34	976	2.5	8	1	1	2	3	5	9	11
35–49	218	2.9	14	1	1	2	3	4	10	15
50–64	1	12.0	0	12	12	12	12	12	12	12
65+	0									
GRAND TOTAL	1357	2.6	10	1	1	2	3	4	9	12

Length of Stay by Diagnosis and Operation, United States, 1997

United States, October 1995–September 1996 Data, by Operation

72.52: PART BREECH EXTRACT NEC. Formerly included in operation group(s) 706.

Type of Patients	Observed Patients	Avg. Stay	Variance	10th	25th	50th	75th	90th	95th	99th
1. SINGLE DX										
0–19 Years	8	1.3	<1	1	1	1	2	2	2	2
20–34	51	1.5	<1	1	1	1	2	2	3	4
35–49	16	1.6	<1	1	1	2	2	2	2	3
50–64	0									
65+	0									
2. MULTIPLE DX										
0–19 Years	66	2.2	11	1	1	2	2	3	4	18
20–34	416	3.1	14	1	1	2	3	8	11	14
35–49	91	2.4	5	1	1	2	3	4	7	10
50–64	0									
65+	0									
TOTAL SINGLE DX	75	1.5	<1	1	1	1	2	2	3	4
MULTIPLE DX	573	2.9	13	1	1	2	3	6	11	15
TOTAL										
0–19 Years	74	2.1	10	1	1	1	2	3	4	18
20–34	467	2.9	13	1	1	2	3	8	11	13
35–49	107	2.3	4	1	1	2	3	4	6	10
50–64	0									
65+	0									
GRAND TOTAL	648	2.7	12	1	1	2	3	6	11	14

72.54: TOT BREECH EXTRACT NEC. Formerly included in operation group(s) 706.

Type of Patients	Observed Patients	Avg. Stay	Variance	10th	25th	50th	75th	90th	95th	99th
1. SINGLE DX										
0–19 Years	8	1.4	<1	1	1	1	2	2	2	2
20–34	46	1.5	<1	1	1	1	2	2	3	3
35–49	6	1.3	<1	1	1	1	2	2	2	2
50–64	0									
65+	0									
2. MULTIPLE DX										
0–19 Years	61	2.5	10	1	1	2	2	4	7	22
20–34	339	2.3	3	1	1	2	3	4	5	9
35–49	79	3.6	24	1	1	2	3	9	12	32
50–64	1	12.0	0	12	12	12	12	12	12	12
65+	0									
TOTAL SINGLE DX	60	1.4	<1	1	1	1	2	2	2	3
MULTIPLE DX	480	2.5	8	1	1	2	3	4	6	12
TOTAL										
0–19 Years	69	2.4	9	1	1	2	2	4	7	22
20–34	385	2.2	3	1	1	2	3	4	5	9
35–49	85	3.5	23	1	1	2	3	9	12	32
50–64	1	12.0	0	12	12	12	12	12	12	12
65+	0									
GRAND TOTAL	540	2.4	7	1	1	2	3	4	5	12

72.6: FORCEPS-AFTERCOMING HEAD. Formerly included in operation group(s) 706.

Type of Patients	Observed Patients	Avg. Stay	Variance	10th	25th	50th	75th	90th	95th	99th
1. SINGLE DX										
0–19 Years	3	1.7	<1	1	1	2	2	2	2	2
20–34	11	3.2	2	1	2	4	4	4	4	4
35–49	1	2.0	0	2	2	2	2	2	2	2
50–64	0									
65+	0									
2. MULTIPLE DX										
0–19 Years	3	1.6	<1	1	1	1	2	3	3	3
20–34	28	2.1	3	1	2	2	2	3	3	17
35–49	8	1.7	<1	1	1	2	2	3	3	3
50–64	0									
65+	0									
TOTAL SINGLE DX	15	3.1	2	1	2	4	4	4	4	4
MULTIPLE DX	39	2.1	2	1	2	2	2	2	3	4
TOTAL										
0–19 Years	6	1.7	<1	1	1	2	2	3	3	3
20–34	39	2.4	3	1	2	2	3	4	4	4
35–49	9	1.8	<1	1	1	2	2	3	3	3
50–64	0									
65+	0									
GRAND TOTAL	54	2.3	2	1	2	2	2	4	4	4

72.7: VACUUM EXTRACTION DEL. Formerly included in operation group(s) 707.

Type of Patients	Observed Patients	Avg. Stay	Variance	10th	25th	50th	75th	90th	95th	99th
1. SINGLE DX										
0–19 Years	2958	1.7	<1	1	1	2	2	2	3	3
20–34	14233	1.7	<1	1	1	2	2	2	3	3
35–49	1326	1.7	<1	1	1	2	2	2	3	3
50–64	2	2.0	0	2	2	2	2	2	2	2
65+	0									
2. MULTIPLE DX										
0–19 Years	6538	1.9	1	1	1	2	2	3	3	6
20–34	41813	1.9	1	1	1	2	2	3	3	5
35–49	6307	1.9	1	1	1	2	2	3	3	4
50–64	8	3.0	5	2	2	3	3	3	3	13
65+	0									
TOTAL SINGLE DX	18519	1.7	<1	1	1	2	2	2	3	3
MULTIPLE DX	54666	1.9	1	1	1	2	2	3	3	5
TOTAL										
0–19 Years	9496	1.9	1	1	1	2	2	3	3	6
20–34	56046	1.8	1	1	1	2	2	3	3	4
35–49	7633	1.9	1	1	1	2	3	3	3	4
50–64	10	2.9	5	2	2	3	3	3	3	13
65+	0									
GRAND TOTAL	73185	1.8	1	1	1	2	2	3	3	4

Length of Stay by Diagnosis and Operation, United States, 1997

United States, October 1995–September 1996 Data, by Operation

72.71: VED W EPISIOTOMY. Formerly included in operation group(s) 707.

Type of Patients	Observed Patients	Avg. Stay	Vari-ance	Percentiles						
				10th	25th	50th	75th	90th	95th	99th
1. SINGLE DX										
0–19 Years	2429	1.7	<1	1	1	2	2	2	3	3
20–34	11745	1.7	<1	1	1	2	2	2	3	3
35–49	1074	1.8	<1	1	1	2	2	2	3	3
50–64	2	2.0	0	2	2	2	2	2	2	2
65+	0									
2. MULTIPLE DX										
0–19 Years	4657	2.0	1	1	1	2	2	3	3	6
20–34	29384	1.9	1	1	1	2	2	3	3	5
35–49	4223	2.0	<1	1	1	2	2	3	3	4
50–64	6	3.2	15	2	2	2	2	13	13	13
65+	0									
TOTAL SINGLE DX	15250	1.7	<1	1	1	2	2	2	3	3
MULTIPLE DX	38270	1.9	1	1	1	2	2	3	3	5
TOTAL										
0–19 Years	7086	1.9	<1	1	1	2	2	3	3	6
20–34	41129	1.9	1	1	1	2	2	3	3	4
35–49	5297	1.9	<1	1	1	2	2	3	3	4
50–64	8	2.9	11	2	2	2	2	13	13	13
65+	0									
GRAND TOTAL	53520	1.9	1	1	1	2	2	3	3	4

72.8: INSTRUMENTAL DEL NEC. Formerly included in operation group(s) 707.

Type of Patients	Observed Patients	Avg. Stay	Vari-ance	Percentiles						
				10th	25th	50th	75th	90th	95th	99th
1. SINGLE DX										
0–19 Years	2	1.6	1	1	1	1	3	3	3	3
20–34	5	1.1		1	1	1	1	1	3	3
35–49	0									
50–64	0									
65+	0									
2. MULTIPLE DX										
0–19 Years	1	1.0	0	1	1	1	1	1	1	1
20–34	8	1.9	<1	1	1	2	3	3	3	5
35–49	3	1.8	<1	1	2	2	2	2	2	3
50–64	0									
65+	0									
TOTAL SINGLE DX	7	1.2	<1	1	1	1	1	3	3	3
MULTIPLE DX	12	1.8	<1	1	1	2	2	3	3	3
TOTAL										
0–19 Years	3	1.2	<1	1	1	1	1	3	3	3
20–34	13	1.6	<1	1	1	1	2	3	3	3
35–49	3	1.8	<1	1	2	2	2	2	2	2
50–64	0									
65+	0									
GRAND TOTAL	19	1.6	<1	1	1	1	2	3	3	3

72.79: VACUUM EXTRACT DEL NEC. Formerly included in operation group(s) 707.

Type of Patients	Observed Patients	Avg. Stay	Vari-ance	Percentiles						
				10th	25th	50th	75th	90th	95th	99th
1. SINGLE DX										
0–19 Years	529	1.7	<1	1	1	2	2	2	3	3
20–34	2488	1.6	<1	1	1	1	2	2	3	3
35–49	252	1.6	<1	1	1	1	2	2	3	3
50–64	0									
65+	0									
2. MULTIPLE DX										
0–19 Years	1881	1.8	<1	1	1	2	2	3	3	5
20–34	12429	1.8	1	1	1	2	2	3	3	5
35–49	2084	1.8	2	1	1	2	2	3	3	4
50–64	2	2.9	<1	3	3	3	3	3	3	3
65+	0									
TOTAL SINGLE DX	3269	1.6	<1	1	1	1	2	2	3	3
MULTIPLE DX	16396	1.8	1	1	1	2	2	3	3	5
TOTAL										
0–19 Years	2410	1.8	<1	1	1	2	2	3	3	4
20–34	14917	1.8	1	1	1	2	2	3	3	4
35–49	2336	1.8	2	1	1	2	3	3	3	3
50–64	2	2.9	<1	3	3	3	3	3	3	3
65+	0									
GRAND TOTAL	19665	1.8	1	1	1	2	2	3	3	4

72.9: INSTRUMENTAL DEL NOS. Formerly included in operation group(s) 707.

Type of Patients	Observed Patients	Avg. Stay	Vari-ance	Percentiles						
				10th	25th	50th	75th	90th	95th	99th
1. SINGLE DX										
0–19 Years	9	1.9	<1	1	1	2	2	3	3	3
20–34	29	2.0	<1	2	2	2	2	2	3	3
35–49	3	1.7	<1	1	1	2	2	2	2	2
50–64	0									
65+	0									
2. MULTIPLE DX										
0–19 Years	15	1.9	<1	1	1	2	2	3	4	4
20–34	92	1.9	<1	1	1	2	2	3	3	4
35–49	10	2.0	<1	2	2	2	3	3	3	3
50–64	0									
65+	0									
TOTAL SINGLE DX	41	2.0	<1	1	2	2	2	2	3	3
MULTIPLE DX	117	1.9	<1	1	1	2	2	3	3	4
TOTAL										
0–19 Years	24	1.9	<1	1	1	2	2	3	3	4
20–34	121	2.0	<1	1	2	2	2	3	3	4
35–49	13	1.9	<1	1	2	2	2	3	3	3
50–64	0									
65+	0									
GRAND TOTAL	158	1.9	<1	1	2	2	2	3	3	4

Length of Stay by Diagnosis and Operation, United States, 1997

United States, October 1995–September 1996 Data, by Operation

73.0: ARTIFICIAL RUPT MEMBRANE. Formerly included in operation group(s) 708.

Type of Patients	Observed Patients	Avg. Stay	Variance	10th	25th	50th	75th	90th	95th	99th
1. SINGLE DX										
0–19 Years	1494	1.6	<1	1	1	2	2	2	3	3
20–34	9045	1.5	<1	1	1	1	2	2	2	3
35–49	807	1.5	<1	1	1	1	2	2	2	3
50–64	1	1.0	0	1	1	1	1	1	1	1
65+	0									
2. MULTIPLE DX										
0–19 Years	1433	1.9	2	1	1	2	2	3	3	6
20–34	8655	1.7	1	1	1	2	2	2	3	4
35–49	1262	1.7	<1	1	1	2	2	3	3	4
50–64	1	1.0	0	1	1	1	1	1	1	1
65+	0									
TOTAL SINGLE DX	11347	1.5	<1	1	1	1	2	2	2	3
MULTIPLE DX	11351	1.7	1	1	1	2	2	2	3	4
TOTAL										
0–19 Years	2927	1.7	1	1	1	2	2	3	3	4
20–34	17700	1.6	<1	1	1	1	2	2	3	4
35–49	2069	1.7	<1	1	1	2	2	2	3	4
50–64	2	1.0	0	1	1	1	1	1	1	1
65+	0									
GRAND TOTAL	22698	1.6	<1	1	1	1	2	2	3	4

73.09: ARTIF RUPT MEMBRANES NEC. Formerly included in operation group(s) 708.

Type of Patients	Observed Patients	Avg. Stay	Variance	10th	25th	50th	75th	90th	95th	99th
1. SINGLE DX										
0–19 Years	1376	1.6	<1	1	1	2	2	2	3	3
20–34	8030	1.5	<1	1	1	1	2	2	3	3
35–49	693	1.5	<1	1	1	1	2	2	2	3
50–64	1	1.0	0	1	1	1	1	1	1	1
65+	0									
2. MULTIPLE DX										
0–19 Years	1258	1.9	3	1	1	2	2	3	3	6
20–34	6996	1.7	1	1	1	2	2	2	3	4
35–49	980	1.7	<1	1	1	2	2	2	3	4
50–64	1	1.0	0	1	1	1	1	1	1	1
65+	0									
TOTAL SINGLE DX	10100	1.5	<1	1	1	1	2	2	2	3
MULTIPLE DX	9235	1.7	1	1	1	2	2	2	3	4
TOTAL										
0–19 Years	2634	1.7	2	1	1	2	2	2	3	4
20–34	15026	1.6	<1	1	1	1	2	2	3	3
35–49	1673	1.6	<1	1	1	2	2	2	3	4
50–64	2	1.0	0	1	1	1	1	1	1	1
65+	0									
GRAND TOTAL	19335	1.6	<1	1	1	1	2	2	3	4

73.01: INDUCTION LABOR BY AROM. Formerly included in operation group(s) 708.

Type of Patients	Observed Patients	Avg. Stay	Variance	10th	25th	50th	75th	90th	95th	99th
1. SINGLE DX										
0–19 Years	118	1.5	<1	1	1	1	2	2	3	3
20–34	1015	1.5	<1	1	1	1	2	2	2	3
35–49	114	1.5	<1	1	1	1	2	2	2	3
50–64	0									
65+	0									
2. MULTIPLE DX										
0–19 Years	175	1.8	<1	1	1	2	2	3	3	4
20–34	1659	1.7	1	1	1	2	2	2	3	4
35–49	282	1.8	<1	1	1	2	2	3	3	5
50–64	0									
65+	0									
TOTAL SINGLE DX	1247	1.5	<1	1	1	1	2	2	2	3
MULTIPLE DX	2116	1.7	<1	1	1	2	2	3	3	4
TOTAL										
0–19 Years	293	1.6	<1	1	1	1	2	3	3	4
20–34	2674	1.6	<1	1	1	2	2	2	3	4
35–49	396	1.7	<1	1	1	2	2	3	3	4
50–64	0									
65+	0									
GRAND TOTAL	3363	1.6	<1	1	1	2	2	2	3	4

73.1: SURG INDUCTION LABOR NEC. Formerly included in operation group(s) 708.

Type of Patients	Observed Patients	Avg. Stay	Variance	10th	25th	50th	75th	90th	95th	99th
1. SINGLE DX										
0–19 Years	11	2.0	<1	1	2	2	2	2	4	4
20–34	73	1.6	<1	1	1	2	2	2	3	4
35–49	14	2.2	<1	1	1	2	3	3	3	3
50–64	0									
65+	0									
2. MULTIPLE DX										
0–19 Years	26	2.4	2	1	1	2	3	5	5	7
20–34	163	2.4	2	1	1	2	3	4	5	7
35–49	29	2.0	2	1	1	2	2	3	5	9
50–64	0									
65+	0									
TOTAL SINGLE DX	98	1.7	<1	1	1	2	2	3	3	4
MULTIPLE DX	218	2.3	2	1	1	2	3	4	5	7
TOTAL										
0–19 Years	37	2.3	2	1	1	2	3	4	5	7
20–34	236	2.1	2	1	1	2	3	4	5	7
35–49	43	2.1	2	1	1	2	2	3	3	9
50–64	0									
65+	0									
GRAND TOTAL	316	2.1	2	1	1	2	3	4	5	7

Length of Stay by Diagnosis and Operation, United States, 1997

United States, October 1995–September 1996 Data, by Operation

73.2: INT/COMB VERSION/EXTRACT. Formerly included in operation group(s) 707.

Type of Patients	Observed Patients	Avg. Stay	Vari-ance	Percentiles						
				10th	25th	50th	75th	90th	95th	99th
1. SINGLE DX										
0–19 Years	1	1.0	0	1	1	1	1	1	1	1
20–34	13	1.2	<1	1	1	1	1	2	2	2
35–49	1	1.0	0	1	1	1	1	1	1	1
50–64	0									
65+										
2. MULTIPLE DX										
0–19 Years	6	2.1	<1	1	1	2	3	3	4	4
20–34	56	2.3	12	1	1	2	3	3	3	8
35–49	11	1.8	<1	1	1	2	2	3	3	3
50–64	0									
65+	0									
TOTAL SINGLE DX	15	1.2	<1	1	1	1	1	2	2	2
MULTIPLE DX	73	2.3	11	1	1	2	3	3	3	8
TOTAL										
0–19 Years	7	2.0	<1	1	1	2	3	3	3	4
20–34	69	2.2	11	1	1	2	3	3	3	8
35–49	12	1.7	<1	1	1	2	2	3	3	3
50–64	0									
65+	0									
GRAND TOTAL	88	2.1	10	1	1	2	3	3	3	8

73.3: FAILED FORCEPS. Formerly included in operation group(s) 708.

Type of Patients	Observed Patients	Avg. Stay	Vari-ance	Percentiles						
				10th	25th	50th	75th	90th	95th	99th
1. SINGLE DX										
0–19 Years	1	2.0	0	2	2	2	2	2	2	2
20–34	3	1.7	<1	1	1	2	2	2	2	2
35–49	0									
50–64	0									
65+	0									
2. MULTIPLE DX										
0–19 Years	1	2.0	0	2	2	2	2	2	2	2
20–34	10	1.9	2	1	1	1	2	3	7	7
35–49	1	2.0	0	2	2	2	2	2	2	2
50–64	0									
65+	0									
TOTAL SINGLE DX	4	1.8	<1	1	2	2	2	2	2	2
MULTIPLE DX	12	1.9	2	1	1	2	2	3	7	7
TOTAL										
0–19 Years	2	2.0	0	2	2	2	2	2	2	2
20–34	13	1.9	2	1	1	1	2	3	7	7
35–49	1	2.0	0	2	2	2	2	2	2	2
50–64	0									
65+	0									
GRAND TOTAL	16	1.9	2	1	1	2	2	3	3	7

73.4: MEDICAL INDUCTION LABOR. Formerly included in operation group(s) 708.

Type of Patients	Observed Patients	Avg. Stay	Vari-ance	Percentiles						
				10th	25th	50th	75th	90th	95th	99th
1. SINGLE DX										
0–19 Years	615	1.7	<1	1	1	2	2	3	3	4
20–34	4893	1.6	<1	1	1	2	2	3	3	4
35–49	597	1.5	<1	1	1	1	2	2	3	4
50–64	1	1.0	0	1	1	1	1	1	1	1
65+	0									
2. MULTIPLE DX										
0–19 Years	1369	2.3	9	1	1	2	3	3	4	14
20–34	10336	2.0	2	1	1	2	2	3	4	8
35–49	1768	2.3	11	1	1	2	2	3	4	29
50–64	2	2.0	0	1	2	2	2	2	2	2
65+	0									
TOTAL SINGLE DX	6106	1.6	<1	1	1	1	2	2	3	4
MULTIPLE DX	13475	2.1	4	1	1	2	2	3	4	9
TOTAL										
0–19 Years	1984	2.2	7	1	1	2	2	3	4	11
20–34	15229	1.9	2	1	1	2	2	3	4	6
35–49	2365	2.1	9	1	2	2	2	3	4	17
50–64	3	2.0	<1	2	2	2	2	2	2	2
65+	0									
GRAND TOTAL	19581	1.9	3	1	1	2	2	3	4	8

73.5: MANUALLY ASSISTED DEL. Formerly included in operation group(s) 708.

Type of Patients	Observed Patients	Avg. Stay	Vari-ance	Percentiles						
				10th	25th	50th	75th	90th	95th	99th
1. SINGLE DX										
0–19 Years	18803	1.6	<1	1	1	1	2	2	3	3
20–34	96840	1.5	<1	1	1	1	2	2	2	3
35–49	10178	1.5	<1	1	1	1	2	2	3	3
50–64	10	1.4	2	1	1	1	1	1	5	5
65+	0									
2. MULTIPLE DX										
0–19 Years	18563	1.9	3	1	1	2	2	3	4	8
20–34	107918	1.8	3	1	1	2	2	3	3	7
35–49	17497	1.9	3	1	1	2	2	3	3	7
50–64	27	1.8	<1	1	1	2	2	3	3	3
65+	0									
TOTAL SINGLE DX	125831	1.5	<1	1	1	1	2	2	2	3
MULTIPLE DX	144005	1.9	3	1	1	2	2	3	3	7
TOTAL										
0–19 Years	37366	1.7	2	1	1	2	2	3	3	6
20–34	204758	1.7	2	1	1	1	2	2	3	5
35–49	27675	1.7	2	1	1	2	2	3	3	5
50–64	37	1.7	<1	1	1	2	2	3	3	5
65+	0									
GRAND TOTAL	269836	1.7	2	1	1	1	2	2	3	5

Length of Stay by Diagnosis and Operation, United States, 1997

United States, October 1995–September 1996 Data, by Operation

73.51: MANUAL ROT FETAL HEAD. Formerly included in operation group(s) 708.

Type of Patients	Observed Patients	Avg. Stay	Vari-ance	10th	25th	50th	75th	90th	95th	99th
1. SINGLE DX										
0–19 Years	18	1.4	<1	1	1	1	2	2	2	2
20–34	89	1.5	<1	1	1	1	2	2	2	2
35–49	10	1.7	<1	1	1	2	2	2	2	2
50–64	0									
65+	0									
2. MULTIPLE DX										
0–19 Years	41	1.9	3	1	1	2	3	3	3	3
20–34	266	1.6	3	1	1	1	3	2	3	3
35–49	40	1.8	<1	1	1	2	2	2	3	4
50–64	0									
65+	0									
TOTAL SINGLE DX	117	1.5	<1	1	1	1	2	2	2	2
MULTIPLE DX	347	1.6	3	1	1	1	2	3	3	3
TOTAL										
0–19 Years	59	1.8	<1	1	1	2	3	3	3	3
20–34	355	1.5	2	1	1	1	2	2	3	3
35–49	50	1.8	<1	1	1	2	2	3	3	4
50–64	0									
65+	0									
GRAND TOTAL	464	1.6	2	1	1	1	2	2	3	3

73.59: MANUAL ASSISTED DEL NEC. Formerly included in operation group(s) 708.

Type of Patients	Observed Patients	Avg. Stay	Vari-ance	10th	25th	50th	75th	90th	95th	99th
1. SINGLE DX										
0–19 Years	18785	1.6	<1	1	1	1	2	2	3	3
20–34	96751	1.5	<1	1	1	1	2	2	2	3
35–49	10168	1.5	<1	1	1	1	2	2	2	3
50–64	10	1.4	2	1	1	1	1	1	5	5
65+	0									
2. MULTIPLE DX										
0–19 Years	18522	1.9	3	1	1	2	2	3	4	8
20–34	107652	1.8	3	1	1	2	2	3	3	7
35–49	17457	1.9	3	1	1	2	2	3	3	7
50–64	27	1.8	<1	1	1	2	2	3	3	3
65+	0									
TOTAL SINGLE DX	125714	1.5	<1	1	1	1	2	2	2	3
MULTIPLE DX	143658	1.9	3	1	1	2	2	3	3	7
TOTAL										
0–19 Years	37307	1.7	2	1	1	2	2	3	3	6
20–34	204403	1.7	2	1	1	1	2	2	3	5
35–49	27625	1.7	<1	1	1	2	2	3	3	5
50–64	37	1.7		1	1	2	2	3	3	5
65+	0									
GRAND TOTAL	269372	1.7	2	1	1	1	2	2	3	5

73.6: EPISIOTOMY. Formerly included in operation group(s) 708.

Type of Patients	Observed Patients	Avg. Stay	Vari-ance	10th	25th	50th	75th	90th	95th	99th
1. SINGLE DX										
0–19 Years	16032	1.6	<1	1	1	2	2	2	3	4
20–34	89023	1.6	<1	1	1	2	2	2	3	3
35–49	10682	1.7	3	1	1	1	2	2	3	3
50–64	9	1.3	<1	1	1	1	1	3	3	3
65+	0									
2. MULTIPLE DX										
0–19 Years	10365	2.0	3	1	1	2	2	3	3	7
20–34	59445	1.9	2	1	1	2	2	3	3	6
35–49	10427	1.9	3	1	1	2	2	3	3	6
50–64	8	2.4	<1	1	2	3	3	3	3	3
65+	0									
TOTAL SINGLE DX	115746	1.6	<1	1	1	2	2	2	3	3
MULTIPLE DX	80245	1.9	3	1	1	2	2	3	3	6
TOTAL										
0–19 Years	26397	1.7	2	1	1	2	2	3	3	5
20–34	148468	1.7	1	1	1	2	2	2	3	4
35–49	21109	1.8	3	1	1	2	2	3	3	5
50–64	17	2.0	<1	1	2	3	3	3	3	3
65+	0									
GRAND TOTAL	195991	1.7	1	1	1	2	2	2	3	4

73.8: FETAL OPS-FACILITATE DEL. Formerly included in operation group(s) 716.

Type of Patients	Observed Patients	Avg. Stay	Vari-ance	10th	25th	50th	75th	90th	95th	99th
1. SINGLE DX										
0–19 Years	0									
20–34	0									
35–49	0									
50–64	0									
65+	0									
2. MULTIPLE DX										
0–19 Years	1	7.0	0	7	7	7	7	7	7	7
20–34	1	1.0	0	1	1	1	1	1	1	1
35–49	0									
50–64	0									
65+	0									
TOTAL SINGLE DX	0									
MULTIPLE DX	2	5.6	8	1	7	7	7	7	7	7
TOTAL										
0–19 Years	1	7.0	0	7	7	7	7	7	7	7
20–34	1	1.0	0	1	1	1	1	1	1	1
35–49	0									
50–64	0									
65+	0									
GRAND TOTAL	2	5.6	8	1	7	7	7	7	7	7

Length of Stay by Diagnosis and Operation, United States, 1997

United States, October 1995–September 1996 Data, by Operation

73.9: OTH OPS ASSISTING DEL. Formerly included in operation group(s) 708, 716.

Type of Patients	Observed Patients	Avg. Stay	Vari- ance	10th	25th	50th	75th	90th	95th	99th
1. SINGLE DX										
0–19 Years	9	1.5	<1	1	1	1	2	2	3	3
20–34	85	1.4	<1	1	1	1	2	2	3	5
35–49	15	1.7	<1	1	1	2	2	2	3	3
50–64	0									
65+	0									
2. MULTIPLE DX										
0–19 Years	26	2.0	<1	1	2	2	2	3	3	4
20–34	197	1.8	5	1	1	1	2	3	3	5
35–49	37	1.5	<1	1	1	1	2	3	3	3
50–64	0									
65+	0									
TOTAL SINGLE DX	109	1.4	<1	1	1	1	2	2	3	5
MULTIPLE DX	260	1.7	4	1	1	1	2	3	3	5
TOTAL										
0–19 Years	35	1.8	<1	1	1	2	2	3	3	4
20–34	282	1.7	4	1	1	1	2	2	3	5
35–49	52	1.6	<1	1	1	1	2	3	3	3
50–64	0									
65+	0									
GRAND TOTAL	369	1.7	3	1	1	1	2	3	3	5

73.91: EXT VERSION-ASSIST DEL. Formerly included in operation group(s) 708.

Type of Patients	Observed Patients	Avg. Stay	Vari- ance	10th	25th	50th	75th	90th	95th	99th
1. SINGLE DX										
0–19 Years	7	1.3	<1	1	1	1	2	2	2	2
20–34	56	1.2	<1	1	1	1	1	2	2	3
35–49	13	1.7	<1	1	1	2	2	3	3	3
50–64	0									
65+	0									
2. MULTIPLE DX										
0–19 Years	15	2.0	<1	1	2	2	2	3	3	4
20–34	100	1.7	7	1	1	1	2	2	3	24
35–49	29	1.5	<1	1	1	1	2	3	3	3
50–64	0									
65+	0									
TOTAL SINGLE DX	76	1.3	<1	1	1	1	1	2	2	3
MULTIPLE DX	144	1.7	5	1	1	1	2	2	3	5
TOTAL										
0–19 Years	22	1.8	<1	1	1	2	2	3	3	4
20–34	156	1.6	5	1	1	1	2	2	3	5
35–49	42	1.6	<1	1	1	1	2	3	3	3
50–64	0									
65+	0									
GRAND TOTAL	220	1.6	4	1	1	1	2	2	3	5

74.0: CLASSICAL CD. Formerly included in operation group(s) 710.

Type of Patients	Observed Patients	Avg. Stay	Vari- ance	10th	25th	50th	75th	90th	95th	99th
1. SINGLE DX										
0–19 Years	24	3.4	1	2	3	3	4	5	6	6
20–34	123	3.0	<1	2	3	3	3	4	4	6
35–49	23	2.8	<1	2	2	3	3	4	4	4
50–64	0									
65+	0									
2. MULTIPLE DX										
0–19 Years	229	7.0	46	3	3	4	7	16	26	30
20–34	2032	5.7	45	3	3	4	5	11	16	37
35–49	647	6.1	63	3	3	4	5	11	19	49
50–64	1	2.0	0	2	2	2	2	2	2	2
65+	0									
TOTAL SINGLE DX	170	3.1	<1	2	3	3	3	4	4	6
MULTIPLE DX	2909	5.9	49	2	3	4	5	11	18	37
TOTAL										
0–19 Years	253	6.7	44	3	3	4	6	15	26	30
20–34	2155	5.5	42	3	3	4	5	10	15	37
35–49	670	6.1	62	3	3	4	5	11	19	49
50–64	1	2.0	0	2	2	2	2	2	2	2
65+	0									
GRAND TOTAL	3079	5.7	47	2	3	4	5	11	17	37

74.1: LOW CERVICAL CD. Formerly included in operation group(s) 709.

Type of Patients	Observed Patients	Avg. Stay	Vari- ance	10th	25th	50th	75th	90th	95th	99th
1. SINGLE DX										
0–19 Years	2548	3.0	1	2	2	3	3	4	5	6
20–34	23446	2.9	2	2	2	3	3	4	4	5
35–49	3505	3.0	3	2	2	3	3	4	4	6
50–64	4	3.8	<1	3	4	4	4	4	4	4
65+	0									
2. MULTIPLE DX										
0–19 Years	14392	3.9	7	2	3	3	4	6	7	13
20–34	136499	3.5	7	2	3	3	4	5	6	12
35–49	31430	3.7	9	2	3	3	4	5	6	16
50–64	41	6.5	156	3	3	3	4	11	16	83
65+	0									
TOTAL SINGLE DX	29503	2.9	2	2	2	3	3	4	4	6
MULTIPLE DX	182362	3.5	7	2	3	3	4	5	6	13
TOTAL										
0–19 Years	16940	3.7	6	2	3	3	4	5	7	13
20–34	159945	3.4	6	2	3	3	4	4	5	11
35–49	34935	3.6	9	2	3	3	4	5	6	15
50–64	45	5.9	124	3	3	4	4	8	16	83
65+	0									
GRAND TOTAL	211865	3.4	7	2	3	3	4	5	6	12

Length of Stay by Diagnosis and Operation, United States, 1997

United States, October 1995–September 1996 Data, by Operation

74.2: EXTRAPERITONEAL CD. Formerly included in operation group(s) 711.

Type of Patients	Observed Patients	Avg. Stay	Vari- ance	10th	25th	50th	75th	90th	95th	99th
1. SINGLE DX										
0–19 Years	0									
20–34	3	2.7	<1	2	2	3	3	3	3	3
35–49	0									
50–64	0									
65+	0									
2. MULTIPLE DX										
0–19 Years	1	3.0	0	3	3	3	3	3	3	3
20–34	30	2.9	<1	2	2	3	3	4	4	5
35–49	3	2.9	1	2	2	3	3	5	5	5
50–64	0									
65+	0									
TOTAL SINGLE DX	3	2.7	<1	2	2	3	3	3	3	3
MULTIPLE DX	34	2.9	<1	2	2	3	3	4	4	5
TOTAL										
0–19 Years	1	3.0	0	3	3	3	3	3	3	3
20–34	33	2.8	<1	2	2	3	3	4	4	5
35–49	3	2.9	1	2	2	3	3	5	5	5
50–64	0									
65+	0									
GRAND TOTAL	37	2.9	<1	2	2	3	3	4	4	5

74.4: CESAREAN SECTION NEC. Formerly included in operation group(s) 711.

Type of Patients	Observed Patients	Avg. Stay	Vari- ance	10th	25th	50th	75th	90th	95th	99th
1. SINGLE DX										
0–19 Years	20	3.3	<1	2	3	3	4	5	5	5
20–34	65	2.9	<1	2	2	3	3	4	4	4
35–49	12	3.1	<1	3	3	3	3	4	4	4
50–64	0									
65+	0									
2. MULTIPLE DX										
0–19 Years	74	4.4	17	2	3	3	5	7	17	27
20–34	497	3.9	12	2	2	3	4	6	8	18
35–49	100	4.3	40	2	3	3	4	6	9	18
50–64	0									
65+	0									
TOTAL SINGLE DX	97	3.0	<1	2	2	3	3	4	4	5
MULTIPLE DX	671	4.0	16	2	3	3	4	6	8	18
TOTAL										
0–19 Years	94	4.2	14	2	3	3	4	7	8	27
20–34	562	3.8	11	2	2	3	4	6	8	18
35–49	112	4.1	35	2	3	3	4	6	8	12
50–64	0									
65+	0									
GRAND TOTAL	768	3.9	14	2	3	3	4	6	8	18

74.3: RMVL EXTRATUBAL PREG. Formerly included in operation group(s) 712.

Type of Patients	Observed Patients	Avg. Stay	Vari- ance	10th	25th	50th	75th	90th	95th	99th
1. SINGLE DX										
0–19 Years	8	1.4	<1	1	1	1	2	2	2	2
20–34	48	1.5	<1	1	1	1	2	2	2	3
35–49	10	1.8	1	1	1	1	3	3	3	4
50–64	0									
65+	0									
2. MULTIPLE DX										
0–19 Years	8	3.5	<1	3	3	4	4	4	4	4
20–34	130	2.7	3	1	2	2	3	4	5	12
35–49	30	2.8	3	1	2	2	4	6	6	9
50–64	0									
65+	0									
TOTAL SINGLE DX	66	1.5	<1	1	1	1	2	2	3	4
MULTIPLE DX	168	2.8	3	1	2	3	4	4	5	9
TOTAL										
0–19 Years	16	2.4	1	1	1	2	4	4	4	4
20–34	178	2.2	2	1	1	2	3	4	4	8
35–49	40	2.6	3	1	1	2	3	5	6	9
50–64	0									
65+	0									
GRAND TOTAL	234	2.3	2	1	1	2	3	4	4	7

74.9: CESAREAN SECTION NOS. Formerly included in operation group(s) 711, 712.

Type of Patients	Observed Patients	Avg. Stay	Vari- ance	10th	25th	50th	75th	90th	95th	99th
1. SINGLE DX										
0–19 Years	8	2.6	<1	2	2	2	3	4	4	4
20–34	58	3.1	4	2	2	3	3	4	6	14
35–49	5	2.7	<1	2	2	3	3	3	4	4
50–64	0									
65+	0									
2. MULTIPLE DX										
0–19 Years	42	4.8	44	2	3	3	4	6	12	44
20–34	207	3.3	3	2	2	3	4	5	7	10
35–49	59	3.6	5	2	3	3	4	5	9	15
50–64	0									
65+	0									
TOTAL SINGLE DX	71	3.0	3	2	2	3	3	4	4	14
MULTIPLE DX	308	3.6	10	2	2	3	4	5	8	15
TOTAL										
0–19 Years	50	4.4	38	2	2	3	4	5	12	44
20–34	265	3.3	3	2	2	3	4	5	6	13
35–49	64	3.6	5	2	3	3	3	5	9	15
50–64	0									
65+	0									
GRAND TOTAL	379	3.5	9	2	2	3	4	5	7	14

Length of Stay by Diagnosis and Operation, United States, 1997

United States, October 1995–September 1996 Data, by Operation

74.99: OTHER CD TYPE NOS. Formerly included in operation group(s) 711.

Type of Patients	Observed Patients	Avg. Stay	Vari-ance	10th	25th	50th	75th	90th	95th	99th
1. SINGLE DX										
0–19 Years	8	2.6	<1	2	2	2	3	4	4	4
20–34	57	3.1	4	2	2	2	3	4	6	14
35–49	5	2.7	<1	2	2	3	3	3	4	4
50–64	0									
65+	0									
2. MULTIPLE DX										
0–19 Years	40	4.8	45	2	3	3	4	6	12	44
20–34	192	3.2	2	2	2	3	4	5	6	8
35–49	44	3.3	3	2	2	3	4	5	5	15
50–64	0									
65+	0									
TOTAL SINGLE DX	70	3.0	3	2	2	3	3	4	4	14
MULTIPLE DX	276	3.5	10	2	2	3	4	5	6	15
TOTAL										
0–19 Years	48	4.4	38	2	2	3	4	5	12	44
20–34	249	3.2	2	2	2	3	3	4	6	8
35–49	49	3.3	3	2	2	3	4	5	5	15
50–64	0									
65+	0									
GRAND TOTAL	346	3.4	9	2	2	3	4	5	6	14

75.0: INTRA-AMNIO INJECT-AB. Formerly included in operation group(s) 713.

Type of Patients	Observed Patients	Avg. Stay	Vari-ance	10th	25th	50th	75th	90th	95th	99th
1. SINGLE DX										
0–19 Years	62	1.4	<1	1	1	1	2	2	2	3
20–34	108	1.3	<1	1	1	1	2	2	2	3
35–49	23	1.3	<1	1	1	1	1	2	2	2
50–64	0									
65+	0									
2. MULTIPLE DX										
0–19 Years	24	2.8	6	1	1	2	4	4	9	15
20–34	83	1.8	3	1	1	1	2	4	4	11
35–49	25	1.2	<1	1	1	1	1	2	2	2
50–64	0									
65+	0									
TOTAL SINGLE DX	193	1.3	<1	1	1	1	2	2	2	3
MULTIPLE DX	132	1.9	3	1	1	1	2	4	4	11
TOTAL										
0–19 Years	86	1.8	3	1	1	1	2	4	4	9
20–34	191	1.7	2	1	1	1	2	2	4	11
35–49	48	1.2	<1	1	1	1	1	2	2	2
50–64	0									
65+	0									
GRAND TOTAL	325	1.7	2	1	1	1	2	3	4	9

75.1: DIAGNOSTIC AMNIOCENTESIS. Formerly included in operation group(s) 714.

Type of Patients	Observed Patients	Avg. Stay	Vari-ance	10th	25th	50th	75th	90th	95th	99th
1. SINGLE DX										
0–19 Years	134	3.6	12	1	1	2	4	10	11	15
20–34	478	3.6	12	1	1	2	4	8	12	15
35–49	57	3.6	4	2	2	4	5	5	5	10
50–64	0									
65+	0									
2. MULTIPLE DX										
0–19 Years	237	4.0	21	1	2	3	4	7	13	24
20–34	1020	5.3	60	1	2	3	5	11	28	30
35–49	205	4.1	18	1	1	2	5	10	12	20
50–64	0									
65+	0									
TOTAL SINGLE DX	669	3.6	11	1	1	2	5	8	11	15
MULTIPLE DX	1462	5.0	49	1	2	3	5	10	26	28
TOTAL										
0–19 Years	371	3.9	18	1	2	3	4	7	11	23
20–34	1498	4.9	48	1	1	3	5	10	24	28
35–49	262	3.9	13	1	1	3	5	7	11	20
50–64	0									
65+	0									
GRAND TOTAL	2131	4.6	39	1	2	3	5	9	17	28

75.2: INTRAUTERINE TRANSFUSION. Formerly included in operation group(s) 715.

Type of Patients	Observed Patients	Avg. Stay	Vari-ance	10th	25th	50th	75th	90th	95th	99th
1. SINGLE DX										
0–19 Years	1	2.0	0	2	2	2	2	2	2	2
20–34	2	1.5	<1	1	1	2	2	2	2	2
35–49	0									
50–64	0									
65+	0									
2. MULTIPLE DX										
0–19 Years	2	1.0	<1	1	1	1	1	1	1	2
20–34	5	1.1	<1	1	1	1	1	1	1	6
35–49	4	2.1	2	1	1	1	4	4	4	4
50–64	0									
65+	0									
TOTAL SINGLE DX	3	1.6	<1	1	1	2	2	2	2	2
MULTIPLE DX	11	1.2	<1	1	1	1	1	1	1	6
TOTAL										
0–19 Years	3	1.1	<1	1	1	1	1	1	2	2
20–34	7	1.2	<1	1	1	1	1	1	1	6
35–49	4	2.1	2	1	1	1	4	4	4	4
50–64	0									
65+	0									
GRAND TOTAL	14	1.2	<1	1	1	1	1	1	2	6

Length of Stay by Diagnosis and Operation, United States, 1997

United States, October 1995–September 1996 Data, by Operation

75.3: IU OPS FETUS & AMNIO NEC. Formerly included in operation group(s) 715.

Type of Patients	Observed Patients	Avg. Stay	Variance	10th	25th	50th	75th	90th	95th	99th
1. SINGLE DX										
0–19 Years	1293	1.7	2	1	1	1	2	3	4	9
20–34	7621	1.7	4	1	1	1	2	3	4	8
35–49	892	1.6	2	1	1	1	2	3	3	9
50–64	3	1.3	<1	1	1	1	2	2	2	2
65+	0									
2. MULTIPLE DX										
0–19 Years	1389	2.8	9	1	1	2	3	5	8	17
20–34	7768	2.6	13	1	1	2	3	4	7	23
35–49	1206	2.7	19	1	1	2	3	5	7	18
50–64	3	1.7	1	1	1	1	3	3	3	3
65+	0									
TOTAL SINGLE DX	9809	1.7	3	1	1	1	2	3	4	9
MULTIPLE DX	10366	2.6	13	1	1	2	3	5	7	22
TOTAL										
0–19 Years	2682	2.2	6	1	1	2	2	4	5	12
20–34	15389	2.2	9	1	1	1	2	4	5	14
35–49	2098	2.2	11	1	1	1	2	4	6	11
50–64	6	1.5	<1	1	1	1	2	3	3	3
65+	0									
GRAND TOTAL	20175	2.2	9	1	1	1	2	4	5	14

75.34: FETAL MONITORING NOS. Formerly included in operation group(s) 715.

Type of Patients	Observed Patients	Avg. Stay	Variance	10th	25th	50th	75th	90th	95th	99th
1. SINGLE DX										
0–19 Years	963	1.8	2	1	1	1	2	3	4	8
20–34	5625	1.7	3	1	1	1	2	3	4	8
35–49	678	1.8	2	1	1	1	2	3	4	9
50–64	3	1.3	<1	1	1	1	2	2	2	2
65+	0									
2. MULTIPLE DX										
0–19 Years	908	3.0	11	1	1	2	3	5	9	19
20–34	5244	2.5	12	1	1	2	3	4	6	15
35–49	841	2.8	24	1	1	1	3	6	8	18
50–64	3	1.7	1	1	1	1	3	3	3	3
65+	0									
TOTAL SINGLE DX	7269	1.7	3	1	1	1	2	3	4	9
MULTIPLE DX	6996	2.6	14	1	1	2	3	5	7	17
TOTAL										
0–19 Years	1871	2.3	6	1	1	2	3	4	5	13
20–34	10869	2.1	8	1	1	1	2	4	5	12
35–49	1519	2.3	14	1	1	1	2	4	7	11
50–64	6	1.5	<1	1	1	1	2	3	3	3
65+	0									
GRAND TOTAL	14265	2.1	8	1	1	1	2	4	5	12

75.32: FETAL EKG (SCALP). Formerly included in operation group(s) 715.

Type of Patients	Observed Patients	Avg. Stay	Variance	10th	25th	50th	75th	90th	95th	99th
1. SINGLE DX										
0–19 Years	202	1.7	<1	1	1	2	2	3	3	4
20–34	1326	1.6	<1	1	1	2	2	2	3	5
35–49	121	1.6	<1	1	1	1	2	2	3	4
50–64	0									
65+	0									
2. MULTIPLE DX										
0–19 Years	285	2.3	2	1	1	2	3	4	5	8
20–34	1561	2.5	15	1	1	2	2	3	4	23
35–49	193	2.0	1	1	1	2	2	3	3	6
50–64	0									
65+	0									
TOTAL SINGLE DX	1649	1.6	<1	1	1	2	2	2	3	4
MULTIPLE DX	2039	2.4	12	1	1	2	2	3	4	23
TOTAL										
0–19 Years	487	2.0	2	1	1	2	2	3	4	8
20–34	2887	2.1	9	1	1	2	2	3	4	23
35–49	314	1.9	<1	1	1	2	2	3	3	5
50–64	0									
65+	0									
GRAND TOTAL	3688	2.1	8	1	1	2	2	3	4	23

75.35: DXTIC PX FETUS/AMNIO NEC. Formerly included in operation group(s) 715.

Type of Patients	Observed Patients	Avg. Stay	Variance	10th	25th	50th	75th	90th	95th	99th
1. SINGLE DX										
0–19 Years	125	1.5	3	1	1	1	1	2	3	9
20–34	654	1.9	12	1	1	1	2	3	5	12
35–49	92	1.3	<1	1	1	1	1	2	3	5
50–64	0									
65+	0									
2. MULTIPLE DX										
0–19 Years	195	2.7	9	1	1	2	3	5	6	15
20–34	934	3.0	15	1	1	2	3	6	9	21
35–49	166	2.8	13	1	1	2	3	6	6	19
50–64	0									
65+	0									
TOTAL SINGLE DX	871	1.7	8	1	1	1	2	3	4	10
MULTIPLE DX	1295	2.9	14	1	1	2	3	6	8	19
TOTAL										
0–19 Years	320	2.0	6	1	1	1	2	4	5	14
20–34	1588	2.5	14	1	1	1	2	5	7	17
35–49	258	2.1	8	1	1	1	2	4	6	14
50–64	0									
65+	0									
GRAND TOTAL	2166	2.3	11	1	1	1	2	4	7	16

Length of Stay by Diagnosis and Operation, United States, 1997

United States, October 1995–September 1996 Data, by Operation

75.51: REP CURRENT OB LAC CERV. Formerly included in operation group(s) 716.

Type of Patients	Observed Patients	Avg. Stay	Variance	10th	25th	50th	75th	90th	95th	99th
1. SINGLE DX										
0–19 Years	26	1.5	<1	1	1	1	2	2	2	3
20–34	158	1.6	<1	1	1	2	2	2	2	3
35–49	16	1.8	<1	2	2	2	2	2	2	3
50–64	0									
65+	0									
2. MULTIPLE DX										
0–19 Years	162	2.1	<1	1	2	2	2	3	3	4
20–34	875	2.3	5	1	1	2	2	4	4	8
35–49	143	3.7	3	1	2	5	5	5	5	5
50–64	0									
65+	0									
TOTAL SINGLE DX	200	1.6	<1	1	1	2	2	2	2	3
MULTIPLE DX	1180	2.6	4	1	2	2	3	5	5	6
TOTAL										
0–19 Years	188	2.0	<1	1	2	2	2	3	3	4
20–34	1033	2.2	4	1	1	2	2	3	4	7
35–49	159	3.6	3	1	2	5	5	5	5	5
50–64	0									
65+	0									
GRAND TOTAL	1380	2.5	4	1	2	2	3	5	5	6

75.6: REP OTH CURRENT OB LAC. Formerly included in operation group(s) 716.

Type of Patients	Observed Patients	Avg. Stay	Variance	10th	25th	50th	75th	90th	95th	99th
1. SINGLE DX										
0–19 Years	5958	1.6	<1	1	1	1	2	2	3	3
20–34	39875	1.5	<1	1	1	1	2	2	3	3
35–49	5154	1.6	<1	1	1	1	2	2	3	3
50–64	4	1.5	<1	1	1	1	1	3	3	3
65+	0									
2. MULTIPLE DX										
0–19 Years	10308	1.9	2	1	1	2	2	3	3	6
20–34	70925	1.8	2	1	1	2	2	3	3	5
35–49	12259	1.9	3	1	1	2	2	3	3	5
50–64	6	1.2	<1	1	1	1	1	2	2	2
65+	0									
TOTAL SINGLE DX	50991	1.5	<1	1	1	1	2	2	2	3
MULTIPLE DX	93498	1.8	2	1	1	2	2	3	3	5
TOTAL										
0–19 Years	16266	1.8	2	1	1	2	2	3	3	5
20–34	110800	1.7	1	1	1	2	2	3	3	4
35–49	17413	1.8	2	1	1	2	2	2	3	4
50–64	10	1.3	<1	1	1	1	1	2	3	3
65+	0									
GRAND TOTAL	144489	1.7	1	1	1	2	2	2	3	4

75.4: MAN RMVL OF RET PLACENTA. Formerly included in operation group(s) 716.

Type of Patients	Observed Patients	Avg. Stay	Variance	10th	25th	50th	75th	90th	95th	99th
1. SINGLE DX										
0–19 Years	57	1.4	<1	1	1	1	2	2	2	3
20–34	372	1.5	<1	1	1	1	2	2	3	3
35–49	57	1.6	2	1	1	1	2	2	3	15
50–64	0									
65+	0									
2. MULTIPLE DX										
0–19 Years	130	1.8	<1	1	1	2	2	3	3	6
20–34	892	2.0	3	1	1	2	2	3	6	6
35–49	221	1.7	<1	1	1	2	2	3	3	5
50–64	0									
65+	0									
TOTAL SINGLE DX	486	1.5	<1	1	1	1	2	2	3	3
MULTIPLE DX	1243	1.9	2	1	1	2	2	3	4	6
TOTAL										
0–19 Years	187	1.6	<1	1	1	1	2	3	3	4
20–34	1264	1.9	2	1	1	2	2	3	4	6
35–49	278	1.7	<1	1	1	1	2	3	3	5
50–64	0									
65+	0									
GRAND TOTAL	1729	1.8	2	1	1	2	2	3	4	6

75.5: REP CURRENT OB LAC UTER. Formerly included in operation group(s) 716.

Type of Patients	Observed Patients	Avg. Stay	Variance	10th	25th	50th	75th	90th	95th	99th
1. SINGLE DX										
0–19 Years	26	1.5	<1	1	1	1	2	2	2	3
20–34	164	1.6	<1	1	1	2	2	2	3	3
35–49	16	1.8	<1	1	2	2	2	2	3	3
50–64	0									
65+	0									
2. MULTIPLE DX										
0–19 Years	165	2.1	<1	2	2	2	2	3	3	4
20–34	898	2.3	6	1	1	2	2	4	4	8
35–49	149	3.7	3	1	2	5	5	5	5	5
50–64	0									
65+	0									
TOTAL SINGLE DX	206	1.6	<1	1	1	2	2	2	2	3
MULTIPLE DX	1212	2.6	4	1	2	2	3	5	5	6
TOTAL										
0–19 Years	191	2.1	<1	1	2	2	2	3	3	4
20–34	1062	2.2	5	1	1	2	2	4	4	7
35–49	165	3.7	3	1	2	5	5	5	5	5
50–64	0									
65+	0									
GRAND TOTAL	1418	2.5	4	2	2	2	3	5	5	6

Length of Stay by Diagnosis and Operation, United States, 1997

United States, October 1995–September 1996 Data, by Operation

75.61: REP OB LAC BLAD/URETHRA. Formerly included in operation group(s) 716.

Type of Patients	Observed Patients	Avg. Stay	Vari-ance	Percentiles						
				10th	25th	50th	75th	90th	95th	99th
1. SINGLE DX										
0–19 Years	249	1.6	<1	1	1	2	2	2	2	3
20–34	1144	1.5	<1	1	1	1	2	2	2	3
35–49	66	1.6	<1	1	1	2	2	2	2	2
50–64	0									
65+	0									
2. MULTIPLE DX										
0–19 Years	799	2.3	10	1	1	2	2	3	4	21
20–34	3635	1.8	2	1	1	2	2	3	3	7
35–49	406	2.1	7	1	1	2	2	3	4	21
50–64	0									
65+	0									
TOTAL SINGLE DX	1459	1.5	<1	1	1	1	2	2	2	3
MULTIPLE DX	4840	1.9	4	1	1	2	2	3	3	8
TOTAL										
0–19 Years	1048	2.1	7	1	1	2	2	3	3	21
20–34	4779	1.7	1	1	1	2	2	2	3	5
35–49	472	2.1	6	1	1	2	2	3	4	21
50–64	0									
65+	0									
GRAND TOTAL	6299	1.8	3	1	1	2	2	2	3	7

75.62: REP OB LAC RECTUM/ANUS. Formerly included in operation group(s) 716.

Type of Patients	Observed Patients	Avg. Stay	Vari-ance	Percentiles						
				10th	25th	50th	75th	90th	95th	99th
1. SINGLE DX										
0–19 Years	431	1.7	<1	1	1	2	2	2	3	4
20–34	2619	1.7	<1	1	1	2	2	2	3	3
35–49	225	1.8	<1	1	1	2	2	2	3	3
50–64	0									
65+	0									
2. MULTIPLE DX										
0–19 Years	937	1.8	<1	1	1	2	2	3	3	5
20–34	6410	2.0	2	1	1	2	2	3	3	6
35–49	849	2.0	<1	1	1	2	2	3	3	5
50–64	1	1.0	0	1	1	1	1	1	1	1
65+	0									
TOTAL SINGLE DX	3275	1.7	<1	1	1	2	2	2	3	3
MULTIPLE DX	8197	2.0	1	1	1	2	2	3	3	5
TOTAL										
0–19 Years	1368	1.8	<1	1	1	2	2	3	3	5
20–34	9029	1.9	1	1	1	2	2	3	3	5
35–49	1074	2.0	<1	1	1	2	2	3	3	4
50–64	1	1.0	0	1	1	1	1	1	1	1
65+	0									
GRAND TOTAL	11472	1.9	1	1	1	2	2	3	3	5

75.69: REP CURRENT OB LAC NEC. Formerly included in operation group(s) 716.

Type of Patients	Observed Patients	Avg. Stay	Vari-ance	Percentiles						
				10th	25th	50th	75th	90th	95th	99th
1. SINGLE DX										
0–19 Years	5278	1.5	<1	1	1	1	2	2	3	3
20–34	36112	1.5	<1	1	1	1	2	2	3	3
35–49	4863	1.5	<1	1	1	1	2	2	3	3
50–64	4	1.5	<1	1	1	1	1	3	3	3
65+	0									
2. MULTIPLE DX										
0–19 Years	8572	1.8	2	1	1	2	2	3	3	5
20–34	60880	1.7	2	1	1	2	2	3	3	5
35–49	11004	1.8	3	1	1	2	2	3	3	5
50–64	5	1.2	<1	1	1	1	1	2	2	2
65+	0									
TOTAL SINGLE DX	46257	1.5	<1	1	1	1	2	2	2	3
MULTIPLE DX	80461	1.8	2	1	1	2	2	3	3	5
TOTAL										
0–19 Years	13850	1.7	1	1	1	2	2	2	3	5
20–34	96992	1.6	1	1	1	2	2	2	3	4
35–49	15867	1.7	2	1	1	2	2	2	3	4
50–64	9	1.3	<1	1	1	1	1	3	3	3
65+	0									
GRAND TOTAL	126718	1.7	1	1	1	2	2	2	3	4

75.7: PP MANUAL EXPLOR UTERUS. Formerly included in operation group(s) 716.

Type of Patients	Observed Patients	Avg. Stay	Vari-ance	Percentiles						
				10th	25th	50th	75th	90th	95th	99th
1. SINGLE DX										
0–19 Years	33	1.8	<1	1	1	2	2	2	3	3
20–34	145	1.8	<1	1	1	2	2	2	3	3
35–49	19	1.9	<1	1	1	2	2	3	3	3
50–64	0									
65+	0									
2. MULTIPLE DX										
0–19 Years	36	1.3	<1	1	1	1	1	2	3	3
20–34	210	1.9	4	1	1	2	2	3	3	14
35–49	37	1.8	1	1	1	2	2	3	4	5
50–64	0									
65+	0									
TOTAL SINGLE DX	197	1.8	<1	1	1	2	2	2	3	3
MULTIPLE DX	283	1.8	3	1	1	2	2	3	3	7
TOTAL										
0–19 Years	69	1.4	<1	1	1	1	1	2	3	3
20–34	355	1.9	2	1	1	2	2	3	3	5
35–49	56	1.8	1	1	1	2	2	3	4	5
50–64	0									
65+	0									
GRAND TOTAL	480	1.8	2	1	1	2	2	3	3	5

Length of Stay by Diagnosis and Operation, United States, 1997

United States, October 1995–September 1996 Data, by Operation

75.8: OB TAMPONADE UTERUS/VAG. Formerly included in operation group(s) 716.

Type of Patients	Observed Patients	Avg. Stay	Vari- ance	Percentiles						
				10th	25th	50th	75th	90th	95th	99th
1. SINGLE DX										
0–19 Years	0									
20–34	1	1.0	0	1	1	1	1	1	1	1
35–49	0									
50–64	0									
65+	0									
2. MULTIPLE DX										
0–19 Years	0									
20–34	4	2.4	<1	2	2	2	3	3	3	3
35–49	0									
50–64	0									
65+	0									
TOTAL SINGLE DX	1	1.0	0	1	1	1	1	1	1	1
MULTIPLE DX	4	2.4	<1	2	2	2	3	3	3	3
TOTAL										
0–19 Years	0									
20–34	5	2.2	<1	1	2	2	3	3	3	3
35–49	0									
50–64	0									
65+	0									
GRAND TOTAL	5	2.2	<1	1	2	2	3	3	3	3

75.9: OTHER OBSTETRICAL OPS. Formerly included in operation group(s) 716.

Type of Patients	Observed Patients	Avg. Stay	Vari- ance	Percentiles						
				10th	25th	50th	75th	90th	95th	99th
1. SINGLE DX										
0–19 Years	3	2.8	2	2	2	2	5	5	5	5
20–34	38	2.0	1	1	1	2	2	4	5	5
35–49	4	1.1	<1	1	1	1	1	1	2	2
50–64	0									
65+	0									
2. MULTIPLE DX										
0–19 Years	21	2.8	2	1	2	2	4	4	5	8
20–34	126	3.3	10	1	2	2	4	5	6	20
35–49	16	3.5	6	1	2	2	5	7	9	9
50–64	0									
65+	0									
TOTAL SINGLE DX	45	1.8	1	1	1	2	2	3	5	5
MULTIPLE DX	163	3.3	9	1	2	2	4	5	7	20
TOTAL										
0–19 Years	24	2.8	2	1	2	2	4	5	5	8
20–34	164	3.0	8	1	2	2	3	5	6	20
35–49	20	2.2	4	1	1	1	2	5	7	9
50–64	0									
65+	0									
GRAND TOTAL	208	2.8	7	1	2	2	3	5	6	20

76.0: FACIAL BONE INCISION. Formerly included in operation group(s) 721.

Type of Patients	Observed Patients	Avg. Stay	Vari- ance	Percentiles						
				10th	25th	50th	75th	90th	95th	99th
1. SINGLE DX										
0–19 Years	0									
20–34	3	2.2	2	1	1	2	4	4	4	4
35–49	7	2.2	3	1	2	2	2	2	7	7
50–64	1	2.0	0	2	2	2	2	2	2	2
65+	1	2.0	0	2	2	2	2	2	2	2
2. MULTIPLE DX										
0–19 Years	12	3.7	10	1	1	2	5	8	12	12
20–34	15	5.3	98	1	1	1	4	6	35	35
35–49	17	3.4	13	1	1	3	3	6	14	14
50–64	8	2.5	2	1	1	3	3	5	5	5
65+	8	5.4	40	1	1	2	14	19	>99	>99
TOTAL SINGLE DX	12	2.2	2	1	1	2	2	4	4	7
MULTIPLE DX	60	4.0	35	1	1	2	4	8	14	35
TOTAL										
0–19 Years	12	3.7	10	1	1	2	5	8	12	12
20–34	18	3.9	57	1	1	1	4	5	35	35
35–49	24	3.2	11	1	1	2	3	6	14	14
50–64	9	2.4	2	1	1	3	3	5	5	5
65+	9	5.2	37	1	1	2	14	19	>99	>99
GRAND TOTAL	72	3.6	28	1	1	2	4	6	14	35

76.1: DXTIC PX FACIAL BONE/JT. Formerly included in operation group(s) 717, 767.

Type of Patients	Observed Patients	Avg. Stay	Vari- ance	Percentiles						
				10th	25th	50th	75th	90th	95th	99th
1. SINGLE DX										
0–19 Years	4	1.0	0	1	1	1	1	1	1	1
20–34	2	2.2	2	1	1	3	3	3	3	3
35–49	3	1.0	0	1	1	1	1	1	1	1
50–64	2	2.1	1	3	3	3	3	3	3	3
65+	1	4.0	0	4	4	4	4	4	4	4
2. MULTIPLE DX										
0–19 Years	14	4.7	38	1	1	1	7	11	12	37
20–34	11	7.0	88	1	3	4	4	28	28	28
35–49	7	10.2	305	1	1	7	5	48	48	48
50–64	12	5.2	10	2	2	7	8	8	11	11
65+	10	11.4	214	1	1	2	29	40	40	40
TOTAL SINGLE DX	12	1.5	1	1	1	1	1	3	4	4
MULTIPLE DX	54	7.3	111	1	1	3	7	28	34	48
TOTAL										
0–19 Years	18	3.9	32	1	1	1	7	10	12	37
20–34	13	6.7	84	1	2	4	4	28	28	28
35–49	10	8.7	264	1	1	7	5	48	48	48
50–64	14	4.9	10	1	1	7	5	7	11	11
65+	11	11.1	209	1	1	2	20	40	40	40
GRAND TOTAL	66	6.7	102	1	1	2	7	20	29	48

Length of Stay by Diagnosis and Operation, United States, 1997

United States, October 1995–September 1996 Data, by Operation

76.2: DESTR FACIAL BONE LES. Formerly included in operation group(s) 717.

Type of Patients	Observed Patients	Avg. Stay	Variance				Percentiles			
				10th	25th	50th	75th	90th	95th	99th
1. SINGLE DX										
0–19 Years	29	2.4	4	1	1	2	3	5	9	9
20–34	25	3.0	4	1	2	2	4	6	6	13
35–49	21	2.2	2	1	1	2	3	3	4	9
50–64	8	1.4	<1	1	1	1	1	3	3	3
65+	5	2.0	0	2	2	2	2	2	2	2
2. MULTIPLE DX										
0–19 Years	60	4.2	36	1	1	3	5	8	10	>99
20–34	58	3.6	30	1	1	2	4	7	11	13
35–49	74	4.8	29	1	2	3	4	11	20	26
50–64	64	5.3	48	1	1	2	7	10	27	27
65+	80	3.9	48	1	1	2	4	9	11	43
TOTAL SINGLE DX	88	2.4	3	1	1	2	3	4	6	9
MULTIPLE DX	336	4.4	38	1	1	3	5	10	13	40
TOTAL										
0–19 Years	89	3.6	27	1	1	2	5	8	10	54
20–34	83	3.4	23	1	1	2	4	7	10	13
35–49	95	4.0	22	1	2	3	4	9	15	26
50–64	72	5.0	46	1	1	2	6	10	21	27
65+	85	3.8	46	1	1	2	4	9	11	43
GRAND TOTAL	424	4.0	31	1	1	2	4	9	11	27

76.3: PARTIAL FACIAL OSTECTOMY. Formerly included in operation group(s) 717.

Type of Patients	Observed Patients	Avg. Stay	Variance				Percentiles			
				10th	25th	50th	75th	90th	95th	99th
1. SINGLE DX										
0–19 Years	18	2.2	2	1	1	2	2	2	6	6
20–34	21	1.8	1	1	1	1	2	3	4	7
35–49	25	3.2	10	1	1	2	5	8	11	14
50–64	21	2.5	5	1	1	1	4	4	8	11
65+	20	4.0	13	1	2	4	4	7	7	18
2. MULTIPLE DX										
0–19 Years	36	3.4	7	1	2	3	3	7	9	14
20–34	46	5.3	23	1	2	4	6	15	17	24
35–49	75	5.3	22	1	2	4	8	10	14	25
50–64	118	6.5	38	1	2	4	7	14	22	31
65+	172	5.2	22	1	2	4	7	11	13	23
TOTAL SINGLE DX	105	2.6	6	1	1	2	3	5	7	14
MULTIPLE DX	447	5.3	25	1	2	4	7	11	17	24
TOTAL										
0–19 Years	54	2.9	6	1	2	2	3	5	8	14
20–34	67	4.3	19	1	2	3	5	9	17	17
35–49	100	4.8	20	1	2	3	7	10	14	25
50–64	139	6.0	36	1	2	4	7	13	22	31
65+	192	5.1	21	1	2	4	7	11	13	23
GRAND TOTAL	552	4.8	22	1	2	3	6	10	14	24

76.31: PARTIAL MANDIBULECTOMY. Formerly included in operation group(s) 717.

Type of Patients	Observed Patients	Avg. Stay	Variance				Percentiles			
				10th	25th	50th	75th	90th	95th	99th
1. SINGLE DX										
0–19 Years	10	2.0	1	1	1	2	2	3	5	5
20–34	14	2.2	3	1	1	2	2	5	7	7
35–49	17	3.4	13	1	1	2	5	7	11	14
50–64	17	2.6	5	1	1	1	4	4	8	11
65+	16	4.4	13	1	2	4	4	7	18	18
2. MULTIPLE DX										
0–19 Years	27	3.8	11	2	2	2	3	9	12	14
20–34	31	5.9	25	2	2	5	6	17	17	24
35–49	61	5.3	26	1	2	4	7	10	16	25
50–64	84	7.4	48	1	2	6	9	17	22	31
65+	111	6.2	23	1	2	5	9	12	14	22
TOTAL SINGLE DX	74	2.9	8	1	1	2	4	5	7	18
MULTIPLE DX	314	6.0	30	1	2	4	8	13	17	25
TOTAL										
0–19 Years	37	3.1	8	1	2	2	3	7	9	14
20–34	45	5.3	23	1	2	4	6	17	17	24
35–49	78	4.8	24	1	2	3	7	10	14	25
50–64	101	6.6	44	1	2	4	8	17	22	31
65+	127	6.0	22	1	2	5	9	12	14	22
GRAND TOTAL	388	5.4	27	1	2	4	7	12	17	24

76.4: FACIAL BONE EXC/RECONST. Formerly included in operation group(s) 718.

Type of Patients	Observed Patients	Avg. Stay	Variance				Percentiles			
				10th	25th	50th	75th	90th	95th	99th
1. SINGLE DX										
0–19 Years	56	3.4	3	1	2	4	5	5	6	9
20–34	13	2.1	4	1	1	1	2	3	7	11
35–49	22	3.1	9	1	1	2	4	7	12	12
50–64	8	4.4	8	1	2	5	5	11	11	11
65+	5	5.6	32	1	1	3	13	13	13	13
2. MULTIPLE DX										
0–19 Years	114	4.1	10	1	2	4	5	6	8	17
20–34	44	3.6	24	1	1	2	3	8	13	27
35–49	74	5.7	55	1	1	3	6	17	28	29
50–64	83	9.7	334	1	2	4	24	24	51	84
65+	29	6.2	48	1	2	4	6	14	15	36
TOTAL SINGLE DX	104	3.4	6	1	1	3	5	5	9	13
MULTIPLE DX	344	5.6	95	1	2	3	5	11	17	51
TOTAL										
0–19 Years	170	3.9	8	1	2	4	5	6	8	17
20–34	57	3.3	21	1	1	3	3	8	13	23
35–49	96	5.2	47	1	1	3	4	13	19	29
50–64	91	9.5	319	1	2	3	8	22	51	84
65+	34	6.1	44	1	2	3	10	14	15	36
GRAND TOTAL	448	5.2	77	1	1	3	5	10	16	51

Length of Stay by Diagnosis and Operation, United States, 1997

United States, October 1995–September 1996 Data, by Operation

76.5: TMJ ARTHROPLASTY. Formerly included in operation group(s) 718.

Type of Patients	Observed Patients	Avg. Stay	Variance	Percentiles 10th	25th	50th	75th	90th	95th	99th
1. SINGLE DX										
0–19 Years	23	1.8	<1	1	1	1	3	3	3	4
20–34	209	1.5	<1	1	1	1	2	2	3	4
35–49	152	1.6	<1	1	1	1	2	2	3	5
50–64	30	1.3	<1	1	1	1	1	2	3	4
65+	5	1.2	<1	1	1	1	1	2	2	2
2. MULTIPLE DX										
0–19 Years	46	2.6	3	1	1	2	4	5	5	9
20–34	232	1.6	<1	1	1	1	2	3	3	5
35–49	258	1.8	1	1	1	1	2	3	3	6
50–64	98	1.8	1	1	1	1	2	3	3	5
65+	26	2.1	3	1	2	2	2	3	4	11
TOTAL SINGLE DX	419	1.5	<1	1	1	1	2	2	3	5
MULTIPLE DX	660	1.8	1	1	1	1	2	3	4	6
TOTAL										
0–19 Years	69	2.5	2	1	1	2	4	4	5	9
20–34	441	1.6	<1	1	1	1	2	2	3	5
35–49	410	1.7	1	1	1	1	2	3	3	5
50–64	128	1.6	1	1	1	1	2	2	3	5
65+	31	2.0	3	1	2	2	2	3	4	11
GRAND TOTAL	1079	1.7	1	1	1	1	2	3	4	5

76.62: OPN OSTY MAND RAMUS. Formerly included in operation group(s) 718.

Type of Patients	Observed Patients	Avg. Stay	Variance	Percentiles 10th	25th	50th	75th	90th	95th	99th
1. SINGLE DX										
0–19 Years	124	1.7	<1	1	1	2	2	2	2	3
20–34	115	1.7	<1	1	1	2	2	2	2	3
35–49	76	1.5	<1	1	1	1	2	2	3	3
50–64	4	1.6	<1	1	1	2	2	2	2	2
65+	0									
2. MULTIPLE DX										
0–19 Years	208	1.8	<1	1	1	2	2	3	4	5
20–34	137	2.0	1	1	1	2	2	3	3	7
35–49	128	1.9	1	1	1	2	2	3	4	6
50–64	25	1.8	1	1	1	2	2	2	3	3
65+	6	3.4	8	2	2	2	6	9	9	9
TOTAL SINGLE DX	319	1.7	<1	1	1	2	2	2	3	3
MULTIPLE DX	504	1.9	1	1	1	2	2	3	4	6
TOTAL										
0–19 Years	332	1.7	<1	1	1	2	2	3	3	5
20–34	252	1.9	<1	1	1	2	2	3	3	7
35–49	204	1.7	1	1	1	2	2	3	3	5
50–64	29	1.8	1	1	1	2	2	2	3	3
65+	6	3.4	8	2	2	2	6	9	9	9
GRAND TOTAL	823	1.8	<1	1	1	2	2	3	3	5

76.6: OTHER FACIAL BONE REPAIR. Formerly included in operation group(s) 718.

Type of Patients	Observed Patients	Avg. Stay	Variance	Percentiles 10th	25th	50th	75th	90th	95th	99th
1. SINGLE DX										
0–19 Years	408	1.9	1	1	1	2	2	3	4	5
20–34	386	1.7	<1	1	1	2	2	3	3	4
35–49	232	1.7	<1	1	1	2	2	3	3	4
50–64	27	1.3	<1	1	1	1	1	1	2	2
65+	1	1.0	0	1	1	1	1	1	1	1
2. MULTIPLE DX										
0–19 Years	1125	2.3	3	1	1	2	3	4	5	8
20–34	914	2.2	2	1	1	2	3	3	5	10
35–49	541	2.0	1	1	1	2	2	3	3	6
50–64	129	1.7	2	1	1	1	2	3	3	6
65+	27	5.7	42	1	1	2	9	18	18	18
TOTAL SINGLE DX	1054	1.8	<1	1	1	2	2	3	3	5
MULTIPLE DX	2736	2.2	3	1	1	2	3	4	4	9
TOTAL										
0–19 Years	1533	2.2	3	1	1	2	2	4	4	7
20–34	1300	2.1	2	1	1	2	2	3	4	10
35–49	773	2.0	1	1	1	2	2	3	3	5
50–64	156	1.7	2	1	1	1	2	3	3	6
65+	28	5.6	42	1	2	2	9	18	18	18
GRAND TOTAL	3790	2.1	2	1	1	2	2	3	4	8

76.64: MAND ORTHOGNATHIC OP NEC. Formerly included in operation group(s) 718.

Type of Patients	Observed Patients	Avg. Stay	Variance	Percentiles 10th	25th	50th	75th	90th	95th	99th
1. SINGLE DX										
0–19 Years	110	1.7	<1	1	1	2	2	3	3	5
20–34	105	1.6	<1	1	1	1	2	2	3	3
35–49	66	1.6	<1	1	1	2	2	2	3	6
50–64	12	1.4	<1	1	1	1	2	2	2	2
65+	0									
2. MULTIPLE DX										
0–19 Years	180	2.4	3	1	2	2	3	3	5	10
20–34	139	2.1	1	1	1	2	3	3	4	10
35–49	124	2.0	2	1	1	2	2	3	3	6
50–64	30	1.2	2	1	1	1	1	2	2	18
65+	5	12.9	56	1	2	18	18	18	18	18
TOTAL SINGLE DX	293	1.7	<1	1	1	2	2	2	3	5
MULTIPLE DX	478	2.2	4	1	1	2	2	3	5	18
TOTAL										
0–19 Years	290	2.2	3	1	1	2	2	3	4	7
20–34	244	1.9	<1	1	1	2	2	3	3	5
35–49	190	1.9	2	1	1	1	1	2	2	6
50–64	42	1.2	2	1	1	1	1	2	2	7
65+	5	12.9	56	1	2	18	18	18	18	18
GRAND TOTAL	771	2.0	3	1	1	2	2	3	4	7

Length of Stay by Diagnosis and Operation, United States, 1997

United States, October 1995–September 1996 Data, by Operation

76.65: SEG OSTEOPLASTY MAXILLA. Formerly included in operation group(s) 718.

Type of Patients	Observed Patients	Avg. Stay	Vari-ance	Percentiles 10th	25th	50th	75th	90th	95th	99th
1. SINGLE DX										
0–19 Years	98	2.2	2	1	1	2	2	3	4	8
20–34	84	1.5	<1	1	1	1	2	3	3	4
35–49	47	2.2	<1	1	2	2	3	3	3	3
50–64	5	1.0	0	1	1	1	1	1	1	1
65+	1	1.0	0	1	1	1	1	1	1	1
2. MULTIPLE DX										
0–19 Years	465	2.2	2	1	2	2	3	3	4	5
20–34	413	2.3	2	1	2	2	3	3	5	10
35–49	175	2.2	<1	1	2	2	3	3	4	3
50–64	34	2.3	1	1	2	2	2	4	5	7
65+	4	6.7	9	1	7	7	8	9	9	9
TOTAL SINGLE DX	235	1.8	1	1	1	2	2	3	3	5
MULTIPLE DX	1091	2.3	2	1	2	2	3	3	4	10
TOTAL										
0–19 Years	563	2.2	2	1	2	2	3	3	4	6
20–34	497	2.1	2	1	1	2	2	3	4	10
35–49	222	2.2	<1	1	2	2	3	3	3	4
50–64	39	2.1	1	1	2	2	2	3	3	7
65+	5	5.7	12	1	7	7	8	9	9	9
GRAND TOTAL	1326	2.2	2	1	2	2	3	3	4	8

76.7: REDUCTION OF FACIAL FX. Formerly included in operation group(s) 719, 720.

Type of Patients	Observed Patients	Avg. Stay	Vari-ance	Percentiles 10th	25th	50th	75th	90th	95th	99th
1. SINGLE DX										
0–19 Years	360	2.1	2	1	1	2	3	4	4	6
20–34	649	2.2	2	1	1	2	3	4	4	7
35–49	344	2.4	5	1	1	2	3	4	5	12
50–64	55	2.3	7	1	1	1	2	4	8	17
65+	11	2.2	1	1	2	2	2	4	5	5
2. MULTIPLE DX										
0–19 Years	1203	4.0	46	1	1	2	4	8	10	29
20–34	2487	3.7	18	1	1	3	4	7	11	23
35–49	1684	3.9	15	1	2	3	5	7	10	18
50–64	440	6.1	54	1	2	4	7	16	16	43
65+	372	6.1	32	1	3	4	8	14	17	23
TOTAL SINGLE DX	1419	2.2	3	1	1	2	3	4	5	8
MULTIPLE DX	6186	4.0	26	1	1	3	5	8	11	25
TOTAL										
0–19 Years	1563	3.5	36	1	1	2	4	7	9	28
20–34	3136	3.4	15	1	1	2	4	6	10	19
35–49	2028	3.6	13	1	1	3	5	7	9	17
50–64	495	5.9	52	1	2	4	7	16	16	43
65+	383	6.0	32	1	2	4	8	14	17	23
GRAND TOTAL	7605	3.7	22	1	1	2	4	7	10	20

76.66: TOT OSTEOPLASTY MAXILLA. Formerly included in operation group(s) 718.

Type of Patients	Observed Patients	Avg. Stay	Vari-ance	Percentiles 10th	25th	50th	75th	90th	95th	99th
1. SINGLE DX										
0–19 Years	24	3.2	2	1	2	3	5	5	5	5
20–34	32	2.1	<1	1	1	2	2	4	4	4
35–49	14	1.7	<1	1	1	2	2	2	2	3
50–64	0									
65+	0									
2. MULTIPLE DX										
0–19 Years	147	2.3	1	1	2	2	3	4	5	6
20–34	150	2.2	2	1	1	2	3	4	5	6
35–49	57	2.0	<1	1	1	2	2	3	3	4
50–64	12	2.1	<1	1	1	2	3	3	3	3
65+	1	1.0	0	1	1	1	1	1	1	1
TOTAL SINGLE DX	70	2.5	2	1	2	2	3	5	5	5
MULTIPLE DX	367	2.3	1	1	2	2	3	4	5	6
TOTAL										
0–19 Years	171	2.4	2	1	2	2	3	4	5	6
20–34	182	2.2	2	1	1	2	3	4	5	6
35–49	71	1.9	<1	1	1	2	2	3	3	4
50–64	12	2.1	<1	1	1	2	3	3	3	3
65+	1	1.0	0	1	1	1	1	1	1	1
GRAND TOTAL	437	2.3	2	1	2	2	3	4	5	6

76.72: OPEN RED MALAR/ZMC FX. Formerly included in operation group(s) 720.

Type of Patients	Observed Patients	Avg. Stay	Vari-ance	Percentiles 10th	25th	50th	75th	90th	95th	99th
1. SINGLE DX										
0–19 Years	34	1.4	5	1	1	1	1	2	2	4
20–34	84	2.0	2	1	1	1	3	2	4	4
35–49	70	1.4	<1	1	1	2	2	2	3	7
50–64	20	2.0	2	2	1	2	2	5	5	7
65+	1	2.0	0	2	2	2	2	2	2	2
2. MULTIPLE DX										
0–19 Years	127	6.1	262	1	1	1	4	8	13	87
20–34	366	3.7	24	1	1	2	4	8	13	28
35–49	305	3.7	12	1	3	3	4	8	11	18
50–64	120	8.8	49	1	3	7	16	16	16	29
65+	78	4.4	13	1	1	3	7	10	12	15
TOTAL SINGLE DX	209	1.7	2	1	1	1	2	4	4	5
MULTIPLE DX	996	4.6	62	1	1	2	5	10	16	33
TOTAL										
0–19 Years	161	4.9	202	1	1	1	3	7	10	87
20–34	450	3.4	20	1	1	2	4	7	11	28
35–49	375	3.2	11	1	1	2	4	7	10	16
50–64	140	8.2	49	1	2	7	16	16	16	29
65+	79	4.4	13	1	1	3	7	10	12	15
GRAND TOTAL	1205	4.0	52	1	1	2	4	8	15	29

Length of Stay by Diagnosis and Operation, United States, 1997

United States, October 1995–September 1996 Data, by Operation

76.74: OPEN RED MAXILLARY FX. Formerly included in operation group(s) 720.

Type of Patients	Observed Patients	Avg. Stay	Variance	10th	25th	50th	75th	90th	95th	99th
1. SINGLE DX										
0–19 Years	5	2.0	<1	2	2	2	2	2	2	3
20–34	23	3.1	5	1	1	3	3	7	8	9
35–49	13	3.5	14	1	2	2	3	12	12	12
50–64	2	1.2	<1	1	1	1	1	1	3	3
65+	0									
2. MULTIPLE DX										
0–19 Years	72	3.8	17	1	1	2	4	9	12	18
20–34	186	5.1	18	1	3	4	6	10	13	24
35–49	139	4.6	17	1	2	3	5	10	13	25
50–64	40	6.2	11	2	4	7	7	8	10	18
65+	36	6.8	30	3	3	3	11	16	17	21
TOTAL SINGLE DX	43	2.8	6	1	1	2	3	6	8	12
MULTIPLE DX	473	5.0	18	1	2	4	7	10	14	20
TOTAL										
0–19 Years	77	3.6	15	1	1	2	4	9	12	18
20–34	209	5.0	17	1	2	4	6	10	13	24
35–49	152	4.5	17	1	2	3	5	10	13	25
50–64	42	5.9	12	1	3	7	7	8	10	18
65+	36	6.8	30	3	3	3	11	16	17	21
GRAND TOTAL	516	4.9	18	1	2	4	7	10	13	20

76.75: CLSD RED MANDIBULAR FX. Formerly included in operation group(s) 719.

Type of Patients	Observed Patients	Avg. Stay	Variance	10th	25th	50th	75th	90th	95th	99th
1. SINGLE DX										
0–19 Years	122	1.8	<1	1	1	2	2	3	3	5
20–34	156	1.7	1	1	1	1	2	3	3	6
35–49	62	2.3	1	1	1	2	3	4	4	5
50–64	4	1.3	<1	1	1	1	2	2	3	3
65+	1	2.0	0	2	2	2	2	2	2	2
2. MULTIPLE DX										
0–19 Years	257	2.4	5	1	1	2	3	4	5	14
20–34	356	2.9	10	1	1	2	3	6	8	16
35–49	182	4.4	8	1	2	5	6	6	12	12
50–64	41	2.2	3	1	2	3	6	6	6	8
65+	36	4.6	10	1	3	3	7	8	12	15
TOTAL SINGLE DX	345	1.9	1	1	1	2	2	3	4	5
MULTIPLE DX	872	3.3	9	1	1	2	5	6	7	12
TOTAL										
0–19 Years	379	2.2	3	1	1	2	3	4	5	9
20–34	512	2.5	8	1	1	2	3	5	7	12
35–49	244	4.0	8	1	2	3	6	5	7	10
50–64	45	2.2	3	1	1	3	3	5	6	10
65+	37	4.6	10	1	3	3	7	8	12	15
GRAND TOTAL	1217	2.9	7	1	1	2	3	6	7	12

76.76: OPEN RED MANDIBULAR FX. Formerly included in operation group(s) 720.

Type of Patients	Observed Patients	Avg. Stay	Variance	10th	25th	50th	75th	90th	95th	99th
1. SINGLE DX										
0–19 Years	152	2.8	2	1	1	2	4	4	5	6
20–34	310	2.5	3	1	2	2	3	4	5	8
35–49	165	3.2	7	1	2	2	4	5	8	16
50–64	22	3.4	16	1	1	2	4	11	11	17
65+	6	2.1	<1	1	2	2	2	4	4	4
2. MULTIPLE DX										
0–19 Years	533	4.1	18	1	2	3	5	7	11	28
20–34	1214	3.5	14	1	2	3	6	7	10	19
35–49	787	3.7	13	1	2	3	5	7	9	19
50–64	161	7.0	108	1	2	4	6	12	43	43
65+	147	5.9	28	2	3	4	7	12	20	23
TOTAL SINGLE DX	655	2.7	4	1	1	2	4	4	5	12
MULTIPLE DX	2842	3.9	20	1	2	3	4	7	11	25
TOTAL										
0–19 Years	685	3.8	15	1	2	3	4	7	9	28
20–34	1524	3.2	12	1	1	2	4	6	8	17
35–49	952	3.6	12	1	2	3	5	7	9	18
50–64	183	6.7	102	1	2	4	6	12	43	43
65+	153	5.8	28	2	3	4	6	11	20	23
GRAND TOTAL	3497	3.6	17	1	2	3	4	7	10	20

76.79: OPEN RED FACIAL FX NEC. Formerly included in operation group(s) 720.

Type of Patients	Observed Patients	Avg. Stay	Variance	10th	25th	50th	75th	90th	95th	99th
1. SINGLE DX										
0–19 Years	33	1.8	2	1	1	1	3	3	5	6
20–34	56	1.7	1	1	1	1	2	3	4	4
35–49	23	1.4	2	1	1	1	1	3	4	12
50–64	6	3.1	5	1	1	3	5	8	8	8
65+	3	2.9	4	2	1	3	5	5	5	5
2. MULTIPLE DX										
0–19 Years	148	4.7	19	1	1	3	8	8	13	19
20–34	269	4.4	26	1	1	3	6	9	12	26
35–49	213	3.9	28	1	1	2	4	8	10	19
50–64	68	3.5	15	1	1	2	4	8	11	19
65+	58	8.3	75	2	2	6	13	18	21	54
TOTAL SINGLE DX	121	1.7	2	1	1	1	2	3	4	6
MULTIPLE DX	756	4.3	27	1	1	3	6	8	12	26
TOTAL										
0–19 Years	181	4.2	17	1	1	3	6	8	11	15
20–34	325	4.0	24	1	1	3	5	8	12	26
35–49	236	3.6	26	1	1	2	4	8	10	18
50–64	74	3.4	15	1	1	2	4	8	11	19
65+	61	8.2	74	2	2	5	13	18	21	54
GRAND TOTAL	877	4.0	24	1	1	3	5	8	11	26

Length of Stay by Diagnosis and Operation, United States, 1997

United States, October 1995–September 1996 Data, by Operation

76.9: OTH OPS FACIAL BONE/JT. Formerly included in operation group(s) 721, 729, 767.

Type of Patients	Observed Patients	Avg. Stay	Variance	10th	25th	50th	75th	90th	95th	99th
1. SINGLE DX										
0–19 Years	62	2.3	3	1	1	2	3	5	7	7
20–34	37	1.6	<1	1	1	1	2	2	4	6
35–49	38	1.7	1	1	1	1	2	3	4	6
50–64	30	1.5	<1	1	1	1	2	3	3	6
65+	7	2.1	<1	1	1	2	3	3	3	3
2. MULTIPLE DX										
0–19 Years	151	2.8	7	1	1	2	3	6	8	11
20–34	160	3.7	19	1	1	3	4	8	10	16
35–49	170	5.2	72	1	1	3	5	11	28	48
50–64	105	3.8	31	1	1	2	4	8	12	21
65+	93	6.5	51	1	1	3	14	14	18	>99
TOTAL SINGLE DX	174	1.9	2	1	1	1	2	3	5	7
MULTIPLE DX	679	4.2	37	1	1	2	4	9	14	28
TOTAL										
0–19 Years	213	2.6	6	1	1	2	3	6	7	11
20–34	197	3.2	15	1	1	2	4	6	10	15
35–49	208	4.3	58	1	1	2	3	9	17	28
50–64	135	3.3	25	1	1	2	4	7	9	21
65+	100	6.2	49	1	1	3	12	14	15	54
GRAND TOTAL	853	3.6	29	1	1	2	4	7	13	28

77.1: OTHER BONE INC W/O DIV. Formerly included in operation group(s) 722, 723.

Type of Patients	Observed Patients	Avg. Stay	Variance	10th	25th	50th	75th	90th	95th	99th
1. SINGLE DX										
0–19 Years	64	3.3	12	1	1	2	4	8	13	13
20–34	45	2.7	12	1	1	2	3	5	6	11
35–49	35	2.6	10	1	1	2	3	6	9	22
50–64	18	2.1	<1	1	1	2	3	3	3	4
65+	9	3.2	7	1	1	4	4	4	4	14
2. MULTIPLE DX										
0–19 Years	146	6.6	52	1	2	5	8	15	17	39
20–34	69	5.6	36	1	2	3	8	14	14	32
35–49	110	5.2	57	1	2	4	6	9	15	26
50–64	69	7.7	90	2	3	5	8	15	26	41
65+	87	9.7	165	1	2	4	13	31	31	33
TOTAL SINGLE DX	171	2.9	11	1	1	2	3	6	9	13
MULTIPLE DX	481	6.8	75	1	2	4	7	15	26	33
TOTAL										
0–19 Years	210	5.6	42	1	2	4	7	13	17	31
20–34	114	4.1	25	1	1	3	5	10	14	32
35–49	145	4.4	44	1	1	3	5	9	11	26
50–64	87	6.6	78	1	2	3	7	15	24	29
65+	96	9.1	154	1	1	4	10	31	31	33
GRAND TOTAL	652	5.6	59	1	2	3	6	13	20	31

77.0: SEQUESTRECTOMY. Formerly included in operation group(s) 722, 723.

Type of Patients	Observed Patients	Avg. Stay	Variance	10th	25th	50th	75th	90th	95th	99th
1. SINGLE DX										
0–19 Years	3	2.9	<1	2	2	3	3	4	4	4
20–34	6	4.6	4	2	3	4	7	7	7	7
35–49	6	1.9	2	3	3	2	2	3	3	12
50–64	2	2.4	<1	2	2	2	3	3	3	3
65+	0									
2. MULTIPLE DX										
0–19 Years	3	10.4	49	3	6	6	17	17	17	17
20–34	30	5.1	17	1	3	4	6	9	11	22
35–49	48	8.9	142	3	3	5	7	17	37	68
50–64	38	8.0	60	1	2	6	10	13	25	37
65+	42	9.4	63	2	4	7	11	19	33	34
TOTAL SINGLE DX	17	2.6	3	1	2	2	3	4	7	12
MULTIPLE DX	161	7.9	82	2	3	6	8	16	28	37
TOTAL										
0–19 Years	6	5.5	28	2	3	3	6	17	17	17
20–34	36	5.0	15	2	3	4	6	7	11	22
35–49	54	7.0	113	1	2	4	6	13	37	68
50–64	40	7.6	58	2	2	6	10	13	25	37
65+	42	9.4	63	2	4	7	11	19	33	34
GRAND TOTAL	178	7.0	72	2	2	5	7	13	22	37

77.2: WEDGE OSTEOTOMY. Formerly included in operation group(s) 722, 723.

Type of Patients	Observed Patients	Avg. Stay	Variance	10th	25th	50th	75th	90th	95th	99th
1. SINGLE DX										
0–19 Years	199	2.3	2	1	1	2	3	4	4	6
20–34	31	3.2	1	2	2	4	4	4	4	5
35–49	68	2.3	1	1	2	2	3	4	4	6
50–64	45	2.6	<1	2	1	2	3	3	4	6
65+	5	1.3	<1	1	1	1	2	2	2	2
2. MULTIPLE DX										
0–19 Years	480	2.8	4	1	2	2	3	5	5	9
20–34	77	2.7	3	1	2	2	3	5	7	8
35–49	227	2.7	3	1	2	2	3	5	7	9
50–64	183	2.8	2	1	2	3	3	4	5	7
65+	49	3.0	4	1	2	3	3	5	7	11
TOTAL SINGLE DX	348	2.4	1	1	1	2	3	4	4	6
MULTIPLE DX	1016	2.8	3	1	2	2	3	5	5	9
TOTAL										
0–19 Years	679	2.6	3	1	2	2	3	4	5	8
20–34	108	2.9	2	1	2	3	4	4	6	8
35–49	295	2.6	3	1	2	2	3	4	5	9
50–64	228	2.7	1	1	2	3	3	4	5	7
65+	54	2.5	4	1	1	2	3	5	6	11
GRAND TOTAL	1364	2.7	3	1	2	2	3	4	5	8

United States, October 1995–September 1996 Data, by Operation

77.25: FEMORAL WEDGE OSTEOTOMY. Formerly included in operation group(s) 722.

Type of Patients	Observed Patients	Avg. Stay	Variance	10th	25th	50th	75th	90th	95th	99th
1. SINGLE DX										
0–19 Years	74	2.5	1	1	2	3	3	4	4	5
20–34	6	4.3	<1	4	4	4	5	5	5	8
35–49	1	6.0	<1	6	6	6	6	6	6	6
50–64	1	2.0	0	2	2	2	2	2	2	2
65+	1	1.0	0	1	1	1	1	1	1	1
2. MULTIPLE DX										
0–19 Years	247	3.2	2	2	2	3	4	5	6	9
20–34	20	4.2	6	2	2	4	6	8	9	9
35–49	29	4.4	5	2	3	3	7	8	8	9
50–64	16	3.6	2	2	3	4	5	6	6	6
65+	7	4.2	2	3	3	4	5	7	7	7
TOTAL SINGLE DX	83	2.6	1	1	2	3	3	4	4	6
MULTIPLE DX	319	3.4	3	2	2	3	4	5	7	9
TOTAL										
0–19 Years	321	3.1	2	2	2	3	4	5	5	9
20–34	26	4.2	4	2	3	4	5	7	8	9
35–49	30	4.4	5	2	3	3	7	8	8	9
50–64	17	3.6	2	2	3	4	5	5	6	6
65+	8	1.8	3	1	1	1	3	5	5	7
GRAND TOTAL	402	3.2	3	2	2	3	4	5	7	9

77.27: TIB & FIB WEDGE OSTY. Formerly included in operation group(s) 723.

Type of Patients	Observed Patients	Avg. Stay	Variance	10th	25th	50th	75th	90th	95th	99th
1. SINGLE DX										
0–19 Years	54	2.1	1	1	1	2	3	4	4	5
20–34	12	3.4	<1	2	3	4	4	4	4	4
35–49	58	2.3	1	1	1	2	4	4	5	7
50–64	42	2.6	<1	1	2	2	3	3	5	6
65+	4	2.0	0	2	2	2	2	2	2	2
2. MULTIPLE DX										
0–19 Years	108	2.5	10	1	1	2	3	4	5	9
20–34	36	2.6	1	1	2	3	3	3	5	6
35–49	171	2.4	2	1	2	2	3	4	5	9
50–64	146	2.7	1	1	2	3	3	4	5	7
65+	30	2.6	1	2	2	3	3	4	5	6
TOTAL SINGLE DX	170	2.4	1	1	2	2	3	4	4	6
MULTIPLE DX	491	2.5	4	1	2	2	3	4	5	7
TOTAL										
0–19 Years	162	2.4	7	1	1	2	3	4	5	7
20–34	48	2.8	1	1	2	3	4	4	4	6
35–49	229	2.4	2	1	2	2	3	4	5	9
50–64	188	2.7	1	1	2	3	3	4	5	7
65+	34	2.5	1	2	2	2	3	4	5	6
GRAND TOTAL	661	2.5	3	2	2	2	3	4	5	7

77.3: OTHER DIVISION OF BONE. Formerly included in operation group(s) 722, 723.

Type of Patients	Observed Patients	Avg. Stay	Variance	10th	25th	50th	75th	90th	95th	99th
1. SINGLE DX										
0–19 Years	799	2.4	5	1	1	2	3	4	5	7
20–34	87	2.5	4	1	1	2	3	5	6	10
35–49	157	2.4	4	1	1	2	3	4	5	7
50–64	94	2.5	2	1	2	2	3	4	4	8
65+	16	3.0	4	1	1	3	4	5	7	7
2. MULTIPLE DX										
0–19 Years	1532	3.3	6	1	2	3	4	6	7	12
20–34	230	4.0	26	1	2	3	5	7	9	24
35–49	410	3.4	7	1	2	3	4	6	7	15
50–64	299	3.2	8	1	2	3	4	5	7	13
65+	131	6.8	87	2	3	4	8	12	16	56
TOTAL SINGLE DX	1153	2.4	4	1	1	2	3	4	5	8
MULTIPLE DX	2602	3.4	11	1	2	3	4	6	8	14
TOTAL										
0–19 Years	2331	3.0	6	1	2	3	4	5	7	10
20–34	317	3.6	20	1	2	3	4	7	8	18
35–49	567	3.2	6	1	2	3	4	6	7	14
50–64	393	3.1	7	1	2	3	4	5	6	14
65+	147	6.5	82	2	3	4	8	12	15	56
GRAND TOTAL	3755	3.2	9	1	2	3	4	5	7	13

77.35: FEMORAL DIVISION NEC. Formerly included in operation group(s) 722.

Type of Patients	Observed Patients	Avg. Stay	Variance	10th	25th	50th	75th	90th	95th	99th
1. SINGLE DX										
0–19 Years	285	2.8	10	1	2	2	3	4	6	7
20–34	12	3.0	2	2	2	2	5	5	6	6
35–49	15	3.5	2	1	2	4	4	5	6	6
50–64	1	3.0	1	2	2	4	4	5	5	5
65+	1	2.0	0	2	2	2	2	2	2	2
2. MULTIPLE DX										
0–19 Years	863	3.7	5	2	2	3	4	6	8	13
20–34	73	5.1	19	1	2	4	6	8	14	27
35–49	60	4.6	4	2	4	5	5	7	7	15
50–64	26	4.6	1	3	4	5	5	5	5	8
65+	26	7.0	33	3	4	4	8	16	25	27
TOTAL SINGLE DX	317	2.9	10	1	2	2	3	4	6	7
MULTIPLE DX	1048	3.9	7	2	2	3	5	7	8	14
TOTAL										
0–19 Years	1148	3.5	6	2	2	3	4	6	7	12
20–34	85	4.8	17	2	2	4	6	8	12	24
35–49	75	4.4	4	2	3	4	6	7	7	15
50–64	30	4.5	1	3	3	5	5	5	5	8
65+	27	6.9	33	3	4	4	11	25	25	27
GRAND TOTAL	1365	3.7	7	2	2	3	4	6	8	14

Length of Stay by Diagnosis and Operation, United States, 1997

United States, October 1995–September 1996 Data, by Operation

77.37: TIBIA/FIBULA DIV NEC. Formerly included in operation group(s) 723.

Type of Patients	Observed Patients	Avg. Stay	Vari- ance	10th	25th	50th	75th	90th	95th	99th
1. SINGLE DX										
0–19 Years	263	2.2	1	1	1	2	3	4	4	5
20–34	47	3.0	4	1	2	3	3	4	8	10
35–49	117	2.2	1	1	2	2	3	4	5	6
50–64	77	2.5	1	1	2	2	3	4	4	5
65+	8	3.5	2	1	3	4	5	5	5	5
2. MULTIPLE DX										
0–19 Years	414	2.6	3	1	1	2	3	5	5	8
20–34	94	3.1	37	1	2	2	3	5	5	14
35–49	265	3.0	3	1	2	3	4	5	6	11
50–64	205	2.7	3	1	2	2	3	4	6	9
65+	35	3.7	3	2	2	3	4	6	8	8
TOTAL SINGLE DX	512	2.3	1	1	1	2	3	4	4	6
MULTIPLE DX	1013	2.8	6	1	2	2	3	5	6	10
TOTAL										
0–19 Years	677	2.4	3	1	1	2	3	4	5	7
20–34	141	3.1	26	1	2	2	3	4	6	14
35–49	382	2.8	3	1	2	3	3	4	5	9
50–64	282	2.6	3	1	2	2	3	4	5	8
65+	43	3.6	3	2	2	3	4	6	7	8
GRAND TOTAL	1525	2.6	5	1	2	2	3	4	5	8

77.4: BIOPSY OF BONE. Formerly included in operation group(s) 725, 726.

Type of Patients	Observed Patients	Avg. Stay	Vari- ance	10th	25th	50th	75th	90th	95th	99th
1. SINGLE DX										
0–19 Years	260	2.9	9	1	1	2	3	7	8	14
20–34	68	2.6	8	1	1	2	3	5	8	17
35–49	74	2.9	9	1	1	2	3	7	8	18
50–64	49	2.3	7	1	1	1	3	4	6	16
65+	42	4.7	18	1	2	5	5	7	10	24
2. MULTIPLE DX										
0–19 Years	293	5.9	33	1	2	4	8	12	16	26
20–34	161	8.6	91	1	3	5	12	19	28	49
35–49	411	9.3	102	2	3	7	12	17	24	47
50–64	663	10.0	97	2	4	7	13	19	28	46
65+	1739	9.4	67	3	4	7	12	18	25	46
TOTAL SINGLE DX	493	2.9	10	1	1	2	3	7	8	16
MULTIPLE DX	3267	9.1	78	2	4	7	12	18	25	46
TOTAL										
0–19 Years	553	4.4	23	1	1	3	6	10	13	24
20–34	229	6.9	75	1	2	4	8	17	28	48
35–49	485	8.2	92	1	3	6	10	16	22	46
50–64	712	9.3	94	1	3	7	12	19	27	46
65+	1781	9.3	67	2	4	7	12	18	25	45
GRAND TOTAL	3760	8.0	72	1	3	6	10	17	23	46

77.39: BONE DIVISION NEC. Formerly included in operation group(s) 723.

Type of Patients	Observed Patients	Avg. Stay	Vari- ance	10th	25th	50th	75th	90th	95th	99th
1. SINGLE DX										
0–19 Years	140	2.8	4	1	1	2	3	5	6	10
20–34	12	3.8	4	1	2	4	5	7	8	8
35–49	7	5.1	5	1	5	5	6	8	8	8
50–64	1	1.0	0	1	1	1	1	1	1	1
65+	1	1.0	0	1	1	1	1	1	1	1
2. MULTIPLE DX										
0–19 Years	136	3.9	18	2	2	3	4	6	9	22
20–34	28	6.1	13	2	4	6	7	12	12	18
35–49	21	8.3	30	3	3	7	13	14	22	22
50–64	5	7.7	77	3	3	3	4	23	23	23
65+	11	23.3	905	2	3	5	49	88	88	88
TOTAL SINGLE DX	161	2.9	4	1	1	2	4	5	6	10
MULTIPLE DX	201	5.0	50	2	2	3	5	9	13	41
TOTAL										
0–19 Years	276	3.4	12	1	2	3	4	5	8	22
20–34	40	5.6	12	2	4	5	7	11	12	18
35–49	28	7.7	27	2	3	6	12	14	14	22
50–64	6	7.2	74	3	3	3	4	23	23	23
65+	12	20.4	841	1	2	3	28	56	88	88
GRAND TOTAL	362	4.1	32	1	2	3	4	7	10	23

77.45: FEMORAL BIOPSY. Formerly included in operation group(s) 725.

Type of Patients	Observed Patients	Avg. Stay	Vari- ance	10th	25th	50th	75th	90th	95th	99th
1. SINGLE DX										
0–19 Years	81	2.7	6	1	1	1	4	7	8	10
20–34	14	2.8	1	1	3	3	3	4	4	6
35–49	21	3.0	5	3	1	3	3	7	7	13
50–64	12	2.0	13	1	1	1	1	2	16	16
65+	10	6.5	25	4	5	5	5	7	24	24
2. MULTIPLE DX										
0–19 Years	95	5.6	36	1	2	4	7	12	14	20
20–34	35	6.2	58	1	2	4	7	12	17	41
35–49	79	6.7	50	2	2	4	8	14	17	36
50–64	118	8.3	71	3	4	7	11	12	18	61
65+	321	7.8	39	3	4	6	9	15	20	29
TOTAL SINGLE DX	138	2.9	8	1	1	2	4	7	7	16
MULTIPLE DX	648	7.3	48	2	3	6	9	14	17	36
TOTAL										
0–19 Years	176	3.8	20	1	2	3	5	8	11	16
20–34	49	5.3	46	1	2	3	6	12	12	41
35–49	100	5.3	36	1	2	3	7	13	16	25
50–64	130	7.0	66	1	2	6	11	12	17	61
65+	331	7.7	38	3	4	6	9	15	20	29
GRAND TOTAL	786	5.9	40	1	2	4	8	12	16	30

Length of Stay by Diagnosis and Operation, United States, 1997

United States, October 1995–September 1996 Data, by Operation

77.47: TIBIA & FIBULA BIOPSY. Formerly included in operation group(s) 726.

Type of Patients	Observed Patients	Avg. Stay	Vari-ance	10th	25th	50th	75th	90th	95th	99th
1. SINGLE DX										
0–19 Years	66	2.9	17	1	1	2	3	4	9	35
20–34	13	2.9	12	1	1	2	2	3	17	17
35–49	5	1.7	<1	1	1	2	2	2	2	2
50–64	6	2.9	2	1	2	3	4	4	5	5
65+	5	2.1	1	1	2	2	2	2	6	6
2. MULTIPLE DX										
0–19 Years	67	6.3	31	2	2	5	9	13	14	28
20–34	23	7.6	41	1	4	5	12	15	18	30
35–49	38	8.9	75	1	2	7	12	16	33	38
50–64	39	7.0	96	1	2	5	8	14	16	77
65+	61	11.0	67	3	5	9	14	25	31	36
TOTAL SINGLE DX	95	2.8	14	1	1	2	3	4	8	17
MULTIPLE DX	228	7.8	56	2	2	6	11	15	23	34
TOTAL										
0–19 Years	133	4.7	27	1	2	2	6	12	14	28
20–34	36	6.5	38	1	2	5	9	15	17	30
35–49	43	7.7	70	1	2	6	11	13	33	38
50–64	45	6.4	85	1	2	5	8	12	16	77
65+	66	9.9	67	2	3	7	13	23	26	36
GRAND TOTAL	323	6.2	48	1	2	4	8	13	17	34

77.49: BONE BIOPSY NEC. Formerly included in operation group(s) 726.

Type of Patients	Observed Patients	Avg. Stay	Vari-ance	10th	25th	50th	75th	90th	95th	99th
1. SINGLE DX										
0–19 Years	50	3.7	13	1	1	2	4	8	11	18
20–34	25	2.4	10	1	1	1	2	4	14	17
35–49	30	3.5	22	1	1	2	3	6	18	21
50–64	26	2.4	4	1	1	1	3	6	7	9
65+	22	4.0	10	1	1	2	7	8	10	11
2. MULTIPLE DX										
0–19 Years	67	6.2	23	1	3	5	9	12	16	22
20–34	62	12.0	152	1	2	7	18	28	45	>99
35–49	215	9.9	134	1	5	7	11	19	29	56
50–64	364	11.9	122	2	5	9	15	23	37	52
65+	1046	10.2	80	3	4	8	13	19	27	48
TOTAL SINGLE DX	153	3.2	12	1	1	2	4	7	11	18
MULTIPLE DX	1754	10.4	99	2	4	8	13	20	28	50
TOTAL										
0–19 Years	117	5.1	20	1	2	4	7	10	13	21
20–34	87	8.7	124	1	3	6	14	28	28	65
35–49	245	9.3	128	1	3	6	10	18	26	56
50–64	390	11.3	120	2	4	8	15	22	37	52
65+	1068	10.1	79	3	4	8	13	19	26	48
GRAND TOTAL	1907	9.9	96	2	4	7	13	19	28	49

77.5: TOE DEFORMITY EXC/REP. Formerly included in operation group(s) 724.

Type of Patients	Observed Patients	Avg. Stay	Vari-ance	10th	25th	50th	75th	90th	95th	99th
1. SINGLE DX										
0–19 Years	40	1.3	<1	1	1	1	1	2	3	3
20–34	33	1.9	<1	1	1	1	2	3	3	7
35–49	40	1.5	<1	1	1	1	2	2	4	5
50–64	39	1.8	2	1	1	1	2	3	4	8
65+	19	1.6	<1	1	1	1	2	3	4	4
2. MULTIPLE DX										
0–19 Years	77	1.6	1	1	1	1	2	3	3	5
20–34	71	2.2	14	1	1	1	2	3	7	15
35–49	221	1.9	5	1	1	1	2	3	5	10
50–64	328	2.1	7	1	1	1	2	3	5	19
65+	419	3.5	16	1	1	2	4	8	10	17
TOTAL SINGLE DX	171	1.6	1	1	1	1	2	3	3	7
MULTIPLE DX	1116	2.4	10	1	1	2	2	4	8	16
TOTAL										
0–19 Years	117	1.5	<1	1	1	1	2	3	3	5
20–34	104	2.2	11	1	1	1	2	3	7	15
35–49	261	1.8	5	1	1	1	2	3	5	10
50–64	367	2.0	7	1	1	1	2	3	5	18
65+	438	3.4	16	1	1	2	4	8	10	17
GRAND TOTAL	1287	2.3	9	1	1	1	2	4	8	15

77.51: BUNIONECT/STC/OSTY. Formerly included in operation group(s) 724.

Type of Patients	Observed Patients	Avg. Stay	Vari-ance	10th	25th	50th	75th	90th	95th	99th
1. SINGLE DX										
0–19 Years	21	1.6	<1	1	1	1	2	3	3	3
20–34	19	1.7	<1	1	1	1	3	3	3	3
35–49	24	1.4	<1	1	1	1	2	2	2	3
50–64	14	1.5	2	1	1	1	2	3	3	7
65+	5	2.1	<1	1	1	2	3	3	3	3
2. MULTIPLE DX										
0–19 Years	38	1.6	<1	1	1	1	2	2	3	3
20–34	33	1.6	2	1	1	1	2	2	3	10
35–49	105	1.8	5	1	1	1	2	3	3	9
50–64	124	1.8	4	1	1	1	2	3	3	5
65+	114	1.9	3	1	1	2	2	3	4	13
TOTAL SINGLE DX	83	1.5	<1	1	1	1	2	3	3	3
MULTIPLE DX	414	1.7	4	1	1	1	2	3	3	8
TOTAL										
0–19 Years	59	1.6	<1	1	1	1	2	2	3	3
20–34	52	1.6	1	1	1	1	2	3	3	10
35–49	129	1.6	4	1	1	1	2	2	3	9
50–64	138	1.8	4	1	1	1	2	2	3	5
65+	119	1.9	3	1	1	2	2	3	4	13
GRAND TOTAL	497	1.7	3	1	1	1	2	3	3	8

Length of Stay by Diagnosis and Operation, United States, 1997

United States, October 1995–September 1996 Data, by Operation

77.6: LOC EXC BONE LESION. Formerly included in operation group(s) 725, 726.

Type of Patients	Observed Patients	Avg. Stay	Variance	10th	25th	50th	75th	90th	95th	99th
1. SINGLE DX										
0–19 Years	596	2.1	5	1	1	1	2	4	6	12
20–34	211	2.4	8	1	1	2	3	4	6	15
35–49	220	2.4	9	1	1	2	3	5	6	11
50–64	75	3.4	16	1	1	2	4	7	11	20
65+	42	4.0	37	1	1	2	5	8	14	21
2. MULTIPLE DX										
0–19 Years	433	5.1	76	1	1	3	6	10	15	45
20–34	412	5.4	49	1	2	3	7	10	16	35
35–49	777	5.2	47	1	2	3	6	11	18	35
50–64	697	7.3	68	1	2	4	10	15	23	42
65+	830	8.8	91	1	3	6	10	20	27	51
TOTAL SINGLE DX	1144	2.3	7	1	1	1	3	4	6	15
MULTIPLE DX	3149	6.4	68	1	2	4	8	14	22	42
TOTAL										
0–19 Years	1029	3.3	36	1	1	2	3	7	10	27
20–34	623	4.5	39	1	1	3	6	9	13	33
35–49	997	4.6	40	1	1	3	5	10	16	34
50–64	772	7.0	65	1	2	4	9	15	21	42
65+	872	8.6	89	1	3	6	10	20	27	51
GRAND TOTAL	4293	5.2	53	1	1	3	6	12	17	39

77.62: LOC EXC BONE LES HUMERUS. Formerly included in operation group(s) 726.

Type of Patients	Observed Patients	Avg. Stay	Variance	10th	25th	50th	75th	90th	95th	99th
1. SINGLE DX										
0–19 Years	72	1.8	<1	1	1	2	2	2	4	6
20–34	11	3.7	8		2	3	3	5	5	9
35–49	13	3.2	48		1	1	3	7	11	36
50–64	1	2.0	0	2	2	2	2	2	2	2
65+	2	14.6	129	1	1	21	21	21	21	21
2. MULTIPLE DX										
0–19 Years	42	3.4	20	1	1	3	4	8	13	25
20–34	18	4.8	8	1	2	6	6	8	8	17
35–49	26	3.1	8	1	1	2	3	7	11	12
50–64	32	2.5	7	1	1	2	3	5	6	11
65+	38	6.8	30	1	2	5	11	15	17	18
TOTAL SINGLE DX	99	2.1	7	1	1	2	2	3	4	9
MULTIPLE DX	156	4.0	15	1	1	3	6	8	12	18
TOTAL										
0–19 Years	114	2.2	6	1	1	2	2	4	6	13
20–34	29	4.6	8	1	2	6	6	8	8	17
35–49	39	3.1	22	1	1	2	3	7	11	36
50–64	33	2.5	7	1	1	2	3	5	6	11
65+	40	7.1	34	1	2	5	12	17	17	21
GRAND TOTAL	255	3.1	12	1	1	2	3	7	9	17

77.61: EXC CHEST CAGE BONE LES. Formerly included in operation group(s) 726.

Type of Patients	Observed Patients	Avg. Stay	Variance	10th	25th	50th	75th	90th	95th	99th
1. SINGLE DX										
0–19 Years	27	2.2	4	1	1	2	3	4	7	13
20–34	11	2.3	2	1	1	3	3	3	3	7
35–49	11	1.9	2	1	1	1	2	3	3	7
50–64	3	5.5	37		2	2	13	13	13	13
65+	8	4.1	87	1	1	1	2	14	14	49
2. MULTIPLE DX										
0–19 Years	15	9.4	451	1	1	2	3	20	73	73
20–34	14	5.8	58	1	1	2	7	14	27	27
35–49	53	5.4	42	1	1	3	10	13	19	26
50–64	129	7.8	52	1	1	4	14	15	19	27
65+	173	12.7	161	1	3	8	17	33	42	51
TOTAL SINGLE DX	60	2.4	13	1	1	2	3	3	7	14
MULTIPLE DX	384	9.3	116	1	1	5	14	20	33	51
TOTAL										
0–19 Years	42	4.3	139	1	1	2	3	4	13	73
20–34	25	3.9	30	1	1	3	3	7	14	27
35–49	64	4.5	34	1	1	2	5	13	15	26
50–64	132	7.8	52	1	1	4	14	15	19	27
65+	181	12.1	160	1	2	8	16	33	42	51
GRAND TOTAL	444	8.0	104	1	1	3	13	18	27	51

77.65: LOC EXC BONE LES FEMUR. Formerly included in operation group(s) 725.

Type of Patients	Observed Patients	Avg. Stay	Variance	10th	25th	50th	75th	90th	95th	99th
1. SINGLE DX										
0–19 Years	128	2.2	7	1	1	1	3	3	6	15
20–34	67	2.3	5	1	1	2	3	3	5	15
35–49	84	1.9	4	1	1	1	2	3	4	7
50–64	21	1.5	1	1	1	1	2	3	4	7
65+	8	2.7	2			3	4	4	4	4
2. MULTIPLE DX										
0–19 Years	95	5.6	150	1	1	2	5	9	17	90
20–34	89	4.4	35	1	1	3	4	8	16	33
35–49	157	3.5	39	1	1	2	4	9	9	45
50–64	99	9.6	181	1	1	2	10	42	42	44
65+	98	7.3	95	1	2	5	8	15	29	56
TOTAL SINGLE DX	308	2.1	5	1	1	1	2	3	6	15
MULTIPLE DX	538	5.5	97	1	1	2	5	10	24	45
TOTAL										
0–19 Years	223	3.6	69	1	1	2	3	6	10	37
20–34	156	3.4	23	1	1	2	3	7	12	28
35–49	241	3.0	28	1	1	2	3	6	8	24
50–64	120	8.5	164	1	1	4	10	42	42	44
65+	106	7.1	91	2	2	4	8	15	29	56
GRAND TOTAL	846	4.2	64	1	1	2	4	8	15	43

Length of Stay by Diagnosis and Operation, United States, 1997

United States, October 1995–September 1996 Data, by Operation

77.67: LOC EXC LES TIBIA/FIBULA. Formerly included in operation group(s) 726.

Type of Patients	Observed Patients	Avg. Stay	Variance	10th	25th	50th	75th	90th	95th	99th
1. SINGLE DX										
0–19 Years	175	1.7	2	1	1	1	2	3	4	8
20–34	44	2.7	18	1	1	1	2	4	6	32
35–49	38	3.7	19	1	1	2	4	7	11	23
50–64	17	4.7	9	1	2	4	6	10	10	11
65+	3	5.4	<1	5	5	5	5	7	7	7
2. MULTIPLE DX										
0–19 Years	99	5.0	44	1	1	3	7	8	14	30
20–34	80	5.6	17	1	3	5	7	11	14	21
35–49	158	5.5	42	1	2	3	8	13	19	34
50–64	72	5.6	24	1	2	4	8	13	15	25
65+	86	7.8	52	2	4	5	9	19	22	27
TOTAL SINGLE DX	277	2.2	7	1	1	1	2	4	6	13
MULTIPLE DX	495	5.7	39	1	2	4	7	12	18	30
TOTAL										
0–19 Years	274	2.8	19	1	1	1	3	8	8	24
20–34	124	4.5	20	1	2	3	6	10	13	26
35–49	196	5.3	40	1	2	4	6	12	19	27
50–64	89	5.5	22	1	2	4	8	12	14	25
65+	89	7.8	50	2	4	5	9	19	22	27
GRAND TOTAL	772	4.3	29	1	1	2	5	9	14	25

77.68: LOC EXC LES MT/TARSAL. Formerly included in operation group(s) 726.

Type of Patients	Observed Patients	Avg. Stay	Variance	10th	25th	50th	75th	90th	95th	99th
1. SINGLE DX										
0–19 Years	41	2.4	6	1	1	2	2	8	8	10
20–34	7	2.2	7	1	1	1	2	3	11	11
35–49	11	1.6	2	1	1	1	16	5	5	5
50–64	5	5.4	46	1	1	1	16	16	16	16
65+	5	4.0	4	1	3	5	5	6	6	6
2. MULTIPLE DX										
0–19 Years	46	4.0	20	1	1	4	4	9	9	15
20–34	40	4.5	26	1	1	3	7	10	12	25
35–49	106	6.2	36	1	3	4	7	14	18	35
50–64	112	7.8	37	2	4	7	9	14	19	43
65+	143	8.1	53	2	4	7	10	16	19	30
TOTAL SINGLE DX	69	2.4	7	1	1	1	2	8	8	11
MULTIPLE DX	447	6.5	39	1	3	5	8	13	18	35
TOTAL										
0–19 Years	87	3.1	13	1	1	2	4	8	9	10
20–34	47	4.2	24	1	2	4	6	10	11	25
35–49	117	5.7	34	1	2	4	6	12	18	35
50–64	117	7.8	37	2	4	7	9	14	19	43
65+	148	8.0	51	2	4	5	10	15	19	30
GRAND TOTAL	516	5.7	35	1	2	4	7	13	16	30

77.69: LOC EXC BONE LESION NEC. Formerly included in operation group(s) 726.

Type of Patients	Observed Patients	Avg. Stay	Variance	10th	25th	50th	75th	90th	95th	99th
1. SINGLE DX										
0–19 Years	94	2.9	9	1	1	2	3	5	6	22
20–34	39	2.4	10	1	1	2	3	4	5	28
35–49	38	2.2	2	1	1	1	3	4	5	7
50–64	20	3.0	5	1	1	2	4	5	7	7
65+	10	2.3	4	1	1	2	2	5	8	8
2. MULTIPLE DX										
0–19 Years	86	6.3	46	1	2	5	8	13	19	39
20–34	119	6.5	91	1	2	4	7	12	30	86
35–49	186	6.6	67	1	2	4	7	13	31	39
50–64	201	7.1	66	1	3	4	9	15	24	38
65+	231	8.3	70	1	3	6	10	23	24	42
TOTAL SINGLE DX	201	2.7	8	1	1	2	3	5	7	12
MULTIPLE DX	823	7.1	69	1	2	4	9	15	24	40
TOTAL										
0–19 Years	180	4.8	32	1	2	3	6	10	14	33
20–34	158	5.7	78	1	2	4	6	10	22	45
35–49	224	5.9	59	1	2	4	6	12	26	34
50–64	221	6.7	61	1	3	4	9	14	21	38
65+	241	8.1	69	1	3	6	10	23	24	42
GRAND TOTAL	1024	6.3	61	1	2	4	7	13	23	39

77.7: EXC BONE FOR GRAFT. Formerly included in operation group(s) 725, 726.

Type of Patients	Observed Patients	Avg. Stay	Variance	10th	25th	50th	75th	90th	95th	99th
1. SINGLE DX										
0–19 Years	62	2.0	2	1	1	1	3	4	5	7
20–34	122	2.2	3	1	1	2	2	3	5	10
35–49	130	2.3	2	1	2	2	3	4	6	6
50–64	64	2.3	2	1	1	2	3	4	6	6
65+	39	3.1	10	1	1	2	3	5	12	15
2. MULTIPLE DX										
0–19 Years	151	2.7	7	1	2	2	3	5	6	16
20–34	226	2.9	7	1	1	2	3	6	6	11
35–49	332	2.5	3	1	1	2	3	4	6	11
50–64	258	2.8	8	1	2	2	3	4	7	16
65+	138	3.4	6	2	2	2	5	8	9	9
TOTAL SINGLE DX	417	2.3	3	1	1	2	3	4	5	9
MULTIPLE DX	1105	2.8	6	1	2	2	3	5	7	14
TOTAL										
0–19 Years	213	2.5	6	1	1	2	3	4	6	16
20–34	348	2.7	6	1	1	2	3	4	6	11
35–49	462	2.4	3	1	2	2	3	4	6	9
50–64	322	2.7	7	1	2	2	3	4	7	15
65+	177	3.4	6	1	2	2	5	8	9	12
GRAND TOTAL	1522	2.7	5	1	1	2	3	5	6	12

Length of Stay by Diagnosis and Operation, United States, 1997

United States, October 1995–September 1996 Data, by Operation

77.79: EXC BONE FOR GRAFT NEC. Formerly included in operation group(s) 726.

Type of Patients	Observed Patients	Avg. Stay	Vari-ance	Percentiles						
				10th	25th	50th	75th	90th	95th	99th
1. SINGLE DX										
0–19 Years	54	1.7	2	1	1	1	2	3	4	7
20–34	115	2.2	4	1	1	1	2	3	5	10
35–49	114	2.3	2	1	1	2	3	4	6	7
50–64	56	2.3	1	1	2	2	2	4	4	9
65+	35	3.3	11	1	1	3	3	5	12	15
2. MULTIPLE DX										
0–19 Years	120	2.4	5	1	2	2	2	4	5	15
20–34	207	2.9	7	1	1	2	3	6	6	11
35–49	291	2.5	4	1	1	2	3	4	5	11
50–64	223	2.6	6	1	2	2	3	4	7	14
65+	111	3.8	7	1	2	3	5	9	9	10
TOTAL SINGLE DX	374	2.2	3	1	1	2	3	4	5	9
MULTIPLE DX	952	2.8	6	1	1	2	3	6	7	12
TOTAL										
0–19 Years	174	2.2	4	1	1	2	2	4	5	11
20–34	322	2.7	6	1	1	2	3	6	6	11
35–49	405	2.4	3	1	1	2	3	4	6	9
50–64	279	2.6	5	1	2	2	3	4	6	14
65+	146	3.8	8	1	2	3	5	8	9	14
GRAND TOTAL	1326	2.6	5	1	1	2	3	5	6	12

77.81: OTH CHEST CAGE OSTECTOMY. Formerly included in operation group(s) 726.

Type of Patients	Observed Patients	Avg. Stay	Vari-ance	Percentiles						
				10th	25th	50th	75th	90th	95th	99th
1. SINGLE DX										
0–19 Years	18	1.6	<1	1	1	1	2	3	4	4
20–34	46	1.3	1	1	1	1	2	3	3	7
35–49	95	1.4	<1	1	1	1	2	2	3	3
50–64	38	1.2	<1	1	1	1	1	2	2	3
65+	16	1.7	1	1	1	1	2	4	4	5
2. MULTIPLE DX										
0–19 Years	16	4.2	10	1	1	2	8	8	8	8
20–34	81	3.2	32	1	1	2	2	4	13	35
35–49	193	2.4	18	1	1	2	2	6	19	>99
50–64	193	2.8	22	1	1	1	2	5	10	28
65+	150	6.4	37	1	2	4	9	13	16	28
TOTAL SINGLE DX	213	1.4	<1	1	1	1	1	2	3	7
MULTIPLE DX	633	3.5	27	1	1	2	3	10	14	>99
TOTAL										
0–19 Years	34	3.1	8	1	1	2	6	8	8	8
20–34	127	2.3	18	1	1	2	2	3	5	35
35–49	288	2.1	13	1	1	1	2	3	11	>99
50–64	231	2.5	19	1	1	1	2	4	9	28
65+	166	6.2	37	1	2	3	9	13	16	28
GRAND TOTAL	846	3.0	22	1	1	1	2	9	13	>99

77.8: OTHER PARTIAL OSTECTOMY. Formerly included in operation group(s) 725, 726.

Type of Patients	Observed Patients	Avg. Stay	Vari-ance	Percentiles						
				10th	25th	50th	75th	90th	95th	99th
1. SINGLE DX										
0–19 Years	199	1.7	2	1	1	1	2	3	4	7
20–34	153	1.7	2	1	1	1	2	3	5	7
35–49	272	1.9	1	1	1	2	2	3	5	5
50–64	171	2.0	2	1	1	2	2	3	5	8
65+	78	2.5	4	1	1	3	3	4	4	15
2. MULTIPLE DX										
0–19 Years	227	3.8	24	1	1	3	4	7	9	22
20–34	383	4.6	48	1	1	2	5	9	16	37
35–49	768	5.3	69	1	1	3	6	13	19	>99
50–64	853	4.6	41	1	2	3	5	9	15	30
65+	1140	7.1	55	1	3	6	9	13	17	34
TOTAL SINGLE DX	873	1.9	2	1	1	2	2	3	4	7
MULTIPLE DX	3371	5.3	51	1	2	3	6	12	16	43
TOTAL										
0–19 Years	426	2.7	13	1	1	2	3	6	7	13
20–34	536	3.7	35	1	1	2	4	7	12	35
35–49	1040	4.1	46	1	1	2	4	9	14	65
50–64	1024	4.2	36	1	2	2	4	9	14	28
65+	1218	6.8	52	1	2	5	9	13	17	32
GRAND TOTAL	4244	4.4	41	1	1	2	5	10	14	33

77.83: PART OSTECTOMY RAD/ULNA. Formerly included in operation group(s) 726.

Type of Patients	Observed Patients	Avg. Stay	Vari-ance	Percentiles						
				10th	25th	50th	75th	90th	95th	99th
1. SINGLE DX										
0–19 Years	8	1.2	<1	1	1	1	1	2	3	3
20–34	18	1.3	<1	1	1	1	1	2	3	5
35–49	39	1.6	<1	1	1	2	2	2	2	4
50–64	20	1.7	<1	1	1	2	2	3	3	3
65+	10	1.8	<1	1	1	2	2	3	3	3
2. MULTIPLE DX										
0–19 Years	16	1.4	<1	1	1	1	2	2	3	3
20–34	47	1.9	2	1	1	1	2	4	5	6
35–49	59	3.3	13	1	2	2	3	7	13	15
50–64	65	2.4	6	1	2	2	3	5	9	9
65+	81	3.1	15	1	2	2	3	6	8	14
TOTAL SINGLE DX	95	1.5	<1	1	1	1	2	2	3	4
MULTIPLE DX	268	2.5	9	1	1	2	3	5	7	15
TOTAL										
0–19 Years	24	1.3	<1	1	1	1	2	2	3	3
20–34	65	1.7	2	1	1	1	2	4	5	6
35–49	98	2.4	7	1	1	2	3	5	7	15
50–64	85	2.3	5	1	2	2	3	4	5	9
65+	91	3.0	14	1	2	2	3	6	8	14
GRAND TOTAL	363	2.2	6	1	1	1	2	4	6	14

Length of Stay by Diagnosis and Operation, United States, 1997

United States, October 1995–September 1996 Data, by Operation

77.85: PART OSTECTOMY-FEMUR. Formerly included in operation group(s) 725.

Type of Patients	Observed Patients	Avg. Stay	Variance	10th	25th	50th	75th	90th	95th	99th
1. SINGLE DX										
0–19 Years	23	2.6	4	1	1	2	3	6	7	8
20–34	10	2.3	4	1	1	2	5	6	6	6
35–49	7	4.6	5	3	3	5	5	5	12	12
50–64	3	5.4	1	5	5	5	5	8	8	8
65+	3	6.7	21	4	4	4	10	15	15	15
2. MULTIPLE DX										
0–19 Years	71	5.5	35	2	3	4	6	9	13	51
20–34	50	9.7	134	2	3	5	12	24	35	51
35–49	80	13.2	226	3	4	7	15	27	46	70
50–64	67	13.9	217	4	6	8	21	27	32	96
65+	161	8.7	44	4	6	6	9	15	25	44
TOTAL SINGLE DX	46	3.4	7	1	1	3	5	6	7	15
MULTIPLE DX	429	9.7	120	3	4	6	10	22	28	51
TOTAL										
0–19 Years	94	4.9	30	1	2	4	6	8	13	22
20–34	60	8.6	121	2	2	5	10	18	33	51
35–49	87	12.6	215	3	4	7	14	27	46	70
50–64	70	13.5	210	4	6	8	20	27	32	96
65+	164	8.7	44	4	5	6	9	15	25	44
GRAND TOTAL	475	9.1	113	2	4	6	9	21	27	51

77.86: PARTIAL PATELLECTOMY. Formerly included in operation group(s) 726.

Type of Patients	Observed Patients	Avg. Stay	Variance	10th	25th	50th	75th	90th	95th	99th
1. SINGLE DX										
0–19 Years	4	1.5	<1	1	1	1	2	2	2	2
20–34	26	2.2	2	1	1	2	3	3	5	6
35–49	49	2.1	1	2	2	2	3	4	4	6
50–64	43	2.2	1	1	1	2	3	4	4	5
65+	25	2.7	<1	2	3	3	3	4	4	4
2. MULTIPLE DX										
0–19 Years	8	2.1	<1	1	1	2	3	3	3	3
20–34	61	3.9	4	2	3	4	4	6	6	12
35–49	90	3.3	5	2	2	3	5	6	8	10
50–64	113	2.7	4	2	2	3	4	4	5	11
65+	211	4.6	10	2	3	4	6	8	10	16
TOTAL SINGLE DX	147	2.2	1	2	2	2	2	3	4	6
MULTIPLE DX	483	3.3	6	2	2	2	4	6	8	13
TOTAL										
0–19 Years	12	1.8	<1	1	1	2	2	3	3	3
20–34	87	3.4	4	1	2	3	4	6	6	11
35–49	139	2.9	2	2	2	3	5	6	6	10
50–64	156	2.7	4	2	2	2	2	4	5	11
65+	236	4.2	9	2	2	3	5	7	10	16
GRAND TOTAL	630	2.9	5	2	2	2	4	5	6	12

77.87: PART OSTECTOMY TIB/FIB. Formerly included in operation group(s) 726.

Type of Patients	Observed Patients	Avg. Stay	Variance	10th	25th	50th	75th	90th	95th	99th
1. SINGLE DX										
0–19 Years	52	2.1	3	1	1	1	2	6	6	9
20–34	10	3.0	3	1	2	2	5	6	6	9
35–49	14	2.4	<1	1	2	3	3	3	3	3
50–64	9	3.3	4	1	2	2	6	6	6	8
65+	0									
2. MULTIPLE DX										
0–19 Years	33	2.8	5	1	2	3	4	7	7	8
20–34	27	3.9	10	1	2	5	5	8	11	16
35–49	31	6.0	28	1	3	4	8	16	16	18
50–64	27	5.0	7	3	4	4	5	8	11	12
65+	21	8.9	23	4	8	8	11	15	17	26
TOTAL SINGLE DX	85	2.4	3	1	1	2	3	6	6	9
MULTIPLE DX	139	5.1	16	1	3	4	6	11	15	19
TOTAL										
0–19 Years	85	2.3	4	1	1	2	2	6	7	9
20–34	37	3.7	8	1	2	3	5	7	8	16
35–49	45	5.1	23	1	2	4	8	16	16	18
50–64	36	4.8	7	2	4	5	5	8	11	12
65+	21	8.9	23	4	8	8	11	15	17	26
GRAND TOTAL	224	4.2	13	1	2	3	5	8	11	16

77.88: PART OSTECTOMY-MT/TARSAL. Formerly included in operation group(s) 726.

Type of Patients	Observed Patients	Avg. Stay	Variance	10th	25th	50th	75th	90th	95th	99th
1. SINGLE DX										
0–19 Years	54	1.1	<1	1	1	1	1	1	2	3
20–34	4	1.3	<1	1	1	1	2	2	2	2
35–49	4	1.4	<1	1	1	1	3	3	3	3
50–64	12	3.2	9	1	1	2	5	10	10	10
65+	11	1.6	5	1	1	1	1	2	9	13
2. MULTIPLE DX										
0–19 Years	29	2.6	1	1	2	3	3	3	3	8
20–34	36	6.2	37	1	2	4	8	16	18	29
35–49	127	7.5	27	2	4	7	10	13	14	22
50–64	185	6.1	22	2	3	5	10	11	14	25
65+	263	7.5	31	2	3	6	10	14	20	30
TOTAL SINGLE DX	85	1.3	2	1	1	1	1	2	2	10
MULTIPLE DX	640	6.3	26	2	3	5	8	13	16	25
TOTAL										
0–19 Years	83	1.8	1	1	1	2	3	3	3	6
20–34	40	5.3	34	1	2	3	7	16	16	29
35–49	131	7.4	27	2	4	7	10	13	14	22
50–64	197	5.9	22	2	3	5	8	10	14	25
65+	274	7.1	32	1	3	6	9	14	20	30
GRAND TOTAL	725	5.4	26	1	2	4	8	12	14	25

Length of Stay by Diagnosis and Operation, United States, 1997

United States, October 1995–September 1996 Data, by Operation

77.89: PARTIAL OSTECTOMY NEC. Formerly included in operation group(s) 726.

Type of Patients	Observed Patients	Avg. Stay	Vari-ance	Percentiles						
				10th	25th	50th	75th	90th	95th	99th
1. SINGLE DX										
0–19 Years	27	2.4	2	1	1	2	3	4	4	7
20–34	33	2.2	1	1	1	2	3	4	5	5
35–49	46	2.2	1	1	1	2	3	4	4	4
50–64	38	2.0	<1	1	1	2	2	3	4	7
65+	10	2.7	2		2	2	3	3	7	7
2. MULTIPLE DX										
0–19 Years	40	5.0	78	1	1	1	5	12	13	60
20–34	58	6.8	98	1	1	3	8	14	32	56
35–49	152	7.0	148	1	2	3	6	14	21	65
50–64	178	7.5	91	1	2	4	9	19	23	68
65+	222	9.9	150	2	3	7	12	16	28	70
TOTAL SINGLE DX	154	2.2	2	1	1	2	3	4	4	7
MULTIPLE DX	650	7.8	125	1	2	4	9	16	24	66
TOTAL										
0–19 Years	67	3.4	33	1	1	2	3	7	11	21
20–34	91	5.5	75	1	1	3	7	12	19	47
35–49	198	5.5	106	1	1	3	5	9	17	65
50–64	216	5.7	69	1	2	3	6	13	20	34
65+	232	9.7	148	2	3	7	12	16	28	70
GRAND TOTAL	804	6.2	96	1	2	3	7	13	20	65

77.91: TOT CHEST CAGE OSTECTOMY. Formerly included in operation group(s) 726.

Type of Patients	Observed Patients	Avg. Stay	Vari-ance	Percentiles						
				10th	25th	50th	75th	90th	95th	99th
1. SINGLE DX										
0–19 Years	13	2.2	1	1	1	2	3	4	5	5
20–34	105	2.0	<1	1	1	2	3	3	5	5
35–49	94	2.0	<1	1	1	2	2	3	3	4
50–64	18	2.5	2	1	2	2	4	4	5	5
65+	6	4.9	5	4	4	5	5	6	13	13
2. MULTIPLE DX										
0–19 Years	30	5.9	66	1	1	3	8	8	35	35
20–34	124	3.2	12	1	1	3	4	5	9	17
35–49	190	4.0	17	2	2	3	4	8	10	22
50–64	54	3.8	15	2	2	2	5	11	14	14
65+	31	7.0	138	1	1	2	5	38	38	38
TOTAL SINGLE DX	236	2.0	<1	1	1	2	3	3	3	5
MULTIPLE DX	429	4.1	31	1	2	2	4	8	14	37
TOTAL										
0–19 Years	43	5.3	58	1	1	2	8	8	35	35
20–34	229	2.7	8	1	2	2	3	4	5	17
35–49	284	3.2	12	1	2	2	4	6	10	20
50–64	72	3.6	13	1	2	2	4	8	13	14
65+	37	6.8	125	1	1	2	5	37	38	38
GRAND TOTAL	665	3.4	21	1	1	2	3	6	10	29

77.9: TOTAL OSTECTOMY. Formerly included in operation group(s) 725, 726.

Type of Patients	Observed Patients	Avg. Stay	Vari-ance	Percentiles						
				10th	25th	50th	75th	90th	95th	99th
1. SINGLE DX										
0–19 Years	26	1.7	1	1	1	1	2	3	3	5
20–34	135	2.1	1	1	1	2	3	3	4	7
35–49	128	2.0	1	1	1	2	3	4	4	5
50–64	42	2.1	<1	1	1	2	3	4	4	5
65+	22	4.5	5	2	4	5	5	7	7	13
2. MULTIPLE DX										
0–19 Years	65	4.5	46	1	1	2	4	8	16	35
20–34	183	3.5	22	1	1	2	4	6	12	25
35–49	313	4.3	26	1	2	3	4	6	13	29
50–64	168	4.0	18	1	2	2	4	9	14	23
65+	211	7.2	72	1	2	4	8	21	25	38
TOTAL SINGLE DX	353	2.1	1	1	1	2	3	3	4	6
MULTIPLE DX	940	4.6	36	1	2	3	5	10	16	35
TOTAL										
0–19 Years	91	4.0	39	1	1	2	3	8	13	35
20–34	318	2.9	14	1	2	2	3	4	8	21
35–49	441	3.6	20	1	2	2	4	6	10	23
50–64	210	3.7	16	1	2	2	4	8	13	23
65+	233	7.1	69	1	2	4	8	18	25	38
GRAND TOTAL	1293	4.0	28	1	2	2	4	8	14	29

77.96: TOTAL PATELLECTOMY. Formerly included in operation group(s) 726.

Type of Patients	Observed Patients	Avg. Stay	Vari-ance	Percentiles						
				10th	25th	50th	75th	90th	95th	99th
1. SINGLE DX										
0–19 Years	2	2.8	<1	2	3	3	3	3	3	3
20–34	16	3.1	4	1	1	3	4	4	9	9
35–49	20	2.1	1	1	1	2	3	4	4	4
50–64	13	2.4	<1	1	2	3	3	4	4	4
65+	12	3.7	3	2	2	4	5	6	7	7
2. MULTIPLE DX										
0–19 Years	8	2.9	4	2	2	2	2	4	7	11
20–34	28	2.8	6	1	1	2	3	8	8	12
35–49	49	3.7	19	2	2	3	4	6	7	38
50–64	39	2.8	5	2	2	3	4	4	8	13
65+	98	4.6	10	2	3	3	6	8	11	16
TOTAL SINGLE DX	63	2.7	2	1	1	3	4	4	5	9
MULTIPLE DX	222	3.6	11	2	2	3	4	7	8	15
TOTAL										
0–19 Years	10	2.9	4	2	2	2	3	4	7	11
20–34	44	2.9	5	1	1	2	4	6	8	12
35–49	69	3.4	16	2	2	2	3	6	7	38
50–64	52	2.8	9	2	2	2	3	3	7	13
65+	110	4.6	9	2	3	3	6	8	10	16
GRAND TOTAL	285	3.5	10	2	2	3	4	7	8	15

Length of Stay by Diagnosis and Operation, United States, 1997

299

United States, October 1995–September 1996 Data, by Operation

78.0: BONE GRAFT. Formerly included in operation group(s) 727, 728.

Type of Patients	Observed Patients	Avg. Stay	Vari- ance	Percentiles						
				10th	25th	50th	75th	90th	95th	99th
1. SINGLE DX										
0–19 Years	150	1.9	2	1	1	1	2	4	5	6
20–34	141	2.3	2	1	1	2	2	4	4	9
35–49	128	2.2	2	1	1	2	3	4	5	7
50–64	56	2.2	3	1	1	2	2	3	4	9
65+	13	3.0	4	1	1	2	6	6	6	6
2. MULTIPLE DX										
0–19 Years	175	3.0	6	1	1	2	4	6	7	9
20–34	328	3.3	13	1	2	3	4	6	8	12
35–49	377	3.4	8	1	2	3	4	6	8	20
50–64	211	4.0	14	1	2	3	5	9	12	17
65+	191	5.8	52	2	3	4	6	9	13	47
TOTAL SINGLE DX	488	2.2	2	1	1	2	3	4	5	7
MULTIPLE DX	1282	3.7	17	1	2	3	4	7	9	19
TOTAL										
0–19 Years	325	2.6	5	1	1	2	3	5	6	8
20–34	469	3.0	10	1	2	2	3	5	7	12
35–49	505	3.1	7	1	1	3	4	6	8	15
50–64	267	3.5	12	1	2	3	4	7	10	17
65+	204	5.8	50	2	3	4	6	9	12	47
GRAND TOTAL	1770	3.3	14	1	2	2	4	6	8	16

78.05: BONE GRAFT TO FEMUR. Formerly included in operation group(s) 727.

Type of Patients	Observed Patients	Avg. Stay	Vari- ance	Percentiles						
				10th	25th	50th	75th	90th	95th	99th
1. SINGLE DX										
0–19 Years	49	2.3	2	1	1	2	3	4	5	10
20–34	34	2.9	6	1	2	3	4	5	5	16
35–49	38	3.4	3	1	2	3	4	6	7	9
50–64	16	2.8	8	1	2	2	4	6	7	18
65+	3	2.4	<1	2	2	2	3	3	3	3
2. MULTIPLE DX										
0–19 Years	54	3.8	7	1	2	3	4	6	8	18
20–34	102	3.6	13	2	2	3	4	5	7	11
35–49	125	3.7	6	1	2	3	5	7	8	14
50–64	57	4.6	11	2	3	3	6	9	11	14
65+	91	6.0	46	3	4	4	7	10	11	45
TOTAL SINGLE DX	140	2.7	4	1	1	2	4	4	5	10
MULTIPLE DX	429	4.4	19	1	2	4	5	7	10	16
TOTAL										
0–19 Years	103	3.1	5	1	1	3	4	5	6	13
20–34	136	3.5	12	1	2	3	4	5	8	11
35–49	163	3.6	5	1	2	3	5	6	8	11
50–64	73	4.2	11	1	2	3	5	9	11	18
65+	94	5.9	46	2	4	4	7	10	11	45
GRAND TOTAL	569	4.0	16	1	2	3	5	7	9	15

78.07: BONE GRAFT TIBIA/FIBULA. Formerly included in operation group(s) 727, 728.

Type of Patients	Observed Patients	Avg. Stay	Vari- ance	Percentiles						
				10th	25th	50th	75th	90th	95th	99th
1. SINGLE DX										
0–19 Years	50	1.9	2	1	1	1	2	3	6	6
20–34	60	2.3	2	1	2	2	3	3	4	9
35–49	60	2.3	2	1	2	2	3	3	6	6
50–64	28	2.1	1	1	1	2	2	2	3	9
65+	7	3.8	5		2	3	6	6		6
2. MULTIPLE DX										
0–19 Years	68	3.2	3	1	2	3	4	6	6	8
20–34	150	3.2	17	1	2	3	3	5	7	14
35–49	186	3.2	10	1	2	3	3	5	7	20
50–64	102	3.9	15	1	2	3	4	8	9	17
65+	46	5.6	52	2	3	4	7	7	13	56
TOTAL SINGLE DX	205	2.2	2	1	1	2	3	3	6	7
MULTIPLE DX	552	3.5	15	1	2	3	4	6	8	20
TOTAL										
0–19 Years	118	2.6	3	1	1	2	4	6	6	7
20–34	210	2.9	12	1	2	2	3	4	7	9
35–49	246	3.0	8	1	2	2	4	5	7	20
50–64	130	3.3	11	1	2	3	4	6	9	17
65+	53	5.4	48	2	3	4	6	7	12	56
GRAND TOTAL	757	3.1	12	1	2	2	3	6	7	17

78.1: APPL EXT FIXATION DEVICE. Formerly included in operation group(s) 727, 728.

Type of Patients	Observed Patients	Avg. Stay	Vari- ance	Percentiles						
				10th	25th	50th	75th	90th	95th	99th
1. SINGLE DX										
0–19 Years	216	5.6	56	1	2	3	6	15	23	43
20–34	65	2.7	6	1	1	2	3	5	12	13
35–49	86	2.9	6	1	1	2	4	5	8	14
50–64	56	2.4	3	1	1	2	3	5	4	12
65+	34	2.4	5	1	1	2	3	5	6	11
2. MULTIPLE DX										
0–19 Years	235	6.4	65	2	2	4	7	13	19	45
20–34	174	7.1	95	1	1	3	8	21	32	44
35–49	222	6.3	75	1	2	3	8	13	19	38
50–64	171	6.4	80	1	1	3	6	15	24	48
65+	339	6.2	99	1	2	4	6	12	19	66
TOTAL SINGLE DX	457	4.1	33	1	1	2	4	8	15	25
MULTIPLE DX	1141	6.5	83	1	2	4	7	14	22	52
TOTAL										
0–19 Years	451	6.1	61	1	2	3	7	13	23	43
20–34	239	6.1	80	1	1	3	7	14	26	44
35–49	308	5.4	59	1	2	3	6	11	18	36
50–64	227	5.0	57	1	1	3	5	10	17	45
65+	373	6.0	94	1	2	4	6	11	19	66
GRAND TOTAL	1598	5.8	70	1	2	3	6	13	21	44

Length of Stay by Diagnosis and Operation, United States, 1997

United States, October 1995–September 1996 Data, by Operation

78.13: APPL EXT FIX RAD/ULNA. Formerly included in operation group(s) 728.

Type of Patients	Observed Patients	Avg. Stay	Variance	10th	25th	50th	75th	90th	95th	99th
1. SINGLE DX										
0–19 Years	6	1.0	0	1	1	1	1	1	1	1
20–34	23	1.5	<1	1	1	1	2	3	3	4
35–49	48	2.3	3	1	1	2	4	5	5	5
50–64	38	2.1	1	1	1	2	3	3	3	4
65+	27	2.1	4	1	1	1	3	3	6	11
2. MULTIPLE DX										
0–19 Years	7	1.9	<1	1	2	2	2	2	2	3
20–34	49	3.4	19	1	1	2	4	9	11	20
35–49	53	3.0	9	1	2	2	3	6	12	13
50–64	84	2.9	6	1	1	2	4	5	7	16
65+	211	3.9	30	1	1	3	5	7	11	18
TOTAL SINGLE DX	142	2.0	2	1	1	1	3	4	5	5
MULTIPLE DX	404	3.4	19	1	1	2	4	6	10	16
TOTAL										
0–19 Years	13	1.7	<1	1	1	2	2	2	2	3
20–34	72	2.9	15	1	1	2	3	5	10	20
35–49	101	2.7	6	1	1	2	3	6	6	13
50–64	122	2.5	4	1	1	2	3	4	6	11
65+	238	3.8	28	1	1	3	5	7	10	18
GRAND TOTAL	546	3.0	15	1	1	2	3	5	9	16

78.15: APPL EXT FIX DEV FEMUR. Formerly included in operation group(s) 727.

Type of Patients	Observed Patients	Avg. Stay	Variance	10th	25th	50th	75th	90th	95th	99th
1. SINGLE DX										
0–19 Years	167	6.4	65	1	2	3	7	20	23	44
20–34	3	2.4	2	1	1	2	4	4	4	4
35–49	4	5.5	8	1	5	5	9	9	9	9
50–64	1	3.0	0	3	3	3	3	3	3	3
65+	2	3.3	3	2	2	2	5	5	5	5
2. MULTIPLE DX										
0–19 Years	141	7.2	73	2	3	4	9	13	20	67
20–34	17	8.5	82	3	4	4	14	14	15	57
35–49	20	11.5	95	2	5	7	18	36	38	>99
50–64	11	15.2	239	3	3	10	15	44	56	56
65+	50	10.5	102	4	5	8	10	20	47	>99
TOTAL SINGLE DX	177	6.3	63	1	2	3	7	20	23	44
MULTIPLE DX	239	8.1	86	2	3	5	10	18	23	67
TOTAL										
0–19 Years	308	6.8	69	1	3	4	8	16	23	44
20–34	20	8.0	78	3	4	4	14	14	15	57
35–49	24	10.6	87	2	5	7	18	20	36	>99
50–64	12	11.1	192	3	3	10	11	40	44	>99
65+	52	10.3	100	4	5	8	10	20	47	>99
GRAND TOTAL	416	7.3	76	1	3	4	9	18	23	51

78.17: APPL EXT FIX DEV TIB/FIB. Formerly included in operation group(s) 728.

Type of Patients	Observed Patients	Avg. Stay	Variance	10th	25th	50th	75th	90th	95th	99th
1. SINGLE DX										
0–19 Years	28	3.5	13	1	2	3	3	7	7	20
20–34	27	3.7	12	1	2	2	5	12	12	12
35–49	26	4.1	14	1	2	2	4	8	14	15
50–64	16	3.8	8	2	2	3	4	7	12	14
65+	3	6.0	6	4	4	6	9	9	9	9
2. MULTIPLE DX										
0–19 Years	62	5.9	58	2	2	4	6	14	18	30
20–34	73	8.9	111	2	2	4	8	26	32	44
35–49	110	6.7	71	2	2	4	8	12	21	34
50–64	55	9.9	125	1	3	5	12	24	36	52
65+	49	17.5	429	3	5	9	23	60	74	84
TOTAL SINGLE DX	100	3.8	12	1	2	2	4	8	12	20
MULTIPLE DX	349	8.5	128	2	3	5	8	22	32	62
TOTAL										
0–19 Years	90	5.1	44	2	2	3	5	9	15	30
20–34	100	7.8	95	1	2	3	8	21	32	44
35–49	136	6.3	63	2	3	4	8	12	20	34
50–64	71	8.6	106	3	3	5	9	24	33	48
65+	52	17.1	418	3	5	8	23	60	74	84
GRAND TOTAL	449	7.5	107	2	2	4	8	19	26	60

78.2: LIMB SHORTENING PX. Formerly included in operation group(s) 727, 728.

Type of Patients	Observed Patients	Avg. Stay	Variance	10th	25th	50th	75th	90th	95th	99th
1. SINGLE DX										
0–19 Years	217	1.5	<1	1	1	1	2	3	3	5
20–34	7	2.2	3	1	1	1	5	5	5	5
35–49	16	1.7	2	1	1	1	2	3	4	9
50–64	0									
65+	1	1.0	0	1	1	1	1	1	1	1
2. MULTIPLE DX										
0–19 Years	335	2.2	4	1	1	2	3	4	6	9
20–34	36	5.0	239	1	1	2	3	6	8	98
35–49	21	1.6	1	1	1	2	1	4	5	5
50–64	14	3.1	8	1	2	2	4	6	6	13
65+	2	2.8	2	2	2	2	4	4	4	4
TOTAL SINGLE DX	241	1.6	<1	1	1	1	2	3	3	5
MULTIPLE DX	408	2.4	18	1	1	2	3	4	6	9
TOTAL										
0–19 Years	552	1.9	2	1	1	1	2	3	4	7
20–34	43	4.4	195	1	1	2	3	5	7	98
35–49	37	1.7	2	1	1	1	1	3	5	5
50–64	14	3.1	8	1	1	2	4	6	6	13
65+	3	2.1	2	1	1	2	2	4	4	4
GRAND TOTAL	649	2.0	11	1	1	1	2	3	5	8

Length of Stay by Diagnosis and Operation, United States, 1997

United States, October 1995–September 1996 Data, by Operation

78.25: LIMB SHORT PX FEMUR. Formerly included in operation group(s) 727.

Type of Patients	Observed Patients	Avg. Stay	Vari-ance	10th	25th	50th	75th	90th	95th	99th
1. SINGLE DX										
0–19 Years	145	1.6	<1	1	1	1	2	3	3	4
20–34	3	3.9	<1	2	2	5	4	5	5	5
35–49	3	3.3	<1	2	3	4	4	4	4	4
50–64	0									
65+	0									
2. MULTIPLE DX										
0–19 Years	229	2.3	4	1	1	2	3	4	6	9
20–34	16	11.0	623	2	3	3	6	10	98	98
35–49	9	3.2	2	1	1	4	4	5	5	5
50–64	1	6.0	0	6	6	6	6	6	6	6
65+	0									
TOTAL SINGLE DX	151	1.7	<1	1	1	1	2	3	3	5
MULTIPLE DX	255	2.7	28	1	1	2	3	5	6	9
TOTAL										
0–19 Years	374	2.0	3	1	1	2	3	3	5	7
20–34	19	9.4	494	3	3	3	5	8	98	98
35–49	12	3.2	2	2	2	4	4	4	5	5
50–64	1	6.0	0	6	6	6	6	6	6	6
65+	0									
GRAND TOTAL	406	2.2	16	1	1	2	3	4	5	9

78.4: OTHER BONE REPAIR. Formerly included in operation group(s) 727, 728.

Type of Patients	Observed Patients	Avg. Stay	Vari-ance	10th	25th	50th	75th	90th	95th	99th
1. SINGLE DX										
0–19 Years	60	2.6	7	1	1	2	3	4	5	17
20–34	39	2.1	2	1	1	2	3	4	5	7
35–49	46	2.3	2	1	1	2	3	5	5	6
50–64	12	2.6	1	1	2	3	3	3	3	5
65+	7	2.3	<1	2	2	2	3	3	3	3
2. MULTIPLE DX										
0–19 Years	85	3.2	18	1	1	2	3	8	8	23
20–34	84	4.8	124	1	1	2	4	7	9	72
35–49	133	3.1	16	1	1	2	4	6	9	22
50–64	82	4.4	24	1	2	3	4	7	13	22
65+	107	6.7	82	2	3	4	7	12	21	64
TOTAL SINGLE DX	164	2.4	4	1	1	2	3	4	5	16
MULTIPLE DX	491	4.2	49	1	1	2	4	8	10	40
TOTAL										
0–19 Years	145	2.9	13	1	1	2	3	6	8	22
20–34	123	4.0	90	1	1	2	3	7	7	72
35–49	179	2.9	13	1	1	2	4	5	8	22
50–64	94	4.2	22	1	2	3	4	7	11	22
65+	114	6.5	79	2	3	4	7	12	17	64
GRAND TOTAL	655	3.7	38	1	1	2	4	7	9	23

78.3: LIMB LENGTHENING PX. Formerly included in operation group(s) 727, 728.

Type of Patients	Observed Patients	Avg. Stay	Vari-ance	10th	25th	50th	75th	90th	95th	99th
1. SINGLE DX										
0–19 Years	85	2.1	2	1	1	2	3	4	5	6
20–34	8	2.3	2	1	1	2	4	5	5	5
35–49	8	2.8	4	1	1	3	4	4	9	9
50–64	0									
65+	1	3.0	0	3	3	3	3	3	3	3
2. MULTIPLE DX										
0–19 Years	169	2.9	3	1	2	3	3	5	6	7
20–34	22	3.6	3	2	2	3	4	6	7	8
35–49	35	2.9	6	1	1	2	3	7	7	13
50–64	10	3.2	<1	2	3	3	3	5	5	5
65+	10	5.0	17	3	3	3	3	10	16	16
TOTAL SINGLE DX	102	2.2	2	1	1	2	3	4	5	6
MULTIPLE DX	246	3.0	4	1	2	3	3	5	7	13
TOTAL										
0–19 Years	254	2.7	3	1	2	2	3	5	6	7
20–34	30	3.2	3	2	2	3	4	5	7	8
35–49	43	2.9	6	1	1	2	3	6	7	13
50–64	10	3.2	<1	2	3	3	3	5	5	5
65+	11	4.7	15	3	3	3	3	10	16	16
GRAND TOTAL	348	2.8	4	2	2	3	3	4	6	9

78.5: INT FIX W/O FX REDUCTION. Formerly included in operation group(s) 727, 728.

Type of Patients	Observed Patients	Avg. Stay	Vari-ance	10th	25th	50th	75th	90th	95th	99th
1. SINGLE DX										
0–19 Years	833	3.0	18	1	2	2	3	5	11	23
20–34	315	3.2	7	2	2	3	4	5	6	17
35–49	228	2.8	4	1	2	2	4	6	6	10
50–64	164	3.4	4	1	3	4	5	6	6	8
65+	192	4.5	13	2	3	4	5	6	7	29
2. MULTIPLE DX										
0–19 Years	709	5.9	60	1	2	3	6	15	20	36
20–34	671	6.1	29	1	3	4	8	14	17	25
35–49	759	6.0	56	1	2	5	7	12	18	54
50–64	888	6.5	51	2	4	5	7	13	21	37
65+	4355	6.7	26	3	4	5	8	11	14	25
TOTAL SINGLE DX	1732	3.1	12	1	1	2	4	6	7	20
MULTIPLE DX	7382	6.4	38	2	3	5	7	12	17	33
TOTAL										
0–19 Years	1542	4.3	40	1	2	2	4	11	19	31
20–34	986	5.1	23	1	2	4	6	11	15	25
35–49	987	5.0	41	1	2	4	7	10	15	37
50–64	1052	5.9	43	2	4	4	8	11	18	35
65+	4547	6.6	26	3	4	5	8	11	14	26
GRAND TOTAL	9114	5.6	33	1	2	4	7	11	15	30

Length of Stay by Diagnosis and Operation, United States, 1997

United States, October 1995–September 1996 Data, by Operation

78.52: INT FIX W/O RED HUMERUS. Formerly included in operation group(s) 728.

Type of Patients	Observed Patients	Avg. Stay	Vari-ance	10th	25th	50th	75th	90th	95th	99th
1. SINGLE DX										
0–19 Years	35	2.1	10	1	1	1	2	2	2	14
20–34	17	2.0	2	1	1	2	2	4	13	5
35–49	16	2.6	2	1	1	3	4	5	5	5
50–64	19	1.9	<1	1	2	3	3	3	3	4
65+	10	3.1	4	1	2	3	3	7	7	7
2. MULTIPLE DX										
0–19 Years	33	4.9	68	1	2	2	4	14	14	51
20–34	37	2.8	5	1	1	2	4	5	5	13
35–49	53	11.2	322	1	2	3	8	54	54	54
50–64	108	5.7	63	1	2	2	3	21	25	30
65+	219	5.1	25	2	2	4	7	10	14	20
TOTAL SINGLE DX	97	2.2	5	1	1	2	2	4	5	13
MULTIPLE DX	450	5.7	76	1	2	3	5	14	25	54
TOTAL										
0–19 Years	68	3.6	43	1	1	2	3	13	14	51
20–34	54	2.6	4	1	1	2	4	5	5	13
35–49	69	9.6	274	1	2	3	8	54	54	54
50–64	127	5.5	60	1	2	2	3	21	25	30
65+	229	5.1	25	2	2	4	7	10	14	20
GRAND TOTAL	547	5.3	68	1	2	2	5	11	23	54

78.55: INT FIX W/O RED FEMUR. Formerly included in operation group(s) 727.

Type of Patients	Observed Patients	Avg. Stay	Vari-ance	10th	25th	50th	75th	90th	95th	99th
1. SINGLE DX										
0–19 Years	680	3.1	20	1	1	2	3	5	14	24
20–34	95	3.9	7	2	2	3	5	7	9	18
35–49	67	3.1	5	1	3	2	5	5	6	13
50–64	76	4.1	3	1	3	4	6	6	7	8
65+	161	4.7	14	2	3	5	5	6	8	29
2. MULTIPLE DX										
0–19 Years	470	7.0	69	1	2	4	9	20	23	37
20–34	333	8.4	37	3	4	7	11	15	18	30
35–49	336	7.2	41	2	3	6	8	14	18	37
50–64	547	7.4	56	3	4	5	8	13	20	51
65+	3850	6.7	23	3	4	6	8	11	14	24
TOTAL SINGLE DX	1079	3.5	15	1	1	2	4	6	8	22
MULTIPLE DX	5536	7.0	34	3	4	5	8	12	17	33
TOTAL										
0–19 Years	1150	4.7	44	1	1	2	5	12	20	33
20–34	428	7.4	34	2	3	6	10	15	18	25
35–49	403	6.1	34	2	2	5	7	12	17	32
50–64	623	6.7	46	2	4	5	7	12	15	44
65+	4011	6.6	23	3	4	5	8	11	14	25
GRAND TOTAL	6615	6.2	32	2	3	5	7	12	16	31

78.57: INT FIX W/O RED TIB/FIB. Formerly included in operation group(s) 728.

Type of Patients	Observed Patients	Avg. Stay	Vari-ance	10th	25th	50th	75th	90th	95th	99th
1. SINGLE DX										
0–19 Years	62	2.8	11	1	1	2	3	4	7	16
20–34	165	3.0	3	1	2	2	3	5	5	9
35–49	117	2.7	4	1	1	2	3	6	6	6
50–64	46	3.2	4	1	2	3	4	5	7	12
65+	12	3.3	3	2	2	3	4	5	9	9
2. MULTIPLE DX										
0–19 Years	105	3.4	22	1	1	2	3	6	10	29
20–34	215	4.4	18	1	2	3	5	9	12	19
35–49	251	4.3	28	1	2	3	5	7	12	23
50–64	138	5.2	33	1	2	3	7	10	14	35
65+	135	6.0	33	3	3	4	7	11	14	42
TOTAL SINGLE DX	402	2.9	4	1	2	2	3	5	6	9
MULTIPLE DX	844	4.6	26	1	2	3	5	8	13	28
TOTAL										
0–19 Years	167	3.2	19	1	1	2	3	6	10	29
20–34	380	3.7	11	1	2	3	4	7	11	17
35–49	368	3.6	17	1	2	3	4	6	7	22
50–64	184	4.8	28	2	3	3	6	8	14	35
65+	147	5.8	32	3	3	4	7	9	13	42
GRAND TOTAL	1246	3.9	19	1	2	3	4	7	11	22

78.59: INT FIX W/O FX RED NEC. Formerly included in operation group(s) 728.

Type of Patients	Observed Patients	Avg. Stay	Vari-ance	10th	25th	50th	75th	90th	95th	99th
1. SINGLE DX										
0–19 Years	32	2.0	3	1	1	1	2	5	6	8
20–34	16	3.6	48	1	1	1	2	5	26	26
35–49	10	3.8	14	1	1	2	6	10	10	10
50–64	7	1.3	2	1	1	1	3	7	4	10
65+	5	4.3	4	2	3	3	3	7	7	7
2. MULTIPLE DX										
0–19 Years	76	3.7	53	1	1	2	4	5	12	30
20–34	41	5.6	14	1	4	5	7	9	13	23
35–49	64	3.8	28	1	1	7	4	14	12	39
50–64	42	6.6	22	2	4	7	7	10	13	26
65+	60	8.2	65	2	3	6	9	20	23	44
TOTAL SINGLE DX	70	2.5	17	1	1	1	2	5	8	26
MULTIPLE DX	283	5.2	38	1	2	4	7	9	15	30
TOTAL										
0–19 Years	108	3.2	38	1	1	2	4	5	8	30
20–34	57	5.0	25	1	2	5	7	9	14	26
35–49	74	3.8	27	1	1	5	7	12	12	32
50–64	49	4.9	22	1	1	5	7	7	12	21
65+	65	8.0	62	2	3	5	8	20	23	44
GRAND TOTAL	353	4.5	34	1	1	2	6	9	14	26

Length of Stay by Diagnosis and Operation, United States, 1997

United States, October 1995–September 1996 Data, by Operation

78.6: RMVL IMPL DEV FROM BONE. Formerly included in operation group(s) 729.

Type of Patients	Observed Patients	Avg. Stay	Vari-ance	10th	25th	50th	75th	90th	95th	99th
1. SINGLE DX										
0–19 Years	359	1.8	9	1	1	1	2	3	4	18
20–34	449	2.0	3	1	1	2	3	3	5	6
35–49	460	2.2	2	1	1	2	3	4	5	5
50–64	231	1.9	2	1	1	1	2	4	4	7
65+	146	2.9	5	1	2	2	3	6	7	10
2. MULTIPLE DX										
0–19 Years	829	3.9	45	1	1	2	4	7	17	36
20–34	847	3.7	30	1	1	2	4	8	10	34
35–49	1196	3.7	32	1	2	2	4	7	10	30
50–64	838	4.5	40	1	2	3	5	9	14	39
65+	1315	5.7	40	2	2	4	8	11	15	24
TOTAL SINGLE DX	1645	2.1	4	1	1	2	2	4	5	8
MULTIPLE DX	5025	4.3	38	1	1	3	5	9	13	31
TOTAL										
0–19 Years	1188	3.2	35	1	1	1	3	5	11	30
20–34	1296	3.1	21	1	1	2	3	6	10	28
35–49	1656	3.3	23	1	1	2	4	5	8	22
50–64	1069	3.9	33	1	1	2	4	7	12	31
65+	1461	5.4	37	1	2	4	7	10	14	24
GRAND TOTAL	6670	3.7	29	1	1	2	4	7	10	28

78.65: RMVL IMPL DEV FEMUR. Formerly included in operation group(s) 729.

Type of Patients	Observed Patients	Avg. Stay	Vari-ance	10th	25th	50th	75th	90th	95th	99th
1. SINGLE DX										
0–19 Years	203	1.9	13	1	1	1	1	2	4	28
20–34	125	1.3	<1	1	1	1	2	2	3	4
35–49	66	1.4	1	1	1	1	2	2	2	4
50–64	41	1.4	1	1	1	1	2	2	2	6
65+	76	3.2	6	1	2	2	4	6	7	14
2. MULTIPLE DX										
0–19 Years	425	3.5	52	1	1	1	3	5	18	31
20–34	158	2.6	10	1	2	2	3	5	10	11
35–49	192	3.3	31	1	2	2	3	6	8	27
50–64	159	4.9	38	1	2	3	6	10	17	29
65+	637	5.5	27	1	2	5	7	11	13	20
TOTAL SINGLE DX	511	1.7	7	1	1	1	2	2	4	12
MULTIPLE DX	1571	4.2	36	1	1	2	5	8	13	30
TOTAL										
0–19 Years	628	2.9	38	1	1	1	2	5	13	30
20–34	283	2.0	6	1	1	1	2	3	7	11
35–49	258	2.8	24	1	1	2	3	4	7	24
50–64	200	4.1	31	1	2	2	6	8	15	26
65+	713	5.4	25	1	2	4	7	10	13	20
GRAND TOTAL	2082	3.5	29	1	1	2	4	8	11	28

78.63: RMVL IMPL DEV RAD/ULNA. Formerly included in operation group(s) 729.

Type of Patients	Observed Patients	Avg. Stay	Vari-ance	10th	25th	50th	75th	90th	95th	99th
1. SINGLE DX										
0–19 Years	11	2.2	2	1	1	2	3	5	5	5
20–34	19	2.8	5	1	2	3	3	3	3	20
35–49	17	2.2	2	1	1	2	3	3	6	6
50–64	12	1.6	<1	1	1	1	3	3	3	6
65+	10	3.0	3	1	3	3	3	3	8	9
2. MULTIPLE DX										
0–19 Years	28	2.8	6	1	1	2	4	5	6	15
20–34	46	4.3	48	1	1	2	5	7	30	>99
35–49	63	2.9	19	1	1	2	3	4	8	30
50–64	39	2.4	2	1	1	2	3	5	6	6
65+	52	6.8	73	2	3	4	6	24	24	51
TOTAL SINGLE DX	69	2.5	3	1	1	3	3	3	5	8
MULTIPLE DX	228	3.9	35	1	1	2	4	6	18	30
TOTAL										
0–19 Years	39	2.6	5	1	1	2	4	5	5	15
20–34	65	3.7	31	1	1	2	3	6	20	>99
35–49	80	2.8	15	1	1	2	3	4	7	30
50–64	51	2.3	2	1	1	2	2	5	6	6
65+	62	5.8	58	2	2	4	5	16	24	51
GRAND TOTAL	297	3.5	27	1	1	2	4	6	13	30

78.67: RMVL IMPL DEV TIB & FIB. Formerly included in operation group(s) 729.

Type of Patients	Observed Patients	Avg. Stay	Vari-ance	10th	25th	50th	75th	90th	95th	99th
1. SINGLE DX										
0–19 Years	45	1.4	<1	1	1	1	2	2	2	3
20–34	86	2.2	8	1	1	1	2	5	5	26
35–49	95	2.0	3	1	2	2	2	3	4	6
50–64	40	1.9	1	1	1	2	2	3	4	7
65+	14	2.4	4	1	2	2	2	3	6	12
2. MULTIPLE DX										
0–19 Years	91	4.6	49	1	1	3	5	5	16	43
20–34	207	5.6	58	1	2	3	6	10	18	44
35–49	259	6.1	94	1	2	3	7	12	18	54
50–64	192	5.3	64	1	2	4	7	14	22	41
65+	159	6.3	21	1	2	6	10	10	13	20
TOTAL SINGLE DX	280	1.9	4	1	1	2	2	3	5	7
MULTIPLE DX	908	5.6	63	1	2	3	6	11	18	43
TOTAL										
0–19 Years	136	3.6	36	1	1	2	5	5	11	43
20–34	293	4.7	48	1	1	2	6	10	16	43
35–49	354	4.9	70	1	2	2	5	10	14	43
50–64	232	4.9	58	1	1	2	4	14	22	41
65+	173	5.8	20	1	2	4	10	10	12	20
GRAND TOTAL	1188	4.8	51	1	1	2	5	10	15	43

Length of Stay by Diagnosis and Operation, United States, 1997

United States, October 1995–September 1996 Data, by Operation

78.69: RMVL IMPL DEV SITE NEC. Formerly included in operation group(s) 729.

Type of Patients	Observed Patients	Avg. Stay	Vari-ance	10th	25th	50th	75th	90th	95th	99th
1. SINGLE DX										
0–19 Years	76	2.2	2	1	1	2	3	4	4	6
20–34	184	2.4	2	1	1	2	3	4	5	6
35–49	250	2.6	2	1	2	2	4	4	5	5
50–64	112	2.1	2	1	1	2	3	4	4	7
65+	30	2.7	4	1	1	2	3	7	7	7
2. MULTIPLE DX										
0–19 Years	222	4.1	26	1	1	3	5	7	12	27
20–34	339	3.2	18	1	1	3	3	5	8	14
35–49	546	3.1	7	2	2	2	3	5	7	12
50–64	340	3.9	18	1	2	3	5	6	9	21
65+	264	5.3	43	1	2	3	6	11	15	37
TOTAL SINGLE DX	652	2.4	2	1	1	2	3	4	5	7
MULTIPLE DX	1711	3.6	18	1	2	3	4	6	9	20
TOTAL										
0–19 Years	298	3.7	22	1	1	3	4	7	10	21
20–34	523	2.9	12	1	1	2	3	5	6	12
35–49	796	2.9	6	1	2	2	3	5	6	10
50–64	452	3.4	14	1	2	3	4	6	7	17
65+	294	4.8	37	1	2	3	6	9	15	26
GRAND TOTAL	2363	3.2	13	1	2	2	4	6	7	17

78.8: OTHER BONE DIAGNOSTIC PX. Formerly included in operation group(s) 727, 728.

Type of Patients	Observed Patients	Avg. Stay	Vari-ance	10th	25th	50th	75th	90th	95th	99th
1. SINGLE DX										
0–19 Years	4	2.7	1	2	2	2	3	3	6	6
20–34	0									
35–49	0									
50–64	0									
65+	0									
2. MULTIPLE DX										
0–19 Years	6	11.2	164	3	3	5	15	35	35	35
20–34	1	4.0	0	4	4	4	4	4	4	4
35–49	1	4.0	0	4	4	4	4	4	4	4
50–64	0									
65+	3	6.5	54	1	1	4	4	18	18	18
TOTAL SINGLE DX	4	2.7	1	2	2	2	3	3	6	6
MULTIPLE DX	11	8.5	109	3	3	4	5	35	35	35
TOTAL										
0–19 Years	10	7.0	100	2	2	3	5	35	35	35
20–34	1	4.0	0	4	4	4	4	4	4	4
35–49	1	4.0	0	4	4	4	4	4	4	4
50–64	0									
65+	3	6.5	54	1	1	4	4	18	18	18
GRAND TOTAL	15	6.5	78	2	3	3	5	18	35	35

78.7: OSTEOCLASIS. Formerly included in operation group(s) 727, 728.

Type of Patients	Observed Patients	Avg. Stay	Vari-ance	10th	25th	50th	75th	90th	95th	99th
1. SINGLE DX										
0–19 Years	13	1.3	<1	1	1	1	1	2	3	4
20–34	1	3.0	0	3	3	3	3	3	3	3
35–49	0									
50–64	0									
65+	0									
2. MULTIPLE DX										
0–19 Years	9	6.4	102	1	1	1	7	26	30	30
20–34	3	6.7	50	1	1	5	16	16	16	16
35–49	3	1.7	<1	1	1	2	2	2	2	2
50–64	2	6.1	3	4	4	7	7	7	7	7
65+	3	6.3	15	5	5	5	5	17	17	17
TOTAL SINGLE DX	14	1.3	<1	1	1	1	1	2	3	4
MULTIPLE DX	20	6.0	66	1	1	2	7	26	26	30
TOTAL										
0–19 Years	22	2.6	32	1	1	1	1	3	9	30
20–34	4	6.0	42	1	1	3	16	16	16	16
35–49	3	1.7	<1	1	1	2	2	2	2	2
50–64	2	6.1	3	4	4	7	7	7	7	7
65+	3	6.3	15	5	5	5	5	17	17	17
GRAND TOTAL	34	3.1	31	1	1	1	2	5	7	17

78.9: INSERT BONE GROWTH STIM. Formerly included in operation group(s) 727, 728.

Type of Patients	Observed Patients	Avg. Stay	Vari-ance	10th	25th	50th	75th	90th	95th	99th
1. SINGLE DX										
0–19 Years	3	2.5	3	1	1	2	5	5	5	5
20–34	0									
35–49	2	1.4	<1	1	1	1	2	2	2	2
50–64	2	1.5	<1	1	1	2	2	2	2	2
65+	0									
2. MULTIPLE DX										
0–19 Years	1	5.0	0	5	5	5	5	5	5	5
20–34	2	3.6	4	2	2	5	5	5	5	5
35–49	12	2.0	5	1	1	1	2	4	9	9
50–64	9	3.5	6	1	2	2	3	8	8	8
65+	7	2.4	1	1	1	3	3	4	4	4
TOTAL SINGLE DX	7	2.1	2	1	1	2	2	5	5	5
MULTIPLE DX	31	2.7	5	1	1	2	4	5	8	9
TOTAL										
0–19 Years	4	3.4	4	1	1	5	5	5	5	5
20–34	2	3.6	4	2	2	5	5	5	5	5
35–49	14	2.0	5	1	1	1	2	4	9	9
50–64	11	3.2	5	1	1	3	3	8	8	8
65+	7	2.4	1	1	1	3	3	4	4	4
GRAND TOTAL	38	2.6	5	1	1	2	4	5	8	9

Length of Stay by Diagnosis and Operation, United States, 1997

United States, October 1995–September 1996 Data, by Operation

79.0: CLSD FX RED W/O INT FIX. Formerly included in operation group(s) 732, 735.

Type of Patients	Observed Patients	Avg. Stay	Vari-ance	10th	25th	50th	75th	90th	95th	99th
1. SINGLE DX										
0–19 Years	3434	2.0	8	1	1	1	2	3	4	18
20–34	526	2.0	3	1	1	1	2	3	4	8
35–49	464	2.0	2	1	1	2	2	4	5	6
50–64	297	2.0	2	1	1	2	2	4	5	8
65+	257	2.2	3	1	1	2	3	4	5	11
2. MULTIPLE DX										
0–19 Years	1719	4.4	48	1	1	2	4	10	18	32
20–34	837	4.0	18	1	1	3	5	11	12	19
35–49	1042	3.7	17	1	2	3	4	7	10	20
50–64	928	4.7	39	1	2	4	6	10	13	27
65+	3317	5.1	29	1	2	4	6	10	13	28
TOTAL SINGLE DX	4978	2.0	7	1	1	1	2	3	5	15
MULTIPLE DX	7843	4.5	32	1	2	3	5	9	13	27
TOTAL										
0–19 Years	5153	2.7	22	1	1	1	2	5	9	23
20–34	1363	3.3	14	1	1	2	4	7	12	17
35–49	1506	3.2	13	1	1	2	4	6	10	17
50–64	1225	3.9	30	1	2	3	5	8	11	22
65+	3574	5.0	28	1	2	4	6	10	13	28
GRAND TOTAL	12821	3.4	22	1	1	2	4	7	11	23

79.01: CLSD FX RED HUMERUS. Formerly included in operation group(s) 735.

Type of Patients	Observed Patients	Avg. Stay	Vari-ance	10th	25th	50th	75th	90th	95th	99th
1. SINGLE DX										
0–19 Years	400	1.5	2	1	1	1	2	2	3	8
20–34	52	1.3	<1	1	1	1	1	2	3	3
35–49	22	1.4	<1	1	1	1	2	2	3	4
50–64	21	1.8	2	1	2	1	2	4	5	5
65+	45	2.0	3	1	1	1	3	5	6	8
2. MULTIPLE DX										
0–19 Years	160	2.9	8	1	1	2	4	6	8	13
20–34	85	3.2	21	1	1	2	3	6	10	16
35–49	101	3.4	18	1	2	2	3	6	10	20
50–64	117	3.5	18	1	2	2	3	10	10	17
65+	572	4.3	14	1	2	3	5	8	11	21
TOTAL SINGLE DX	540	1.5	2	1	1	1	2	2	3	8
MULTIPLE DX	1035	3.7	15	1	1	3	4	7	10	19
TOTAL										
0–19 Years	560	1.8	4	1	1	1	2	3	6	10
20–34	137	2.7	16	1	1	2	3	4	6	16
35–49	123	3.0	15	1	1	2	3	4	10	20
50–64	138	3.2	16	1	2	2	3	8	12	17
65+	617	4.1	13	1	2	3	5	8	11	21
GRAND TOTAL	1575	2.8	10	1	1	2	3	6	8	16

79.02: CLSD RED FX RADIUS/ULNA. Formerly included in operation group(s) 735.

Type of Patients	Observed Patients	Avg. Stay	Vari-ance	10th	25th	50th	75th	90th	95th	99th
1. SINGLE DX										
0–19 Years	1018	1.2	<1	1	1	1	1	2	2	4
20–34	67	1.8	<1	1	1	1	2	2	3	5
35–49	86	1.5	<1	1	1	1	2	2	3	5
50–64	81	1.7	<1	1	1	1	3	3	3	3
65+	95	1.7	2	1	1	1	2	3	4	6
2. MULTIPLE DX										
0–19 Years	356	2.4	14	1	1	2	2	5	7	15
20–34	200	3.0	11	1	1	2	3	6	10	18
35–49	245	2.8	11	1	1	2	3	6	8	14
50–64	291	3.7	34	1	2	2	4	8	10	18
65+	1203	4.5	23	1	2	3	5	9	11	20
TOTAL SINGLE DX	1347	1.3	<1	1	1	1	1	2	3	4
MULTIPLE DX	2295	3.6	20	1	1	2	4	7	10	18
TOTAL										
0–19 Years	1374	1.5	4	1	1	1	2	2	4	8
20–34	267	2.7	9	1	1	2	3	5	9	18
35–49	331	2.5	9	1	1	2	3	6	8	14
50–64	372	3.3	27	1	2	2	4	7	8	18
65+	1298	4.3	22	1	2	3	5	9	11	20
GRAND TOTAL	3642	2.6	13	1	1	1	3	5	8	15

79.05: CLSD FX RED FEMUR. Formerly included in operation group(s) 732.

Type of Patients	Observed Patients	Avg. Stay	Vari-ance	10th	25th	50th	75th	90th	95th	99th
1. SINGLE DX										
0–19 Years	1052	3.6	24	1	1	2	3	8	15	24
20–34	11	5.1	98	1	2	3	4	5	44	44
35–49	12	2.6	3	2	2	2	3	4	5	10
50–64	10	2.4	2	1	2	2	3	4	6	7
65+	22	3.5	4	1	2	3	4	6	6	8
2. MULTIPLE DX										
0–19 Years	688	6.8	73	1	2	3	7	19	23	44
20–34	58	5.1	34	1	2	4	5	12	16	20
35–49	47	7.5	47	2	3	7	9	14	14	48
50–64	62	7.4	93	1	2	4	9	22	22	54
65+	356	6.7	46	1	3	5	9	14	21	30
TOTAL SINGLE DX	1107	3.5	24	1	1	2	3	8	15	24
MULTIPLE DX	1211	6.8	64	1	2	4	8	18	23	42
TOTAL										
0–19 Years	1740	4.8	45	1	1	2	5	14	20	32
20–34	69	5.1	38	1	2	4	5	12	16	44
35–49	59	6.6	42	2	2	6	7	14	14	48
50–64	72	5.8	69	1	2	3	6	11	22	54
65+	378	6.6	45	1	3	5	9	13	21	30
GRAND TOTAL	2318	5.1	46	1	1	3	5	13	20	32

Length of Stay by Diagnosis and Operation, United States, 1997

United States, October 1995–September 1996 Data, by Operation

79.06: CLSD FX RED TIBIA/FIBULA. Formerly included in operation group(s) 735.

Type of Patients	Observed Patients	Avg. Stay	Vari-ance	10th	25th	50th	75th	90th	95th	99th
1. SINGLE DX										
0–19 Years	923	1.6	<1	1	1	1	2	3	3	5
20–34	343	2.0	3	1	1	1	2	4	5	8
35–49	309	2.1	2	1	1	1	3	4	5	6
50–64	165	2.2	3	1	1	2	3	5	6	9
65+	86	2.6	5	1	1	2	3	5	6	13
2. MULTIPLE DX										
0–19 Years	444	2.9	39	1	1	2	3	4	8	22
20–34	345	3.9	13	1	1	2	5	8	11	17
35–49	507	3.8	15	1	1	3	5	7	11	20
50–64	377	5.1	39	1	2	3	6	10	13	38
65+	1000	5.7	37	2	3	4	7	11	14	34
TOTAL SINGLE DX	1826	1.8	2	1	1	1	2	3	4	6
MULTIPLE DX	2673	4.3	30	1	2	3	5	9	12	28
TOTAL										
0–19 Years	1367	2.0	13	1	1	2	2	3	4	9
20–34	688	3.0	9	1	1	2	4	6	9	15
35–49	816	3.1	11	1	1	2	4	6	9	17
50–64	542	4.1	29	1	1	3	5	9	10	21
65+	1086	5.5	35	2	3	4	7	11	14	34
GRAND TOTAL	4499	3.2	19	1	1	2	4	6	9	17

79.1: CLSD FX RED W INT FIX. Formerly included in operation group(s) 730, 733.

Type of Patients	Observed Patients	Avg. Stay	Vari-ance	10th	25th	50th	75th	90th	95th	99th
1. SINGLE DX										
0–19 Years	2454	1.9	9	1	1	1	2	3	5	20
20–34	552	2.4	3	1	1	2	3	4	6	8
35–49	537	2.6	5	1	1	2	3	5	5	17
50–64	340	3.3	4	1	2	3	5	6	7	8
65+	351	4.0	10	1	2	4	5	9	9	10
2. MULTIPLE DX										
0–19 Years	1144	5.5	49	1	1	3	6	14	24	32
20–34	1162	5.6	30	1	3	4	7	11	14	26
35–49	1131	5.6	34	1	2	4	6	11	18	30
50–64	1208	5.6	24	2	3	4	7	11	14	23
65+	7299	6.5	19	3	4	5	8	11	14	23
TOTAL SINGLE DX	4234	2.3	8	1	1	1	3	4	6	17
MULTIPLE DX	11944	6.0	26	2	3	5	7	11	15	26
TOTAL										
0–19 Years	3598	3.1	24	1	1	3	3	6	13	26
20–34	1714	4.5	22	1	2	3	5	9	12	25
35–49	1668	4.5	25	1	2	3	5	9	13	26
50–64	1548	5.1	20	1	2	4	6	10	13	21
65+	7650	6.3	19	3	4	5	8	11	14	23
GRAND TOTAL	16178	4.8	24	1	2	4	6	10	13	25

79.07: CLSD FX RED MT/TARSAL. Formerly included in operation group(s) 735.

Type of Patients	Observed Patients	Avg. Stay	Vari-ance	10th	25th	50th	75th	90th	95th	99th
1. SINGLE DX										
0–19 Years	10	2.9	6	1	2	2	2	8	8	8
20–34	21	1.7	3	1	1	1	2	2	5	11
35–49	19	2.0	1	1	1	2	2	3	3	7
50–64	12	2.2	1	1	1	2	2	3	6	7
65+	4	3.4	2	2	2	4	5	5	5	5
2. MULTIPLE DX										
0–19 Years	9	2.5	2	1	2	3	3	3	3	8
20–34	48	5.6	17	2	2	4	10	12	12	15
35–49	39	4.0	7	1	1	4	6	7	9	10
50–64	19	6.6	123	1	3	4	7	8	8	70
65+	30	4.6	10	2	2	4	7	7	7	20
TOTAL SINGLE DX	66	2.1	3	1	1	2	2	3	6	9
MULTIPLE DX	145	5.1	22	1	2	4	7	12	12	15
TOTAL										
0–19 Years	19	2.8	4	2	2	2	3	8	8	8
20–34	69	4.6	16	1	2	3	7	12	12	15
35–49	58	3.3	6	1	1	2	5	7	9	10
50–64	31	3.8	51	1	2	4	7	8	8	70
65+	34	4.5	9	2	2	4	7	7	7	20
GRAND TOTAL	211	4.1	18	2	2	2	5	11	12	12

79.11: CRIF HUMERUS. Formerly included in operation group(s) 733.

Type of Patients	Observed Patients	Avg. Stay	Vari-ance	10th	25th	50th	75th	90th	95th	99th
1. SINGLE DX										
0–19 Years	1577	1.3	2	1	1	1	1	2	2	5
20–34	27	2.0	11	1	1	1	2	3	4	20
35–49	32	2.0	1	1	2	2	2	2	3	4
50–64	22	3.6	3	1	1	5	5	5	5	5
65+	42	1.7	1	1	1	1	2	3	4	6
2. MULTIPLE DX										
0–19 Years	339	1.8	6	1	1	1	2	3	6	14
20–34	54	5.7	33	1	2	2	9	14	14	27
35–49	56	4.3	23	1	2	2	5	10	17	23
50–64	97	4.3	20	1	2	3	5	8	13	32
65+	411	4.9	21	2	2	4	6	10	13	28
TOTAL SINGLE DX	1700	1.4	2	1	1	1	1	2	2	5
MULTIPLE DX	957	3.4	17	1	1	2	4	8	13	18
TOTAL										
0–19 Years	1916	1.4	3	1	1	1	1	2	2	9
20–34	81	4.9	30	1	1	2	7	14	14	27
35–49	88	3.4	15	1	2	2	3	7	10	20
50–64	119	4.1	15	1	2	3	5	7	8	19
65+	453	4.4	19	1	2	3	5	9	11	24
GRAND TOTAL	2657	2.0	7	1	1	1	2	4	6	14

Length of Stay by Diagnosis and Operation, United States, 1997

United States, October 1995–September 1996 Data, by Operation

79.12: CRIF RADIUS/ULNA. Formerly included in operation group(s) 733.

Type of Patients	Observed Patients	Avg. Stay	Vari-ance	10th	25th	50th	75th	90th	95th	99th
1. SINGLE DX										
0–19 Years	184	1.3	<1	1	1	1	1	2	2	3
20–34	78	1.4	<1	1	1	1	1	3	3	4
35–49	100	1.2	<1	1	1	1	1	2	2	3
50–64	92	1.5	<1	1	1	1	2	2	2	4
65+	74	1.8	3	1	1	1	2	4	4	6
2. MULTIPLE DX										
0–19 Years	83	2.5	16	1	1	1	2	5	12	22
20–34	100	4.3	94	1	1	2	4	7	11	74
35–49	155	2.9	10	1	1	2	4	5	10	18
50–64	184	3.8	22	1	1	2	4	7	11	26
65+	425	3.6	14	1	1	3	4	9	12	18
TOTAL SINGLE DX	528	1.4	<1	1	1	1	2	2	3	4
MULTIPLE DX	947	3.5	25	1	1	2	4	7	11	24
TOTAL										
0–19 Years	267	1.7	6	1	1	1	2	3	4	13
20–34	178	3.1	58	1	1	1	3	4	8	74
35–49	255	2.3	7	1	1	1	4	5	5	15
50–64	276	3.0	16	1	1	2	3	7	8	16
65+	499	3.4	13	1	1	2	4	8	11	14
GRAND TOTAL	1475	2.7	17	1	1	1	3	5	8	15

79.16: CRIF TIBIA & FIBULA. Formerly included in operation group(s) 733.

Type of Patients	Observed Patients	Avg. Stay	Vari-ance	10th	25th	50th	75th	90th	95th	99th
1. SINGLE DX										
0–19 Years	186	2.1	1	1	1	2	3	3	5	5
20–34	233	2.5	2	1	1	2	3	5	6	7
35–49	230	3.1	7	1	2	2	4	5	6	17
50–64	82	4.0	5	2	2	3	5	8	8	9
65+	25	3.9	4	2	2	4	5	6	6	12
2. MULTIPLE DX										
0–19 Years	117	4.6	24	1	2	3	5	9	13	28
20–34	311	4.3	17	1	2	3	5	8	10	20
35–49	368	4.7	20	2	2	4	6	8	12	21
50–64	211	4.9	21	2	3	5	7	10	13	18
65+	230	6.0	24	2	3	5	7	11	15	30
TOTAL SINGLE DX	756	2.7	4	1	1	2	3	5	6	9
MULTIPLE DX	1237	4.8	20	2	2	4	6	9	12	23
TOTAL										
0–19 Years	303	3.0	11	1	1	2	3	5	9	19
20–34	544	3.4	11	1	2	3	4	6	8	15
35–49	598	4.0	14	1	2	3	5	7	9	17
50–64	293	4.7	17	2	2	3	6	8	13	17
65+	255	5.7	22	2	3	5	7	11	14	29
GRAND TOTAL	1993	3.9	14	1	2	3	5	7	9	17

79.15: CRIF FEMUR. Formerly included in operation group(s) 730.

Type of Patients	Observed Patients	Avg. Stay	Vari-ance	10th	25th	50th	75th	90th	95th	99th
1. SINGLE DX										
0–19 Years	442	5.1	40	1	2	3	5	15	21	27
20–34	131	3.0	2	2	2	2	4	5	6	8
35–49	119	3.1	3	1	2	3	4	5	7	11
50–64	126	4.1	2	2	3	4	5	6	7	8
65+	198	5.4	11	3	4	4	7	9	9	11
2. MULTIPLE DX										
0–19 Years	540	9.0	64	2	3	6	13	24	26	32
20–34	537	7.1	25	3	4	6	9	13	15	28
35–49	395	8.0	53	3	4	6	8	17	26	33
50–64	648	6.7	21	3	4	6	8	12	14	23
65+	6147	6.8	18	3	4	6	8	11	15	23
TOTAL SINGLE DX	1016	4.4	20	1	2	3	5	7	11	25
MULTIPLE DX	8267	7.1	25	3	4	6	8	13	16	27
TOTAL										
0–19 Years	982	7.3	58	2	2	4	9	20	25	32
20–34	668	6.0	22	2	3	5	7	11	14	26
35–49	514	6.6	43	2	4	5	8	12	23	30
50–64	774	6.3	19	3	4	5	7	11	14	23
65+	6345	6.7	18	3	4	6	8	11	14	23
GRAND TOTAL	9283	6.7	25	3	4	5	8	12	16	26

79.17: CRIF METATARSAL/TARSAL. Formerly included in operation group(s) 733.

Type of Patients	Observed Patients	Avg. Stay	Vari-ance	10th	25th	50th	75th	90th	95th	99th
1. SINGLE DX										
0–19 Years	14	2.6	18	1	1	2	2	4	4	24
20–34	25	1.9	2	1	1	2	2	2	3	9
35–49	34	2.1	2	1	1	1	3	5	5	5
50–64	10	2.0	<1	2	2	2	3	5	5	5
65+	7	3.3	4	1	1	3	4	7	7	7
2. MULTIPLE DX										
0–19 Years	10	5.0	9	2	2	6	7	7	12	12
20–34	52	4.0	8	2	2	3	7	7	7	16
35–49	66	4.5	20	1	3	3	4	8	18	18
50–64	25	4.5	6	1	3	4	7	8	8	8
65+	27	3.7	6	1	3	3	4	6	7	17
TOTAL SINGLE DX	90	2.1	4	1	1	2	2	4	5	8
MULTIPLE DX	180	4.3	11	2	2	3	5	7	11	18
TOTAL										
0–19 Years	24	3.7	15	1	1	2	6	7	12	24
20–34	77	3.7	7	1	3	3	5	5	14	16
35–49	100	3.7	15	1	2	3	4	5	18	18
50–64	35	3.3	5	1	2	2	4	8	8	8
65+	34	3.6	6	1	3	3	4	6	7	17
GRAND TOTAL	270	3.6	10	1	2	3	4	7	8	18

Length of Stay by Diagnosis and Operation, United States, 1997

United States, October 1995–September 1996 Data, by Operation

79.2: OPEN FRACTURE REDUCTION. Formerly included in operation group(s) 732, 735.

Type of Patients	Observed Patients	Avg. Stay	Vari-ance	10th	25th	50th	75th	90th	95th	99th
1. SINGLE DX										
0–19 Years	213	2.0	2	1	1	2	2	3	4	6
20–34	77	2.3	2	1	1	2	3	3	5	7
35–49	85	3.4	7	1	2	2	4	7	7	14
50–64	39	2.4	3	1	1	2	4	4	6	7
65+	26	2.9	3	1	1	2	5	5	5	7
2. MULTIPLE DX										
0–19 Years	144	5.2	26	1	2	4	7	14	15	17
20–34	139	5.1	49	1	2	3	5	10	21	40
35–49	152	4.8	22	1	2	4	5	10	14	23
50–64	105	5.4	36	1	2	3	6	11	18	26
65+	243	6.3	34	2	3	4	8	12	14	32
TOTAL SINGLE DX	440	2.3	3	1	1	2	3	4	6	8
MULTIPLE DX	783	5.4	34	1	2	4	7	12	16	26
TOTAL										
0–19 Years	357	3.2	13	1	1	2	4	7	9	17
20–34	216	4.0	32	1	2	3	4	7	11	35
35–49	237	4.3	17	1	2	3	5	8	13	22
50–64	144	4.8	31	1	2	3	6	8	18	26
65+	269	6.0	32	2	3	4	7	12	14	28
GRAND TOTAL	1223	4.2	24	1	2	3	5	9	14	24

79.26: OPEN RED TIBIA/FIB FX. Formerly included in operation group(s) 735.

Type of Patients	Observed Patients	Avg. Stay	Vari-ance	10th	25th	50th	75th	90th	95th	99th
1. SINGLE DX										
0–19 Years	60	2.6	3	1	1	2	3	5	5	13
20–34	27	2.8	<1	2	2	3	3	5	4	6
35–49	43	3.7	7	1	2	3	6	7	7	14
50–64	11	2.9	5	1	1	2	5	7	7	7
65+	12	3.5	2	2	2	4	5	5	5	7
2. MULTIPLE DX										
0–19 Years	54	6.7	21	2	4	5	9	14	17	17
20–34	54	5.8	67	2	2	5	7	21	21	46
35–49	70	6.6	27	2	3	5	8	13	22	24
50–64	46	8.5	53	3	5	6	8	18	26	38
65+	49	7.3	25	2	3	7	10	12	12	34
TOTAL SINGLE DX	153	3.0	4	1	2	3	3	5	6	13
MULTIPLE DX	273	6.9	40	2	3	5	8	14	21	26
TOTAL										
0–19 Years	114	4.8	17	1	2	3	5	9	14	17
20–34	81	4.6	42	2	2	3	4	8	21	21
35–49	113	5.2	20	2	2	4	7	11	14	23
50–64	57	7.7	50	1	4	6	7	18	26	26
65+	61	6.8	24	2	3	7	10	12	12	34
GRAND TOTAL	426	5.4	30	1	2	4	7	12	17	26

79.22: OPEN RED RADIUS/ULNA FX. Formerly included in operation group(s) 735.

Type of Patients	Observed Patients	Avg. Stay	Vari-ance	10th	25th	50th	75th	90th	95th	99th
1. SINGLE DX										
0–19 Years	96	1.7	1	1	1	1	2	3	4	5
20–34	18	1.6	1	1	1	1	2	3	4	5
35–49	13	2.9	5	1	1	2	3	7	7	7
50–64	12	1.9	1	1	1	1	3	3	4	4
65+	9	1.4	<1	1	1	1	2	2	3	3
2. MULTIPLE DX										
0–19 Years	31	2.4	7	1	1	1	3	5	6	16
20–34	18	4.6	8	2	2	5	6	8	11	11
35–49	28	3.3	18	1	1	2	3	6	14	21
50–64	18	2.6	2	1	2	2	3	4	7	7
65+	64	3.5	14	1	2	2	3	6	12	25
TOTAL SINGLE DX	148	1.8	1	1	1	1	2	3	4	5
MULTIPLE DX	159	3.1	10	1	1	2	3	6	8	21
TOTAL										
0–19 Years	127	1.9	2	1	1	1	2	3	4	6
20–34	36	3.1	7	1	1	2	5	7	8	11
35–49	41	3.2	15	1	1	2	3	7	7	21
50–64	30	2.4	2	1	2	2	2	4	7	7
65+	73	3.2	12	1	2	2	3	6	12	25
GRAND TOTAL	307	2.4	6	1	1	2	3	4	6	12

79.3: OPEN FX REDUCT W INT FIX. Formerly included in operation group(s) 731, 734.

Type of Patients	Observed Patients	Avg. Stay	Vari-ance	10th	25th	50th	75th	90th	95th	99th
1. SINGLE DX										
0–19 Years	4488	1.9	2	1	1	2	2	3	4	7
20–34	5812	2.3	3	1	1	2	3	3	5	9
35–49	5901	2.4	3	1	1	2	3	4	5	9
50–64	3621	2.6	3	1	2	2	3	5	6	12
65+	2372	3.8	5	1	2	3	5	7	8	12
2. MULTIPLE DX										
0–19 Years	3669	4.3	24	1	2	3	6	9	11	23
20–34	8227	4.7	25	1	2	3	6	10	13	25
35–49	10454	4.9	31	1	2	3	6	10	13	27
50–64	10728	5.2	29	1	3	4	6	10	14	29
65+	48181	6.9	27	3	4	6	8	11	15	29
TOTAL SINGLE DX	22194	2.4	3	1	1	2	3	4	6	9
MULTIPLE DX	81259	5.9	29	2	3	5	7	11	14	28
TOTAL										
0–19 Years	8157	2.9	13	1	1	2	3	6	8	15
20–34	14039	3.7	18	1	2	3	4	7	10	20
35–49	16355	3.9	22	1	2	3	4	8	11	22
50–64	14349	4.5	23	1	2	3	5	9	12	25
65+	50553	6.7	26	3	4	6	8	11	15	28
GRAND TOTAL	103453	4.9	24	2	2	4	6	9	13	25

Length of Stay by Diagnosis and Operation, United States, 1997

United States, October 1995–September 1996 Data, by Operation

79.31: ORIF HUMERUS. Formerly included in operation group(s) 734.

Type of Patients	Observed Patients	Avg. Stay	Variance	10th	25th	50th	75th	90th	95th	99th
1. SINGLE DX										
0–19 Years	1091	1.5	<1	1	1	1	2	2	3	4
20–34	270	2.3	3	1	1	2	3	5	5	8
35–49	241	2.3	2	1	1	2	3	4	5	6
50–64	227	2.2	2	1	1	2	3	4	4	8
65+	210	2.6	2	1	2	2	3	4	5	7
2. MULTIPLE DX										
0–19 Years	482	3.2	16	1	1	2	3	6	10	22
20–34	561	4.0	20	1	2	3	4	8	11	27
35–49	695	4.5	26	1	2	3	5	10	16	25
50–64	791	4.3	21	1	2	3	5	9	13	23
65+	2368	5.2	25	2	2	4	6	10	14	24
TOTAL SINGLE DX	2039	1.8	1	1	1	1	2	3	4	6
MULTIPLE DX	4897	4.5	23	1	2	3	5	9	13	24
TOTAL										
0–19 Years	1573	2.0	5	1	1	1	2	3	4	11
20–34	831	3.4	14	1	1	2	4	6	9	19
35–49	936	4.0	21	1	2	3	4	7	13	23
50–64	1018	3.8	17	1	2	3	5	8	12	20
65+	2578	4.9	23	2	2	4	6	10	14	24
GRAND TOTAL	6936	3.5	17	1	1	2	4	7	10	20

79.32: ORIF RADIUS/ULNA. Formerly included in operation group(s) 734.

Type of Patients	Observed Patients	Avg. Stay	Variance	10th	25th	50th	75th	90th	95th	99th
1. SINGLE DX										
0–19 Years	923	1.7	<1	1	1	1	2	2	4	5
20–34	735	1.8	2	1	1	1	2	3	4	6
35–49	541	1.6	1	1	1	1	2	3	3	6
50–64	331	1.7	1	1	1	1	2	3	3	5
65+	212	2.0	1	1	2	2	3	4	5	5
2. MULTIPLE DX										
0–19 Years	490	2.8	27	1	1	2	3	5	7	18
20–34	990	3.7	14	1	2	3	4	7	11	19
35–49	1012	3.6	19	1	2	2	4	7	11	19
50–64	769	3.2	13	1	2	2	4	7	9	19
65+	1508	4.1	21	2	2	3	5	8	11	21
TOTAL SINGLE DX	2742	1.7	1	1	1	1	2	3	4	6
MULTIPLE DX	4769	3.6	19	1	2	2	4	7	10	19
TOTAL										
0–19 Years	1413	2.1	10	1	1	2	2	3	4	10
20–34	1725	2.9	10	1	1	2	3	5	9	18
35–49	1553	2.8	13	1	2	2	3	7	7	16
50–64	1100	2.8	10	1	2	2	3	5	7	16
65+	1720	3.8	19	2	2	3	5	7	10	20
GRAND TOTAL	7511	2.8	12	1	1	2	3	5	7	16

79.33: ORIF CARPALS/METACARPALS. Formerly included in operation group(s) 734.

Type of Patients	Observed Patients	Avg. Stay	Variance	10th	25th	50th	75th	90th	95th	99th
1. SINGLE DX										
0–19 Years	49	1.4	<1	1	1	1	2	2	2	3
20–34	140	1.4	<1	1	1	1	1	2	3	5
35–49	50	1.4	<1	1	1	1	1	3	5	5
50–64	8	1.0	0	1	1	1	1	1	1	1
65+	9	1.7	<1	1	1	2	2	2	4	4
2. MULTIPLE DX										
0–19 Years	84	3.3	51	1	1	2	2	5	8	50
20–34	224	3.2	10	1	1	2	4	5	11	13
35–49	143	4.0	45	1	1	2	3	8	22	45
50–64	72	3.7	17	1	1	2	4	12	14	15
65+	40	3.5	8	2	2	3	4	7	14	14
TOTAL SINGLE DX	256	1.4	<1	1	1	1	2	2	3	5
MULTIPLE DX	563	3.5	26	1	1	2	4	8	13	22
TOTAL										
0–19 Years	133	2.6	33	1	1	1	2	3	6	50
20–34	364	2.5	7	1	1	1	3	5	9	13
35–49	193	3.1	30	1	1	1	2	5	10	25
50–64	80	3.5	16	1	1	2	4	5	14	15
65+	49	3.2	8	2	2	3	4	5	10	14
GRAND TOTAL	819	2.8	18	1	1	1	3	5	9	22

79.34: ORIF FINGER. Formerly included in operation group(s) 734.

Type of Patients	Observed Patients	Avg. Stay	Variance	10th	25th	50th	75th	90th	95th	99th
1. SINGLE DX										
0–19 Years	70	1.5	1	1	1	1	2	2	4	6
20–34	140	2.0	2	1	1	2	3	3	4	6
35–49	89	1.6	1	1	1	1	2	3	5	5
50–64	38	2.7	3	1	2	2	5	5	5	5
65+	13	2.2	<1	2	2	2	3	3	3	3
2. MULTIPLE DX										
0–19 Years	145	2.7	5	1	1	2	3	6	7	12
20–34	280	2.9	7	1	1	2	3	8	9	13
35–49	286	2.9	9	1	1	2	3	6	12	12
50–64	136	1.4	2	1	1	2	3	6	6	6
65+	88	2.9	8	2	2	2	3	6	8	16
TOTAL SINGLE DX	350	1.8	2	1	1	1	2	3	5	6
MULTIPLE DX	935	2.4	7	1	1	2	3	5	8	12
TOTAL										
0–19 Years	215	2.2	4	1	1	1	3	6	6	12
20–34	420	2.6	6	1	2	2	3	5	8	13
35–49	375	2.6	8	1	1	1	3	5	9	12
50–64	174	1.5	2	1	1	2	3	3	4	6
65+	101	2.8	6	2	2	2	3	6	7	16
GRAND TOTAL	1285	2.3	5	1	1	1	3	5	7	12

Length of Stay by Diagnosis and Operation, United States, 1997

United States, October 1995–September 1996 Data, by Operation

79.37: ORIF METATARSAL/TARSAL. Formerly included in operation group(s) 734.

Type of Patients	Observed Patients	Avg. Stay	Vari-ance	10th	25th	50th	75th	90th	95th	99th
1. SINGLE DX										
0–19 Years	91	1.9	2	1	1	2	2	3	3	10
20–34	297	2.4	3	1	1	2	3	5	5	7
35–49	369	2.7	4	1	2	2	3	5	7	10
50–64	161	2.9	2	1	2	2	4	5	5	7
65+	33	2.8	4	1	2	2	3	4	8	10
2. MULTIPLE DX										
0–19 Years	98	3.8	20	1	1	3	4	9	10	30
20–34	364	4.8	19	1	2	3	6	9	14	20
35–49	441	3.9	17	1	2	3	5	8	10	25
50–64	288	4.5	17	1	2	3	7	13	13	18
65+	180	4.1	13	2	2	3	4	8	11	23
TOTAL SINGLE DX	951	2.5	3	1	1	2	3	5	5	10
MULTIPLE DX	1371	4.3	18	1	2	3	5	9	13	20
TOTAL										
0–19 Years	189	2.8	11	1	1	2	3	5	9	17
20–34	661	3.6	13	1	2	3	4	6	10	20
35–49	810	3.4	12	1	2	3	4	7	9	16
50–64	449	4.0	13	1	2	3	5	9	13	17
65+	213	3.9	12	2	2	3	4	7	10	23
GRAND TOTAL	2322	3.5	12	1	2	2	4	7	10	20

79.39: ORIF BONE NEC X FACIAL. Formerly included in operation group(s) 734.

Type of Patients	Observed Patients	Avg. Stay	Vari-ance	10th	25th	50th	75th	90th	95th	99th
1. SINGLE DX										
0–19 Years	70	2.5	4	1	1	2	3	6	7	10
20–34	149	2.7	14	1	1	2	3	5	7	12
35–49	142	2.8	10	1	2	3	3	5	9	20
50–64	50	3.2	4	2	2	3	4	6	7	12
65+	24	3.0	6	1	3	3	3	5	10	12
2. MULTIPLE DX										
0–19 Years	130	6.2	52	1	1	2	10	15	23	26
20–34	436	7.9	42	1	3	7	11	15	18	33
35–49	439	9.0	122	1	2	6	12	18	27	79
50–64	270	8.1	59	1	2	6	11	19	26	36
65+	263	7.1	49	1	3	5	9	16	21	28
TOTAL SINGLE DX	435	2.7	10	1	1	2	3	5	7	15
MULTIPLE DX	1538	7.9	70	1	2	6	11	16	23	39
TOTAL										
0–19 Years	200	5.2	41	1	2	2	7	13	19	26
20–34	585	6.2	39	1	2	5	10	13	17	28
35–49	581	7.5	101	1	2	4	10	15	23	79
50–64	320	7.2	53	1	2	5	10	17	20	36
65+	287	6.8	47	1	3	5	9	15	20	28
GRAND TOTAL	1973	6.7	60	1	2	4	10	15	20	36

79.35: ORIF FEMUR. Formerly included in operation group(s) 731.

Type of Patients	Observed Patients	Avg. Stay	Vari-ance	10th	25th	50th	75th	90th	95th	99th
1. SINGLE DX										
0–19 Years	467	3.8	7	1	2	3	4	6	7	15
20–34	350	3.9	4	2	3	3	5	6	8	11
35–49	299	4.2	10	2	2	4	5	7	9	15
50–64	329	4.7	7	2	3	4	6	8	9	13
65+	847	5.4	6	3	4	5	6	8	9	15
2. MULTIPLE DX										
0–19 Years	1041	6.5	28	2	3	5	8	11	14	29
20–34	1631	8.0	56	3	4	6	9	14	20	41
35–49	1899	7.7	56	3	4	6	9	13	20	39
50–64	3245	8.2	46	3	5	6	9	14	22	34
65+	37200	7.4	27	4	5	6	8	12	16	30
TOTAL SINGLE DX	2292	4.5	7	2	3	4	5	7	9	13
MULTIPLE DX	45016	7.5	32	3	5	6	8	12	16	32
TOTAL										
0–19 Years	1508	5.6	23	2	3	4	7	10	13	26
20–34	1981	7.2	48	2	3	5	9	12	18	39
35–49	2198	7.2	51	3	4	5	8	13	18	37
50–64	3574	7.8	43	3	4	6	9	13	20	34
65+	38047	7.4	27	4	5	6	8	12	16	30
GRAND TOTAL	47308	7.3	31	3	4	6	8	12	16	31

79.36: ORIF TIBIA & FIBULA. Formerly included in operation group(s) 734.

Type of Patients	Observed Patients	Avg. Stay	Vari-ance	10th	25th	50th	75th	90th	95th	99th
1. SINGLE DX										
0–19 Years	1698	2.0	1	1	1	2	2	3	4	6
20–34	3711	2.3	3	1	1	2	3	4	5	8
35–49	4156	2.4	2	1	1	2	3	4	5	8
50–64	2471	2.5	3	1	2	2	3	4	5	8
65+	1024	3.0	3	1	2	3	4	5	7	8
2. MULTIPLE DX										
0–19 Years	1181	3.9	14	1	2	3	5	8	10	16
20–34	3707	3.9	14	1	2	3	5	7	10	20
35–49	5511	4.1	17	1	2	3	5	8	11	20
50–64	5138	4.2	17	1	2	3	5	8	11	21
65+	6518	5.1	20	2	3	4	6	9	11	25
TOTAL SINGLE DX	13060	2.4	3	1	1	2	3	4	5	8
MULTIPLE DX	22055	4.3	17	1	2	3	5	8	11	21
TOTAL										
0–19 Years	2879	2.8	8	1	1	2	3	6	7	12
20–34	7418	3.1	9	1	2	2	4	6	8	15
35–49	9667	3.3	11	1	2	2	4	6	9	16
50–64	7609	3.6	12	1	2	3	4	7	9	19
65+	7542	4.8	18	2	3	4	6	8	11	22
GRAND TOTAL	35115	3.5	12	1	2	3	4	7	9	17

Length of Stay by Diagnosis and Operation, United States, 1997

United States, October 1995–September 1996 Data, by Operation

79.4: CR SEP EPIPHYSIS. Formerly included in operation group(s) 732, 735.

Type of Patients	Observed Patients	Avg. Stay	Variance	10th	25th	50th	75th	90th	95th	99th
1. SINGLE DX										
0–19 Years	294	1.7	2	1	1	1	2	3	4	8
20–34	12	2.2	1	1	1	2	3	3	4	5
35–49	11	2.2	3	1	1	1	3	4	4	9
50–64	4	3.6	<1	2	3	4	4	4	10	10
65+	5	4.3	14	1	1	4	10	10	10	10
2. MULTIPLE DX										
0–19 Years	92	2.7	6	1	2	2	3	5	6	12
20–34	8	4.7	9	1	3	3	9	9	9	9
35–49	24	6.1	26	2	3	5	8	12	22	22
50–64	8	10.0	31	3	5	15	15	15	15	15
65+	32	6.1	31	2	3	5	7	9	14	46
TOTAL SINGLE DX	326	1.8	2	1	1	1	2	3	4	8
MULTIPLE DX	164	3.9	17	1	2	2	5	8	12	22
TOTAL										
0–19 Years	386	2.0	3	1	1	2	2	3	4	11
20–34	20	3.6	7	1	2	3	4	9	9	9
35–49	35	3.5	14	1	1	2	4	8	12	22
50–64	12	7.4	29	2	4	15	15	15	15	15
65+	37	5.9	30	2	3	5	7	10	14	46
GRAND TOTAL	490	2.5	8	1	1	2	3	4	7	15

79.45: CR SEP EPIPH FEMUR. Formerly included in operation group(s) 732.

Type of Patients	Observed Patients	Avg. Stay	Variance	10th	25th	50th	75th	90th	95th	99th
1. SINGLE DX										
0–19 Years	221	1.9	2	1	1	1	2	3	4	11
20–34	1	5.0	0	5	5	5	5	5	5	5
35–49	1	4.0	0	4	4	4	4	4	4	4
50–64	0									
65+	2	3.1	1	2	2	4	4	4	4	4
2. MULTIPLE DX										
0–19 Years	66	3.0	10	1	1	2	3	5	9	22
20–34	1	1.0	0	1	1	1	1	1	1	1
35–49	4	6.6	21	2	3	3	12	12	12	12
50–64	1	3.0	0	3	3	3	3	3	3	3
65+	10	5.8	5	2	4	7	7	7	7	9
TOTAL SINGLE DX	225	1.9	2	1	1	2	2	4	4	11
MULTIPLE DX	82	3.6	11	1	2	2	5	7	9	22
TOTAL										
0–19 Years	287	2.1	4	1	1	2	2	4	5	11
20–34	2	2.2	6	1	1	1	5	5	5	5
35–49	5	5.3	12	3	3	4	4	12	12	12
50–64	1	3.0		3	3	3	3	3	3	3
65+	12	5.6	5	2	4	7	7	7	7	9
GRAND TOTAL	307	2.4	5	1	1	2	3	4	7	12

79.5: OPEN RED SEP EPIPHYSIS. Formerly included in operation group(s) 731, 734.

Type of Patients	Observed Patients	Avg. Stay	Variance	10th	25th	50th	75th	90th	95th	99th
1. SINGLE DX										
0–19 Years	168	2.7	3	1	1	2	3	6	6	9
20–34	34	2.2	1	1	1	2	3	3	4	9
35–49	18	5.0	3	3	3	6	6	6	6	9
50–64	10	1.8	<1	1	1	2	2	3	3	3
65+	4	5.7	39	2	2	2	15	15	15	15
2. MULTIPLE DX										
0–19 Years	90	2.6	6	1	1	2	3	5	6	18
20–34	32	3.3	7	1	2	2	4	8	8	12
35–49	50	5.2	54	2	2	3	5	10	15	44
50–64	27	7.0	28	2	3	5	12	17	17	22
65+	57	7.0	28	2	3	6	9	13	18	33
TOTAL SINGLE DX	234	2.9	4	1	2	2	3	6	6	9
MULTIPLE DX	256	3.9	21	1	2	2	5	8	12	22
TOTAL										
0–19 Years	258	2.6	5	1	1	2	3	6	6	11
20–34	66	2.7	4	1	2	2	3	6	8	9
35–49	68	5.1	28	2	2	4	6	7	10	44
50–64	37	5.4	25	2	3	6	9	13	17	22
65+	61	7.0	29	2	3	6	9	14	18	33
GRAND TOTAL	490	3.4	12	1	2	2	4	6	8	18

79.6: OPEN FX SITE DEBRIDEMENT. Formerly included in operation group(s) 725, 726.

Type of Patients	Observed Patients	Avg. Stay	Variance	10th	25th	50th	75th	90th	95th	99th
1. SINGLE DX										
0–19 Years	396	2.5	3	1	1	2	3	4	6	9
20–34	318	2.8	5	1	1	2	3	5	7	10
35–49	224	3.0	7	1	2	3	4	6	8	14
50–64	75	3.4	4	1	2	3	4	6	7	11
65+	31	3.3	4	2	2	3	4	6	8	8
2. MULTIPLE DX										
0–19 Years	483	5.5	34	1	2	4	7	11	18	27
20–34	819	5.4	35	1	2	3	6	11	18	27
35–49	664	6.6	61	1	2	4	8	14	19	46
50–64	316	6.8	59	1	3	4	8	14	23	41
65+	330	7.3	44	2	3	5	8	16	19	32
TOTAL SINGLE DX	1044	2.8	5	1	1	2	3	5	7	12
MULTIPLE DX	2612	6.0	45	1	2	4	7	13	19	35
TOTAL										
0–19 Years	879	4.1	22	1	2	3	5	8	12	23
20–34	1137	4.7	28	1	2	3	5	10	16	26
35–49	888	5.7	49	2	2	5	7	13	17	41
50–64	391	6.1	50	2	2	4	8	12	20	41
65+	361	7.1	43	2	3	5	8	16	19	32
GRAND TOTAL	3656	5.1	35	1	2	3	6	11	17	30

Length of Stay by Diagnosis and Operation, United States, 1997

United States, October 1995–September 1996 Data, by Operation

79.62: DEBRIDE OPEN FX RAD/ULNA. Formerly included in operation group(s) 726.

Type of Patients	Observed Patients	Avg. Stay	Variance	10th	25th	50th	75th	90th	95th	99th
1. SINGLE DX										
0–19 Years	141	1.8	<1	1	1	2	2	3	3	4
20–34	31	2.5	3	1	1	2	2	3	3	13
35–49	26	2.5	2	1	2	3	3	4	5	11
50–64	14	2.0	2	1	1	3	3	3	3	7
65+	9	3.2	1	3	3	3	4	4	5	5
2. MULTIPLE DX										
0–19 Years	76	3.2	14	1	1	2	3	6	10	13
20–34	71	3.6	4	2	3	3	4	6	6	14
35–49	80	5.2	27	1	2	4	6	10	17	32
50–64	43	3.7	6	2	2	3	5	7	8	13
65+	98	6.3	32	2	3	4	8	19	19	20
TOTAL SINGLE DX	221	2.1	1	1	1	2	3	3	4	5
MULTIPLE DX	368	4.4	17	2	2	3	4	8	11	20
TOTAL										
0–19 Years	217	2.4	6	1	1	2	3	4	5	11
20–34	102	3.5	4	1	3	3	4	5	8	14
35–49	106	4.5	22	1	2	3	5	10	11	22
50–64	57	3.4	5	1	2	3	4	7	7	13
65+	107	6.1	30	2	3	4	7	19	19	20
GRAND TOTAL	589	3.6	13	1	2	3	4	7	10	19

79.64: DEBRIDE OPEN FX FINGER. Formerly included in operation group(s) 726.

Type of Patients	Observed Patients	Avg. Stay	Variance	10th	25th	50th	75th	90th	95th	99th
1. SINGLE DX										
0–19 Years	19	1.8	<1	1	1	2	2	3	3	5
20–34	30	1.7	1	1	1	2	2	2	2	9
35–49	47	1.7	<1	1	1	2	3	3	3	4
50–64	10	2.2	5	1	1	1	3	3	10	10
65+	4	1.8	<1	1	2	2	4	2	2	2
2. MULTIPLE DX										
0–19 Years	62	2.4	6	1	1	2	3	4	6	17
20–34	99	1.9	3	1	1	1	2	4	5	11
35–49	73	2.8	4	1	1	2	4	6	6	10
50–64	50	3.6	55	1	1	3	4	6	14	41
65+	30	2.6	3	1	2	2	4	4	5	8
TOTAL SINGLE DX	110	1.8	<1	1	1	2	2	3	3	5
MULTIPLE DX	314	2.4	10	1	1	1	3	4	6	11
TOTAL										
0–19 Years	81	2.2	5	1	1	2	3	4	5	17
20–34	129	1.8	2	1	1	2	2	3	5	11
35–49	120	2.2	2	1	1	2	4	6	6	10
50–64	60	3.4	49	1	1	2	3	5	12	41
65+	34	2.4	2	1	1	2	4	4	5	8
GRAND TOTAL	424	2.2	7	1	2	2	4	5	11

79.65: DEBRIDE OPEN FX FEMUR. Formerly included in operation group(s) 725.

Type of Patients	Observed Patients	Avg. Stay	Variance	10th	25th	50th	75th	90th	95th	99th
1. SINGLE DX										
0–19 Years	17	3.5	5	1	3	3	3	6	9	9
20–34	16	4.3	12	2	2	3	5	7	7	18
35–49	7	3.1	4	1	2	2	5	6	6	6
50–64	0									
65+	0									
2. MULTIPLE DX										
0–19 Years	56	11.8	79	3	4	9	20	22	27	42
20–34	102	8.8	66	2	4	7	10	20	23	40
35–49	61	11.5	139	2	6	7	14	19	46	67
50–64	21	15.3	138	7	9	13	21	24	25	69
65+	17	10.3	31	6	7	9	14	20	23	23
TOTAL SINGLE DX	40	3.7	7	1	2	3	5	6	9	18
MULTIPLE DX	257	10.7	98	3	6	7	14	22	26	60
TOTAL										
0–19 Years	73	10.0	74	3	3	7	14	22	26	42
20–34	118	8.4	62	2	3	6	10	19	21	36
35–49	68	11.1	135	2	6	6	13	18	46	67
50–64	21	15.3	138	7	9	13	21	24	25	69
65+	17	10.3	31	6	7	9	14	20	23	23
GRAND TOTAL	297	10.0	93	2	4	7	12	21	24	54

79.66: DEBRIDE OPN FX TIBIA/FIB. Formerly included in operation group(s) 726.

Type of Patients	Observed Patients	Avg. Stay	Variance	10th	25th	50th	75th	90th	95th	99th
1. SINGLE DX										
0–19 Years	147	3.0	5	1	2	2	3	6	6	17
20–34	146	3.6	6	1	2	3	4	6	9	14
35–49	88	4.3	11	2	2	4	6	8	12	17
50–64	34	4.4	6	2	3	4	5	8	10	11
65+	10	4.7	4	2	3	5	6	7	8	8
2. MULTIPLE DX										
0–19 Years	167	6.5	31	2	3	6	8	11	16	25
20–34	339	7.1	52	2	3	5	9	18	22	39
35–49	310	8.2	62	2	3	6	9	15	21	44
50–64	119	10.0	80	2	4	7	12	23	28	45
65+	120	9.7	61	3	5	8	13	17	23	53
TOTAL SINGLE DX	425	3.5	7	1	2	3	4	6	8	17
MULTIPLE DX	1055	7.8	56	2	3	6	9	16	22	41
TOTAL										
0–19 Years	314	4.7	21	1	2	3	6	9	12	21
20–34	485	6.2	42	2	2	4	7	13	20	35
35–49	398	7.4	54	2	3	6	9	14	19	41
50–64	153	8.8	70	2	4	6	11	19	26	41
65+	130	9.5	60	3	5	8	12	16	23	53
GRAND TOTAL	1480	6.5	45	2	3	4	8	14	19	36

© 1997 by HCIA Inc.

Length of Stay by Diagnosis and Operation, United States, 1997

United States, October 1995–September 1996 Data, by Operation

79.7: CLOSED RED DISLOCATION. Formerly included in operation group(s) 736, 737.

Type of Patients	Observed Patients	Avg. Stay	Variance	Percentiles						
				10th	25th	50th	75th	90th	95th	99th
1. SINGLE DX										
0–19 Years	213	1.8	6	1	1	1	2	3	4	15
20–34	154	1.5	1	1	1	1	2	3	4	7
35–49	189	1.5	1	1	1	1	2	2	4	6
50–64	186	1.7	2	1	1	1	2	3	4	6
65+	415	2.1	2	1	1	2	2	4	5	8
2. MULTIPLE DX										
0–19 Years	224	3.7	24	1	1	2	4	7	7	26
20–34	350	3.4	17	1	1	2	4	6	8	20
35–49	413	3.0	14	1	1	2	3	6	8	19
50–64	543	3.6	16	1	2	2	4	9	10	18
65+	2147	4.1	24	1	1	3	5	8	12	24
TOTAL SINGLE DX	1157	1.8	3	1	1	1	2	3	4	8
MULTIPLE DX	3677	3.7	21	1	1	2	4	8	10	23
TOTAL										
0–19 Years	437	2.8	16	1	1	2	3	6	7	19
20–34	504	2.8	13	1	1	2	4	5	7	20
35–49	602	2.6	11	1	1	1	3	6	8	16
50–64	729	3.0	12	1	1	2	4	8	10	14
65+	2562	3.7	21	1	1	2	4	7	10	23
GRAND TOTAL	4834	3.2	16	1	1	2	4	7	9	20

79.71: CLSD RED DISLOC SHOULDER. Formerly included in operation group(s) 737.

Type of Patients	Observed Patients	Avg. Stay	Variance	Percentiles						
				10th	25th	50th	75th	90th	95th	99th
1. SINGLE DX										
0–19 Years	14	1.1	<1	1	1	1	1	1	1	3
20–34	29	1.3	<1	1	1	1	2	2	2	2
35–49	21	1.1	<1	1	1	1	1	1	2	2
50–64	15	1.6	<1	1	1	1	2	2	2	3
65+	16	1.9	<1	1	2	2	2	2	2	6
2. MULTIPLE DX										
0–19 Years	16	2.2	<1	1	1	3	3	3	3	3
20–34	70	2.1	2	1	1	2	3	5	6	7
35–49	75	2.5	8	1	1	2	3	5	7	16
50–64	84	5.8	27	1	1	3	10	11	12	22
65+	376	5.0	23	1	2	4	6	10	14	19
TOTAL SINGLE DX	95	1.4	<1	1	1	1	2	2	2	3
MULTIPLE DX	621	4.3	20	1	1	3	5	10	11	19
TOTAL										
0–19 Years	30	1.4	<1	1	1	1	2	3	3	3
20–34	99	1.9	2	1	1	1	2	4	5	7
35–49	96	2.2	7	1	1	1	2	4	6	14
50–64	99	5.3	26	1	1	3	10	11	12	22
65+	392	4.5	21	1	2	3	6	9	14	19
GRAND TOTAL	716	3.7	17	1	1	2	5	9	10	18

79.75: CLSD RED DISLOC HIP. Formerly included in operation group(s) 736.

Type of Patients	Observed Patients	Avg. Stay	Variance	Percentiles						
				10th	25th	50th	75th	90th	95th	99th
1. SINGLE DX										
0–19 Years	139	2.0	9	1	1	1	2	3	6	18
20–34	50	2.1	3	1	1	1	2	5	7	6
35–49	124	1.7	1	1	1	1	2	3	5	6
50–64	152	1.7	2	1	1	1	2	3	4	8
65+	382	2.1	2	1	1	2	3	4	5	8
2. MULTIPLE DX										
0–19 Years	154	4.0	13	1	2	3	5	7	11	19
20–34	158	3.9	27	1	1	3	4	8	9	34
35–49	225	3.1	18	1	1	2	3	6	8	24
50–64	389	2.7	11	1	1	2	3	5	7	19
65+	1610	3.6	19	1	1	2	4	7	10	23
TOTAL SINGLE DX	847	1.9	3	1	1	1	2	4	5	9
MULTIPLE DX	2536	3.5	18	1	1	2	4	7	10	22
TOTAL										
0–19 Years	293	3.0	12	1	1	2	3	7	8	19
20–34	208	3.6	23	1	1	3	4	7	9	25
35–49	349	2.6	12	1	1	1	3	5	7	16
50–64	541	2.4	8	1	1	2	3	5	6	14
65+	1992	3.3	16	1	1	2	4	6	10	20
GRAND TOTAL	3383	3.0	14	1	1	2	3	6	8	20

79.8: OPEN RED DISLOCATION. Formerly included in operation group(s) 736, 737.

Type of Patients	Observed Patients	Avg. Stay	Variance	Percentiles						
				10th	25th	50th	75th	90th	95th	99th
1. SINGLE DX										
0–19 Years	247	2.3	8	1	1	2	2	4	6	16
20–34	115	2.1	3	1	1	2	2	4	6	7
35–49	64	2.6	5	1	1	2	4	7	7	11
50–64	16	2.5	7	1	1	2	4	10	10	10
65+	22	3.2	3	1	2	3	4	6	6	7
2. MULTIPLE DX										
0–19 Years	282	3.4	11	1	2	3	4	5	8	14
20–34	129	4.3	17	1	2	3	5	9	12	15
35–49	132	4.6	53	1	1	3	4	8	15	27
50–64	101	5.7	28	1	3	4	6	17	17	18
65+	185	8.5	29	2	4	7	13	15	20	22
TOTAL SINGLE DX	464	2.3	6	1	1	2	2	4	7	11
MULTIPLE DX	829	4.9	27	1	2	3	5	12	14	27
TOTAL										
0–19 Years	529	2.9	10	1	1	2	3	5	7	14
20–34	244	3.2	11	1	1	2	4	7	9	15
35–49	196	3.7	34	1	1	3	4	7	10	27
50–64	117	5.4	26	1	3	3	6	17	17	18
65+	207	8.2	29	2	4	7	13	14	20	22
GRAND TOTAL	1293	4.0	21	1	1	3	4	8	13	20

Length of Stay by Diagnosis and Operation, United States, 1997

United States, October 1995–September 1996 Data, by Operation

79.85: OPEN RED DISLOC HIP. Formerly included in operation group(s) 736.

Type of Patients	Observed Patients	Avg. Stay	Variance	10th	25th	50th	75th	90th	95th	99th
1. SINGLE DX										
0–19 Years	191	2.5	10	1	1	2	2	4	7	17
20–34	6	3.0	3	2	2	2	4	7	7	8
35–49	4	3.5	2	2	3	3	3	7	7	7
50–64	2	4.8	13	3	3	3	10	10	10	10
65+	9	4.5	2	2	4	4	6	6	7	7
2. MULTIPLE DX										
0–19 Years	244	3.4	6	1	2	3	4	5	7	14
20–34	24	7.1	13	4	4	7	9	12	15	15
35–49	20	6.7	99	2	3	5	8	8	15	68
50–64	20	12.2	44	4	5	12	17	17	18	39
65+	113	9.6	30	3	5	8	13	20	20	23
TOTAL SINGLE DX	**212**	**2.6**	**9**	**1**	**1**	**2**	**3**	**5**	**7**	**17**
MULTIPLE DX	**421**	**5.5**	**25**	**2**	**2**	**4**	**6**	**13**	**17**	**20**
TOTAL										
0–19 Years	435	3.0	7	1	2	2	4	5	7	14
20–34	30	5.1	12	3	2	4	7	10	12	15
35–49	24	5.3	59	1	3	3	6	8	10	68
50–64	22	11.9	44	4	5	12	17	17	18	39
65+	122	9.4	29	3	5	8	13	19	20	23
GRAND TOTAL	**633**	**4.6**	**21**	**1**	**2**	**3**	**5**	**12**	**14**	**20**

79.9: BONE INJURY OP NOS. Formerly included in operation group(s) 727, 728.

Type of Patients	Observed Patients	Avg. Stay	Variance	10th	25th	50th	75th	90th	95th	99th
1. SINGLE DX										
0–19 Years	1	1.0	0	1	1	1	1	1	1	1
20–34	0									
35–49	2	1.0	0	1	1	1	1	1	1	1
50–64	0									
65+	0									
2. MULTIPLE DX										
0–19 Years	1	1.0	0	1	1	1	1	1	1	1
20–34	1	3.0	0	3	3	3	3	3	3	3
35–49	0									
50–64	1	2.0	0	2	2	2	2	2	2	2
65+	0									
TOTAL SINGLE DX	**3**	**1.0**	**0**	**1**	**1**	**1**	**1**	**1**	**1**	**1**
MULTIPLE DX	**3**	**2.0**	**<1**	**1**	**1**	**2**	**3**	**3**	**3**	**3**
TOTAL										
0–19 Years	2	1.0	0	1	1	1	1	1	1	1
20–34	1	3.0	0	3	3	3	3	3	3	3
35–49	2	1.0	0	1	1	1	1	1	1	1
50–64	1	2.0	0	2	2	2	2	2	2	2
65+	0									
GRAND TOTAL	**6**	**1.7**	**<1**	**1**	**1**	**1**	**3**	**3**	**3**	**3**

80.0: ARTHROTOMY RMVL PROSTH. Formerly included in operation group(s) 738.

Type of Patients	Observed Patients	Avg. Stay	Variance	10th	25th	50th	75th	90th	95th	99th
1. SINGLE DX										
0–19 Years	1	1.0	0	1	1	1	1	1	1	1
20–34	8	2.4	3	1	1	2	3	6	6	6
35–49	9	4.1	10	1	2	4	6	7	11	11
50–64	20	4.0	6	2	2	3	5	7	10	10
65+	19	2.7	6	1	1	2	2	8	9	11
2. MULTIPLE DX										
0–19 Years	10	6.7	187	1	2	3	5	9	63	63
20–34	38	7.4	88	1	2	4	8	20	30	44
35–49	147	9.2	75	2	4	7	11	19	23	43
50–64	270	8.9	68	4	5	7	10	14	26	51
65+	812	11.2	122	3	5	7	13	25	28	68
TOTAL SINGLE DX	**57**	**3.0**	**6**	**1**	**1**	**2**	**4**	**6**	**9**	**11**
MULTIPLE DX	**1277**	**10.2**	**104**	**3**	**4**	**7**	**12**	**23**	**28**	**52**
TOTAL										
0–19 Years	11	5.6	155	1	1	3	4	9	9	63
20–34	46	6.5	77	1	2	3	6	16	30	44
35–49	156	9.1	73	2	4	7	11	19	23	43
50–64	290	8.6	66	3	5	7	10	13	23	51
65+	831	10.9	120	3	5	7	13	25	28	68
GRAND TOTAL	**1334**	**9.9**	**101**	**3**	**4**	**7**	**11**	**22**	**27**	**51**

80.05: RMVL PROSTH HIP INC. Formerly included in operation group(s) 738.

Type of Patients	Observed Patients	Avg. Stay	Variance	10th	25th	50th	75th	90th	95th	99th
1. SINGLE DX										
0–19 Years	0									
20–34	0									
35–49	1	2.0	0	2	2	2	2	2	2	2
50–64	6	4.9	11	2	2	5	7	10	10	10
65+	4	2.9	17	1	1	1	1	11	11	11
2. MULTIPLE DX										
0–19 Years	3	2.4	1	1	2	2	2	4	4	4
20–34	18	12.2	136	4	4	6	16	30	30	44
35–49	72	12.9	96	4	6	9	15	23	41	45
50–64	95	12.3	112	5	7	8	13	21	44	51
65+	390	12.4	157	4	5	8	14	25	40	70
TOTAL SINGLE DX	**11**	**3.9**	**12**	**1**	**1**	**2**	**5**	**10**	**11**	**11**
MULTIPLE DX	**578**	**12.4**	**137**	**4**	**6**	**8**	**14**	**25**	**41**	**67**
TOTAL										
0–19 Years	3	2.4	1	1	2	2	2	4	4	4
20–34	18	12.2	136	4	4	6	16	30	30	44
35–49	73	12.7	97	4	6	9	15	23	41	45
50–64	101	11.9	109	4	6	8	13	21	44	51
65+	394	12.3	156	4	5	8	14	25	40	70
GRAND TOTAL	**589**	**12.2**	**136**	**4**	**5**	**8**	**14**	**25**	**40**	**67**

Length of Stay by Diagnosis and Operation, United States, 1997

United States, October 1995–September 1996 Data, by Operation

80.06: RMVL PROSTH KNEE INC. Formerly included in operation group(s) 738.

Type of Patients	Observed Patients	Avg. Stay	Variance	10th	25th	50th	75th	90th	95th	99th
1. SINGLE DX										
0–19 Years	0									
20–34	2	4.2	3	5	5	5	6	6	6	6
35–49	2	5.4	<1	5	5	5	6	6	6	6
50–64	7	4.2	2	3	3	4	5	6	6	6
65+	11	5.9	5	3	4	6	8	9	9	9
2. MULTIPLE DX										
0–19 Years	1	63.0	0	63	63	63	63	63	63	63
20–34	4	2.5	3	1	2	2	2	6	6	6
35–49	34	9.1	57	2	6	7	9	15	34	34
50–64	138	7.8	41	4	5	6	8	12	18	36
65+	364	10.8	99	3	5	7	14	26	26	68
TOTAL SINGLE DX	22	5.0	4	3	3	5	6	8	9	9
MULTIPLE DX	541	9.8	84	3	5	7	11	23	26	60
TOTAL										
0–19 Years	1	63.0	0	63	63	63	63	63	63	63
20–34	6	3.0	4	2	2	2	3	6	6	9
35–49	36	9.0	56	2	6	7	9	15	34	34
50–64	145	7.7	40	4	5	6	8	12	16	36
65+	375	10.8	98	3	5	7	14	26	26	68
GRAND TOTAL	563	9.7	83	3	5	7	11	22	26	51

80.11: OTH ARTHROTOMY SHOULDER. Formerly included in operation group(s) 738.

Type of Patients	Observed Patients	Avg. Stay	Variance	10th	25th	50th	75th	90th	95th	99th
1. SINGLE DX										
0–19 Years	6	6.0	5	1	7	7	7	7	8	8
20–34	6	1.7		1	1	1	2	4	4	4
35–49	9	1.4	<1	1	1	1	2	2	3	5
50–64	7	3.0	7	1	1	2	5	5	11	11
65+	9	2.5	3	1	2	2	2	7	7	7
2. MULTIPLE DX										
0–19 Years	21	5.3	8	1	2	6	8	8	8	11
20–34	33	4.0	13	1	2	3	8	8	14	14
35–49	58	7.8	48	1	3	4	11	19	20	23
50–64	60	6.9	52	1	2	4	10	17	24	31
65+	96	10.6	75	3	4	7	14	26	28	30
TOTAL SINGLE DX	37	3.6	7	1	1	2	7	7	7	8
MULTIPLE DX	268	7.7	54	1	2	5	10	19	26	31
TOTAL										
0–19 Years	27	5.7	7	1	4	7	7	8	8	11
20–34	39	3.7	12	1	1	2	5	7	14	14
35–49	67	6.8	46	1	2	4	11	19	19	23
50–64	67	6.6	49	1	2	4	9	17	24	31
65+	105	10.0	74	2	4	7	13	26	28	30
GRAND TOTAL	305	7.0	49	1	2	4	8	19	25	30

80.1: OTHER ARTHROTOMY. Formerly included in operation group(s) 738.

Type of Patients	Observed Patients	Avg. Stay	Variance	10th	25th	50th	75th	90th	95th	99th
1. SINGLE DX										
0–19 Years	325	4.0	11	1	2	3	5	7	10	18
20–34	210	3.3	6	1	1	2	5	7	8	9
35–49	153	3.2	14	1	1	3	5	6	6	9
50–64	63	2.8	4	1	1	2	4	6	6	10
65+	35	2.7	4	2	2	2	2	5	8	13
2. MULTIPLE DX										
0–19 Years	648	5.7	22	1	3	5	8	11	14	21
20–34	572	4.5	28	1	2	3	5	9	12	25
35–49	688	6.2	37	1	3	4	8	12	18	30
50–64	621	6.3	48	2	2	4	8	14	18	33
65+	870	8.7	55	3	4	7	11	18	25	35
TOTAL SINGLE DX	786	3.5	10	1	1	3	5	7	8	16
MULTIPLE DX	3399	6.3	40	1	2	4	8	13	18	31
TOTAL										
0–19 Years	973	5.2	19	1	2	4	7	10	13	21
20–34	782	4.2	23	1	2	3	5	8	10	25
35–49	841	5.4	33	1	2	3	5	11	15	27
50–64	684	6.0	46	1	2	4	7	14	18	33
65+	905	8.4	54	2	4	6	11	17	24	35
GRAND TOTAL	4185	5.7	35	1	2	4	7	11	16	28

80.12: OTH ARTHROTOMY ELBOW. Formerly included in operation group(s) 738.

Type of Patients	Observed Patients	Avg. Stay	Variance	10th	25th	50th	75th	90th	95th	99th
1. SINGLE DX										
0–19 Years	20	3.1	6	1	1	2	4	7	8	9
20–34	14	4.2	9	1	2	2	8	8	8	8
35–49	10	2.0	<1	1	1	2	2	3	4	4
50–64	5	1.5	<1	1	1	2	2	5	4	4
65+	7	2.5	3	1	1	2	3	5	5	5
2. MULTIPLE DX										
0–19 Years	47	4.4	26	1	1	3	5	9	18	27
20–34	32	3.6	21	1	1	3	4	6	7	27
35–49	58	4.6	11	1	2	4	6	8	11	13
50–64	58	3.8	12	1	2	3	4	8	13	14
65+	78	5.8	76	1	1	3	7	12	20	41
TOTAL SINGLE DX	56	3.1	6	1	1	2	4	8	8	9
MULTIPLE DX	273	4.5	31	1	1	3	6	9	13	27
TOTAL										
0–19 Years	67	4.0	20	1	1	3	4	8	13	27
20–34	46	3.8	16	1	2	2	5	8	8	27
35–49	68	4.0	9	1	2	3	5	11	11	13
50–64	63	3.7	12	1	2	3	4	8	13	14
65+	85	5.7	73	1	1	3	6	12	20	41
GRAND TOTAL	329	4.2	26	1	1	3	5	8	13	27

Length of Stay by Diagnosis and Operation, United States, 1997

United States, October 1995–September 1996 Data, by Operation

80.14: OTH ARTHROTOMY HAND. Formerly included in operation group(s) 738.

Type of Patients	Observed Patients	Avg. Stay	Vari-ance	10th	25th	50th	75th	90th	95th	99th
1. SINGLE DX										
0–19 Years	8	3.6	5	1	2	2	6	7	7	7
20–34	42	3.1	6	1	2	2	4	7	7	12
35–49	33	2.5	4	1	1	1	4	5	6	7
50–64	6	1.4	<1	1	1	1	1	3	3	4
65+	1	2.0	0	2	2	2	2	2	2	2
2. MULTIPLE DX										
0–19 Years	36	4.9	21	2	3	3	4	15	15	21
20–34	96	4.5	12	2	3	4	5	7	8	20
35–49	104	4.4	19	1	2	3	5	9	14	27
50–64	56	4.7	10	2	3	4	6	8	12	15
65+	37	5.7	19	1	2	4	8	14	15	16
TOTAL SINGLE DX	90	2.6	4	1	1	2	4	6	7	9
MULTIPLE DX	329	4.6	16	2	2	3	5	8	14	21
TOTAL										
0–19 Years	44	4.7	19	2	3	3	4	7	15	21
20–34	138	4.0	10	1	2	3	5	7	8	20
35–49	137	3.7	14	1	1	3	4	7	11	27
50–64	62	3.9	10	1	2	3	5	8	11	15
65+	38	5.6	19	1	2	4	8	14	15	16
GRAND TOTAL	419	4.1	13	2	2	3	5	8	12	21

80.16: OTH ARTHROTOMY KNEE. Formerly included in operation group(s) 738.

Type of Patients	Observed Patients	Avg. Stay	Vari-ance	10th	25th	50th	75th	90th	95th	99th
1. SINGLE DX										
0–19 Years	129	3.0	5	1	1	2	4	6	7	10
20–34	97	3.5	5	1	1	2	4	7	7	7
35–49	68	3.1	4	1	1	3	5	5	5	6
50–64	32	3.4	4	1	2	4	4	5	6	10
65+	14	3.6	9	1	2	2	4	8	13	13
2. MULTIPLE DX										
0–19 Years	220	4.6	23	1	1	3	6	10	13	21
20–34	235	4.3	22	1	2	3	5	8	11	25
35–49	284	6.1	43	2	3	4	8	11	21	35
50–64	254	6.9	62	1	2	5	8	17	21	33
65+	380	9.1	56	3	4	6	11	18	25	35
TOTAL SINGLE DX	340	3.2	5	1	1	3	5	6	7	10
MULTIPLE DX	1373	6.2	45	1	2	4	8	13	19	33
TOTAL										
0–19 Years	349	4.0	17	1	1	3	5	9	10	21
20–34	332	4.1	19	1	2	3	5	7	10	25
35–49	352	5.3	35	1	2	4	6	10	15	34
50–64	286	6.6	59	1	2	5	7	16	19	33
65+	394	9.0	56	3	4	6	11	18	24	35
GRAND TOTAL	1713	5.6	38	1	2	4	7	11	18	31

80.15: OTH ARTHROTOMY HIP. Formerly included in operation group(s) 738.

Type of Patients	Observed Patients	Avg. Stay	Vari-ance	10th	25th	50th	75th	90th	95th	99th
1. SINGLE DX										
0–19 Years	121	5.6	19	2	3	4	6	11	18	21
20–34	18	4.2	5	1	2	4	6	8	8	8
35–49	11	6.9	120	2	4	6	6	6	7	61
50–64	4	5.5	5	3	4	4	8	8	8	8
65+	2	2.3	2	2	2	2	2	2	2	9
2. MULTIPLE DX										
0–19 Years	226	7.5	21	3	4	7	10	11	15	24
20–34	68	7.1	27	2	3	6	9	11	17	31
35–49	78	8.4	32	2	5	6	11	15	18	30
50–64	88	6.9	54	2	2	5	7	16	24	27
65+	175	8.1	36	3	4	7	9	15	20	35
TOTAL SINGLE DX	156	5.3	28	2	2	4	6	9	16	21
MULTIPLE DX	635	7.6	32	2	4	7	9	14	18	28
TOTAL										
0–19 Years	347	6.9	21	3	4	6	9	11	16	22
20–34	86	6.4	23	2	3	6	9	10	15	28
35–49	89	8.1	55	2	4	6	10	15	18	48
50–64	92	6.9	53	2	2	5	8	15	24	27
65+	177	7.6	36	2	4	6	9	13	20	35
GRAND TOTAL	791	7.1	32	2	4	6	9	13	18	27

80.17: OTH ARTHROTOMY ANKLE. Formerly included in operation group(s) 738.

Type of Patients	Observed Patients	Avg. Stay	Vari-ance	10th	25th	50th	75th	90th	95th	99th
1. SINGLE DX										
0–19 Years	22	3.6	5	1	1	3	5	6	8	8
20–34	16	1.7	3	1	1	1	1	4	4	9
35–49	10	3.8	4	1	2	3	6	6	6	6
50–64	4	3.2	1	2	3	3	3	3	6	6
65+	2	2.4	<1	2	2	2	3	3	3	3
2. MULTIPLE DX										
0–19 Years	54	6.4	15	2	4	6	10	11	11	20
20–34	45	3.1	5	1	1	2	4	7	7	10
35–49	45	6.3	24	2	2	5	8	14	15	27
50–64	38	4.9	21	1	1	3	8	11	12	28
65+	29	10.8	46	3	4	11	13	22	24	26
TOTAL SINGLE DX	54	3.0	5	1	1	3	5	6	8	9
MULTIPLE DX	211	5.6	22	1	2	4	8	11	14	24
TOTAL										
0–19 Years	76	5.8	14	1	3	5	8	11	11	20
20–34	61	2.8	5	1	1	2	4	6	7	10
35–49	55	5.8	21	1	2	5	8	12	14	27
50–64	42	4.8	20	1	2	3	8	11	12	14
65+	31	10.6	46	3	4	11	13	22	24	26
GRAND TOTAL	265	5.1	20	1	2	4	7	11	13	24

Length of Stay by Diagnosis and Operation, United States, 1997

United States, October 1995–September 1996 Data, by Operation

80.2: ARTHROSCOPY. Formerly included in operation group(s) 742.

Type of Patients	Observed Patients	Avg. Stay	Vari-ance	Percentiles						
				10th	25th	50th	75th	90th	95th	99th
1. SINGLE DX										
0–19 Years	94	1.8	3	1	1	1	2	3	5	13
20–34	172	1.5	1	1	1	1	2	3	3	6
35–49	105	1.7	1	1	1	1	2	4	4	5
50–64	40	2.5	5	1	1	2	4	4	8	8
65+	17	2.4	3	1	1	1	4	6	6	6
2. MULTIPLE DX										
0–19 Years	99	3.4	16	1	1	1	5	10	12	20
20–34	229	2.8	23	1	1	1	5	5	10	23
35–49	228	3.0	32	1	1	2	3	6	8	14
50–64	187	3.1	16	1	1	2	3	7	11	18
65+	216	5.6	44	1	2	4	7	12	16	35
TOTAL SINGLE DX	428	1.7	2	1	1	1	2	3	4	8
MULTIPLE DX	959	3.4	27	1	1	2	3	7	12	23
TOTAL										
0–19 Years	193	2.6	10	1	1	1	3	5	10	16
20–34	401	2.4	17	1	1	1	2	3	6	23
35–49	333	2.6	23	1	1	1	3	4	7	13
50–64	227	3.0	15	1	1	2	3	7	11	17
65+	233	5.5	42	1	2	4	7	12	15	35
GRAND TOTAL	1387	3.0	21	1	1	1	3	6	10	23

80.26: KNEE ARTHROSCOPY. Formerly included in operation group(s) 742.

Type of Patients	Observed Patients	Avg. Stay	Vari-ance	Percentiles						
				10th	25th	50th	75th	90th	95th	99th
1. SINGLE DX										
0–19 Years	72	1.8	4	1	1	1	2	3	5	13
20–34	108	1.7	2	1	1	1	2	3	3	9
35–49	67	1.9	1	1	1	2	2	4	4	5
50–64	13	3.8	6	1	1	4	4	8	8	8
65+	8	2.6	4	1	1	1	4	6	6	6
2. MULTIPLE DX										
0–19 Years	83	3.1	16	1	1	1	3	7	14	16
20–34	179	2.0	10	1	1	1	3	5	5	14
35–49	140	3.0	7	1	1	2	3	6	9	13
50–64	101	4.8	24	1	1	3	6	11	14	27
65+	128	7.2	51	2	3	5	9	13	17	35
TOTAL SINGLE DX	268	1.9	3	1	1	1	2	4	5	9
MULTIPLE DX	631	3.5	21	1	1	2	4	9	12	21
TOTAL										
0–19 Years	155	2.5	10	1	1	1	2	5	12	16
20–34	287	1.9	7	1	1	1	2	3	5	11
35–49	207	2.7	6	1	1	2	3	6	7	13
50–64	114	4.7	22	1	1	3	6	11	12	19
65+	136	7.1	50	2	3	5	9	13	17	35
GRAND TOTAL	899	3.1	17	1	1	2	3	7	11	17

80.21: SHOULDER ARTHROSCOPY. Formerly included in operation group(s) 742.

Type of Patients	Observed Patients	Avg. Stay	Vari-ance	Percentiles						
				10th	25th	50th	75th	90th	95th	99th
1. SINGLE DX										
0–19 Years	18	1.4	<1	1	1	1	2	2	2	3
20–34	60	1.2	<1	1	1	1	1	2	2	6
35–49	33	1.3	<1	1	1	1	1	2	2	4
50–64	27	1.6	1	1	1	1	2	2	3	8
65+	9	2.2	2	1	1	1	4	4	4	4
2. MULTIPLE DX										
0–19 Years	11	2.8	8	1	1	2	2	7	10	10
20–34	40	5.5	67	1	1	1	6	23	23	23
35–49	75	2.2	6	1	1	2	3	3	4	12
50–64	82	1.8	7	1	1	1	2	3	4	13
65+	78	2.3	10	1	1	1	2	5	6	26
TOTAL SINGLE DX	147	1.3	<1	1	1	1	1	2	2	4
MULTIPLE DX	286	2.8	21	1	1	1	2	5	10	23
TOTAL										
0–19 Years	29	1.9	3	1	1	1	2	2	7	10
20–34	100	3.5	41	1	1	1	2	6	23	23
35–49	108	2.0	5	1	1	1	2	3	4	11
50–64	109	1.8	6	1	1	1	2	2	3	13
65+	87	2.3	9	1	1	1	2	4	6	26
GRAND TOTAL	433	2.4	16	1	1	1	2	3	7	23

80.3: BIOPSY JOINT STRUCTURE. Formerly included in operation group(s) 743.

Type of Patients	Observed Patients	Avg. Stay	Vari-ance	Percentiles						
				10th	25th	50th	75th	90th	95th	99th
1. SINGLE DX										
0–19 Years	27	5.2	20	1	2	3	7	13	13	13
20–34	13	2.8	5	1	2	2	3	6	9	9
35–49	17	4.1	5	1	2	5	5	5	9	10
50–64	6	2.4	7	1	1	1	3	4	6	
65+	5	4.2	5	6	6	6	6	6	6	6
2. MULTIPLE DX										
0–19 Years	35	4.2	15	1	2	2	5	11	11	15
20–34	27	7.3	34	3	5	5	8	15	19	31
35–49	48	9.3	31	3	4	8	14	18	18	18
50–64	58	13.2	241	4	6	6	14	30	30	91
65+	111	8.4	37	3	5	6	13	15	25	29
TOTAL SINGLE DX	68	4.3	13	1	2	3	5	13	13	13
MULTIPLE DX	279	9.4	99	2	4	6	11	18	30	34
TOTAL										
0–19 Years	62	4.7	18	1	2	3	7	13	13	14
20–34	40	5.6	28	2	3	5	7	10	15	31
35–49	65	7.8	29	2	3	6	11	18	18	18
50–64	64	12.6	235	3	5	6	13	30	30	91
65+	116	8.3	36	3	5	6	12	14	25	29
GRAND TOTAL	347	8.3	85	2	3	6	10	18	30	30

Length of Stay by Diagnosis and Operation, United States, 1997

United States, October 1995–September 1996 Data, by Operation

80.4: JT CAPSULE/LIG/CART DIV. Formerly included in operation group(s) 738.

Type of Patients	Observed Patients	Avg. Stay	Variance	Percentiles 10th	25th	50th	75th	90th	95th	99th
1. SINGLE DX										
0–19 Years	377	1.5	<1	1	1	1	2	2	3	3
20–34	78	2.0	1	1	1	1	2	2	3	6
35–49	74	1.8	2	1	1	2	2	3	4	8
50–64	33	1.7	1	1	1	1	2	3	3	5
65+	23	2.1	1	1	1	2	3	4	5	5
2. MULTIPLE DX										
0–19 Years	384	2.7	9	1	1	2	3	5	6	18
20–34	163	2.3	3	1	1	2	3	4	5	8
35–49	247	2.4	4	1	1	2	3	5	6	11
50–64	175	2.8	6	1	1	2	3	5	7	13
65+	196	3.8	11	1	2	3	4	8	9	19
TOTAL SINGLE DX	585	1.6	1	1	1	1	2	3	3	6
MULTIPLE DX	1165	2.7	7	1	1	2	3	5	7	13
TOTAL										
0–19 Years	761	2.1	5	1	1	2	2	4	6	10
20–34	241	2.2	3	1	1	2	3	4	5	8
35–49	321	2.3	4	1	1	2	3	5	6	10
50–64	208	2.7	6	1	1	2	3	5	7	13
65+	219	3.6	10	1	2	3	4	8	9	19
GRAND TOTAL	1750	2.4	5	1	1	2	3	4	6	11

80.46: KNEE STRUCTURE DIVISION. Formerly included in operation group(s) 738.

Type of Patients	Observed Patients	Avg. Stay	Variance	Percentiles 10th	25th	50th	75th	90th	95th	99th
1. SINGLE DX										
0–19 Years	56	1.7	<1	1	1	1	2	3	3	5
20–34	52	2.1	2	1	1	2	3	4	4	7
35–49	39	2.0	2	1	1	2	2	4	4	9
50–64	18	2.4	2	1	1	2	2	4	5	5
65+	15	2.8	1	2	2	2	3	5	5	5
2. MULTIPLE DX										
0–19 Years	123	2.5	8	1	1	2	3	5	7	9
20–34	106	2.3	2	1	1	2	3	4	4	5
35–49	124	2.5	4	1	1	2	3	5	6	13
50–64	101	3.3	5	1	2	3	4	5	7	12
65+	133	3.8	12	1	3	3	4	6	9	19
TOTAL SINGLE DX	180	2.0	1	1	1	2	2	4	4	7
MULTIPLE DX	587	2.8	6	1	1	2	3	5	7	13
TOTAL										
0–19 Years	179	2.2	6	1	1	2	3	4	6	9
20–34	158	2.2	2	1	1	2	3	4	4	7
35–49	163	2.5	4	1	1	2	3	4	6	11
50–64	119	3.2	5	1	2	3	4	5	7	12
65+	148	3.8	11	1	2	3	4	6	9	19
GRAND TOTAL	767	2.6	5	1	1	2	3	5	6	12

80.48: FOOT JOINT STRUCT DIV. Formerly included in operation group(s) 738.

Type of Patients	Observed Patients	Avg. Stay	Variance	Percentiles 10th	25th	50th	75th	90th	95th	99th
1. SINGLE DX										
0–19 Years	253	1.5	<1	1	1	1	2	2	3	3
20–34	0									
35–49	0									
50–64	0									
65+	0									
2. MULTIPLE DX										
0–19 Years	96	1.8	1	1	1	1	2	4	4	4
20–34	2	2.0	0	2	2	2	2	2	2	2
35–49	1	1.0	0	1	1	1	1	1	1	1
50–64	1	1.0	0	1	1	1	1	1	1	1
65+	6	6.5	8	8	7	8	8	8	9	9
TOTAL SINGLE DX	253	1.5	<1	1	1	1	2	2	3	3
MULTIPLE DX	106	2.1	3	1	1	2	2	4	6	8
TOTAL										
0–19 Years	349	1.6	<1	1	1	2	2	3	3	4
20–34	2	2.0	0	2	2	2	2	2	2	2
35–49	1	1.0	0	1	1	1	1	1	1	1
50–64	1	1.0	0	1	1	1	1	1	1	1
65+	6	6.5	8	8	7	8	8	8	9	9
GRAND TOTAL	359	1.7	1	1	1	1	2	3	3	8

80.5: IV DISC EXC/DESTRUCTION. Formerly included in operation group(s) 739, 740.

Type of Patients	Observed Patients	Avg. Stay	Variance	Percentiles 10th	25th	50th	75th	90th	95th	99th
1. SINGLE DX										
0–19 Years	329	1.7	2	1	1	1	2	3	4	7
20–34	8017	1.8	1	1	1	1	2	3	4	6
35–49	16532	1.8	1	1	1	1	2	3	4	7
50–64	5989	1.9	2	1	1	2	2	3	4	7
65+	1386	2.3	2	1	1	2	3	4	5	7
2. MULTIPLE DX										
0–19 Years	229	4.5	27	1	1	2	6	9	14	22
20–34	4879	2.6	10	1	1	2	3	5	7	11
35–49	16026	2.7	11	1	1	2	3	5	7	13
50–64	12120	3.0	10	1	1	2	3	5	7	14
65+	9518	4.3	17	1	2	3	5	8	12	20
TOTAL SINGLE DX	32253	1.8	2	1	1	1	2	3	4	7
MULTIPLE DX	42772	3.1	12	1	1	2	4	6	8	15
TOTAL										
0–19 Years	558	2.8	14	1	1	2	3	6	9	17
20–34	12896	2.1	5	1	1	2	2	4	5	9
35–49	32558	2.2	6	1	1	2	3	4	6	9
50–64	18109	2.6	8	1	1	2	3	5	7	12
65+	10904	4.0	15	1	2	3	5	8	11	19
GRAND TOTAL	75025	2.5	8	1	1	2	3	4	6	12

Length of Stay by Diagnosis and Operation, United States, 1997

United States, October 1995–September 1996 Data, by Operation

80.51: IV DISC EXCISION. Formerly included in operation group(s) 740.

Type of Patients	Observed Patients	Avg. Stay	Vari-ance	10th	25th	50th	75th	90th	95th	99th
1. SINGLE DX										
0–19 Years	326	1.7	2	1	1	1	2	3	4	7
20–34	7959	1.8	1	1	1	1	2	3	4	6
35–49	16442	1.8	1	1	1	1	2	3	4	7
50–64	5935	1.9	2	1	1	2	2	3	4	7
65+	1368	2.3	2	1	1	2	3	4	5	7
2. MULTIPLE DX										
0–19 Years	223	4.5	26	1	1	2	6	9	14	22
20–34	4844	2.6	10	1	1	2	3	5	5	11
35–49	15914	2.7	11	1	1	2	3	5	7	13
50–64	12037	3.0	10	1	2	2	3	5	7	14
65+	9449	4.3	17	1	2	3	5	8	12	20
TOTAL SINGLE DX	32030	1.8	2	1	1	1	2	3	4	7
MULTIPLE DX	42467	3.1	12	1	1	2	4	6	8	15
TOTAL										
0–19 Years	549	2.8	13	1	1	2	3	6	9	17
20–34	12803	2.1	5	1	1	2	2	4	5	9
35–49	32356	2.2	6	1	1	2	2	5	5	9
50–64	17972	2.6	8	1	1	2	3	5	7	12
65+	10817	4.0	15	1	2	3	5	8	11	19
GRAND TOTAL	74497	2.5	8	1	1	2	3	5	6	12

80.6: EXC KNEE SEMILUNAR CART. Formerly included in operation group(s) 741.

Type of Patients	Observed Patients	Avg. Stay	Vari-ance	10th	25th	50th	75th	90th	95th	99th
1. SINGLE DX										
0–19 Years	79	1.5	<1	1	1	1	2	2	3	4
20–34	137	1.4	<1	1	1	1	2	2	3	4
35–49	76	2.2	<1	1	1	2	3	3	3	4
50–64	21	1.5	<1	1	1	1	2	2	2	5
65+	10	2.1	2	1	1	1	3	5	5	5
2. MULTIPLE DX										
0–19 Years	200	1.4	<1	1	1	1	2	2	3	4
20–34	528	1.8	3	1	1	1	2	3	5	11
35–49	545	2.1	4	1	1	1	3	4	5	12
50–64	428	3.0	17	1	1	2	3	5	7	32
65+	356	4.1	29	1	1	3	5	8	12	37
TOTAL SINGLE DX	323	1.7	<1	1	1	1	2	3	3	4
MULTIPLE DX	2057	2.4	10	1	1	1	3	4	6	14
TOTAL										
0–19 Years	279	1.4	<1	1	1	1	2	2	3	4
20–34	665	1.8	2	1	1	1	2	3	4	11
35–49	621	2.1	3	1	1	2	3	4	5	12
50–64	449	2.9	16	1	1	2	3	5	7	32
65+	366	4.1	29	1	1	3	5	8	11	37
GRAND TOTAL	2380	2.3	8	1	1	1	2	4	6	12

80.59: IV DISC DESTRUCTION NEC. Formerly included in operation group(s) 740.

Type of Patients	Observed Patients	Avg. Stay	Vari-ance	10th	25th	50th	75th	90th	95th	99th
1. SINGLE DX										
0–19 Years	2	1.1	<1	1	1	1	1	1	2	2
20–34	44	1.3	<1	1	1	1	1	2	2	4
35–49	64	1.5	1	1	1	1	2	2	4	5
50–64	36	1.6	2	1	1	1	2	3	4	9
65+	10	2.0	3	1	2	2	3	4	6	6
2. MULTIPLE DX										
0–19 Years	1	7.0	0	7	7	7	7	7	7	7
20–34	25	1.7	2	1	1	1	2	4	4	8
35–49	70	2.0	4	1	1	2	2	4	4	9
50–64	50	2.7	6	1	2	2	3	5	7	14
65+	43	4.0	9	1	2	3	5	7	10	15
TOTAL SINGLE DX	156	1.4	1	1	1	1	2	2	3	6
MULTIPLE DX	189	2.4	5	1	1	2	3	5	7	14
TOTAL										
0–19 Years	3	1.6	3	1	1	1	1	2	7	7
20–34	69	1.4	1	1	1	1	1	2	4	8
35–49	134	1.8	3	1	1	1	2	3	4	9
50–64	86	2.4	9	1	2	2	3	5	7	14
65+	53	3.7	9	1	2	3	5	7	10	15
GRAND TOTAL	345	2.1	4	1	1	1	2	4	6	10

80.7: SYNOVECTOMY. Formerly included in operation group(s) 743.

Type of Patients	Observed Patients	Avg. Stay	Vari-ance	10th	25th	50th	75th	90th	95th	99th
1. SINGLE DX										
0–19 Years	32	2.8	1	2	2	3	3	4	4	6
20–34	41	2.3	4	2	1	2	3	5	7	9
35–49	44	2.5	3	1	1	2	4	4	5	9
50–64	22	2.8	2	1	2	3	4	4	5	6
65+	8	3.1	3	1	2	3	3	6	6	8
2. MULTIPLE DX										
0–19 Years	96	4.0	16	1	1	3	5	7	9	25
20–34	116	4.4	30	1	1	2	6	9	11	28
35–49	249	5.7	40	1	2	4	6	13	14	41
50–64	236	5.4	35	1	2	4	6	11	17	27
65+	371	8.2	55	2	3	5	11	19	26	30
TOTAL SINGLE DX	147	2.6	2	1	1	2	3	4	6	8
MULTIPLE DX	1068	6.0	41	1	2	4	7	12	20	30
TOTAL										
0–19 Years	128	3.5	10	1	2	3	4	6	7	23
20–34	157	3.8	23	1	1	2	5	8	10	28
35–49	293	5.3	36	2	2	4	6	12	14	41
50–64	258	5.3	34	1	2	4	6	10	17	27
65+	379	8.0	54	2	3	5	11	19	26	30
GRAND TOTAL	1215	5.5	37	1	2	4	6	12	18	30

Length of Stay by Diagnosis and Operation, United States, 1997

United States, October 1995–September 1996 Data, by Operation

80.76: KNEE SYNOVECTOMY. Formerly included in operation group(s) 743.

Type of Patients	Observed Patients	Avg. Stay	Vari-ance	10th	25th	50th	75th	90th	95th	99th
1. SINGLE DX										
0–19 Years	23	2.8	1	2	2	3	3	4	4	7
20–34	31	2.4	4	1	1	3	3	4	8	9
35–49	30	2.8	4	1	1	3	4	5	7	9
50–64	15	3.2	1	2	2	3	4	4	5	6
65+	6	3.1	3	2	2	2	6	6	6	6
2. MULTIPLE DX										
0–19 Years	66	4.3	22	1	1	3	5	8	12	25
20–34	84	5.0	39	1	2	3	6	10	14	28
35–49	177	6.0	41	1	2	4	7	11	17	42
50–64	174	6.0	39	2	3	4	6	12	20	28
65+	299	8.7	59	2	4	6	11	22	26	30
TOTAL SINGLE DX	105	2.7	3	1	2	3	3	4	6	9
MULTIPLE DX	800	6.6	46	1	3	4	8	14	22	31
TOTAL										
0–19 Years	89	3.5	11	1	2	3	4	7	8	25
20–34	115	4.2	30	1	1	2	5	9	11	28
35–49	207	5.6	37	1	2	4	7	11	14	41
50–64	189	5.8	37	2	3	4	6	12	20	28
65+	305	8.5	58	2	4	5	11	22	26	30
GRAND TOTAL	905	5.9	41	1	2	4	7	12	20	30

80.81: DESTR SHOULDER LES NEC. Formerly included in operation group(s) 743.

Type of Patients	Observed Patients	Avg. Stay	Vari-ance	10th	25th	50th	75th	90th	95th	99th
1. SINGLE DX										
0–19 Years	11	1.2	<1	1	1	1	1	1	2	7
20–34	21	1.4	1	1	1	1	2	1	6	9
35–49	54	2.6	3	1	1	2	4	5	5	8
50–64	41	2.0	<1	1	1	2	3	3	3	4
65+	21	2.3	2	1	1	3	3	3	3	8
2. MULTIPLE DX										
0–19 Years	22	4.3	32	1	1	1	5	13	22	22
20–34	92	2.1	5	1	1	1	2	4	6	10
35–49	237	2.7	33	1	1	1	2	5	9	23
50–64	319	2.9	18	1	1	1	2	6	11	18
65+	353	4.0	37	1	1	2	4	8	13	40
TOTAL SINGLE DX	148	1.9	2	1	1	1	3	4	5	7
MULTIPLE DX	1023	3.1	26	1	1	2	3	7	11	24
TOTAL										
0–19 Years	33	2.2	13	1	1	1	1	5	7	22
20–34	113	2.0	4	1	1	1	2	4	4	10
35–49	291	2.7	27	1	1	2	3	5	5	17
50–64	360	2.8	16	1	1	2	2	6	11	18
65+	374	3.8	34	1	1	2	4	8	12	40
GRAND TOTAL	1171	2.9	22	1	1	1	3	6	10	22

80.8: OTH EXC/DESTR JOINT LES. Formerly included in operation group(s) 743.

Type of Patients	Observed Patients	Avg. Stay	Vari-ance	10th	25th	50th	75th	90th	95th	99th
1. SINGLE DX										
0–19 Years	142	3.1	11	1	1	1	4	7	9	17
20–34	139	3.7	11	1	1	2	5	9	12	12
35–49	160	2.5	5	1	1	2	3	5	5	8
50–64	94	3.1	9	1	1	2	3	8	11	13
65+	48	4.2	9	1	2	4	4	8	8	17
2. MULTIPLE DX										
0–19 Years	254	5.2	28	1	2	4	7	10	17	25
20–34	479	4.0	19	1	1	2	5	9	12	20
35–49	794	4.7	41	1	1	3	5	10	16	29
50–64	791	4.9	45	1	1	2	6	11	17	38
65+	1024	6.9	57	1	2	5	9	15	22	42
TOTAL SINGLE DX	583	3.2	9	1	1	2	4	7	9	15
MULTIPLE DX	3342	5.2	42	1	1	3	6	12	17	37
TOTAL										
0–19 Years	396	4.3	22	1	1	3	6	9	15	22
20–34	618	3.9	17	1	1	2	5	9	12	17
35–49	954	4.3	35	1	1	2	5	9	15	29
50–64	885	4.7	41	1	1	2	5	11	16	38
65+	1072	6.7	54	1	2	4	9	15	22	42
GRAND TOTAL	3925	4.9	37	1	1	3	6	11	16	33

80.85: DESTR HIP LESION NEC. Formerly included in operation group(s) 743.

Type of Patients	Observed Patients	Avg. Stay	Vari-ance	10th	25th	50th	75th	90th	95th	99th
1. SINGLE DX										
0–19 Years	13	4.6	5	2	3	4	5	8	10	10
20–34	11	8.7	18	2	5	12	12	12	12	12
35–49	10	2.1	<1	2	2	2	2	3	3	5
50–64	5	2.0	<1	1	2	2	2	3	3	3
65+	3	4.7	7	2	2	7	7	7	7	7
2. MULTIPLE DX										
0–19 Years	34	5.8	17	2	2	5	9	13	15	17
20–34	34	8.5	41	2	3	9	12	14	17	43
35–49	67	6.0	30	1	3	5	7	15	16	44
50–64	48	8.0	70	2	3	6	9	15	26	56
65+	91	11.9	96	3	5	8	18	28	28	49
TOTAL SINGLE DX	42	4.5	14	2	2	2	5	12	12	12
MULTIPLE DX	274	7.9	55	2	3	5	9	17	20	47
TOTAL										
0–19 Years	47	5.4	13	2	2	5	7	10	13	17
20–34	45	8.6	32	2	4	9	12	14	14	26
35–49	77	4.9	25	2	2	3	5	13	16	37
50–64	53	7.3	66	2	2	5	7	14	21	56
65+	94	11.7	94	3	5	8	18	27	28	49
GRAND TOTAL	316	7.1	48	2	2	5	9	16	18	44

Length of Stay by Diagnosis and Operation, United States, 1997

United States, October 1995–September 1996 Data, by Operation

80.86: DESTR KNEE LESION NEC. Formerly included in operation group(s) 743.

Type of Patients	Observed Patients	Avg. Stay	Vari-ance	Percentiles						
				10th	25th	50th	75th	90th	95th	99th
1. SINGLE DX										
0–19 Years	69	4.0	16	1	1	3	5	7	17	17
20–34	61	3.1	5	1	1	3	5	5	7	12
35–49	58	2.7	4	1	1	2	4	5	7	9
50–64	24	5.8	24	2	2	3	12	13	13	13
65+	16	5.5	9	3	4	4	8	8	12	17
2. MULTIPLE DX										
0–19 Years	108	5.1	16	1	2	5	7	8	11	19
20–34	188	4.2	23	1	2	5	5	10	12	33
35–49	278	5.7	47	1	2	4	6	11	22	29
50–64	247	7.5	83	1	2	4	9	17	29	38
65+	407	8.7	61	2	4	7	11	17	25	42
TOTAL SINGLE DX	228	3.9	11	1	1	3	5	8	12	17
MULTIPLE DX	1228	6.4	52	1	2	4	8	13	21	38
TOTAL										
0–19 Years	177	4.6	16	1	2	4	6	8	12	19
20–34	249	3.9	19	1	1	2	5	8	12	24
35–49	336	5.3	42	1	2	3	5	11	21	29
50–64	271	7.4	79	1	2	4	10	16	29	38
65+	423	8.3	56	2	4	6	11	16	22	42
GRAND TOTAL	1456	6.0	46	1	2	4	7	13	18	38

81.0: SPINAL FUSION. Formerly included in operation group(s) 744.

Type of Patients	Observed Patients	Avg. Stay	Vari-ance	Percentiles						
				10th	25th	50th	75th	90th	95th	99th
1. SINGLE DX										
0–19 Years	1074	5.1	3	3	4	5	6	7	8	12
20–34	1176	3.1	4	1	1	2	4	5	7	9
35–49	3693	2.6	3	1	1	2	3	5	6	9
50–64	1476	2.6	3	1	2	2	4	5	5	7
65+	274	3.3	5	1	2	3	4	7	7	10
2. MULTIPLE DX										
0–19 Years	2591	8.0	38	4	5	6	9	14	18	37
20–34	2367	5.5	30	2	3	4	7	9	13	29
35–49	7848	4.2	14	1	2	3	5	8	10	18
50–64	5863	5.0	24	2	2	4	6	9	12	24
65+	4338	6.9	53	2	4	5	8	12	17	35
TOTAL SINGLE DX	7693	3.0	4	1	2	2	4	6	7	9
MULTIPLE DX	23007	5.5	29	2	3	4	6	10	13	27
TOTAL										
0–19 Years	3665	7.2	31	4	5	6	8	12	16	29
20–34	3543	4.8	23	1	2	4	6	8	11	25
35–49	11541	3.6	11	1	2	3	4	7	9	16
50–64	7339	4.5	21	1	3	4	6	8	11	22
65+	4612	6.6	51	2	3	5	7	12	17	35
GRAND TOTAL	30700	4.8	24	1	2	4	6	8	12	24

80.9: OTHER JOINT EXCISION. Formerly included in operation group(s) 743.

Type of Patients	Observed Patients	Avg. Stay	Vari-ance	Percentiles						
				10th	25th	50th	75th	90th	95th	99th
1. SINGLE DX										
0–19 Years	15	3.1	3	1	1	3	5	5	5	5
20–34	18	1.7	3	1	1	1	2	2	3	10
35–49	22	1.4	<1	1	1	1	2	2	3	3
50–64	10	2.6	<1	1	3	3	3	3	3	4
65+	5	7.1	55	1	2	3	17	17	17	17
2. MULTIPLE DX										
0–19 Years	26	3.4	36	1	1	2	2	9	20	28
20–34	35	4.4	32	1	2	2	5	8	19	28
35–49	63	5.9	57	1	2	6	6	8	8	21
50–64	76	3.6	41	1	2	5	5	6	12	35
65+	82	7.2	59	1	2	5	9	15	22	41
TOTAL SINGLE DX	70	2.4	5	1	1	2	3	5	5	17
MULTIPLE DX	282	5.1	51	1	1	3	8	9	15	32
TOTAL										
0–19 Years	41	3.3	27	1	1	2	3	5	10	28
20–34	53	3.2	21	1	1	2	4	7	10	28
35–49	85	5.1	51	1	2	4	8	8	8	21
50–64	86	3.4	34	1	2	2	3	6	9	17
65+	87	7.2	59	1	2	5	9	15	22	41
GRAND TOTAL	352	4.6	43	1	1	2	6	8	14	28

81.01: ATLAS-AXIS SP FUSION. Formerly included in operation group(s) 744.

Type of Patients	Observed Patients	Avg. Stay	Vari-ance	Percentiles						
				10th	25th	50th	75th	90th	95th	99th
1. SINGLE DX										
0–19 Years	21	4.5	11	2	3	3	5	7	12	20
20–34	19	3.0	2	2	2	3	3	5	5	8
35–49	18	3.1	7	1	1	2	4	7	7	14
50–64	10	2.2	3	1	1	1	3	4	7	7
65+	6	4.6	5	2	2	6	6	6	9	9
2. MULTIPLE DX										
0–19 Years	88	7.6	90	3	4	5	8	14	19	63
20–34	53	7.1	50	2	3	5	9	14	22	31
35–49	72	6.1	14	2	3	5	8	10	15	16
50–64	91	6.0	23	3	3	6	8	10	15	22
65+	175	9.2	50	3	6	8	10	15	23	45
TOTAL SINGLE DX	74	3.5	7	1	2	3	4	6	7	14
MULTIPLE DX	479	7.6	49	3	4	6	9	14	18	38
TOTAL										
0–19 Years	109	7.0	76	3	3	4	7	11	18	63
20–34	72	6.0	41	2	3	4	5	11	17	31
35–49	90	5.6	14	2	3	4	8	10	15	16
50–64	101	5.6	22	1	3	5	6	10	14	17
65+	181	9.1	49	3	5	8	10	15	23	45
GRAND TOTAL	553	7.1	45	2	3	6	8	13	17	36

Length of Stay by Diagnosis and Operation, United States, 1997

United States, October 1995–September 1996 Data, by Operation

81.02: ANTERIOR CERV FUSION NEC. Formerly included in operation group(s) 744.

Type of Patients	Observed Patients	Avg. Stay	Variance	10th	25th	50th	75th	90th	95th	99th
1. SINGLE DX										
0–19 Years	20	4.6	9	1	2	3	6	11	11	11
20–34	635	2.0	1	1	1	2	3	3	3	12
35–49	2780	1.9	<1	1	1	2	2	3	3	5
50–64	1122	2.0	1	1	1	2	2	3	4	6
65+	191	2.6	4	1	2	2	3	3	4	8
2. MULTIPLE DX										
0–19 Years	67	9.1	56	3	4	6	14	21	23	36
20–34	646	4.1	46	1	2	2	4	7	17	45
35–49	3742	2.6	8	1	1	2	3	4	6	13
50–64	2614	3.0	14	1	1	2	3	5	9	20
65+	1138	4.8	31	1	2	3	5	10	16	28
TOTAL SINGLE DX	4748	2.0	1	1	1	2	2	3	4	6
MULTIPLE DX	8207	3.1	17	1	1	2	3	5	9	23
TOTAL										
0–19 Years	87	8.4	51	2	3	6	11	21	23	36
20–34	1281	3.1	26	1	1	2	3	5	8	23
35–49	6522	2.3	5	1	1	2	3	4	5	10
50–64	3736	2.7	11	1	1	2	3	4	7	15
65+	1329	4.4	27	1	2	3	5	9	14	27
GRAND TOTAL	12955	2.7	11	1	1	2	3	4	6	17

81.03: POST CERVICAL FUSION NEC. Formerly included in operation group(s) 744.

Type of Patients	Observed Patients	Avg. Stay	Variance	10th	25th	50th	75th	90th	95th	99th
1. SINGLE DX										
0–19 Years	42	3.9	3	3	3	3	4	6	9	9
20–34	53	4.4	6	2	2	4	6	8	10	12
35–49	71	3.8	4	2	3	3	4	6	7	12
50–64	30	4.1	3	2	3	5	5	5	7	8
65+	10	4.6	8	2	3	4	5	10	11	11
2. MULTIPLE DX										
0–19 Years	76	7.2	61	2	3	4	8	14	21	39
20–34	148	6.8	39	2	4	7	7	9	19	36
35–49	264	5.0	33	2	3	3	5	8	13	37
50–64	221	5.8	34	2	3	4	7	10	14	26
65+	275	7.2	38	3	4	5	8	14	18	31
TOTAL SINGLE DX	206	4.0	4	2	3	4	5	6	8	11
MULTIPLE DX	984	6.2	38	2	3	4	7	11	16	36
TOTAL										
0–19 Years	118	6.1	44	2	3	4	7	9	16	39
20–34	201	6.4	35	2	3	6	7	9	14	36
35–49	335	4.8	29	2	3	4	5	8	12	36
50–64	251	5.5	28	2	3	4	7	10	14	26
65+	285	7.2	37	3	4	5	8	14	18	31
GRAND TOTAL	1190	5.8	34	2	3	4	7	10	14	36

81.04: ANTERIOR DORSAL FUSION. Formerly included in operation group(s) 744.

Type of Patients	Observed Patients	Avg. Stay	Variance	10th	25th	50th	75th	90th	95th	99th
1. SINGLE DX										
0–19 Years	147	6.2	5	4	5	5	7	8	12	14
20–34	15	4.8	2	4	4	5	5	5	6	12
35–49	10	7.2	15	4	4	6	10	12	15	15
50–64	6	8.3	65	4	4	7	7	10	34	34
65+	1	1.0	0	1	1	1	1	1	1	1
2. MULTIPLE DX										
0–19 Years	513	9.9	43	5	6	8	13	20	22	29
20–34	77	9.5	38	5	7	8	10	13	17	37
35–49	91	11.4	64	4	5	9	20	21	27	35
50–64	84	11.1	44	5	8	9	14	19	21	45
65+	67	11.0	39	6	6	9	14	18	20	41
TOTAL SINGLE DX	179	5.9	6	4	5	5	6	8	10	15
MULTIPLE DX	832	10.2	45	5	6	8	13	21	22	34
TOTAL										
0–19 Years	660	9.2	38	5	6	7	11	16	22	29
20–34	92	7.6	29	4	5	7	9	11	14	36
35–49	101	11.2	62	5	5	9	18	21	24	35
50–64	90	10.9	46	5	8	9	14	19	21	34
65+	68	11.0	40	6	6	9	14	18	20	41
GRAND TOTAL	1011	9.4	41	4	5	7	11	18	22	32

81.05: POSTERIOR DORSAL FUSION. Formerly included in operation group(s) 744.

Type of Patients	Observed Patients	Avg. Stay	Variance	10th	25th	50th	75th	90th	95th	99th
1. SINGLE DX										
0–19 Years	645	5.2	2	4	4	5	6	7	7	9
20–34	46	5.5	9	2	4	5	7	8	9	9
35–49	28	7.1	34	4	4	6	9	11	11	37
50–64	7	5.2	14	2	3	4	8	13	13	13
65+	1	10.0	0	10	10	10	10	10	10	10
2. MULTIPLE DX										
0–19 Years	1337	7.6	30	4	5	6	8	12	16	32
20–34	233	9.7	59	4	5	8	10	16	25	38
35–49	196	8.2	48	3	5	6	10	15	22	34
50–64	172	10.2	58	3	5	8	16	16	22	38
65+	181	19.1	496	4	7	10	19	75	75	75
TOTAL SINGLE DX	727	5.3	3	4	4	5	6	7	8	10
MULTIPLE DX	2119	8.8	75	4	5	6	9	15	19	61
TOTAL										
0–19 Years	1982	6.9	23	4	5	6	7	10	13	29
20–34	279	9.1	54	4	5	7	10	15	25	34
35–49	224	8.0	46	3	4	6	9	14	19	34
50–64	179	10.1	58	3	5	8	16	16	22	38
65+	182	19.1	495	4	7	10	19	75	75	75
GRAND TOTAL	2846	7.9	60	4	5	6	8	13	17	40

Length of Stay by Diagnosis and Operation, United States, 1997

United States, October 1995–September 1996 Data, by Operation

81.06: ANTERIOR LUMBAR FUSION. Formerly included in operation group(s) 744.

Type of Patients	Observed Patients	Avg. Stay	Vari-ance	Percentiles						
				10th	25th	50th	75th	90th	95th	99th
1. SINGLE DX										
0–19 Years	24	5.1	2	4	4	5	6	7	7	8
20–34	56	3.5	3	2	3	3	5	6	6	7
35–49	100	4.7	3	2	4	5	6	7	7	7
50–64	21	3.7	1	3	3	3	5	5	6	8
65+	3	4.4	3	3	3	4	4	7	7	7
2. MULTIPLE DX										
0–19 Years	71	8.8	50	4	5	6	10	16	22	51
20–34	188	5.2	10	3	3	4	6	7	9	15
35–49	497	6.5	10	4	5	6	7	12	12	17
50–64	265	11.0	112	4	5	7	10	21	43	43
65+	135	9.1	30	5	6	8	9	14	17	31
TOTAL SINGLE DX	204	4.3	3	2	3	4	5	6	7	8
MULTIPLE DX	1156	7.4	39	3	4	6	8	12	16	43
TOTAL										
0–19 Years	95	8.0	41	4	5	6	9	14	18	51
20–34	244	4.8	9	2	3	4	6	7	8	15
35–49	597	6.0	9	4	4	6	7	10	12	16
50–64	286	9.9	103	3	5	7	10	21	43	43
65+	138	9.0	30	5	6	8	9	14	17	31
GRAND TOTAL	1360	6.7	32	3	4	6	7	11	14	43

81.08: POSTERIOR LUMBAR FUSION. Formerly included in operation group(s) 744.

Type of Patients	Observed Patients	Avg. Stay	Vari-ance	Percentiles						
				10th	25th	50th	75th	90th	95th	99th
1. SINGLE DX										
0–19 Years	122	4.2	3	2	3	4	5	7	8	9
20–34	212	4.2	3	2	3	4	5	7	7	7
35–49	385	4.3	5	2	3	4	5	6	9	9
50–64	173	4.2	2	3	3	4	5	6	7	9
65+	32	5.6	3	4	4	5	7	8	8	8
2. MULTIPLE DX										
0–19 Years	258	6.9	41	3	4	6	7	11	14	44
20–34	608	5.4	10	3	4	5	7	8	9	14
35–49	1624	5.1	6	3	4	5	6	8	10	14
50–64	1424	5.6	8	3	4	5	7	8	11	15
65+	1538	6.1	12	3	4	5	7	9	13	22
TOTAL SINGLE DX	924	4.3	3	2	3	4	5	7	7	9
MULTIPLE DX	5452	5.6	11	3	4	5	6	8	11	17
TOTAL										
0–19 Years	380	6.0	30	3	3	5	7	9	11	44
20–34	820	5.0	8	3	4	5	6	8	8	14
35–49	2009	4.9	6	3	4	4	6	8	9	14
50–64	1597	5.4	8	3	4	5	7	8	10	14
65+	1570	6.1	12	3	4	5	7	9	13	22
GRAND TOTAL	6376	5.4	10	3	4	5	6	8	10	17

81.07: LAT TRANS LUMBAR FUSION. Formerly included in operation group(s) 744.

Type of Patients	Observed Patients	Avg. Stay	Vari-ance	Percentiles						
				10th	25th	50th	75th	90th	95th	99th
1. SINGLE DX										
0–19 Years	14	3.3	1	3	3	3	3	4	7	7
20–34	59	4.2	5	2	3	3	5	5	6	12
35–49	126	4.6	2	3	4	5	6	6	7	8
50–64	45	4.2	6	2	2	4	5	6	13	13
65+	18	4.3	2	3	3	4	5	7	7	9
2. MULTIPLE DX										
0–19 Years	31	6.8	38	3	3	5	10	10	13	42
20–34	155	4.6	6	3	3	4	6	7	7	14
35–49	464	5.3	8	3	4	5	6	8	11	13
50–64	418	6.1	13	4	5	6	7	9	11	17
65+	510	7.0	27	3	5	6	7	11	13	28
TOTAL SINGLE DX	262	4.4	3	2	3	4	5	6	6	12
MULTIPLE DX	1578	5.8	15	3	4	5	7	8	11	28
TOTAL										
0–19 Years	45	5.7	29	3	3	3	7	10	10	33
20–34	214	4.5	6	2	3	4	5	7	7	14
35–49	590	5.1	7	3	4	5	6	7	9	13
50–64	463	6.0	13	3	4	6	7	8	11	16
65+	528	6.9	26	3	5	6	7	10	13	28
GRAND TOTAL	1840	5.6	13	3	4	5	6	8	11	21

81.09: REFUSION OF SPINE. Formerly included in operation group(s) 744.

Type of Patients	Observed Patients	Avg. Stay	Vari-ance	Percentiles						
				10th	25th	50th	75th	90th	95th	99th
1. SINGLE DX										
0–19 Years	26	4.6	4	2	3	5	5	7	10	11
20–34	74	3.5	2	2	3	3	4	5	7	10
35–49	165	3.4	3	2	2	3	4	5	7	9
50–64	58	2.6	3	1	2	2	3	5	6	9
65+	8	2.5	2	2	2	2	2	4	7	7
2. MULTIPLE DX										
0–19 Years	115	5.6	11	2	4	5	7	10	13	16
20–34	252	4.8	7	3	3	4	6	7	10	16
35–49	880	4.6	9	2	3	4	5	7	10	17
50–64	561	5.3	12	2	4	5	6	8	12	17
65+	303	7.2	38	3	4	6	8	10	24	37
TOTAL SINGLE DX	331	3.3	3	2	2	3	4	5	6	9
MULTIPLE DX	2111	5.2	14	2	3	4	6	8	11	23
TOTAL										
0–19 Years	141	5.4	10	2	4	5	7	10	12	16
20–34	326	4.6	7	2	3	4	5	7	10	15
35–49	1045	4.4	9	2	3	4	6	8	10	16
50–64	619	5.0	12	2	3	4	6	8	11	17
65+	311	7.0	38	3	4	6	7	10	22	37
GRAND TOTAL	2442	4.9	13	2	3	4	6	8	11	22

Length of Stay by Diagnosis and Operation, United States, 1997

United States, October 1995–September 1996 Data, by Operation

81.1: FOOT & ANKLE ARTHRODESIS. Formerly included in operation group(s) 745.

Type of Patients	Observed Patients	Avg. Stay	Vari-ance	Percentiles						
				10th	25th	50th	75th	90th	95th	99th
1. SINGLE DX										
0–19 Years	66	1.7	<1	1	1	2	2	3	3	4
20–34	142	2.0	<1	1	1	2	2	3	3	4
35–49	286	2.1	1	1	1	2	2	3	4	5
50–64	233	2.4	1	1	2	2	3	4	4	5
65+	100	2.6	2	1	2	2	3	5	5	5
2. MULTIPLE DX										
0–19 Years	222	2.6	3	1	2	2	3	4	7	10
20–34	403	2.7	3	1	2	2	3	4	5	9
35–49	806	2.7	4	1	1	2	3	4	6	12
50–64	899	3.1	5	1	2	3	4	5	7	10
65+	740	3.6	6	1	2	3	4	6	8	12
TOTAL SINGLE DX	827	2.2	1	1	1	2	3	4	4	5
MULTIPLE DX	3070	3.0	5	1	2	2	4	5	7	12
TOTAL										
0–19 Years	288	2.4	2	1	1	2	3	4	5	8
20–34	545	2.5	3	1	2	2	3	4	5	8
35–49	1092	2.5	4	1	1	2	3	4	5	12
50–64	1132	2.9	4	1	2	3	4	5	6	9
65+	840	3.4	6	1	2	3	4	6	8	11
GRAND TOTAL	3897	2.8	4	1	2	2	3	5	6	10

81.11: ANKLE FUSION. Formerly included in operation group(s) 745.

Type of Patients	Observed Patients	Avg. Stay	Vari-ance	Percentiles						
				10th	25th	50th	75th	90th	95th	99th
1. SINGLE DX										
0–19 Years	6	1.5	<1	1	1	1	2	2	2	3
20–34	60	2.2	1	1	1	2	3	3	4	5
35–49	138	2.3	1	1	1	2	3	4	4	5
50–64	118	2.6	<1	1	2	3	3	4	4	5
65+	52	2.8	2	1	2	2	4	5	5	5
2. MULTIPLE DX										
0–19 Years	17	3.0	8	1	1	2	3	8	8	15
20–34	174	2.8	3	1	2	2	3	5	6	11
35–49	377	2.5	3	1	1	2	3	4	6	8
50–64	410	3.3	6	2	2	3	4	5	6	13
65+	345	4.1	7	2	2	3	5	8	8	13
TOTAL SINGLE DX	374	2.4	1	1	2	2	3	4	4	5
MULTIPLE DX	1323	3.2	5	1	2	3	4	6	7	11
TOTAL										
0–19 Years	23	2.2	4	1	1	2	2	3	8	15
20–34	234	2.6	3	1	2	2	3	4	5	9
35–49	515	2.4	2	1	1	2	3	4	5	7
50–64	528	3.2	5	1	2	3	4	5	6	11
65+	397	3.9	7	2	2	3	5	7	8	12
GRAND TOTAL	1697	3.0	4	1	2	2	4	5	7	9

81.12: TRIPLE ARTHRODESIS. Formerly included in operation group(s) 745.

Type of Patients	Observed Patients	Avg. Stay	Vari-ance	Percentiles						
				10th	25th	50th	75th	90th	95th	99th
1. SINGLE DX										
0–19 Years	45	1.9	<1	1	1	2	2	3	4	4
20–34	27	2.1	1	1	1	2	2	3	4	6
35–49	50	2.3	1	1	2	2	2	4	5	7
50–64	37	2.1	<1	1	1	2	2	4	4	4
65+	15	3.3	<1	2	3	3	4	4	4	5
2. MULTIPLE DX										
0–19 Years	141	2.8	3	1	2	2	3	5	7	10
20–34	119	2.8	4	2	2	2	3	4	5	17
35–49	160	2.8	6	1	2	2	3	4	5	12
50–64	210	2.9	3	1	2	2	4	5	6	7
65+	196	3.0	3	2	2	3	4	5	5	9
TOTAL SINGLE DX	174	2.2	1	1	2	2	2	4	4	6
MULTIPLE DX	826	2.8	4	1	2	2	3	5	6	10
TOTAL										
0–19 Years	186	2.6	3	1	2	2	3	4	7	10
20–34	146	2.7	3	2	2	2	3	4	5	17
35–49	210	2.6	4	1	2	2	3	4	5	8
50–64	247	2.8	3	1	2	2	3	5	5	7
65+	211	3.1	3	2	2	3	4	5	5	9
GRAND TOTAL	1000	2.7	3	1	2	2	3	4	5	9

81.13: SUBTALAR FUSION. Formerly included in operation group(s) 745.

Type of Patients	Observed Patients	Avg. Stay	Vari-ance	Percentiles						
				10th	25th	50th	75th	90th	95th	99th
1. SINGLE DX										
0–19 Years	7	1.3	<1	1	1	1	2	2	3	3
20–34	29	1.9	<1	1	1	1	2	3	4	4
35–49	66	1.6	<1	1	1	1	2	3	4	4
50–64	41	2.4	<1	1	2	3	3	3	3	3
65+	12	2.0	<1	2	2	2	2	2	3	4
2. MULTIPLE DX										
0–19 Years	50	2.1	<1	1	1	2	3	4	4	4
20–34	66	2.4	2	1	1	2	3	4	4	6
35–49	149	3.0	7	2	2	2	3	4	12	13
50–64	104	2.8	4	1	1	2	3	6	7	8
65+	66	3.6	6	1	2	3	5	6	6	6
TOTAL SINGLE DX	155	1.9	<1	1	1	2	2	3	3	4
MULTIPLE DX	435	2.8	5	1	1	2	3	5	6	13
TOTAL										
0–19 Years	57	2.0	<1	1	1	2	3	3	4	4
20–34	95	2.2	1	1	1	2	3	4	4	6
35–49	215	2.5	5	1	2	2	3	4	6	13
50–64	145	2.6	2	1	2	2	3	4	7	8
65+	78	3.3	5	1	2	3	5	6	6	6
GRAND TOTAL	590	2.5	4	1	1	2	3	4	6	12

Length of Stay by Diagnosis and Operation, United States, 1997

United States, October 1995–September 1996 Data, by Operation

81.4: LOW LIMB JOINT REP NEC. Formerly included in operation group(s) 747, 749, 751.

Type of Patients	Observed Patients	Avg. Stay	Variance	10th	25th	50th	75th	90th	95th	99th
1. SINGLE DX										
0–19 Years	1367	1.5	<1	1	1	1	2	3	3	4
20–34	1794	1.5	<1	1	1	1	2	2	3	4
35–49	772	1.5	<1	1	1	1	2	2	3	5
50–64	108	2.4	3	1	1	2	3	5	6	9
65+	39	4.1	4	2	3	4	4	7	8	11
2. MULTIPLE DX										
0–19 Years	1417	2.0	5	1	1	1	2	3	5	11
20–34	2690	1.9	11	1	1	1	2	3	4	8
35–49	1722	2.0	3	1	1	1	2	3	5	10
50–64	467	3.6	16	1	1	2	4	7	10	27
65+	421	5.9	27	2	3	5	7	11	15	22
TOTAL SINGLE DX	4080	1.5	<1	1	1	1	2	3	3	5
MULTIPLE DX	6717	2.2	9	1	1	1	2	4	6	12
TOTAL										
0–19 Years	2784	1.8	3	1	1	1	2	3	4	10
20–34	4484	1.7	7	1	1	1	2	3	3	7
35–49	2494	1.8	2	1	1	1	2	3	5	8
50–64	575	3.4	14	1	1	2	4	7	9	20
65+	460	5.8	26	2	3	4	7	10	15	22
GRAND TOTAL	10797	1.9	6	1	1	1	2	3	5	10

81.40: REPAIR OF HIP NEC. Formerly included in operation group(s) 747.

Type of Patients	Observed Patients	Avg. Stay	Variance	10th	25th	50th	75th	90th	95th	99th
1. SINGLE DX										
0–19 Years	85	2.8	4	1	2	2	3	3	4	13
20–34	3	3.6	1	3	3	3	5	5	5	5
35–49	1	5.0	0	5	5	5	5	5	5	5
50–64	6	7.1	9	1	6	8	9	12	12	12
65+	2	4.2	1	3	3	5	5	5	5	5
2. MULTIPLE DX										
0–19 Years	99	4.7	18	2	2	3	5	11	16	22
20–34	12	7.1	68	3	4	6	6	7	18	58
35–49	7	7.6	5	4	8	8	8	8	13	13
50–64	18	9.5	102	5	8	3	17	27	27	45
65+	68	9.4	54	5	5	7	11	17	20	64
TOTAL SINGLE DX	97	2.9	5	1	2	3	3	4	7	13
MULTIPLE DX	204	6.4	41	2	3	4	8	13	18	28
TOTAL										
0–19 Years	184	4.0	14	2	2	3	4	6	12	20
20–34	15	6.7	61	3	4	6	6	7	18	58
35–49	8	7.5	5	4	7	8	8	8	13	13
50–64	24	9.3	95	5	5	5	12	27	27	45
65+	70	9.4	54	5	5	7	11	17	20	64
GRAND TOTAL	301	5.4	33	2	2	3	6	11	16	27

81.2: ARTHRODESIS OF OTH JOINT. Formerly included in operation group(s) 745.

Type of Patients	Observed Patients	Avg. Stay	Variance	10th	25th	50th	75th	90th	95th	99th
1. SINGLE DX										
0–19 Years	23	1.6	<1	1	1	1	2	2	4	4
20–34	88	2.0	1	1	1	2	2	3	4	5
35–49	97	2.0	1	1	1	2	3	3	4	7
50–64	51	1.9	1	1	1	2	2	3	3	4
65+	25	2.2	<1	1	2	2	3	3	3	4
2. MULTIPLE DX										
0–19 Years	46	4.2	12	1	2	4	5	6	8	22
20–34	120	3.0	24	1	1	2	3	6	7	16
35–49	244	3.2	8	1	1	2	4	7	9	14
50–64	200	2.9	14	1	1	2	3	6	8	20
65+	202	4.9	21	1	2	4	7	10	11	20
TOTAL SINGLE DX	284	2.0	1	1	1	2	2	3	4	7
MULTIPLE DX	812	3.6	16	1	1	2	5	7	9	20
TOTAL										
0–19 Years	69	3.7	11	1	2	3	5	6	6	22
20–34	208	2.5	14	1	1	2	3	5	6	11
35–49	341	2.8	6	1	1	2	3	7	9	14
50–64	251	2.7	11	1	1	2	3	5	8	20
65+	227	4.6	20	1	2	3	7	9	11	16
GRAND TOTAL	1096	3.1	12	1	1	2	4	7	8	16

81.26: METACARPOCARPAL FUSION. Formerly included in operation group(s) 745.

Type of Patients	Observed Patients	Avg. Stay	Variance	10th	25th	50th	75th	90th	95th	99th
1. SINGLE DX										
0–19 Years	4	1.7	<1	1	1	2	2	2	2	2
20–34	43	1.7	<1	1	1	1	2	3	4	4
35–49	53	1.6	<1	1	1	1	2	3	4	4
50–64	27	1.8	<1	1	1	2	2	3	4	4
65+	15	2.0	<1	1	2	2	2	3	3	3
2. MULTIPLE DX										
0–19 Years	2	2.3	<1	2	2	2	3	3	3	3
20–34	46	1.5	<1	1	1	1	2	3	3	3
35–49	101	1.9	1	1	1	2	2	3	3	6
50–64	85	1.7	2	1	1	1	2	3	4	8
65+	48	3.6	7	1	2	2	7	7	7	7
TOTAL SINGLE DX	142	1.7	<1	1	1	1	2	2	3	4
MULTIPLE DX	282	2.1	3	1	1	2	2	5	7	7
TOTAL										
0–19 Years	6	1.8	<1	1	2	2	2	2	3	3
20–34	89	1.6	<1	1	1	1	2	3	3	4
35–49	154	1.8	1	1	1	2	2	3	4	6
50–64	112	1.7	1	1	1	1	2	3	4	7
65+	63	3.5	6	1	2	2	7	7	7	7
GRAND TOTAL	424	2.0	2	1	1	2	2	4	7	7

Length of Stay by Diagnosis and Operation, United States, 1997

United States, October 1995–September 1996 Data, by Operation

81.44: PATELLAR STABILIZATION. Formerly included in operation group(s) 749.

Type of Patients	Observed Patients	Avg. Stay	Vari-ance	10th	25th	50th	75th	90th	95th	99th
1. SINGLE DX										
0–19 Years	93	1.9	<1	1	1	2	2	4	4	4
20–34	78	1.5	<1	1	1	1	2	2	3	3
35–49	38	1.9	<1	1	1	2	2	3	3	3
50–64	6	1.6	<1	1	1	1	2	3	3	5
65+	7	3.5	2	3	3	3	4	4	8	8
2. MULTIPLE DX										
0–19 Years	108	1.9	1	1	1	2	2	3	4	5
20–34	112	2.2	2	1	1	2	2	4	4	7
35–49	60	2.2	2	1	1	2	3	4	5	7
50–64	30	3.0	3	2	2	2	4	4	6	10
65+	66	4.1	4	2	3	3	5	7	8	10
TOTAL SINGLE DX	222	1.8	<1	1	1	2	2	3	3	4
MULTIPLE DX	376	2.4	3	1	1	2	3	4	5	8
TOTAL										
0–19 Years	201	1.9	<1	1	1	2	2	3	4	5
20–34	190	1.9	1	1	1	2	2	3	4	7
35–49	98	2.1	2	1	1	2	3	3	4	7
50–64	36	2.8	3	1	2	2	4	4	6	10
65+	73	4.1	4	2	3	3	5	7	8	10
GRAND TOTAL	598	2.1	2	1	1	2	2	4	4	7

81.46: COLLATERAL LIG REP NEC. Formerly included in operation group(s) 749.

Type of Patients	Observed Patients	Avg. Stay	Vari-ance	10th	25th	50th	75th	90th	95th	99th
1. SINGLE DX										
0–19 Years	10	2.0	<1	1	1	2	3	3	3	3
20–34	22	2.5	1	1	2	3	3	3	3	5
35–49	8	2.7	<1	1	2	2	3	3	4	4
50–64	4	2.0	<1	2	2	2	2	2	3	3
65+	2	3.6	<1	3	3	4	4	4	4	4
2. MULTIPLE DX										
0–19 Years	36	4.5	17	1	1	3	7	10	10	16
20–34	75	3.1	10	1	1	2	4	7	7	16
35–49	47	3.3	7	1	2	2	5	9	9	11
50–64	27	4.3	8	2	3	3	5	9	11	12
65+	18	4.5	9	1	3	4	4	8	8	15
TOTAL SINGLE DX	46	2.4	<1	1	2	2	3	3	4	5
MULTIPLE DX	203	3.7	11	1	1	2	5	9	10	16
TOTAL										
0–19 Years	46	4.3	15	1	1	2	7	10	10	16
20–34	97	3.0	9	1	1	2	3	6	8	16
35–49	55	3.3	7	1	2	2	4	8	9	11
50–64	31	3.8	7	2	2	3	4	9	11	11
65+	20	4.5	9	1	3	4	4	8	8	15
GRAND TOTAL	249	3.5	10	1	1	2	4	9	10	16

81.45: CRUCIATE LIG REPAIR NEC. Formerly included in operation group(s) 749.

Type of Patients	Observed Patients	Avg. Stay	Vari-ance	10th	25th	50th	75th	90th	95th	99th
1. SINGLE DX										
0–19 Years	1051	1.4	<1	1	1	2	2	2	3	4
20–34	1467	1.4	<1	1	1	2	2	2	3	3
35–49	587	1.4	<1	1	1	2	2	2	3	3
50–64	40	2.0	2	1	1	2	2	3	3	5
65+	0									
2. MULTIPLE DX										
0–19 Years	1041	1.6	1	1	1	2	2	3	4	5
20–34	2122	1.8	13	1	1	2	2	3	4	7
35–49	1170	1.7	2	1	1	2	3	4	5	7
50–64	132	2.1	2	1	2	2	4	4	6	10
65+	15	6.6	18	2	3	3	5	7	8	10
TOTAL SINGLE DX	3145	1.4	<1	1	1	2	2	2	3	4
MULTIPLE DX	4480	1.7	7	1	1	2	3	4	5	8
TOTAL										
0–19 Years	2092	1.5	<1	1	1	2	2	3	3	4
20–34	3589	1.6	8	1	1	2	2	3	3	5
35–49	1757	1.6	2	1	1	2	3	3	3	6
50–64	172	2.0	2	1	1	2	2	4	5	9
65+	15	6.6	18	2	5	6	6	16	16	16
GRAND TOTAL	7625	1.6	4	1	1	2	2	3	3	5

81.47: OTHER REPAIR OF KNEE. Formerly included in operation group(s) 749.

Type of Patients	Observed Patients	Avg. Stay	Vari-ance	10th	25th	50th	75th	90th	95th	99th
1. SINGLE DX										
0–19 Years	97	1.7	1	1	1	1	2	3	3	5
20–34	127	1.6	<1	1	1	1	2	3	4	4
35–49	100	1.8	1	1	1	1	2	3	4	6
50–64	42	3.3	4	1	2	3	4	7	7	9
65+	24	4.5	4	2	4	4	5	8	8	11
2. MULTIPLE DX										
0–19 Years	99	2.0	8	1	1	1	2	3	9	11
20–34	300	2.5	5	1	2	2	3	5	7	10
35–49	343	2.5	4	1	2	2	3	5	6	12
50–64	227	4.1	11	2	2	3	6	6	10	20
65+	239	5.2	20	2	3	4	6	8	11	22
TOTAL SINGLE DX	390	1.9	2	1	1	1	2	4	4	7
MULTIPLE DX	1208	3.0	9	1	1	2	4	6	7	15
TOTAL										
0–19 Years	196	1.9	5	1	1	1	2	3	4	11
20–34	427	2.2	4	1	2	2	3	4	7	8
35–49	443	2.4	4	1	1	2	3	5	6	12
50–64	269	4.0	10	2	3	3	6	7	10	20
65+	263	5.1	19	2	3	4	6	8	11	22
GRAND TOTAL	1598	2.7	7	1	1	2	3	6	7	13

Length of Stay by Diagnosis and Operation, United States, 1997

United States, October 1995–September 1996 Data, by Operation

81.49: OTHER REPAIR OF ANKLE. Formerly included in operation group(s) 751.

Type of Patients	Observed Patients	Avg. Stay	Vari-ance	Percentiles						
				10th	25th	50th	75th	90th	95th	99th
1. SINGLE DX										
0–19 Years	26	1.3	<1	1	1	1	2	2	2	3
20–34	88	1.4	<1	1	1	1	2	2	3	3
35–49	35	1.4	<1	1	1	1	1	2	2	6
50–64	10	1.7	<1	1	1	2	2	3	4	4
65+	4	3.2	2	1	3	4	4	4	4	4
2. MULTIPLE DX										
0–19 Years	25	1.2	<1	1	1	1	1	2	2	2
20–34	52	2.0	1	1	1	1	1	2	2	3
35–49	81	2.1	2	1	1	2	3	3	4	9
50–64	29	1.8	<1	1	1	2	2	3	3	6
65+	14	4.7	9	2	2	4	7	11	11	11
TOTAL SINGLE DX	163	1.4	<1	1	1	1	2	2	3	4
MULTIPLE DX	201	2.0	2	1	1	2	2	4	4	7
TOTAL										
0–19 Years	51	1.3	<1	1	1	1	1	2	2	3
20–34	140	1.6	<1	1	1	1	2	3	4	4
35–49	116	1.8	2	1	1	1	2	3	3	6
50–64	39	1.8	<1	1	1	2	2	3	3	6
65+	18	4.2	7	2	3	4	5	7	11	11
GRAND TOTAL	364	1.7	1	1	1	1	2	3	4	6

81.51: TOTAL HIP REPLACEMENT. Formerly included in operation group(s) 746.

Type of Patients	Observed Patients	Avg. Stay	Vari-ance	Percentiles						
				10th	25th	50th	75th	90th	95th	99th
1. SINGLE DX										
0–19 Years	11	6.1	30	3	4	4	5	20	20	20
20–34	141	4.3	15	3	3	4	5	5	6	8
35–49	734	4.4	2	3	3	4	5	6	7	8
50–64	1381	4.4	2	3	3	4	5	6	7	9
65+	2328	4.6	3	3	4	4	5	6	7	11
2. MULTIPLE DX										
0–19 Years	45	5.4	6	3	3	5	8	8	10	12
20–34	664	4.8	5	3	4	4	6	7	9	15
35–49	3205	5.0	7	3	4	4	6	7	8	13
50–64	7625	5.3	8	3	4	5	6	7	9	15
65+	23685	5.8	10	3	4	5	6	8	11	19
TOTAL SINGLE DX	4595	4.5	3	3	3	4	5	6	7	9
MULTIPLE DX	35224	5.5	10	3	4	5	6	8	10	17
TOTAL										
0–19 Years	56	5.5	9	3	3	5	8	8	10	20
20–34	805	4.8	7	3	3	4	5	7	9	15
35–49	3939	4.9	6	3	4	5	5	7	8	13
50–64	9006	5.2	8	3	4	5	6	8	10	14
65+	26013	5.6	10	3	4	5	6	8	11	18
GRAND TOTAL	39819	5.4	9	3	4	5	6	8	10	16

81.5: JOINT REPL LOWER EXT. Formerly included in operation group(s) 746, 747, 748, 749, 750.

Type of Patients	Observed Patients	Avg. Stay	Vari-ance	Percentiles						
				10th	25th	50th	75th	90th	95th	99th
1. SINGLE DX										
0–19 Years	24	4.6	16	1	1	3	8	8	16	16
20–34	93	4.2	3	3	3	4	5	6	8	9
35–49	811	4.5	3	3	3	4	5	6	7	11
50–64	3067	4.6	3	3	4	4	5	6	7	10
65+	6631	4.8	3	3	4	4	6	7	8	11
2. MULTIPLE DX										
0–19 Years	57	7.2	12	3	4	7	10	10	10	20
20–34	435	6.1	21	3	4	5	7	10	12	21
35–49	3156	5.4	13	3	4	5	6	8	10	20
50–64	16729	5.4	8	3	4	5	6	8	10	16
65+	74315	6.1	14	3	4	5	7	9	12	21
TOTAL SINGLE DX	10626	4.7	3	3	4	4	5	7	8	10
MULTIPLE DX	94692	5.9	13	3	4	5	7	9	11	19
TOTAL										
0–19 Years	81	6.5	14	2	4	6	9	10	10	16
20–34	528	5.7	18	3	4	5	6	9	12	19
35–49	3967	5.2	11	3	4	5	6	8	10	18
50–64	19796	5.2	8	3	4	5	6	8	10	15
65+	80946	6.0	13	3	4	5	7	9	12	20
GRAND TOTAL	105318	5.8	12	3	4	5	7	9	11	19

81.52: PARTIAL HIP REPLACEMENT. Formerly included in operation group(s) 747.

Type of Patients	Observed Patients	Avg. Stay	Vari-ance	Percentiles						
				10th	25th	50th	75th	90th	95th	99th
1. SINGLE DX										
0–19 Years	4	3.2	<1	3	3	3	3	4	4	6
20–34	12	5.8	6	4	5	6	6	9	9	9
35–49	49	4.9	6	3	3	4	5	9	10	12
50–64	132	5.3	3	3	4	5	6	7	10	12
65+	953	5.8	7	3	4	5	7	9	10	14
2. MULTIPLE DX										
0–19 Years	18	8.4	10	5	6	10	10	10	10	12
20–34	65	7.5	63	3	4	5	7	12	15	47
35–49	282	7.5	49	3	4	5	8	12	19	42
50–64	1278	7.6	21	4	5	6	9	13	17	27
65+	23845	7.6	26	4	5	6	8	12	15	29
TOTAL SINGLE DX	1150	5.6	6	3	4	5	6	8	10	14
MULTIPLE DX	25488	7.6	26	4	5	6	9	12	16	30
TOTAL										
0–19 Years	22	7.6	12	3	5	9	10	10	10	12
20–34	77	7.2	53	3	4	6	7	12	13	47
35–49	331	7.1	43	3	4	5	8	11	17	40
50–64	1410	7.4	20	4	5	6	8	13	16	27
65+	24798	7.5	25	4	5	6	8	12	15	29
GRAND TOTAL	26638	7.5	25	4	5	6	8	12	15	29

Length of Stay by Diagnosis and Operation, United States, 1997

United States, October 1995–September 1996 Data, by Operation

81.53: HIP REPLACEMENT REVISION. Formerly included in operation group(s) 747.

Type of Patients	Observed Patients	Avg. Stay	Vari-ance	10th	25th	50th	75th	90th	95th	99th
1. SINGLE DX										
0–19 Years	0									
20–34	35	4.6	3	3	4	4	5	7	8	8
35–49	164	4.3	6	2	3	4	5	7	9	12
50–64	201	4.9	8	3	3	4	6	7	9	20
65+	362	4.8	4	3	4	4	5	7	8	12
2. MULTIPLE DX										
0–19 Years	5	5.3	2	3	4	6	6	8	8	8
20–34	166	5.9	13	3	4	5	6	8	10	21
35–49	822	6.0	20	3	4	5	7	9	12	24
50–64	1341	6.0	17	3	4	5	7	10	12	20
65+	4516	6.4	16	4	4	5	7	10	13	21
TOTAL SINGLE DX	762	4.7	6	3	3	4	6	7	8	13
MULTIPLE DX	6850	6.2	17	3	4	5	7	10	12	21
TOTAL										
0–19 Years	5	5.3	2	3	4	6	6	8	8	8
20–34	201	5.7	12	3	4	5	6	8	10	21
35–49	986	5.8	18	3	4	5	7	9	11	23
50–64	1542	5.8	16	3	4	5	7	9	12	20
65+	4878	6.3	15	3	4	5	7	10	12	21
GRAND TOTAL	7612	6.1	16	3	4	5	7	9	12	20

81.54: TOTAL KNEE REPLACEMENT. Formerly included in operation group(s) 748.

Type of Patients	Observed Patients	Avg. Stay	Vari-ance	10th	25th	50th	75th	90th	95th	99th
1. SINGLE DX										
0–19 Years	12	5.9	22	1	1	6	8	16	16	16
20–34	39	3.6	2	3	3	3	4	5	6	8
35–49	532	4.6	2	3	4	4	5	6	7	10
50–64	2561	4.6	3	3	4	4	6	6	7	9
65+	4970	4.7	3	3	4	4	6	7	7	9
2. MULTIPLE DX										
0–19 Years	22	6.7	8	4	4	7	7	9	9	20
20–34	161	5.5	7	3	4	5	6	8	10	18
35–49	1798	4.9	5	3	4	5	6	7	8	11
50–64	12994	5.2	6	3	4	5	6	7	8	13
65+	42256	5.3	6	3	4	5	6	8	9	14
TOTAL SINGLE DX	8114	4.6	3	3	4	4	5	7	7	9
MULTIPLE DX	57231	5.3	6	3	4	5	6	8	9	14
TOTAL										
0–19 Years	34	6.3	14	1	4	7	8	9	16	20
20–34	200	5.0	6	3	3	5	6	7	10	13
35–49	2330	4.8	4	3	4	5	5	7	8	11
50–64	15555	5.1	5	3	4	5	6	7	8	13
65+	47226	5.3	6	3	4	5	6	7	9	14
GRAND TOTAL	65345	5.2	6	3	4	5	6	7	9	14

81.55: KNEE REPLACEMENT REV. Formerly included in operation group(s) 749.

Type of Patients	Observed Patients	Avg. Stay	Vari-ance	10th	25th	50th	75th	90th	95th	99th
1. SINGLE DX										
0–19 Years	1	1.0	0	1	1	1	1	1	1	1
20–34	4	3.9	<1	3	3	4	5	5	5	5
35–49	48	4.3	3	3	3	4	5	6	7	12
50–64	161	4.4	1	3	4	4	5	5	7	8
65+	338	4.2	3	2	3	4	5	6	7	8
2. MULTIPLE DX										
0–19 Years	8	3.0	<1	2	3	3	4	4	4	4
20–34	39	6.2	12	3	3	5	11	11	11	13
35–49	226	4.8	6	3	4	4	6	7	9	13
50–64	1080	4.9	7	3	4	4	6	7	9	14
65+	3637	5.4	12	3	4	5	6	8	10	17
TOTAL SINGLE DX	552	4.3	2	3	3	4	5	6	7	8
MULTIPLE DX	4990	5.3	10	3	4	5	6	8	10	17
TOTAL										
0–19 Years	9	2.9	<1	1	3	3	3	4	4	4
20–34	43	6.0	11	3	3	5	8	11	11	13
35–49	274	4.8	5	3	3	4	6	7	9	13
50–64	1241	4.8	6	3	4	4	6	7	8	14
65+	3975	5.3	11	3	4	5	6	8	10	17
GRAND TOTAL	5542	5.1	9	3	4	4	6	8	9	17

81.7: HAND/FINGER ARTHROPLASTY. Formerly included in operation group(s) 750, 751.

Type of Patients	Observed Patients	Avg. Stay	Vari-ance	10th	25th	50th	75th	90th	95th	99th
1. SINGLE DX										
0–19 Years	20	1.1	<1	1	1	1	1	2	2	3
20–34	38	1.6	<1	1	1	1	2	3	4	4
35–49	60	1.2	<1	1	1	1	1	2	2	3
50–64	98	1.3	<1	1	1	1	2	2	2	3
65+	75	1.5	<1	1	1	1	2	2	3	3
2. MULTIPLE DX										
0–19 Years	21	2.4	12	1	1	1	1	5	14	14
20–34	53	2.3	17	1	1	1	1	3	12	20
35–49	140	2.2	15	1	1	1	2	3	4	32
50–64	215	1.4	<1	1	1	1	2	3	4	4
65+	261	1.8	3	1	1	1	2	3	4	7
TOTAL SINGLE DX	291	1.3	<1	1	1	1	2	2	3	4
MULTIPLE DX	690	1.8	6	1	1	1	2	3	4	14
TOTAL										
0–19 Years	41	1.8	7	1	1	1	1	3	5	14
20–34	91	2.1	12	1	1	1	2	3	5	20
35–49	200	1.9	11	1	1	1	2	3	4	32
50–64	313	1.4	<1	1	1	1	2	2	3	4
65+	336	1.7	2	1	1	1	2	3	4	7
GRAND TOTAL	981	1.7	5	1	1	1	2	3	3	10

Length of Stay by Diagnosis and Operation, United States, 1997

United States, October 1995–September 1996 Data, by Operation

81.75: CARPAL/CMC ARTHROPLASTY. Formerly included in operation group(s) 751.

Type of Patients	Observed Patients	Avg. Stay	Variance	Percentiles						
				10th	25th	50th	75th	90th	95th	99th
1. SINGLE DX										
0–19 Years	4	1.1	<1	1	1	1	1	2	2	2
20–34	11	1.2	<1	1	1	1	1	2	2	2
35–49	22	1.1	<1	1	1	1	1	1	2	2
50–64	36	1.3	<1	1	1	1	1	2	2	2
65+	17	1.4	<1	1	1	1	2	2	2	3
2. MULTIPLE DX										
0–19 Years	4	1.2	<1	1	1	1	1	1	3	3
20–34	24	3.2	33	1	1	1	1	10	20	20
35–49	52	2.7	28	1	1	2	2	3	5	32
50–64	74	1.2	<1	1	1	1	1	1	3	3
65+	59	1.6	1	1	1	1	2	3	3	7
TOTAL SINGLE DX	90	1.2	<1	1	1	1	1	2	2	3
MULTIPLE DX	213	1.9	12	1	1	1	2	2	3	20
TOTAL										
0–19 Years	8	1.1	<1	1	1	1	1	2	2	3
20–34	35	2.6	24	1	1	1	1	2	20	20
35–49	74	2.2	21	1	1	1	1	3	4	32
50–64	110	1.2	<1	1	1	1	1	2	2	3
65+	76	1.5	1	1	1	1	2	2	3	7
GRAND TOTAL	303	1.7	9	1	1	1	2	2	3	20

81.8: SHOULD/ELB ARTHROPLASTY. Formerly included in operation group(s) 750, 751.

Type of Patients	Observed Patients	Avg. Stay	Variance	Percentiles						
				10th	25th	50th	75th	90th	95th	99th
1. SINGLE DX										
0–19 Years	409	1.3	<1	1	1	1	1	2	2	3
20–34	1005	1.3	<1	1	1	1	1	2	2	3
35–49	870	1.4	<1	1	1	1	2	2	2	3
50–64	859	1.6	<1	1	1	1	2	3	3	5
65+	747	2.3	2	1	1	2	3	3	4	7
2. MULTIPLE DX										
0–19 Years	181	1.6	<1	1	1	1	2	2	3	4
20–34	769	1.7	2	1	1	1	2	3	4	5
35–49	1718	1.8	4	1	1	1	2	3	4	9
50–64	2961	1.9	3	1	1	2	2	3	4	8
65+	4877	3.3	9	1	2	2	4	6	8	19
TOTAL SINGLE DX	3890	1.5	<1	1	1	1	2	2	3	5
MULTIPLE DX	10506	2.4	6	1	1	2	3	4	6	13
TOTAL										
0–19 Years	590	1.4	<1	1	1	1	2	2	2	3
20–34	1774	1.5	<1	1	1	1	2	2	3	5
35–49	2588	1.7	3	1	1	2	2	3	4	6
50–64	3820	1.9	8	1	1	2	3	3	4	7
65+	5624	3.2	8	1	2	2	4	6	8	18
GRAND TOTAL	14396	2.1	4	1	1	2	2	4	5	10

81.80: TOTAL SHOULDER REPL. Formerly included in operation group(s) 750.

Type of Patients	Observed Patients	Avg. Stay	Variance	Percentiles						
				10th	25th	50th	75th	90th	95th	99th
1. SINGLE DX										
0–19 Years	1	2.0	0	2	2	2	2	2	2	2
20–34	9	1.8	<1	1	1	2	2	2	2	4
35–49	25	2.3	<1	2	2	2	3	3	3	7
50–64	101	2.4	1	2	2	2	3	3	4	9
65+	194	2.8	<1	2	2	3	3	4	5	7
2. MULTIPLE DX										
0–19 Years	0									
20–34	28	3.5	10	1	2	3	4	5	12	21
35–49	94	3.0	3	2	2	3	3	4	4	9
50–64	350	2.8	2	2	2	3	3	4	5	9
65+	1186	3.5	7	2	2	3	4	6	7	15
TOTAL SINGLE DX	330	2.6	1	2	2	2	3	4	4	7
MULTIPLE DX	1658	3.3	5	2	2	3	4	5	7	14
TOTAL										
0–19 Years	1	2.0	0	2	2	2	2	2	2	2
20–34	37	3.1	8	1	2	2	3	5	9	21
35–49	119	2.9	3	2	2	3	3	4	4	9
50–64	451	2.7	2	2	2	3	3	4	5	9
65+	1380	3.4	6	2	2	3	4	5	7	15
GRAND TOTAL	1988	3.2	5	2	2	3	4	5	6	13

81.81: PARTIAL SHOULDER REPL. Formerly included in operation group(s) 750.

Type of Patients	Observed Patients	Avg. Stay	Variance	Percentiles						
				10th	25th	50th	75th	90th	95th	99th
1. SINGLE DX										
0–19 Years	4	2.2	4	2	1	1	3	6	6	6
20–34	18	2.5	4	1	2	2	2	4	5	10
35–49	30	2.4	4	2	1	1	3	4	5	8
50–64	89	2.6	3	2	2	2	3	4	5	8
65+	161	3.0	3	2	3	3	3	5	6	9
2. MULTIPLE DX										
0–19 Years	1	3.0	0	3	3	3	3	3	3	3
20–34	35	2.9	3	1	2	3	3	5	5	10
35–49	136	3.1	3	1	3	3	4	6	8	11
50–64	345	3.3	12	2	2	3	4	6	8	14
65+	1391	4.7	17	2	3	4	6	8	12	20
TOTAL SINGLE DX	302	2.8	3	2	2	2	3	5	6	10
MULTIPLE DX	1908	4.3	15	2	2	3	5	8	11	19
TOTAL										
0–19 Years	5	2.8	<1	2	3	3	3	3	3	6
20–34	53	2.8	3	1	2	2	3	5	5	10
35–49	166	3.0	3	1	2	3	3	5	6	9
50–64	434	3.1	10	2	2	2	4	5	8	14
65+	1552	4.6	16	2	2	3	5	8	12	20
GRAND TOTAL	2210	4.1	13	2	2	3	5	7	10	19

Length of Stay by Diagnosis and Operation, United States, 1997

United States, October 1995–September 1996 Data, by Operation

81.82: REP RECUR SHOULD DISLOC. Formerly included in operation group(s) 751.

Type of Patients	Observed Patients	Avg. Stay	Vari-ance	Percentiles						
				10th	25th	50th	75th	90th	95th	99th
1. SINGLE DX										
0–19 Years	336	1.2	<1	1	1	1	1	2	2	3
20–34	670	1.3	<1	1	1	1	1	2	2	3
35–49	216	1.3	<1	1	1	1	2	2	2	3
50–64	37	1.7	2	1	1	1	2	2	6	6
65+	13	2.1	6	1	1	2	2	3	3	14
2. MULTIPLE DX										
0–19 Years	131	1.5	<1	1	1	1	2	2	2	4
20–34	364	1.4	<1	1	1	1	2	2	3	5
35–49	179	1.6	<1	1	1	1	2	3	3	4
50–64	79	1.5	<1	1	1	1	2	3	3	5
65+	78	4.1	9	1	2	3	7	9	9	9
TOTAL SINGLE DX	1272	1.3	<1	1	1	1	1	2	2	3
MULTIPLE DX	831	1.7	2	1	1	1	2	3	4	9
TOTAL										
0–19 Years	467	1.3	<1	1	1	1	1	2	2	4
20–34	1034	1.3	<1	1	1	1	2	2	2	4
35–49	395	1.4	<1	1	1	1	2	2	3	3
50–64	116	1.6	<1	1	1	1	2	3	3	6
65+	91	4.0	9	1	2	2	7	9	9	9
GRAND TOTAL	2103	1.4	1	1	1	1	2	2	3	7

81.83: SHOULD ARTHROPLASTY NEC. Formerly included in operation group(s) 751.

Type of Patients	Observed Patients	Avg. Stay	Vari-ance	Percentiles						
				10th	25th	50th	75th	90th	95th	99th
1. SINGLE DX										
0–19 Years	62	1.4	<1	1	1	1	2	2	2	3
20–34	287	1.3	<1	1	1	1	1	2	2	3
35–49	572	1.3	<1	1	1	1	2	2	2	3
50–64	591	1.4	<1	1	1	1	2	2	2	3
65+	357	1.7	<1	1	1	2	2	3	3	5
2. MULTIPLE DX										
0–19 Years	40	1.6	<1	1	1	1	2	2	3	3
20–34	300	1.6	1	1	1	1	2	2	3	5
35–49	1247	1.6	4	1	1	1	2	3	3	5
50–64	2103	1.6	1	1	1	1	2	3	3	5
65+	2103	2.2	3	1	2	2	2	3	4	9
TOTAL SINGLE DX	1869	1.4	<1	1	1	1	2	2	2	3
MULTIPLE DX	5793	1.8	2	1	1	1	2	3	4	7
TOTAL										
0–19 Years	102	1.5	<1	1	1	1	2	2	2	3
20–34	587	1.5	<1	1	1	1	2	2	3	5
35–49	1819	1.5	3	1	1	1	2	2	3	5
50–64	2694	1.6	<1	1	1	1	2	2	3	5
65+	2460	2.1	3	1	1	2	2	3	4	9
GRAND TOTAL	7662	1.7	2	1	1	1	2	3	3	6

81.84: TOTAL ELBOW REPLACEMENT. Formerly included in operation group(s) 750.

Type of Patients	Observed Patients	Avg. Stay	Vari-ance	Percentiles						
				10th	25th	50th	75th	90th	95th	99th
1. SINGLE DX										
0–19 Years	1	1.0	0	1	1	1	1	1	1	1
20–34	5	1.4	<1	1	1	1	1	2	2	2
35–49	19	1.5	<1	1	1	1	2	2	3	4
50–64	34	2.2	<1	1	2	2	3	3	3	4
65+	19	2.2	<1	2	2	2	2	3	3	5
2. MULTIPLE DX										
0–19 Years	2	2.0	0	2	2	2	2	3	2	2
20–34	19	2.6	7	1	2	2	2	3	6	15
35–49	44	3.7	15	1	2	2	3	13	13	13
50–64	68	3.3	4	2	2	3	4	6	6	11
65+	92	3.0	3	2	2	3	4	5	5	9
TOTAL SINGLE DX	78	1.9	<1	1	1	2	2	3	3	4
MULTIPLE DX	225	3.2	6	1	2	2	3	6	7	13
TOTAL										
0–19 Years	3	1.9	<1	1	2	2	2	2	2	2
20–34	24	2.5	6	1	2	2	2	3	6	15
35–49	63	2.8	10	1	1	2	3	5	13	13
50–64	102	2.9	3	2	2	3	3	6	6	6
65+	111	2.9	3	2	2	3	3	5	5	7
GRAND TOTAL	303	2.8	5	1	2	2	3	5	6	13

81.9: OTHER JOINT STRUCTURE OP. Formerly included in operation group(s) 750, 751, 767.

Type of Patients	Observed Patients	Avg. Stay	Vari-ance	Percentiles						
				10th	25th	50th	75th	90th	95th	99th
1. SINGLE DX										
0–19 Years	524	3.1	6	1	2	2	4	6	8	12
20–34	163	2.1	3	1	1	2	4	4	5	10
35–49	148	2.6	3	1	1	2	3	5	6	8
50–64	78	3.9	6	1	2	5	5	5	7	14
65+	95	3.2	6	1	2	3	4	6	7	13
2. MULTIPLE DX										
0–19 Years	676	5.0	33	1	2	4	6	9	12	28
20–34	617	5.0	34	1	2	3	6	9	13	41
35–49	1083	5.7	42	2	2	4	6	11	16	38
50–64	1419	6.1	32	2	3	4	8	12	15	30
65+	5082	7.0	36	2	3	5	9	13	18	27
TOTAL SINGLE DX	1008	2.9	5	1	1	2	4	6	7	12
MULTIPLE DX	8877	6.4	36	2	3	5	8	12	17	30
TOTAL										
0–19 Years	1200	4.2	23	1	2	3	5	8	10	21
20–34	780	4.5	30	1	2	3	5	8	12	33
35–49	1231	5.4	38	1	2	4	6	10	16	38
50–64	1497	6.0	31	2	3	4	8	11	15	30
65+	5177	7.0	36	2	3	5	9	13	18	27
GRAND TOTAL	9885	6.0	34	2	3	4	7	12	16	29

Length of Stay by Diagnosis and Operation, United States, 1997

81.91: ARTHROCENTESIS. Formerly included in operation group(s) 767.

Type of Patients	Observed Patients	Avg. Stay	Vari-ance	Percentiles						
				10th	25th	50th	75th	90th	95th	99th
1. SINGLE DX										
0–19 Years	456	3.3	6	1	2	2	4	6	8	12
20–34	83	2.9	5	1	1	2	4	5	7	11
35–49	100	3.1	3	1	2	3	4	6	6	8
50–64	55	4.3	6	2	2	5	5	6	9	14
65+	66	3.1	6	1	2	3	3	6	8	16
2. MULTIPLE DX										
0–19 Years	607	5.4	36	1	2	4	7	9	13	28
20–34	487	5.4	40	2	2	4	6	9	13	41
35–49	881	5.8	34	2	3	4	7	11	16	27
50–64	1084	6.4	34	2	3	5	8	12	15	30
65+	3515	7.0	34	2	4	5	9	13	17	27
TOTAL SINGLE DX	760	3.3	6	1	2	3	4	6	8	12
MULTIPLE DX	6574	6.4	35	2	3	5	8	12	16	30
TOTAL										
0–19 Years	1063	4.5	24	1	2	3	5	8	10	21
20–34	570	5.1	36	1	3	4	6	9	13	41
35–49	981	5.6	32	2	3	4	7	11	16	27
50–64	1139	6.3	33	2	3	5	8	12	15	30
65+	3581	6.9	34	2	4	5	9	13	17	27
GRAND TOTAL	7334	6.1	33	2	3	5	8	12	16	28

81.92: INJECTION INTO JOINT. Formerly included in operation group(s) 767.

Type of Patients	Observed Patients	Avg. Stay	Vari-ance	Percentiles						
				10th	25th	50th	75th	90th	95th	99th
1. SINGLE DX										
0–19 Years	21	1.0	0	1	1	1	1	1	1	1
20–34	6	1.4	<1	1	1	1	2	3	3	3
35–49	6	2.3	1	1	1	2	4	6	6	6
50–64	8	2.9	3	1	2	2	4	6	6	6
65+	13	4.2	5	2	4	4	6	7	8	8
2. MULTIPLE DX										
0–19 Years	9	8.1	77	2	5	7	7	9	39	39
20–34	32	7.0	23	2	3	9	9	11	13	36
35–49	116	7.4	109	2	3	4	6	18	38	45
50–64	277	5.8	29	2	3	5	6	11	15	25
65+	1459	7.6	42	2	4	6	9	15	21	29
TOTAL SINGLE DX	54	2.2	3	1	1	1	3	5	6	8
MULTIPLE DX	1893	7.3	46	2	3	5	9	14	21	38
TOTAL										
0–19 Years	30	4.2	47	1	1	1	6	8	8	39
20–34	38	6.4	23	2	3	5	6	9	13	30
35–49	122	7.0	104	2	3	3	6	13	38	45
50–64	285	5.8	29	2	3	4	7	11	15	25
65+	1472	7.5	42	2	4	6	9	15	21	29
GRAND TOTAL	1947	7.2	45	2	3	5	9	14	21	38

82.0: INC HAND SOFT TISSUE. Formerly included in operation group(s) 752.

Type of Patients	Observed Patients	Avg. Stay	Vari-ance	Percentiles						
				10th	25th	50th	75th	90th	95th	99th
1. SINGLE DX										
0–19 Years	34	2.8	3	1	1	3	4	5	6	8
20–34	79	3.0	3	1	2	2	4	5	7	9
35–49	72	2.9	5	1	2	2	4	6	9	10
50–64	25	2.6	4	1	1	2	3	7	7	8
65+	4	2.6	7	2	2	2	2	2	13	13
2. MULTIPLE DX										
0–19 Years	80	4.3	15	2	2	3	5	7	10	18
20–34	202	3.9	8	2	2	3	5	7	10	15
35–49	242	4.3	11	2	2	4	5	7	9	20
50–64	152	5.9	23	1	3	5	8	10	12	30
65+	136	6.2	18	2	3	5	8	12	14	19
TOTAL SINGLE DX	214	2.9	4	1	1	2	4	6	7	10
MULTIPLE DX	812	4.7	14	2	2	4	6	8	10	20
TOTAL										
0–19 Years	114	4.0	13	1	2	3	5	7	8	18
20–34	281	3.6	6	1	2	3	5	7	8	14
35–49	314	4.0	10	1	2	4	5	7	8	13
50–64	177	5.4	22	1	2	5	8	10	12	30
65+	140	5.9	18	2	3	5	8	11	14	19
GRAND TOTAL	1026	4.3	12	1	2	3	5	8	10	18

82.01: EXPLOR TEND SHEATH HAND. Formerly included in operation group(s) 752.

Type of Patients	Observed Patients	Avg. Stay	Vari-ance	Percentiles						
				10th	25th	50th	75th	90th	95th	99th
1. SINGLE DX										
0–19 Years	23	2.8	4	1	1	3	3	5	6	10
20–34	39	2.9	2	2	2	2	3	5	7	9
35–49	35	3.1	5	1	2	3	3	4	7	9
50–64	11	2.4	1	1	1	3	3	4	4	5
65+	4	2.6	7	2	2	2	2	2	13	13
2. MULTIPLE DX										
0–19 Years	28	3.9	15	2	2	3	5	7	7	36
20–34	102	3.6	7	2	2	3	4	6	9	12
35–49	122	4.2	8	2	2	4	5	7	7	20
50–64	78	5.1	12	2	3	4	7	10	12	14
65+	62	5.8	19	2	3	5	7	10	13	30
TOTAL SINGLE DX	112	2.9	3	1	2	2	3	5	7	9
MULTIPLE DX	392	4.4	11	1	2	3	6	8	10	16
TOTAL										
0–19 Years	51	3.5	11	1	2	3	5	6	7	11
20–34	141	3.4	5	2	2	3	4	6	7	12
35–49	157	4.0	8	2	2	3	5	9	8	20
50–64	89	4.8	12	2	3	4	7	10	12	14
65+	66	5.5	19	2	3	4	7	10	13	30
GRAND TOTAL	504	4.0	10	2	3	3	5	7	10	16

Length of Stay by Diagnosis and Operation, United States, 1997

United States, October 1995–September 1996 Data, by Operation

82.09: INC SOFT TISSUE HAND NEC. Formerly included in operation group(s) 752.

Type of Patients	Observed Patients	Avg. Stay	Vari-ance	Percentiles						
				10th	25th	50th	75th	90th	95th	99th
1. SINGLE DX										
0–19 Years	10	2.8	3	1	1	2	4	5	5	7
20–34	35	3.2	4	1	2	3	4	6	7	9
35–49	25	2.4	6	1	1	1	3	6	10	10
50–64	12	2.7	6	1	1	1	4	7	8	8
65+	0									
2. MULTIPLE DX										
0–19 Years	35	4.9	20	1	3	4	5	9	18	20
20–34	74	3.9	7	2	2	4	5	7	7	7
35–49	94	4.4	13	2	2	4	5	8	9	13
50–64	53	7.2	40	2	3	8	8	10	22	30
65+	56	6.9	19	2	3	7	8	13	14	19
TOTAL SINGLE DX	82	2.8	5	1	1	2	4	6	7	10
MULTIPLE DX	312	5.1	19	2	3	4	6	8	12	22
TOTAL										
0–19 Years	45	4.5	17	1	2	4	4	8	18	20
20–34	109	3.7	6	1	2	3	5	6	7	15
35–49	119	3.9	12	1	2	3	5	7	9	13
50–64	65	6.2	36	1	3	5	8	9	22	30
65+	56	6.9	19	2	3	7	8	13	14	19
GRAND TOTAL	394	4.6	17	1	2	4	6	8	10	22

82.1: DIV HAND MUSC/TEND/FASC. Formerly included in operation group(s) 754.

Type of Patients	Observed Patients	Avg. Stay	Vari-ance	Percentiles						
				10th	25th	50th	75th	90th	95th	99th
1. SINGLE DX										
0–19 Years	1	1.0	0	1	1	1	1	1	1	1
20–34	13	2.8	2	1	2	2	4	4	4	8
35–49	6	1.3	<1	1	1	1	1	2	3	4
50–64	5	1.9	1	1	1	2	2	4	4	4
65+	4	6.4	36	1	1	13	13	13	13	13
2. MULTIPLE DX										
0–19 Years	14	6.0	30	2	2	4	6	19	19	19
20–34	33	4.3	26	1	2	3	5	8	9	39
35–49	38	4.0	7	2	2	4	5	7	8	15
50–64	21	5.2	18	1	2	5	5	11	15	19
65+	21	5.7	38	2	3	7	7	16	16	28
TOTAL SINGLE DX	29	2.3	5	1	1	2	3	4	8	13
MULTIPLE DX	127	4.7	21	2	2	3	5	8	13	28
TOTAL										
0–19 Years	15	5.3	29	1	2	3	6	19	19	19
20–34	46	3.9	21	1	2	3	4	7	8	39
35–49	44	3.2	7	1	1	3	4	6	8	15
50–64	26	4.9	17	1	2	5	5	11	15	19
65+	25	5.8	37	1	2	3	7	13	16	28
GRAND TOTAL	156	4.2	19	1	2	3	5	8	11	19

82.2: EXC LES HAND SOFT TISSUE. Formerly included in operation group(s) 753.

Type of Patients	Observed Patients	Avg. Stay	Vari-ance	Percentiles						
				10th	25th	50th	75th	90th	95th	99th
1. SINGLE DX										
0–19 Years	13	1.4	<1	1	1	1	1	3	3	3
20–34	5	2.0	<1	1	1	1	2	3	3	3
35–49	8	3.5	5	1	1	4	6	7	7	7
50–64	3	1.1	<1	1	1	1	1	1	2	2
65+	1	13.0	0	13	13	13	13	13	13	13
2. MULTIPLE DX										
0–19 Years	5	3.3	3	1	2	4	4	7	7	7
20–34	9	5.6	28	1	3	4	8	8	24	24
35–49	20	4.5	13	1	1	3	7	11	11	12
50–64	11	1.6	4	1	1	1	1	3	5	13
65+	15	3.9	15	1	1	3	4	8	15	15
TOTAL SINGLE DX	30	1.9	3	1	1	1	2	4	6	7
MULTIPLE DX	60	3.4	13	1	1	2	4	8	11	15
TOTAL										
0–19 Years	18	1.8	2	1	1	1	3	4	4	7
20–34	14	4.6	23	1	2	3	6	8	8	24
35–49	28	4.3	12	1	1	3	6	11	11	12
50–64	14	1.5	4	1	1	1	1	2	5	13
65+	16	4.3	17	1	1	3	4	13	15	15
GRAND TOTAL	90	2.9	11	1	1	1	4	7	11	13

82.3: OTH EXC HAND SOFT TISS. Formerly included in operation group(s) 754.

Type of Patients	Observed Patients	Avg. Stay	Vari-ance	Percentiles						
				10th	25th	50th	75th	90th	95th	99th
1. SINGLE DX										
0–19 Years	3	4.9	<1	5	5	5	5	5	5	5
20–34	5	1.7	<1	1	1	1	3	3	3	3
35–49	7	6.0	15	1	1	9	9	9	9	9
50–64	14	1.1	<1	1	1	1	1	1	2	2
65+	12	1.2	<1	1	1	1	1	3	3	3
2. MULTIPLE DX										
0–19 Years	9	3.3	1	2	2	4	4	4	4	6
20–34	17	5.8	7	2	3	8	8	8	8	8
35–49	34	4.0	16	1	1	2	5	10	15	15
50–64	45	2.4	6	1	1	1	3	5	7	7
65+	52	4.2	48	1	1	1	3	20	20	31
TOTAL SINGLE DX	41	3.4	8	1	1	1	5	9	9	9
MULTIPLE DX	157	4.1	18	1	1	2	6	8	13	20
TOTAL										
0–19 Years	12	3.9	2	2	4	4	5	5	5	6
20–34	22	5.5	8	2	3	8	8	8	8	8
35–49	41	4.2	17	1	1	2	6	9	15	15
50–64	59	2.2	5	1	1	1	2	5	7	13
65+	64	3.6	40	1	1	1	3	9	20	31
GRAND TOTAL	198	4.0	17	1	1	2	5	8	10	20

Length of Stay by Diagnosis and Operation, United States, 1997

United States, October 1995–September 1996 Data, by Operation

82.4: SUTURE HAND SOFT TISSUE. Formerly included in operation group(s) 755.

Type of Patients	Observed Patients	Avg. Stay	Variance	10th	25th	50th	75th	90th	95th	99th
1. SINGLE DX										
0–19 Years	57	1.5	<1	1	1	1	2	2	3	4
20–34	143	1.6	<1	1	1	1	2	2	3	5
35–49	63	2.5	6	1	1	1	3	7	9	9
50–64	13	1.6	<1	1	1	2	2	2	2	2
65+	8	2.0	<1	2	2	2	2	3	3	5
2. MULTIPLE DX										
0–19 Years	138	1.7	2	1	1	2	2	3	4	7
20–34	320	2.1	3	1	1	2	3	4	5	11
35–49	162	2.2	4	1	1	2	3	4	6	10
50–64	65	2.4	5	1	1	1	3	6	8	10
65+	62	3.6	19	1	1	2	5	7	17	17
TOTAL SINGLE DX	284	1.7	2	1	1	1	2	3	4	8
MULTIPLE DX	747	2.1	4	1	1	1	3	4	6	10
TOTAL										
0–19 Years	195	1.6	1	1	1	1	2	3	4	7
20–34	463	2.0	3	1	1	1	2	3	5	9
35–49	225	2.3	4	1	1	2	2	4	7	10
50–64	78	2.3	5	1	1	2	2	6	8	10
65+	70	3.3	16	1	1	2	4	6	17	17
GRAND TOTAL	1031	2.0	3	1	1	1	2	4	5	10

82.45: SUTURE HAND TENDON NEC. Formerly included in operation group(s) 755.

Type of Patients	Observed Patients	Avg. Stay	Variance	10th	25th	50th	75th	90th	95th	99th
1. SINGLE DX										
0–19 Years	24	1.3	<1	1	1	1	2	2	2	3
20–34	62	1.7	<1	1	1	1	3	3	3	5
35–49	29	2.6	6	1	1	1	4	7	7	12
50–64	5	1.6	<1	1	1	2	2	2	2	2
65+	3	2.9	2	1	1	3	3	5	5	5
2. MULTIPLE DX										
0–19 Years	51	1.9	3	1	1	1	2	3	4	9
20–34	139	2.2	4	1	1	2	3	4	5	13
35–49	71	2.2	2	1	1	2	3	4	5	8
50–64	22	2.9	6	1	1	2	3	8	8	8
65+	30	4.9	32	1	1	2	5	17	17	17
TOTAL SINGLE DX	123	1.8	2	1	1	1	2	3	5	7
MULTIPLE DX	313	2.3	5	1	1	2	3	4	6	13
TOTAL										
0–19 Years	75	1.7	2	1	1	1	2	3	4	9
20–34	201	2.1	3	1	1	2	2	4	5	13
35–49	100	2.3	3	1	1	2	3	6	6	9
50–64	27	2.7	5	1	1	2	3	8	8	8
65+	33	4.8	30	1	1	2	5	17	17	17
GRAND TOTAL	436	2.2	4	1	1	2	3	4	6	13

82.44: SUT FLEXOR TEND HAND NEC. Formerly included in operation group(s) 755.

Type of Patients	Observed Patients	Avg. Stay	Variance	10th	25th	50th	75th	90th	95th	99th
1. SINGLE DX										
0–19 Years	23	1.6	<1	1	1	1	2	2	3	5
20–34	62	1.6	1	1	1	1	2	3	3	8
35–49	26	2.7	6	1	1	2	3	7	9	9
50–64	7	1.7	<1	1	1	2	2	2	2	2
65+	5	1.9	<1	2	2	2	2	3	3	3
2. MULTIPLE DX										
0–19 Years	66	1.4	2	1	1	1	1	3	4	7
20–34	150	2.2	3	1	1	2	3	4	6	9
35–49	75	1.9	1	1	1	1	2	3	4	10
50–64	32	1.6	1	1	1	1	2	3	4	6
65+	20	2.9	4	1	2	2	5	5	7	7
TOTAL SINGLE DX	123	1.8	2	1	1	1	2	3	4	9
MULTIPLE DX	343	1.9	2	1	1	1	2	3	5	7
TOTAL										
0–19 Years	89	1.4	<1	1	1	1	1	3	4	6
20–34	212	2.0	2	1	1	1	2	3	6	8
35–49	101	2.0	4	1	1	1	2	3	6	10
50–64	39	1.6	1	1	1	1	2	3	4	6
65+	25	2.6	3	1	1	2	5	5	5	7
GRAND TOTAL	466	1.9	2	1	1	1	2	3	5	9

82.5: HAND MUSC/TEND TRANSPL. Formerly included in operation group(s) 755.

Type of Patients	Observed Patients	Avg. Stay	Variance	10th	25th	50th	75th	90th	95th	99th
1. SINGLE DX										
0–19 Years	11	1.1	<1	1	1	1	1	2	2	2
20–34	5	2.7	4	1	1	1	5	5	5	5
35–49	2	1.0	0	1	1	1	1	1	1	1
50–64	2	1.0	0	1	1	1	1	1	1	1
65+	1	1.0	0	1	1	1	1	1	1	1
2. MULTIPLE DX										
0–19 Years	28	1.4	<1	1	1	1	1	3	4	4
20–34	12	5.2	185	1	1	1	4	4	58	58
35–49	18	2.1	2	1	1	2	4	4	4	4
50–64	19	1.6	<1	1	1	1	2	2	3	3
65+	29	3.3	4	2	2	4	4	4	7	8
TOTAL SINGLE DX	21	1.4	<1	1	1	1	1	2	5	5
MULTIPLE DX	106	2.4	17	1	1	1	3	4	4	8
TOTAL										
0–19 Years	39	1.3	<1	1	1	1	1	2	3	4
20–34	17	4.5	133	1	1	1	4	5	5	58
35–49	20	2.0	1	1	1	2	2	3	3	4
50–64	21	1.5	<1	1	1	1	2	2	3	3
65+	30	3.2	4	2	2	4	4	4	6	8
GRAND TOTAL	127	2.3	15	1	1	1	3	4	4	8

Length of Stay by Diagnosis and Operation, United States, 1997

United States, October 1995–September 1996 Data, by Operation

82.6: RECONSTRUCTION OF THUMB. Formerly included in operation group(s) 755.

Type of Patients	Observed Patients	Avg. Stay	Vari-ance	10th	25th	50th	75th	90th	95th	99th
1. SINGLE DX										
0–19 Years	15	1.2	<1	1	1	1	1	2	2	2
20–34	1	3.0	0	3	3	3	3	3	3	3
35–49	3	5.8	9	1	3	8	8	8	8	8
50–64	3	1.0	0	1	1	1	1	1	1	1
65+	0									
2. MULTIPLE DX										
0–19 Years	32	3.0	33	1	1	1	1	6	23	23
20–34	10	4.5	10	1	2	2	9	9	9	9
35–49	7	10.4	37	6	6	9	11	21	21	21
50–64	3	5.8	1	5	5	5	7	7	7	7
65+	4	1.2	<1	1	1	1	1	2	2	2
TOTAL SINGLE DX	22	1.8	4	1	1	1	2	3	8	8
MULTIPLE DX	56	4.2	32	1	1	1	6	9	21	23
TOTAL										
0–19 Years	47	2.2	20	1	1	1	1	3	7	23
20–34	11	4.4	10	1	2	2	6	9	9	9
35–49	10	8.6	31	2	6	8	9	21	21	21
50–64	6	3.4	7	1	1	5	5	7	7	7
65+	4	1.2	<1	1	1	1	1	2	2	2
GRAND TOTAL	78	3.3	23	1	1	1	3	9	11	23

82.7: PLASTIC OP HND GRFT/IMPL. Formerly included in operation group(s) 755.

Type of Patients	Observed Patients	Avg. Stay	Vari-ance	10th	25th	50th	75th	90th	95th	99th
1. SINGLE DX										
0–19 Years	9	1.4	<1	1	1	1	1	2	2	2
20–34	10	1.3	<1	1	1	1	1	2	2	3
35–49	9	1.1	<1	1	1	1	1	1	1	3
50–64	0									
65+	0									
2. MULTIPLE DX										
0–19 Years	14	2.9	24	1	1	1	1	16	16	16
20–34	16	1.7	3	1	1	1	2	3	3	10
35–49	14	2.2	2	1	1	2	6	5	5	5
50–64	8	4.0	5	2	3	3	6	8	8	8
65+	4	2.9	8	1	1	1	7	7	7	7
TOTAL SINGLE DX	28	1.2	<1	1	1	1	1	2	2	3
MULTIPLE DX	56	2.5	9	1	1	1	3	5	8	16
TOTAL										
0–19 Years	23	2.4	16	1	1	1	2	2	16	16
20–34	26	1.5	2	1	1	1	2	3	3	10
35–49	23	1.7	1	1	1	1	1	3	3	5
50–64	8	4.0	5	2	3	3	6	8	8	8
65+	4	2.9	8	1	1	1	7	7	7	7
GRAND TOTAL	84	2.0	6	1	1	1	2	3	7	16

82.8: OTHER PLASTIC OPS HAND. Formerly included in operation group(s) 755.

Type of Patients	Observed Patients	Avg. Stay	Vari-ance	10th	25th	50th	75th	90th	95th	99th
1. SINGLE DX										
0–19 Years	22	1.7	2	1	1	1	1	5	5	5
20–34	23	1.4	<1	1	1	1	1	3	5	6
35–49	17	2.1	2	1	1	2	3	3	3	7
50–64	3	1.1	<1	1	1	1	1	1	1	3
65+	0									
2. MULTIPLE DX										
0–19 Years	30	2.2	4	1	1	2	2	4	7	10
20–34	36	2.4	2	1	2	2	3	5	6	6
35–49	26	4.3	53	1	1	2	4	8	14	36
50–64	8	9.6	145	1	1	3	28	28	28	28
65+	10	2.8	7	1	1	1	3	7	8	8
TOTAL SINGLE DX	65	1.6	1	1	1	1	2	3	5	6
MULTIPLE DX	110	3.4	28	1	1	2	3	5	10	28
TOTAL										
0–19 Years	52	1.9	3	1	1	1	2	5	5	10
20–34	59	2.2	2	1	1	2	2	5	6	6
35–49	43	3.3	32	1	1	2	3	4	14	36
50–64	11	3.8	61	1	1	1	1	3	28	28
65+	10	2.8	7	2	1	1	3	7	8	8
GRAND TOTAL	175	2.6	17	1	1	1	2	5	6	6

82.9: OTH HAND SOFT TISSUE OPS. Formerly included in operation group(s) 767.

Type of Patients	Observed Patients	Avg. Stay	Vari-ance	10th	25th	50th	75th	90th	95th	99th
1. SINGLE DX										
0–19 Years	5	3.4	5	1	1	3	6	6	6	6
20–34	4	2.9	<1	2	3	3	3	3	3	3
35–49	6	1.4	<1	1	1	1	2	2	3	3
50–64	1	1.0	0	1	1	1	1	1	1	1
65+	1	1.0	0	1	1	1	1	1	1	1
2. MULTIPLE DX										
0–19 Years	8	3.6	17	1	1	1	6	11	11	11
20–34	23	3.3	38	1	1	1	3	4	6	31
35–49	22	3.4	9	1	1	2	5	9	10	10
50–64	11	7.1	26	1	1	12	12	12	12	12
65+	13	4.2	8	2	2	3	5	8	10	10
TOTAL SINGLE DX	17	2.8	2	1	2	3	3	3	6	6
MULTIPLE DX	77	4.1	26	1	1	2	5	12	12	31
TOTAL										
0–19 Years	13	3.5	10	1	1	1	6	6	11	11
20–34	27	3.1	22	1	3	3	3	4	5	31
35–49	28	3.0	8	1	1	2	5	7	10	10
50–64	12	6.9	26	1	1	5	12	12	12	12
65+	14	4.0	8	2	2	3	5	8	10	10
GRAND TOTAL	94	3.7	18	1	1	3	4	10	12	31

Length of Stay by Diagnosis and Operation, United States, 1997

United States, October 1995–September 1996 Data, by Operation

83.0: INC MUSC/TEND/FASC/BURSA. Formerly included in operation group(s) 752.

Type of Patients	Observed Patients	Avg. Stay	Variance	Percentiles						
				10th	25th	50th	75th	90th	95th	99th
1. SINGLE DX										
0–19 Years	109	2.9	5	1	1	2	4	5	8	11
20–34	86	3.0	5	1	1	3	4	5	7	11
35–49	80	3.6	6	1	1	3	6	7	7	7
50–64	35	2.6	5	1	1	2	3	6	7	7
65+	16	2.7	4	1	2	2	3	4	5	11
2. MULTIPLE DX										
0–19 Years	255	4.5	26	1	2	4	5	8	10	31
20–34	280	5.4	38	1	2	3	6	11	17	37
35–49	473	7.9	97	1	3	5	8	17	26	65
50–64	414	7.5	43	2	3	6	9	17	19	34
65+	464	9.4	82	2	3	6	11	23	27	37
TOTAL SINGLE DX	326	3.1	5	1	1	2	4	7	7	11
MULTIPLE DX	1886	7.2	65	1	3	5	8	16	23	40
TOTAL										
0–19 Years	364	4.1	21	1	2	3	5	8	10	31
20–34	366	4.9	32	1	2	3	5	10	16	29
35–49	553	7.4	87	1	3	5	8	16	22	65
50–64	449	7.1	59	1	3	5	9	17	19	34
65+	480	9.2	81	2	3	6	11	23	27	37
GRAND TOTAL	2212	6.6	58	1	2	4	8	14	21	37

83.03: BURSOTOMY. Formerly included in operation group(s) 752.

Type of Patients	Observed Patients	Avg. Stay	Variance	Percentiles						
				10th	25th	50th	75th	90th	95th	99th
1. SINGLE DX										
0–19 Years	9	3.1	2	1	2	3	4	6	6	6
20–34	11	4.1	<1	3	4	3	4	5	6	6
35–49	21	5.5	4	2	4	7	7	7	7	7
50–64	10	3.2	7	2	2	2	3	7	7	14
65+	10	3.6	6	2	2	3	4	5	11	11
2. MULTIPLE DX										
0–19 Years	27	3.7	5	1	2	3	5	8	8	8
20–34	55	4.5	7	2	2	3	5	7	7	24
35–49	148	5.2	19	1	2	4	7	10	11	21
50–64	123	6.5	24	3	3	5	8	11	18	27
65+	167	7.5	33	3	4	6	10	12	16	36
TOTAL SINGLE DX	61	4.4	5	2	2	4	7	7	7	11
MULTIPLE DX	520	5.8	22	2	3	5	7	11	13	26
TOTAL										
0–19 Years	36	3.7	5	1	2	3	5	8	8	8
20–34	66	4.5	6	3	3	4	5	6	7	17
35–49	169	5.3	16	2	3	5	7	10	10	18
50–64	133	6.2	24	2	3	5	8	11	18	27
65+	177	7.4	33	3	4	6	10	12	16	35
GRAND TOTAL	581	5.7	20	2	3	5	7	10	12	24

83.02: MYOTOMY. Formerly included in operation group(s) 752.

Type of Patients	Observed Patients	Avg. Stay	Variance	Percentiles						
				10th	25th	50th	75th	90th	95th	99th
1. SINGLE DX										
0–19 Years	16	2.1	5	1	1	1	2	2	10	11
20–34	8	2.8	2	1	1	3	4	4	5	5
35–49	8	3.1	5	1	1	3	3	7	7	7
50–64	6	1.3	2	1	1	1	1	1	1	9
65+	2	1.6	<1	1	1	2	2	2	2	2
2. MULTIPLE DX										
0–19 Years	48	6.8	101	1	3	4	9	10	57	>99
20–34	42	8.3	47	2	3	7	11	16	19	37
35–49	49	15.2	374	1	5	8	13	65	65	65
50–64	53	9.5	59	1	3	7	13	19	22	>99
65+	51	10.2	85	2	3	7	14	22	28	46
TOTAL SINGLE DX	40	2.1	4	1	1	1	2	4	7	11
MULTIPLE DX	243	10.5	166	2	3	7	12	22	40	65
TOTAL										
0–19 Years	64	5.4	77	1	3	4	7	10	11	>99
20–34	50	7.6	45	2	3	6	10	16	19	37
35–49	57	14.1	353	2	5	8	13	65	65	65
50–64	59	7.5	57	1	3	5	13	17	19	39
65+	53	10.1	84	2	3	7	14	21	28	46
GRAND TOTAL	283	9.1	149	2	3	6	10	19	37	65

83.09: SOFT TISSUE INCISION NEC. Formerly included in operation group(s) 752.

Type of Patients	Observed Patients	Avg. Stay	Variance	Percentiles						
				10th	25th	50th	75th	90th	95th	99th
1. SINGLE DX										
0–19 Years	80	3.2	5	1	1	3	5	5	8	13
20–34	56	3.0	5	1	1	3	5	6	7	9
35–49	37	2.1	2	1	1	2	2	5	6	6
50–64	12	3.5	5	1	2	4	6	6	6	6
65+	3	2.2	<1	2	2	2	2	4	4	4
2. MULTIPLE DX										
0–19 Years	161	4.3	15	1	2	3	6	8	10	24
20–34	158	5.5	50	1	2	3	6	12	19	39
35–49	232	8.4	78	2	3	6	9	17	32	44
50–64	204	8.2	51	2	3	7	10	18	24	44
65+	223	11.8	117	2	4	7	14	26	37	37
TOTAL SINGLE DX	188	2.9	5	1	1	2	4	5	7	8
MULTIPLE DX	978	7.6	67	1	3	5	9	18	25	37
TOTAL										
0–19 Years	241	4.0	12	1	2	3	5	7	10	17
20–34	214	4.9	41	1	2	3	5	10	17	39
35–49	269	7.8	73	1	3	5	8	17	32	44
50–64	216	8.1	50	1	3	7	10	17	24	44
65+	226	11.5	116	2	4	7	19	26	37	37
GRAND TOTAL	1166	7.0	61	1	2	4	8	17	24	37

United States, October 1995–September 1996 Data, by Operation

83.1: MUSC/TEND/FASC DIVISION. Formerly included in operation group(s) 752.

Type of Patients	Observed Patients	Avg. Stay	Vari-ance	Percentiles						
				10th	25th	50th	75th	90th	95th	99th
1. SINGLE DX										
0–19 Years	306	1.9	4	1	1	1	2	4	5	13
20–34	48	2.6	3	1	1	2	3	4	5	8
35–49	54	2.8	5	1	1	2	3	7	7	7
50–64	13	2.0	<1	1	2	2	2	3	3	3
65+	4	2.8	<1	2	3	3	3	3	3	3
2. MULTIPLE DX										
0–19 Years	1282	3.0	15	1	1	2	3	5	8	20
20–34	266	5.8	31	1	2	5	8	11	15	30
35–49	249	5.6	34	1	2	4	7	12	17	29
50–64	147	10.1	172	1	3	6	11	22	47	60
65+	185	7.4	51	2	3	7	8	13	18	27
TOTAL SINGLE DX	425	2.2	4	1	1	2	2	4	7	13
MULTIPLE DX	2129	4.3	33	1	2	3	5	9	12	27
TOTAL										
0–19 Years	1588	2.8	13	1	1	2	3	5	8	16
20–34	314	5.2	27	1	2	4	7	10	15	28
35–49	303	4.9	28	1	2	3	6	11	14	27
50–64	160	9.6	165	1	4	5	10	22	47	60
65+	189	7.0	49	2	3	6	8	13	18	27
GRAND TOTAL	2554	3.9	28	1	2	3	4	8	12	24

83.13: OTHER TENOTOMY. Formerly included in operation group(s) 752.

Type of Patients	Observed Patients	Avg. Stay	Vari-ance	Percentiles						
				10th	25th	50th	75th	90th	95th	99th
1. SINGLE DX										
0–19 Years	99	1.6	1	1	1	1	2	3	3	7
20–34	8	2.1	2	1	1	1	3	3	6	6
35–49	12	1.7	<1	1	1	2	2	3	3	7
50–64	3	1.7	<1	1	1	2	2	3	3	3
65+	2	3.0	<1	3	3	3	3	3	3	3
2. MULTIPLE DX										
0–19 Years	421	2.8	27	1	1	2	3	4	5	21
20–34	49	1.9	4	1	1	2	2	4	5	7
35–49	30	3.1	29	1	1	2	3	4	10	36
50–64	26	3.6	15	1	2	3	4	9	9	26
65+	50	4.3	49	1	2	3	4	7	9	44
TOTAL SINGLE DX	124	1.8	1	1	1	1	2	3	3	6
MULTIPLE DX	576	2.8	26	1	1	2	3	4	6	21
TOTAL										
0–19 Years	520	2.6	23	1	1	2	3	4	5	19
20–34	57	1.9	4	1	1	1	2	3	5	7
35–49	42	2.8	23	1	1	2	3	4	6	36
50–64	29	3.4	14	1	2	3	4	9	9	26
65+	52	4.0	37	1	2	3	4	7	9	44
GRAND TOTAL	700	2.6	22	1	1	2	3	4	6	20

83.12: ADDUCTOR TENOTOMY OF HIP. Formerly included in operation group(s) 752.

Type of Patients	Observed Patients	Avg. Stay	Vari-ance	Percentiles						
				10th	25th	50th	75th	90th	95th	99th
1. SINGLE DX										
0–19 Years	90	2.3	7	1	1	1	2	4	9	13
20–34	0									
35–49	0									
50–64	0									
65+	0									
2. MULTIPLE DX										
0–19 Years	502	2.9	7	1	2	2	3	4	6	20
20–34	17	3.2	3	2	2	3	4	5	7	9
35–49	6	1.4	<1	1	1	1	2	3	3	3
50–64	11	5.7	11	2	4	6	6	11	11	16
65+	35	8.7	68	3	8	8	8	13	18	19
TOTAL SINGLE DX	90	2.3	7	1	1	1	2	4	9	13
MULTIPLE DX	571	3.3	14	1	2	2	4	7	8	20
TOTAL										
0–19 Years	592	2.8	7	1	2	2	3	4	6	15
20–34	17	3.2	3	2	2	3	4	5	7	9
35–49	6	1.4	<1	1	1	1	2	3	3	3
50–64	11	5.7	11	2	4	6	6	11	11	16
65+	35	8.7	68	3	8	8	8	13	18	19
GRAND TOTAL	661	3.2	13	1	2	2	3	6	8	18

83.14: FASCIOTOMY. Formerly included in operation group(s) 752.

Type of Patients	Observed Patients	Avg. Stay	Vari-ance	Percentiles						
				10th	25th	50th	75th	90th	95th	99th
1. SINGLE DX										
0–19 Years	76	2.5	4	1	1	2	3	5	7	9
20–34	26	3.0	4	1	2	3	4	5	8	14
35–49	14	4.1	8	1	1	4	7	7	7	7
50–64	6	2.3	<1	1	2	3	3	3	3	3
65+	0									
2. MULTIPLE DX										
0–19 Years	217	4.3	16	1	2	3	5	9	11	24
20–34	169	7.2	32	1	4	6	9	13	15	37
35–49	168	6.7	39	2	3	4	9	13	18	29
50–64	84	13.7	236	3	4	8	14	32	55	68
65+	78	8.9	34	2	4	8	12	17	21	26
TOTAL SINGLE DX	122	3.1	6	1	1	2	4	7	7	8
MULTIPLE DX	716	6.7	52	1	2	5	8	13	18	45
TOTAL										
0–19 Years	293	3.9	15	1	1	3	5	9	11	19
20–34	195	6.5	30	1	3	6	8	12	15	37
35–49	182	6.2	34	1	3	4	7	12	17	29
50–64	90	13.2	232	2	4	8	14	32	55	68
65+	78	8.9	34	2	4	8	12	17	21	26
GRAND TOTAL	838	6.1	46	1	2	4	8	12	16	37

Length of Stay by Diagnosis and Operation, United States, 1997

United States, October 1995–September 1996 Data, by Operation

83.19: SOFT TISSUE DIVISION NEC. Formerly included in operation group(s) 752.

Type of Patients	Observed Patients	Avg. Stay	Vari-ance	Percentiles						
				10th	25th	50th	75th	90th	95th	99th
1. SINGLE DX										
0–19 Years	38	1.1	<1	1	1	1	1	2	2	2
20–34	13	1.8	<1	1	1	2	2	2	3	3
35–49	28	1.9	<1	1	2	2	2	2	3	5
50–64	3	2.0	0	2	2	2	2	2	2	2
65+	2	1.3	<1	1	1	1	2	2	2	2
2. MULTIPLE DX										
0–19 Years	118	2.5	3	1	2	2	3	4	5	9
20–34	30	4.8	41	1	1	2	5	12	17	30
35–49	42	4.1	14	1	2	2	6	12	19	21
50–64	22	5.7	32	1	1	4	10	15	19	19
65+	21	5.7	15	2	2	5	8	13	13	13
TOTAL SINGLE DX	84	1.5	<1	1	1	1	2	2	2	3
MULTIPLE DX	233	3.5	13	1	2	2	4	7	10	19
TOTAL										
0–19 Years	156	2.0	3	1	1	2	2	4	4	9
20–34	43	3.3	23	1	1	2	3	7	12	30
35–49	70	3.2	9	1	2	2	2	6	7	21
50–64	25	5.0	28	2	2	2	6	15	16	16
65+	23	5.3	16	2	2	5	7	13	13	13
GRAND TOTAL	317	2.8	10	1	1	2	3	6	8	17

83.2: SOFT TISSUE DXTIC PX. Formerly included in operation group(s) 753, 767.

Type of Patients	Observed Patients	Avg. Stay	Vari-ance	Percentiles						
				10th	25th	50th	75th	90th	95th	99th
1. SINGLE DX										
0–19 Years	112	2.9	6	1	1	2	4	7	8	11
20–34	42	4.2	22	1	1	2	6	9	16	19
35–49	33	3.8	32	1	1	2	3	9	23	23
50–64	34	1.7	2	2	1	1	1	1	5	5
65+	26	2.0	32	1	1	1	2	1	4	41
2. MULTIPLE DX										
0–19 Years	269	10.4	150	1	3	6	14	22	43	63
20–34	161	9.0	61	1	3	7	16	22	64	>99
35–49	301	9.0	60	2	4	7	11	18	28	33
50–64	334	7.1	71	1	1	5	9	18	24	41
65+	797	9.0	87	1	2	7	11	17	24	52
TOTAL SINGLE DX	247	2.3	13	1	1	1	2	5	7	17
MULTIPLE DX	1946	8.8	86	1	3	6	11	19	28	52
TOTAL										
0–19 Years	381	8.4	123	1	2	5	11	17	31	62
20–34	203	8.2	58	1	3	6	14	21	33	>99
35–49	334	8.8	60	2	4	7	11	18	28	33
50–64	452	5.4	56	1	1	5	7	14	22	39
65+	823	8.3	86	1	2	6	11	16	23	52
GRAND TOTAL	2193	7.7	79	1	1	5	10	17	24	51

83.21: SOFT TISSUE BIOPSY. Formerly included in operation group(s) 753.

Type of Patients	Observed Patients	Avg. Stay	Vari-ance	Percentiles						
				10th	25th	50th	75th	90th	95th	99th
1. SINGLE DX										
0–19 Years	112	2.9	6	1	1	2	4	7	8	11
20–34	42	4.2	22	1	1	2	6	9	16	19
35–49	32	3.8	33	1	1	2	4	10	23	23
50–64	34	1.7	2	1	1	1	1	5	5	5
65+	26	2.0	32	1	1	1	1	1	4	41
2. MULTIPLE DX										
0–19 Years	269	10.4	150	1	3	6	14	22	43	63
20–34	161	9.0	61	1	3	7	16	22	64	>99
35–49	301	9.0	60	2	4	7	11	18	28	33
50–64	418	7.1	71	1	1	5	9	18	24	41
65+	793	9.0	87	1	2	7	11	17	24	52
TOTAL SINGLE DX	246	2.3	13	1	1	1	2	5	7	17
MULTIPLE DX	1942	8.8	86	1	3	6	11	18	28	52
TOTAL										
0–19 Years	381	8.4	123	1	2	5	11	17	31	62
20–34	203	8.2	58	1	3	6	14	21	33	>99
35–49	333	8.8	60	2	4	7	11	18	28	33
50–64	452	5.4	56	1	1	5	7	14	22	39
65+	819	8.3	86	1	2	6	11	16	23	52
GRAND TOTAL	2188	7.6	79	1	1	5	10	17	24	51

83.3: EXC LES SOFT TISSUE. Formerly included in operation group(s) 753.

Type of Patients	Observed Patients	Avg. Stay	Vari-ance	Percentiles						
				10th	25th	50th	75th	90th	95th	99th
1. SINGLE DX										
0–19 Years	168	2.4	5	1	1	1	3	5	9	9
20–34	96	1.6	2	1	1	1	2	3	4	10
35–49	124	2.4	6	1	1	1	3	5	8	12
50–64	96	2.6	5	2	1	2	4	4	5	10
65+	51	1.7	2	1	1	1	2	4	4	7
2. MULTIPLE DX										
0–19 Years	125	3.2	23	1	2	2	4	6	9	19
20–34	145	5.1	17	1	2	3	8	11	12	16
35–49	288	4.5	49	1	2	2	5	9	12	31
50–64	339	4.2	36	1	2	2	4	8	15	33
65+	547	6.4	71	1	2	4	8	15	20	58
TOTAL SINGLE DX	535	2.2	5	1	1	1	3	5	7	12
MULTIPLE DX	1444	4.9	48	1	2	2	6	11	15	33
TOTAL										
0–19 Years	293	2.8	14	1	1	1	3	6	9	14
20–34	241	3.5	13	1	2	2	5	9	11	16
35–49	412	3.8	37	1	1	2	4	9	11	30
50–64	435	3.8	30	1	2	2	7	9	14	29
65+	598	6.0	66	1	3	3	7	14	18	58
GRAND TOTAL	1979	4.1	37	1	1	2	5	9	14	30

Length of Stay by Diagnosis and Operation, United States, 1997

United States, October 1995–September 1996 Data, by Operation

83.32: EXC LESION OF MUSCLE. Formerly included in operation group(s) 753.

Type of Patients	Observed Patients	Avg. Stay	Vari-ance	10th	25th	50th	75th	90th	95th	99th
1. SINGLE DX										
0–19 Years	41	2.0	2	1	1	1	3	4	5	9
20–34	25	1.5	<1	1	1	1	2	2	4	5
35–49	33	2.5	1	1	2	1	3	4	5	5
50–64	28	1.9	2	1	1	1	2	5	5	5
65+	14	1.2	<1	1	1	1	1	2	3	3
2. MULTIPLE DX										
0–19 Years	27	3.5	24	1	2	2	4	5	7	32
20–34	45	4.7	15	1	2	4	6	9	15	17
35–49	63	3.9	15	1	1	2	5	8	12	20
50–64	84	4.8	46	1	2	3	5	9	15	41
65+	100	9.9	234	1	2	4	8	39	58	58
TOTAL SINGLE DX	141	1.9	2	1	1	1	3	4	5	5
MULTIPLE DX	319	5.6	82	1	2	3	6	11	22	58
TOTAL										
0–19 Years	68	2.6	12	1	1	2	3	4	5	22
20–34	70	3.5	12	1	1	2	4	8	10	15
35–49	96	3.5	11	1	1	2	4	7	11	14
50–64	112	4.1	37	1	1	2	4	8	11	41
65+	114	7.4	181	1	2	2	5	22	39	58
GRAND TOTAL	460	4.3	56	1	1	2	4	8	13	41

83.4: OTHER EXC MUSC/TEND/FASC. Formerly included in operation group(s) 756.

Type of Patients	Observed Patients	Avg. Stay	Vari-ance	10th	25th	50th	75th	90th	95th	99th
1. SINGLE DX										
0–19 Years	32	2.3	5	1	1	1	3	5	6	13
20–34	41	2.8	5	1	1	2	3	7	7	10
35–49	57	1.9	1	1	1	2	2	3	4	5
50–64	30	2.0	2	1	1	1	2	4	5	6
65+	9	2.8	3	1	2	2	3	6	6	6
2. MULTIPLE DX										
0–19 Years	60	7.8	88	1	1	5	9	21	24	49
20–34	105	4.7	31	1	2	3	5	8	15	31
35–49	169	8.3	95	1	1	4	11	27	28	33
50–64	158	7.9	96	1	2	4	9	24	24	38
65+	205	7.7	58	1	2	5	11	14	22	42
TOTAL SINGLE DX	169	2.2	3	1	1	2	3	5	5	7
MULTIPLE DX	697	7.3	75	1	2	4	9	20	27	38
TOTAL										
0–19 Years	92	5.7	63	1	1	2	6	15	24	49
20–34	146	4.4	27	1	2	3	5	8	15	27
35–49	226	6.7	79	1	1	3	7	22	28	33
50–64	188	6.7	83	1	1	3	8	23	24	38
65+	214	7.5	57	1	2	5	11	14	22	42
GRAND TOTAL	866	6.3	65	1	1	3	8	16	24	38

83.39: EXC LES SOFT TISSUE NEC. Formerly included in operation group(s) 753.

Type of Patients	Observed Patients	Avg. Stay	Vari-ance	10th	25th	50th	75th	90th	95th	99th
1. SINGLE DX										
0–19 Years	119	2.6	6	1	1	2	3	4	9	10
20–34	65	1.7	3	1	1	1	2	2	4	11
35–49	87	2.3	7	1	2	2	3	4	9	12
50–64	65	3.0	6	1	1	2	2	5	9	10
65+	36	2.5	2	1	1	2	3	2	6	7
2. MULTIPLE DX										
0–19 Years	93	3.1	23	1	1	1	4	6	9	18
20–34	88	5.6	18	1	2	5	8	11	12	16
35–49	213	4.6	56	1	1	2	5	9	13	31
50–64	247	4.2	37	1	1	2	4	13	15	29
65+	432	5.9	43	1	2	4	8	15	15	27
TOTAL SINGLE DX	372	2.4	6	1	1	1	3	5	9	12
MULTIPLE DX	1073	4.8	42	1	1	3	6	11	15	29
TOTAL										
0–19 Years	212	2.9	15	1	1	1	3	6	9	14
20–34	153	3.7	15	1	2	2	5	10	11	16
35–49	300	3.9	42	1	1	2	4	8	12	31
50–64	312	4.0	30	1	1	2	4	9	15	29
65+	468	5.8	42	1	2	3	8	14	15	27
GRAND TOTAL	1445	4.2	33	1	1	2	5	10	14	29

83.45: OTHER MYECTOMY. Formerly included in operation group(s) 756.

Type of Patients	Observed Patients	Avg. Stay	Vari-ance	10th	25th	50th	75th	90th	95th	99th
1. SINGLE DX										
0–19 Years	12	3.2	13	1	1	2	3	7	13	13
20–34	21	1.7	5	1	1	1	2	3	5	5
35–49	29	1.9	<1	1	1	2	2	3	5	5
50–64	15	1.5	1	1	1	1	2	3	5	5
65+	4	1.7	<1	1	1	1	2	3	3	3
2. MULTIPLE DX										
0–19 Years	27	8.4	51	1	3	6	9	20	21	31
20–34	58	4.8	32	1	2	3	5	9	21	31
35–49	90	9.4	103	1	2	4	15	28	31	33
50–64	72	9.1	88	2	3	6	23	23	35	38
65+	80	10.3	63	2	4	10	13	18	30	42
TOTAL SINGLE DX	81	1.9	2	1	1	1	2	3	5	7
MULTIPLE DX	327	8.3	76	1	3	5	10	22	28	38
TOTAL										
0–19 Years	39	7.0	46	1	2	5	9	20	20	31
20–34	79	4.4	29	1	1	3	4	8	18	27
35–49	119	7.3	85	1	1	3	8	28	28	33
50–64	87	7.1	76	1	3	4	8	21	31	38
65+	84	9.9	63	2	3	9	12	18	30	42
GRAND TOTAL	408	6.9	67	1	2	3	9	20	28	37

Length of Stay by Diagnosis and Operation, United States, 1997

United States, October 1995–September 1996 Data, by Operation

83.5: BURSECTOMY. Formerly included in operation group(s) 756.

Type of Patients	Observed Patients	Avg. Stay	Variance	10th	25th	50th	75th	90th	95th	99th
1. SINGLE DX										
0–19 Years	2	1.2	<1	1	1	1	1	2	2	2
20–34	16	1.9	1	1	1	1	1	2	2	4
35–49	39	2.1	3	1	1	1	3	3	4	9
50–64	34	1.7	3	1	1	1	2	3	4	10
65+	15	1.7	2	1	1	1	2	3	3	10
2. MULTIPLE DX										
0–19 Years	15	5.1	15	2	3	3	8	13	13	13
20–34	57	2.5	3	1	1	1	4	7	7	8
35–49	192	3.6	15	1	1	2	4	10	13	16
50–64	222	3.5	18	1	1	2	5	7	8	27
65+	255	4.1	16	1	1	3	5	10	13	18
TOTAL SINGLE DX	106	1.8	2	1	1	1	2	3	4	9
MULTIPLE DX	741	3.6	15	1	1	2	5	8	12	18
TOTAL										
0–19 Years	17	4.6	15	1	2	3	4	11	13	13
20–34	73	2.4	3	1	1	2	4	4	7	8
35–49	231	3.3	13	1	1	2	4	7	13	16
50–64	256	3.1	15	1	1	2	4	7	8	23
65+	270	3.8	15	1	1	2	5	9	13	18
GRAND TOTAL	847	3.3	13	1	1	2	4	7	11	16

83.6: SUTURE MUSC/TENDON/FASC. Formerly included in operation group(s) 756.

Type of Patients	Observed Patients	Avg. Stay	Variance	10th	25th	50th	75th	90th	95th	99th
1. SINGLE DX										
0–19 Years	135	1.6	<1	1	1	1	2	3	3	4
20–34	432	1.7	1	1	1	1	2	3	4	7
35–49	808	1.5	<1	1	1	1	2	3	3	4
50–64	932	1.6	<1	1	1	1	2	3	3	4
65+	489	1.8	1	1	1	1	2	3	4	6
2. MULTIPLE DX										
0–19 Years	200	2.3	3	1	1	2	3	5	5	8
20–34	541	2.7	8	1	1	2	3	6	7	14
35–49	1203	2.0	5	1	1	1	2	3	4	8
50–64	2247	1.9	2	1	1	2	2	3	4	11
65+	2694	2.4	5	1	1	2	3	4	6	10
TOTAL SINGLE DX	2796	1.6	<1	1	1	1	2	3	3	5
MULTIPLE DX	6885	2.2	4	1	1	2	2	4	5	11
TOTAL										
0–19 Years	335	2.0	3	1	1	2	2	4	5	7
20–34	973	2.3	6	1	1	2	3	4	6	12
35–49	2011	1.8	3	1	1	1	2	3	4	6
50–64	3179	1.8	2	1	1	2	2	3	4	8
65+	3183	2.3	5	1	1	2	3	4	5	9
GRAND TOTAL	9681	2.0	3	1	1	2	2	3	4	9

83.63: ROTATOR CUFF REPAIR. Formerly included in operation group(s) 756.

Type of Patients	Observed Patients	Avg. Stay	Variance	10th	25th	50th	75th	90th	95th	99th
1. SINGLE DX										
0–19 Years	6	1.8	<1	1	1	2	2	2	3	3
20–34	58	1.5	<1	1	1	1	2	2	3	3
35–49	433	1.3	<1	1	1	1	2	2	2	3
50–64	793	1.6	<1	1	1	1	2	3	3	3
65+	446	1.6	<1	1	1	1	2	3	3	4
2. MULTIPLE DX										
0–19 Years	3	1.4	<1	1	1	1	2	2	2	3
20–34	59	1.5	<1	1	1	1	2	2	2	3
35–49	706	1.6	<1	1	1	1	2	2	3	4
50–64	1912	1.7	<1	1	1	2	2	3	3	4
65+	2362	2.1	3	1	1	2	3	3	4	7
TOTAL SINGLE DX	1736	1.5	<1	1	1	1	2	2	3	4
MULTIPLE DX	5042	1.8	2	1	1	2	2	3	4	6
TOTAL										
0–19 Years	9	1.7	<1	1	1	2	2	3	3	3
20–34	117	1.5	<1	1	1	1	2	2	3	3
35–49	1139	1.5	<1	1	1	1	2	2	3	3
50–64	2705	1.7	<1	1	1	2	2	3	3	4
65+	2808	2.0	3	1	1	2	3	3	4	7
GRAND TOTAL	6778	1.8	1	1	1	2	2	3	3	6

83.64: OTHER SUTURE OF TENDON. Formerly included in operation group(s) 756.

Type of Patients	Observed Patients	Avg. Stay	Variance	10th	25th	50th	75th	90th	95th	99th
1. SINGLE DX										
0–19 Years	88	1.6	<1	1	1	1	2	3	3	4
20–34	285	1.7	1	1	1	1	2	3	4	7
35–49	308	1.6	<1	1	1	1	2	3	4	4
50–64	109	1.8	2	1	1	1	2	3	4	10
65+	31	3.4	7	1	1	3	5	6	6	14
2. MULTIPLE DX										
0–19 Years	113	2.0	4	1	1	1	2	4	4	11
20–34	272	2.9	11	1	1	2	3	7	11	19
35–49	278	2.3	3	1	1	2	4	6	6	8
50–64	202	3.4	11	1	1	2	4	8	11	14
65+	208	4.1	19	1	2	3	5	8	9	15
TOTAL SINGLE DX	821	1.7	1	1	1	1	2	3	4	7
MULTIPLE DX	1073	2.9	10	1	1	2	3	6	9	14
TOTAL										
0–19 Years	201	1.7	2	1	1	1	2	3	4	6
20–34	557	2.3	7	1	1	2	3	4	7	12
35–49	586	1.9	2	1	1	1	3	4	4	6
50–64	311	2.8	8	1	1	2	3	6	11	12
65+	239	4.0	18	1	2	3	5	7	9	15
GRAND TOTAL	1894	2.3	6	1	1	2	3	4	6	12

Length of Stay by Diagnosis and Operation, United States, 1997

United States, October 1995–September 1996 Data, by Operation

83.65: OTHER MUSCLE/FASC SUTURE. Formerly included in operation group(s) 756.

Type of Patients	Observed Patients	Avg. Stay	Vari-ance	10th	25th	50th	75th	90th	95th	99th
1. SINGLE DX										
0–19 Years	31	1.5	1	1	1	1	2	2	4	7
20–34	54	1.7	1	1	1	1	2	2	4	5
35–49	33	1.7	2	1	1	1	2	3	5	7
50–64	17	2.7	2	1	1	3	4	4	4	4
65+	7	2.5	<1	1	2	3	3	3	3	6
2. MULTIPLE DX										
0–19 Years	74	2.4	2	1	1	2	3	4	4	8
20–34	187	2.9	6	1	1	2	4	6	6	12
35–49	183	2.8	24	1	1	2	3	4	8	15
50–64	107	3.9	11	1	2	3	4	9	11	14
65+	77	4.1	16	1	1	3	5	7	12	19
TOTAL SINGLE DX	142	1.9	1	1	1	1	2	4	4	5
MULTIPLE DX	628	3.0	13	1	1	2	4	5	7	14
TOTAL										
0–19 Years	105	2.2	2	1	1	2	3	4	4	8
20–34	241	2.6	5	1	1	2	3	5	6	12
35–49	216	2.6	22	1	1	2	3	4	7	11
50–64	124	3.6	9	1	2	3	4	8	11	14
65+	84	3.9	14	1	1	3	5	7	12	19
GRAND TOTAL	770	2.8	11	1	1	2	3	5	7	14

83.75: TENDON TRANSF/TRANSPL. Formerly included in operation group(s) 757.

Type of Patients	Observed Patients	Avg. Stay	Vari-ance	10th	25th	50th	75th	90th	95th	99th
1. SINGLE DX										
0–19 Years	78	1.5	<1	1	1	1	2	2	3	4
20–34	32	1.5	<1	1	1	1	2	3	3	5
35–49	22	2.1	<1	1	1	2	2	4	4	4
50–64	14	1.3	<1	1	1	1	2	2	2	2
65+	3	1.7	<1	1	1	2	2	2	2	2
2. MULTIPLE DX										
0–19 Years	207	1.7	3	1	1	1	2	3	3	6
20–34	59	1.8	1	1	1	1	2	3	3	6
35–49	70	2.0	3	1	1	2	2	3	4	8
50–64	50	2.6	3	1	2	2	3	3	3	9
65+	50	2.6	2	1	2	2	3	4	7	9
TOTAL SINGLE DX	149	1.6	<1	1	1	1	2	2	4	5
MULTIPLE DX	436	1.9	3	1	1	2	2	3	4	8
TOTAL										
0–19 Years	285	1.6	2	1	1	1	2	3	3	5
20–34	91	1.6	1	1	1	1	2	3	4	5
35–49	92	2.0	2	1	1	2	3	3	3	8
50–64	64	2.3	3	1	2	2	3	3	3	9
65+	53	2.6	2	1	2	2	3	4	7	9
GRAND TOTAL	585	1.8	2	1	1	1	2	3	4	7

83.7: MUSCLE/TENDON RECONST. Formerly included in operation group(s) 757.

Type of Patients	Observed Patients	Avg. Stay	Vari-ance	10th	25th	50th	75th	90th	95th	99th
1. SINGLE DX										
0–19 Years	107	1.6	<1	1	1	1	2	3	3	4
20–34	49	1.8	5	1	1	1	2	3	4	19
35–49	41	2.1	2	1	1	2	2	4	5	9
50–64	23	1.4	<1	1	1	1	4	4	4	9
65+	8	2.6	<1	1	2	3	3	3	4	4
2. MULTIPLE DX										
0–19 Years	309	1.8	3	1	1	1	2	3	4	6
20–34	82	2.7	18	1	1	2	3	4	5	>99
35–49	104	2.2	3	1	1	2	3	4	8	11
50–64	85	3.7	20	1	2	2	3	9	15	15
65+	96	3.5	8	1	2	3	4	7	9	13
TOTAL SINGLE DX	228	1.7	2	1	1	1	2	3	4	5
MULTIPLE DX	676	2.3	8	1	1	2	3	4	5	15
TOTAL										
0–19 Years	416	1.7	2	1	1	1	2	3	4	6
20–34	131	2.3	12	1	1	2	2	4	5	28
35–49	145	2.1	3	1	1	2	2	4	5	9
50–64	108	3.3	17	1	2	2	3	6	15	15
65+	104	3.4	7	1	2	3	3	7	8	13
GRAND TOTAL	904	2.2	6	1	1	2	2	4	5	15

83.8: MUSC/TEND/FASC OP NEC. Formerly included in operation group(s) 757.

Type of Patients	Observed Patients	Avg. Stay	Vari-ance	10th	25th	50th	75th	90th	95th	99th
1. SINGLE DX										
0–19 Years	955	1.6	1	1	1	1	2	3	3	5
20–34	211	1.9	2	1	1	2	2	3	5	9
35–49	306	1.9	1	1	1	2	2	3	4	6
50–64	146	1.7	1	1	1	1	2	3	4	6
65+	80	2.5	2	1	1	2	3	4	5	7
2. MULTIPLE DX										
0–19 Years	1335	2.2	6	1	1	2	2	4	5	12
20–34	272	3.4	57	1	1	2	3	5	8	53
35–49	413	3.8	48	1	1	2	5	7	13	27
50–64	431	5.5	101	1	1	2	5	14	25	>99
65+	509	5.7	56	1	2	4	6	11	20	44
TOTAL SINGLE DX	1698	1.7	1	1	1	1	2	3	4	7
MULTIPLE DX	2960	3.4	38	1	1	2	3	6	12	35
TOTAL										
0–19 Years	2290	1.9	4	1	1	1	2	3	4	9
20–34	483	2.8	35	1	1	2	3	5	6	20
35–49	719	3.0	30	1	1	2	3	5	10	21
50–64	577	4.4	75	1	1	3	3	12	18	90
65+	589	5.3	50	1	2	3	6	9	17	38
GRAND TOTAL	4658	2.8	26	1	1	2	3	5	7	25

Length of Stay by Diagnosis and Operation, United States, 1997

United States, October 1995–September 1996 Data, by Operation

83.84: CLUBFOOT RELEASE NEC. Formerly included in operation group(s) 757.

Type of Patients	Observed Patients	Avg. Stay	Variance	10th	25th	50th	75th	90th	95th	99th
1. SINGLE DX										
0–19 Years	691	1.5	<1	1	1	1	2	2	3	7
20–34	1	2.0	0	2	1	2	2	2	2	2
35–49	0									
50–64	0									
65+	0									
2. MULTIPLE DX										
0–19 Years	298	2.1	6	1	1	2	2	3	4	7
20–34	1	1.0	0	1	1	1	1	1	1	1
35–49	2	2.9	<1	2	3	3	3	3	3	3
50–64	1	2.0	0	2	2	2	2	2	2	2
65+	1	9.0	0	9	9	9	9	9	9	9
TOTAL SINGLE DX	692	1.5	1	1	1	1	2	2	3	7
MULTIPLE DX	303	2.1	6	1	1	2	2	3	4	9
TOTAL										
0–19 Years	989	1.7	3	1	1	1	2	3	3	7
20–34	2	1.2	<1	1	1	1	1	2	2	2
35–49	2	2.9	<1	2	3	3	3	3	3	3
50–64	1	2.0	0	2	2	2	2	2	2	2
65+	1	9.0	0	9	9	9	9	9	9	9
GRAND TOTAL	995	1.7	3	1	1	1	2	3	3	9

83.85: CHANGE IN M/T LENGTH NEC. Formerly included in operation group(s) 757.

Type of Patients	Observed Patients	Avg. Stay	Variance	10th	25th	50th	75th	90th	95th	99th
1. SINGLE DX										
0–19 Years	209	1.6	<1	1	1	1	2	3	4	4
20–34	8	2.0	1	1	1	2	2	3	5	5
35–49	16	1.8	<1	1	2	2	2	3	3	5
50–64	4	2.0	<1	2	2	2	2	3	3	3
65+	1	1.0	0	1	1	1	1	1	1	1
2. MULTIPLE DX										
0–19 Years	944	1.9	2	1	1	2	2	3	4	7
20–34	75	2.7	7	1	1	2	3	4	6	20
35–49	65	3.2	35	1	2	2	3	5	5	34
50–64	51	3.8	25	1	1	2	3	11	11	23
65+	43	3.1	5	1	1	3	4	6	6	16
TOTAL SINGLE DX	238	1.6	<1	1	1	1	2	3	4	4
MULTIPLE DX	1178	2.1	5	1	1	2	2	4	4	11
TOTAL										
0–19 Years	1153	1.9	2	1	1	1	2	3	4	7
20–34	83	2.7	7	1	1	2	3	4	6	20
35–49	81	3.0	31	1	2	2	3	5	5	34
50–64	55	3.6	23	1	1	2	3	11	11	23
65+	44	3.1	5	1	1	3	4	6	6	16
GRAND TOTAL	1416	2.0	4	1	1	2	2	3	4	10

83.86: QUADRICEPSPLASTY. Formerly included in operation group(s) 757.

Type of Patients	Observed Patients	Avg. Stay	Variance	10th	25th	50th	75th	90th	95th	99th
1. SINGLE DX										
0–19 Years	11	1.7	1	1	1	1	2	4	4	4
20–34	11	2.8	1	1	2	3	3	5	7	7
35–49	28	2.7	1	2	2	3	3	4	5	6
50–64	17	3.0	2	2	2	3	4	6	6	6
65+	24	3.0	4	1	1	3	4	7	7	7
2. MULTIPLE DX										
0–19 Years	17	2.3	3	1	2	2	2	4	6	10
20–34	17	2.5	3	1	1	2	3	4	5	6
35–49	50	3.1	5	1	1	2	5	6	8	10
50–64	75	3.8	7	1	2	3	5	8	9	12
65+	103	4.6	17	1	2	4	6	7	15	25
TOTAL SINGLE DX	91	2.7	2	1	2	3	3	4	6	7
MULTIPLE DX	262	3.7	10	1	2	3	5	7	9	18
TOTAL										
0–19 Years	28	2.1	2	1	1	2	2	4	4	10
20–34	28	2.6	2	1	2	3	3	4	5	7
35–49	78	3.0	3	1	2	3	4	5	6	8
50–64	92	3.6	7	1	2	3	4	8	9	9
65+	127	4.3	15	1	2	4	5	7	14	25
GRAND TOTAL	353	3.4	8	1	2	3	4	7	8	17

83.88: OTHER PLASTIC OPS TENDON. Formerly included in operation group(s) 757.

Type of Patients	Observed Patients	Avg. Stay	Variance	10th	25th	50th	75th	90th	95th	99th
1. SINGLE DX										
0–19 Years	25	1.4	<1	1	1	1	2	3	3	6
20–34	161	1.9	2	1	1	1	2	3	4	7
35–49	226	1.8	1	1	1	2	2	3	3	6
50–64	102	1.5	<1	1	1	1	2	3	3	5
65+	45	2.5	2	1	3	3	3	4	4	6
2. MULTIPLE DX										
0–19 Years	39	4.0	22	1	1	2	5	9	12	28
20–34	121	2.3	15	1	1	1	2	4	6	8
35–49	194	2.5	7	1	1	2	3	4	6	16
50–64	208	2.3	3	1	1	2	3	5	6	>99
65+	251	4.4	23	1	2	3	6	7	11	19
TOTAL SINGLE DX	559	1.8	1	1	1	1	2	3	4	6
MULTIPLE DX	813	3.0	13	1	1	2	3	6	8	44
TOTAL										
0–19 Years	64	3.1	16	1	1	1	3	9	9	22
20–34	282	2.1	8	1	1	1	2	4	5	8
35–49	420	2.1	4	1	1	1	3	4	5	10
50–64	310	2.0	2	1	1	1	3	4	5	>99
65+	296	4.1	21	1	2	3	6	7	10	17
GRAND TOTAL	1372	2.5	8	1	1	2	3	5	6	15

United States, October 1995–September 1996 Data, by Operation

83.9: OTHER CONN TISSUE OPS. Formerly included in operation group(s) 757, 767.

Type of Patients	Observed Patients	Avg. Stay	Vari-ance	10th	25th	50th	75th	90th	95th	99th
1. SINGLE DX										
0–19 Years	27	2.9	4	1	1	2	4	7	7	8
20–34	17	2.0	2	1	1	1	3	4	7	5
35–49	25	3.5	7	1	2	3	4	5	6	15
50–64	10	3.1	4	1	1	3	4	5	8	8
65+	7	3.8	3	2	2	4	5	5	7	7
2. MULTIPLE DX										
0–19 Years	53	4.9	55	2	2	2	4	10	15	41
20–34	111	5.7	25	2	2	4	8	13	13	21
35–49	207	8.2	95	2	3	4	8	32	32	32
50–64	242	6.2	50	1	3	4	7	15	15	44
65+	544	7.1	40	2	3	5	9	16	20	30
TOTAL SINGLE DX	86	2.7	4	1	1	2	4	5	6	8
MULTIPLE DX	1157	6.8	54	2	3	4	8	15	21	35
TOTAL										
0–19 Years	80	4.5	46	1	2	2	4	10	15	41
20–34	128	4.9	22	1	2	3	5	13	13	21
35–49	232	7.7	89	2	3	4	7	32	32	32
50–64	252	6.2	49	1	3	4	7	15	15	44
65+	551	7.1	40	2	3	5	9	16	20	30
GRAND TOTAL	1243	6.5	51	1	2	4	8	15	21	32

83.95: SOFT TISSUE ASP NEC. Formerly included in operation group(s) 767.

Type of Patients	Observed Patients	Avg. Stay	Vari-ance	10th	25th	50th	75th	90th	95th	99th
1. SINGLE DX										
0–19 Years	20	3.2	4	1	2	2	4	7	7	8
20–34	12	1.7	1	1	1	1	2	3	5	5
35–49	6	4.3	2	2	2	5	5	6	6	6
50–64	6	4.2	3	2	3	4	4	8	8	8
65+	2	3.6	3	2	2	5	5	5	5	5
2. MULTIPLE DX										
0–19 Years	27	3.7	13	2	2	2	3	10	11	18
20–34	41	6.4	26	2	2	5	8	12	19	25
35–49	64	16.0	162	3	5	8	32	32	32	66
50–64	57	10.0	121	1	2	7	15	15	23	66
65+	144	7.9	58	1	3	5	10	18	22	29
TOTAL SINGLE DX	46	2.5	3	1	1	2	3	5	6	8
MULTIPLE DX	333	9.0	94	1	2	5	11	22	32	33
TOTAL										
0–19 Years	47	3.6	11	2	2	2	4	8	10	18
20–34	53	4.2	19	1	1	2	5	9	12	21
35–49	70	15.1	160	3	5	8	32	32	32	32
50–64	63	9.8	118	1	2	7	15	15	23	66
65+	146	7.9	58	1	3	5	10	18	22	29
GRAND TOTAL	379	8.1	87	1	2	5	10	21	32	32

83.94: ASPIRATION OF BURSA. Formerly included in operation group(s) 767.

Type of Patients	Observed Patients	Avg. Stay	Vari-ance	10th	25th	50th	75th	90th	95th	99th
1. SINGLE DX										
0–19 Years	3	4.4	8	1	1	6	7	7	7	7
20–34	2	3.2	2	1	1	4	4	4	4	4
35–49	6	2.4	3	1	2	2	4	5	5	5
50–64	1	3.0	0	3	3	3	3	3	3	3
65+	0									
2. MULTIPLE DX										
0–19 Years	13	4.3	4	3	4	4	4	5	7	13
20–34	26	3.1	2	1	2	3	4	5	5	6
35–49	76	3.9	7	2	3	3	5	5	8	18
50–64	71	4.1	6	2	3	4	5	6	8	11
65+	120	6.9	27	3	4	5	9	16	19	23
TOTAL SINGLE DX	12	3.1	3	1	1	4	4	5	6	7
MULTIPLE DX	306	4.7	13	2	3	4	5	8	11	20
TOTAL										
0–19 Years	16	4.3	4	3	4	4	4	7	7	13
20–34	28	3.1	2	1	2	3	4	5	5	6
35–49	82	3.8	7	2	3	3	5	5	5	18
50–64	72	4.1	6	2	3	4	5	6	8	11
65+	120	6.9	27	3	4	5	9	16	19	23
GRAND TOTAL	318	4.6	13	2	3	4	5	8	11	19

84.0: AMPUTATION OF UPPER LIMB. Formerly included in operation group(s) 758, 759.

Type of Patients	Observed Patients	Avg. Stay	Vari-ance	10th	25th	50th	75th	90th	95th	99th
1. SINGLE DX										
0–19 Years	66	1.3	2	1	1	1	1	2	2	9
20–34	124	1.8	2	1	1	1	2	4	5	8
35–49	96	1.5	1	1	1	1	2	3	4	6
50–64	62	1.8	1	1	1	1	3	3	6	6
65+	25	2.6	3	1	1	3	3	6	6	6
2. MULTIPLE DX										
0–19 Years	105	3.7	48	1	1	2	3	7	11	32
20–34	214	4.2	17	1	2	3	5	9	12	19
35–49	376	5.2	38	1	1	3	6	11	17	33
50–64	391	7.4	84	1	2	4	7	24	29	37
65+	342	6.3	50	1	2	4	8	15	22	33
TOTAL SINGLE DX	373	1.7	2	1	1	1	2	3	4	8
MULTIPLE DX	1428	5.8	53	1	1	3	7	14	23	36
TOTAL										
0–19 Years	171	2.5	26	1	1	1	2	4	9	31
20–34	338	3.4	13	1	1	2	5	8	10	17
35–49	472	4.4	32	1	1	3	5	10	15	29
50–64	453	6.7	77	1	1	3	6	20	27	36
65+	367	5.9	47	1	2	3	8	15	21	33
GRAND TOTAL	1801	4.9	44	1	1	2	6	11	18	33

United States, October 1995–September 1996 Data, by Operation

84.01: FINGER AMPUTATION. Formerly included in operation group(s) 758.

Type of Patients	Observed Patients	Avg. Stay	Variance	Percentiles						
				10th	25th	50th	75th	90th	95th	99th
1. SINGLE DX										
0–19 Years	49	1.3	2	1	1	1	1	2	2	9
20–34	95	1.7	2	1	1	1	2	4	5	6
35–49	77	1.5	1	1	1	1	2	2	4	6
50–64	51	1.6	<1	1	1	1	2	3	3	4
65+	15	1.8	<1	1	1	1	3	3	3	3
2. MULTIPLE DX										
0–19 Years	75	3.3	43	1	1	1	2	7	11	32
20–34	159	3.7	12	1	1	2	5	8	10	16
35–49	297	4.6	33	1	1	3	6	10	13	30
50–64	294	5.6	52	1	2	3	8	12	23	36
65+	256	6.2	47	1	2	3	8	15	22	33
TOTAL SINGLE DX	287	1.5	2	1	1	1	2	3	4	7
MULTIPLE DX	1081	5.0	39	1	1	3	6	11	16	36
TOTAL										
0–19 Years	124	2.2	21	1	1	1	1	3	9	28
20–34	254	3.1	10	1	1	1	4	7	9	16
35–49	374	4.0	28	1	1	2	5	9	13	29
50–64	345	5.1	47	1	1	3	6	11	19	36
65+	271	5.8	44	1	2	3	8	15	19	30
GRAND TOTAL	1368	4.2	33	1	1	2	5	9	15	32

84.1: AMPUTATION OF LOWER LIMB. Formerly included in operation group(s) 760, 761, 762, 763.

Type of Patients	Observed Patients	Avg. Stay	Variance	Percentiles						
				10th	25th	50th	75th	90th	95th	99th
1. SINGLE DX										
0–19 Years	93	3.2	5	1	1	4	4	6	8	9
20–34	55	2.9	6	1	1	2	4	7	8	9
35–49	77	5.0	26	2	2	3	6	10	13	34
50–64	101	6.3	44	1	2	4	8	10	10	38
65+	188	6.2	28	1	3	5	8	12	17	26
2. MULTIPLE DX										
0–19 Years	159	10.3	223	1	2	4	15	26	43	80
20–34	564	10.8	103	3	5	8	13	25	31	57
35–49	2792	11.0	104	3	5	8	13	22	30	57
50–64	7056	12.7	128	3	6	10	16	24	33	63
65+	16967	11.3	104	3	5	8	14	22	29	56
TOTAL SINGLE DX	514	4.8	24	1	2	4	6	9	12	26
MULTIPLE DX	27538	11.7	112	3	5	9	14	23	31	59
TOTAL										
0–19 Years	252	7.8	157	1	2	4	7	19	30	72
20–34	619	10.1	99	2	4	8	11	23	30	53
35–49	2869	10.8	103	3	5	8	13	22	30	56
50–64	7157	12.7	128	3	6	10	16	24	33	63
65+	17155	11.3	104	3	5	8	14	22	29	56
GRAND TOTAL	28052	11.5	112	3	5	9	14	22	30	58

84.11: TOE AMPUTATION. Formerly included in operation group(s) 760.

Type of Patients	Observed Patients	Avg. Stay	Variance	Percentiles						
				10th	25th	50th	75th	90th	95th	99th
1. SINGLE DX										
0–19 Years	42	3.2	3	1	1	4	4	4	4	9
20–34	22	2.1	5	1	1	2	2	5	9	9
35–49	44	4.2	11	2	2	3	4	10	13	14
50–64	48	4.9	48	1	1	3	6	9	10	38
65+	56	4.0	9	1	1	3	6	8	10	12
2. MULTIPLE DX										
0–19 Years	60	5.6	45	1	2	2	7	15	19	33
20–34	245	8.6	59	3	4	7	10	14	24	44
35–49	1174	9.0	50	3	4	8	12	16	24	35
50–64	2548	9.7	64	3	5	8	12	18	25	43
65+	3868	9.4	76	2	4	7	12	18	23	51
TOTAL SINGLE DX	212	3.6	15	1	1	3	4	7	9	14
MULTIPLE DX	7895	9.3	66	2	4	7	12	18	24	48
TOTAL										
0–19 Years	102	4.5	28	1	2	3	4	9	15	25
20–34	267	7.9	57	1	4	7	9	13	23	44
35–49	1218	8.8	49	2	4	8	11	15	24	35
50–64	2596	9.6	64	2	4	8	12	18	25	43
65+	3924	9.3	75	2	4	7	12	18	23	51
GRAND TOTAL	8107	9.1	65	2	4	7	12	18	23	46

84.12: AMPUTATION THROUGH FOOT. Formerly included in operation group(s) 763.

Type of Patients	Observed Patients	Avg. Stay	Variance	Percentiles						
				10th	25th	50th	75th	90th	95th	99th
1. SINGLE DX										
0–19 Years	9	3.9	9	1	1	2	7	8	8	8
20–34	3	2.1	2	1	1	2	2	5	5	5
35–49	4	10.4	160	3	3	3	23	33	33	33
50–64	9	10.8	109	2	5	7	18	22	35	35
65+	14	10.0	42	3	5	7	17	19	19	23
2. MULTIPLE DX										
0–19 Years	11	6.3	45	1	1	2	13	14	22	22
20–34	72	11.1	77	2	5	10	13	19	29	40
35–49	465	12.3	134	3	5	9	16	27	34	57
50–64	1109	13.2	101	4	6	11	17	26	31	59
65+	1651	13.4	159	3	6	10	16	27	32	73
TOTAL SINGLE DX	39	7.5	59	1	2	5	8	19	23	35
MULTIPLE DX	3308	13.1	134	3	6	10	16	26	32	63
TOTAL										
0–19 Years	20	4.9	25	1	2	2	8	13	13	22
20–34	75	10.9	77	2	5	10	13	19	29	40
35–49	469	12.3	134	3	5	9	16	27	34	57
50–64	1118	13.2	101	4	6	11	17	26	31	59
65+	1665	13.3	158	3	6	10	16	27	32	71
GRAND TOTAL	3347	13.0	133	3	6	10	16	26	32	62

Length of Stay by Diagnosis and Operation, United States, 1997

United States, October 1995–September 1996 Data, by Operation

84.15: BK AMPUTATION NEC. Formerly included in operation group(s) 761.

Type of Patients	Observed Patients	Avg. Stay	Vari-ance	10th	25th	50th	75th	90th	95th	99th
1. SINGLE DX										
0–19 Years	8	4.2	14	1	2	2	7	12	12	12
20–34	15	4.0	4	2	3	4	4	6	7	7
35–49	21	6.4	55	2	3	4	7	10	34	34
50–64	32	6.9	23	3	4	5	9	12	19	23
65+	57	7.6	49	1	3	5	11	13	24	38
2. MULTIPLE DX										
0–19 Years	30	21.4	409	2	4	22	26	44	72	80
20–34	158	12.3	102	3	4	10	16	30	31	>99
35–49	785	13.1	148	3	6	9	16	27	39	74
50–64	2212	15.0	184	4	7	12	18	27	38	99
65+	5099	12.3	102	4	6	9	15	23	31	56
TOTAL SINGLE DX	133	6.5	35	2	3	4	9	12	19	34
MULTIPLE DX	8284	13.3	136	4	6	10	17	25	34	66
TOTAL										
0–19 Years	38	18.7	386	2	2	11	26	43	64	80
20–34	173	11.7	100	3	4	8	14	30	30	>99
35–49	806	12.9	148	3	6	9	15	27	39	74
50–64	2244	14.9	183	4	7	12	18	27	38	99
65+	5156	12.2	102	4	6	9	15	23	31	55
GRAND TOTAL	8417	13.2	135	4	6	10	17	25	34	65

84.2: EXTREMITY REATTACHMENT. Formerly included in operation group(s) 764.

Type of Patients	Observed Patients	Avg. Stay	Vari-ance	10th	25th	50th	75th	90th	95th	99th
1. SINGLE DX										
0–19 Years	56	4.0	9	1	1	3	7	8	10	11
20–34	46	3.7	7	1	2	3	5	7	9	17
35–49	45	3.5	7	1	1	4	5	7	8	13
50–64	14	2.8	4	1	1	2	4	6	6	8
65+	9	7.2	42	3	4	5	6	24	24	24
2. MULTIPLE DX										
0–19 Years	40	5.2	31	1	3	4	5	9	11	34
20–34	66	5.9	8	3	3	6	7	9	11	16
35–49	55	5.9	20	2	3	5	7	13	14	25
50–64	44	5.7	14	1	3	5	7	13	14	14
65+	10	5.5	5	3	4	5	7	7	11	11
TOTAL SINGLE DX	170	3.7	8	1	1	3	5	7	9	13
MULTIPLE DX	215	5.7	18	2	3	5	7	10	13	25
TOTAL										
0–19 Years	96	4.6	19	1	2	4	6	9	10	34
20–34	112	4.7	9	1	3	4	6	8	10	16
35–49	100	4.5	14	1	2	4	5	8	13	19
50–64	58	5.0	13	1	2	5	6	10	14	14
65+	19	6.2	20	3	4	5	7	8	11	24
GRAND TOTAL	385	4.7	14	1	2	4	6	9	11	17

84.17: ABOVE KNEE AMPUTATION. Formerly included in operation group(s) 762.

Type of Patients	Observed Patients	Avg. Stay	Vari-ance	10th	25th	50th	75th	90th	95th	99th
1. SINGLE DX										
0–19 Years	9	3.6	2	2	3	4	5	5	5	5
20–34	11	4.8	8	2	2	4	8	9	9	9
35–49	6	4.0	3	1	4	4	5	6	6	6
50–64	9	7.9	29	4	5	8	10	12	26	26
65+	58	6.2	13	3	4	6	7	11	12	21
2. MULTIPLE DX										
0–19 Years	22	20.4	662	4	4	6	30	44	70	88
20–34	60	15.3	183	6	7	11	21	31	37	72
35–49	273	11.2	117	3	4	8	13	22	33	83
50–64	1066	14.4	139	4	7	11	19	30	38	68
65+	6145	11.0	90	4	5	8	14	21	28	55
TOTAL SINGLE DX	93	5.9	14	2	3	5	7	10	12	21
MULTIPLE DX	7566	11.6	104	4	6	8	14	23	31	60
TOTAL										
0–19 Years	31	17.8	596	3	4	5	13	70	70	88
20–34	71	14.0	174	3	6	9	18	30	37	72
35–49	279	11.1	116	3	4	7	13	22	33	83
50–64	1075	14.4	139	4	7	10	19	30	38	68
65+	6203	10.9	90	4	5	8	13	21	28	54
GRAND TOTAL	7659	11.5	104	4	5	8	14	23	31	60

84.3: AMPUTATION STUMP REV. Formerly included in operation group(s) 765.

Type of Patients	Observed Patients	Avg. Stay	Vari-ance	10th	25th	50th	75th	90th	95th	99th
1. SINGLE DX										
0–19 Years	5	1.2	<1	1	1	1	1	3	3	3
20–34	15	6.4	138	1	1	2	3	36	36	36
35–49	15	4.8	30	1	1	3	4	16	16	16
50–64	19	2.5	5	1	1	1	4	6	7	9
65+	11	8.1	31	1	4	7	12	14	21	21
2. MULTIPLE DX										
0–19 Years	53	4.2	77	1	1	1	5	7	10	59
20–34	99	7.9	57	2	4	7	11	13	17	46
35–49	276	8.7	75	1	2	5	13	25	25	30
50–64	494	7.8	65	2	3	5	9	17	23	41
65+	860	8.5	95	2	4	6	9	17	24	77
TOTAL SINGLE DX	65	4.7	54	1	1	2	5	12	16	36
MULTIPLE DX	1782	8.1	80	1	3	6	10	18	25	44
TOTAL										
0–19 Years	58	4.1	73	1	1	1	5	7	10	59
20–34	114	7.8	66	1	3	6	10	14	18	46
35–49	291	8.5	74	1	2	5	12	23	25	30
50–64	513	7.6	64	2	3	5	9	17	23	39
65+	871	8.5	95	2	4	6	9	17	24	77
GRAND TOTAL	1847	8.0	79	1	3	5	10	17	25	43

Length of Stay by Diagnosis and Operation, United States, 1997

United States, October 1995–September 1996 Data, by Operation

84.4: IMPL OR FIT PROSTH LIMB. Formerly included in operation group(s) 766, 767.

Type of Patients	Observed Patients	Avg. Stay	Vari- ance	Percentiles 10th	25th	50th	75th	90th	95th	99th
1. SINGLE DX										
0–19 Years	1	2.0	0	2	2	2	2	2	2	2
20–34	1	3.0	0	3	3	3	3	3	3	3
35–49	0									
50–64	0									
65+	1	9.0	0	9	9	9	9	9	9	9
2. MULTIPLE DX										
0–19 Years	0									
20–34	1	81.0	0	81	81	81	81	81	81	81
35–49	0									
50–64	4	2.2	<1	2	2	2	2	3	4	4
65+	8	8.2	33	2	3	7	16	16	16	16
TOTAL SINGLE DX	3	3.4	5	2	2	3	3	9	9	9
MULTIPLE DX	13	11.7	550	2	2	2	7	16	81	81
TOTAL										
0–19 Years	1	2.0	0	2	2	2	2	2	2	2
20–34	2	38.4	>999	3	3	3	81	81	81	81
35–49	0									
50–64	4	2.2	<1	2	2	2	2	3	4	4
65+	9	8.3	30	2	3	9	16	16	16	16
GRAND TOTAL	16	10.1	453	2	2	2	4	16	81	81

85.0: MASTOTOMY. Formerly included in operation group(s) 771.

Type of Patients	Observed Patients	Avg. Stay	Vari- ance	Percentiles 10th	25th	50th	75th	90th	95th	99th
1. SINGLE DX										
0–19 Years	52	2.5	2	1	1	2	3	4	5	9
20–34	110	2.1	2	1	1	2	3	4	5	9
35–49	69	2.1	2	1	1	2	2	4	5	8
50–64	33	2.5	3	1	1	2	4	5	5	8
65+	6	2.1	2	1	1	1	3	4	4	4
2. MULTIPLE DX										
0–19 Years	31	4.3	11	2	2	3	5	8	10	20
20–34	147	2.8	3	1	2	3	4	5	6	8
35–49	209	3.3	15	1	2	2	4	6	8	16
50–64	127	4.7	10	2	2	3	7	9	10	13
65+	116	4.8	8	1	2	5	6	8	10	14
TOTAL SINGLE DX	270	2.2	2	1	1	2	3	4	5	8
MULTIPLE DX	630	3.7	10	1	2	3	5	7	9	14
TOTAL										
0–19 Years	83	3.2	7	1	2	3	4	6	8	10
20–34	257	2.5	3	1	1	2	4	5	5	8
35–49	278	2.9	11	1	2	3	3	6	7	15
50–64	160	4.3	10	2	2	3	6	8	10	13
65+	122	4.7	8	1	2	5	6	8	10	14
GRAND TOTAL	900	3.3	8	1	1	2	4	6	8	13

84.9: OTHER MUSCULOSKELETAL OP. Formerly included in operation group(s) 766.

Type of Patients	Observed Patients	Avg. Stay	Vari- ance	Percentiles 10th	25th	50th	75th	90th	95th	99th
1. SINGLE DX										
0–19 Years	2	3.6	<1	3	3	4	4	4	4	4
20–34	0									
35–49	0									
50–64	0									
65+										
2. MULTIPLE DX										
0–19 Years	8	39.6	769	1	7	41	67	67	67	67
20–34	2	2.8	3	2	2	2	2	7	7	7
35–49	2	5.7	71	1	1	1	17	17	17	17
50–64	3	2.6	0	1	1	4	4	4	4	4
65+	1	3.0	0	3	3	3	3	3	3	3
TOTAL SINGLE DX	2	3.6	<1	3	3	4	4	4	4	4
MULTIPLE DX	16	13.2	484	1	2	2	7	67	67	67
TOTAL										
0–19 Years	10	29.0	814	2	3	8	67	67	67	67
20–34	2	2.8	3	2	2	2	2	7	7	7
35–49	2	5.7	71	1	1	1	17	17	17	17
50–64	3	2.6	<1	1	1	4	4	4	4	4
65+	1	3.0	0	3	3	3	3	3	3	3
GRAND TOTAL	18	12.2	442	1	2	2	7	67	67	67

85.1: BREAST DIAGNOSTIC PX. Formerly included in operation group(s) 768, 780.

Type of Patients	Observed Patients	Avg. Stay	Vari- ance	Percentiles 10th	25th	50th	75th	90th	95th	99th
1. SINGLE DX										
0–19 Years	4	4.6	17	1	1	4	11	11	11	11
20–34	22	3.0	6	2	2	3	3	4	12	12
35–49	56	2.1	2	1	1	2	2	4	7	7
50–64	38	3.4	9	1	1	2	3	4	9	9
65+	24	2.2	3	1	1	2	3	3	6	9
2. MULTIPLE DX										
0–19 Years	3	3.1	7	1	1	2	6	6	6	6
20–34	59	6.3	48	2	3	4	6	12	23	41
35–49	230	5.9	58	2	2	4	6	14	18	38
50–64	300	5.8	51	2	2	4	7	12	15	30
65+	649	8.5	58	2	4	7	11	16	22	40
TOTAL SINGLE DX	144	2.6	5	1	1	2	3	6	9	11
MULTIPLE DX	1241	7.2	57	1	2	5	9	15	20	38
TOTAL										
0–19 Years	7	4.2	15	1	1	4	6	11	11	11
20–34	81	5.1	35	2	2	3	6	11	16	41
35–49	286	5.2	50	1	1	3	6	12	18	32
50–64	338	5.5	47	1	2	4	7	11	15	30
65+	673	8.3	57	2	3	6	11	16	22	40
GRAND TOTAL	1385	6.7	54	1	2	5	8	14	18	36

Length of Stay by Diagnosis and Operation

United States, October 1995–September 1996 Data, by Operation

85.11: PERC BREAST BIOPSY. Formerly included in operation group(s) 768.

Type of Patients	Observed Patients	Vari-ance	Avg. Stay	Percentiles						
				10th	25th	50th	75th	90th	95th	99th
1. SINGLE DX										
0–19 Years	0									
20–34	5	19	4.5	1	2	2	7	12	12	12
35–49	14	2	1.6	1	1	1	2	3	5	5
50–64	11	13	5.4	1	2	7	9	9	9	9
65+	3	6	3.3	1	1	5	5	6	6	6
2. MULTIPLE DX										
0–19 Years	2	7	4.2	2	2	6	6	6	6	6
20–34	26	19	5.6	1	3	5	6	10	12	28
35–49	99	73	6.9	2	2	5	6	18	18	38
50–64	131	92	7.4	2	2	5	8	14	17	82
65+	325	62	8.2	3	5	6	9	14	19	58
TOTAL SINGLE DX	33	12	3.6	1	1	2	7	9	9	12
MULTIPLE DX	583	68	7.7	2	4	6	9	15	19	54
TOTAL										
0–19 Years	2	7	4.2	2	2	6	6	6	6	6
20–34	31	19	5.4	1	3	5	6	12	12	28
35–49	113	69	6.4	2	2	4	6	18	18	31
50–64	142	84	7.2	2	2	6	8	14	17	38
65+	328	61	8.2	3	4	6	9	14	19	58
GRAND TOTAL	616	66	7.4	2	3	6	8	14	18	42

85.2: EXC/DESTR BREAST TISS. Formerly included in operation group(s) 768, 771.

Type of Patients	Observed Patients	Vari-ance	Avg. Stay	Percentiles						
				10th	25th	50th	75th	90th	95th	99th
1. SINGLE DX										
0–19 Years	10	<1	1.2	1	1	1	1	2	2	2
20–34	99	<1	1.4	1	1	1	2	2	3	4
35–49	575	<1	1.3	1	1	1	1	2	3	4
50–64	703	1	1.6	1	1	1	2	2	4	5
65+	490	1	1.5	1	1	1	2	2	3	5
2. MULTIPLE DX										
0–19 Years	19	208	5.1	1	1	2	4	4	10	86
20–34	157	16	3.2	1	1	1	4	10	14	15
35–49	1068	16	2.4	1	1	1	4	5	8	20
50–64	1638	14	2.4	1	1	1	2	4	8	22
65+	2485	19	3.1	1	1	2	3	7	11	24
TOTAL SINGLE DX	1877	<1	1.4	1	1	1	2	2	3	5
MULTIPLE DX	5367	18	2.7	1	1	1	2	5	9	22
TOTAL										
0–19 Years	29	157	4.1	1	1	2	3	4	5	86
20–34	256	11	2.5	1	1	1	2	6	11	15
35–49	1643	10	2.0	1	1	1	2	3	5	15
50–64	2341	11	2.2	1	1	1	2	3	6	15
65+	2975	16	2.8	1	1	2	3	6	10	21
GRAND TOTAL	7244	13	2.3	1	1	1	2	4	8	18

85.12: OPEN BIOPSY OF BREAST. Formerly included in operation group(s) 768.

Type of Patients	Observed Patients	Vari-ance	Avg. Stay	Percentiles						
				10th	25th	50th	75th	90th	95th	99th
1. SINGLE DX										
0–19 Years	4	17	4.6	1	1	4	11	11	11	11
20–34	17	2	2.6	1	2	3	3	4	4	12
35–49	42	2	2.2	1	1	2	2	4	7	7
50–64	27	3	2.4	1	1	2	3	6	8	8
65+	21	2	2.1	1	1	2	3	3	4	9
2. MULTIPLE DX										
0–19 Years	1	0	1.0	1	1	1	1	1	1	1
20–34	33	81	7.1	2	3	4	6	23	23	41
35–49	131	42	5.0	1	2	3	5	12	14	39
50–64	169	25	4.8	1	2	3	5	10	13	25
65+	324	53	8.9	1	3	7	14	18	23	34
TOTAL SINGLE DX	111	3	2.4	1	1	2	3	4	7	11
MULTIPLE DX	658	47	6.8	1	2	4	10	16	22	32
TOTAL										
0–19 Years	5	17	4.3	1	1	4	4	11	11	11
20–34	50	47	4.9	1	2	3	4	8	23	41
35–49	173	33	4.3	1	1	2	4	10	14	32
50–64	196	23	4.5	1	2	3	5	10	13	24
65+	345	52	8.3	1	3	6	13	16	23	34
GRAND TOTAL	769	43	6.1	1	2	3	8	14	18	30

85.21: LOCAL EXC BREAST LESION. Formerly included in operation group(s) 768.

Type of Patients	Observed Patients	Vari-ance	Avg. Stay	Percentiles						
				10th	25th	50th	75th	90th	95th	99th
1. SINGLE DX										
0–19 Years	5	<1	1.5	1	1	1	2	2	2	2
20–34	60	<1	1.6	1	1	1	2	3	3	7
35–49	315	<1	1.2	1	1	1	1	2	2	3
50–64	363	2	1.6	1	1	1	2	2	5	7
65+	259	2	1.6	1	1	1	2	2	4	11
2. MULTIPLE DX										
0–19 Years	12	4	3.0	1	1	3	4	4	5	10
20–34	116	21	4.0	1	1	1	5	13	15	15
35–49	667	25	2.9	1	1	1	2	6	10	36
50–64	919	23	3.0	1	1	2	3	6	9	25
65+	1408	25	3.7	1	1	2	4	10	13	27
TOTAL SINGLE DX	1002	1	1.4	1	1	1	2	2	3	5
MULTIPLE DX	3122	24	3.3	1	2	2	3	8	12	25
TOTAL										
0–19 Years	17	4	2.7	1	1	2	4	4	5	10
20–34	176	17	3.3	1	1	1	4	10	14	15
35–49	982	17	2.3	1	1	1	2	4	7	19
50–64	1282	18	2.6	1	1	2	2	5	8	25
65+	1667	22	3.3	1	2	2	3	8	12	24
GRAND TOTAL	4124	19	2.8	1	1	1	3	6	10	23

Length of Stay by Diagnosis and Operation, United States, 1997

United States, October 1995–September 1996 Data, by Operation

85.22: QUADRANT RESECT BREAST. Formerly included in operation group(s) 768.

Type of Patients	Observed Patients	Avg. Stay	Vari-ance	10th	25th	50th	75th	90th	95th	99th
1. SINGLE DX										
0–19 Years	1	1.0	0	1	1	1	1	1	1	1
20–34	10	1.9	<1	1	1	2	2	3	3	3
35–49	61	1.4	<1	1	1	1	2	2	3	3
50–64	83	1.6	<1	1	1	2	2	2	2	3
65+	52	1.6	<1	1	1	1	2	2	3	5
2. MULTIPLE DX										
0–19 Years	0									
20–34	11	1.8	1	1	1	1	2	3	5	5
35–49	87	2.4	3	1	1	2	3	5	5	8
50–64	170	2.0	4	1	1	1	2	3	5	11
65+	268	1.9	4	1	1	1	2	3	4	12
TOTAL SINGLE DX	207	1.5	<1	1	1	1	2	2	2	3
MULTIPLE DX	536	2.0	4	1	1	1	2	3	5	11
TOTAL										
0–19 Years	1	1.0	0	1	1	1	1	1	1	1
20–34	21	1.8	1	1	1	2	2	3	5	5
35–49	148	1.9	2	1	1	1	2	3	5	8
50–64	253	1.8	3	1	1	2	2	2	3	11
65+	320	1.9	3	1	1	1	2	3	4	10
GRAND TOTAL	743	1.9	3	1	1	1	2	3	4	11

85.23: SUBTOTAL MASTECTOMY. Formerly included in operation group(s) 768.

Type of Patients	Observed Patients	Avg. Stay	Vari-ance	10th	25th	50th	75th	90th	95th	99th
1. SINGLE DX										
0–19 Years	1	1.0	0	1	1	1	1	1	1	1
20–34	24	1.3	<1	1	1	1	1	2	2	8
35–49	195	1.4	<1	1	1	1	1	2	2	6
50–64	253	1.5	1	1	1	1	2	3	4	4
65+	179	1.4	<1	1	1	1	2	2	2	4
2. MULTIPLE DX										
0–19 Years	2	1.2	<1	1	1	1	1	2	2	2
20–34	25	1.4	1	1	1	1	1	2	2	7
35–49	299	1.5	2	1	1	1	2	2	2	6
50–64	538	1.6	2	1	1	1	2	3	3	5
65+	790	2.4	14	1	1	1	2	4	7	21
TOTAL SINGLE DX	652	1.4	<1	1	1	1	2	2	3	5
MULTIPLE DX	1654	1.9	7	1	1	1	2	3	4	15
TOTAL										
0–19 Years	3	1.2	<1	1	1	1	1	2	2	2
20–34	49	1.4	1	1	1	1	1	2	2	7
35–49	494	1.5	2	1	1	1	2	2	3	6
50–64	791	1.6	2	1	1	1	2	3	3	5
65+	969	2.2	11	1	1	1	2	4	5	20
GRAND TOTAL	2306	1.8	5	1	1	1	2	3	4	12

85.3: RED MAMMOPLASTY/ECTOMY. Formerly included in operation group(s) 771.

Type of Patients	Observed Patients	Avg. Stay	Vari-ance	10th	25th	50th	75th	90th	95th	99th
1. SINGLE DX										
0–19 Years	340	1.3	<1	1	1	1	1	2	.	3
20–34	1219	1.4	2	1	1	1	2	2	2	3
35–49	636	1.3	<1	1	1	1	2	2	2	3
50–64	229	1.3	<1	1	1	1	1	2	2	3
65+	48	2.0	2	1	2	2	2	3	6	6
2. MULTIPLE DX										
0–19 Years	208	1.2	<1	1	1	1	1	2	2	3
20–34	981	1.5	<1	1	1	1	2	2	3	5
35–49	957	1.9	9	1	1	1	2	3	4	11
50–64	572	2.1	8	1	1	1	2	3	4	25
65+	175	2.1	4	1	1	1	2	4	7	8
TOTAL SINGLE DX	2472	1.4	1	1	1	1	2	2	2	3
MULTIPLE DX	2893	1.8	5	1	1	1	2	3	4	7
TOTAL										
0–19 Years	548	1.3	<1	1	1	1	1	2	2	3
20–34	2200	1.5	2	1	1	1	2	2	3	4
35–49	1593	1.7	6	1	1	1	2	3	3	7
50–64	801	1.9	6	1	1	1	2	3	4	6
65+	223	2.1	3	1	1	2	2	4	7	7
GRAND TOTAL	5365	1.6	3	1	1	1	2	2	3	5

85.32: BILAT RED MAMMOPLASTY. Formerly included in operation group(s) 771.

Type of Patients	Observed Patients	Avg. Stay	Vari-ance	10th	25th	50th	75th	90th	95th	99th
1. SINGLE DX										
0–19 Years	305	1.2	<1	1	1	1	1	2	2	3
20–34	1177	1.4	2	1	1	1	2	2	2	3
35–49	602	1.3	<1	1	1	1	2	2	2	3
50–64	213	1.3	<1	1	1	1	1	2	2	3
65+	44	2.0	2	1	2	2	2	3	6	6
2. MULTIPLE DX										
0–19 Years	188	1.2	<1	1	1	1	1	2	2	3
20–34	934	1.5	<1	1	1	1	2	2	3	5
35–49	817	1.8	8	1	1	1	2	3	3	10
50–64	467	1.5	<1	1	1	1	2	3	3	5
65+	125	1.6	<1	1	1	1	2	2	3	5
TOTAL SINGLE DX	2341	1.4	2	1	1	1	2	2	2	3
MULTIPLE DX	2531	1.6	3	1	1	1	2	2	3	5
TOTAL										
0–19 Years	493	1.2	<1	1	1	1	1	2	2	3
20–34	2111	1.5	2	1	1	1	2	2	3	4
35–49	1419	1.6	5	1	1	1	2	3	3	4
50–64	680	1.5	<1	1	1	1	2	2	3	4
65+	169	1.7	1	1	1	2	2	2	3	6
GRAND TOTAL	4872	1.5	2	1	1	1	2	2	3	4

Length of Stay by Diagnosis and Operation, United States, 1997

United States, October 1995–September 1996 Data, by Operation

85.4: MASTECTOMY. Formerly included in operation group(s) 769, 770.

Type of Patients	Observed Patients	Avg. Stay	Vari-ance	10th	25th	50th	75th	90th	95th	99th
1. SINGLE DX										
0–19 Years	5	1.3	<1	1	1	1	1	3	3	4
20–34	184	2.0	2	1	1	2	2	4	5	6
35–49	1501	2.1	1	1	1	2	3	3	4	6
50–64	1866	2.1	1	1	1	2	2	3	4	7
65+	1633	2.1	1	1	1	2	2	3	4	6
2. MULTIPLE DX										
0–19 Years	5	1.7	2	1	1	2	2	5	5	5
20–34	442	2.8	3	1	2	3	4	5	5	8
35–49	3931	2.9	4	1	2	2	4	5	6	9
50–64	5788	2.6	7	1	1	2	3	4	6	10
65+	10647	3.0	8	1	2	2	3	5	7	14
TOTAL SINGLE DX	5189	2.1	1	1	1	2	2	3	4	6
MULTIPLE DX	20813	2.8	7	1	2	2	3	5	6	12
TOTAL										
0–19 Years	10	1.5	2	1	1	2	2	5	5	5
20–34	626	2.5	3	1	1	2	3	5	5	7
35–49	5432	2.7	3	1	2	2	3	5	6	9
50–64	7654	2.5	5	1	1	2	3	4	5	9
65+	12280	2.8	7	1	2	2	3	5	7	14
GRAND TOTAL	26002	2.7	6	1	1	2	3	5	6	11

85.41: UNILAT SIMPLE MASTECTOMY. Formerly included in operation group(s) 769.

Type of Patients	Observed Patients	Avg. Stay	Vari-ance	10th	25th	50th	75th	90th	95th	99th
1. SINGLE DX										
0–19 Years	1	1.0	0	1	1	1	1	1	1	1
20–34	19	1.3	<1	1	1	1	1	2	2	4
35–49	179	2.0	2	1	1	1	3	4	5	6
50–64	215	1.9	2	1	1	2	2	3	4	7
65+	171	2.0	1	1	1	2	2	4	4	5
2. MULTIPLE DX										
0–19 Years	1	5.0	0	5	5	5	5	5	5	5
20–34	50	3.1	6	1	1	2	4	7	8	9
35–49	430	3.0	7	1	1	2	4	6	7	13
50–64	599	2.3	6	1	1	2	3	4	5	11
65+	1178	3.2	15	1	1	2	3	5	11	21
TOTAL SINGLE DX	585	1.9	1	1	1	2	2	4	4	6
MULTIPLE DX	2258	2.9	11	1	1	2	3	5	8	20
TOTAL										
0–19 Years	2	3.7	4	1	1	5	5	5	5	5
20–34	69	2.0	3	1	1	1	2	4	7	9
35–49	609	2.7	6	1	1	2	3	5	7	11
50–64	814	2.2	5	1	2	2	3	4	5	10
65+	1349	3.0	14	1	1	2	3	6	10	21
GRAND TOTAL	2843	2.7	9	1	1	2	3	5	7	15

85.42: BILAT SIMPLE MASTECTOMY. Formerly included in operation group(s) 769.

Type of Patients	Observed Patients	Avg. Stay	Vari-ance	10th	25th	50th	75th	90th	95th	99th
1. SINGLE DX										
0–19 Years	4	1.3	<1	1	1	1	1	3	3	4
20–34	6	2.4	7	1	1	1	2	9	9	9
35–49	48	2.5	1	1	2	2	3	4	5	6
50–64	24	2.8	2	1	2	2	3	5	5	8
65+	8	2.4	1	1	2	2	3	5	5	5
2. MULTIPLE DX										
0–19 Years	4	1.0	0	1	1	1	1	1	1	1
20–34	33	2.5	7	1	1	3	3	3	4	6
35–49	153	2.6	6	1	1	2	3	5	8	9
50–64	123	2.9	6	1	2	3	4	5	7	13
65+	56	3.1	14	1	2	3	3	5	6	32
TOTAL SINGLE DX	90	2.5	2	1	2	2	3	4	5	8
MULTIPLE DX	369	2.7	7	1	1	2	3	5	7	13
TOTAL										
0–19 Years	8	1.1	<1	1	1	1	1	1	3	4
20–34	39	2.5	7	1	1	2	3	3	4	9
35–49	201	2.6	5	1	2	2	3	4	6	8
50–64	147	2.9	5	1	2	3	3	5	7	13
65+	64	3.0	13	1	2	3	3	5	6	32
GRAND TOTAL	459	2.7	6	1	1	2	3	5	6	11

85.43: UNILAT EXTEN SMP MAST. Formerly included in operation group(s) 770.

Type of Patients	Observed Patients	Avg. Stay	Vari-ance	10th	25th	50th	75th	90th	95th	99th
1. SINGLE DX										
0–19 Years	0									
20–34	153	2.2	2	1	1	2	3	5	6	6
35–49	1223	2.1	1	1	1	2	3	3	4	6
50–64	1572	2.1	1	1	1	2	2	3	4	6
65+	1417	2.1	1	1	1	2	2	3	4	6
2. MULTIPLE DX										
0–19 Years	0									
20–34	340	2.7	2	1	2	3	4	5	5	6
35–49	3175	2.8	3	1	2	2	4	5	6	9
50–64	4784	2.6	5	1	1	2	3	4	6	9
65+	9036	2.9	6	1	2	2	3	5	7	13
TOTAL SINGLE DX	4365	2.1	1	1	1	2	2	3	4	6
MULTIPLE DX	17335	2.8	5	1	2	2	3	5	6	11
TOTAL										
0–19 Years	0									
20–34	493	2.6	2	1	1	2	3	5	5	6
35–49	4398	2.6	3	1	1	2	3	5	6	8
50–64	6356	2.4	4	1	1	2	3	4	5	9
65+	10453	2.8	6	1	2	2	3	5	6	12
GRAND TOTAL	21700	2.6	4	1	2	2	3	5	6	10

Length of Stay by Diagnosis and Operation, United States, 1997

United States, October 1995–September 1996 Data, by Operation

85.44: BILAT EXTEN SMP MAST. Formerly included in operation group(s) 770.

Type of Patients	Observed Patients	Avg. Stay	Vari-ance	10th	25th	50th	75th	90th	95th	99th
1. SINGLE DX										
0–19 Years	0									
20–34	2	2.3	<1	2	2	2	3	3	3	3
35–49	20	3.1	1	1	2	3	4	4	5	6
50–64	34	2.6	<1	2	2	2	3	4	4	4
65+	15	2.7	<1	2	2	3	3	3	4	4
2. MULTIPLE DX										
0–19 Years	0									
20–34	10	4.3	4	2	3	3	6	7	7	7
35–49	107	3.1	3	2	2	3	4	5	6	9
50–64	140	4.0	64	1	2	3	4	6	8	16
65+	181	3.6	7	2	2	3	4	6	8	17
TOTAL SINGLE DX	71	2.8	<1	2	2	3	4	4	4	5
MULTIPLE DX	438	3.6	23	2	2	3	4	6	8	16
TOTAL										
0–19 Years	0									
20–34	12	3.7	3	2	2	3	5	7	7	7
35–49	127	3.1	2	2	2	3	4	5	6	9
50–64	174	3.6	49	2	2	3	3	5	7	16
65+	196	3.5	6	2	2	3	4	6	8	17
GRAND TOTAL	509	3.4	20	2	2	3	4	5	7	16

85.45: UNILAT RAD MASTECTOMY. Formerly included in operation group(s) 770.

Type of Patients	Observed Patients	Avg. Stay	Vari-ance	10th	25th	50th	75th	90th	95th	99th
1. SINGLE DX										
0–19 Years	0									
20–34	3	1.7	<1	1	1	2	2	3	3	3
35–49	20	2.0	<1	1	1	2	3	3	3	4
50–64	18	2.1	2	2	2	2	2	3	3	11
65+	21	1.9	1	1	1	2	2	4	5	5
2. MULTIPLE DX										
0–19 Years	0									
20–34	9	3.0	3	1	1	3	5	5	5	5
35–49	56	4.5	12	2	2	4	6	7	8	20
50–64	119	3.4	23	1	2	3	3	5	9	30
65+	166	3.9	30	1	1	3	4	8	11	26
TOTAL SINGLE DX	62	2.0	1	1	2	2	2	3	4	5
MULTIPLE DX	350	3.8	23	1	2	3	4	7	11	30
TOTAL										
0–19 Years	0									
20–34	12	2.6	3	1	1	2	4	5	5	5
35–49	76	4.1	11	1	2	3	6	7	7	20
50–64	137	3.3	20	1	2	2	3	5	9	30
65+	187	3.6	27	1	1	3	4	7	11	26
GRAND TOTAL	412	3.6	20	1	2	2	4	6	9	26

85.5: AUGMENTATION MAMMOPLASTY. Formerly included in operation group(s) 771.

Type of Patients	Observed Patients	Avg. Stay	Vari-ance	10th	25th	50th	75th	90th	95th	99th
1. SINGLE DX										
0–19 Years	5	1.4	<1	1	1	1	2	2	2	2
20–34	33	1.1	<1	1	1	1	1	2	2	2
35–49	14	1.1	<1	1	1	1	1	2	2	2
50–64	7	1.0	<1	1	1	1	1	1	1	1
65+	0									
2. MULTIPLE DX										
0–19 Years	5	1.3	<1	1	1	1	2	2	2	2
20–34	35	1.4	<1	1	1	1	2	2	3	4
35–49	88	1.6	<1	1	1	1	2	3	3	5
50–64	49	1.8	2	1	1	1	2	3	3	7
65+	11	1.5	<1	1	1	1	2	2	3	3
TOTAL SINGLE DX	59	1.1	<1	1	1	1	1	2	2	2
MULTIPLE DX	188	1.6	<1	1	1	1	2	3	3	5
TOTAL										
0–19 Years	10	1.4	<1	1	1	1	2	2	2	2
20–34	68	1.3	<1	1	1	1	1	2	3	3
35–49	102	1.5	<1	1	1	1	2	3	3	4
50–64	56	1.6	1	1	1	1	2	3	3	7
65+	11	1.5	<1	1	1	1	2	2	3	3
GRAND TOTAL	247	1.4	<1	1	1	1	2	2	3	4

85.6: MASTOPEXY. Formerly included in operation group(s) 771.

Type of Patients	Observed Patients	Avg. Stay	Vari-ance	10th	25th	50th	75th	90th	95th	99th
1. SINGLE DX										
0–19 Years	1	2.0	0	2	2	2	2	2	2	2
20–34	7	1.4	2	1	1	1	1	2	6	6
35–49	3	1.0	0	1	1	1	1	1	1	1
50–64	0									
65+	0									
2. MULTIPLE DX										
0–19 Years	0									
20–34	9	1.4	<1	1	1	1	2	2	2	2
35–49	25	1.7	2	1	1	1	2	3	3	8
50–64	8	2.4	<1	1	2	2	3	3	3	3
65+	0									
TOTAL SINGLE DX	11	1.3	<1	1	1	1	1	2	2	6
MULTIPLE DX	42	1.7	1	1	1	1	2	3	3	8
TOTAL										
0–19 Years	1	2.0	0	2	2	2	2	2	2	2
20–34	16	1.4	1	1	1	1	1	2	3	6
35–49	28	1.5	1	1	1	1	2	3	3	8
50–64	8	2.4	<1	1	2	2	3	3	3	3
65+	0									
GRAND TOTAL	53	1.6	1	1	1	1	2	3	3	6

Length of Stay by Diagnosis and Operation, United States, 1997

United States, October 1995–September 1996 Data, by Operation

85.7: TOTAL BREAST RECONST. Formerly included in operation group(s) 771.

Type of Patients	Observed Patients	Vari-ance	Avg. Stay	10th	25th	50th	75th	90th	95th	99th
1. SINGLE DX										
0–19 Years	1	0	1.0	1	1	1	1	1	1	1
20–34	7	4	3.1	1	1	4	4	6	6	6
35–49	27	3	3.9	2	3	4	4	5	7	11
50–64	22	3	4.1	3	3	4	4	5	8	14
65+	3	4	2.9	1	2	2	5	5	5	5
2. MULTIPLE DX										
0–19 Years	3	<1	2.7	2	2	2	4	4	4	4
20–34	61	2	3.5	2	3	4	4	5	6	6
35–49	573	4	4.1	2	3	4	5	6	7	11
50–64	496	6	4.1	2	3	4	5	6	7	17
65+	78	5	3.8	2	2	3	5	6	8	16
TOTAL SINGLE DX	60	4	3.7	1	3	4	4	5	7	11
MULTIPLE DX	1211	5	4.1	2	3	4	5	6	7	11
TOTAL										
0–19 Years	4	1	1.7	1	1	1	2	4	4	4
20–34	68	2	3.5	1	2	4	4	5	6	6
35–49	600	4	4.1	2	3	4	5	6	7	11
50–64	518	6	4.1	2	3	4	5	6	7	17
65+	81	5	3.8	2	2	3	5	6	8	16
GRAND TOTAL	1271	5	4.1	2	3	4	5	6	7	11

85.8: OTHER BREAST REPAIR. Formerly included in operation group(s) 771.

Type of Patients	Observed Patients	Vari-ance	Avg. Stay	10th	25th	50th	75th	90th	95th	99th
1. SINGLE DX										
0–19 Years	6	1	1.6	1	1	1	2	4	4	4
20–34	4	5	2.6	1	1	4	4	6	6	6
35–49	21	1	2.7	1	3	3	3	3	4	6
50–64	16	<1	2.2	2	3	2	2	3	4	5
65+	4	<1	1.5	1	1	1	2	3	3	3
2. MULTIPLE DX										
0–19 Years	6	164	11.0	1	1	3	28	28	28	28
20–34	47	37	3.3	1	1	2	3	6	8	44
35–49	212	66	4.4	1	2	3	4	5	9	43
50–64	174	19	2.6	1	1	2	3	4	4	12
65+	64	14	3.9	1	2	3	4	7	11	20
TOTAL SINGLE DX	51	1	2.4	1	2	3	3	3	4	6
MULTIPLE DX	503	46	3.7	1	2	3	5	7	7	43
TOTAL										
0–19 Years	12	61	4.2	1	1	1	3	5	28	28
20–34	51	36	3.2	1	2	2	3	6	8	44
35–49	233	57	4.1	1	2	3	4	6	7	43
50–64	190	17	2.5	1	2	3	3	4	5	10
65+	68	13	3.8	1	2	3	3	7	11	20
GRAND TOTAL	554	40	3.6	1	3	2	3	5	7	43

85.85: BREAST MUSCLE FLAP GRAFT. Formerly included in operation group(s) 771.

Type of Patients	Observed Patients	Vari-ance	Avg. Stay	10th	25th	50th	75th	90th	95th	99th
1. SINGLE DX										
0–19 Years	0									
20–34	0									
35–49	9	<1	3.0	3	3	3	3	3	3	6
50–64	7	<1	2.3	2	2	2	2	4	4	5
65+	2	0	2.0	2	2	2	2	2	2	2
2. MULTIPLE DX										
0–19 Years	3	4	2.5	1	1	2	5	5	5	5
20–34	13	2	2.8	2	2	2	3	4	8	8
35–49	76	1	3.0	2	2	3	4	4	5	5
50–64	68	44	3.5	2	2	2	4	5	6	14
65+	16	1	3.4	3	3	3	3	5	5	10
TOTAL SINGLE DX	18	<1	2.8	2	2	3	3	3	4	6
MULTIPLE DX	176	10	3.2	2	2	3	4	5	5	8
TOTAL										
0–19 Years	3	4	2.5	1	2	2	5	5	5	5
20–34	13	2	2.8	2	2	2	3	4	8	8
35–49	85	<1	3.0	2	2	3	3	4	5	6
50–64	75	34	3.2	2	3	3	3	5	6	14
65+	18	1	3.3	3	3	3	3	5	5	10
GRAND TOTAL	194	9	3.1	2	2	3	3	4	5	8

85.9: OTHER BREAST OPERATIONS. Formerly included in operation group(s) 771, 780.

Type of Patients	Observed Patients	Vari-ance	Avg. Stay	10th	25th	50th	75th	90th	95th	99th
1. SINGLE DX										
0–19 Years	6	<1	1.7	1	1	1	3	3	3	4
20–34	23	1	1.8	1	1	1	2	3	3	9
35–49	63	<1	1.6	1	1	1	2	3	3	5
50–64	36	2	1.9	2	1	2	2	3	5	6
65+	8	2	2.1	1	1	1	4	4	5	5
2. MULTIPLE DX										
0–19 Years	15	3	3.4	2	2	3	5	6	6	6
20–34	74	11	3.7	1	1	2	6	7	8	17
35–49	322	13	3.1	1	1	2	4	6	8	18
50–64	332	5	2.7	1	1	3	4	5	7	14
65+	146	15	4.2	1	3	3	5	11	14	16
TOTAL SINGLE DX	136	1	1.7	1	1	1	2	3	4	6
MULTIPLE DX	889	10	3.2	1	1	2	4	6	9	17
TOTAL										
0–19 Years	21	2	2.3	1	1	2	3	5	5	6
20–34	97	10	3.3	1	1	2	6	7	8	17
35–49	385	11	2.9	1	1	2	4	6	7	17
50–64	368	5	2.7	1	1	2	3	5	6	12
65+	154	14	4.1	1	3	3	5	9	14	16
GRAND TOTAL	1025	9	3.0	1	2	2	4	6	8	16

United States, October 1995–September 1996 Data, by Operation

85.94: BREAST IMPLANT REMOVAL. Formerly included in operation group(s) 771.

Type of Patients	Observed Patients	Avg. Stay	Vari-ance	10th	25th	50th	75th	90th	95th	99th
1. SINGLE DX										
0–19 Years	0									
20–34	4	1.0	0	1	1	1	1	1	1	1
35–49	32	1.4	<1	1	1	1	3	3	3	6
50–64	18	2.1	2	1	1	2	5	5	6	6
65+	3	2.1	2	1	1	1	4	4	4	4
2. MULTIPLE DX										
0–19 Years	0									
20–34	23	2.8	4	1	1	2	5	6	6	6
35–49	114	3.2	21	1	1	1	4	6	10	22
50–64	147	2.8	7	1	1	2	4	6	7	14
65+	37	2.6	6	1	1	1	3	7	7	11
TOTAL SINGLE DX	57	1.7	1	1	1	1	2	3	4	6
MULTIPLE DX	321	2.9	12	1	1	2	4	6	7	17
TOTAL										
0–19 Years	0									
20–34	27	2.6	4	1	1	1	4	6	6	6
35–49	146	2.8	17	1	1	1	3	5	8	22
50–64	165	2.7	6	1	1	2	4	6	7	14
65+	40	2.5	6	1	1	1	3	6	7	11
GRAND TOTAL	378	2.7	10	1	1	1	4	6	7	17

86.0: INCISION SKIN & SUBCU. Formerly included in operation group(s) 772, 775, 776, 779, 780.

Type of Patients	Observed Patients	Avg. Stay	Vari-ance	10th	25th	50th	75th	90th	95th	99th
1. SINGLE DX										
0–19 Years	1735	3.8	15	1	2	3	5	8	12	22
20–34	1025	2.8	7	1	1	2	3	5	7	14
35–49	855	3.6	9	2	2	3	5	7	7	14
50–64	381	3.7	13	1	2	3	5	6	9	23
65+	194	4.4	16	1	2	3	5	11	11	22
2. MULTIPLE DX										
0–19 Years	5603	8.0	97	2	3	5	9	18	26	59
20–34	5447	6.8	44	2	3	5	8	14	22	35
35–49	9526	7.5	61	2	3	5	9	15	24	38
50–64	8927	7.7	48	2	4	6	10	15	20	36
65+	12012	9.4	74	2	4	7	12	20	27	44
TOTAL SINGLE DX	4190	3.5	11	1	2	3	4	7	9	17
MULTIPLE DX	41515	8.0	65	2	3	6	10	17	24	42
TOTAL										
0–19 Years	7338	7.1	81	1	2	4	8	15	22	51
20–34	6472	6.1	40	2	2	4	7	13	20	31
35–49	10381	7.1	58	2	3	5	8	14	23	37
50–64	9308	7.5	47	2	3	6	10	15	20	36
65+	12206	9.4	74	2	4	7	12	20	27	44
GRAND TOTAL	45705	7.5	61	2	3	5	9	16	23	40

86.01: ASPIRATION SKIN & SUBCU. Formerly included in operation group(s) 780.

Type of Patients	Observed Patients	Avg. Stay	Vari-ance	10th	25th	50th	75th	90th	95th	99th
1. SINGLE DX										
0–19 Years	70	3.4	3	2	2	3	4	5	6	11
20–34	27	4.3	10	2	2	3	4	5	6	11
35–49	36	4.1	4	2	3	3	5	5	8	9
50–64	19	2.7	5	1	2	2	3	6	9	9
65+	9	3.5	4	1	2	3	5	6	7	7
2. MULTIPLE DX										
0–19 Years	191	4.4	10	1	3	3	5	10	11	14
20–34	165	5.3	23	1	2	5	7	9	12	19
35–49	291	6.2	33	2	2	5	7	14	18	30
50–64	286	7.1	37	3	3	6	9	12	14	38
65+	549	8.9	56	3	4	6	11	19	25	36
TOTAL SINGLE DX	161	3.6	5	2	2	3	4	7	9	11
MULTIPLE DX	1482	6.8	39	2	3	5	8	14	19	36
TOTAL										
0–19 Years	261	4.1	9	1	3	3	5	7	11	14
20–34	192	5.1	21	2	3	4	6	10	11	18
35–49	327	6.0	31	2	2	4	7	14	17	30
50–64	305	6.8	36	2	3	5	9	12	14	38
65+	558	8.8	55	3	4	6	11	19	25	36
GRAND TOTAL	1643	6.5	37	2	3	5	8	13	18	36

86.03: INCISION PILONIDAL SINUS. Formerly included in operation group(s) 772.

Type of Patients	Observed Patients	Avg. Stay	Vari-ance	10th	25th	50th	75th	90th	95th	99th
1. SINGLE DX										
0–19 Years	86	2.3	4	1	1	2	3	4	5	12
20–34	77	1.9	1	1	1	2	2	3	4	5
35–49	11	3.2	2	1	2	4	4	4	4	6
50–64	2	3.0	0	3						3
65+	0									
2. MULTIPLE DX										
0–19 Years	52	2.7	13	1	1	2	3	5	5	29
20–34	58	2.9	7	1	2	2	3	4	5	19
35–49	39	5.2	48	1	1	3	5	10	31	32
50–64	15	10.4	4	11	11	11	11	11	11	11
65+	11	8.6	141	2	3	4	8	11	44	44
TOTAL SINGLE DX	176	2.2	2	1	1	2	3	4	5	6
MULTIPLE DX	175	7.8	24	1	3	11	11	11	11	19
TOTAL										
0–19 Years	138	2.4	7	1	1	2	3	5	5	12
20–34	135	2.4	4	1	1	2	3	4	5	9
35–49	50	4.7	37	1	3	3	5	15	15	32
50–64	17	10.4	5	11	11	11	11	11	11	36
65+	11	8.6	141	2	3	4	8	11	44	44
GRAND TOTAL	351	6.1	24	1	2	4	11	11	11	14

Length of Stay by Diagnosis and Operation, United States, 1997

United States, October 1995–September 1996 Data, by Operation

86.04: OTHER SKIN & SUBCU I&D. Formerly included in operation group(s) 775.

Type of Patients	Observed Patients	Avg. Stay	Variance	Percentiles						
				10th	25th	50th	75th	90th	95th	99th
1. SINGLE DX										
0–19 Years	773	3.2	7	1	2	3	4	6	7	14
20–34	587	2.8	4	1	1	2	4	5	6	12
35–49	514	3.7	5	2	2	3	5	7	7	10
50–64	207	3.6	5	2	2	3	5	5	7	13
65+	88	4.5	12	1	2	4	5	11	11	13
2. MULTIPLE DX										
0–19 Years	1770	4.7	29	2	2	4	5	8	10	21
20–34	2402	4.8	18	2	2	4	5	9	12	24
35–49	3948	6.0	30	2	3	4	7	10	15	31
50–64	2949	6.0	25	2	3	5	7	11	14	25
65+	3588	7.7	55	2	3	6	9	14	22	44
TOTAL SINGLE DX	2169	3.3	6	1	2	3	4	6	7	12
MULTIPLE DX	14657	6.0	33	2	3	4	7	11	15	32
TOTAL										
0–19 Years	2543	4.3	23	1	2	3	5	7	10	20
20–34	2989	4.4	16	1	2	3	5	8	11	20
35–49	4462	5.7	28	2	3	4	7	9	14	29
50–64	3156	5.8	24	2	3	5	7	11	14	25
65+	3676	7.6	54	2	3	6	9	14	21	44
GRAND TOTAL	16826	5.6	30	2	3	4	7	10	14	32

86.06: INSERTION INFUSION PUMP. Formerly included in operation group(s) 775.

Type of Patients	Observed Patients	Avg. Stay	Variance	Percentiles						
				10th	25th	50th	75th	90th	95th	99th
1. SINGLE DX										
0–19 Years	18	3.6	5	2	2	3	5	6	9	10
20–34	36	3.5	33	1	2	2	3	4	9	30
35–49	51	2.7	2	1	2	2	3	4	4	8
50–64	25	2.7	7	1	2	3	3	5	5	20
65+	9	2.8	1	1	3	3	3	4	6	>99
2. MULTIPLE DX										
0–19 Years	63	7.0	61	2	2	4	8	18	18	51
20–34	114	8.7	145	1	2	5	8	24	30	85
35–49	293	4.7	22	1	2	3	5	11	15	24
50–64	297	7.6	54	1	2	5	9	20	22	35
65+	339	8.3	70	2	2	5	11	23	23	44
TOTAL SINGLE DX	139	2.9	11	1	2	2	3	4	6	30
MULTIPLE DX	1106	7.1	61	1	2	4	8	19	23	36
TOTAL										
0–19 Years	81	6.7	56	2	2	4	8	17	18	51
20–34	150	6.9	112	1	2	3	7	19	30	37
35–49	344	4.3	19	1	2	3	5	9	15	24
50–64	322	6.9	50	2	2	4	9	19	22	35
65+	348	8.0	68	2	2	5	11	23	23	44
GRAND TOTAL	1245	6.5	56	1	2	4	8	18	23	36

86.05: INC W RMVL FB SKIN/SUBCU. Formerly included in operation group(s) 775.

Type of Patients	Observed Patients	Avg. Stay	Variance	Percentiles						
				10th	25th	50th	75th	90th	95th	99th
1. SINGLE DX										
0–19 Years	154	1.9	3	1	1	2	2	3	4	7
20–34	87	1.6	1	1	1	1	2	3	3	8
35–49	48	2.1	2	1	1	2	2	6	6	6
50–64	11	1.2	2	1	1	1	1	2	2	15
65+	4	1.1	<1	1	1	1	1	2	2	2
2. MULTIPLE DX										
0–19 Years	577	7.2	60	1	2	4	9	15	22	32
20–34	359	6.3	40	1	3	4	7	12	19	39
35–49	482	7.7	64	2	3	5	10	16	21	35
50–64	414	7.9	61	2	4	6	9	17	22	39
65+	396	8.5	40	3	4	6	11	17	21	30
TOTAL SINGLE DX	304	1.8	2	1	1	1	2	3	4	7
MULTIPLE DX	2228	7.5	55	2	3	5	9	16	21	39
TOTAL										
0–19 Years	731	6.0	52	1	2	4	8	14	20	32
20–34	446	5.3	36	1	3	3	7	11	15	39
35–49	530	7.2	61	1	3	5	9	16	21	35
50–64	425	7.4	60	1	3	5	9	16	22	39
65+	400	8.4	40	2	4	6	11	17	21	30
GRAND TOTAL	2532	6.7	52	2	3	5	9	15	20	35

86.07: VAD INSERTION. Formerly included in operation group(s) 776.

Type of Patients	Observed Patients	Avg. Stay	Variance	Percentiles						
				10th	25th	50th	75th	90th	95th	99th
1. SINGLE DX										
0–19 Years	487	5.6	27	1	2	4	8	13	14	25
20–34	120	4.8	22	1	1	3	6	10	17	22
35–49	108	5.0	40	1	1	3	6	9	23	25
50–64	86	6.1	50	1	1	3	6	23	23	26
65+	72	5.8	32	1	2	4	8	15	18	22
2. MULTIPLE DX										
0–19 Years	2313	11.7	150	2	4	8	14	26	38	73
20–34	1759	9.9	68	3	5	6	13	23	25	38
35–49	3479	10.4	106	2	4	7	13	25	35	47
50–64	4110	9.2	68	2	4	7	12	18	25	45
65+	6200	10.9	90	2	4	8	14	23	31	44
TOTAL SINGLE DX	873	5.5	30	1	2	4	7	13	16	25
MULTIPLE DX	17861	10.4	95	2	4	7	13	23	31	49
TOTAL										
0–19 Years	2800	10.5	132	1	4	7	13	22	34	66
20–34	1879	9.6	67	3	4	6	13	23	25	38
35–49	3587	10.2	105	2	4	7	12	25	35	46
50–64	4196	9.2	68	2	4	7	12	18	25	45
65+	6272	10.9	90	2	4	8	14	23	31	44
GRAND TOTAL	18734	10.2	93	2	4	7	13	23	30	48

Length of Stay by Diagnosis and Operation, United States, 1997

United States, October 1995–September 1996 Data, by Operation

86.09: SKIN/SUBCU INCISION NEC. Formerly included in operation group(s) 775.

Type of Patients	Observed Patients	Avg. Stay	Vari-ance	10th	25th	50th	75th	90th	95th	99th
1. SINGLE DX										
0–19 Years	146	3.1	5	1	2	2	4	5	8	13
20–34	90	2.0	3	1	1	2	4	4	6	9
35–49	86	2.4	4	1	1	2	3	6	6	10
50–64	31	5.8	28	1	2	3	8	15	15	15
65+	12	3.2	5	2	2	2	3	7	9	9
2. MULTIPLE DX										
0–19 Years	636	7.0	91	1	2	4	9	14	18	72
20–34	587	7.6	36	2	3	7	11	11	17	29
35–49	991	7.2	47	2	3	5	9	15	18	38
50–64	853	7.4	39	2	4	6	8	15	22	30
65+	928	7.9	45	2	3	6	10	18	20	35
TOTAL SINGLE DX	365	2.7	6	1	1	2	3	5	7	15
MULTIPLE DX	3995	7.4	50	2	3	6	10	15	20	34
TOTAL										
0–19 Years	782	6.3	77	1	2	4	8	13	16	47
20–34	677	6.5	35	1	2	5	11	11	15	28
35–49	1077	6.7	45	1	3	5	8	14	18	36
50–64	884	7.3	39	2	3	6	8	15	22	30
65+	940	7.8	45	2	3	6	10	18	20	35
GRAND TOTAL	4360	6.9	47	1	3	5	9	14	19	31

86.1: SKIN & SUBCU DXTIC PX. Formerly included in operation group(s) 773, 780.

Type of Patients	Observed Patients	Avg. Stay	Vari-ance	10th	25th	50th	75th	90th	95th	99th
1. SINGLE DX										
0–19 Years	64	4.0	43	1	1	3	5	7	8	59
20–34	27	5.0	13	1	3	4	8	11	11	11
35–49	36	4.8	6	2	4	4	5	8	9	15
50–64	16	4.9	9	1	2	6	7	15	15	9
65+	16	5.1	30	1	1	2	7	14	14	23
2. MULTIPLE DX										
0–19 Years	355	7.4	66	2	3	5	9	16	22	50
20–34	370	7.2	42	2	3	7	11	15	20	34
35–49	718	8.1	75	2	3	5	9	21	25	32
50–64	641	7.0	41	2	3	6	8	13	16	29
65+	1308	8.7	49	3	5	6	10	15	20	35
TOTAL SINGLE DX	159	4.7	22	1	2	4	6	9	11	15
MULTIPLE DX	3392	8.0	55	2	4	6	10	15	22	34
TOTAL										
0–19 Years	419	7.0	64	2	3	4	8	15	22	50
20–34	397	7.0	40	2	3	5	11	14	20	33
35–49	754	7.9	72	2	3	5	8	21	25	32
50–64	657	6.9	40	2	3	6	8	13	16	29
65+	1324	8.6	49	3	5	7	11	15	20	34
GRAND TOTAL	3551	7.8	54	2	3	6	10	15	22	34

86.11: SKIN & SUBCU BIOPSY. Formerly included in operation group(s) 773.

Type of Patients	Observed Patients	Avg. Stay	Vari-ance	10th	25th	50th	75th	90th	95th	99th
1. SINGLE DX										
0–19 Years	63	4.1	44	1	1	3	5	7	8	59
20–34	27	5.0	13	1	4	4	8	8	11	11
35–49	36	4.8	6	1	4	4	5	8	9	15
50–64	16	4.9	9	1	2	6	7	9	9	9
65+	16	5.1	30	1	1	2	7	14	14	23
2. MULTIPLE DX										
0–19 Years	352	7.4	66	2	3	5	9	16	22	50
20–34	369	7.2	43	2	3	7	9	15	20	34
35–49	716	8.1	75	2	3	5	10	21	25	32
50–64	638	7.0	41	2	3	6	8	13	16	29
65+	1300	8.7	49	3	5	7	11	15	20	34
TOTAL SINGLE DX	158	4.7	22	1	2	4	6	9	11	15
MULTIPLE DX	3375	8.0	56	2	4	6	10	15	22	34
TOTAL										
0–19 Years	415	7.0	65	1	3	4	8	15	22	50
20–34	396	7.1	41	2	3	5	9	14	20	33
35–49	752	7.9	72	2	3	5	9	21	25	32
50–64	654	7.0	40	2	3	6	8	13	16	30
65+	1316	8.6	49	3	5	7	11	15	20	34
GRAND TOTAL	3533	7.8	55	2	3	6	10	15	22	34

86.2: EXC/DESTR SKIN LESION. Formerly included in operation group(s) 772, 774, 779, 780.

Type of Patients	Observed Patients	Avg. Stay	Vari-ance	10th	25th	50th	75th	90th	95th	99th
1. SINGLE DX										
0–19 Years	1098	2.9	12	1	1	2	3	6	9	15
20–34	1136	3.2	11	1	1	2	4	6	9	15
35–49	863	3.9	16	1	2	3	4	7	11	23
50–64	407	4.7	29	1	1	3	5	10	15	30
65+	303	5.0	32	1	2	3	6	12	18	30
2. MULTIPLE DX										
0–19 Years	5173	5.6	56	2	2	3	6	13	19	41
20–34	6287	7.3	78	1	2	5	8	17	24	48
35–49	9922	9.9	109	3	3	6	12	22	29	56
50–64	11664	10.6	108	3	4	8	13	23	31	58
65+	24521	11.6	114	3	5	8	14	23	34	62
TOTAL SINGLE DX	3807	3.6	17	1	1	2	4	7	11	22
MULTIPLE DX	57567	9.9	105	2	4	7	12	21	30	57
TOTAL										
0–19 Years	6271	5.2	50	1	2	3	6	12	19	37
20–34	7423	6.7	71	1	2	4	8	15	22	45
35–49	10785	9.3	104	2	3	6	11	21	29	56
50–64	12071	10.4	106	2	4	7	13	21	30	58
65+	24824	11.5	114	3	5	8	14	23	34	61
GRAND TOTAL	61374	9.5	102	2	3	6	12	21	29	56

Length of Stay by Diagnosis and Operation, United States, 1997

United States, October 1995–September 1996 Data, by Operation

86.21: EXCISION OF PILONID CYST. Formerly included in operation group(s) 772.

Type of Patients	Observed Patients	Avg. Stay	Variance	10th	25th	50th	75th	90th	95th	99th
1. SINGLE DX										
0–19 Years	114	1.9	2	1	1	1	2	3	5	8
20–34	132	1.6	<1	1	1	1	2	3	4	4
35–49	41	1.7	<1	1	1	1	2	2	3	7
50–64	10	2.0	1	1	1	2	3	4	4	4
65+	2	1.0	0	1	1	1	1	1	1	1
2. MULTIPLE DX										
0–19 Years	69	2.5	5	1	1	1	3	8	8	8
20–34	79	4.6	77	1	1	2	4	13	13	66
35–49	41	3.4	16	1	1	2	4	8	12	24
50–64	22	3.1	19	1	1	3	3	4	4	28
65+	9	4.9	4	3	3	4	7	7	7	7
TOTAL SINGLE DX	299	1.7	1	1	1	1	2	3	4	6
MULTIPLE DX	220	3.4	32	1	1	2	4	8	11	31
TOTAL										
0–19 Years	183	2.1	4	1	1	1	2	4	8	8
20–34	211	2.7	30	1	1	1	2	4	8	31
35–49	82	2.5	9	1	1	2	2	6	8	15
50–64	32	2.8	15	1	1	2	3	4	4	28
65+	11	4.4	6	3	3	4	7	7	7	7
GRAND TOTAL	519	2.5	16	1	1	1	3	4	8	15

86.23: NAIL REMOVAL. Formerly included in operation group(s) 779.

Type of Patients	Observed Patients	Avg. Stay	Variance	10th	25th	50th	75th	90th	95th	99th
1. SINGLE DX										
0–19 Years	18	3.1	18	1	1	1	3	5	17	17
20–34	4	1.9	<1	2	2	2	2	2	2	2
35–49	7	2.3	0	1	2	2	2	3	7	7
50–64	1	1.0	0	1	1	1	1	1	1	1
65+	1	4.0	0	4	4	4	4	4	4	4
2. MULTIPLE DX										
0–19 Years	53	3.2	13	1	1	2	4	7	12	>99
20–34	42	6.7	36	2	3	5	8	13	14	51
35–49	83	7.0	59	2	3	5	7	13	24	42
50–64	124	6.1	39	2	3	4	7	11	19	34
65+	323	8.9	76	2	4	6	11	20	29	39
TOTAL SINGLE DX	31	2.6	10	1	1	2	2	5	7	17
MULTIPLE DX	625	7.2	58	2	3	5	9	14	24	43
TOTAL										
0–19 Years	71	3.2	14	1	1	2	4	7	12	>99
20–34	46	5.9	33	2	2	4	8	11	14	19
35–49	90	6.7	56	2	3	4	7	13	19	42
50–64	125	6.1	39	2	3	4	7	10	19	34
65+	324	8.9	75	2	4	6	11	20	29	39
GRAND TOTAL	656	6.9	57	1	3	5	9	14	22	42

86.22: EXC DEBRIDE WND/INFECT. Formerly included in operation group(s) 774.

Type of Patients	Observed Patients	Avg. Stay	Variance	10th	25th	50th	75th	90th	95th	99th
1. SINGLE DX										
0–19 Years	759	3.2	15	1	1	2	4	6	9	15
20–34	888	3.6	13	1	1	2	4	7	10	19
35–49	734	4.0	17	1	2	3	4	8	11	21
50–64	358	4.8	31	1	1	3	6	10	15	30
65+	272	5.3	35	1	2	3	6	13	18	30
2. MULTIPLE DX										
0–19 Years	2965	6.9	75	1	2	4	8	17	23	45
20–34	5528	7.5	83	1	2	5	9	16	26	50
35–49	8701	10.3	115	2	4	7	13	23	31	56
50–64	10066	10.9	110	3	5	8	14	22	31	61
65+	19405	12.2	124	3	5	9	15	25	36	63
TOTAL SINGLE DX	3011	3.9	19	1	1	3	5	8	11	23
MULTIPLE DX	46665	10.4	113	2	4	7	13	22	31	60
TOTAL										
0–19 Years	3724	6.3	66	1	2	4	7	15	21	43
20–34	6416	7.0	76	1	3	4	8	15	23	47
35–49	9435	9.8	110	2	3	6	12	22	29	56
50–64	10424	10.7	108	2	4	8	13	22	31	60
65+	19677	12.1	124	3	5	9	15	25	35	63
GRAND TOTAL	49676	10.0	109	2	4	7	13	21	30	58

86.26: LIG DERMAL APPENDAGE. Formerly included in operation group(s) 780.

Type of Patients	Observed Patients	Avg. Stay	Variance	10th	25th	50th	75th	90th	95th	99th
1. SINGLE DX										
0–19 Years	46	1.5	2	1	1	1	1	3	3	7
20–34	1	2.0	0	2	2	2	2	2	2	2
35–49	0									
50–64	0									
65+	0									
2. MULTIPLE DX										
0–19 Years	1263	2.4	9	1	1	2	3	3	5	18
20–34	0									
35–49	0									
50–64	0									
65+	3	6.5	<1	5	7	7	7	7	7	7
TOTAL SINGLE DX	47	1.5	2	1	1	1	1	3	3	7
MULTIPLE DX	1266	2.4	9	1	1	2	3	4	6	18
TOTAL										
0–19 Years	1309	2.4	9	1	1	2	3	3	5	18
20–34	1	2.0	0	2	2	2	2	2	2	2
35–49	0									
50–64	0									
65+	3	6.5	<1	5	7	7	7	7	7	7
GRAND TOTAL	1313	2.4	9	1	1	2	3	3	6	18

Length of Stay by Diagnosis and Operation, United States, 1997

86.27: DEBRIDEMENT OF NAIL. Formerly included in operation group(s) 780.

Type of Patients	Observed Patients	Avg. Stay	Variance	10th	25th	50th	75th	90th	95th	99th
1. SINGLE DX										
0–19 Years	7	1.7	<1	1	1	1	2	3	4	4
20–34	1	2.0	0	2	2	2	2	3	4	4
35–49	1	6.0	0	6	6	6	6	6	6	6
50–64	2	4.9	<1	5	5	5	5	5	5	5
65+	3	6.7	2	5	6	6	8	8	8	8
2. MULTIPLE DX										
0–19 Years	13	6.4	120	1	2	4	5	22	22	51
20–34	27	11.3	129	3	6	7	13	30	60	>99
35–49	153	10.6	156	2	2	5	15	39	39	92
50–64	380	13.5	172	4	6	9	18	29	31	95
65+	2404	11.3	97	4	5	8	14	23	31	62
TOTAL SINGLE DX	14	4.1	3	1	2	5	5	5	6	8
MULTIPLE DX	2977	11.5	112	4	5	8	14	24	33	66
TOTAL										
0–19 Years	20	4.5	74	1	1	2	4	5	22	51
20–34	28	11.1	128	3	6	7	12	30	60	>99
35–49	154	10.6	156	2	2	5	15	39	39	92
50–64	382	13.3	169	4	6	9	17	29	31	95
65+	2407	11.3	97	4	5	8	14	23	31	62
GRAND TOTAL	2991	11.5	112	3	5	8	14	24	33	66

86.3: OTH LOC EXC/DESTR SKIN. Formerly included in operation group(s) 773.

Type of Patients	Observed Patients	Avg. Stay	Variance	10th	25th	50th	75th	90th	95th	99th
1. SINGLE DX										
0–19 Years	295	1.5	1	1	1	1	2	3	4	5
20–34	140	2.7	10	1	1	2	2	3	7	15
35–49	141	2.2	10	1	1	1	2	4	6	14
50–64	82	2.3	4	1	1	1	3	6	6	9
65+	40	2.9	7	1	1	1	5	8	8	13
2. MULTIPLE DX										
0–19 Years	372	4.5	47	1	1	2	5	10	24	54
20–34	315	7.9	89	1	2	5	9	22	27	54
35–49	575	5.9	52	1	2	4	8	11	18	40
50–64	605	7.5	106	1	2	5	9	18	21	86
65+	1355	7.9	68	1	3	6	10	17	20	48
TOTAL SINGLE DX	698	2.1	5	1	1	1	2	4	6	13
MULTIPLE DX	3222	7.0	74	1	2	4	8	16	21	50
TOTAL										
0–19 Years	667	3.2	29	1	1	1	3	8	11	28
20–34	455	6.3	70	1	1	3	8	14	27	54
35–49	716	5.2	46	1	2	3	7	10	16	31
50–64	687	6.8	96	1	2	5	9	16	21	68
65+	1395	7.7	66	1	3	6	10	17	20	46
GRAND TOTAL	3920	6.0	64	1	1	3	8	14	20	42

86.28: NONEXC DEBRIDEMENT WOUND. Formerly included in operation group(s) 779.

Type of Patients	Observed Patients	Avg. Stay	Variance	10th	25th	50th	75th	90th	95th	99th
1. SINGLE DX										
0–19 Years	153	2.7	8	1	1	2	3	6	7	14
20–34	109	2.4	3	1	1	2	3	4	5	13
35–49	77	3.8	17	2	2	2	4	6	10	25
50–64	34	4.7	16	1	2	3	6	12	12	17
65+	22	3.2	6	1	2	2	4	6	8	>99
2. MULTIPLE DX										
0–19 Years	795	5.1	25	1	2	4	6	11	13	22
20–34	607	5.8	31	1	2	4	8	18	18	20
35–49	942	6.1	33	1	3	5	9	12	15	32
50–64	1060	7.4	58	2	3	6	9	12	18	53
65+	2363	8.7	54	3	5	7	10	16	22	42
TOTAL SINGLE DX	395	3.0	9	1	1	2	3	6	7	21
MULTIPLE DX	5767	7.2	46	2	3	5	9	14	18	39
TOTAL										
0–19 Years	948	4.7	23	1	2	3	6	10	12	22
20–34	716	5.4	28	1	2	3	7	16	18	18
35–49	1019	6.0	32	1	3	4	8	12	15	32
50–64	1094	7.3	57	2	3	6	9	12	18	53
65+	2385	8.6	53	3	4	7	10	16	21	43
GRAND TOTAL	6162	6.9	45	2	3	5	9	14	18	38

86.4: RAD EXCISION SKIN LESION. Formerly included in operation group(s) 775.

Type of Patients	Observed Patients	Avg. Stay	Variance	10th	25th	50th	75th	90th	95th	99th
1. SINGLE DX										
0–19 Years	55	1.7	2	1	1	1	2	3	4	10
20–34	73	2.6	10	1	1	1	3	6	9	19
35–49	121	2.6	8	1	1	2	5	6	7	13
50–64	114	3.3	5	1	2	2	5	6	5	10
65+	96	3.4	7	1	2	3	4	5	8	13
2. MULTIPLE DX										
0–19 Years	86	7.9	87	2	2	3	9	20	35	35
20–34	177	7.5	116	1	2	4	8	15	28	58
35–49	344	8.0	104	1	3	4	9	18	28	62
50–64	433	6.1	50	2	2	4	8	12	19	39
65+	1175	7.4	76	2	2	4	9	18	27	41
TOTAL SINGLE DX	459	2.8	7	1	1	2	4	5	7	13
MULTIPLE DX	2215	7.3	81	1	2	4	8	16	26	46
TOTAL										
0–19 Years	141	4.7	53	1	1	2	4	15	18	35
20–34	250	6.2	92	1	2	3	8	14	22	58
35–49	465	6.7	87	1	2	4	7	15	25	49
50–64	547	5.5	42	1	2	4	6	10	15	38
65+	1271	7.0	71	1	2	4	8	16	26	38
GRAND TOTAL	2674	6.4	69	1	2	4	8	15	23	42

United States, October 1995–September 1996 Data, by Operation

86.5: SKIN & SUBCU SUTURE. Formerly included in operation group(s) 775.

Type of Patients	Observed Patients	Avg. Stay	Vari-ance	Percentiles						
				10th	25th	50th	75th	90th	95th	99th
1. SINGLE DX										
0–19 Years	297	1.6	2	1	1	1	2	3	4	8
20–34	253	1.6	2	1	1	1	2	3	4	6
35–49	151	2.3	4	1	1	2	3	5	7	7
50–64	58	2.8	8	1	1	2	4	6	7	12
65+	49	3.0	6	1	1	2	5	7	8	8
2. MULTIPLE DX										
0–19 Years	2283	2.8	15	1	1	2	3	6	7	17
20–34	4045	2.9	20	1	1	2	3	6	9	18
35–49	3156	3.7	25	1	1	2	4	9	12	28
50–64	1662	3.9	23	1	1	2	5	8	14	24
65+	5523	5.6	36	1	2	4	7	11	16	36
TOTAL SINGLE DX	808	1.9	3	1	1	1	2	4	6	8
MULTIPLE DX	16669	3.9	26	1	1	2	5	8	12	26
TOTAL										
0–19 Years	2580	2.6	14	1	1	2	3	6	7	17
20–34	4298	2.8	19	1	1	2	3	6	8	18
35–49	3307	3.6	24	1	1	2	4	8	12	26
50–64	1720	3.9	23	1	1	2	5	8	14	24
65+	5572	5.6	36	1	2	4	7	11	16	36
GRAND TOTAL	17477	3.8	25	1	1	2	4	8	12	25

86.6: FREE SKIN GRAFT. Formerly included in operation group(s) 777.

Type of Patients	Observed Patients	Avg. Stay	Vari-ance	Percentiles						
				10th	25th	50th	75th	90th	95th	99th
1. SINGLE DX										
0–19 Years	189	3.8	19	1	1	2	5	9	13	23
20–34	183	4.4	15	1	1	3	7	8	13	18
35–49	184	4.2	10	1	3	3	5	5	10	19
50–64	114	5.3	20	1	2	4	8	12	17	17
65+	129	6.2	33	1	3	5	7	13	13	35
2. MULTIPLE DX										
0–19 Years	994	11.3	119	2	4	7	15	25	32	57
20–34	887	11.9	127	2	5	9	15	27	31	63
35–49	1280	10.7	132	2	4	7	14	24	31	86
50–64	1153	10.6	139	2	4	7	13	24	30	70
65+	1804	11.5	128	2	4	7	16	26	32	57
TOTAL SINGLE DX	799	4.5	18	1	2	3	6	9	13	19
MULTIPLE DX	6118	11.2	130	2	4	7	14	25	32	63
TOTAL										
0–19 Years	1183	9.8	108	1	3	6	14	23	30	53
20–34	1070	10.0	109	1	3	7	12	23	29	62
35–49	1464	9.7	118	1	3	6	13	22	31	85
50–64	1267	10.2	132	1	4	7	12	23	30	59
65+	1933	11.2	124	2	4	7	15	26	32	57
GRAND TOTAL	6917	10.3	120	2	3	7	13	24	30	59

86.59: SKIN SUTURE NEC. Formerly included in operation group(s) 775.

Type of Patients	Observed Patients	Avg. Stay	Vari-ance	Percentiles						
				10th	25th	50th	75th	90th	95th	99th
1. SINGLE DX										
0–19 Years	296	1.6	2	1	1	1	2	3	4	8
20–34	253	1.6	2	1	1	1	2	2	3	6
35–49	151	2.3	4	1	1	2	3	5	7	7
50–64	58	2.8	8	1	1	2	4	6	7	12
65+	49	3.0	6	1	1	2	5	7	8	8
2. MULTIPLE DX										
0–19 Years	2280	2.8	15	1	1	2	3	6	7	18
20–34	4032	2.9	20	1	1	2	3	6	9	18
35–49	3149	3.7	25	1	1	2	4	9	12	28
50–64	1657	3.9	23	1	1	2	5	8	14	24
65+	5508	5.6	36	1	2	4	7	11	16	36
TOTAL SINGLE DX	807	1.9	3	1	1	1	2	4	6	8
MULTIPLE DX	16626	3.9	26	1	1	2	5	8	12	26
TOTAL										
0–19 Years	2576	2.6	14	1	1	2	3	6	7	17
20–34	4285	2.8	19	1	1	2	3	6	8	18
35–49	3300	3.6	24	1	1	2	4	8	12	26
50–64	1715	3.9	23	1	1	2	5	8	14	24
65+	5557	5.6	36	1	2	4	7	11	16	36
GRAND TOTAL	17433	3.8	25	1	1	2	4	8	12	25

86.62: HAND SKIN GRAFT NEC. Formerly included in operation group(s) 777.

Type of Patients	Observed Patients	Avg. Stay	Vari-ance	Percentiles						
				10th	25th	50th	75th	90th	95th	99th
1. SINGLE DX										
0–19 Years	7	3.5	4	1	2	4	4	4	9	9
20–34	11	2.4	3	1	1	2	3	6	6	7
35–49	13	3.2	9	1	2	2	3	4	13	13
50–64	1	2.0	0	2	2	2	2	2	2	2
65+	5	2.8	1	1	2	3	4	4	4	4
2. MULTIPLE DX										
0–19 Years	80	10.0	67	3	6	6	13	22	30	41
20–34	85	13.2	184	2	5	11	14	33	43	63
35–49	102	8.6	99	2	2	6	11	17	21	45
50–64	37	8.9	66	1	3	7	11	19	22	37
65+	41	16.5	553	1	2	9	14	41	91	91
TOTAL SINGLE DX	37	3.1	5	1	2	2	4	4	8	13
MULTIPLE DX	345	10.7	148	2	4	7	13	21	33	63
TOTAL										
0–19 Years	87	9.2	64	3	6	6	11	21	30	37
20–34	96	12.0	176	1	3	9	13	30	41	63
35–49	115	8.0	92	2	2	4	10	17	21	45
50–64	38	8.8	66	1	3	7	11	19	22	37
65+	46	14.2	484	1	2	6	14	34	91	91
GRAND TOTAL	382	9.8	138	1	3	6	12	21	32	63

Length of Stay by Diagnosis and Operation, United States, 1997

United States, October 1995–September 1996 Data, by Operation

86.63: FTHICK SKIN GRAFT NEC. Formerly included in operation group(s) 777.

Type of Patients	Observed Patients	Avg. Stay	Vari-ance	10th	25th	50th	75th	90th	95th	99th
1. SINGLE DX										
0–19 Years	26	1.6	2	1	1	1	2	2	3	8
20–34	14	5.0	18	3	3	3	5	10	18	18
35–49	12	5.9	15	4	4	5	6	10	15	22
50–64	5	4.7	25	1	1	3	6	16	16	16
65+	7	4.4	10	1	2	3	6	10	10	10
2. MULTIPLE DX										
0–19 Years	67	5.7	37	1	2	5	7	16	19	24
20–34	33	12.2	294	1	2	7	11	27	56	78
35–49	57	6.7	42	1	2	4	10	16	23	24
50–64	46	7.3	66	2	2	4	8	16	29	46
65+	117	6.0	46	2	2	4	6	13	15	31
TOTAL SINGLE DX	64	3.6	14	1	1	3	4	8	10	18
MULTIPLE DX	320	6.7	66	1	2	4	7	14	19	53
TOTAL										
0–19 Years	93	4.3	29	1	1	2	5	11	18	24
20–34	47	8.0	147	2	3	3	9	18	27	56
35–49	69	6.6	36	1	2	4	9	15	22	24
50–64	51	7.1	64	2	2	4	8	16	19	46
65+	124	5.9	45	2	2	4	6	13	15	31
GRAND TOTAL	384	6.0	57	1	2	4	7	14	18	36

86.7: PEDICLE GRAFTS OR FLAPS. Formerly included in operation group(s) 778.

Type of Patients	Observed Patients	Avg. Stay	Vari-ance	10th	25th	50th	75th	90th	95th	99th
1. SINGLE DX										
0–19 Years	91	2.3	6	1	1	1	3	6	6	8
20–34	69	2.5	9	1	1	1	3	7	7	13
35–49	87	3.4	16	1	1	2	4	8	13	17
50–64	43	3.2	14	1	1	2	4	6	7	26
65+	21	4.4	53	1	2	2	3	9	19	37
2. MULTIPLE DX										
0–19 Years	244	7.6	138	1	1	3	9	22	29	85
20–34	359	10.3	143	1	2	6	14	28	37	58
35–49	558	12.0	217	1	3	8	15	29	58	64
50–64	488	9.1	92	1	2	6	11	24	28	48
65+	739	11.0	121	2	4	7	15	26	33	53
TOTAL SINGLE DX	311	2.9	15	1	1	1	3	6	8	19
MULTIPLE DX	2388	10.5	149	1	2	6	14	26	36	59
TOTAL										
0–19 Years	335	6.0	104	1	1	2	6	17	27	69
20–34	428	8.7	126	2	2	4	13	22	37	57
35–49	645	11.1	202	1	2	7	14	28	47	64
50–64	531	8.8	89	2	2	5	11	22	27	47
65+	760	10.7	120	2	3	7	15	26	33	53
GRAND TOTAL	2699	9.5	138	1	2	5	12	25	33	58

86.69: FREE SKIN GRAFT NEC. Formerly included in operation group(s) 777.

Type of Patients	Observed Patients	Avg. Stay	Vari-ance	10th	25th	50th	75th	90th	95th	99th
1. SINGLE DX										
0–19 Years	143	4.5	25	1	1	2	5	11	14	23
20–34	143	4.4	15	1	1	3	7	8	13	18
35–49	145	4.2	9	1	2	3	5	7	10	15
50–64	100	5.6	20	1	2	4	9	12	17	17
65+	115	6.5	35	1	3	5	7	13	13	35
2. MULTIPLE DX										
0–19 Years	725	12.2	123	2	5	9	16	25	33	60
20–34	711	12.0	113	3	5	9	15	27	30	63
35–49	1047	11.0	140	2	4	8	14	26	33	86
50–64	1007	10.8	149	2	4	7	13	24	31	90
65+	1573	11.8	121	2	4	8	16	26	32	57
TOTAL SINGLE DX	646	4.7	18	1	2	3	7	10	13	19
MULTIPLE DX	5063	11.5	130	2	4	8	15	26	32	63
TOTAL										
0–19 Years	868	10.7	113	1	3	7	15	23	30	57
20–34	854	10.0	99	1	3	7	13	24	29	51
35–49	1192	9.9	124	2	4	7	12	23	31	86
50–64	1107	10.4	141	2	4	7	12	24	30	70
65+	1688	11.5	118	2	4	7	16	26	32	57
GRAND TOTAL	5709	10.6	121	2	4	7	14	25	31	60

86.72: PEDICLE GRAFT ADV. Formerly included in operation group(s) 778.

Type of Patients	Observed Patients	Avg. Stay	Vari-ance	10th	25th	50th	75th	90th	95th	99th
1. SINGLE DX										
0–19 Years	15	1.3	<1	1	1	1	1	2	3	4
20–34	10	2.2	9	1	1	2	2	5	5	9
35–49	16	3.1	6	1	2	3	3	5	7	13
50–64	5	1.4	<1	1	1	1	2	2	2	2
65+	2	3.0	0	3	3	3	3	3	3	3
2. MULTIPLE DX										
0–19 Years	41	8.9	348	1	3	3	5	22	69	85
20–34	45	8.0	52	1	5	5	13	16	16	52
35–49	66	8.0	110	2	5	5	8	20	35	46
50–64	41	9.1	121	1	3	4	9	25	27	72
65+	88	10.5	122	1	3	7	15	30	30	55
TOTAL SINGLE DX	48	2.2	3	1	1	2	3	4	5	13
MULTIPLE DX	281	9.0	134	1	2	5	13	21	30	55
TOTAL										
0–19 Years	56	7.2	279	1	2	2	4	16	22	85
20–34	55	7.2	49	1	3	3	13	16	16	52
35–49	82	7.4	98	1	3	3	8	19	33	46
50–64	46	8.5	116	1	3	4	9	25	27	72
65+	90	10.3	120	1	3	6	15	30	30	55
GRAND TOTAL	329	8.3	124	1	2	4	11	19	30	55

United States, October 1995–September 1996 Data, by Operation

86.74: ATTACH PEDICLE GRAFT NEC. Formerly included in operation group(s) 778.

Type of Patients	Observed Patients	Avg. Stay	Variance	10th	25th	50th	75th	90th	95th	99th
1. SINGLE DX										
0–19 Years	36	2.4	8	1	1	1	2	5	8	14
20–34	22	2.7	6	1	1	2	4	4	8	13
35–49	26	3.8	14	1	1	3	4	10	10	17
50–64	17	3.8	12	1	2	3	4	7	16	16
65+	9	1.7	1	1	1	1	2	3	5	5
2. MULTIPLE DX										
0–19 Years	126	7.6	107	1	2	4	9	27	33	>99
20–34	183	10.1	110	2	2	6	14	24	33	59
35–49	285	14.2	205	2	5	8	16	32	58	58
50–64	247	10.0	96	2	2	7	15	24	30	47
65+	453	11.2	107	2	4	7	16	26	33	46
TOTAL SINGLE DX	110	2.8	10	1	1	2	4	6	8	16
MULTIPLE DX	1294	11.3	137	2	3	7	15	28	34	58
TOTAL										
0–19 Years	162	6.2	86	1	1	3	7	17	29	60
20–34	205	9.4	104	2	2	6	14	22	32	59
35–49	311	13.6	199	2	4	8	16	29	58	58
50–64	264	9.7	93	2	2	6	14	24	29	47
65+	462	11.1	107	2	4	7	16	26	32	46
GRAND TOTAL	1404	10.6	132	1	3	7	15	26	33	58

86.8: OTHER SKIN & SUBCU REP. Formerly included in operation group(s) 779.

Type of Patients	Observed Patients	Avg. Stay	Variance	10th	25th	50th	75th	90th	95th	99th
1. SINGLE DX										
0–19 Years	100	1.8	5	1	1	1	1	3	7	12
20–34	123	1.5	1	1	1	1	2	3	7	9
35–49	216	1.6	<1	1	1	1	2	3	3	5
50–64	186	1.4	<1	1	1	1	2	2	3	4
65+	72	1.4	<1	1	1	1	2	3	3	5
2. MULTIPLE DX										
0–19 Years	241	3.0	22	1	1	1	3	6	9	28
20–34	378	3.0	11	1	1	2	4	6	7	18
35–49	800	2.6	7	1	2	2	3	4	5	14
50–64	649	2.6	16	1	1	1	3	5	7	21
65+	327	3.3	19	1	2	2	4	7	11	19
TOTAL SINGLE DX	697	1.5	1	1	1	1	2	3	3	7
MULTIPLE DX	2395	2.8	13	1	1	2	3	5	8	18
TOTAL										
0–19 Years	341	2.7	18	1	1	1	2	6	8	27
20–34	501	2.6	8	1	1	2	3	5	7	18
35–49	1016	2.4	6	1	1	2	3	4	5	12
50–64	835	2.3	13	1	1	1	2	4	6	14
65+	399	2.9	16	1	1	2	3	6	9	18
GRAND TOTAL	3092	2.5	11	1	1	2	3	5	7	18

86.75: REV PEDICLE/FLAP GRAFT. Formerly included in operation group(s) 778.

Type of Patients	Observed Patients	Avg. Stay	Variance	10th	25th	50th	75th	90th	95th	99th
1. SINGLE DX										
0–19 Years	12	2.3	4	1	1	1	4	6	6	7
20–34	14	4.4	33	1	1	2	7	10	10	35
35–49	14	2.7	19	1	1	1	3	4	9	30
50–64	10	2.4	3	1	1	1	4	6	6	6
65+	6	4.8	70	2	2	2	2	16	30	37
2. MULTIPLE DX										
0–19 Years	35	3.1	13	1	1	2	3	10	12	21
20–34	65	14.3	268	1	2	5	21	43	43	64
35–49	112	6.2	51	1	2	4	8	12	16	45
50–64	112	7.7	75	1	1	4	9	19	24	33
65+	104	8.8	137	1	3	5	9	18	32	88
TOTAL SINGLE DX	56	3.6	34	1	1	2	3	7	10	37
MULTIPLE DX	428	8.3	121	1	2	4	9	21	37	50
TOTAL										
0–19 Years	47	2.9	11	1	1	2	3	6	12	12
20–34	79	12.6	241	1	2	5	16	43	43	58
35–49	126	5.8	48	1	2	4	8	12	15	45
50–64	122	7.2	71	1	1	4	9	19	24	33
65+	110	8.0	125	1	2	4	9	18	32	88
GRAND TOTAL	484	7.5	110	1	2	4	8	18	36	48

86.82: FACIAL RHYTIDECTOMY. Formerly included in operation group(s) 779.

Type of Patients	Observed Patients	Avg. Stay	Variance	10th	25th	50th	75th	90th	95th	99th
1. SINGLE DX										
0–19 Years	0									
20–34	2	1.0	0	1	1	1	1	1	1	1
35–49	33	1.3	<1	1	1	1	2	2	2	3
50–64	106	1.2	<1	1	1	1	1	2	2	3
65+	53	1.2	<1	1	1	1	1	2	2	3
2. MULTIPLE DX										
0–19 Years	1	2.0	0	2	2	2	2	2	2	2
20–34	1	2.0	0	2	2	2	2	2	2	2
35–49	78	1.3	<1	1	1	1	2	2	3	3
50–64	222	1.3	<1	1	1	1	1	2	3	4
65+	96	1.3	<1	1	1	1	1	2	3	4
TOTAL SINGLE DX	194	1.2	<1	1	1	1	1	2	2	3
MULTIPLE DX	398	1.3	<1	1	1	1	2	2	2	4
TOTAL										
0–19 Years	1	2.0	0	2	2	2	2	2	2	2
20–34	3	1.6	<1	1	1	2	2	2	2	3
35–49	111	1.3	<1	1	1	1	1	2	2	3
50–64	328	1.3	<1	1	1	1	1	2	2	4
65+	149	1.3	<1	1	1	1	1	2	3	4
GRAND TOTAL	592	1.3	<1	1	1	1	1	2	2	3

Length of Stay by Diagnosis and Operation, United States, 1997

United States, October 1995–September 1996 Data, by Operation

86.83: SIZE RED PLASTIC OP. Formerly included in operation group(s) 779.

Type of Patients	Observed Patients	Avg. Stay	Variance	Percentiles						
				10th	25th	50th	75th	90th	95th	99th
1. SINGLE DX										
0–19 Years	4	2.2	<1	1	1	3	3	3	3	3
20–34	90	1.5	<1	1	1	1	2	2	3	3
35–49	162	1.6	<1	1	1	1	2	3	3	5
50–64	71	1.7	<1	1	1	1	2	3	3	4
65+	14	2.2	1	1	1	2	2	4	5	5
2. MULTIPLE DX										
0–19 Years	13	3.2	7	1	1	2	5	9	9	9
20–34	221	2.4	4	1	1	2	3	5	5	6
35–49	577	2.5	5	1	1	2	3	4	5	12
50–64	339	3.4	26	1	1	2	3	6	9	22
65+	98	3.9	10	1	2	3	5	7	9	15
TOTAL SINGLE DX	341	1.6	<1	1	1	1	2	3	3	5
MULTIPLE DX	1248	2.8	11	1	1	2	3	5	6	13
TOTAL										
0–19 Years	17	3.0	6	1	1	2	4	9	9	9
20–34	311	2.1	3	1	1	1	3	4	5	6
35–49	739	2.4	4	1	1	2	3	4	5	11
50–64	410	3.2	23	1	1	2	3	6	8	22
65+	112	3.6	9	1	2	3	5	6	9	15
GRAND TOTAL	1589	2.6	9	1	1	2	3	5	6	12

86.89: SKIN REP & RECONST NEC. Formerly included in operation group(s) 779.

Type of Patients	Observed Patients	Avg. Stay	Variance	Percentiles						
				10th	25th	50th	75th	90th	95th	99th
1. SINGLE DX										
0–19 Years	21	3.0	11	1	1	2	3	7	12	12
20–34	20	1.8	4	1	1	1	1	4	7	9
35–49	9	1.7	2	1	1	1	2	2	4	8
50–64	3	2.8	3	1	1	4	4	4	4	4
65+	3	2.1	1	1	1	3	3	3	3	3
2. MULTIPLE DX										
0–19 Years	82	3.8	29	1	1	2	5	7	10	40
20–34	108	2.9	6	1	1	2	4	7	8	11
35–49	86	4.6	26	1	2	3	5	12	16	21
50–64	54	3.9	24	1	2	3	5	8	14	25
65+	95	5.2	43	1	2	3	7	14	15	24
TOTAL SINGLE DX	56	2.1	5	1	1	1	2	4	7	12
MULTIPLE DX	425	4.0	25	1	1	2	5	8	14	24
TOTAL										
0–19 Years	103	3.6	26	1	1	2	5	7	10	40
20–34	128	2.6	6	1	1	2	3	6	8	11
35–49	95	4.0	23	1	2	3	4	12	16	21
50–64	57	3.8	24	1	2	3	5	8	14	25
65+	98	5.1	42	1	2	3	7	12	15	24
GRAND TOTAL	481	3.7	23	1	1	2	4	8	12	22

86.9: OTHER SKIN & SUBCU OPS. Formerly included in operation group(s) 777, 779, 780.

Type of Patients	Observed Patients	Avg. Stay	Variance	Percentiles						
				10th	25th	50th	75th	90th	95th	99th
1. SINGLE DX										
0–19 Years	35	1.7	1	1	1	1	2	3	4	5
20–34	9	3.3	16	1	1	1	2	4	12	12
35–49	5	1.7	<1	1	1	2	2	2	2	5
50–64	3	1.0	0	1	1	1	1	1	1	1
65+	1	1.0	0	1	1	1	1	1	1	1
2. MULTIPLE DX										
0–19 Years	80	15.7	338	1	2	2	41	41	41	41
20–34	18	3.4	7	1	1	2	5	5	8	8
35–49	22	3.8	22	1	1	3	4	6	13	33
50–64	8	3.4	9	1	1	1	7	7	7	9
65+	13	7.7	28	1	4	7	7	15	19	20
TOTAL SINGLE DX	53	1.9	3	1	1	1	2	3	5	12
MULTIPLE DX	141	10.5	223	1	1	3	8	41	41	41
TOTAL										
0–19 Years	115	12.2	290	1	1	2	41	41	41	41
20–34	27	3.3	9	1	1	2	5	8	8	12
35–49	27	3.0	15	1	1	2	3	5	7	33
50–64	11	3.3	9	1	1	2	7	7	7	9
65+	14	7.2	29	1	3	7	7	15	19	20
GRAND TOTAL	194	8.4	183	1	1	2	7	41	41	41

87.0: HEAD/NECK SFT TISS X-RAY. Formerly included in operation group(s) 781, 786, 787.

Type of Patients	Observed Patients	Avg. Stay	Variance	Percentiles						
				10th	25th	50th	75th	90th	95th	99th
1. SINGLE DX										
0–19 Years	1908	2.0	4	1	1	1	2	4	5	8
20–34	764	2.8	12	1	1	2	3	5	7	18
35–49	630	3.6	19	1	1	2	6	6	7	27
50–64	421	3.0	13	1	1	2	3	6	7	16
65+	525	3.6	17	1	2	3	4	6	9	20
2. MULTIPLE DX										
0–19 Years	5327	3.5	20	1	1	2	4	7	11	22
20–34	4654	4.0	23	1	1	2	5	8	14	24
35–49	6888	4.5	26	1	2	3	6	9	13	25
50–64	10238	5.0	26	1	2	4	7	10	14	26
65+	37591	6.1	33	2	3	5	7	12	15	30
TOTAL SINGLE DX	4248	2.7	11	1	1	2	3	6	7	16
MULTIPLE DX	64698	5.3	30	1	2	4	7	11	14	27
TOTAL										
0–19 Years	7235	3.2	16	1	1	2	4	6	10	19
20–34	5418	3.9	22	1	1	2	5	8	12	24
35–49	7518	4.4	25	1	2	3	6	9	13	25
50–64	10659	4.9	26	1	2	4	6	10	14	26
65+	38116	6.1	33	2	3	5	7	12	15	30
GRAND TOTAL	68946	5.2	29	1	2	4	6	10	14	27

Length of Stay by Diagnosis and Operation, United States, 1997

United States, October 1995–September 1996 Data, by Operation

87.03: CAT SCAN HEAD. Formerly included in operation group(s) 786.

Type of Patients	Observed Patients	Avg. Stay	Vari-ance	10th	25th	50th	75th	90th	95th	99th
1. SINGLE DX										
0–19 Years	1886	2.0	4	1	1	1	2	4	5	8
20–34	756	2.8	12	1	1	2	3	5	7	18
35–49	625	3.6	19	1	1	2	3	6	7	27
50–64	419	3.0	13	1	1	2	3	6	9	16
65+	521	3.6	17	1	2	3	4	6	9	20
2. MULTIPLE DX										
0–19 Years	5227	3.5	20	1	1	2	4	7	11	21
20–34	4605	4.0	22	1	1	3	5	8	14	24
35–49	6798	4.5	25	1	2	3	6	9	13	25
50–64	10169	5.0	26	1	2	4	6	10	14	26
65+	37453	6.1	33	2	3	5	7	12	15	30
TOTAL SINGLE DX	4207	2.7	11	1	1	2	3	6	7	16
MULTIPLE DX	64252	5.3	30	1	2	4	7	11	14	27
TOTAL										
0–19 Years	7113	3.1	16	1	1	2	3	6	9	19
20–34	5361	3.8	21	1	1	2	5	8	12	24
35–49	7423	4.4	25	1	2	3	6	9	13	25
50–64	10588	4.9	26	1	2	4	6	10	14	26
65+	37974	6.1	33	2	3	5	7	12	15	30
GRAND TOTAL	68459	5.2	29	1	2	4	6	10	14	27

87.2: X-RAY OF SPINE. Formerly included in operation group(s) 782, 787.

Type of Patients	Observed Patients	Avg. Stay	Vari-ance	10th	25th	50th	75th	90th	95th	99th
1. SINGLE DX										
0–19 Years	20	1.7	2	1	1	1	2	4	4	5
20–34	157	2.7	6	1	1	2	4	6	7	9
35–49	279	2.4	3	1	1	2	3	5	6	9
50–64	138	2.5	5	1	1	1	4	4	6	9
65+	73	2.2	2	1	1	2	3	4	5	6
2. MULTIPLE DX										
0–19 Years	45	2.3	5	1	1	1	3	5	6	11
20–34	293	3.4	19	1	1	2	4	7	10	31
35–49	753	3.9	24	1	1	2	5	8	12	28
50–64	600	4.1	17	1	2	3	5	9	11	19
65+	932	5.8	31	2	2	4	8	13	15	21
TOTAL SINGLE DX	667	2.5	4	1	1	2	3	5	6	9
MULTIPLE DX	2623	4.4	24	1	1	3	5	9	13	23
TOTAL										
0–19 Years	65	2.1	4	1	1	1	2	5	6	11
20–34	450	3.1	14	1	1	2	4	6	8	21
35–49	1032	3.5	19	1	1	2	4	7	10	23
50–64	738	3.8	15	1	2	3	5	8	10	17
65+	1005	5.6	30	1	2	4	7	13	15	21
GRAND TOTAL	3290	4.0	21	1	1	3	5	8	12	22

87.1: OTHER HEAD/NECK X-RAY. Formerly included in operation group(s) 787.

Type of Patients	Observed Patients	Avg. Stay	Vari-ance	10th	25th	50th	75th	90th	95th	99th
1. SINGLE DX										
0–19 Years	6	2.1	6	1	1	2	2	2	10	10
20–34	0									
35–49	0									
50–64	0									
65+	1	32.0	0	32	32	32	32	32	32	32
2. MULTIPLE DX										
0–19 Years	47	3.5	18	1	2	2	4	5	11	21
20–34	12	4.9	7	2	3	3	8	8	8	24
35–49	23	5.7	22	1	2	5	10	13	14	19
50–64	19	2.9	2	2	2	3	3	4	4	4
65+	26	4.5	7	3	3	4	5	7	10	16
TOTAL SINGLE DX	7	6.4	121	1	1	2	2	32	32	32
MULTIPLE DX	127	4.2	14	1	2	3	4	8	11	19
TOTAL										
0–19 Years	53	3.4	17	2	2	2	3	5	11	24
20–34	12	4.9	7	2	3	3	8	8	8	8
35–49	23	5.7	22	2	2	5	10	13	14	19
50–64	19	2.9	2	2	2	3	3	4	4	9
65+	27	5.0	21	3	3	4	5	8	14	32
GRAND TOTAL	134	4.2	17	1	2	3	4	8	11	24

87.21: CONTRAST MYELOGRAM. Formerly included in operation group(s) 782.

Type of Patients	Observed Patients	Avg. Stay	Vari-ance	10th	25th	50th	75th	90th	95th	99th
1. SINGLE DX										
0–19 Years	11	2.0	2	1	1	1	4	4	5	5
20–34	146	2.4	4	1	1	2	3	5	7	9
35–49	261	2.4	3	1	1	2	3	5	6	9
50–64	128	2.6	6	1	1	2	4	5	7	8
65+	71	2.2	2	1	1	1	3	4	5	8
2. MULTIPLE DX										
0–19 Years	20	2.9	6	1	1	2	4	6	9	13
20–34	237	3.6	20	1	1	2	4	7	10	31
35–49	696	3.9	22	1	1	2	5	8	12	28
50–64	555	4.2	18	1	1	3	5	8	11	19
65+	846	6.1	34	1	2	4	8	13	16	22
TOTAL SINGLE DX	617	2.4	4	1	1	2	3	5	7	9
MULTIPLE DX	2354	4.6	25	1	1	3	6	10	14	23
TOTAL										
0–19 Years	31	2.7	5	1	1	2	4	6	6	11
20–34	383	3.1	14	1	1	2	4	7	8	20
35–49	957	3.5	18	1	1	2	4	7	10	22
50–64	683	3.9	16	1	1	3	5	8	10	19
65+	917	5.9	32	2	2	4	8	13	15	22
GRAND TOTAL	2971	4.1	21	1	1	3	5	9	13	22

Length of Stay by Diagnosis and Operation, United States, 1997

United States, October 1995–September 1996 Data, by Operation

87.3: THORAX SOFT TISSUE X-RAY. Formerly included in operation group(s) 787.

Type of Patients	Observed Patients	Avg. Stay	Variance	Percentiles						
				10th	25th	50th	75th	90th	95th	99th
1. SINGLE DX										
0–19 Years	15	1.3	<1	1	1	1	1	2	3	6
20–34	5	6.9	6	4	8	8	8	8	8	10
35–49	4	3.4	<1	3	3	3	4	5	5	5
50–64	8	6.3	16	4	4	4	12	12	12	12
65+	3	21.8	547	4	4	9	48	48	48	48
2. MULTIPLE DX										
0–19 Years	55	11.9	670	1	1	2	7	20	97	99
20–34	24	7.0	42	1	3	5	9	17	17	30
35–49	77	8.9	106	2	4	5	10	20	32	53
50–64	83	6.4	21	2	4	6	8	12	12	24
65+	136	8.0	47	2	3	6	9	23	23	26
TOTAL SINGLE DX	29	4.3	36	1	1	3	8	8	8	48
MULTIPLE DX	375	8.3	149	2	3	5	9	17	23	97
TOTAL										
0–19 Years	70	9.8	555	1	1	2	4	20	97	99
20–34	29	7.0	29	1	3	5	8	17	17	22
35–49	81	8.7	103	2	3	5	8	20	32	53
50–64	85	6.4	21	2	4	6	8	12	12	24
65+	139	8.1	51	2	3	6	9	23	23	28
GRAND TOTAL	404	8.1	142	2	3	5	9	17	23	97

87.41: CAT SCAN THORAX. Formerly included in operation group(s) 786.

Type of Patients	Observed Patients	Avg. Stay	Variance	Percentiles						
				10th	25th	50th	75th	90th	95th	99th
1. SINGLE DX										
0–19 Years	32	4.1	24	1	2	3	5	5	12	28
20–34	42	5.5	7	1	2	7	7	7	9	11
35–49	54	5.0	14	1	4	5	5	8	9	23
50–64	43	3.4	2	1	2	4	4	5	6	8
65+	45	2.4	5	1	1	1	4	4	6	9
2. MULTIPLE DX										
0–19 Years	253	5.0	30	1	1	3	7	11	14	28
20–34	354	6.2	44	1	2	4	8	13	16	34
35–49	751	6.2	29	2	3	5	8	11	16	26
50–64	1359	6.1	25	1	3	5	8	12	16	23
65+	3497	7.0	32	2	4	6	9	13	16	26
TOTAL SINGLE DX	216	4.1	11	1	1	4	5	7	8	20
MULTIPLE DX	6214	6.6	31	2	3	5	9	12	16	27
TOTAL										
0–19 Years	285	4.9	29	1	1	3	7	11	14	28
20–34	396	6.1	38	1	3	4	7	12	16	34
35–49	805	6.1	28	2	3	5	8	11	16	24
50–64	1402	6.0	24	1	3	5	8	12	16	23
65+	3542	6.9	32	2	4	6	9	13	16	26
GRAND TOTAL	6430	6.5	30	2	3	5	8	12	16	27

87.4: OTHER X-RAY OF THORAX. Formerly included in operation group(s) 786, 787.

Type of Patients	Observed Patients	Avg. Stay	Variance	Percentiles						
				10th	25th	50th	75th	90th	95th	99th
1. SINGLE DX										
0–19 Years	195	3.2	10	1	1	2	4	6	9	16
20–34	126	5.1	11	1	2	7	7	7	9	16
35–49	117	4.8	16	2	2	5	5	8	11	23
50–64	98	3.5	4	1	2	4	4	5	7	10
65+	85	2.7	12	1	1	1	4	5	7	13
2. MULTIPLE DX										
0–19 Years	907	4.6	25	1	2	3	6	10	13	28
20–34	600	6.1	50	1	2	4	7	12	16	34
35–49	1066	6.1	29	2	3	5	8	11	16	27
50–64	1794	6.0	25	2	3	5	8	12	16	23
65+	4307	7.0	32	2	4	6	9	13	16	27
TOTAL SINGLE DX	621	3.9	12	1	1	3	5	7	9	17
MULTIPLE DX	8674	6.4	31	2	3	5	8	12	16	28
TOTAL										
0–19 Years	1102	4.4	23	1	2	3	5	10	12	28
20–34	726	5.9	43	1	2	4	7	12	16	34
35–49	1183	6.0	28	2	3	5	8	11	15	27
50–64	1892	5.9	24	2	3	5	8	12	15	23
65+	4392	6.8	32	2	4	6	9	13	16	27
GRAND TOTAL	9295	6.2	31	2	3	5	8	12	15	28

87.44: ROUTINE CHEST X-RAY. Formerly included in operation group(s) 787.

Type of Patients	Observed Patients	Avg. Stay	Variance	Percentiles						
				10th	25th	50th	75th	90th	95th	99th
1. SINGLE DX										
0–19 Years	139	2.8	4	1	1	2	3	5	7	10
20–34	58	3.6	13	1	1	2	5	7	14	14
35–49	49	4.0	23	1	2	2	5	10	15	23
50–64	48	3.5	6	1	2	2	5	6	7	13
65+	35	4.3	53	1	1	2	4	6	11	44
2. MULTIPLE DX										
0–19 Years	479	3.5	13	1	2	3	4	6	8	13
20–34	165	5.3	73	1	2	3	6	11	13	58
35–49	208	5.4	27	2	2	4	7	10	16	29
50–64	351	5.2	25	1	2	4	7	10	14	23
65+	590	5.9	35	2	3	4	7	11	15	34
TOTAL SINGLE DX	329	3.3	13	1	1	2	4	7	10	15
MULTIPLE DX	1793	5.0	30	1	2	3	6	10	13	29
TOTAL										
0–19 Years	618	3.4	11	1	2	3	4	6	8	13
20–34	223	4.9	58	1	2	3	5	11	13	58
35–49	257	5.1	26	2	2	3	6	10	15	29
50–64	399	5.0	23	2	2	3	7	10	14	21
65+	625	5.8	36	2	3	4	7	11	15	36
GRAND TOTAL	2122	4.7	28	1	2	3	5	9	13	28

Length of Stay by Diagnosis and Operation, United States, 1997

United States, October 1995–September 1996 Data, by Operation

87.49: CHEST X-RAY NEC. Formerly included in operation group(s) 787.

Type of Patients	Observed Patients	Avg. Stay	Vari-ance	10th	25th	50th	75th	90th	95th	99th
1. SINGLE DX										
0–19 Years	23	4.0	11	1	1	3	5	10	10	10
20–34	25	6.1	26	2	3	5	7	17	17	26
35–49	13	3.9	11	1	1	2	6	9	11	11
50–64	7	3.3	11	1	2	2	4	4	15	15
65+	5	4.6	18	1	1	5	5	13	13	13
2. MULTIPLE DX										
0–19 Years	152	6.7	43	2	3	5	7	13	18	35
20–34	77	5.9	45	2	3	4	6	9	17	37
35–49	91	7.4	40	2	4	6	9	11	20	33
50–64	71	5.5	30	1	2	4	6	10	17	33
65+	195	7.5	33	3	4	6	10	15	16	23
TOTAL SINGLE DX	73	4.6	17	1	2	3	6	10	13	17
MULTIPLE DX	586	6.9	38	2	3	5	8	14	17	33
TOTAL										
0–19 Years	175	6.4	40	2	3	5	7	13	16	33
20–34	102	6.0	40	2	3	4	6	9	17	37
35–49	104	7.0	39	2	3	5	9	11	14	33
50–64	78	5.3	28	1	2	4	6	10	17	33
65+	200	7.4	33	3	4	6	10	15	16	23
GRAND TOTAL	659	6.7	36	2	3	5	8	13	17	33

87.51: PERC HEPAT CHOLANGIOGRAM. Formerly included in operation group(s) 787.

Type of Patients	Observed Patients	Avg. Stay	Vari-ance	10th	25th	50th	75th	90th	95th	99th
1. SINGLE DX										
0–19 Years	5	1.6	1	1	1	1	1	4	4	4
20–34	4	1.7	1	1	1	1	3	3	3	3
35–49	6	3.0	4	2	2	2	4	5	8	8
50–64	5	3.2	23	2	2	2	2	2	21	21
65+	7	4.6	23	1	1	2	9	9	15	15
2. MULTIPLE DX										
0–19 Years	15	2.5	5	1	1	3	3	7	7	7
20–34	25	5.9	16	2	2	5	9	12	13	15
35–49	67	6.1	24	2	3	5	7	11	18	27
50–64	101	5.9	25	2	3	5	6	14	15	30
65+	243	7.1	34	2	3	5	10	15	20	29
TOTAL SINGLE DX	27	3.0	15	1	2	2	2	5	9	21
MULTIPLE DX	451	6.4	29	2	3	5	9	14	17	29
TOTAL										
0–19 Years	20	2.3	4	1	1	1	3	6	7	7
20–34	29	5.5	16	1	2	4	7	12	13	15
35–49	73	5.7	23	2	3	5	6	11	18	24
50–64	106	5.5	26	2	3	4	6	13	15	27
65+	250	7.1	34	2	3	5	9	15	20	29
GRAND TOTAL	478	6.1	29	2	3	4	8	13	16	29

87.5: BILIARY TRACT X-RAY. Formerly included in operation group(s) 787.

Type of Patients	Observed Patients	Avg. Stay	Vari-ance	10th	25th	50th	75th	90th	95th	99th
1. SINGLE DX										
0–19 Years	6	2.4	8	1	1	1	3	4	10	10
20–34	14	2.4	2	1	2	2	2	5	5	5
35–49	18	2.6	2	2	2	2	2	5	6	8
50–64	10	3.0	19	1	2	2	2	3	21	21
65+	9	3.6	16	1	1	2	4	9	15	15
2. MULTIPLE DX										
0–19 Years	54	3.9	9	1	1	4	5	7	11	15
20–34	73	5.6	51	2	2	3	7	10	13	26
35–49	141	4.6	17	1	3	3	5	10	11	20
50–64	213	5.3	21	2	3	4	5	10	15	28
65+	463	7.2	36	2	3	6	9	14	18	29
TOTAL SINGLE DX	57	2.7	7	1	2	2	2	5	6	21
MULTIPLE DX	944	6.0	30	1	3	5	8	12	15	27
TOTAL										
0–19 Years	60	3.8	9	1	1	4	5	7	10	15
20–34	87	4.9	42	1	2	3	5	10	12	26
35–49	159	4.2	15	1	2	3	5	9	11	19
50–64	223	5.1	21	1	3	4	5	10	15	28
65+	472	7.1	36	2	3	6	9	14	18	29
GRAND TOTAL	1001	5.7	29	1	2	4	8	12	15	26

87.6: OTH DIGESTIVE SYST X-RAY. Formerly included in operation group(s) 787.

Type of Patients	Observed Patients	Avg. Stay	Vari-ance	10th	25th	50th	75th	90th	95th	99th
1. SINGLE DX										
0–19 Years	432	1.9	2	1	1	1	2	3	5	8
20–34	87	2.1	4	1	1	2	2	4	5	14
35–49	101	3.0	5	2	2	3	4	6	6	8
50–64	66	2.7	2	2	2	3	3	4	5	9
65+	55	3.8	20	1	2	3	4	5	7	27
2. MULTIPLE DX										
0–19 Years	1256	4.4	27	1	2	3	5	9	12	33
20–34	366	6.0	96	2	3	4	5	8	16	62
35–49	688	4.6	33	1	2	4	6	8	12	45
50–64	975	4.7	21	1	2	4	6	8	11	24
65+	2656	6.1	25	2	3	5	8	11	15	24
TOTAL SINGLE DX	741	2.3	4	1	1	2	3	4	6	8
MULTIPLE DX	5941	5.3	31	1	2	4	6	10	14	28
TOTAL										
0–19 Years	1688	3.7	22	1	2	2	4	7	11	23
20–34	453	5.2	81	1	3	3	5	7	14	62
35–49	789	4.3	28	1	2	3	5	8	11	45
50–64	1041	4.6	20	1	3	3	6	8	11	22
65+	2711	6.0	25	2	3	5	8	11	15	24
GRAND TOTAL	6682	4.9	28	1	2	3	6	9	13	26

Length of Stay by Diagnosis and Operation, United States, 1997

United States, October 1995–September 1996 Data, by Operation

87.61: BARIUM SWALLOW. Formerly included in operation group(s) 787.

Type of Patients	Observed Patients	Avg. Stay	Variance	10th	25th	50th	75th	90th	95th	99th
1. SINGLE DX										
0–19 Years	54	2.5	2	1	1	2	4	4	5	9
20–34	6	1.8	<1	1	1	2	2	2	2	2
35–49	10	1.8	<1	1	1	1	3	4	4	4
50–64	3	1.7	<1	1	1	2	2	2	2	4
65+	2	19.3	122	5	5	27	27	27	27	27
2. MULTIPLE DX										
0–19 Years	169	4.6	18	2	2	4	5	8	10	19
20–34	47	17.3	531	3	4	5	13	62	62	62
35–49	71	4.0	13	1	2	4	5	8	10	29
50–64	150	5.9	49	2	2	4	7	10	14	50
65+	593	7.3	36	2	4	6	9	14	18	30
TOTAL SINGLE DX	75	3.0	19	1	1	2	3	4	7	27
MULTIPLE DX	1030	7.0	63	2	3	5	8	13	18	62
TOTAL										
0–19 Years	223	4.1	15	1	2	3	5	7	9	17
20–34	53	16.2	509	2	4	5	11	62	62	62
35–49	81	3.7	12	1	1	3	4	8	10	29
50–64	153	5.8	48	2	2	4	7	10	14	50
65+	595	7.4	37	2	4	6	9	14	19	30
GRAND TOTAL	1105	6.7	61	2	3	5	8	12	18	62

87.62: UPPER GI SERIES. Formerly included in operation group(s) 787.

Type of Patients	Observed Patients	Avg. Stay	Variance	10th	25th	50th	75th	90th	95th	99th
1. SINGLE DX										
0–19 Years	232	2.4	4	1	1	2	3	5	6	8
20–34	37	2.4	6	1	1	2	2	5	6	14
35–49	53	2.2	2	2	2	2	3	4	4	11
50–64	31	2.9	<1	1	3	3	3	4	4	6
65+	21	2.1	2	1	1	1	3	5	5	5
2. MULTIPLE DX										
0–19 Years	862	4.7	29	1	2	3	6	9	13	25
20–34	227	4.7	21	2	3	4	5	7	11	32
35–49	439	4.8	43	2	2	3	6	8	13	45
50–64	541	4.3	16	1	2	3	6	8	9	16
65+	1154	5.7	25	2	3	4	7	11	14	22
TOTAL SINGLE DX	374	2.4	3	1	1	2	3	4	5	8
MULTIPLE DX	3223	5.0	27	1	2	4	6	9	13	25
TOTAL										
0–19 Years	1094	4.2	24	1	2	3	5	9	12	23
20–34	264	4.3	20	1	2	3	5	7	11	27
35–49	492	4.4	38	1	2	3	5	8	12	45
50–64	572	4.2	15	1	2	3	6	8	9	16
65+	1175	5.7	25	2	3	4	7	11	14	22
GRAND TOTAL	3597	4.7	25	1	2	3	6	9	12	23

87.63: SMALL BOWEL SERIES. Formerly included in operation group(s) 787.

Type of Patients	Observed Patients	Avg. Stay	Variance	10th	25th	50th	75th	90th	95th	99th
1. SINGLE DX										
0–19 Years	3	2.4	<1	2	2	2	3	3	3	3
20–34	5	2.6	<1	1	2	2	3	3	4	4
35–49	19	4.2	3	3	3	4	6	6	6	7
50–64	9	3.5	7	2	2	2	3	9	9	9
65+	10	3.8	<1	2	4	4	4	4	4	7
2. MULTIPLE DX										
0–19 Years	23	5.5	38	2	2	3	4	16	17	29
20–34	30	4.0	7	1	3	4	5	6	6	14
35–49	52	4.7	19	2	2	4	5	8	11	34
50–64	73	5.3	23	2	2	3	7	12	13	19
65+	169	4.8	18	1	2	3	6	11	12	19
TOTAL SINGLE DX	46	4.0	3	2	3	4	6	6	6	9
MULTIPLE DX	347	4.8	19	1	2	3	6	11	13	19
TOTAL										
0–19 Years	26	5.3	37	2	2	3	4	16	17	29
20–34	35	4.0	7	2	3	4	5	6	6	14
35–49	71	4.5	11	2	3	4	6	7	8	13
50–64	82	5.1	21	2	2	3	6	12	13	19
65+	179	4.6	16	1	2	3	5	10	12	19
GRAND TOTAL	393	4.6	16	1	2	4	6	9	12	19

87.64: LOWER GI SERIES. Formerly included in operation group(s) 787.

Type of Patients	Observed Patients	Avg. Stay	Variance	10th	25th	50th	75th	90th	95th	99th
1. SINGLE DX										
0–19 Years	130	1.3	<1	1	1	1	2	2	3	3
20–34	36	1.8	<1	1	1	2	2	3	3	6
35–49	18	4.0	36	1	2	3	4	5	5	39
50–64	22	2.3	<1	2	2	2	2	4	5	6
65+	22	3.3	3	2	2	3	4	5	7	8
2. MULTIPLE DX										
0–19 Years	177	3.3	26	1	2	2	3	4	11	36
20–34	46	3.8	17	1	2	3	4	6	10	19
35–49	101	4.6	15	2	2	4	5	6	9	28
50–64	177	5.0	16	2	3	4	7	8	12	24
65+	649	5.7	15	2	3	5	7	11	12	19
TOTAL SINGLE DX	228	1.6	2	1	1	1	2	3	3	5
MULTIPLE DX	1150	4.9	19	1	2	4	6	9	11	24
TOTAL										
0–19 Years	307	2.4	15	1	1	2	2	3	4	36
20–34	82	2.7	9	1	1	3	5	5	6	19
35–49	119	4.6	17	2	3	4	6	8	8	30
50–64	199	4.7	15	2	3	5	7	10	10	24
65+	671	5.6	15	2	3	5	7	11	12	19
GRAND TOTAL	1378	4.2	17	1	2	3	5	8	11	23

Length of Stay by Diagnosis and Operation, United States, 1997

United States, October 1995–September 1996 Data, by Operation

87.7: X-RAY OF URINARY SYSTEM. Formerly included in operation group(s) 786, 787.

Type of Patients	Observed Patients	Avg. Stay	Variance	10th	25th	50th	75th	90th	95th	99th
1. SINGLE DX										
0–19 Years	321	2.2	2	1	1	2	3	4	5	7
20–34	877	1.6	1	1	1	1	2	3	3	5
35–49	958	1.6	1	1	1	1	2	3	3	6
50–64	460	1.7	1	1	1	1	2	3	3	5
65+	122	1.7	1	1	1	1	2	3	4	7
2. MULTIPLE DX										
0–19 Years	1552	4.3	24	1	2	3	5	8	10	20
20–34	2187	2.8	10	1	1	2	3	5	7	14
35–49	3046	2.8	9	1	1	2	3	5	7	15
50–64	2594	3.2	10	1	1	2	4	6	8	15
65+	4099	5.7	26	1	2	4	7	11	14	26
TOTAL SINGLE DX	2738	1.7	1	1	1	1	2	3	4	6
MULTIPLE DX	13478	3.7	16	1	1	3	5	7	10	19
TOTAL										
0–19 Years	1873	3.9	20	1	2	3	5	7	10	17
20–34	3064	2.4	7	1	1	2	3	4	6	11
35–49	4004	2.4	7	1	1	2	3	5	6	13
50–64	3054	2.9	9	1	1	2	4	6	8	13
65+	4221	5.6	26	1	2	4	7	11	14	26
GRAND TOTAL	16216	3.3	14	1	1	2	4	7	9	17

87.74: RETROGRADE PYELOGRAM. Formerly included in operation group(s) 787.

Type of Patients	Observed Patients	Avg. Stay	Variance	10th	25th	50th	75th	90th	95th	99th
1. SINGLE DX										
0–19 Years	37	2.1	3	1	1	1	3	4	7	7
20–34	182	2.1	2	1	1	2	3	4	4	6
35–49	221	1.9	2	1	1	2	2	3	4	8
50–64	113	1.7	1	1	1	2	2	3	4	6
65+	28	2.3	2	1	1	2	3	3	5	10
2. MULTIPLE DX										
0–19 Years	115	3.3	20	1	2	2	3	6	7	12
20–34	516	3.5	12	1	2	3	4	7	7	13
35–49	922	3.6	9	1	2	3	5	6	9	16
50–64	870	4.1	13	1	2	3	5	8	10	19
65+	1735	7.0	33	2	3	6	9	13	17	35
TOTAL SINGLE DX	581	2.0	2	1	1	2	2	4	4	7
MULTIPLE DX	4158	4.9	22	1	2	4	6	10	13	24
TOTAL										
0–19 Years	152	3.1	17	1	2	2	3	6	7	11
20–34	698	3.1	9	1	2	2	4	6	7	10
35–49	1143	3.3	8	1	2	2	4	6	9	16
50–64	983	3.7	12	1	2	3	5	8	9	18
65+	1763	6.9	33	2	3	5	9	13	17	35
GRAND TOTAL	4739	4.5	20	1	2	3	6	9	12	22

87.73: IV PYELOGRAM. Formerly included in operation group(s) 787.

Type of Patients	Observed Patients	Avg. Stay	Variance	10th	25th	50th	75th	90th	95th	99th
1. SINGLE DX										
0–19 Years	148	1.9	1	1	1	1	3	3	4	6
20–34	620	1.5	1	1	1	1	2	3	3	5
35–49	678	1.5	<1	1	1	1	2	3	3	5
50–64	320	1.6	<1	1	1	1	2	3	3	4
65+	84	1.5	<1	1	1	1	2	2	3	5
2. MULTIPLE DX										
0–19 Years	341	3.0	5	1	1	2	4	6	9	9
20–34	1416	2.4	5	1	1	2	3	4	5	10
35–49	1814	2.4	5	1	1	2	3	5	6	9
50–64	1420	2.6	6	1	1	2	3	5	6	11
65+	1642	4.3	15	2	2	3	5	8	10	18
TOTAL SINGLE DX	1850	1.5	<1	1	1	1	2	3	3	5
MULTIPLE DX	6633	2.8	7	1	1	2	3	5	7	12
TOTAL										
0–19 Years	489	2.7	4	1	1	2	3	5	8	9
20–34	2036	2.1	4	1	1	1	3	4	5	9
35–49	2492	2.1	4	1	1	1	2	5	6	8
50–64	1740	2.4	5	1	1	2	3	5	6	10
65+	1726	4.1	14	1	2	3	5	7	10	18
GRAND TOTAL	8483	2.5	6	1	1	2	3	5	6	11

87.76: RETRO CYSTOURETHROGRAM. Formerly included in operation group(s) 787.

Type of Patients	Observed Patients	Avg. Stay	Variance	10th	25th	50th	75th	90th	95th	99th
1. SINGLE DX										
0–19 Years	74	3.1	2	2	2	3	4	5	5	7
20–34	3	4.1	1	2	3	5	5	5	5	5
35–49	1	1.0	0	1	1	1	1	1	1	1
50–64	0									
65+	0									
2. MULTIPLE DX										
0–19 Years	849	5.2	32	2	3	4	6	9	11	26
20–34	33	5.1	31	1	3	3	6	9	20	29
35–49	39	4.1	21	1	2	3	5	7	12	14
50–64	36	7.5	124	1	2	4	8	20	22	84
65+	68	7.6	32	3	4	5	10	15	20	23
TOTAL SINGLE DX	78	3.1	2	1	2	3	4	5	5	7
MULTIPLE DX	1025	5.3	35	2	3	4	6	10	11	29
TOTAL										
0–19 Years	923	5.0	30	2	3	4	6	8	10	23
20–34	36	5.1	28	1	3	3	5	8	20	29
35–49	40	4.1	21	1	2	3	5	7	12	14
50–64	36	7.5	124	1	2	4	8	20	22	84
65+	68	7.6	32	3	4	5	10	15	20	23
GRAND TOTAL	1103	5.2	33	2	3	4	6	9	11	26

Length of Stay by Diagnosis and Operation, United States, 1997

United States, October 1995–September 1996 Data, by Operation

87.77: CYSTOGRAM NEC. Formerly included in operation group(s) 787.

Type of Patients	Observed Patients	Avg. Stay	Variance	10th	25th	50th	75th	90th	95th	99th
1. SINGLE DX										
0–19 Years	14	3.8	16	1	1	1	5	12	12	12
20–34	7	2.2	2	1	1	2	5	5	5	5
35–49	6	3.3	4	1	1	2	5	5	7	7
50–64	0									
65+	3	4.8	3	4	4	4	4	8	8	8
2. MULTIPLE DX										
0–19 Years	100	5.7	54	1	2	4	7	10	15	22
20–34	69	5.5	47	1	3	4	5	11	12	27
35–49	55	5.4	26	2	2	4	8	10	11	39
50–64	41	5.7	14	2	4	5	7	10	16	18
65+	156	6.8	28	1	4	5	8	11	19	32
TOTAL SINGLE DX	30	3.4	8	1	1	2	5	7	8	12
MULTIPLE DX	421	6.0	37	1	3	4	7	11	15	27
TOTAL										
0–19 Years	114	5.5	50	1	2	4	7	10	13	22
20–34	76	5.4	46	1	3	4	5	11	12	27
35–49	61	4.8	20	1	2	4	6	9	10	28
50–64	41	5.7	14	2	4	5	7	10	16	18
65+	159	6.8	28	1	4	5	8	11	19	32
GRAND TOTAL	451	5.8	35	1	3	4	7	11	14	27

87.8: FEMALE GENITAL X-RAY. Formerly included in operation group(s) 787.

Type of Patients	Observed Patients	Avg. Stay	Variance	10th	25th	50th	75th	90th	95th	99th
1. SINGLE DX										
0–19 Years	0									
20–34	0									
35–49	0									
50–64	0									
65+	0									
2. MULTIPLE DX										
0–19 Years	2	2.5	<1	2	2	3	3	3	3	3
20–34	4	3.6	1	2	2	4	4	5	5	5
35–49	2	2.1	1	1	1	3	3	3	3	3
50–64	0									
65+	2	8.2	9	5	5	10	10	10	10	10
TOTAL SINGLE DX	0									
MULTIPLE DX	10	3.3	5	1	2	3	4	5	10	10
TOTAL										
0–19 Years	2	2.5	<1	2	2	3	3	3	3	3
20–34	4	3.6	1	2	2	4	4	5	5	5
35–49	2	2.1	1	1	1	3	3	3	3	3
50–64	0									
65+	2	8.2	9	5	5	10	10	10	10	10
GRAND TOTAL	10	3.3	5	1	2	3	4	5	10	10

87.79: URINARY SYSTEM X-RAY NEC. Formerly included in operation group(s) 787.

Type of Patients	Observed Patients	Avg. Stay	Variance	10th	25th	50th	75th	90th	95th	99th
1. SINGLE DX										
0–19 Years	38	1.8	1	1	1	1	2	4	4	6
20–34	52	1.6	<1	1	1	1	2	2	4	5
35–49	44	1.7	2	1	1	1	2	3	5	7
50–64	20	2.6	3	1	1	2	4	5	6	6
65+	2	1.8	<1	1	2	2	2	2	2	2
2. MULTIPLE DX										
0–19 Years	115	3.1	10	1	1	2	4	6	8	16
20–34	105	5.0	35	1	2	3	5	10	18	40
35–49	139	5.2	53	1	1	3	5	14	17	35
50–64	141	4.8	14	1	2	4	7	9	10	20
65+	359	6.3	25	2	3	5	8	12	16	24
TOTAL SINGLE DX	156	1.7	1	1	1	1	2	4	4	6
MULTIPLE DX	859	5.3	30	1	2	4	7	11	15	34
TOTAL										
0–19 Years	153	2.7	8	1	1	2	3	6	6	16
20–34	157	3.5	23	1	1	3	5	6	18	19
35–49	183	4.3	42	1	1	2	5	14	15	35
50–64	161	4.5	13	2	2	4	6	9	10	20
65+	361	6.3	25	2	3	5	8	12	16	24
GRAND TOTAL	1015	4.6	26	1	1	3	6	9	14	25

87.9: MALE GENITAL X-RAY. Formerly included in operation group(s) 787.

Type of Patients	Observed Patients	Avg. Stay	Variance	10th	25th	50th	75th	90th	95th	99th
1. SINGLE DX										
0–19 Years	0									
20–34	0									
35–49	0									
50–64	0									
65+	0									
2. MULTIPLE DX										
0–19 Years	0									
20–34	0									
35–49	3	4.9	2	4	4	4	5	7	7	7
50–64	0									
65+	3	4.6	19	1	1	3	10	10	10	10
TOTAL SINGLE DX	0									
MULTIPLE DX	6	4.8	10	1	3	4	7	10	10	10
TOTAL										
0–19 Years	0									
20–34	0									
35–49	3	4.9	2	4	4	4	5	7	7	7
50–64	0									
65+	3	4.6	19	1	1	3	10	10	10	10
GRAND TOTAL	6	4.8	10	1	3	4	7	10	10	10

Length of Stay by Diagnosis and Operation, United States, 1997

United States, October 1995–September 1996 Data, by Operation

88.0: SOFT TISSUE X-RAY ABD. Formerly included in operation group(s) 786, 787.

Type of Patients	Observed Patients	Avg. Stay	Variance	10th	25th	50th	75th	90th	95th	99th
1. SINGLE DX										
0–19 Years	498	2.4	5	1	1	2	3	5	7	9
20–34	601	2.7	3	1	1	2	4	5	7	8
35–49	596	3.3	5	1	2	3	4	6	8	10
50–64	349	3.4	5	1	2	3	5	6	8	10
65+	200	3.9	5	1	3	3	5	7	8	10
2. MULTIPLE DX										
0–19 Years	1265	4.2	17	1	2	3	6	8	11	20
20–34	2365	4.8	26	1	2	3	6	9	14	32
35–49	3602	4.7	18	1	2	4	6	9	12	21
50–64	3833	5.2	15	2	3	4	6	9	12	20
65+	8087	6.2	26	2	3	5	8	11	15	25
TOTAL SINGLE DX	2244	3.0	5	1	1	3	4	6	7	10
MULTIPLE DX	19152	5.3	22	1	2	4	7	10	13	22
TOTAL										
0–19 Years	1763	3.7	14	1	1	2	5	7	9	18
20–34	2966	4.4	22	1	2	3	5	8	12	21
35–49	4198	4.5	16	1	2	4	6	8	11	20
50–64	4182	5.0	14	2	3	4	6	9	11	20
65+	8287	6.2	26	2	3	5	8	11	15	25
GRAND TOTAL	21396	5.1	20	1	2	4	6	10	13	21

88.01: CAT SCAN OF ABDOMEN. Formerly included in operation group(s) 786.

Type of Patients	Observed Patients	Avg. Stay	Variance	10th	25th	50th	75th	90th	95th	99th
1. SINGLE DX										
0–19 Years	497	2.4	5	1	1	2	3	5	7	9
20–34	596	2.7	3	1	2	2	4	5	6	8
35–49	594	3.3	5	1	2	3	4	6	8	10
50–64	347	3.4	5	1	2	3	5	6	8	10
65+	198	4.0	5	1	3	3	5	7	8	10
2. MULTIPLE DX										
0–19 Years	1256	4.1	17	1	2	3	6	8	11	20
20–34	2351	4.8	26	1	2	3	6	9	14	32
35–49	3566	4.7	18	1	2	4	6	9	12	21
50–64	3807	5.2	15	2	3	4	6	9	12	20
65+	8036	6.2	26	2	3	5	8	11	15	25
TOTAL SINGLE DX	2232	3.0	5	1	1	3	4	6	7	10
MULTIPLE DX	19016	5.3	22	1	2	4	7	10	13	22
TOTAL										
0–19 Years	1753	3.7	14	1	1	2	5	7	9	18
20–34	2947	4.4	22	1	2	3	5	8	12	21
35–49	4160	4.5	16	1	2	4	6	8	11	20
50–64	4154	5.0	14	2	3	4	6	9	11	20
65+	8234	6.2	26	2	3	5	8	11	15	25
GRAND TOTAL	21248	5.0	20	1	2	4	6	10	13	21

88.1: OTHER X-RAY OF ABDOMEN. Formerly included in operation group(s) 787.

Type of Patients	Observed Patients	Avg. Stay	Variance	10th	25th	50th	75th	90th	95th	99th
1. SINGLE DX										
0–19 Years	50	1.6	2	1	1	1	2	2	5	7
20–34	15	2.4	3	1	1	2	3	6	6	7
35–49	16	2.3	1	2	2	2	3	3	6	7
50–64	12	3.3	3	2	3	3	3	5	6	14
65+	10	3.6	3	2	3	3	4	4	4	11
2. MULTIPLE DX										
0–19 Years	153	2.9	13	1	1	2	3	5	8	22
20–34	81	3.9	7	1	2	4	4	6	8	20
35–49	143	4.3	28	1	2	4	4	10	15	30
50–64	109	4.0	5	2	3	3	4	7	8	13
65+	325	4.3	11	1	2	3	6	8	10	15
TOTAL SINGLE DX	103	2.4	3	1	1	2	3	4	6	9
MULTIPLE DX	811	4.0	13	1	2	3	5	8	10	20
TOTAL										
0–19 Years	203	2.5	10	1	1	2	3	5	7	22
20–34	96	3.8	7	1	2	4	4	6	8	20
35–49	159	4.0	25	1	2	3	4	9	13	29
50–64	121	3.9	5	2	3	3	4	7	8	13
65+	335	4.2	10	1	2	3	6	8	10	15
GRAND TOTAL	914	3.8	12	1	2	3	4	8	10	17

88.19: ABDOMINAL X-RAY NEC. Formerly included in operation group(s) 787.

Type of Patients	Observed Patients	Avg. Stay	Variance	10th	25th	50th	75th	90th	95th	99th
1. SINGLE DX										
0–19 Years	42	1.4	<1	1	1	1	2	2	2	7
20–34	10	2.3	2	1	1	2	3	3	7	7
35–49	10	2.2	<1	2	2	2	2	3	3	6
50–64	9	3.1	<1	2	3	3	3	4	5	6
65+	10	3.6	3	2	3	3	4	4	4	11
2. MULTIPLE DX										
0–19 Years	120	2.5	7	1	1	2	3	4	7	13
20–34	50	3.7	5	1	2	4	4	4	8	10
35–49	90	3.8	26	1	2	2	3	6	13	30
50–64	82	3.9	5	2	3	3	4	6	8	13
65+	300	4.2	10	1	2	3	6	8	10	14
TOTAL SINGLE DX	81	2.3	2	1	1	2	3	4	4	7
MULTIPLE DX	642	3.8	12	1	2	3	4	8	9	16
TOTAL										
0–19 Years	162	2.2	6	1	1	2	2	4	6	13
20–34	60	3.5	5	1	2	4	4	4	8	10
35–49	100	3.6	23	1	2	2	3	6	12	30
50–64	91	3.8	4	2	3	3	4	6	8	13
65+	310	4.2	10	1	2	3	5	8	10	14
GRAND TOTAL	723	3.6	11	1	2	3	4	7	8	15

Length of Stay by Diagnosis and Operation, United States, 1997

United States, October 1995–September 1996 Data, by Operation

88.2: SKEL X-RAY-EXT & PELVIS. Formerly included in operation group(s) 787.

Type of Patients	Observed Patients	Avg. Stay	Vari-ance	Percentiles						
				10th	25th	50th	75th	90th	95th	99th
1. SINGLE DX										
0–19 Years	15	2.3	4	1	1	1	3	6	6	6
20–34	7	1.9	<1	1	1	2	4	6	3	3
35–49	11	27.9	187	1	35	35	35	35	35	35
50–64	3	4.3	16	2	2	2	4	12	12	12
65+	8	2.5	4	1	2	2	2	8	8	8
2. MULTIPLE DX										
0–19 Years	50	4.1	16	1	2	4	4	8	15	>99
20–34	52	3.9	14	1	1	2	5	9	15	17
35–49	71	6.3	34	1	4	5	6	13	22	23
50–64	56	4.8	20	2	3	3	7	11	13	22
65+	196	6.9	42	2	3	6	9	12	15	33
TOTAL SINGLE DX	44	16.7	267	1	2	4	35	35	35	35
MULTIPLE DX	425	6.1	34	2	3	5	8	11	15	23
TOTAL										
0–19 Years	65	3.7	14	1	1	3	4	6	11	29
20–34	59	3.8	13	1	1	2	5	8	11	17
35–49	82	10.1	128	1	4	5	9	35	35	35
50–64	59	4.8	20	2	3	4	7	11	13	22
65+	204	6.8	41	2	3	5	9	12	15	33
GRAND TOTAL	469	7.0	62	1	3	5	8	13	22	35

88.3: OTHER X-RAY. Formerly included in operation group(s) 786, 787.

Type of Patients	Observed Patients	Avg. Stay	Vari-ance	Percentiles						
				10th	25th	50th	75th	90th	95th	99th
1. SINGLE DX										
0–19 Years	246	2.6	4	1	1	2	3	5	6	10
20–34	169	3.2	4	1	2	3	4	6	6	8
35–49	180	3.2	9	1	1	3	4	6	7	14
50–64	70	3.9	26	1	1	3	6	6	9	28
65+	35	4.9	7	2	3	5	6	8	10	12
2. MULTIPLE DX										
0–19 Years	517	4.4	15	1	2	3	6	9	12	22
20–34	485	4.1	13	1	2	3	5	9	12	16
35–49	713	4.7	21	2	2	4	6	8	11	32
50–64	715	5.2	23	2	2	4	6	10	12	21
65+	1587	5.9	27	2	3	5	7	12	15	27
TOTAL SINGLE DX	700	3.1	7	1	1	2	4	6	7	12
MULTIPLE DX	4017	5.1	22	1	2	4	6	10	12	24
TOTAL										
0–19 Years	763	3.8	12	1	2	3	5	7	10	22
20–34	654	3.8	10	1	2	3	5	8	10	14
35–49	893	4.4	19	2	2	4	5	8	11	27
50–64	785	5.1	23	2	3	4	6	10	12	28
65+	1622	5.9	27	2	3	5	7	12	15	27
GRAND TOTAL	4717	4.8	20	1	2	4	6	9	12	22

88.38: OTHER C.A.T. SCAN. Formerly included in operation group(s) 786.

Type of Patients	Observed Patients	Avg. Stay	Vari-ance	Percentiles						
				10th	25th	50th	75th	90th	95th	99th
1. SINGLE DX										
0–19 Years	187	2.6	3	1	1	2	3	5	6	9
20–34	164	3.1	4	1	2	3	4	6	6	7
35–49	180	3.2	9	1	2	3	4	6	7	14
50–64	69	4.1	27	1	2	3	4	6	11	28
65+	34	4.9	7	2	3	5	6	8	10	12
2. MULTIPLE DX										
0–19 Years	435	4.3	11	1	2	3	6	8	10	18
20–34	475	4.1	13	1	2	3	5	9	12	16
35–49	696	4.6	21	2	2	4	6	8	11	32
50–64	698	5.2	23	2	2	4	6	10	12	21
65+	1526	5.9	27	2	3	5	7	12	15	27
TOTAL SINGLE DX	634	3.1	7	1	1	2	4	6	7	12
MULTIPLE DX	3830	5.1	21	2	2	4	6	10	12	24
TOTAL										
0–19 Years	622	3.8	9	1	2	3	5	7	9	18
20–34	639	3.8	10	1	2	3	5	8	10	14
35–49	876	4.3	19	1	2	4	5	8	11	27
50–64	767	5.1	23	2	3	5	7	10	12	28
65+	1560	5.9	26	2	3	5	7	12	15	27
GRAND TOTAL	4464	4.8	20	1	2	4	6	9	12	22

88.4: CONTRAST ARTERIOGRAPHY. Formerly included in operation group(s) 783, 785.

Type of Patients	Observed Patients	Avg. Stay	Vari-ance	Percentiles						
				10th	25th	50th	75th	90th	95th	99th
1. SINGLE DX										
0–19 Years	190	2.2	4	1	1	1	2	4	8	12
20–34	457	2.6	5	1	1	2	4	5	8	10
35–49	519	3.0	7	1	1	2	3	6	8	14
50–64	412	2.8	7	1	1	2	3	6	8	15
65+	420	2.6	6	1	1	2	3	6	7	11
2. MULTIPLE DX										
0–19 Years	386	5.3	30	1	2	4	8	12	20	>99
20–34	1270	4.3	15	1	2	3	6	8	11	19
35–49	3058	5.2	21	1	2	4	7	10	13	21
50–64	5372	5.3	23	2	2	4	7	11	14	26
65+	11594	5.6	23	2	3	5	7	11	14	22
TOTAL SINGLE DX	1998	2.7	6	1	1	2	3	6	8	13
MULTIPLE DX	21680	5.4	23	1	2	4	7	10	14	23
TOTAL										
0–19 Years	576	4.2	23	1	1	2	6	9	13	>99
20–34	1727	3.9	13	1	1	3	5	8	11	16
35–49	3577	4.9	20	1	2	4	7	10	13	20
50–64	5784	5.1	22	1	2	4	6	11	14	26
65+	12014	5.5	23	1	2	4	7	11	14	22
GRAND TOTAL	23678	5.2	22	2	2	4	7	10	13	23

Length of Stay by Diagnosis and Operation, United States, 1997

United States, October 1995–September 1996 Data, by Operation

88.41: CEREBRAL ARTERIOGRAM. Formerly included in operation group(s) 783.

Type of Patients	Observed Patients	Avg. Stay	Variance	10th	25th	50th	75th	90th	95th	99th
1. SINGLE DX										
0–19 Years	86	2.3	4	1	1	1	3	4	8	8
20–34	191	2.7	6	1	1	1	4	6	9	11
35–49	269	3.7	10	1	1	3	5	8	11	14
50–64	216	3.2	11	1	1	3	3	6	11	15
65+	216	3.1	8	1	1	2	4	6	7	13
2. MULTIPLE DX										
0–19 Years	166	6.0	42	1	2	4	8	13	18	39
20–34	485	5.1	22	1	2	3	6	11	14	28
35–49	1337	5.8	23	2	3	5	8	11	13	21
50–64	2364	5.4	19	1	2	5	7	10	13	22
65+	4804	5.4	19	1	3	5	7	10	12	21
TOTAL SINGLE DX	978	3.1	9	1	1	2	4	6	9	15
MULTIPLE DX	9156	5.5	20	1	3	5	7	10	13	21
TOTAL										
0–19 Years	252	4.6	31	1	1	3	6	9	14	30
20–34	676	4.4	18	1	1	3	6	10	12	26
35–49	1606	5.5	22	2	2	4	7	11	13	19
50–64	2580	5.2	19	1	2	5	6	10	13	22
65+	5020	5.4	19	1	3	5	7	10	12	21
GRAND TOTAL	10134	5.3	20	1	2	4	7	10	13	21

88.42: CONTRAST AORTOGRAM. Formerly included in operation group(s) 785.

Type of Patients	Observed Patients	Avg. Stay	Variance	10th	25th	50th	75th	90th	95th	99th
1. SINGLE DX										
0–19 Years	10	4.1	11	1	1	3	9	9	9	9
20–34	28	2.8	3	1	1	3	4	5	5	6
35–49	44	1.9	3	1	1	1	2	4	7	10
50–64	54	2.0	1	1	1	2	2	3	4	6
65+	72	1.7	2	1	1	1	2	3	4	8
2. MULTIPLE DX										
0–19 Years	47	4.9	12	1	1	5	7	10	10	13
20–34	147	3.7	10	1	1	3	5	8	11	14
35–49	390	4.5	10	1	2	4	6	9	11	14
50–64	904	5.1	27	2	2	4	7	10	15	29
65+	2268	5.2	23	1	2	4	7	11	14	22
TOTAL SINGLE DX	208	2.1	2	1	1	2	2	4	5	9
MULTIPLE DX	3756	5.0	22	1	2	4	7	10	14	22
TOTAL										
0–19 Years	57	4.8	12	1	1	4	8	10	10	13
20–34	175	3.5	8	1	1	3	5	6	10	14
35–49	434	4.3	10	1	2	3	6	9	10	14
50–64	958	4.8	26	1	2	3	6	10	15	29
65+	2340	5.0	22	1	2	4	7	10	14	22
GRAND TOTAL	3964	4.8	21	1	2	3	6	10	13	22

88.43: PULMONARY ARTERIOGRAM. Formerly included in operation group(s) 785.

Type of Patients	Observed Patients	Avg. Stay	Variance	10th	25th	50th	75th	90th	95th	99th
1. SINGLE DX										
0–19 Years	1	1.0	0	1	1	1	1	1	1	1
20–34	48	3.9	9	1	1	3	6	10	10	10
35–49	71	3.2	5	1	2	2	5	6	7	9
50–64	33	3.9	6	1	2	4	5	8	8	11
65+	18	4.0	7	1	2	3	6	7	8	11
2. MULTIPLE DX										
0–19 Years	31	6.1	26	2	2	8	9	>99	>99	>99
20–34	296	4.7	13	1	2	4	7	8	9	15
35–49	579	5.1	15	1	2	4	7	10	14	15
50–64	675	5.4	13	2	3	4	7	10	11	16
65+	1014	6.3	20	2	3	5	8	12	16	22
TOTAL SINGLE DX	171	3.2	6	1	1	2	5	7	9	10
MULTIPLE DX	2595	5.6	17	2	3	5	8	10	14	22
TOTAL										
0–19 Years	32	4.6	24	1	1	3	9	25	>99	>99
20–34	344	4.6	13	1	2	4	7	8	9	15
35–49	650	4.9	15	1	2	4	7	9	14	15
50–64	708	5.3	13	2	3	5	7	10	11	16
65+	1032	6.2	20	2	3	5	8	12	16	22
GRAND TOTAL	2766	5.4	16	1	2	5	7	10	13	21

88.45: RENAL ARTERIOGRAM. Formerly included in operation group(s) 785.

Type of Patients	Observed Patients	Avg. Stay	Variance	10th	25th	50th	75th	90th	95th	99th
1. SINGLE DX										
0–19 Years	14	2.2	3	1	1	1	2	6	6	6
20–34	41	2.4	2	1	2	2	3	4	6	8
35–49	58	2.3	4	1	1	2	3	4	6	17
50–64	28	1.6	<1	1	1	1	2	3	3	5
65+	15	1.4	<1	1	1	1	2	2	2	3
2. MULTIPLE DX										
0–19 Years	39	4.5	14	1	2	3	6	12	12	12
20–34	67	5.1	14	1	2	4	7	12	12	15
35–49	192	4.8	15	1	2	4	8	8	13	19
50–64	248	5.0	23	1	3	3	7	10	14	30
65+	404	6.1	35	1	4	4	8	13	18	26
TOTAL SINGLE DX	156	2.0	2	1	1	2	2	4	5	6
MULTIPLE DX	950	5.4	26	1	2	4	7	12	15	26
TOTAL										
0–19 Years	53	3.8	12	1	1	2	5	11	12	12
20–34	108	4.3	12	1	2	3	6	10	12	15
35–49	250	4.3	14	1	2	4	5	7	11	17
50–64	276	4.7	22	1	2	3	6	10	14	30
65+	419	5.8	34	1	2	4	7	12	17	26
GRAND TOTAL	1106	5.0	24	1	2	3	6	11	14	26

Length of Stay by Diagnosis and Operation, United States, 1997

United States, October 1995–September 1996 Data, by Operation

88.47: ABD ARTERIOGRAM NEC. Formerly included in operation group(s) 785.

Type of Patients	Observed Patients	Avg. Stay	Vari-ance	10th	25th	50th	75th	90th	95th	99th
1. SINGLE DX										
0–19 Years	6	2.1	6	1	1	1	1	8	8	8
20–34	4	1.2	<1	1	1	1	1	2	2	2
35–49	9	1.5	<1	1	1	1	1	2	3	3
50–64	16	2.3	4	1	1	1	4	5	5	8
65+	8	1.2	<1	1	1	1	1	2	2	2
2. MULTIPLE DX										
0–19 Years	24	6.7	49	1	2	5	7	15	25	29
20–34	38	5.0	21	1	2	4	6	9	13	25
35–49	112	8.3	114	1	2	4	8	29	29	36
50–64	215	4.5	19	1	2	3	5	8	14	26
65+	469	6.5	37	2	3	6	8	11	14	38
TOTAL SINGLE DX	43	1.7	2	1	1	1	2	3	5	8
MULTIPLE DX	858	6.2	41	1	3	5	7	11	15	30
TOTAL										
0–19 Years	30	5.6	42	1	1	3	7	15	25	29
20–34	42	4.5	20	1	1	3	6	9	11	25
35–49	121	7.6	106	1	2	3	8	29	29	36
50–64	231	4.4	19	1	2	3	5	8	14	26
65+	477	6.4	37	2	3	6	8	11	14	38
GRAND TOTAL	901	6.0	40	1	3	5	7	11	15	29

88.48: CONTRAST ARTERIOGRAM-LEG. Formerly included in operation group(s) 785.

Type of Patients	Observed Patients	Avg. Stay	Vari-ance	10th	25th	50th	75th	90th	95th	99th
1. SINGLE DX										
0–19 Years	51	2.3	6	1	1	1	2	3	12	12
20–34	83	2.1	2	1	1	1	3	4	5	7
35–49	39	1.8	2	1	1	1	2	4	5	8
50–64	46	2.3	5	1	1	1	3	7	8	8
65+	79	2.9	6	1	1	2	4	6	9	11
2. MULTIPLE DX										
0–19 Years	44	3.5	28	1	1	2	3	9	11	23
20–34	125	3.1	7	1	1	2	4	5	8	16
35–49	278	3.6	14	1	2	2	5	8	11	19
50–64	759	5.7	38	1	2	4	7	11	18	39
65+	2328	5.7	27	2	2	4	8	12	15	25
TOTAL SINGLE DX	298	2.3	5	1	1	1	3	5	7	11
MULTIPLE DX	3534	5.3	28	1	2	4	7	11	15	26
TOTAL										
0–19 Years	95	2.8	17	1	1	1	3	7	11	12
20–34	208	2.7	6	1	1	2	4	5	7	13
35–49	317	3.3	13	1	1	2	5	8	10	17
50–64	805	5.4	36	1	2	4	6	11	18	39
65+	2407	5.6	27	1	2	4	8	12	15	25
GRAND TOTAL	3832	5.1	27	1	2	4	7	11	14	26

88.49: CONTRAST ARTERIOGRAM NEC. Formerly included in operation group(s) 785.

Type of Patients	Observed Patients	Avg. Stay	Vari-ance	10th	25th	50th	75th	90th	95th	99th
1. SINGLE DX										
0–19 Years	16	2.2	3	1	1	2	2	6	7	7
20–34	55	2.2	4	1	1	2	3	6	5	11
35–49	25	2.6	4	1	2	2	2	6	7	14
50–64	18	2.3	4	1	1	2	3	4	6	9
65+	11	2.3	4	1	1	1	3	7	7	7
2. MULTIPLE DX										
0–19 Years	31	2.6	7	1	1	2	3	7	9	11
20–34	86	2.7	5	1	2	2	3	6	6	13
35–49	148	5.5	18	1	2	6	6	10	14	15
50–64	176	4.3	24	1	1	3	4	15	15	22
65+	260	5.4	25	1	2	4	7	12	15	21
TOTAL SINGLE DX	125	2.4	4	1	1	2	3	5	7	11
MULTIPLE DX	701	4.5	20	1	1	3	6	10	15	19
TOTAL										
0–19 Years	47	2.5	6	1	1	2	3	6	9	11
20–34	141	2.6	5	1	1	2	3	6	6	13
35–49	173	5.0	17	1	2	5	6	9	11	15
50–64	194	4.2	24	1	1	3	4	15	15	22
65+	271	5.3	24	1	2	4	7	12	15	21
GRAND TOTAL	826	4.2	19	1	1	2	6	10	15	18

88.5: CONTRAST ANGIOCARDIOGRAM. Formerly included in operation group(s) 784, 785.

Type of Patients	Observed Patients	Avg. Stay	Vari-ance	10th	25th	50th	75th	90th	95th	99th
1. SINGLE DX										
0–19 Years	7	3.3	27	1	1	1	2	16	16	16
20–34	3	1.6	<1	1	1	1	2	3	3	
35–49	50	1.6	2	1	1	1	2	3	3	10
50–64	71	3.0	32	1	1	1	2	6	8	38
65+	33	1.4	<1	1	1	2	1	3	3	4
2. MULTIPLE DX										
0–19 Years	62	4.0	50	1	1	3	7	8	15	16
20–34	79	4.4	17	1	3	3	6	9	11	18
35–49	601	4.2	62	1	2	2	4	8	11	53
50–64	1274	3.1	11	1	2	2	4	7	9	15
65+	1753	3.6	15	1	2	2	5	8	11	19
TOTAL SINGLE DX	164	2.2	16	1	1	1	2	4	6	24
MULTIPLE DX	3769	3.5	22	1	1	2	4	8	10	19
TOTAL										
0–19 Years	69	3.9	49	1	1	1	7	8	15	16
20–34	82	4.4	17	1	3	3	6	9	11	18
35–49	651	4.1	60	1	2	2	4	8	11	53
50–64	1345	3.1	11	1	1	2	4	7	9	15
65+	1786	3.5	14	1	2	2	5	8	11	19
GRAND TOTAL	3933	3.5	21	1	1	2	4	8	10	19

Length of Stay by Diagnosis and Operation, United States, 1997

United States, October 1995–September 1996 Data, by Operation

88.53: LT HEART ANGIOCARDIOGRAM. Formerly included in operation group(s) 785.

Type of Patients	Observed Patients	Avg. Stay	Vari-ance	Percentiles						
				10th	25th	50th	75th	90th	95th	99th
1. SINGLE DX										
0–19 Years	1	1.0	0	1	1	1	1	1	1	1
20–34	0									
35–49	6	1.8	<1	1	1	1	3	3	3	3
50–64	17	2.7	8	1	1	1	4	8	9	9
65+	3	2.7	<1	3	3	3	3	3	3	3
2. MULTIPLE DX										
0–19 Years	3	1.3	1	1	1	1	2	4	5	5
20–34	7	1.7	2	1	1	1	2	4	5	5
35–49	79	3.4	6	1	2	3	4	5	9	13
50–64	156	5.7	41	1	2	3	7	14	23	23
65+	180	4.4	22	1	2	3	5	8	9	23
TOTAL SINGLE DX	27	2.5	6	1	1	1	3	6	8	9
MULTIPLE DX	425	4.6	26	1	2	3	5	8	12	23
TOTAL										
0–19 Years	4	1.3	1	1	1	1	1	1	1	5
20–34	7	1.7	2	1	1	1	2	4	5	5
35–49	85	3.3	6	1	2	3	4	5	9	13
50–64	173	5.4	38	1	2	3	6	11	23	23
65+	183	4.3	22	1	2	3	5	8	9	23
GRAND TOTAL	452	4.5	25	1	2	3	5	8	12	23

88.56: COR ARTERIOGRAM-2 CATH. Formerly included in operation group(s) 784.

Type of Patients	Observed Patients	Avg. Stay	Vari-ance	Percentiles						
				10th	25th	50th	75th	90th	95th	99th
1. SINGLE DX										
0–19 Years	0									
20–34	1	1.0	0	1	1	1	1	1	1	1
35–49	30	1.5	2	1	1	1	1	2	2	10
50–64	38	3.5	45	1	1	1	2	6	24	38
65+	10	1.1	<1	1	1	1	1	1	2	3
2. MULTIPLE DX										
0–19 Years	1	1.0	0	1	1	1	1	1	1	1
20–34	36	4.4	18	1	2	3	6	9	18	18
35–49	351	2.7	5	1	2	2	4	6	8	11
50–64	746	2.8	7	1	2	2	4	7	8	12
65+	992	3.3	12	1	2	3	4	8	10	17
TOTAL SINGLE DX	79	2.4	23	1	1	1	2	3	6	24
MULTIPLE DX	2126	3.1	9	1	2	2	4	7	9	14
TOTAL										
0–19 Years	1	1.0	0	1	1	1	1	1	1	1
20–34	37	4.4	18	1	2	3	6	9	18	18
35–49	381	2.7	5	1	2	2	3	6	7	11
50–64	784	2.8	8	1	1	2	4	7	8	12
65+	1002	3.3	12	1	1	2	4	8	10	16
GRAND TOTAL	2205	3.0	10	1	1	2	4	7	9	14

88.57: CORONARY ARTERIOGRAM NEC. Formerly included in operation group(s) 784.

Type of Patients	Observed Patients	Avg. Stay	Vari-ance	Percentiles						
				10th	25th	50th	75th	90th	95th	99th
1. SINGLE DX										
0–19 Years	0									
20–34	0									
35–49	7	1.4	<1	1	1	1	1	3	3	3
50–64	10	1.7	<1	1	1	1	2	4	4	4
65+	18	1.0	0	1	1	1	1	1	1	1
2. MULTIPLE DX										
0–19 Years	3	8.1	54	1	1	10	14	14	14	14
20–34	5	2.0	3	1	1	1	4	5	5	5
35–49	96	3.3	7	1	2	2	4	7	9	12
50–64	265	3.6	14	1	2	2	5	9	9	15
65+	392	4.1	18	1	2	3	5	9	13	23
TOTAL SINGLE DX	35	1.2	<1	1	1	1	1	2	3	4
MULTIPLE DX	761	3.9	16	1	1	3	5	9	10	18
TOTAL										
0–19 Years	3	8.1	54	1	1	10	14	14	14	14
20–34	5	2.0	3	1	1	1	2	4	5	5
35–49	103	3.1	7	1	1	2	4	7	9	12
50–64	275	3.6	14	1	1	2	5	9	9	15
65+	410	4.0	18	1	1	3	5	9	13	23
GRAND TOTAL	796	3.8	15	1	1	2	5	9	10	18

88.6: PHLEBOGRAPHY. Formerly included in operation group(s) 785.

Type of Patients	Observed Patients	Avg. Stay	Vari-ance	Percentiles						
				10th	25th	50th	75th	90th	95th	99th
1. SINGLE DX										
0–19 Years	14	4.2	8	1	1	5	6	8	8	9
20–34	80	4.2	6	1	2	5	6	8	8	11
35–49	97	4.2	4	2	3	4	6	6	8	10
50–64	43	3.3	4	1	2	3	4	6	7	8
65+	43	5.7	15	2	3	5	7	13	13	20
2. MULTIPLE DX										
0–19 Years	52	6.6	33	1	3	7	7	8	12	35
20–34	244	5.4	27	1	3	5	6	9	11	23
35–49	524	5.8	21	2	3	5	7	9	13	23
50–64	628	5.4	14	1	3	5	7	9	12	17
65+	1122	6.9	27	2	4	6	8	13	19	26
TOTAL SINGLE DX	277	4.1	6	1	2	4	6	7	8	13
MULTIPLE DX	2570	6.1	23	2	3	5	7	10	15	23
TOTAL										
0–19 Years	66	6.2	29	1	3	7	7	8	11	35
20–34	324	5.0	21	1	2	5	6	8	10	18
35–49	621	5.6	19	2	3	5	7	9	12	23
50–64	671	5.2	14	1	3	5	7	9	12	16
65+	1165	6.8	26	2	4	6	8	13	19	26
GRAND TOTAL	2847	5.9	21	2	3	5	7	10	14	23

Length of Stay by Diagnosis and Operation, United States, 1997

United States, October 1995–September 1996 Data, by Operation

88.66: CONTRAST PHLEBOGRAM-LEG. Formerly included in operation group(s) 785.

Type of Patients	Observed Patients	Avg. Stay	Vari-ance	10th	25th	50th	75th	90th	95th	99th
1. SINGLE DX										
0–19 Years	5	3.2	4	1	1	5	5	5	5	5
20–34	55	3.4	6	1	1	3	5	6	7	11
35–49	78	4.2	4	2	3	4	6	6	8	10
50–64	35	3.3	4	1	2	3	4	6	7	8
65+	39	5.5	11	2	3	5	7	13	13	13
2. MULTIPLE DX										
0–19 Years	21	4.8	45	1	1	3	5	11	13	35
20–34	170	5.2	27	1	2	5	6	9	11	18
35–49	362	5.1	8	2	3	5	6	8	10	15
50–64	441	5.5	9	2	3	5	7	8	10	15
65+	902	6.9	26	2	4	6	8	13	20	25
TOTAL SINGLE DX	212	3.9	6	1	2	4	5	6	8	13
MULTIPLE DX	1896	5.9	19	2	3	5	7	10	14	21
TOTAL										
0–19 Years	26	4.3	33	1	1	3	5	10	13	35
20–34	225	4.8	23	1	1	5	6	9	10	16
35–49	440	5.0	7	2	3	5	7	8	10	15
50–64	476	5.2	9	2	3	5	7	8	10	15
65+	941	6.9	26	2	4	6	8	13	20	23
GRAND TOTAL	2108	5.7	18	2	3	5	7	10	13	21

88.67: CONTRAST PHLEBOGRAM NEC. Formerly included in operation group(s) 785.

Type of Patients	Observed Patients	Avg. Stay	Vari-ance	10th	25th	50th	75th	90th	95th	99th
1. SINGLE DX										
0–19 Years	6	5.9	9	1	6	6	8	9	9	9
20–34	21	5.1	3	2	4	6	6	6	7	8
35–49	16	4.2	4	2	3	4	6	6	7	8
50–64	7	3.0	4	1	1	2	5	5	5	5
65+	3	4.1	15	1	1	4	9	9	9	9
2. MULTIPLE DX										
0–19 Years	22	7.9	28	5	7	7	8	8	12	35
20–34	57	5.5	10	2	4	5	6	9	10	17
35–49	119	6.4	26	1	3	6	7	10	12	23
50–64	148	6.0	25	2	3	5	7	12	14	19
65+	150	6.9	24	2	4	6	9	11	15	31
TOTAL SINGLE DX	53	4.9	5	1	4	6	6	7	8	9
MULTIPLE DX	496	6.5	24	2	4	6	8	11	14	23
TOTAL										
0–19 Years	28	7.7	26	5	7	7	8	8	10	35
20–34	78	5.3	7	2	4	5	6	8	10	17
35–49	135	6.3	25	1	3	6	7	10	12	23
50–64	155	5.9	25	1	3	5	7	12	14	19
65+	153	6.9	24	2	4	6	9	11	15	31
GRAND TOTAL	549	6.3	22	2	4	6	8	10	13	23

88.7: DIAGNOSTIC ULTRASOUND. Formerly included in operation group(s) 787.

Type of Patients	Observed Patients	Avg. Stay	Vari-ance	10th	25th	50th	75th	90th	95th	99th
1. SINGLE DX										
0–19 Years	1969	2.4	4	1	1	2	3	4	5	9
20–34	2828	2.3	3	1	1	2	3	4	6	9
35–49	1487	2.8	6	1	1	2	4	5	7	8
50–64	909	2.6	6	1	1	2	3	5	8	11
65+	706	3.8	9	1	2	3	5	7	9	14
2. MULTIPLE DX										
0–19 Years	8843	5.7	60	1	2	3	5	14	20	41
20–34	9738	4.1	21	1	2	3	5	8	11	22
35–49	12917	4.4	20	1	2	3	6	8	11	21
50–64	18951	5.4	22	1	2	4	7	11	14	21
65+	49798	5.8	23	2	3	5	7	11	14	24
TOTAL SINGLE DX	7899	2.6	5	1	1	2	3	5	6	9
MULTIPLE DX	100247	5.3	26	1	2	4	6	10	14	26
TOTAL										
0–19 Years	10812	5.1	52	1	2	3	5	11	17	39
20–34	12566	3.7	17	1	1	3	4	7	10	22
35–49	14404	4.2	18	1	2	3	5	8	11	20
50–64	19860	5.2	22	1	2	4	7	10	14	21
65+	50504	5.7	23	2	3	5	7	11	14	23
GRAND TOTAL	108146	5.1	25	1	2	4	6	10	14	25

88.71: DXTIC US-HEAD/NECK. Formerly included in operation group(s) 787.

Type of Patients	Observed Patients	Avg. Stay	Vari-ance	10th	25th	50th	75th	90th	95th	99th
1. SINGLE DX										
0–19 Years	75	3.4	11	1	2	3	4	6	7	10
20–34	8	2.9	9	1	2	2	3	3	12	12
35–49	24	1.4	<1	1	1	1	2	3	4	5
50–64	60	2.2	2	1	1	2	2	4	4	8
65+	91	2.7	4	1	1	2	4	5	6	12
2. MULTIPLE DX										
0–19 Years	1058	14.1	164	2	4	9	23	30	39	60
20–34	77	3.9	24	2	2	2	3	7	19	22
35–49	335	3.7	13	1	1	3	6	7	8	17
50–64	1200	5.3	23	1	2	3	6	14	14	14
65+	4482	5.0	19	2	2	4	6	9	12	20
TOTAL SINGLE DX	258	2.6	6	1	1	2	3	5	6	9
MULTIPLE DX	7152	6.5	55	1	2	4	7	14	21	39
TOTAL										
0–19 Years	1133	13.3	161	2	3	8	20	30	39	60
20–34	85	3.8	23	1	1	2	3	7	19	22
35–49	359	3.4	12	1	1	2	5	7	8	15
50–64	1260	5.2	22	1	2	3	6	14	14	15
65+	4573	4.9	18	2	2	4	6	9	12	20
GRAND TOTAL	7410	6.3	54	1	2	4	7	14	20	39

Length of Stay by Diagnosis and Operation, United States, 1997

United States, October 1995–September 1996 Data, by Operation

88.72: DXTIC ULTRASOUND-HEART. Formerly included in operation group(s) 787.

Type of Patients	Observed Patients	Avg. Stay	Variance	10th	25th	50th	75th	90th	95th	99th
1. SINGLE DX										
0–19 Years	416	2.8	9	1	1	2	3	4	6	13
20–34	237	2.8	6	1	1	2	3	5	6	11
35–49	435	2.2	3	1	1	2	3	4	5	8
50–64	407	2.4	8	1	1	1	3	5	8	11
65+	353	3.8	11	1	2	3	5	7	9	14
2. MULTIPLE DX										
0–19 Years	2639	6.3	74	1	2	3	7	14	23	50
20–34	1984	4.6	28	1	2	3	6	9	13	29
35–49	5956	4.3	21	1	2	3	5	8	11	23
50–64	11517	5.4	25	1	2	4	7	10	16	21
65+	31923	5.7	21	2	3	5	7	11	13	22
TOTAL SINGLE DX	1848	2.7	8	1	1	2	3	5	7	13
MULTIPLE DX	54019	5.5	25	1	2	4	7	10	14	24
TOTAL										
0–19 Years	3055	5.8	67	1	2	3	6	12	20	50
20–34	2221	4.4	26	1	2	3	5	8	12	29
35–49	6391	4.1	20	1	2	3	5	8	11	22
50–64	11924	5.3	25	1	2	4	7	10	16	21
65+	32276	5.7	21	2	3	5	7	11	13	22
GRAND TOTAL	55867	5.4	25	1	2	4	7	10	14	24

88.73: DXTIC US-THORAX NEC. Formerly included in operation group(s) 787.

Type of Patients	Observed Patients	Avg. Stay	Variance	10th	25th	50th	75th	90th	95th	99th
1. SINGLE DX										
0–19 Years	5	4.0	8	2	2	3	5	10	10	10
20–34	8	1.7	1	1	1	1	2	3	5	5
35–49	5	1.7	2	1	1	1	2	2	5	5
50–64	2	3.0	0	3	3	3	3	3	3	3
65+	4	7.7	2	6	6	9	9	9	9	9
2. MULTIPLE DX										
0–19 Years	13	3.2	8	2	2	2	2	9	10	15
20–34	32	4.5	8	2	3	3	6	8	10	15
35–49	38	4.9	40	1	2	3	5	8	9	41
50–64	49	4.8	20	2	2	4	6	8	11	27
65+	138	6.5	12	2	4	6	9	9	11	17
TOTAL SINGLE DX	24	3.9	9	1	1	2	6	9	9	10
MULTIPLE DX	270	5.5	16	2	3	5	8	9	11	21
TOTAL										
0–19 Years	18	3.3	8	2	2	2	2	9	10	15
20–34	40	3.6	7	1	3	3	4	8	9	13
35–49	43	4.7	38	1	2	3	5	8	9	41
50–64	51	4.7	19	2	2	4	6	8	11	27
65+	142	6.5	11	2	4	6	9	9	11	17
GRAND TOTAL	294	5.3	16	2	2	4	8	9	11	21

88.74: DXTIC ULTRASOUND-DIGEST. Formerly included in operation group(s) 787.

Type of Patients	Observed Patients	Avg. Stay	Variance	10th	25th	50th	75th	90th	95th	99th
1. SINGLE DX										
0–19 Years	49	2.4	2	1	1	2	3	6	6	7
20–34	126	2.2	4	1	1	2	3	4	5	15
35–49	92	1.8	1	1	1	1	2	3	4	4
50–64	54	2.0	1	1	1	2	3	3	5	6
65+	35	2.4	2	1	1	2	3	4	5	7
2. MULTIPLE DX										
0–19 Years	152	3.6	11	1	2	2	4	7	11	18
20–34	479	3.2	11	1	1	2	4	7	8	11
35–49	704	3.7	8	1	2	3	5	7	8	14
50–64	641	4.3	16	1	3	3	6	8	10	25
65+	1090	5.5	47	1	3	4	6	9	14	47
TOTAL SINGLE DX	356	2.1	2	1	1	2	3	4	5	7
MULTIPLE DX	3066	4.2	22	1	2	3	5	8	10	20
TOTAL										
0–19 Years	201	3.3	9	1	2	2	4	6	11	11
20–34	605	3.0	7	1	1	2	4	6	7	11
35–49	796	3.4	7	1	2	3	4	7	8	13
50–64	695	4.1	16	1	3	3	5	8	10	25
65+	1125	5.4	46	1	3	4	6	9	14	39
GRAND TOTAL	3422	4.0	20	1	2	3	5	8	10	18

88.75: DXTIC ULTRASOUND-URINARY. Formerly included in operation group(s) 787.

Type of Patients	Observed Patients	Avg. Stay	Variance	10th	25th	50th	75th	90th	95th	99th
1. SINGLE DX										
0–19 Years	335	2.7	2	1	2	2	3	4	5	7
20–34	118	2.6	10	1	1	2	3	4	5	11
35–49	70	2.6	3	1	2	2	3	4	6	10
50–64	31	2.2	4	1	1	2	2	4	5	14
65+	6	4.7	36	2	2	2	2	20	20	20
2. MULTIPLE DX										
0–19 Years	2390	3.5	7	1	2	3	4	6	7	14
20–34	962	3.8	8	1	2	3	5	6	8	14
35–49	919	4.0	19	1	2	3	5	7	10	19
50–64	981	4.8	16	1	3	4	6	9	11	20
65+	2432	6.5	29	2	3	5	8	13	16	26
TOTAL SINGLE DX	560	2.6	4	1	2	3	3	4	5	10
MULTIPLE DX	7684	4.5	17	1	2	4	5	8	11	21
TOTAL										
0–19 Years	2725	3.4	7	1	2	3	4	6	7	13
20–34	1080	3.7	8	1	2	3	5	6	8	13
35–49	989	3.9	18	1	2	3	5	7	10	18
50–64	1012	4.7	15	1	2	4	6	8	11	20
65+	2438	6.5	30	2	3	5	8	13	16	26
GRAND TOTAL	8244	4.4	17	1	2	3	5	8	11	21

Length of Stay by Diagnosis and Operation, United States, 1997

United States, October 1995–September 1996 Data, by Operation

88.76: DXTIC ULTRASOUND-ABD. Formerly included in operation group(s) 787.

Type of Patients	Observed Patients	Avg. Stay	Vari- ance	10th	25th	50th	75th	90th	95th	99th
1. SINGLE DX										
0–19 Years	700	2.0	2	1	1	1	2	4	5	8
20–34	764	2.1	2	1	1	1	3	4	4	7
35–49	415	3.2	6	1	1	3	5	5	6	7
50–64	175	2.5	2	1	1	2	3	4	5	8
65+	75	3.5	10	1	1	2	6	9	9	15
2. MULTIPLE DX										
0–19 Years	1631	3.9	19	1	2	3	4	8	15	17
20–34	2351	4.2	27	1	1	3	5	8	17	22
35–49	2748	4.4	14	1	2	4	6	8	10	19
50–64	2272	5.1	18	1	2	4	7	11	11	21
65+	4222	5.5	23	2	3	4	7	10	15	27
TOTAL SINGLE DX	2129	2.4	3	1	1	2	3	5	5	8
MULTIPLE DX	13224	4.7	21	1	2	3	6	9	13	22
TOTAL										
0–19 Years	2331	3.4	15	1	1	2	4	7	12	16
20–34	3115	3.6	21	1	1	2	4	7	11	22
35–49	3163	4.2	12	1	2	4	6	8	11	16
50–64	2447	4.9	17	1	2	4	6	11	11	21
65+	4297	5.5	23	2	3	4	7	10	15	27
GRAND TOTAL	15353	4.4	19	1	2	3	5	9	12	22

88.77: DXTIC ULTRASOUND-VASC. Formerly included in operation group(s) 787.

Type of Patients	Observed Patients	Avg. Stay	Vari- ance	10th	25th	50th	75th	90th	95th	99th
1. SINGLE DX										
0–19 Years	20	3.2	7	1	1	1	5	8	8	12
20–34	157	4.1	5	1	3	4	5	7	8	9
35–49	175	4.0	5	1	2	4	5	7	8	10
50–64	146	3.8	6	2	2	3	5	8	8	12
65+	130	4.4	5	2	3	4	5	7	8	13
2. MULTIPLE DX										
0–19 Years	87	5.0	40	1	2	3	6	9	12	43
20–34	642	5.9	30	2	3	4	6	11	16	34
35–49	1346	5.4	34	2	2	4	7	10	11	28
50–64	2056	5.9	19	2	4	5	7	9	12	24
65+	5062	6.7	33	2	4	5	8	12	16	33
TOTAL SINGLE DX	628	4.0	5	1	2	4	5	7	8	12
MULTIPLE DX	9193	6.2	30	2	3	5	7	11	15	33
TOTAL										
0–19 Years	107	4.6	33	1	1	3	5	9	12	39
20–34	799	5.5	26	2	3	4	6	10	16	34
35–49	1521	5.3	31	2	2	4	7	10	11	23
50–64	2202	5.7	18	2	4	5	7	9	12	23
65+	5192	6.7	33	2	4	5	8	12	16	33
GRAND TOTAL	9821	6.1	29	2	3	5	7	10	14	33

88.78: DXTIC US-GRAVID UTERUS. Formerly included in operation group(s) 787.

Type of Patients	Observed Patients	Avg. Stay	Vari- ance	10th	25th	50th	75th	90th	95th	99th
1. SINGLE DX										
0–19 Years	184	2.8	3	1	1	2	4	4	6	7
20–34	1072	2.2	3	1	1	2	4	4	5	9
35–49	161	2.3	13	1	1	2	3	4	4	8
50–64	0									
65+	0									
2. MULTIPLE DX										
0–19 Years	513	6.4	76	1	2	3	7	17	17	35
20–34	2582	3.5	15	1	2	3	7	7	9	19
35–49	462	3.9	18	1	2	4	4	7	11	24
50–64	5	2.7	<1	2	2	2	4	4	4	4
65+	0									
TOTAL SINGLE DX	1417	2.3	4	1	1	2	3	4	5	8
MULTIPLE DX	3562	4.1	29	1	1	3	5	8	17	24
TOTAL										
0–19 Years	697	5.5	61	1	2	3	4	17	17	27
20–34	3654	3.1	12	1	1	2	4	6	8	16
35–49	623	3.3	17	1	1	2	4	6	9	23
50–64	5	2.7	<1	2	2	2	4	4	4	4
65+	0									
GRAND TOTAL	4979	3.6	22	1	1	2	4	7	11	22

88.79: DXTIC ULTRASOUND NEC. Formerly included in operation group(s) 787.

Type of Patients	Observed Patients	Avg. Stay	Vari- ance	10th	25th	50th	75th	90th	95th	99th
1. SINGLE DX										
0–19 Years	185	2.1	2	1	1	2	3	4	4	9
20–34	338	2.3	3	1	1	2	3	4	6	11
35–49	110	3.2	12	1	2	2	5	6	7	11
50–64	34	2.5	2	1	2	2	5	6	7	11
65+	12	4.4	2	2	4	5	5	6	6	6
2. MULTIPLE DX										
0–19 Years	360	3.5	11	1	1	2	4	7	14	14
20–34	629	3.8	11	1	2	3	5	7	8	18
35–49	409	4.3	15	1	2	5	5	8	12	21
50–64	230	4.9	6	2	4	5	5	9	12	16
65+	449	5.5	15	2	3	4	7	9	12	20
TOTAL SINGLE DX	679	2.4	4	1	1	2	3	5	6	11
MULTIPLE DX	2077	4.4	12	1	2	4	5	8	10	18
TOTAL										
0–19 Years	545	3.0	9	1	1	2	3	6	10	14
20–34	967	3.3	9	1	2	3	4	6	8	17
35–49	519	4.1	15	2	2	3	5	7	11	20
50–64	264	4.7	7	2	3	5	5	7	9	16
65+	461	5.5	15	2	3	4	7	9	12	20
GRAND TOTAL	2756	4.0	11	1	2	3	5	7	10	17

Length of Stay by Diagnosis and Operation, United States, 1997

United States, October 1995–September 1996 Data, by Operation

88.8: THERMOGRAPHY. Formerly included in operation group(s) 787.

Type of Patients	Observed Patients	Avg. Stay	Variance	10th	25th	50th	75th	90th	95th	99th
1. SINGLE DX										
0–19 Years	0									
20–34	0									
35–49	0									
50–64	0									
65+	0									
2. MULTIPLE DX										
0–19 Years	0									
20–34	0									
35–49	1	2.0	0	2	2	2	2	2	2	2
50–64	1	10.0	0	10	10	10	10	10	10	10
65+	1	5.0	0	5	5	5	5	5	5	5
TOTAL SINGLE DX	0									
MULTIPLE DX	3	5.3	15	2	2	5	10	10	10	10
TOTAL										
0–19 Years	0									
20–34	0									
35–49	1	2.0	0	2	2	2	2	2	2	2
50–64	1	10.0	0	10	10	10	10	10	10	10
65+	1	5.0	0	5	5	5	5	5	5	5
GRAND TOTAL	3	5.3	15	2	2	5	10	10	10	10

88.9: OTHER DIAGNOSTIC IMAGING. Formerly included in operation group(s) 787.

Type of Patients	Observed Patients	Avg. Stay	Variance	10th	25th	50th	75th	90th	95th	99th
1. SINGLE DX										
0–19 Years	715	3.1	11	1	1	2	3	5	8	17
20–34	385	3.5	14	1	2	3	4	5	8	14
35–49	446	3.2	8	1	1	2	4	8	9	16
50–64	253	3.8	7	1	2	3	4	7	10	14
65+	216	4.3	27	1	2	2	5	8	20	28
2. MULTIPLE DX										
0–19 Years	2450	5.6	38	1	2	3	7	12	17	32
20–34	1699	5.9	56	2	2	4	7	13	16	43
35–49	3048	5.2	24	2	3	4	6	10	13	26
50–64	4047	6.0	31	2	3	5	8	11	15	27
65+	8931	6.4	32	2	3	5	8	12	16	28
TOTAL SINGLE DX	2015	3.4	12	1	1	2	4	6	9	20
MULTIPLE DX	20175	6.0	34	2	3	4	7	12	16	28
TOTAL										
0–19 Years	3165	5.0	33	1	2	3	6	11	16	29
20–34	2084	5.5	51	1	2	4	6	11	15	38
35–49	3494	4.9	22	1	2	4	6	9	13	24
50–64	4300	6.0	30	2	3	4	8	11	15	27
65+	9147	6.4	32	2	3	5	8	12	16	28
GRAND TOTAL	22190	5.7	32	2	3	4	7	11	15	28

88.91: MRI-BRAIN & BRAIN STEM. Formerly included in operation group(s) 787.

Type of Patients	Observed Patients	Avg. Stay	Variance	10th	25th	50th	75th	90th	95th	99th
1. SINGLE DX										
0–19 Years	457	3.5	15	1	2	3	4	6	10	18
20–34	223	3.6	22	1	2	3	4	6	11	21
35–49	192	3.7	13	1	1	3	5	6	9	19
50–64	135	3.6	9	1	2	3	4	8	10	15
65+	150	4.5	28	1	2	3	5	7	21	22
2. MULTIPLE DX										
0–19 Years	1710	5.7	44	1	2	3	7	13	18	38
20–34	1074	6.6	69	1	2	4	7	14	24	43
35–49	1955	5.3	27	2	2	4	6	10	14	27
50–64	2756	5.7	29	1	2	4	7	11	15	27
65+	6483	6.2	31	2	3	5	7	12	16	27
TOTAL SINGLE DX	1157	3.7	17	1	1	3	4	8	11	21
MULTIPLE DX	13978	5.9	35	2	3	4	7	12	16	29
TOTAL										
0–19 Years	2167	5.2	38	1	2	3	6	12	17	33
20–34	1297	6.1	63	1	2	4	7	14	20	43
35–49	2147	5.1	26	1	2	4	6	10	14	26
50–64	2891	5.6	28	1	2	4	7	11	15	27
65+	6633	6.2	31	2	3	5	7	12	16	27
GRAND TOTAL	15135	5.8	34	2	2	4	7	12	16	28

88.93: MRI-SPINAL CANAL. Formerly included in operation group(s) 787.

Type of Patients	Observed Patients	Avg. Stay	Variance	10th	25th	50th	75th	90th	95th	99th
1. SINGLE DX										
0–19 Years	95	2.5	3	1	1	2	3	5	6	8
20–34	121	3.3	3	1	1	3	5	5	5	7
35–49	215	2.9	5	1	2	2	4	5	8	9
50–64	93	4.1	6	2	3	4	5	8	8	12
65+	44	3.6	26	2	2	2	2	6	8	28
2. MULTIPLE DX										
0–19 Years	247	5.6	24	1	2	4	8	11	16	23
20–34	427	4.4	29	1	2	3	5	7	7	38
35–49	772	4.9	23	2	2	3	5	9	12	28
50–64	900	6.8	41	2	3	5	10	12	17	25
65+	1612	7.2	39	2	3	6	9	14	16	37
TOTAL SINGLE DX	568	3.1	6	1	2	2	4	5	8	10
MULTIPLE DX	3958	6.2	36	2	3	5	8	11	16	33
TOTAL										
0–19 Years	342	4.6	20	1	2	3	6	11	12	22
20–34	548	4.2	25	1	2	3	5	7	8	33
35–49	987	4.4	19	1	2	4	5	8	11	22
50–64	993	6.6	40	2	3	5	10	11	17	24
65+	1656	7.0	39	2	3	5	9	14	16	37
GRAND TOTAL	4526	5.8	33	1	2	4	7	11	15	28

Length of Stay by Diagnosis and Operation, United States, 1997

United States, October 1995–September 1996 Data, by Operation

88.94: MRI-MUSCULOSKELETAL. Formerly included in operation group(s) 787.

Type of Patients	Observed Patients	Avg. Stay	Variance	10th	25th	50th	75th	90th	95th	99th
1. SINGLE DX										
0–19 Years	36	2.9	3	1	1	3	4	5	5	9
20–34	12	4.5	4	3	3	4	5	9	9	9
35–49	14	4.0	4	2	2	4	6	7	7	7
50–64	9	3.9	<1	3	4	4	4	5	6	6
65+	12	5.3	8	2	4	5	9	9	6	9
2. MULTIPLE DX										
0–19 Years	88	7.0	41	2	3	5	8	19	23	23
20–34	65	6.6	47	2	4	5	7	11	18	47
35–49	118	5.0	6	3	3	4	7	7	8	15
50–64	124	7.3	7	4	6	8	8	9	11	18
65+	301	6.9	30	3	4	5	9	14	17	29
TOTAL SINGLE DX	83	3.7	5	1	2	3	5	7	9	9
MULTIPLE DX	696	6.2	17	3	3	6	8	9	13	23
TOTAL										
0–19 Years	124	5.5	31	1	2	4	6	13	21	23
20–34	77	6.1	37	2	3	5	6	9	15	47
35–49	132	5.0	6	3	3	4	7	7	8	15
50–64	133	7.2	7	4	6	8	8	11	11	18
65+	313	6.8	29	3	3	5	9	13	16	29
GRAND TOTAL	779	6.0	17	3	3	6	8	9	13	23

88.97: MRI SITE NEC&NOS. Formerly included in operation group(s) 787.

Type of Patients	Observed Patients	Avg. Stay	Variance	10th	25th	50th	75th	90th	95th	99th
1. SINGLE DX										
0–19 Years	114	2.3	7	1	1	2	3	4	5	15
20–34	25	2.6	6	1	1	2	3	5	5	13
35–49	21	3.4	16	1	2	2	5	5	7	24
50–64	13	2.8	8	1	1	2	3	5	6	16
65+	7	7.5	19	1	3	10	10	14	14	14
2. MULTIPLE DX										
0–19 Years	337	5.2	26	2	2	3	7	11	14	22
20–34	113	5.3	33	1	2	4	6	10	14	36
35–49	167	6.0	27	2	3	4	8	12	17	23
50–64	216	6.0	16	2	3	5	8	11	13	18
65+	420	5.8	25	2	3	4	7	11	14	29
TOTAL SINGLE DX	180	2.6	9	1	1	2	3	5	6	15
MULTIPLE DX	1253	5.7	25	2	3	4	7	12	14	25
TOTAL										
0–19 Years	451	4.5	23	1	2	3	5	11	13	21
20–34	138	4.8	30	1	2	3	6	10	13	36
35–49	188	5.9	27	1	3	4	8	12	17	24
50–64	229	5.9	16	2	3	5	7	11	13	18
65+	427	5.8	25	2	3	4	7	11	14	29
GRAND TOTAL	1433	5.3	24	1	2	4	7	12	14	25

89.0: DX INTERVIEW/CONSUL/EXAM. Formerly included in operation group(s) 796.

Type of Patients	Observed Patients	Avg. Stay	Variance	10th	25th	50th	75th	90th	95th	99th
1. SINGLE DX										
0–19 Years	7	3.2	4	2	2	2	4	7	7	7
20–34	7	1.9	<1	1	1	1	3	3	3	3
35–49	4	2.9	3	1	1	4	4	5	5	5
50–64	8	5.0	37	1	1	1	14	14	14	14
65+	6	1.5	<1	1	1	1	2	2	2	2
2. MULTIPLE DX										
0–19 Years	49	2.9	14	1	1	2	3	5	8	15
20–34	32	4.1	9	1	2	4	5	7	10	19
35–49	33	4.1	5	2	3	3	6	7	8	10
50–64	29	4.0	7	1	2	3	5	7	8	14
65+	80	6.2	18	2	3	5	8	14	18	18
TOTAL SINGLE DX	32	3.2	14	1	1	2	3	7	14	14
MULTIPLE DX	223	4.8	15	1	2	4	6	9	14	18
TOTAL										
0–19 Years	56	2.9	13	1	1	2	3	6	8	15
20–34	39	3.9	8	1	2	4	5	7	8	19
35–49	37	4.1	5	1	3	3	6	7	8	10
50–64	37	4.1	12	1	2	3	5	7	14	14
65+	86	6.1	18	2	3	5	8	14	15	18
GRAND TOTAL	255	4.7	15	1	2	4	6	9	14	18

89.1: NERVOUS SYSTEM EXAMS. Formerly included in operation group(s) 796.

Type of Patients	Observed Patients	Avg. Stay	Variance	10th	25th	50th	75th	90th	95th	99th
1. SINGLE DX										
0–19 Years	1931	2.6	7	1	1	2	3	5	7	14
20–34	384	3.8	16	1	1	3	5	7	9	26
35–49	267	4.2	28	1	2	2	5	8	13	24
50–64	75	4.2	13	1	2	3	5	10	13	15
65+	58	4.8	60	1	1	1	5	12	22	37
2. MULTIPLE DX										
0–19 Years	3907	5.2	54	1	2	3	6	11	17	38
20–34	953	5.2	31	1	2	3	7	10	14	30
35–49	1158	4.8	21	2	2	4	6	10	13	21
50–64	900	7.5	86	2	3	5	9	17	18	55
65+	2259	6.7	38	2	3	5	8	14	19	32
TOTAL SINGLE DX	2715	2.9	12	1	1	2	3	6	8	17
MULTIPLE DX	9177	5.7	48	1	2	4	7	12	17	34
TOTAL										
0–19 Years	5838	4.4	40	1	1	2	5	10	14	31
20–34	1337	4.8	28	1	2	3	6	9	13	28
35–49	1425	4.7	22	1	2	3	6	10	13	22
50–64	975	7.3	83	2	3	4	8	16	18	55
65+	2317	6.6	39	2	3	5	8	14	19	32
GRAND TOTAL	11892	5.1	41	1	2	3	6	11	15	31

Length of Stay by Diagnosis and Operation, United States, 1997

United States, October 1995–September 1996 Data, by Operation

89.14: ELECTROENCEPHALOGRAM. Formerly included in operation group(s) 796.

Type of Patients	Observed Patients	Avg. Stay	Vari-ance	Percentiles						
				10th	25th	50th	75th	90th	95th	99th
1. SINGLE DX										
0–19 Years	854	2.6	10	1	1	2	3	5	7	20
20–34	141	3.7	28	1	1	2	4	7	12	31
35–49	100	4.6	50	1	1	2	4	8	15	46
50–64	46	4.1	17	1	2	2	4	13	13	18
65+	49	5.2	68	1	1	2	5	15	23	37
2. MULTIPLE DX										
0–19 Years	2128	5.9	70	1	2	3	7	13	18	45
20–34	593	4.9	34	1	2	3	6	10	14	30
35–49	784	4.7	23	1	2	3	5	10	13	22
50–64	735	7.8	94	2	3	5	9	17	18	55
65+	2130	6.7	37	2	3	5	8	14	19	32
TOTAL SINGLE DX	1190	3.0	18	1	1	2	3	6	9	24
MULTIPLE DX	6370	6.1	54	1	2	4	7	13	18	37
TOTAL										
0–19 Years	2982	5.0	55	1	1	3	5	11	17	40
20–34	734	4.7	33	1	2	3	6	9	14	30
35–49	884	4.7	26	1	2	3	5	10	13	25
50–64	781	7.6	91	2	3	5	9	17	18	55
65+	2179	6.6	38	2	3	5	8	14	19	32
GRAND TOTAL	7560	5.6	50	1	2	3	7	12	17	35

89.19: VIDEO/TELEMETRIC EEG MON. Formerly included in operation group(s) 796.

Type of Patients	Observed Patients	Avg. Stay	Vari-ance	Percentiles						
				10th	25th	50th	75th	90th	95th	99th
1. SINGLE DX										
0–19 Years	857	2.6	5	1	1	2	3	5	7	11
20–34	185	4.3	6	1	2	4	6	7	8	12
35–49	134	4.9	8	2	3	4	7	8	9	15
50–64	25	4.8	5	2	4	5	6	8	8	10
65+	6	4.2	6	1	3	4	6	7	7	7
2. MULTIPLE DX										
0–19 Years	1363	4.0	28	1	1	3	5	8	12	23
20–34	316	5.7	13	2	3	5	8	10	12	17
35–49	302	5.5	11	2	3	5	7	9	11	18
50–64	114	5.3	11	2	3	5	7	8	10	22
65+	61	5.0	14	2	3	4	7	9	11	24
TOTAL SINGLE DX	1207	3.0	6	1	1	2	4	6	8	12
MULTIPLE DX	2156	4.5	24	1	2	3	6	9	12	22
TOTAL										
0–19 Years	2220	3.5	19	1	1	2	4	7	10	20
20–34	501	5.2	11	2	3	4	7	9	12	15
35–49	436	5.3	10	2	3	4	7	9	11	18
50–64	139	5.3	10	2	3	5	7	8	10	14
65+	67	5.0	13	2	3	4	7	8	11	24
GRAND TOTAL	3363	3.9	18	1	1	3	5	8	10	19

89.17: POLYSOMNOGRAM. Formerly included in operation group(s) 796.

Type of Patients	Observed Patients	Avg. Stay	Vari-ance	Percentiles						
				10th	25th	50th	75th	90th	95th	99th
1. SINGLE DX										
0–19 Years	131	2.2	2	1	1	2	3	4	5	8
20–34	12	1.7	<1	1	1	2	2	2	2	2
35–49	7	1.8	<1	1	2	2	2	2	2	2
50–64	1	1.0	0	1	1	1	1	1	1	1
65+	1	1.0	0	1	1	1	1	1	1	1
2. MULTIPLE DX										
0–19 Years	277	4.6	38	1	2	3	6	10	14	44
20–34	7	3.7	12	2	2	2	3	11	14	14
35–49	30	3.9	14	1	1	1	7	9	12	12
50–64	23	4.9	10	2	3	4	5	9	13	13
65+	27	6.6	38	1	1	4	11	13	23	25
TOTAL SINGLE DX	152	2.1	2	1	1	2	3	3	4	7
MULTIPLE DX	364	4.6	33	1	1	3	6	10	13	42
TOTAL										
0–19 Years	408	3.8	28	1	1	2	4	8	11	33
20–34	19	3.0	9	1	2	2	2	6	11	14
35–49	37	3.4	11	1	1	1	6	9	9	12
50–64	24	4.8	10	2	2	4	5	9	13	13
65+	28	6.4	38	1	1	4	10	13	22	25
GRAND TOTAL	516	3.9	25	1	1	2	4	9	11	32

89.2: GU SYSTEM-EXAMINATION. Formerly included in operation group(s) 796.

Type of Patients	Observed Patients	Avg. Stay	Vari-ance	Percentiles						
				10th	25th	50th	75th	90th	95th	99th
1. SINGLE DX										
0–19 Years	60	2.1	5	1	1	1	2	4	7	11
20–34	93	1.5	1	1	1	1	2	2	3	9
35–49	16	2.0	<1	1	2	2	3	3	3	3
50–64	3	1.8	0	1	1	1	3	3	3	3
65+	1	1.0		1	1	1	1	1	1	1
2. MULTIPLE DX										
0–19 Years	176	3.5	28	1	1	2	4	7	14	24
20–34	204	4.6	67	1	2	2	4	11	18	39
35–49	144	7.8	73	1	2	5	9	25	31	31
50–64	115	10.7	21	4	10	12	12	12	13	27
65+	546	8.9	55	2	5	7	11	18	23	41
TOTAL SINGLE DX	173	1.8	3	1	1	1	2	3	4	11
MULTIPLE DX	1185	8.1	53	1	3	6	12	15	20	34
TOTAL										
0–19 Years	236	3.2	23	1	1	1	3	7	12	24
20–34	297	3.9	53	1	1	2	3	7	16	39
35–49	160	7.5	71	1	2	4	8	22	31	31
50–64	118	10.7	21	4	10	12	12	12	13	27
65+	547	8.9	55	2	5	7	11	18	23	41
GRAND TOTAL	1358	7.6	52	1	2	5	12	14	19	34

Length of Stay by Diagnosis and Operation, United States, 1997

United States, October 1995–September 1996 Data, by Operation

89.22: CYSTOMETROGRAM. Formerly included in operation group(s) 796.

Type of Patients	Observed Patients	Avg. Stay	Variance	10th	25th	50th	75th	90th	95th	99th
1. SINGLE DX										
0–19 Years	12	1.1	<1	1	1	1	1	1	2	2
20–34	2	4.0	0	4	4	4	4	4	4	4
35–49	1	1.0	0	1	1	1	1	1	1	1
50–64	0									
65+	0									
2. MULTIPLE DX										
0–19 Years	61	2.0	7	1	1	1	1	7	7	11
20–34	45	10.6	190	2	2	7	14	24	36	80
35–49	62	11.3	110	2	4	7	11	31	31	31
50–64	73	11.3	17	5	12	12	12	12	12	27
65+	369	10.2	65	4	5	7	13	19	25	42
TOTAL SINGLE DX	15	1.5	1	1	1	1	1	4	4	4
MULTIPLE DX	610	10.3	57	3	5	11	12	18	25	41
TOTAL										
0–19 Years	73	1.9	6	1	1	1	1	7	7	11
20–34	47	10.4	187	2	2	6	14	24	36	80
35–49	63	11.3	110	2	4	7	11	31	31	31
50–64	73	11.3	17	5	12	12	12	12	12	27
65+	369	10.2	65	4	5	7	13	19	25	42
GRAND TOTAL	625	10.3	57	3	5	11	12	17	25	39

89.37: VITAL CAPACITY. Formerly included in operation group(s) 796.

Type of Patients	Observed Patients	Avg. Stay	Variance	10th	25th	50th	75th	90th	95th	99th
1. SINGLE DX										
0–19 Years	22	4.8	11	1	2	3	6	8	12	14
20–34	12	4.0	16	1	2	3	6	7	16	16
35–49	12	4.0	10	2	2	3	5	9	12	12
50–64	14	4.3	3	2	3	5	5	6	7	10
65+	12	6.4	8	1	4	8	8	8	10	10
2. MULTIPLE DX										
0–19 Years	107	6.5	22	2	3	6	9	14	15	23
20–34	82	4.7	19	1	3	3	6	12	14	21
35–49	114	5.0	24	2	3	3	5	8	16	21
50–64	194	4.9	28	2	3	4	6	9	12	21
65+	375	6.1	19	3	3	5	8	11	14	18
TOTAL SINGLE DX	72	4.9	10	1	3	4	7	8	10	16
MULTIPLE DX	872	5.6	23	2	3	4	7	11	14	21
TOTAL										
0–19 Years	129	6.4	22	2	3	6	9	14	14	22
20–34	94	4.6	19	1	2	3	5	12	14	21
35–49	126	5.0	23	2	3	3	5	9	16	21
50–64	208	4.9	26	2	3	4	6	9	12	21
65+	387	6.1	18	3	3	5	8	11	14	18
GRAND TOTAL	944	5.5	22	2	3	4	7	11	14	21

89.3: OTHER EXAMINATIONS. Formerly included in operation group(s) 796.

Type of Patients	Observed Patients	Avg. Stay	Variance	10th	25th	50th	75th	90th	95th	99th
1. SINGLE DX										
0–19 Years	583	2.0	2	1	1	2	2	4	5	8
20–34	25	4.5	17	1	2	3	4	7	16	16
35–49	31	3.3	9	2	2	2	4	9	11	12
50–64	24	3.7	6	1	2	3	5	5	7	15
65+	23	5.4	9	1	2	6	8	8	10	10
2. MULTIPLE DX										
0–19 Years	1651	4.6	26	1	2	3	6	10	14	28
20–34	169	4.1	17	1	2	3	4	10	14	20
35–49	256	4.9	23	2	2	3	5	9	15	21
50–64	359	4.8	24	2	3	4	6	9	11	21
65+	722	6.3	25	2	3	5	8	11	16	23
TOTAL SINGLE DX	686	2.2	4	1	1	2	3	4	5	11
MULTIPLE DX	3157	4.9	26	1	2	3	6	10	14	25
TOTAL										
0–19 Years	2234	4.0	22	1	1	2	5	9	12	23
20–34	194	4.1	17	1	2	3	4	10	14	20
35–49	287	4.8	23	2	2	3	5	10	15	21
50–64	383	4.8	23	2	3	4	6	9	11	21
65+	745	6.3	24	2	3	5	8	11	16	23
GRAND TOTAL	3843	4.4	23	1	2	3	5	9	13	22

89.38: RESPIRATORY MEASURE NEC. Formerly included in operation group(s) 796.

Type of Patients	Observed Patients	Avg. Stay	Variance	10th	25th	50th	75th	90th	95th	99th
1. SINGLE DX										
0–19 Years	247	1.9	1	1	1	2	2	3	4	5
20–34	6	7.5	37	1	3	4	16	16	16	16
35–49	10	3.7	11	2	2	2	4	11	11	11
50–64	5	2.2	2	2	2	2	3	5	5	5
65+	8	3.1	3	2	2	2	4	6	6	6
2. MULTIPLE DX										
0–19 Years	609	4.3	22	1	1	3	5	10	12	19
20–34	36	3.9	11	1	2	3	4	8	15	15
35–49	70	5.1	32	1	2	3	7	10	11	44
50–64	78	4.8	9	1	2	4	6	10	10	14
65+	173	6.2	26	2	3	5	8	11	15	38
TOTAL SINGLE DX	276	2.0	2	1	1	2	2	3	4	7
MULTIPLE DX	966	4.6	22	1	2	3	6	10	12	20
TOTAL										
0–19 Years	856	3.7	18	1	2	2	4	9	12	19
20–34	42	4.5	17	1	3	3	5	8	15	16
35–49	80	4.9	30	1	2	3	6	10	11	44
50–64	83	4.6	9	1	2	4	6	9	10	14
65+	181	6.1	25	2	3	5	8	10	15	38
GRAND TOTAL	1242	4.0	19	1	1	2	5	9	12	19

Length of Stay by Diagnosis and Operation, United States, 1997

United States, October 1995–September 1996 Data, by Operation

89.39: NONOPERATIVE EXAMS NEC. Formerly included in operation group(s) 796.

Type of Patients	Observed Patients	Avg. Stay	Variance	10th	25th	50th	75th	90th	95th	99th
1. SINGLE DX										
0–19 Years	280	1.9	3	1	1	1	2	4	5	8
20–34	4	3.6	<1	3	4	4	4	4	4	4
35–49	6	2.1	2	1	1	2	2	5	5	5
50–64	4	5.2	39	1	1	2	4	15	15	15
65+	2	4.9	13	1	1	7	7	7	7	7
2. MULTIPLE DX										
0–19 Years	860	4.5	30	1	1	3	5	8	13	30
20–34	28	3.0	10	1	1	3	3	4	6	20
35–49	53	4.2	17	2	2	2	5	10	10	29
50–64	55	4.5	29	2	2	2	5	8	8	28
65+	98	6.8	45	1	2	5	8	21	21	25
TOTAL SINGLE DX	**296**	**1.9**	**3**	**1**	**1**	**1**	**2**	**4**	**5**	**8**
MULTIPLE DX	**1094**	**4.5**	**30**	**1**	**1**	**3**	**5**	**9**	**13**	**30**
TOTAL										
0–19 Years	1140	3.9	25	1	1	3	5	8	11	30
20–34	32	3.1	9	1	1	3	3	4	5	20
35–49	59	4.1	17	2	2	2	5	10	10	15
50–64	59	4.5	29	2	2	2	5	8	8	28
65+	100	6.8	45	1	2	5	8	21	21	25
GRAND TOTAL	**1390**	**4.0**	**26**	**1**	**1**	**3**	**5**	**8**	**12**	**30**

89.41: TREADMILL STRESS TEST. Formerly included in operation group(s) 796.

Type of Patients	Observed Patients	Avg. Stay	Variance	10th	25th	50th	75th	90th	95th	99th
1. SINGLE DX										
0–19 Years	7	1.1	<1	1	1	1	1	1	2	2
20–34	49	1.2	<1	1	1	1	1	2	2	2
35–49	308	1.4	<1	1	1	1	1	3	3	3
50–64	309	1.6	2	1	1	1	2	2	4	7
65+	109	1.9	1	1	1	2	3	3	3	5
2. MULTIPLE DX										
0–19 Years	13	2.5	5	1	2	2	2	3	10	10
20–34	203	2.4	4	1	1	2	3	6	6	10
35–49	1749	2.0	2	1	1	1	3	4	5	9
50–64	2970	2.4	3	1	1	2	3	5	6	10
65+	2931	3.2	6	1	1	3	4	6	8	11
TOTAL SINGLE DX	**782**	**1.5**	**<1**	**1**	**1**	**1**	**2**	**3**	**3**	**6**
MULTIPLE DX	**7866**	**2.6**	**4**	**1**	**2**	**2**	**3**	**5**	**6**	**10**
TOTAL										
0–19 Years	20	2.0	4	1	1	2	2	2	3	10
20–34	252	2.2	4	1	1	2	2	5	6	10
35–49	2057	1.9	2	1	1	1	2	4	4	8
50–64	3279	2.3	3	1	1	2	3	5	6	10
65+	3040	3.2	6	1	1	3	4	6	7	11
GRAND TOTAL	**8648**	**2.5**	**4**	**1**	**1**	**2**	**3**	**5**	**6**	**10**

89.4: PACER/CARD STRESS TEST. Formerly included in operation group(s) 796.

Type of Patients	Observed Patients	Avg. Stay	Variance	10th	25th	50th	75th	90th	95th	99th
1. SINGLE DX										
0–19 Years	11	1.2	<1	1	1	1	1	2	2	3
20–34	133	1.4	<1	1	1	1	1	2	3	6
35–49	784	1.4	<1	1	1	1	2	3	3	5
50–64	660	1.7	2	1	1	1	2	3	4	8
65+	274	2.2	2	1	1	2	3	4	4	6
2. MULTIPLE DX										
0–19 Years	35	4.9	7	2	2	5	7	7	10	11
20–34	479	2.4	4	1	1	2	3	4	6	10
35–49	4127	2.2	3	1	1	2	3	4	5	9
50–64	7066	2.7	5	1	1	2	4	5	7	11
65+	9010	3.7	9	1	2	3	5	7	9	14
TOTAL SINGLE DX	**1862**	**1.6**	**1**	**1**	**1**	**1**	**2**	**3**	**4**	**7**
MULTIPLE DX	**20717**	**3.0**	**6**	**1**	**2**	**2**	**4**	**6**	**7**	**12**
TOTAL										
0–19 Years	46	4.0	8	1	1	3	7	7	7	11
20–34	612	2.2	4	1	1	2	3	4	6	10
35–49	4911	2.1	3	1	1	2	3	4	5	8
50–64	7726	2.7	5	1	1	2	3	5	6	10
65+	9284	3.7	8	1	2	3	5	7	9	14
GRAND TOTAL	**22579**	**2.9**	**6**	**1**	**1**	**2**	**4**	**6**	**7**	**12**

89.44: CV STRESS TEST NEC. Formerly included in operation group(s) 796.

Type of Patients	Observed Patients	Avg. Stay	Variance	10th	25th	50th	75th	90th	95th	99th
1. SINGLE DX										
0–19 Years	3	1.2	<1	1	1	1	1	2	2	2
20–34	84	1.6	1	1	1	1	2	3	4	6
35–49	475	1.5	1	1	1	1	2	3	4	6
50–64	347	1.9	3	1	1	1	2	3	4	8
65+	163	2.4	2	1	1	2	3	4	5	6
2. MULTIPLE DX										
0–19 Years	19	5.9	3	3	5	7	7	7	7	9
20–34	265	2.3	5	1	1	2	3	4	5	13
35–49	2367	2.5	3	1	1	2	3	4	6	9
50–64	4049	3.0	6	1	1	2	4	6	7	13
65+	5906	4.0	10	1	2	3	5	7	10	15
TOTAL SINGLE DX	**1072**	**1.8**	**2**	**1**	**1**	**1**	**2**	**3**	**4**	**7**
MULTIPLE DX	**12606**	**3.3**	**8**	**1**	**2**	**3**	**4**	**6**	**8**	**14**
TOTAL										
0–19 Years	22	5.3	6	1	3	7	7	7	7	7
20–34	349	2.2	4	1	1	2	3	4	5	9
35–49	2842	2.4	3	1	1	2	3	4	5	8
50–64	4396	3.0	6	1	1	2	4	6	7	13
65+	6069	4.0	10	1	2	3	5	7	10	15
GRAND TOTAL	**13678**	**3.2**	**7**	**1**	**2**	**3**	**4**	**6**	**8**	**14**

Length of Stay by Diagnosis and Operation, United States, 1997

United States, October 1995–September 1996 Data, by Operation

89.5: OTHER CARDIAC FUNCT TEST. Formerly included in operation group(s) 796.

Type of Patients	Observed Patients	Avg. Stay	Vari-ance	10th	25th	50th	75th	90th	95th	99th
1. SINGLE DX										
0–19 Years	748	2.4	6	1	1	2	3	4	6	13
20–34	256	2.7	8	1	1	2	3	6	10	13
35–49	469	2.6	10	1	1	2	3	5	7	12
50–64	469	3.0	18	1	1	1	3	7	9	31
65+	370	3.1	12	1	1	2	4	7	9	12
2. MULTIPLE DX										
0–19 Years	3198	3.6	14	1	1	2	4	7	10	17
20–34	1542	3.4	14	1	1	2	4	7	7	19
35–49	3718	2.9	9	1	1	2	3	6	8	15
50–64	6682	3.3	9	1	1	2	4	7	9	15
65+	19230	4.3	16	1	2	3	5	8	11	19
TOTAL SINGLE DX	2312	2.6	9	1	1	2	3	5	7	14
MULTIPLE DX	34370	3.8	14	1	2	3	5	8	10	18
TOTAL										
0–19 Years	3946	3.4	13	1	1	2	4	7	10	17
20–34	1798	3.3	13	1	1	2	4	7	9	19
35–49	4187	2.9	10	1	1	2	3	6	8	15
50–64	7151	3.3	10	1	2	2	4	7	9	15
65+	19600	4.3	16	1	2	3	5	8	11	19
GRAND TOTAL	36682	3.7	13	1	2	3	5	7	10	17

89.50: AMBULATORY CARD MONITOR. Formerly included in operation group(s) 796.

Type of Patients	Observed Patients	Avg. Stay	Vari-ance	10th	25th	50th	75th	90th	95th	99th
1. SINGLE DX										
0–19 Years	22	3.0	10	1	1	1	4	9	9	13
20–34	5	3.4	6	2	2	2	2	8	8	8
35–49	11	1.8	<1	1	1	2	2	3	3	3
50–64	11	3.7	10	1	1	3	6	10	10	10
65+	8	2.3	1	1	1	2	3	4	4	5
2. MULTIPLE DX										
0–19 Years	78	3.2	7	1	1	2	4	7	9	13
20–34	55	4.1	40	1	2	3	4	7	13	27
35–49	93	4.3	11	1	3	4	4	8	9	19
50–64	221	4.6	18	2	3	5	6	10	13	27
65+	964	5.6	16	2	3	5	8	11	13	19
TOTAL SINGLE DX	57	2.8	7	1	1	2	3	7	9	13
MULTIPLE DX	1411	5.1	17	1	2	4	7	10	13	19
TOTAL										
0–19 Years	100	3.1	8	1	1	2	4	7	9	13
20–34	60	4.1	38	2	2	3	4	7	9	27
35–49	104	4.1	11	1	2	3	4	8	9	19
50–64	232	4.6	17	2	3	3	6	10	13	19
65+	972	5.5	16	2	3	5	8	10	13	19
GRAND TOTAL	1468	5.0	16	1	2	4	7	10	13	19

89.51: RHYTHM ELECTROCARDIOGRAM. Formerly included in operation group(s) 796.

Type of Patients	Observed Patients	Avg. Stay	Vari-ance	10th	25th	50th	75th	90th	95th	99th
1. SINGLE DX										
0–19 Years	33	1.9	2	1	1	1	2	4	5	6
20–34	0									
35–49	3	3.1	16	1	1	1	6	12	12	12
50–64	4	2.9	2	1	1	3	3	5	5	5
65+	1	1.0	0	1	1	1	1	1	1	1
2. MULTIPLE DX										
0–19 Years	174	1.6	1	1	1	1	2	3	4	6
20–34	16	6.3	38	1	1	4	7	17	18	18
35–49	16	2.1	5	1	1	1	2	5	8	9
50–64	31	3.2	8	2	2	2	3	7	7	17
65+	62	3.8	7	1	2	3	5	7	8	17
TOTAL SINGLE DX	41	1.9	2	1	1	1	2	4	6	6
MULTIPLE DX	299	1.8	3	1	1	1	2	4	5	8
TOTAL										
0–19 Years	207	1.6	1	1	1	1	2	3	4	6
20–34	16	6.3	38	1	1	4	7	17	18	18
35–49	19	2.3	8	1	1	1	2	6	7	12
50–64	35	3.2	8	1	2	2	3	7	8	17
65+	63	3.7	7	1	2	3	4	7	8	17
GRAND TOTAL	340	1.8	3	1	1	1	2	4	5	7

89.52: ELECTROCARDIOGRAM. Formerly included in operation group(s) 796.

Type of Patients	Observed Patients	Avg. Stay	Vari-ance	10th	25th	50th	75th	90th	95th	99th
1. SINGLE DX										
0–19 Years	179	3.3	22	1	1	2	3	6	12	18
20–34	78	4.9	20	1	2	3	9	10	11	22
35–49	130	3.0	7	1	1	2	4	5	6	13
50–64	91	5.1	64	1	1	2	4	14	31	31
65+	63	4.5	53	1	2	2	4	9	18	50
2. MULTIPLE DX										
0–19 Years	1008	5.1	38	1	1	3	6	13	17	34
20–34	449	5.5	30	1	2	3	8	11	19	25
35–49	913	3.8	17	1	1	2	4	8	11	23
50–64	1244	3.6	11	1	2	2	5	7	11	16
65+	2543	4.3	19	1	2	3	5	8	11	22
TOTAL SINGLE DX	541	3.7	26	1	1	2	4	8	10	31
MULTIPLE DX	6157	4.3	22	1	2	3	5	9	13	25
TOTAL										
0–19 Years	1187	4.8	36	1	1	3	5	13	17	33
20–34	527	5.5	29	1	2	3	8	11	19	25
35–49	1043	3.7	16	1	1	2	4	8	10	21
50–64	1335	3.7	14	1	2	2	6	7	10	20
65+	2606	4.3	19	1	2	3	5	8	11	23
GRAND TOTAL	6698	4.3	22	1	2	3	5	9	13	25

Length of Stay by Diagnosis and Operation, United States, 1997

United States, October 1995–September 1996 Data, by Operation

89.54: ECG MONITORING. Formerly included in operation group(s) 796.

Type of Patients	Observed Patients	Avg. Stay	Vari-ance	10th	25th	50th	75th	90th	95th	99th
1. SINGLE DX										
0–19 Years	468	2.2	4	1	1	2	3	4	6	13
20–34	145	1.8	2	1	1	1	2	5	5	7
35–49	300	2.4	13	1	1	1	2	5	7	12
50–64	349	2.5	8	1	1	1	3	7	8	15
65+	280	2.9	6	1	1	2	4	7	9	12
2. MULTIPLE DX										
0–19 Years	1801	3.6	10	1	2	3	5	7	10	17
20–34	933	2.6	5	1	1	2	3	5	7	11
35–49	2527	2.7	7	1	1	2	3	5	7	11
50–64	4978	3.2	8	1	1	2	4	6	8	14
65+	14873	4.2	15	1	2	3	5	8	10	18
TOTAL SINGLE DX	1542	2.3	6	1	1	2	3	4	7	12
MULTIPLE DX	25112	3.7	12	1	2	3	5	7	9	16
TOTAL										
0–19 Years	2269	3.3	9	1	1	2	4	7	9	16
20–34	1078	2.5	5	1	1	2	3	5	7	11
35–49	2827	2.6	8	1	1	2	4	5	7	12
50–64	5327	3.1	8	1	1	2	4	6	8	14
65+	15153	4.2	15	1	2	3	5	8	10	18
GRAND TOTAL	26654	3.6	12	1	1	3	5	7	9	16

89.6: CIRCULATORY MONITORING. Formerly included in operation group(s) 795.

Type of Patients	Observed Patients	Avg. Stay	Vari-ance	10th	25th	50th	75th	90th	95th	99th
1. SINGLE DX										
0–19 Years	671	1.9	2	1	1	1	2	4	5	6
20–34	240	2.8	9	1	2	2	3	4	5	10
35–49	208	3.0	4	1	2	3	4	5	6	11
50–64	175	3.4	4	1	2	3	5	6	6	11
65+	145	4.3	9	2	2	4	5	7	9	18
2. MULTIPLE DX										
0–19 Years	2352	4.2	25	1	2	3	5	8	11	26
20–34	1612	4.6	23	1	2	4	5	9	12	24
35–49	2861	5.7	40	1	2	4	7	11	16	34
50–64	4067	7.6	43	2	3	5	10	17	21	28
65+	11024	7.6	40	2	3	6	10	15	20	32
TOTAL SINGLE DX	1439	2.4	4	1	1	2	3	5	6	9
MULTIPLE DX	21916	6.7	40	2	3	5	8	14	19	31
TOTAL										
0–19 Years	3023	3.5	20	1	1	2	4	7	10	20
20–34	1852	4.4	21	1	2	4	5	8	11	22
35–49	3069	5.5	39	1	2	4	6	10	16	34
50–64	4242	7.4	42	2	3	5	9	17	21	28
65+	11169	7.5	40	2	3	6	10	15	20	32
GRAND TOTAL	23355	6.4	38	1	3	5	8	14	18	30

89.59: NONOP CARD/VASC EXAM NEC. Formerly included in operation group(s) 796.

Type of Patients	Observed Patients	Avg. Stay	Vari-ance	10th	25th	50th	75th	90th	95th	99th
1. SINGLE DX										
0–19 Years	46	3.0	7	1	1	2	3	4	9	9
20–34	27	2.6	2	1	1	3	3	3	6	7
35–49	24	2.7	1	2	2	2	3	4	4	6
50–64	12	2.8	2	1	1	2	4	4	4	5
65+	16	2.6	3	1	1	2	5	5	5	5
2. MULTIPLE DX										
0–19 Years	134	4.0	15	1	2	3	5	7	9	18
20–34	84	3.2	4	1	2	2	5	5	6	8
35–49	160	3.9	13	1	1	2	5	5	8	16
50–64	199	4.0	11	1	2	3	6	9	9	12
65+	757	5.1	19	2	3	4	6	9	10	26
TOTAL SINGLE DX	125	2.8	4	1	2	2	3	5	8	9
MULTIPLE DX	1334	4.5	16	1	2	4	6	8	10	20
TOTAL										
0–19 Years	180	3.8	13	1	2	2	6	7	9	15
20–34	111	3.1	4	1	2	2	5	5	6	8
35–49	184	3.6	10	1	2	3	4	6	9	14
50–64	211	3.9	11	1	2	3	5	9	9	12
65+	773	5.0	19	2	3	4	6	9	10	24
GRAND TOTAL	1459	4.3	15	1	2	3	6	8	10	20

89.62: CVP MONITORING. Formerly included in operation group(s) 795.

Type of Patients	Observed Patients	Avg. Stay	Vari-ance	10th	25th	50th	75th	90th	95th	99th
1. SINGLE DX										
0–19 Years	2	6.3	2	6	6	6	6	6	12	12
20–34	8	9.0	175	1	2	4	5	37	37	37
35–49	5	4.2	12	1	3	3	5	13	13	13
50–64	3	6.8	3	6	6	6	6	11	11	11
65+	6	7.7	38	1	4	7	12	18	18	18
2. MULTIPLE DX										
0–19 Years	59	7.4	32	2	4	7	10	16	16	64
20–34	63	5.3	31	3	4	4	4	8	13	21
35–49	184	10.4	115	3	5	7	11	21	34	69
50–64	168	16.3	48	6	14	17	21	21	23	41
65+	588	14.2	78	5	8	13	19	22	27	45
TOTAL SINGLE DX	24	6.7	36	2	4	6	6	11	13	37
MULTIPLE DX	1062	12.6	80	4	5	11	17	22	24	45
TOTAL										
0–19 Years	61	7.3	29	2	4	6	8	16	16	29
20–34	71	5.4	34	3	4	4	4	8	13	32
35–49	189	10.3	114	3	5	7	10	21	34	69
50–64	171	16.2	49	6	12	17	21	21	23	41
65+	594	14.2	78	5	8	13	19	22	27	45
GRAND TOTAL	1086	12.5	80	4	5	11	17	22	24	44

Length of Stay by Diagnosis and Operation, United States, 1997

United States, October 1995–September 1996 Data, by Operation

89.64: PA WEDGE MONITORING. Formerly included in operation group(s) 795.

Type of Patients	Observed Patients	Avg. Stay	Vari-ance	Percentiles						
				10th	25th	50th	75th	90th	95th	99th
1. SINGLE DX										
0–19 Years	2	3.0	8	1	1	1	6	6	6	6
20–34	4	2.4	<1	2	1	2	3	3	3	3
35–49	3	1.3	<1	1	1	1	2	2	2	2
50–64	9	2.3	4	1	1	1	5	5	5	7
65+	6	12.4	49	8	8	17	17	20	20	20
2. MULTIPLE DX										
0–19 Years	18	13.5	271	1	3	9	12	36	38	73
20–34	102	9.8	78	2	4	8	13	18	26	>99
35–49	314	8.9	59	2	4	7	11	18	27	40
50–64	783	10.1	48	2	5	8	14	20	21	33
65+	2160	11.3	57	4	6	9	14	21	25	40
TOTAL SINGLE DX	24	3.3	18	1	1	1	5	7	17	20
MULTIPLE DX	3377	10.8	57	3	6	9	14	20	25	38
TOTAL										
0–19 Years	20	12.6	256	1	3	9	12	36	38	73
20–34	106	9.7	78	2	4	8	13	18	26	>99
35–49	317	8.8	59	2	4	6	11	18	27	34
50–64	792	9.9	48	2	5	8	14	20	21	33
65+	2166	11.3	57	4	6	9	14	21	25	40
GRAND TOTAL	3401	10.7	57	3	6	9	14	20	25	38

89.65: ARTERIAL BLD GAS MEASURE. Formerly included in operation group(s) 795.

Type of Patients	Observed Patients	Avg. Stay	Vari-ance	Percentiles						
				10th	25th	50th	75th	90th	95th	99th
1. SINGLE DX										
0–19 Years	538	2.1	2	1	1	1	3	5	5	6
20–34	223	2.6	3	1	2	2	3	4	5	8
35–49	195	3.0	3	1	2	3	4	5	5	8
50–64	156	3.3	3	1	2	3	4	5	6	9
65+	130	4.0	5	2	2	3	5	6	7	12
2. MULTIPLE DX										
0–19 Years	1964	4.2	22	1	2	3	5	8	10	26
20–34	1379	3.9	13	1	2	3	5	7	9	16
35–49	2247	4.3	17	1	2	3	5	8	11	21
50–64	2897	5.0	15	2	3	4	6	9	12	21
65+	7745	5.8	21	2	3	5	7	11	14	23
TOTAL SINGLE DX	1242	2.6	3	1	1	2	3	5	6	9
MULTIPLE DX	16232	5.1	19	1	2	4	6	10	13	22
TOTAL										
0–19 Years	2502	3.7	18	1	2	3	5	7	10	23
20–34	1602	3.7	12	1	2	3	4	7	9	15
35–49	2442	4.2	16	1	2	3	5	8	10	20
50–64	3053	4.9	15	2	3	4	6	9	12	20
65+	7875	5.8	20	2	3	5	7	11	14	23
GRAND TOTAL	17474	4.9	19	1	2	4	6	9	12	21

89.66: MIX VENOUS BLD GAS MEAS. Formerly included in operation group(s) 795.

Type of Patients	Observed Patients	Avg. Stay	Vari-ance	Percentiles						
				10th	25th	50th	75th	90th	95th	99th
1. SINGLE DX										
0–19 Years	105	1.3	<1	1	1	1	1	2	3	4
20–34	1	2.0	0	2	2	2	2	2	2	2
35–49	1	2.0	0	2	2	2	2	2	2	2
50–64	0									
65+	0									
2. MULTIPLE DX										
0–19 Years	192	2.6	9	1	1	2	3	5	8	18
20–34	8	3.9	22	1	1	1	5	13	13	13
35–49	10	7.0	26	2	3	5	14	14	14	14
50–64	11	5.4	5	3	3	7	7	7	7	8
65+	23	5.4	7	3	3	5	6	7	15	15
TOTAL SINGLE DX	107	1.3	<1	1	1	1	1	2	3	4
MULTIPLE DX	244	2.9	10	1	1	2	3	5	11	18
TOTAL										
0–19 Years	297	2.0	5	1	1	1	2	4	5	11
20–34	9	3.8	20	1	1	1	3	13	13	13
35–49	11	6.5	25	1	2	4	11	14	14	14
50–64	11	5.4	5	2	3	7	7	7	7	8
65+	23	5.4	7	3	3	5	6	7	15	15
GRAND TOTAL	351	2.2	6	1	1	1	2	5	6	14

89.68: CARDIAC OUTPUT MONIT NEC. Formerly included in operation group(s) 795.

Type of Patients	Observed Patients	Avg. Stay	Vari-ance	Percentiles						
				10th	25th	50th	75th	90th	95th	99th
1. SINGLE DX										
0–19 Years	5	3.2	7	1	1	2	3	5	9	9
20–34	1	4.0	0	4	4	4	4	4	4	4
35–49	3	2.2	<1	2	2	2	2	3	4	4
50–64	3	2.6	<1	2	2	3	3	3	3	3
65+	1	3.0	0	3	3	3	3	3	3	3
2. MULTIPLE DX										
0–19 Years	59	5.3	20	2	2	4	7	12	13	16
20–34	27	5.8	18	2	2	5	8	10	12	28
35–49	73	5.1	20	3	3	5	5	7	10	26
50–64	151	5.3	18	1	3	5	7	10	12	22
65+	358	5.4	13	3	3	5	7	11	11	21
TOTAL SINGLE DX	13	2.9	4	1	2	2	3	7	9	9
MULTIPLE DX	668	5.4	16	2	3	5	7	10	12	22
TOTAL										
0–19 Years	64	5.2	19	1	2	4	7	12	13	16
20–34	28	5.8	18	2	2	5	8	10	12	28
35–49	76	5.0	19	2	3	5	5	7	10	26
50–64	154	5.3	18	1	3	4	7	10	12	22
65+	359	5.4	13	2	3	5	7	10	11	21
GRAND TOTAL	681	5.3	16	2	3	5	7	10	12	22

382

Length of Stay by Diagnosis and Operation, United States, 1997

89.7: GENERAL PHYSICAL EXAM. Formerly included in operation group(s) 796.

Type of Patients	Observed Patients	Avg. Stay	Variance	10th	25th	50th	75th	90th	95th	99th
1. SINGLE DX										
0–19 Years	59	1.9	<1	1	1	2	2	3	3	4
20–34	1	1.0	0	1	1	1	1	1	1	1
35–49	3	10.7	6	8	8	10	13	13	13	13
50–64	1	5.0	0	5	5	5	5	5	5	5
65+	1	1.0	0	1	1	1	1	1	1	1
2. MULTIPLE DX										
0–19 Years	10	2.4	1	1	1	2	3	4	4	4
20–34	16	3.5	13	1	2	3	4	7	12	17
35–49	26	3.8	9	1	1	3	5	6	12	14
50–64	16	3.5	12	1	1	3	5	5	11	16
65+	9	9.9	105	2	3	6	11	35	35	35
TOTAL SINGLE DX	65	2.1	2	1	1	2	2	3	3	10
MULTIPLE DX	77	4.0	22	1	1	3	5	9	12	35
TOTAL										
0–19 Years	69	1.9	<1	1	1	2	2	3	3	4
20–34	17	3.4	12	1	1	2	4	7	12	17
35–49	29	4.3	13	1	2	3	6	10	13	14
50–64	17	3.6	12	1	1	3	5	5	11	16
65+	10	9.0	101	1	2	6	11	17	35	35
GRAND TOTAL	142	2.9	11	1	1	2	3	5	9	17

89.8: AUTOPSY. Formerly included in operation group(s) 796.

Type of Patients	Observed Patients	Avg. Stay	Variance	10th	25th	50th	75th	90th	95th	99th
1. SINGLE DX										
0–19 Years	0									
20–34	0									
35–49	0									
50–64	0									
65+										
2. MULTIPLE DX										
0–19 Years	0									
20–34	0									
35–49	0									
50–64	0									
65+	1	9.0	0	9	9	9	9	9	9	9
TOTAL SINGLE DX	0									
MULTIPLE DX	1	9.0	0	9	9	9	9	9	9	9
TOTAL										
0–19 Years	0									
20–34	0									
35–49	0									
50–64	0									
65+	1	9.0	0	9	9	9	9	9	9	9
GRAND TOTAL	1	9.0	0	9	9	9	9	9	9	9

90.0: MICRO EXAM-NERVOUS SYST. Formerly included in operation group(s) 796.

Type of Patients	Observed Patients	Avg. Stay	Variance	10th	25th	50th	75th	90th	95th	99th
1. SINGLE DX										
0–19 Years	1	1.0	0	1	1	1	1	1	1	1
20–34	0									
35–49	0									
50–64	0									
65+	0									
2. MULTIPLE DX										
0–19 Years	3	2.0	<1	1	2	2	2	2	5	5
20–34	1	2.0	0	2	2	2	2	2	2	2
35–49	2	12.8	144	1	1	22	22	22	22	22
50–64	1	3.0	0	3	3	3	3	3	3	3
65+	2	16.6	199	5	5	5	29	29	29	29
TOTAL SINGLE DX	1	1.0	0	1	1	1	1	1	1	1
MULTIPLE DX	9	4.3	48	1	2	2	2	5	22	29
TOTAL										
0–19 Years	4	1.8	<1	1	1	2	2	2	2	5
20–34	1	2.0	0	2	2	2	2	2	2	2
35–49	2	12.8	144	1	1	22	22	22	22	22
50–64	1	3.0	0	3	3	3	3	3	3	3
65+	2	16.6	199	5	5	5	29	29	29	29
GRAND TOTAL	10	3.9	43	1	2	2	2	5	22	29

90.1: MICRO EXAM-ENDOCRINE NEC. Formerly included in operation group(s) 796.

Type of Patients	Observed Patients	Avg. Stay	Variance	10th	25th	50th	75th	90th	95th	99th
1. SINGLE DX										
0–19 Years	0									
20–34	0									
35–49	0									
50–64	0									
65+	0									
2. MULTIPLE DX										
0–19 Years	0									
20–34	0									
35–49	0									
50–64	0									
65+	0									
TOTAL SINGLE DX	0									
MULTIPLE DX	0									
TOTAL										
0–19 Years	0									
20–34	0									
35–49	0									
50–64	0									
65+	0									
GRAND TOTAL	0									

Length of Stay by Diagnosis and Operation, United States, 1997

United States, October 1995–September 1996 Data, by Operation

90.2: MICRO EXAM-EYE. Formerly included in operation group(s) 796.

Type of Patients	Observed Patients	Avg. Stay	Variance	10th	25th	50th	75th	90th	95th	99th
1. SINGLE DX										
0–19 Years	0									
20–34	0									
35–49	0									
50–64	0									
65+	0									
2. MULTIPLE DX										
0–19 Years	12	4.2	4	2	3	4	5	8	9	9
20–34	0									
35–49	1	5.0	0	5	5	5	5	5	5	5
50–64	1	5.0	0	5	5	5	5	5	5	5
65+	5	6.0	55	1	1	3	5	20	20	20
TOTAL SINGLE DX	0									
MULTIPLE DX	19	4.7	13	2	3	4	5	8	9	20
TOTAL										
0–19 Years	12	4.2	4	2	3	4	5	8	9	9
20–34	0									
35–49	1	5.0	0	5	5	5	5	5	5	5
50–64	1	5.0	0	5	5	5	5	5	5	5
65+	5	6.0	55	1	1	3	5	20	20	20
GRAND TOTAL	19	4.7	13	2	3	4	5	8	9	20

90.3: MICRO EXAM-ENT/LARYNX. Formerly included in operation group(s) 796.

Type of Patients	Observed Patients	Avg. Stay	Variance	10th	25th	50th	75th	90th	95th	99th
1. SINGLE DX										
0–19 Years	10	1.8	1	1	1	1	2	4	4	5
20–34	1	3.0	0	3	3	3	3	3	3	3
35–49	1	7.0	0	7	7	7	7	7	7	7
50–64	0									
65+	1	3.0	0	3	3	3	3	3	3	3
2. MULTIPLE DX										
0–19 Years	28	2.7	4	1	1	2	4	5	5	7
20–34	1	5.0	0	5	5	5	5	5	5	5
35–49	3	4.0	3	1	2	5	5	5	5	5
50–64	2	7.0	1	6	6	6	8	8	8	8
65+	6	3.5	3	2	2	3	4	7	7	7
TOTAL SINGLE DX	13	2.2	2	1	1	2	3	4	5	7
MULTIPLE DX	40	3.1	4	1	1	2	5	5	6	8
TOTAL										
0–19 Years	38	2.6	3	1	1	2	4	5	5	7
20–34	2	4.4	<1	3	3	5	5	5	5	5
35–49	4	4.1	3	1	2	5	5	5	5	7
50–64	2	7.0	1	6	6	6	8	8	8	8
65+	7	3.4	3	2	2	3	4	7	7	7
GRAND TOTAL	53	3.0	4	1	1	2	5	5	6	8

90.4: MICRO EXAM-LOWER RESP. Formerly included in operation group(s) 796.

Type of Patients	Observed Patients	Avg. Stay	Variance	10th	25th	50th	75th	90th	95th	99th
1. SINGLE DX										
0–19 Years	5	1.8	<1	1	1	2	2	2	4	4
20–34	2	1.1	<1	1	1	2	1	2	1	2
35–49	7	3.8	1	3	3	3	5	5	5	5
50–64	2	5.4	<1	5	5	5	6	6	6	6
65+	13	2.5	2	1	2	2	3	4	4	9
2. MULTIPLE DX										
0–19 Years	7	8.0	261	2	2	2	7	7	57	57
20–34	15	4.1	10	3	3	4	4	4	6	22
35–49	36	4.0	6	2	2	4	5	7	7	14
50–64	49	4.2	7	2	3	3	7	9	8	15
65+	140	5.2	11	2	3	4	6	9	11	15
TOTAL SINGLE DX	29	2.5	2	1	1	2	3	4	5	8
MULTIPLE DX	247	4.7	12	2	3	4	6	9	10	15
TOTAL										
0–19 Years	12	4.9	137	1	2	2	7	7	7	57
20–34	17	3.3	9	1	2	3	4	4	5	22
35–49	43	3.9	6	2	2	4	5	7	7	14
50–64	51	4.3	7	2	3	4	7	9	8	15
65+	153	4.8	11	2	3	4	6	9	10	14
GRAND TOTAL	276	4.4	11	2	2	4	5	8	10	15

90.5: MICRO EXAM-BLOOD. Formerly included in operation group(s) 796.

Type of Patients	Observed Patients	Avg. Stay	Variance	10th	25th	50th	75th	90th	95th	99th
1. SINGLE DX										
0–19 Years	110	2.2	5	1	1	2	2	3	4	12
20–34	23	2.6	5	1	2	2	3	4	6	18
35–49	17	3.1	4	2	2	3	3	5	8	12
50–64	9	4.0	2	2	4	4	4	6	6	8
65+	6	3.1	4	1	1	3	6	6	6	6
2. MULTIPLE DX										
0–19 Years	484	4.9	23	2	3	3	5	9	16	22
20–34	61	3.2	6	1	2	3	4	4	7	16
35–49	49	3.7	7	2	2	3	5	5	7	20
50–64	48	4.1	13	2	3	3	5	8	11	20
65+	188	5.2	22	2	3	4	5	10	13	19
TOTAL SINGLE DX	165	2.8	5	1	2	2	3	4	5	12
MULTIPLE DX	830	4.7	19	2	3	3	5	8	12	20
TOTAL										
0–19 Years	594	4.4	21	1	2	3	5	8	14	22
20–34	84	3.1	6	1	2	3	4	5	7	16
35–49	66	3.6	7	2	3	3	4	5	10	15
50–64	57	4.0	10	2	3	3	4	8	10	20
65+	194	5.2	22	2	3	4	5	10	12	19
GRAND TOTAL	995	4.4	17	2	2	3	5	8	11	20

384

Length of Stay by Diagnosis and Operation, United States, 1997

United States, October 1995–September 1996 Data, by Operation

90.52: CULTURE-BLOOD. Formerly included in operation group(s) 796.

Type of Patients	Observed Patients	Avg. Stay	Variance	10th	25th	50th	75th	90th	95th	99th
1. SINGLE DX										
0–19 Years	23	1.6	<1	1	1	1	2	3	3	3
20–34	3	2.6	2	1	1	3	4	4	4	4
35–49	5	2.8	<1	2	3	3	3	3	3	3
50–64	3	4.2	2	4	4	4	4	4	4	4
65+	3	3.3	6	1	1	3	6	6	6	6
2. MULTIPLE DX										
0–19 Years	296	5.3	27	2	3	4	6	10	17	22
20–34	8	3.4	1	2	3	3	4	5	5	6
35–49	15	3.5	1	3	3	3	5	5	5	9
50–64	16	4.6	19	2	3	3	4	10	20	20
65+	95	4.3	4	2	3	4	5	7	8	11
TOTAL SINGLE DX	37	2.9	2	1	2	3	4	4	4	8
MULTIPLE DX	430	4.7	16	2	3	3	5	8	11	20
TOTAL										
0–19 Years	319	5.0	26	1	3	3	6	10	17	22
20–34	11	3.1	2	1	2	3	4	4	5	6
35–49	20	3.3	1	2	3	3	3	5	5	5
50–64	19	4.5	12	2	3	4	4	8	10	20
65+	98	4.3	4	2	3	4	5	7	8	11
GRAND TOTAL	467	4.5	14	2	3	3	5	8	10	20

90.7: MICRO EXAM-LYMPH SYSTEM. Formerly included in operation group(s) 796.

Type of Patients	Observed Patients	Avg. Stay	Variance	10th	25th	50th	75th	90th	95th	99th
1. SINGLE DX										
0–19 Years	0									
20–34	0									
35–49	0									
50–64	0									
65+	0									
2. MULTIPLE DX										
0–19 Years	1	1.0	0	1	1	1	1	1	1	1
20–34	0									
35–49	1	4.0	0	4	4	4	4	4	4	4
50–64	1	11.0	0	11	11	11	11	11	11	11
65+	0									
TOTAL SINGLE DX	0									
MULTIPLE DX	3	3.6	10	1	1	4	4	11	11	11
TOTAL										
0–19 Years	1	1.0	0	1	1	1	1	1	1	1
20–34	0									
35–49	1	4.0	0	4	4	4	4	4	4	4
50–64	1	11.0	0	11	11	11	11	11	11	11
65+	0									
GRAND TOTAL	3	3.6	10	1	1	4	4	11	11	11

90.6: MICRO EXAM-SPLEEN/MARROW. Formerly included in operation group(s) 796.

Type of Patients	Observed Patients	Avg. Stay	Variance	10th	25th	50th	75th	90th	95th	99th
1. SINGLE DX										
0–19 Years	0									
20–34	0									
35–49	0									
50–64	0									
65+	0									
2. MULTIPLE DX										
0–19 Years	0									
20–34	0									
35–49	0									
50–64	0									
65+	0									
TOTAL SINGLE DX	0									
MULTIPLE DX	0									
TOTAL										
0–19 Years	0									
20–34	0									
35–49	0									
50–64	0									
65+	0									
GRAND TOTAL	0									

90.8: MICRO EXAM-UPPER GI. Formerly included in operation group(s) 796.

Type of Patients	Observed Patients	Avg. Stay	Variance	10th	25th	50th	75th	90th	95th	99th
1. SINGLE DX										
0–19 Years	0									
20–34	0									
35–49	0									
50–64	0									
65+	0									
2. MULTIPLE DX										
0–19 Years	0									
20–34	0									
35–49	5	2.7	3	1	1	3	4	5	5	5
50–64	5	3.1	2	1	3	3	3	6	6	6
65+	11	10.7	54	5	6	7	15	22	29	29
TOTAL SINGLE DX	0									
MULTIPLE DX	21	6.8	43	1	3	5	7	20	22	29
TOTAL										
0–19 Years	0									
20–34	0									
35–49	5	2.7	3	1	1	3	4	5	5	5
50–64	5	3.1	2	1	3	3	3	6	6	6
65+	11	10.7	54	5	6	7	15	22	29	29
GRAND TOTAL	21	6.8	43	1	3	5	7	20	22	29

Length of Stay by Diagnosis and Operation, United States, 1997

United States, October 1995–September 1996 Data, by Operation

90.9: MICRO EXAM-LOWER GI. Formerly included in operation group(s) 796.

Type of Patients	Observed Patients	Avg. Stay	Vari-ance	Percentiles						
				10th	25th	50th	75th	90th	95th	99th
1. SINGLE DX										
0–19 Years	5	2.1	2	1	1	1	4	4	4	4
20–34	1	2.0	0	2	2	2	2	2	2	2
35–49	1	1.0	0	1	1	1	1	1	1	1
50–64	2	4.5	<1	4	4	4	6	6	6	6
65+	1	2.0	0	2	2	2	2	2	2	2
2. MULTIPLE DX										
0–19 Years	31	2.6	1	1	2	2	3	4	4	5
20–34	6	2.0	<1	1	2	2	2	2	3	3
35–49	7	3.2	6	2	2	2	5	6	10	10
50–64	11	2.5	2	2	2	2	5	4	5	8
65+	22	4.0	2	3	3	4	5	6	6	7
TOTAL SINGLE DX	10	2.9	3	1	1	4	4	4	6	6
MULTIPLE DX	77	3.0	3	2	2	2	4	6	6	10
TOTAL										
0–19 Years	36	2.5	1	1	2	2	3	4	4	5
20–34	7	2.0	<1	2	2	2	2	2	3	3
35–49	8	3.2	6	1	2	2	5	6	10	10
50–64	13	2.6	2	2	2	2	5	5	6	8
65+	23	4.0	2	3	3	4	5	6	6	7
GRAND TOTAL	87	3.0	3	2	2	2	4	6	6	10

91.0: MICRO EXAM-BIL/PANCREAS. Formerly included in operation group(s) 796.

Type of Patients	Observed Patients	Avg. Stay	Vari-ance	Percentiles						
				10th	25th	50th	75th	90th	95th	99th
1. SINGLE DX										
0–19 Years	0									
20–34	0									
35–49	1	2.0	0	2	2	2	2	2	2	2
50–64	0									
65+	0									
2. MULTIPLE DX										
0–19 Years	0									
20–34	0									
35–49	0									
50–64	0									
65+	0									
TOTAL SINGLE DX	1	2.0	0	2	2	2	2	2	2	2
MULTIPLE DX	0									
TOTAL										
0–19 Years	0									
20–34	0									
35–49	1	2.0	0	2	2	2	2	2	2	2
50–64	0									
65+	0									
GRAND TOTAL	1	2.0	0	2	2	2	2	2	2	2

91.1: MICRO EXAM-PERITONEUM. Formerly included in operation group(s) 796.

Type of Patients	Observed Patients	Avg. Stay	Vari-ance	Percentiles						
				10th	25th	50th	75th	90th	95th	99th
1. SINGLE DX										
0–19 Years	0									
20–34	0									
35–49	0									
50–64	0									
65+	0									
2. MULTIPLE DX										
0–19 Years	0									
20–34	0									
35–49	1	3.0	0	3	3	3	3	3	3	3
50–64	0									
65+	1	8.0	0	8	8	8	8	8	8	8
TOTAL SINGLE DX	0									
MULTIPLE DX	2	4.1	5	3	3	3	3	8	8	8
TOTAL										
0–19 Years	0									
20–34	0									
35–49	1	3.0	0	3	3	3	3	3	3	3
50–64	0									
65+	1	8.0	0	8	8	8	8	8	8	8
GRAND TOTAL	2	4.1	5	3	3	3	3	8	8	8

91.2: MICRO EXAM-UPPER URINARY. Formerly included in operation group(s) 796.

Type of Patients	Observed Patients	Avg. Stay	Vari-ance	Percentiles						
				10th	25th	50th	75th	90th	95th	99th
1. SINGLE DX										
0–19 Years	0									
20–34	0									
35–49	0									
50–64	0									
65+	0									
2. MULTIPLE DX										
0–19 Years	0									
20–34	0									
35–49	1	12.0	0	12	12	12	12	12	12	12
50–64	0									
65+	2	3.3	15	1	1	1	8	8	8	8
TOTAL SINGLE DX	0									
MULTIPLE DX	3	9.1	23	1	8	12	12	12	12	12
TOTAL										
0–19 Years	0									
20–34	0									
35–49	1	12.0	0	12	12	12	12	12	12	12
50–64	0									
65+	2	3.3	15	1	1	1	8	8	8	8
GRAND TOTAL	3	9.1	23	1	8	12	12	12	12	12

Length of Stay by Diagnosis and Operation, United States, 1997

United States, October 1995–September 1996 Data, by Operation

91.3: MICRO EXAM-LOWER URINARY. Formerly included in operation group(s) 796.

Type of Patients	Observed Patients	Avg. Stay	Variance	10th	25th	50th	75th	90th	95th	99th
1. SINGLE DX										
0–19 Years	9	1.3	<1	1	1	1	2	2	2	2
20–34	27	1.9	1	1	1	2	2	3	3	7
35–49	4	4.1	1	2	2	5	5	5	5	5
50–64	4	1.5	<1	1	1	1	2	2	2	6
65+	1	1.0	0	1	1	1	1	1	1	1
2. MULTIPLE DX										
0–19 Years	59	2.8	34	1	2	2	2	3	4	26
20–34	66	4.0	8	1	2	3	5	11	11	11
35–49	56	3.8	9	1	2	2	6	6	9	14
50–64	47	4.2	18	1	2	3	6	7	7	12
65+	249	5.4	52	2	3	4	6	9	10	62
TOTAL SINGLE DX	45	2.0	2	1	1	2	2	5	5	7
MULTIPLE DX	477	4.5	33	1	2	3	6	7	10	21
TOTAL										
0–19 Years	68	2.6	30	1	2	2	2	3	4	26
20–34	93	3.6	8	1	2	3	5	7	11	11
35–49	60	3.9	8	1	2	3	6	6	9	14
50–64	51	3.7	16	1	2	3	4	7	7	12
65+	250	5.4	52	2	3	4	6	9	10	62
GRAND TOTAL	522	4.3	30	1	2	3	5	7	10	21

91.33: C&S-LOWER URINARY. Formerly included in operation group(s) 796.

Type of Patients	Observed Patients	Avg. Stay	Variance	10th	25th	50th	75th	90th	95th	99th
1. SINGLE DX										
0–19 Years	3	1.5	<1	1	1	2	2	2	2	2
20–34	24	1.9	1	1	1	2	2	3	3	7
35–49	4	4.1	2	2	2	5	5	5	5	5
50–64	0									
65+	0									
2. MULTIPLE DX										
0–19 Years	20	2.4	7	2	2	2	2	3	4	7
20–34	29	3.3	3	1	2	2	5	5	5	7
35–49	23	4.0	4	2	2	5	6	6	6	9
50–64	26	3.9	30	1	2	3	3	7	7	38
65+	137	4.6	8	2	3	4	6	8	10	13
TOTAL SINGLE DX	31	2.4	3	1	1	2	3	5	5	7
MULTIPLE DX	235	4.1	10	1	2	3	5	7	9	12
TOTAL										
0–19 Years	23	2.4	6	2	2	2	2	3	4	7
20–34	53	2.8	3	2	2	2	5	5	5	7
35–49	27	4.0	4	2	2	5	6	6	6	9
50–64	26	3.9	30	1	2	3	3	7	7	38
65+	137	4.6	8	2	3	4	6	8	10	13
GRAND TOTAL	266	3.9	10	1	2	3	5	7	9	12

91.32: CULTURE-LOWER URINARY. Formerly included in operation group(s) 796.

Type of Patients	Observed Patients	Avg. Stay	Variance	10th	25th	50th	75th	90th	95th	99th
1. SINGLE DX										
0–19 Years	5	1.2	<1	1	1	1	1	2	2	2
20–34	3	2.1	<1	2	2	2	2	3	3	3
35–49	0									
50–64	4	1.5	<1	1	1	1	2	2	2	6
65+	0									
2. MULTIPLE DX										
0–19 Years	26	2.0	<1	1	2	2	2	3	3	5
20–34	33	4.5	11	1	2	3	5	11	11	11
35–49	26	3.7	11	1	1	2	6	8	12	14
50–64	21	4.4	4	2	3	4	7	7	7	8
65+	112	6.3	104	2	3	4	6	10	13	62
TOTAL SINGLE DX	12	1.6	<1	1	1	2	2	2	2	3
MULTIPLE DX	218	4.9	49	1	2	3	6	9	11	62
TOTAL										
0–19 Years	31	1.9	<1	1	1	2	2	3	3	5
20–34	36	4.3	10	1	2	3	5	11	11	11
35–49	26	3.7	11	1	1	2	6	8	12	14
50–64	25	3.5	5	1	2	3	6	7	7	8
65+	112	6.3	104	2	3	4	6	10	13	62
GRAND TOTAL	230	4.6	46	1	2	3	5	8	11	62

91.4: MICRO EXAM-FEMALE GENIT. Formerly included in operation group(s) 796.

Type of Patients	Observed Patients	Avg. Stay	Variance	10th	25th	50th	75th	90th	95th	99th
1. SINGLE DX										
0–19 Years	1	2.0	0	2	2	2	2	2	2	2
20–34	6	1.8	<1	1	1	2	2	2	3	5
35–49	1	5.0	0	5	5	5	5	5	5	5
50–64	0									
65+	0									
2. MULTIPLE DX										
0–19 Years	9	3.1	4	1	2	2	4	7	7	8
20–34	22	5.8	17	2	4	4	7	12	14	22
35–49	33	4.5	21	2	2	4	4	8	12	34
50–64	13	10.6	41	4	7	10	13	15	32	32
65+	27	8.7	46	2	4	6	12	19	24	28
TOTAL SINGLE DX	8	1.8	<1	1	1	2	2	2	3	5
MULTIPLE DX	104	5.6	27	2	2	4	7	13	15	28
TOTAL										
0–19 Years	10	3.1	4	1	2	2	4	7	7	8
20–34	28	3.3	10	1	2	4	5	6	9	16
35–49	34	4.5	21	2	2	5	5	8	12	34
50–64	13	10.6	41	4	7	10	13	15	32	32
65+	27	8.7	46	2	4	6	12	19	24	28
GRAND TOTAL	112	4.6	23	1	2	3	5	10	14	28

Length of Stay by Diagnosis and Operation, United States, 1997

United States, October 1995–September 1996 Data, by Operation

91.5: MICRO EXAM-MS/JT FLUID. Formerly included in operation group(s) 796.

Type of Patients	Observed Patients	Avg. Stay	Variance	10th	25th	50th	75th	90th	95th	99th
1. SINGLE DX										
0–19 Years	0									
20–34	0									
35–49	0									
50–64	1	3.0	0	3	3	3	3	3	3	3
65+	1	9.0	0	9	9	9	9	9	9	9
2. MULTIPLE DX										
0–19 Years	2	8.1	24	5	5	5	15	15	15	15
20–34	0									
35–49	2	4.6	<1	4	4	5	5	5	5	5
50–64	0									
65+	2	3.2	1	2	2	4	4	4	4	4
TOTAL SINGLE DX	2	6.6	14	3	3	9	9	9	9	9
MULTIPLE DX	6	6.1	18	2	4	5	5	15	15	15
TOTAL										
0–19 Years	2	8.1	24	5	5	5	15	15	15	15
20–34	0									
35–49	2	4.6	<1	4	4	5	5	5	5	5
50–64	1	3.0	0	3	3	3	3	3	3	3
65+	3	4.8	9	2	2	4	9	9	9	9
GRAND TOTAL	8	6.2	17	3	4	5	5	15	15	15

91.6: MICRO EXAM-INTEGUMENT. Formerly included in operation group(s) 796.

Type of Patients	Observed Patients	Avg. Stay	Variance	10th	25th	50th	75th	90th	95th	99th
1. SINGLE DX										
0–19 Years	0									
20–34	0									
35–49	2	3.7	4	2	2	2	6	6	6	6
50–64	0									
65+	1	4.0	0	4	4	4	4	4	4	4
2. MULTIPLE DX										
0–19 Years	3	6.3	7	2	5	8	8	8	8	8
20–34	6	3.5	6	1	1	5	5	5	5	12
35–49	8	5.9	11	1	3	5	7	7	14	14
50–64	10	5.1	13	1	3	6	6	6	7	25
65+	34	5.5	12	2	3	5	7	11	13	16
TOTAL SINGLE DX	3	3.8	4	2	2	4	6	6	6	6
MULTIPLE DX	61	4.7	10	1	2	5	6	8	12	15
TOTAL										
0–19 Years	3	6.3	7	2	5	8	8	8	8	8
20–34	6	3.5	6	1	1	5	5	5	5	12
35–49	10	5.2	10	2	3	5	7	7	14	14
50–64	10	5.1	13	1	3	6	6	6	7	25
65+	35	5.5	12	2	3	5	7	11	13	16
GRAND TOTAL	64	4.6	10	2	2	5	6	8	12	15

91.7: MICRO EXAM-OP WOUND. Formerly included in operation group(s) 796.

Type of Patients	Observed Patients	Avg. Stay	Variance	10th	25th	50th	75th	90th	95th	99th
1. SINGLE DX										
0–19 Years	0									
20–34	0									
35–49	0									
50–64	0									
65+	0									
2. MULTIPLE DX										
0–19 Years	1	3.0	0	3	3	3	3	3	3	3
20–34	0									
35–49	0									
50–64	0									
65+	1	24.0	0	24	24	24	24	24	24	24
TOTAL SINGLE DX	0									
MULTIPLE DX	2	3.9	18	3	3	3	3	3	3	24
TOTAL										
0–19 Years	1	3.0	0	3	3	3	3	3	3	3
20–34	0									
35–49	0									
50–64	0									
65+	1	24.0	0	24	24	24	24	24	24	24
GRAND TOTAL	2	3.9	18	3	3	3	3	3	3	24

91.8: MICRO EXAM NEC. Formerly included in operation group(s) 796.

Type of Patients	Observed Patients	Avg. Stay	Variance	10th	25th	50th	75th	90th	95th	99th
1. SINGLE DX										
0–19 Years	1	8.0	0	8	8	8	8	8	8	8
20–34	2	1.5	1	1	1	1	1	4	4	4
35–49	0									
50–64	0									
65+	1	4.0	0	4	4	4	4	4	4	4
2. MULTIPLE DX										
0–19 Years	2	2.3	<1	2	2	2	2	5	5	5
20–34	3	2.2	<1	2	2	2	2	2	4	5
35–49	1	11.0	0	11	11	11	11	11	11	11
50–64	2	3.1	4	2	2	6	6	6	6	6
65+	5	6.1	1	6	6	6	6	6	9	9
TOTAL SINGLE DX	4	2.7	6	1	1	1	4	8	8	8
MULTIPLE DX	13	3.6	5	2	2	2	6	6	6	11
TOTAL										
0–19 Years	3	2.5	2	2	2	2	2	5	5	8
20–34	5	2.1	<1	2	2	2	2	2	4	5
35–49	1	11.0	0	11	11	11	11	11	11	11
50–64	2	3.1	4	2	2	6	6	6	7	25
65+	6	6.1	1	6	6	6	6	6	9	9
GRAND TOTAL	17	3.5	5	2	2	2	6	6	6	9

Length of Stay by Diagnosis and Operation, United States, 1997

United States, October 1995–September 1996 Data, by Operation

91.9: MICRO EXAM NOS. Formerly included in operation group(s) 796.

Type of Patients	Observed Patients	Avg. Stay	Vari-ance	10th	25th	50th	75th	90th	95th	99th
1. SINGLE DX										
0–19 Years	0									
20–34	0									
35–49	0									
50–64	0									
65+	0									
2. MULTIPLE DX										
0–19 Years	0									
20–34	0									
35–49	0									
50–64	1	3.0	0	3	3	3	3	3	3	3
65+	0									
TOTAL SINGLE DX	**0**									
MULTIPLE DX	**1**	**3.0**	**0**	**3**	**3**	**3**	**3**	**3**	**3**	**3**
TOTAL										
0–19 Years	0									
20–34	0									
35–49	0									
50–64	1	3.0	0	3	3	3	3	3	3	3
65+	0									
GRAND TOTAL	**1**	**3.0**	**0**	**3**	**3**	**3**	**3**	**3**	**3**	**3**

92.02: LIVER SCAN/ISOTOPE FUNCT. Formerly included in operation group(s) 787.

Type of Patients	Observed Patients	Avg. Stay	Vari-ance	10th	25th	50th	75th	90th	95th	99th
1. SINGLE DX										
0–19 Years	13	2.9	5	1	1	2	6	6	7	7
20–34	36	2.1	3	1	1	2	4	6	7	12
35–49	32	3.0	<1	3	3	3	3	3	3	8
50–64	8	1.7	1	1	1	2	2	2	5	5
65+	3	3.0	3	1	1	4	4	4	4	4
2. MULTIPLE DX										
0–19 Years	32	4.6	7	1	2	4	6	9	9	9
20–34	103	3.1	7	1	1	3	4	5	7	18
35–49	194	4.7	12	2	2	3	7	10	11	17
50–64	191	4.1	10	2	2	3	5	8	11	14
65+	350	6.6	19	2	4	6	8	12	15	23
TOTAL SINGLE DX	**92**	**2.8**	**1**	**1**	**2**	**3**	**3**	**3**	**4**	**8**
MULTIPLE DX	**870**	**5.0**	**15**	**1**	**2**	**4**	**7**	**11**	**12**	**18**
TOTAL										
0–19 Years	45	4.1	7	1	2	4	6	8	9	9
20–34	139	2.8	6	1	1	3	4	5	6	12
35–49	226	4.1	8	2	3	3	5	8	11	14
50–64	199	4.1	9	2	2	3	5	8	11	14
65+	353	6.5	19	2	4	6	8	12	15	23
GRAND TOTAL	**962**	**4.6**	**13**	**1**	**2**	**3**	**6**	**9**	**12**	**17**

92.0: ISOTOPE SCAN & FUNCTION. Formerly included in operation group(s) 787.

Type of Patients	Observed Patients	Avg. Stay	Vari-ance	10th	25th	50th	75th	90th	95th	99th
1. SINGLE DX										
0–19 Years	78	2.9	5	1	1	2	4	6	7	11
20–34	86	2.1	2	1	1	2	3	4	4	9
35–49	168	2.7	1	1	2	3	3	3	5	8
50–64	112	2.3	2	1	1	2	3	4	5	8
65+	68	2.8	3	1	2	2	4	6	6	8
2. MULTIPLE DX										
0–19 Years	484	4.7	13	2	3	4	6	9	11	18
20–34	352	4.3	19	1	1	3	5	11	14	18
35–49	1092	5.1	27	1	2	3	7	11	14	23
50–64	1808	4.5	16	1	2	3	5	9	13	18
65+	3879	6.0	23	2	3	5	7	12	15	24
TOTAL SINGLE DX	**512**	**2.6**	**2**	**1**	**1**	**3**	**3**	**4**	**5**	**8**
MULTIPLE DX	**7615**	**5.3**	**22**	**1**	**2**	**4**	**7**	**11**	**14**	**22**
TOTAL										
0–19 Years	562	4.5	12	2	2	4	6	9	11	17
20–34	438	3.8	16	1	1	3	4	9	14	17
35–49	1260	4.7	23	1	2	3	6	9	12	21
50–64	1920	4.4	15	1	2	3	5	9	12	18
65+	3947	5.9	23	2	3	5	7	12	15	24
GRAND TOTAL	**8127**	**5.1**	**21**	**2**	**2**	**4**	**7**	**10**	**14**	**21**

92.03: RENAL SCAN/ISOTOPE STUDY. Formerly included in operation group(s) 787.

Type of Patients	Observed Patients	Avg. Stay	Vari-ance	10th	25th	50th	75th	90th	95th	99th
1. SINGLE DX										
0–19 Years	21	3.3	4	1	2	3	5	5	5	11
20–34	6	1.6	2	1	1	1	2	2	6	6
35–49	6	2.2	5	1	1	1	3	7	7	7
50–64	10	3.6	3	2	3	3	4	7	7	7
65+	2	2.6	<1	2	2	3	3	3	3	3
2. MULTIPLE DX										
0–19 Years	273	4.3	7	2	3	4	5	7	10	14
20–34	56	3.8	21	1	1	3	5	8	8	24
35–49	99	8.1	44	2	3	7	9	21	24	28
50–64	126	5.3	17	2	2	4	7	10	11	19
65+	268	7.6	35	3	4	6	10	13	15	28
TOTAL SINGLE DX	**45**	**2.8**	**4**	**1**	**1**	**3**	**4**	**5**	**7**	**11**
MULTIPLE DX	**822**	**6.0**	**26**	**2**	**3**	**4**	**8**	**12**	**14**	**26**
TOTAL										
0–19 Years	294	4.2	7	2	3	4	5	7	10	14
20–34	62	3.6	19	1	1	2	5	8	8	11
35–49	105	7.7	44	2	3	6	8	21	24	28
50–64	136	5.2	16	2	2	4	7	10	11	19
65+	270	7.6	35	3	4	6	10	13	15	28
GRAND TOTAL	**867**	**5.9**	**26**	**3**	**3**	**4**	**8**	**12**	**14**	**26**

Length of Stay by Diagnosis and Operation, United States, 1997

United States, October 1995–September 1996 Data, by Operation

92.04: GI SCAN & ISOTOPE STUDY. Formerly included in operation group(s) 787.

Type of Patients	Observed Patients	Avg. Stay	Variance	10th	25th	50th	75th	90th	95th	99th
1. SINGLE DX										
0–19 Years	38	2.7	5	1	1	2	3	6	7	11
20–34	18	1.5	<1	1	1	1	2	3	3	5
35–49	21	1.9	2	1	1	1	2	3	4	7
50–64	7	4.6	9	2	2	2	8	8	8	8
65+	7	3.9	5	1	1	3	6	6	6	6
2. MULTIPLE DX										
0–19 Years	147	5.3	26	2	2	4	6	11	16	21
20–34	63	3.6	14	2	2	3	4	6	13	17
35–49	89	6.6	37	2	2	4	13	16	16	20
50–64	94	5.6	17	2	3	5	7	14	14	16
65+	275	6.4	20	1	3	5	8	13	17	22
TOTAL SINGLE DX	91	2.5	4	1	1	2	3	6	7	10
MULTIPLE DX	668	5.8	24	2	3	4	7	14	16	20
TOTAL										
0–19 Years	185	4.7	23	1	2	3	6	10	16	21
20–34	81	3.0	11	1	1	2	3	6	7	17
35–49	110	6.1	36	2	2	3	8	16	16	20
50–64	101	5.5	17	2	3	5	7	14	14	16
65+	282	6.3	20	1	3	5	8	13	17	22
GRAND TOTAL	759	5.5	23	2	2	4	7	13	16	19

92.05: CV SCAN/ISOTOPE STUDY. Formerly included in operation group(s) 787.

Type of Patients	Observed Patients	Avg. Stay	Variance	10th	25th	50th	75th	90th	95th	99th
1. SINGLE DX										
0–19 Years	5	4.4	5	2	2	4	6	7	7	7
20–34	18	2.3	1	1	1	3	3	4	4	4
35–49	100	2.2	2	1	1	2	3	5	5	8
50–64	85	2.0	1	1	1	2	3	4	4	5
65+	53	2.6	2	1	1	2	3	4	5	10
2. MULTIPLE DX										
0–19 Years	16	7.2	13	2	4	9	9	9	15	15
20–34	94	3.6	9	1	1	2	5	9	9	15
35–49	639	4.2	26	1	2	3	5	8	11	20
50–64	1349	4.3	16	2	2	3	5	8	11	18
65+	2885	5.5	20	2	3	4	7	11	14	22
TOTAL SINGLE DX	261	2.3	2	1	1	2	3	4	5	7
MULTIPLE DX	4983	5.0	20	1	2	4	6	10	13	21
TOTAL										
0–19 Years	21	6.6	13	2	4	9	9	9	10	15
20–34	112	3.3	8	1	1	2	4	8	9	13
35–49	739	4.0	23	1	2	3	5	8	10	19
50–64	1434	4.2	15	1	2	3	5	9	11	18
65+	2938	5.4	20	2	3	4	7	11	14	22
GRAND TOTAL	5244	4.9	20	1	2	4	6	10	13	21

92.1: OTHER RADIOISOTOPE SCAN. Formerly included in operation group(s) 787.

Type of Patients	Observed Patients	Avg. Stay	Variance	10th	25th	50th	75th	90th	95th	99th
1. SINGLE DX										
0–19 Years	184	3.6	7	1	2	3	5	7	8	15
20–34	173	2.6	4	1	1	2	4	5	7	10
35–49	212	2.9	4	1	1	3	4	6	6	11
50–64	129	3.1	4	1	1	2	5	6	7	7
65+	140	4.0	6	1	2	3	5	8	9	10
2. MULTIPLE DX										
0–19 Years	453	5.6	23	2	3	5	7	11	15	26
20–34	990	4.8	26	2	3	5	7	11	12	26
35–49	2166	4.7	16	1	2	4	6	8	11	20
50–64	3073	5.4	21	2	3	4	7	11	12	20
65+	8386	6.6	32	2	3	5	8	12	16	28
TOTAL SINGLE DX	838	3.1	5	1	1	2	4	6	7	10
MULTIPLE DX	15068	5.9	27	2	3	5	7	11	14	26
TOTAL										
0–19 Years	637	5.0	19	1	2	4	6	10	13	26
20–34	1163	4.4	23	1	2	3	5	8	11	24
35–49	2378	4.6	15	1	2	4	6	8	10	20
50–64	3202	5.3	20	2	3	4	7	11	12	20
65+	8526	6.6	32	2	3	5	8	12	16	28
GRAND TOTAL	15906	5.8	26	2	3	4	7	11	14	25

92.14: BONE SCAN. Formerly included in operation group(s) 787.

Type of Patients	Observed Patients	Avg. Stay	Variance	10th	25th	50th	75th	90th	95th	99th
1. SINGLE DX										
0–19 Years	144	3.4	7	1	1	3	5	7	8	15
20–34	26	2.2	4	1	1	1	2	5	6	10
35–49	36	4.0	3	3	3	4	4	5	6	12
50–64	17	2.4	1	2	2	2	4	4	4	6
65+	47	4.6	5	2	3	5	6	8	10	10
2. MULTIPLE DX										
0–19 Years	296	5.5	26	2	2	4	7	11	15	28
20–34	167	6.9	33	2	4	5	9	11	20	32
35–49	411	5.8	25	2	3	4	7	10	13	31
50–64	693	7.3	37	3	4	6	12	13	18	30
65+	3039	7.2	43	3	3	5	8	13	18	40
TOTAL SINGLE DX	270	3.4	6	1	2	3	4	6	8	10
MULTIPLE DX	4606	6.9	39	2	3	5	8	12	17	37
TOTAL										
0–19 Years	440	4.8	20	1	2	3	6	10	13	26
20–34	193	6.0	31	1	3	4	7	10	19	28
35–49	447	5.6	24	2	4	4	7	10	13	31
50–64	710	7.2	37	2	4	5	11	12	13	30
65+	3086	7.1	43	3	3	5	8	13	18	40
GRAND TOTAL	4876	6.7	38	2	3	5	8	12	16	35

United States, October 1995–September 1996 Data, by Operation

92.15: PULMONARY SCAN. Formerly included in operation group(s) 787.

Type of Patients	Observed Patients	Avg. Stay	Variance	10th	25th	50th	75th	90th	95th	99th
1. SINGLE DX										
0–19 Years	15	4.5	7	2	2	5	7	7	8	16
20–34	120	2.8	4	1	1	2	4	6	7	8
35–49	154	2.6	4	1	1	2	3	5	6	11
50–64	99	3.0	4	1	1	2	5	6	6	9
65+	78	3.9	6	2	2	3	5	8	9	10
2. MULTIPLE DX										
0–19 Years	66	5.4	11	1	4	5	6	10	10	21
20–34	747	4.1	17	1	2	3	5	8	10	20
35–49	1628	4.3	11	1	2	4	5	8	10	16
50–64	2235	4.6	12	1	2	4	6	8	11	16
65+	4955	6.2	24	2	3	5	8	12	14	25
TOTAL SINGLE DX	466	3.0	5	1	1	2	4	6	7	10
MULTIPLE DX	9631	5.3	19	2	3	4	7	10	13	25
TOTAL										
0–19 Years	81	5.2	10	1	3	5	6	9	10	19
20–34	867	3.8	15	1	2	3	5	8	9	20
35–49	1782	4.2	11	1	2	4	5	7	10	15
50–64	2334	4.5	12	1	2	4	6	8	10	16
65+	5033	6.2	23	2	3	5	8	12	14	25
GRAND TOTAL	10097	5.2	19	1	2	4	7	10	13	25

92.18: TOTAL BODY SCAN. Formerly included in operation group(s) 787.

Type of Patients	Observed Patients	Avg. Stay	Variance	10th	25th	50th	75th	90th	95th	99th
1. SINGLE DX										
0–19 Years	2	4.8	17	2	2	2	8	8	8	8
20–34	4	6.8	29	2	2	5	12	12	12	12
35–49	3	2.6	<1	1	2	3	3	3	3	3
50–64	1	5.0	0	5	5	5	5	5	5	5
65+	4	8.0	5	4	8	8	10	10	10	10
2. MULTIPLE DX										
0–19 Years	16	6.0	24	2	5	5	6	10	13	37
20–34	16	8.9	38	5	5	7	11	15	27	27
35–49	39	8.4	77	2	4	6	8	15	22	47
50–64	54	5.7	19	2	2	4	9	9	11	20
65+	185	8.2	60	3	4	5	10	17	21	37
TOTAL SINGLE DX	14	5.9	14	2	3	5	9	12	12	12
MULTIPLE DX	310	7.4	48	2	3	5	9	15	21	35
TOTAL										
0–19 Years	18	5.9	23	2	5	5	6	10	13	37
20–34	20	8.6	37	5	5	7	11	15	27	27
35–49	42	8.0	74	2	3	6	8	15	22	47
50–64	55	5.7	19	2	2	4	9	9	11	20
65+	189	8.2	59	3	4	5	10	17	21	37
GRAND TOTAL	324	7.4	48	3	3	5	9	15	21	35

92.19: SCAN OF OTHER SITES. Formerly included in operation group(s) 787.

Type of Patients	Observed Patients	Avg. Stay	Variance	10th	25th	50th	75th	90th	95th	99th
1. SINGLE DX										
0–19 Years	13	4.2	7	1	2	2	7	8	8	8
20–34	22	2.5	2	1	2	2	3	3	4	11
35–49	16	3.0	2	1	2	4	4	4	4	4
50–64	9	3.0	<1	2	3	3	3	5	5	5
65+	10	1.8	<1	1	1	2	2	3	3	4
2. MULTIPLE DX										
0–19 Years	32	5.9	31	1	3	4	6	17	20	22
20–34	40	6.3	111	1	2	3	5	10	43	56
35–49	66	5.8	18	2	3	4	7	11	13	20
50–64	54	4.2	16	1	2	3	6	12	12	14
65+	114	5.4	13	2	3	5	6	11	12	17
TOTAL SINGLE DX	70	2.7	3	1	2	2	4	4	6	8
MULTIPLE DX	306	5.4	28	2	3	4	6	11	12	31
TOTAL										
0–19 Years	45	5.5	25	1	2	4	7	15	18	20
20–34	62	4.5	64	1	2	4	4	7	11	43
35–49	82	5.2	18	2	3	4	6	11	12	20
50–64	63	4.0	14	1	2	3	5	9	12	14
65+	124	5.2	13	2	3	4	6	11	12	17
GRAND TOTAL	376	4.9	24	2	2	4	6	11	12	22

92.2: THER RADIOLOGY & NU MED. Formerly included in operation group(s) 788.

Type of Patients	Observed Patients	Avg. Stay	Variance	10th	25th	50th	75th	90th	95th	99th
1. SINGLE DX										
0–19 Years	13	5.0	15	1	1	3	8	8	8	15
20–34	172	1.7	1	1	1	2	2	2	3	11
35–49	463	2.0	2	1	1	2	2	3	3	5
50–64	448	2.1	2	1	1	2	2	3	4	9
65+	417	2.2	6	1	1	2	3	3	4	10
2. MULTIPLE DX										
0–19 Years	243	5.1	23	1	2	4	7	11	16	19
20–34	820	4.3	38	1	2	4	4	8	17	28
35–49	2535	5.0	28	1	2	3	6	11	15	27
50–64	5012	6.9	50	2	3	5	9	15	18	31
65+	8490	7.8	57	2	3	5	10	17	22	44
TOTAL SINGLE DX	1513	2.1	3	1	1	2	2	3	4	9
MULTIPLE DX	17100	6.9	51	2	2	5	9	15	20	37
TOTAL										
0–19 Years	256	5.1	22	1	2	4	7	11	16	19
20–34	992	3.7	31	1	1	2	3	7	14	28
35–49	2998	4.6	25	1	2	3	5	10	14	24
50–64	5460	6.6	48	2	2	4	8	15	18	31
65+	8907	7.6	57	2	3	5	10	16	22	43
GRAND TOTAL	18613	6.5	49	1	2	4	8	15	19	36

Length of Stay by Diagnosis and Operation, United States, 1997

United States, October 1995–September 1996 Data, by Operation

92.23: ISOTOPE TELERADIOTHERAPY. Formerly included in operation group(s) 788.

Type of Patients	Observed Patients	Avg. Stay	Variance	10th	25th	50th	75th	90th	95th	99th
1. SINGLE DX										
0–19 Years	1	1.0	0	1	1	1	1	1	1	1
20–34	19	1.1	<1	1	1	1	1	2	2	2
35–49	24	2.0	2	1	1	2	2	3	3	3
50–64	12	3.1	5	1	1	2	4	7	9	12
65+	5	2.5	3	2	2	2	2	2	8	8
2. MULTIPLE DX										
0–19 Years	12	3.8	12	1	2	3	4	7	14	14
20–34	73	2.8	34	1	1	2	5	5	6	21
35–49	180	4.4	25	1	2	3	6	7	11	23
50–64	278	7.2	41	1	2	5	11	16	19	27
65+	495	11.7	155	2	4	7	13	32	45	45
TOTAL SINGLE DX	61	1.6	2	1	1	1	2	2	4	9
MULTIPLE DX	1038	8.9	107	2	2	6	10	19	44	45
TOTAL										
0–19 Years	13	3.7	12	1	1	3	4	7	14	14
20–34	92	1.9	15	1	1	1	2	2	4	8
35–49	204	4.2	23	1	2	2	5	7	10	23
50–64	290	7.1	41	2	2	5	11	15	19	27
65+	500	11.7	154	2	4	7	13	32	45	45
GRAND TOTAL	1099	8.4	103	1	2	5	10	18	37	45

92.27: RADIOACTIVE ELEMENT IMPL. Formerly included in operation group(s) 788.

Type of Patients	Observed Patients	Avg. Stay	Variance	10th	25th	50th	75th	90th	95th	99th
1. SINGLE DX										
0–19 Years	2	3.0	0	3	3	3	3	3	3	3
20–34	78	2.2	<1	2	2	2	2	3	3	3
35–49	316	2.1	<1	1	2	2	2	3	3	4
50–64	353	1.9	<1	1	1	2	2	3	3	6
65+	354	2.0	3	1	1	2	3	3	3	8
2. MULTIPLE DX										
0–19 Years	3	3.7	19	2	2	2	2	13	15	15
20–34	101	2.2	2	1	2	2	2	4	4	8
35–49	380	3.1	9	1	2	2	4	4	6	13
50–64	689	3.5	31	1	2	2	3	5	9	43
65+	1248	3.0	14	1	1	2	3	5	8	19
TOTAL SINGLE DX	1103	2.0	1	1	1	2	2	3	3	6
MULTIPLE DX	2421	3.1	18	1	2	2	3	5	8	19
TOTAL										
0–19 Years	5	3.5	12	2	2	2	3	3	13	15
20–34	179	2.2	1	1	2	2	2	3	3	7
35–49	696	2.6	5	1	2	2	3	4	8	9
50–64	1042	3.0	22	1	2	2	3	5	8	43
65+	1602	2.8	12	1	1	2	3	4	7	17
GRAND TOTAL	3524	2.8	13	1	2	2	3	4	6	15

92.24: PHOTON TELERADIOTHERAPY. Formerly included in operation group(s) 788.

Type of Patients	Observed Patients	Avg. Stay	Variance	10th	25th	50th	75th	90th	95th	99th
1. SINGLE DX										
0–19 Years	3	5.5	12	1	1	8	8	8	8	8
20–34	2	10.3	4	5	11	11	11	11	11	11
35–49	4	2.3	4	1	1	6	5	6	6	6
50–64	5	4.8	10	1	1	6	7	9	9	9
65+	6	4.6	15	2	2	3	4	12	12	12
2. MULTIPLE DX										
0–19 Years	42	6.3	25	2	3	5	7	14	19	19
20–34	93	6.5	63	2	2	5	8	11	16	26
35–49	409	6.8	33	2	3	5	10	15	19	23
50–64	1039	8.5	67	2	4	6	10	16	22	35
65+	1789	8.7	56	2	4	6	11	20	24	34
TOTAL SINGLE DX	20	5.5	14	1	1	7	8	11	11	12
MULTIPLE DX	3372	8.3	57	2	4	6	10	18	23	33
TOTAL										
0–19 Years	45	6.2	24	1	3	5	7	14	19	19
20–34	95	6.6	62	2	2	5	8	11	15	26
35–49	413	6.7	33	2	3	4	9	15	19	23
50–64	1044	8.5	67	2	4	6	10	16	22	35
65+	1795	8.7	56	2	4	6	11	20	24	34
GRAND TOTAL	3392	8.3	57	2	4	6	10	18	23	33

92.28: ISOTOPE INJECT/INSTILL. Formerly included in operation group(s) 788.

Type of Patients	Observed Patients	Avg. Stay	Variance	10th	25th	50th	75th	90th	95th	99th
1. SINGLE DX										
0–19 Years	3	3.3	10	1	1	2	7	7	7	7
20–34	26	1.3	<1	1	1	1	1	2	3	3
35–49	35	1.5	<1	1	1	1	2	2	3	5
50–64	20	1.4	<1	1	1	1	2	3	3	5
65+	12	2.0	2	1	1	2	3	3	4	4
2. MULTIPLE DX										
0–19 Years	8	3.1	2	2	2	4	4	4	5	5
20–34	63	2.2	1	1	1	2	2	3	4	7
35–49	114	2.4	11	1	1	1	5	4	9	19
50–64	99	3.8	13	1	2	3	5	7	9	19
65+	172	4.5	12	2	2	3	7	8	10	21
TOTAL SINGLE DX	96	1.4	<1	1	1	1	2	2	3	4
MULTIPLE DX	456	3.4	11	1	2	2	4	7	9	17
TOTAL										
0–19 Years	11	3.2	3	1	2	4	4	5	7	7
20–34	89	1.9	1	1	1	2	2	3	3	7
35–49	149	2.2	8	1	1	1	4	7	9	17
50–64	119	3.1	11	2	2	3	7	8	9	16
65+	184	4.3	12	2	2	3	7	8	10	21
GRAND TOTAL	552	2.9	9	1	1	2	3	7	8	17

Length of Stay by Diagnosis and Operation, United States, 1997

United States, October 1995–September 1996 Data, by Operation

92.29: RADIOTHERAPEUTIC PX NEC. Formerly included in operation group(s) 788.

Type of Patients	Observed Patients	Avg. Stay	Vari-ance	10th	25th	50th	75th	90th	95th	99th
1. SINGLE DX										
0–19 Years	4	5.9	50	1	1	1	15	15	15	15
20–34	45	1.7	<1	1	1	1	2	2	2	3
35–49	83	1.9	5	1	1	2	2	2	3	9
50–64	56	3.4	7	2	2	2	4	7	9	13
65+	40	3.5	31	1	1	2	3	8	10	44
2. MULTIPLE DX										
0–19 Years	172	4.5	22	1	2	3	6	9	13	25
20–34	470	4.7	44	1	2	3	5	11	22	28
35–49	1335	5.2	29	1	2	4	7	11	15	30
50–64	2651	6.9	43	2	3	5	9	15	17	30
65+	4408	8.0	45	2	4	6	10	16	21	34
TOTAL SINGLE DX	228	2.4	9	1	1	2	2	4	6	15
MULTIPLE DX	9036	7.0	43	2	3	5	9	15	19	31
TOTAL										
0–19 Years	176	4.5	22	1	2	3	6	9	13	25
20–34	515	4.4	41	1	2	2	4	10	21	28
35–49	1418	4.9	28	1	2	3	6	11	14	29
50–64	2707	6.9	43	2	3	5	9	15	17	30
65+	4448	8.0	45	2	4	6	10	16	21	34
GRAND TOTAL	9264	6.9	43	2	3	5	9	15	19	31

93.0: DXTIC PHYSICAL TX. Formerly included in operation group(s) 791.

Type of Patients	Observed Patients	Avg. Stay	Vari-ance	10th	25th	50th	75th	90th	95th	99th
1. SINGLE DX										
0–19 Years	22	3.3	14	1	1	2	4	5	12	23
20–34	12	3.4	1	3	3	3	3	5	6	8
35–49	15	5.2	17	1	2	4	7	13	13	13
50–64	7	3.5	7	1	2	2	4	9	9	9
65+	7	3.1	3	2	2	2	3	7	7	7
2. MULTIPLE DX										
0–19 Years	66	11.1	127	3	3	8	14	24	46	51
20–34	57	7.3	33	2	3	6	9	15	22	22
35–49	96	12.2	116	2	4	12	15	28	33	47
50–64	195	12.3	149	3	4	10	14	29	36	60
65+	498	11.5	105	3	5	7	15	25	31	49
TOTAL SINGLE DX	63	3.6	8	1	2	3	4	6	9	14
MULTIPLE DX	912	11.6	115	3	4	8	14	27	33	49
TOTAL										
0–19 Years	88	9.0	108	2	2	5	12	16	33	51
20–34	69	5.8	25	2	3	3	8	11	22	22
35–49	111	11.8	113	2	4	11	14	28	33	47
50–64	202	12.1	147	2	4	9	14	29	36	60
65+	505	11.5	105	3	5	7	15	25	31	49
GRAND TOTAL	975	11.1	113	2	4	7	14	25	33	49

92.3: STEREOTACTIC RADIOSURG. Formerly included in operation group(s) 505.

Type of Patients	Observed Patients	Avg. Stay	Vari-ance	10th	25th	50th	75th	90th	95th	99th
1. SINGLE DX										
0–19 Years	31	2.2	1	1	2	2	2	4	4	6
20–34	29	1.5	3	1	1	1	2	3	4	9
35–49	60	1.2	<1	1	1	1	1	1	2	7
50–64	50	1.2	1	1	1	1	1	1	2	9
65+	54	1.1	<1	1	1	1	1	1	2	4
2. MULTIPLE DX										
0–19 Years	44	5.9	192	1	2	2	5	7	28	92
20–34	41	1.7	3	1	1	1	1	3	7	10
35–49	125	1.8	2	1	1	1	2	4	4	8
50–64	151	1.6	5	1	1	1	1	4	6	13
65+	192	1.9	11	1	1	1	1	4	6	16
TOTAL SINGLE DX	224	1.2	<1	1	1	1	1	1	2	6
MULTIPLE DX	553	2.1	24	1	1	1	1	4	6	19
TOTAL										
0–19 Years	75	4.9	144	1	2	2	4	5	7	92
20–34	70	1.6	3	1	1	1	1	3	6	9
35–49	185	1.4	1	1	1	1	1	2	4	7
50–64	201	1.5	4	1	1	1	1	2	4	9
65+	246	1.6	8	1	1	1	1	2	5	15
GRAND TOTAL	777	1.8	16	1	1	1	1	3	5	15

93.01: FUNCTIONAL PT EVALUATION. Formerly included in operation group(s) 791.

Type of Patients	Observed Patients	Avg. Stay	Vari-ance	10th	25th	50th	75th	90th	95th	99th
1. SINGLE DX										
0–19 Years	3	2.1	<1	1	1	2	3	3	3	3
20–34	3	2.9	1	2	2	3	4	4	4	4
35–49	2	12.4	0	11	11	13	13	13	13	13
50–64	1	3.0	0	3	3	3	3	3	3	3
65+	1	2.0	0	2	2	2	2	2	2	2
2. MULTIPLE DX										
0–19 Years	24	10.6	34	2	5	12	16	16	16	33
20–34	8	12.8	47	3	8	11	22	22	22	22
35–49	26	18.3	174	2	6	15	28	39	43	47
50–64	72	17.2	218	3	7	13	26	36	43	87
65+	272	13.7	141	3	5	9	21	30	35	49
TOTAL SINGLE DX	10	4.7	19	1	2	3	4	13	13	13
MULTIPLE DX	402	14.6	157	3	5	11	22	31	38	52
TOTAL										
0–19 Years	27	9.5	38	2	3	11	14	16	16	33
20–34	11	11.6	52	3	6	11	22	22	22	22
35–49	28	18.1	169	2	6	15	28	39	43	47
50–64	73	17.1	218	3	7	13	26	36	43	87
65+	273	13.7	141	3	5	9	21	30	35	49
GRAND TOTAL	412	14.5	156	3	5	11	22	31	37	52

Length of Stay by Diagnosis and Operation, United States, 1997

93.08: ELECTROMYOGRAPHY. Formerly included in operation group(s) 791.

Type of Patients	Observed Patients	Avg. Stay	Variance	10th	25th	50th	75th	90th	95th	99th
1. SINGLE DX										
0–19 Years	18	3.6	17	1	1	2	4	5	12	23
20–34	8	3.4	1	1	2	3	4	5	12	8
35–49	11	3.3	3	1	2	3	5	5	7	7
50–64	4	4.1	9	2	2	3	5	9	9	9
65+	5	3.4	4	2	2	3	4	7	7	7
2. MULTIPLE DX										
0–19 Years	35	12.7	195	2	4	8	15	46	46	51
20–34	47	5.2	11	2	2	5	8	9	12	15
35–49	56	6.8	47	2	2	5	9	13	18	50
50–64	110	8.1	43	2	3	7	10	14	21	27
65+	196	8.2	28	4	5	6	13	13	18	27
TOTAL SINGLE DX	46	3.5	7	2	2	3	4	5	8	14
MULTIPLE DX	444	8.1	45	2	4	6	10	14	19	46
TOTAL										
0–19 Years	53	9.4	150	2	2	4	12	24	46	51
20–34	55	4.4	7	2	3	3	6	8	9	13
35–49	67	6.4	43	2	2	4	9	12	18	26
50–64	114	8.0	42	2	3	6	10	14	21	27
65+	201	8.1	28	4	5	6	13	13	18	27
GRAND TOTAL	490	7.6	43	2	4	5	10	14	18	33

93.2: OTH PT MS MANIPULATION. Formerly included in operation group(s) 791.

Type of Patients	Observed Patients	Avg. Stay	Variance	10th	25th	50th	75th	90th	95th	99th
1. SINGLE DX										
0–19 Years	25	2.1	3	1	1	1	2	5	5	11
20–34	42	2.9	2	1	2	2	3	5	6	6
35–49	58	2.3	5	1	1	2	3	4	7	13
50–64	53	2.1	4	1	1	2	3	4	5	13
65+	64	3.2	9	1	1	2	4	10	10	11
2. MULTIPLE DX										
0–19 Years	96	8.6	155	1	2	3	7	26	43	43
20–34	81	7.1	92	1	2	3	8	15	23	45
35–49	180	5.6	38	1	2	3	6	14	17	38
50–64	397	6.0	63	1	2	4	7	12	18	36
65+	2117	9.6	71	3	4	7	13	20	25	41
TOTAL SINGLE DX	242	2.6	6	1	1	2	3	5	9	11
MULTIPLE DX	2871	8.6	73	2	3	6	11	19	23	43
TOTAL										
0–19 Years	121	7.1	127	1	2	3	5	21	43	43
20–34	123	5.9	69	1	2	3	6	14	17	45
35–49	238	4.7	31	1	2	3	4	12	14	30
50–64	450	5.6	58	1	2	4	6	11	16	34
65+	2181	9.3	70	2	4	7	12	19	24	41
GRAND TOTAL	3113	8.0	70	2	3	5	10	18	23	42

93.1: PT EXERCISES. Formerly included in operation group(s) 791.

Type of Patients	Observed Patients	Avg. Stay	Variance	10th	25th	50th	75th	90th	95th	99th
1. SINGLE DX										
0–19 Years	5	2.3	4	1	1	1	4	4	8	8
20–34	16	3.5	13	1	2	2	3	5	16	16
35–49	16	2.7	3	1	1	3	4	5	9	9
50–64	17	3.7	7	1	1	3	4	9	9	9
65+	17	3.5	19	1	2	2	3	9	13	23
2. MULTIPLE DX										
0–19 Years	29	8.3	248	2	2	3	7	17	73	73
20–34	32	7.9	94	2	2	3	9	26	35	35
35–49	63	7.6	86	1	3	5	10	14	29	49
50–64	108	7.4	100	2	3	7	10	21	28	56
65+	511	10.0	64	2	4	8	13	22	26	38
TOTAL SINGLE DX	71	3.1	10	1	1	2	4	5	9	16
MULTIPLE DX	743	9.2	78	1	3	6	12	21	27	38
TOTAL										
0–19 Years	34	6.8	191	1	2	3	4	13	19	73
20–34	48	6.8	77	1	2	4	7	26	26	35
35–49	79	6.1	65	1	3	4	6	12	24	49
50–64	125	7.1	94	1	4	6	10	21	28	56
65+	528	9.7	64	2	4	8	13	21	25	37
GRAND TOTAL	814	8.6	75	1	3	6	11	21	26	38

93.22: AMB & GAIT TRAINING. Formerly included in operation group(s) 791.

Type of Patients	Observed Patients	Avg. Stay	Variance	10th	25th	50th	75th	90th	95th	99th
1. SINGLE DX										
0–19 Years	4	3.0	9	1	1	1	3	10	10	10
20–34	9	2.8	2	1	1	3	4	10	10	5
35–49	9	3.4	2	2	3	3	4	4	5	10
50–64	5	4.6	26	1	2	2	6	13	13	13
65+	11	5.1	8	2	4	4	6	9	9	14
2. MULTIPLE DX										
0–19 Years	15	8.9	98	2	2	4	14	25	26	45
20–34	36	6.6	91	1	2	4	7	14	30	38
35–49	72	9.1	54	2	3	7	14	19	23	38
50–64	228	8.3	99	2	4	6	14	16	25	64
65+	1725	10.4	76	3	5	8	14	21	27	41
TOTAL SINGLE DX	38	3.9	8	1	2	3	4	9	10	14
MULTIPLE DX	2076	10.0	79	3	4	7	13	21	26	42
TOTAL										
0–19 Years	19	8.1	90	1	2	4	13	18	26	45
20–34	45	6.0	79	1	2	4	5	10	23	38
35–49	81	8.3	51	2	3	5	14	17	22	38
50–64	233	8.3	98	2	3	6	14	16	25	49
65+	1736	10.4	76	3	5	8	14	21	27	41
GRAND TOTAL	2114	9.9	79	3	4	7	13	20	26	42

United States, October 1995–September 1996 Data, by Operation

93.26: MANUAL RUPT JOINT ADHES. Formerly included in operation group(s) 791.

Type of Patients	Observed Patients	Avg. Stay	Vari-ance	10th	25th	50th	75th	90th	95th	99th
1. SINGLE DX										
0–19 Years	5	1.4	<1	1	1	1	2	2	2	2
20–34	20	2.7	2	1	2	2	2	4	6	6
35–49	38	1.4	<1	1	1	1	2	3	3	4
50–64	41	1.8	1	1	1	1	2	3	4	5
65+	28	2.1	<1	1	2	2	3	3	3	4
2. MULTIPLE DX										
0–19 Years	7	2.7	2	1	2	2	3	4	6	6
20–34	22	2.8	10	1	2	2	3	7	8	19
35–49	70	2.9	4	1	2	3	3	4	7	14
50–64	107	2.5	3	1	1	2	3	4	5	9
65+	136	3.3	19	1	2	2	3	7	9	20
TOTAL SINGLE DX	132	1.8	1	1	1	1	2	3	4	5
MULTIPLE DX	342	2.9	9	1	1	2	3	5	8	15
TOTAL										
0–19 Years	12	2.2	2	1	1	2	3	4	6	6
20–34	42	2.8	6	1	2	2	3	4	7	19
35–49	108	2.3	3	1	1	2	3	4	5	9
50–64	148	2.3	2	1	1	2	3	4	5	9
65+	164	3.2	17	1	2	2	3	7	8	20
GRAND TOTAL	474	2.6	7	1	1	2	3	4	7	14

93.32: WHIRLPOOL TREATMENT. Formerly included in operation group(s) 791.

Type of Patients	Observed Patients	Avg. Stay	Vari-ance	10th	25th	50th	75th	90th	95th	99th
1. SINGLE DX										
0–19 Years	14	6.1	14	1	3	5	9	12	12	12
20–34	4	4.4	<1	4	4	4	5	5	5	5
35–49	11	5.3	10	1	4	4	5	11	11	12
50–64	8	10.6	36	5	5	9	15	20	20	20
65+	4	6.3	35	3	3	3	5	17	17	17
2. MULTIPLE DX										
0–19 Years	72	5.1	26	1	3	3	6	9	14	23
20–34	69	5.0	8	2	3	4	7	10	10	11
35–49	165	6.4	35	2	3	4	9	10	15	30
50–64	186	6.2	19	3	3	5	8	11	14	21
65+	393	7.7	32	3	4	6	9	14	16	33
TOTAL SINGLE DX	41	6.6	20	2	4	5	9	12	15	20
MULTIPLE DX	885	6.7	28	2	3	5	8	12	15	30
TOTAL										
0–19 Years	86	5.3	24	1	3	4	6	9	13	23
20–34	73	5.0	7	2	3	4	7	9	10	11
35–49	176	6.4	34	2	3	5	9	10	12	25
50–64	194	6.4	20	3	3	5	8	12	15	21
65+	397	7.7	32	3	4	6	9	14	16	33
GRAND TOTAL	926	6.7	28	2	3	5	9	12	15	29

93.3: OTHER PT THERAPEUTIC PX. Formerly included in operation group(s) 791.

Type of Patients	Observed Patients	Avg. Stay	Vari-ance	10th	25th	50th	75th	90th	95th	99th
1. SINGLE DX										
0–19 Years	83	5.8	22	1	2	4	9	12	14	18
20–34	74	3.0	4	1	2	2	4	6	7	8
35–49	116	3.4	8	1	2	3	4	5	9	14
50–64	61	5.2	24	1	2	4	6	9	20	23
65+	96	4.4	13	2	2	3	5	8	11	20
2. MULTIPLE DX										
0–19 Years	517	11.8	174	2	4	6	15	29	43	60
20–34	750	10.0	143	1	3	6	12	21	34	65
35–49	1472	8.8	87	2	3	6	10	18	27	52
50–64	2804	10.0	75	3	4	7	13	21	28	46
65+	15153	9.7	60	3	4	7	13	20	24	37
TOTAL SINGLE DX	430	4.2	14	1	2	3	5	9	12	20
MULTIPLE DX	20696	9.8	71	3	4	7	13	20	26	42
TOTAL										
0–19 Years	600	11.1	160	2	4	6	13	28	42	60
20–34	824	9.2	132	1	3	5	11	20	33	64
35–49	1588	8.3	82	2	3	5	10	17	25	52
50–64	2865	9.9	74	3	4	7	13	21	28	46
65+	15249	9.7	60	3	4	7	13	20	24	37
GRAND TOTAL	21126	9.6	70	3	4	7	13	20	26	42

93.38: COMBINED PT NOS. Formerly included in operation group(s) 791.

Type of Patients	Observed Patients	Avg. Stay	Vari-ance	10th	25th	50th	75th	90th	95th	99th
1. SINGLE DX										
0–19 Years	1	2.0	0	2	2	2	2	2	2	2
20–34	3	3.2	4	1	2	2	6	6	6	6
35–49	10	2.6	<1	2	2	2	3	4	5	5
50–64	6	5.3	1	3	4	6	6	6	6	6
65+	9	3.1	2	1	3	3	3	4	6	6
2. MULTIPLE DX										
0–19 Years	24	12.7	89	5	5	9	19	32	32	47
20–34	32	12.9	109	2	6	9	21	22	38	51
35–49	59	12.6	125	2	4	11	14	29	33	57
50–64	137	10.9	125	2	3	6	14	27	38	48
65+	681	11.0	73	3	5	8	14	23	30	39
TOTAL SINGLE DX	29	3.3	3	2	2	3	4	6	6	6
MULTIPLE DX	933	11.3	88	3	5	8	15	24	32	45
TOTAL										
0–19 Years	25	12.7	89	5	5	9	19	32	32	47
20–34	35	11.6	106	2	3	7	21	22	25	51
35–49	69	10.9	118	2	3	6	14	26	33	57
50–64	143	10.7	121	2	4	6	14	27	38	48
65+	690	10.9	73	3	5	8	14	23	30	39
GRAND TOTAL	962	11.0	87	3	5	8	15	23	32	45

Length of Stay by Diagnosis and Operation, United States, 1997

United States, October 1995–September 1996 Data, by Operation

93.39: PHYSICAL THERAPY NEC. Formerly included in operation group(s) 791.

Type of Patients	Observed Patients	Avg. Stay	Vari-ance	10th	25th	50th	75th	90th	95th	99th
1. SINGLE DX										
0–19 Years	50	6.2	26	1	2	4	10	12	14	24
20–34	63	2.9	4	1	2	2	3	5	6	8
35–49	83	3.3	8	1	2	2	4	5	9	14
50–64	43	4.3	20	1	2	3	5	7	9	23
65+	80	4.5	14	2	2	3	5	8	11	22
2. MULTIPLE DX										
0–19 Years	375	13.0	207	2	4	6	16	33	49	60
20–34	621	10.6	158	1	3	6	13	23	36	67
35–49	1188	9.4	98	2	3	6	11	19	28	52
50–64	2418	10.4	77	3	5	8	14	21	28	46
65+	13906	9.8	61	3	4	7	13	20	24	37
TOTAL SINGLE DX	319	4.1	14	1	2	3	5	8	12	22
MULTIPLE DX	18508	9.9	72	3	4	7	13	20	26	43
TOTAL										
0–19 Years	425	12.4	194	2	4	6	15	29	45	60
20–34	684	9.7	146	1	3	5	12	21	34	66
35–49	1271	8.8	92	2	3	5	11	19	27	52
50–64	2461	10.3	77	3	5	8	14	21	28	46
65+	13986	9.7	61	3	4	7	13	20	24	37
GRAND TOTAL	18827	9.8	72	3	4	7	13	20	26	42

93.44: OTHER SKELETAL TRACTION. Formerly included in operation group(s) 791.

Type of Patients	Observed Patients	Avg. Stay	Vari-ance	10th	25th	50th	75th	90th	95th	99th
1. SINGLE DX										
0–19 Years	229	14.5	82	1	7	14	21	26	29	33
20–34	7	3.0	4	1	3	3	3	5	5	5
35–49	24	6.7	110	1	3	4	6	7	34	48
50–64	7	3.7	2	3	3	3	5	5	7	7
65+	3	8.5	23	2	2	12	12	12	12	12
2. MULTIPLE DX										
0–19 Years	212	17.5	118	4	10	17	23	30	36	54
20–34	54	14.1	274	2	3	7	22	41	47	81
35–49	61	13.9	417	2	2	4	17	43	63	97
50–64	53	14.3	178	4	7	8	16	35	42	48
65+	124	12.3	166	4	5	7	15	23	43	62
TOTAL SINGLE DX	270	13.4	89	1	4	14	20	25	29	37
MULTIPLE DX	504	15.1	200	2	5	10	21	33	43	68
TOTAL										
0–19 Years	441	15.7	98	2	8	16	22	28	33	46
20–34	61	12.3	246	2	3	5	19	38	45	81
35–49	85	12.0	344	2	3	4	8	43	48	82
50–64	60	13.5	172	2	7	8	15	35	41	48
65+	127	12.3	164	3	5	7	15	23	43	62
GRAND TOTAL	774	14.4	153	2	5	13	21	28	36	62

93.4: SKELETAL & OTH TRACTION. Formerly included in operation group(s) 791.

Type of Patients	Observed Patients	Avg. Stay	Vari-ance	10th	25th	50th	75th	90th	95th	99th
1. SINGLE DX										
0–19 Years	370	11.8	83	1	3	12	19	23	28	33
20–34	32	3.1	2	1	2	3	4	5	6	7
35–49	58	5.2	53	1	3	3	6	7	12	48
50–64	17	4.4	6	1	2	4	6	7	7	7
65+	23	4.5	29	1	1	2	5	12	14	28
2. MULTIPLE DX										
0–19 Years	330	13.9	120	2	4	14	21	27	33	47
20–34	132	9.4	95	2	4	10	10	15	22	62
35–49	164	8.9	212	2	3	4	7	23	43	82
50–64	143	9.3	114	2	3	7	11	19	35	48
65+	561	9.1	103	3	4	6	10	17	26	55
TOTAL SINGLE DX	500	10.1	80	1	2	7	16	23	28	33
MULTIPLE DX	1330	10.3	123	2	3	7	13	23	31	54
TOTAL										
0–19 Years	700	12.7	100	1	3	13	20	25	29	42
20–34	164	8.5	86	2	3	7	10	12	22	51
35–49	222	7.9	170	2	2	4	6	18	39	70
50–64	160	8.8	105	2	2	6	10	16	35	48
65+	584	8.9	101	3	4	6	10	17	26	54
GRAND TOTAL	1830	10.3	110	2	3	7	14	23	28	48

93.46: LIMB SKIN TRACTION NEC. Formerly included in operation group(s) 791.

Type of Patients	Observed Patients	Avg. Stay	Vari-ance	10th	25th	50th	75th	90th	95th	99th
1. SINGLE DX										
0–19 Years	112	7.1	43	1	2	4	13	17	19	22
20–34	7	2.2	4	1	1	2	2	6	9	9
35–49	9	6.6	35	2	2	6	7	12	12	28
50–64	3	6.0	4	2	7	7	7	7	7	7
65+	12	5.1	43	1	1	2	9	9	28	28
2. MULTIPLE DX										
0–19 Years	91	10.7	95	1	2	8	20	22	27	42
20–34	26	7.2	23	3	3	4	12	12	19	20
35–49	45	5.2	31	2	3	4	6	8	21	26
50–64	49	7.3	85	1	3	4	10	16	23	48
65+	367	8.4	93	2	3	6	10	15	26	55
TOTAL SINGLE DX	143	6.7	40	1	2	4	11	16	19	24
MULTIPLE DX	578	8.5	86	2	3	6	10	20	26	48
TOTAL										
0–19 Years	203	9.0	73	1	2	5	15	22	22	38
20–34	33	6.4	23	1	3	4	12	12	13	20
35–49	54	5.4	31	2	2	4	6	14	15	28
50–64	52	7.2	75	2	2	4	9	14	23	48
65+	379	8.3	92	2	3	6	10	15	26	55
GRAND TOTAL	721	8.1	78	1	3	5	10	19	23	42

Length of Stay by Diagnosis and Operation, United States, 1997

United States, October 1995–September 1996 Data, by Operation

93.5: OTH IMMOB/PRESS/WND ATTN. Formerly included in operation group(s) 791.

Type of Patients	Observed Patients	Avg. Stay	Variance	Percentiles						
				10th	25th	50th	75th	90th	95th	99th
1. SINGLE DX										
0–19 Years	872	4.1	29	1	1	2	3	14	18	23
20–34	274	1.9	2	1	1	1	2	4	5	7
35–49	175	1.9	3	1	1	1	2	4	5	8
50–64	99	1.3	2	1	1	1	1	2	3	5
65+	95	4.0	83	1	1	2	3	6	19	27
2. MULTIPLE DX										
0–19 Years	1394	4.3	33	1	1	2	4	12	19	27
20–34	776	4.3	90	1	1	2	4	7	11	83
35–49	844	3.8	22	1	1	3	4	8	11	20
50–64	767	4.5	25	1	2	3	6	8	12	32
65+	2740	6.2	59	1	3	4	7	12	17	56
TOTAL SINGLE DX	1515	3.0	21	1	1	1	3	6	15	22
MULTIPLE DX	6521	5.0	48	1	2	3	6	10	15	34
TOTAL										
0–19 Years	2266	4.2	31	1	1	2	4	13	18	24
20–34	1050	3.6	65	1	1	2	4	6	9	28
35–49	1019	3.4	18	1	1	2	4	7	11	17
50–64	866	3.8	21	1	1	3	5	8	10	28
65+	2835	6.2	60	3	3	4	7	12	17	56
GRAND TOTAL	8036	4.5	42	1	1	3	5	9	15	30

93.51: PLASTER JACKET APPL. Formerly included in operation group(s) 791.

Type of Patients	Observed Patients	Avg. Stay	Variance	Percentiles						
				10th	25th	50th	75th	90th	95th	99th
1. SINGLE DX										
0–19 Years	259	6.7	53	1	1	2	14	18	20	25
20–34	5	3.0	2	1	2	4	4	4	5	5
35–49	3	3.8	<1	4	4	4	4	4	4	4
50–64	1	2.0	0	2	2	2	2	2	2	2
65+	0									
2. MULTIPLE DX										
0–19 Years	188	7.8	73	1	2	3	16	21	22	31
20–34	6	3.4	15	1	1	3	4	13	13	13
35–49	7	4.0	10	1	1	5	6	6	6	14
50–64	9	6.7	28	1	3	4	12	15	15	15
65+	13	5.2	23	3	3	3	4	16	16	18
TOTAL SINGLE DX	268	6.4	50	1	1	3	12	18	20	25
MULTIPLE DX	223	7.4	67	1	2	3	14	20	21	31
TOTAL										
0–19 Years	447	7.2	62	1	1	3	15	20	21	30
20–34	11	3.2	8	1	2	2	4	5	13	13
35–49	10	3.8	3	4	4	4	4	6	6	14
50–64	10	6.1	27	1	3	4	12	15	15	15
65+	13	5.2	23	3	3	3	4	16	16	18
GRAND TOTAL	491	6.9	58	1	1	3	13	19	21	29

93.53: OTHER CAST APPLICATION. Formerly included in operation group(s) 791.

Type of Patients	Observed Patients	Avg. Stay	Variance	Percentiles						
				10th	25th	50th	75th	90th	95th	99th
1. SINGLE DX										
0–19 Years	410	3.0	19	1	1	1	3	8	15	21
20–34	99	1.9	2	1	1	1	2	4	5	7
35–49	65	1.8	2	1	1	1	2	4	5	6
50–64	34	2.0	6	1	1	1	2	4	4	15
65+	35	6.4	79	1	2	3	4	27	27	27
2. MULTIPLE DX										
0–19 Years	462	3.7	24	1	1	2	4	8	15	23
20–34	218	6.1	237	1	1	3	4	7	17	83
35–49	274	3.7	13	1	2	3	5	7	8	20
50–64	284	5.1	27	1	3	4	6	8	12	32
65+	1014	7.3	114	1	3	4	7	14	25	56
TOTAL SINGLE DX	643	2.7	16	1	1	1	2	5	11	22
MULTIPLE DX	2252	5.6	85	1	2	3	6	10	18	56
TOTAL										
0–19 Years	872	3.4	22	1	1	2	3	8	15	22
20–34	317	4.9	175	1	1	2	4	6	8	83
35–49	339	3.4	11	1	1	2	4	7	8	17
50–64	318	4.8	26	1	2	4	6	8	11	32
65+	1049	7.3	114	1	3	4	7	14	26	56
GRAND TOTAL	2895	4.9	71	1	1	3	5	9	16	56

93.54: APPLICATION OF SPLINT. Formerly included in operation group(s) 791.

Type of Patients	Observed Patients	Avg. Stay	Variance	Percentiles						
				10th	25th	50th	75th	90th	95th	99th
1. SINGLE DX										
0–19 Years	99	2.1	8	1	1	1	2	3	5	15
20–34	84	2.1	3	1	1	1	2	3	7	7
35–49	43	1.9	<1	1	1	1	2	2	3	3
50–64	27	1.7	1	1	1	1	2	3	5	5
65+	25	2.4	2	1	1	2	3	5	6	6
2. MULTIPLE DX										
0–19 Years	250	2.9	16	1	1	2	3	6	6	24
20–34	218	2.9	10	1	1	2	4	7	9	19
35–49	219	3.2	9	1	1	3	4	6	9	17
50–64	180	4.0	27	1	2	3	5	8	13	22
65+	677	4.9	24	1	2	4	6	10	13	21
TOTAL SINGLE DX	278	2.0	4	1	1	2	2	3	6	10
MULTIPLE DX	1544	3.9	19	1	1	3	5	7	11	20
TOTAL										
0–19 Years	349	2.7	14	1	1	2	3	6	6	23
20–34	302	2.7	8	1	1	2	3	6	7	19
35–49	262	3.0	8	1	1	3	4	5	8	14
50–64	207	3.8	25	1	1	3	6	7	8	22
65+	702	4.8	23	1	2	4	6	10	13	21
GRAND TOTAL	1822	3.6	17	1	1	2	4	7	10	19

Length of Stay by Diagnosis and Operation, United States, 1997

United States, October 1995–September 1996 Data, by Operation

93.57: APPL OTH WND DRESSING. Formerly included in operation group(s) 791.

Type of Patients	Observed Patients	Avg. Stay	Vari-ance	Percentiles 10th	25th	50th	75th	90th	95th	99th
1. SINGLE DX										
0–19 Years	38	5.1	26	1	2	3	6	9	12	26
20–34	20	2.1	3	1	1	1	3	4	7	8
35–49	17	3.9	39	1	2	2	4	7	7	33
50–64	3	4.1	8	2	2	3	8	8	8	8
65+	3	36.2	>999	3	7	7	85	85	85	85
2. MULTIPLE DX										
0–19 Years	330	4.7	25	1	1	3	6	11	16	23
20–34	143	3.9	15	1	1	3	4	10	13	17
35–49	142	5.2	86	1	2	3	5	10	15	73
50–64	83	4.6	31	1	2	3	5	9	14	34
65+	114	7.5	41	2	3	6	11	14	21	30
TOTAL SINGLE DX	81	5.2	103	1	1	3	5	9	12	85
MULTIPLE DX	812	5.2	41	1	2	3	6	13	15	30
TOTAL										
0–19 Years	368	4.8	25	1	1	3	6	11	16	25
20–34	163	3.6	14	1	1	2	4	9	13	16
35–49	159	5.1	83	1	2	3	5	10	15	73
50–64	86	4.6	30	1	2	3	5	9	14	34
65+	117	7.9	74	2	3	6	11	14	21	41
GRAND TOTAL	893	5.2	46	1	2	3	6	12	15	30

93.6: OSTEOPATHIC MANIPULATION. Formerly included in operation group(s) 791.

Type of Patients	Observed Patients	Avg. Stay	Vari-ance	Percentiles 10th	25th	50th	75th	90th	95th	99th
1. SINGLE DX										
0–19 Years	1	2.0	0	2	2	2	2	2	2	2
20–34	2	2.7	<1	3	3	3	3	3	3	3
35–49	2	5.7	2	5	5	5	5	7	8	8
50–64	2	5.5	2	6	6	6	6	6	6	6
65+	1	1.0	0	1	1	1	1	1	1	1
2. MULTIPLE DX										
0–19 Years	79	2.0	2	1	1	2	3	3	4	7
20–34	65	4.5	7	1	2	3	6	9	9	11
35–49	103	4.0	8	1	2	4	5	7	9	17
50–64	99	5.0	13	2	2	4	6	10	14	18
65+	230	5.5	11	2	3	5	7	10	11	15
TOTAL SINGLE DX	9	4.1	4	2	3	3	6	6	8	8
MULTIPLE DX	576	4.2	10	1	2	3	6	8	10	17
TOTAL										
0–19 Years	80	2.0	2	1	1	2	3	3	4	7
20–34	68	4.4	7	2	2	3	6	9	9	11
35–49	105	4.0	8	1	2	4	5	7	8	17
50–64	101	5.0	12	2	2	4	6	10	14	18
65+	231	5.4	11	2	3	5	7	10	11	15
GRAND TOTAL	585	4.2	10	1	2	3	6	8	10	17

93.59: IMMOB/PRESS/WND ATTN NEC. Formerly included in operation group(s) 791.

Type of Patients	Observed Patients	Avg. Stay	Vari-ance	Percentiles 10th	25th	50th	75th	90th	95th	99th
1. SINGLE DX										
0–19 Years	38	2.9	4	1	1	2	3	7	7	8
20–34	45	1.8	2	1	1	1	2	4	5	7
35–49	32	1.4	1	1	1	1	1	2	2	6
50–64	28	1.1	<1	1	1	1	1	1	2	3
65+	29	2.1	3	1	1	1	3	4	5	11
2. MULTIPLE DX										
0–19 Years	95	4.0	44	1	1	2	4	8	23	38
20–34	118	4.0	20	1	1	3	4	9	12	22
35–49	147	3.9	15	1	2	2	4	11	12	16
50–64	176	4.2	20	1	3	3	6	10	12	21
65+	822	6.0	31	2	3	5	7	11	16	28
TOTAL SINGLE DX	172	1.5	2	1	1	1	1	3	5	7
MULTIPLE DX	1358	5.0	27	1	2	3	6	11	14	24
TOTAL										
0–19 Years	133	3.7	33	1	1	2	4	7	12	38
20–34	163	3.0	14	1	1	2	4	6	10	22
35–49	179	3.0	12	1	1	1	4	10	11	16
50–64	204	2.9	14	1	1	1	3	8	10	16
65+	851	5.7	30	2	3	4	7	11	14	28
GRAND TOTAL	1530	4.1	23	1	1	3	5	9	12	23

93.61: OMT FOR GEN MOBIL. Formerly included in operation group(s) 791.

Type of Patients	Observed Patients	Avg. Stay	Vari-ance	Percentiles 10th	25th	50th	75th	90th	95th	99th
1. SINGLE DX										
0–19 Years	1	2.0	0	2	2	2	2	2	2	2
20–34	0									
35–49	1	8.0	0	8	8	8	8	8	8	8
50–64	0									
65+	0									
2. MULTIPLE DX										
0–19 Years	9	3.0	1	2	2	3	3	4	5	7
20–34	17	4.1	8	2	2	3	5	8	11	11
35–49	32	3.1	5	1	2	2	4	7	8	8
50–64	40	4.9	10	2	3	4	6	10	14	14
65+	91	5.7	11	2	3	5	7	10	12	14
TOTAL SINGLE DX	2	6.0	10	2	2	8	8	8	8	8
MULTIPLE DX	189	4.6	10	2	2	4	6	9	11	14
TOTAL										
0–19 Years	10	3.0	1	2	2	3	3	4	5	7
20–34	17	4.1	8	2	2	3	5	8	11	11
35–49	33	3.2	5	1	2	2	4	8	8	8
50–64	40	4.9	10	2	2	4	6	10	14	14
65+	91	5.7	11	2	3	5	7	10	12	14
GRAND TOTAL	191	4.6	10	2	2	4	6	9	11	14

Length of Stay by Diagnosis and Operation, United States, 1997

United States, October 1995–September 1996 Data, by Operation

93.7: SPEECH/READ/BLIND REHAB. Formerly included in operation group(s) 791.

Type of Patients	Observed Patients	Avg. Stay	Variance	10th	25th	50th	75th	90th	95th	99th
1. SINGLE DX										
0–19 Years	3	2.0	<1	1	1	2	3	3	3	3
20–34	0									
35–49	2	13.4	4	11	11	15	15	15	15	15
50–64	4	3.5	8	1	2	2	7	7	7	7
65+	2	5.0	3	4	4	4	7	7	7	7
2. MULTIPLE DX										
0–19 Years	66	16.2	226	4	4	10	26	38	56	56
20–34	11	15.2	211	3	6	12	22	>99	>99	>99
35–49	39	14.0	269	2	5	8	15	41	76	>99
50–64	99	9.0	53	2	3	7	11	20	22	31
65+	577	9.1	90	3	4	5	11	20	28	53
TOTAL SINGLE DX	11	6.1	28	1	2	3	11	15	15	15
MULTIPLE DX	792	10.1	111	3	4	6	12	22	34	57
TOTAL										
0–19 Years	69	15.7	225	3	4	10	23	38	50	56
20–34	11	15.2	211	3	6	12	22	>99	>99	>99
35–49	41	13.9	248	2	5	10	15	41	76	>99
50–64	103	8.9	52	2	3	7	11	19	22	31
65+	579	9.1	89	3	4	5	11	20	28	53
GRAND TOTAL	803	10.0	111	4	4	6	12	22	34	56

93.8: OTHER REHAB THERAPY. Formerly included in operation group(s) 791.

Type of Patients	Observed Patients	Avg. Stay	Variance	10th	25th	50th	75th	90th	95th	99th
1. SINGLE DX										
0–19 Years	99	6.2	28	1	2	4	8	15	17	23
20–34	169	8.2	53	3	4	5	10	16	20	34
35–49	173	10.6	99	2	4	8	14	24	28	57
50–64	62	12.2	54	4	6	12	15	21	26	43
65+	36	11.0	86	6	7	8	10	18	40	46
2. MULTIPLE DX										
0–19 Years	563	13.5	214	2	4	9	16	36	48	77
20–34	770	10.1	82	2	4	8	13	21	31	92
35–49	1103	11.8	149	3	5	8	14	24	35	80
50–64	1096	13.3	105	4	7	10	16	23	32	52
65+	4103	14.7	109	5	8	12	18	27	35	55
TOTAL SINGLE DX	539	9.3	71	2	4	7	12	17	24	46
MULTIPLE DX	7635	13.6	121	4	7	11	17	26	35	58
TOTAL										
0–19 Years	662	12.8	201	2	4	8	15	35	48	77
20–34	939	9.8	77	3	4	8	12	20	29	58
35–49	1276	11.6	144	3	5	8	14	24	35	80
50–64	1158	13.3	104	4	7	11	16	23	31	52
65+	4139	14.7	109	5	8	12	18	27	35	55
GRAND TOTAL	8174	13.4	120	4	7	11	17	26	35	57

93.75: OTHER SPEECH THERAPY. Formerly included in operation group(s) 791.

Type of Patients	Observed Patients	Avg. Stay	Variance	10th	25th	50th	75th	90th	95th	99th
1. SINGLE DX										
0–19 Years	3	2.0	<1	1	1	2	3	3	3	3
20–34	0									
35–49	2	13.4	4	11	11	15	15	15	15	15
50–64	4	3.5	8	1	2	2	7	7	7	7
65+	2	5.0	3	4	4	4	7	7	7	7
2. MULTIPLE DX										
0–19 Years	65	17.3	232	4	8	10	26	39	56	56
20–34	11	15.2	211	3	6	12	22	>99	>99	>99
35–49	32	12.2	227	2	5	7	15	41	76	>99
50–64	95	8.9	56	2	3	6	12	20	22	31
65+	551	9.0	90	3	4	5	10	20	28	56
TOTAL SINGLE DX	11	6.1	28	1	2	3	11	15	15	15
MULTIPLE DX	754	10.0	111	3	4	6	12	22	34	56
TOTAL										
0–19 Years	68	16.8	232	3	6	10	26	38	56	56
20–34	11	15.2	211	3	6	12	22	>99	>99	>99
35–49	34	12.4	206	2	5	6	15	26	76	>99
50–64	99	8.8	56	2	3	6	12	20	22	31
65+	553	9.0	90	3	4	5	10	20	28	56
GRAND TOTAL	765	9.9	110	3	4	6	12	22	34	56

93.81: RECREATIONAL THERAPY. Formerly included in operation group(s) 791.

Type of Patients	Observed Patients	Avg. Stay	Variance	10th	25th	50th	75th	90th	95th	99th
1. SINGLE DX										
0–19 Years	10	10.7	15	5	7	11	15	15	15	15
20–34	7	4.5	40	1	1	1	5	16	23	23
35–49	13	10.9	104	4	4	4	14	27	37	37
50–64	3	10.2	71	2	2	14	18	18	18	18
65+	2	16.5	5	15	15	17	18	18	18	18
2. MULTIPLE DX										
0–19 Years	40	5.8	49	2	2	3	7	14	16	47
20–34	60	6.8	82	1	4	4	8	13	19	48
35–49	68	6.5	51	1	3	3	7	18	23	31
50–64	57	10.5	46	5	5	8	14	21	23	34
65+	132	14.6	55	6	10	14	20	25	28	35
TOTAL SINGLE DX	35	8.9	67	1	2	5	14	18	27	37
MULTIPLE DX	357	9.9	70	2	3	7	14	21	26	35
TOTAL										
0–19 Years	50	6.1	48	2	2	3	7	14	16	47
20–34	67	6.6	78	1	2	4	8	13	19	48
35–49	81	6.9	56	2	3	3	8	18	25	34
50–64	60	10.5	46	5	5	8	14	21	21	34
65+	134	14.6	55	6	10	14	20	25	28	35
GRAND TOTAL	392	9.8	70	2	3	7	14	21	26	35

Length of Stay by Diagnosis and Operation, United States, 1997

United States, October 1995–September 1996 Data, by Operation

93.83: OCCUPATIONAL THERAPY. Formerly included in operation group(s) 791.

Type of Patients	Observed Patients	Avg. Stay	Variance	10th	25th	50th	75th	90th	95th	99th
1. SINGLE DX										
0–19 Years	75	5.8	31	1	2	3	8	14	18	23
20–34	158	8.2	49	3	4	6	10	16	19	30
35–49	157	10.7	99	2	4	6	14	23	28	57
50–64	57	12.2	52	4	7	12	15	21	26	43
65+	33	10.9	89	6	7	8	10	15	40	46
2. MULTIPLE DX										
0–19 Years	472	14.2	220	2	4	9	17	36	48	77
20–34	643	10.5	78	3	5	8	13	21	31	>99
35–49	906	10.7	97	3	5	8	13	21	30	56
50–64	771	12.5	108	4	7	9	15	23	30	55
65+	2886	13.8	100	4	7	12	17	25	33	50
TOTAL SINGLE DX	480	9.4	71	3	4	8	12	17	24	46
MULTIPLE DX	5678	12.9	110	4	6	10	16	24	33	58
TOTAL										
0–19 Years	547	13.5	209	2	4	9	16	36	48	77
20–34	801	10.1	73	3	4	8	13	20	30	87
35–49	1063	10.7	98	3	5	8	13	21	29	57
50–64	828	12.5	106	4	7	9	15	23	30	50
65+	2919	13.8	100	4	7	12	17	25	33	50
GRAND TOTAL	6158	12.6	109	3	6	10	16	24	33	57

93.9: RESPIRATORY THERAPY. Formerly included in operation group(s) 789, 791.

Type of Patients	Observed Patients	Avg. Stay	Variance	10th	25th	50th	75th	90th	95th	99th
1. SINGLE DX										
0–19 Years	8283	2.4	3	1	1	2	3	4	5	9
20–34	742	3.6	13	1	1	2	4	5	10	17
35–49	598	3.1	6	1	2	2	4	5	8	11
50–64	388	3.3	4	1	2	3	4	6	7	8
65+	333	4.0	8	1	2	3	5	7	9	15
2. MULTIPLE DX										
0–19 Years	21139	4.6	45	1	2	3	5	8	14	37
20–34	2440	5.1	27	1	2	3	6	11	14	24
35–49	3663	4.6	14	2	2	3	6	9	12	21
50–64	5461	5.1	16	2	3	4	6	10	12	20
65+	13247	5.9	23	2	3	5	8	11	14	23
TOTAL SINGLE DX	10344	2.6	4	1	1	2	3	4	6	10
MULTIPLE DX	45950	5.0	33	1	2	3	6	10	14	30
TOTAL										
0–19 Years	29422	4.1	35	1	2	3	4	7	12	32
20–34	3182	4.8	24	1	2	3	6	10	14	22
35–49	4261	4.4	14	1	2	3	5	8	11	20
50–64	5849	5.0	16	2	3	4	6	10	12	20
65+	13580	5.9	22	2	3	5	8	11	14	23
GRAND TOTAL	56294	4.6	29	1	2	3	5	9	13	27

93.89: REHABILITATION NEC. Formerly included in operation group(s) 791.

Type of Patients	Observed Patients	Avg. Stay	Variance	10th	25th	50th	75th	90th	95th	99th
1. SINGLE DX										
0–19 Years	10	7.1	14	3	4	7	8	11	16	16
20–34	4	18.5	372	2	9	13	17	50	50	50
35–49	0									
50–64	1	4.0	0	4	4	4	4	4	4	4
65+	1	10.0	0	10	10	10	10	10	10	10
2. MULTIPLE DX										
0–19 Years	40	22.4	305	6	9	13	46	46	46	76
20–34	48	9.2	112	1	1	4	12	24	34	40
35–49	114	18.4	357	5	6	12	25	36	80	80
50–64	255	15.7	98	7	9	14	20	24	37	52
65+	1074	16.6	126	7	9	14	20	30	43	57
TOTAL SINGLE DX	16	9.3	93	3	4	8	10	16	17	50
MULTIPLE DX	1531	16.5	147	6	8	14	20	33	43	58
TOTAL										
0–19 Years	50	20.1	291	6	8	12	30	46	46	76
20–34	52	9.5	120	1	1	5	12	26	36	48
35–49	114	18.4	357	5	6	12	25	36	80	80
50–64	256	15.7	98	7	9	14	20	24	37	52
65+	1075	16.6	126	7	9	14	20	30	43	57
GRAND TOTAL	1547	16.5	147	6	8	14	20	32	43	58

93.90: CPAP. Formerly included in operation group(s) 789.

Type of Patients	Observed Patients	Avg. Stay	Variance	10th	25th	50th	75th	90th	95th	99th
1. SINGLE DX										
0–19 Years	44	3.5	26	1	2	3	4	4	7	44
20–34	3	3.2	2	1	1	4	4	4	4	4
35–49	4	1.9	1	1	1	1	2	4	4	4
50–64	1	4.0	0	4	4	4	4	4	4	4
65+	4	3.3	6	2	2	2	4	4	13	13
2. MULTIPLE DX										
0–19 Years	2380	12.7	198	2	4	7	16	32	45	68
20–34	117	7.3	49	2	3	5	13	14	14	34
35–49	292	6.6	25	2	3	6	8	13	16	25
50–64	530	7.6	40	3	4	6	10	14	17	31
65+	893	7.3	29	2	4	6	9	13	18	27
TOTAL SINGLE DX	56	3.4	21	1	2	3	4	4	6	44
MULTIPLE DX	4212	10.2	127	2	4	7	11	22	34	60
TOTAL										
0–19 Years	2424	12.5	196	2	4	7	16	32	44	68
20–34	120	7.2	49	1	3	5	13	14	14	34
35–49	296	6.6	25	2	3	6	8	13	16	25
50–64	531	7.6	40	3	4	6	10	14	17	31
65+	897	7.3	29	2	4	6	9	13	18	27
GRAND TOTAL	4268	10.1	127	2	4	6	11	22	34	60

Length of Stay by Diagnosis and Operation, United States, 1997

United States, October 1995–September 1996 Data, by Operation

93.93: NONMECH RESUSCITATION. Formerly included in operation group(s) 791.

Type of Patients	Observed Patients	Avg. Stay	Vari-ance	10th	25th	50th	75th	90th	95th	99th
1. SINGLE DX										
0–19 Years	101	1.8	<1	1	1	2	2	3	3	4
20–34	1	2.0	0	2	2	2	2	2	2	2
35–49	1	2.0	0	2	2	2	2	2	2	2
50–64	1	1.0	0	1	1	1	1	1	1	1
65+	0									
2. MULTIPLE DX										
0–19 Years	628	2.8	8	1	2	2	3	4	7	13
20–34	4	2.7	25	1	1	1	1	4	19	19
35–49	11	4.8	10	2	2	6	6	7	14	14
50–64	17	6.7	33	1	3	6	8	19	19	19
65+	33	6.0	13	3	4	5	5	11	16	18
TOTAL SINGLE DX	104	1.8	<1	1	1	2	2	3	3	4
MULTIPLE DX	693	3.1	10	1	2	2	3	5	8	18
TOTAL										
0–19 Years	729	2.7	7	1	2	2	3	4	7	13
20–34	5	2.6	23	1	1	1	1	4	19	19
35–49	12	4.7	10	2	2	6	6	7	14	14
50–64	18	6.5	33	1	3	6	6	19	19	19
65+	33	6.0	13	3	4	5	5	11	16	18
GRAND TOTAL	797	3.0	9	1	2	2	3	5	7	16

93.95: HYPERBARIC OXYGENATION. Formerly included in operation group(s) 791.

Type of Patients	Observed Patients	Avg. Stay	Vari-ance	10th	25th	50th	75th	90th	95th	99th
1. SINGLE DX										
0–19 Years	11	2.2	5	1	1	1	1	6	6	6
20–34	18	1.2	<1	1	1	1	1	1	3	3
35–49	21	3.2	34	1	1	1	1	7	22	22
50–64	6	1.7	3	1	1	1	1	4	7	7
65+	7	2.5	9	1	1	1	2	6	10	10
2. MULTIPLE DX										
0–19 Years	25	3.7	14	1	1	2	7	10	10	12
20–34	33	3.1	15	1	1	2	3	9	9	20
35–49	60	3.7	14	1	2	2	5	8	15	16
50–64	51	6.7	49	1	1	4	10	14	25	25
65+	76	3.6	22	1	1	1	4	8	15	21
TOTAL SINGLE DX	63	2.3	15	1	1	1	1	6	7	22
MULTIPLE DX	245	4.1	25	1	1	2	6	10	15	25
TOTAL										
0–19 Years	36	3.3	12	1	1	1	4	10	10	12
20–34	51	2.6	12	1	1	1	3	8	9	20
35–49	81	3.6	18	1	2	2	4	8	15	22
50–64	57	6.1	45	1	2	3	8	13	25	25
65+	83	3.5	21	1	1	1	4	8	15	21
GRAND TOTAL	308	3.9	24	1	1	2	5	10	15	25

93.94: NEBULIZER THERAPY. Formerly included in operation group(s) 791.

Type of Patients	Observed Patients	Avg. Stay	Vari-ance	10th	25th	50th	75th	90th	95th	99th
1. SINGLE DX										
0–19 Years	5462	2.3	2	1	1	2	3	4	5	8
20–34	477	2.5	2	1	1	2	3	5	5	8
35–49	398	3.3	4	1	2	3	4	5	8	10
50–64	251	3.5	3	2	2	3	4	6	7	8
65+	206	4.1	8	1	2	3	5	7	8	15
2. MULTIPLE DX										
0–19 Years	10186	3.0	6	1	2	2	4	5	7	12
20–34	1338	3.8	15	1	2	3	5	7	9	18
35–49	1797	4.2	9	2	2	4	5	8	9	15
50–64	2422	4.9	12	2	3	4	6	9	11	16
65+	5620	5.9	21	2	3	5	7	11	13	22
TOTAL SINGLE DX	6794	2.5	3	1	1	2	3	4	5	8
MULTIPLE DX	21363	4.1	12	1	2	3	5	8	10	17
TOTAL										
0–19 Years	15648	2.8	5	1	2	2	3	5	6	10
20–34	1815	3.5	12	1	2	3	4	6	8	15
35–49	2195	4.0	8	1	2	3	5	7	9	14
50–64	2673	4.8	11	2	3	4	6	9	11	16
65+	5826	5.8	21	2	3	5	7	10	13	22
GRAND TOTAL	28157	3.8	11	1	2	3	5	7	9	16

93.96: OXYGEN ENRICHMENT NEC. Formerly included in operation group(s) 791.

Type of Patients	Observed Patients	Avg. Stay	Vari-ance	10th	25th	50th	75th	90th	95th	99th
1. SINGLE DX										
0–19 Years	2353	2.4	2	1	2	2	3	4	5	8
20–34	177	3.8	10	1	2	3	4	10	10	13
35–49	125	2.3	5	1	1	2	3	4	5	8
50–64	95	3.0	4	1	2	2	4	6	7	9
65+	102	3.4	6	1	1	3	5	7	8	10
2. MULTIPLE DX										
0–19 Years	6897	4.6	37	1	2	3	5	9	13	30
20–34	663	5.2	20	1	2	4	7	10	14	20
35–49	1160	4.1	12	1	2	3	5	8	10	15
50–64	1933	4.3	12	1	2	3	6	9	10	17
65+	4889	5.6	19	2	3	4	7	11	13	23
TOTAL SINGLE DX	2852	2.5	3	1	2	2	3	4	5	9
MULTIPLE DX	15542	4.8	29	1	2	3	6	9	13	26
TOTAL										
0–19 Years	9250	4.1	29	1	2	3	4	7	11	26
20–34	840	5.0	19	1	2	4	7	10	14	20
35–49	1285	3.9	11	1	2	3	5	7	10	15
50–64	2028	4.3	12	1	2	3	6	9	10	16
65+	4991	5.6	19	2	3	4	7	11	13	23
GRAND TOTAL	18394	4.4	25	1	2	3	5	9	12	26

Length of Stay by Diagnosis and Operation, United States, 1997

United States, October 1995–September 1996 Data, by Operation

93.99: OTHER RESP PROCEDURES. Formerly included in operation group(s) 791.

Type of Patients	Observed Patients	Avg. Stay	Variance	Percentiles						
				10th	25th	50th	75th	90th	95th	99th
1. SINGLE DX										
0–19 Years	296	4.1	16	1	1	2	4	10	14	19
20–34	63	8.3	37	1	3	8	12	17	20	22
35–49	48	3.8	11	1	3	3	4	10	11	16
50–64	34	2.9	4	1	2	2	3	7	7	7
65+	14	6.7	14	3	4	6	9	10	18	18
2. MULTIPLE DX										
0–19 Years	906	5.1	31	1	2	3	6	13	16	30
20–34	266	8.0	47	2	2	6	12	17	21	29
35–49	331	6.0	29	2	3	4	7	14	19	22
50–64	466	5.0	14	2	3	4	6	10	11	20
65+	1623	5.9	27	2	3	5	7	11	13	23
TOTAL SINGLE DX	455	4.7	21	1	2	3	6	12	14	19
MULTIPLE DX	3592	5.7	29	2	2	4	7	12	16	25
TOTAL										
0–19 Years	1202	4.9	28	1	2	3	6	13	15	29
20–34	329	8.1	45	1	2	6	12	17	21	29
35–49	379	5.8	27	1	3	4	7	14	19	22
50–64	500	4.9	13	2	3	4	6	10	11	17
65+	1637	5.9	27	2	3	5	8	11	13	23
GRAND TOTAL	4047	5.6	28	1	2	4	7	12	15	24

94.08: PSYCH EVAL & TEST NEC. Formerly included in operation group(s) 792.

Type of Patients	Observed Patients	Avg. Stay	Variance	Percentiles						
				10th	25th	50th	75th	90th	95th	99th
1. SINGLE DX										
0–19 Years	7	5.1	4	4	4	4	6	8	8	8
20–34	18	8.7	50	2	3	6	19	19	19	19
35–49	9	11.7	61	3	6	7	21	21	21	21
50–64	3	20.6	71	5	25	25	25	25	25	25
65+	0									
2. MULTIPLE DX										
0–19 Years	81	5.0	8	3	3	5	6	7	8	17
20–34	78	5.0	10	1	4	5	6	7	10	11
35–49	67	5.1	6	3	4	5	7	8	9	13
50–64	21	9.6	34	3	5	8	16	17	21	21
65+	22	10.5	29	3	6	11	15	19	19	21
TOTAL SINGLE DX	37	10.2	63	3	4	6	19	21	25	25
MULTIPLE DX	269	5.4	11	3	3	5	6	8	11	19
TOTAL										
0–19 Years	88	5.0	8	3	3	5	6	7	8	17
20–34	96	5.3	13	1	3	5	6	8	11	19
35–49	76	5.6	13	3	4	4	7	9	10	21
50–64	24	11.1	52	3	5	8	17	25	25	25
65+	22	10.5	29	3	6	11	15	19	19	21
GRAND TOTAL	306	5.6	15	3	3	5	7	9	13	21

94.0: PSYCH EVAL & TESTING. Formerly included in operation group(s) 792.

Type of Patients	Observed Patients	Avg. Stay	Variance	Percentiles						
				10th	25th	50th	75th	90th	95th	99th
1. SINGLE DX										
0–19 Years	11	8.8	95	2	4	4	8	28	28	28
20–34	24	6.9	40	2	3	3	8	19	19	19
35–49	17	12.4	55	3	6	12	21	21	21	26
50–64	4	19.4	70	5	12	25	25	25	25	25
65+	1	2.0	0	2	2	2	2	2	2	2
2. MULTIPLE DX										
0–19 Years	118	5.7	18	3	3	5	6	8	10	28
20–34	111	5.2	11	2	3	5	6	8	10	14
35–49	93	5.8	10	3	4	5	7	8	13	17
50–64	26	8.4	21	3	6	7	8	17	21	21
65+	29	10.2	30	3	6	11	15	17	19	21
TOTAL SINGLE DX	57	9.5	66	2	3	6	19	21	25	28
MULTIPLE DX	377	5.9	16	3	4	5	7	9	13	25
TOTAL										
0–19 Years	129	5.7	19	3	3	5	6	8	10	28
20–34	135	5.3	14	2	3	5	6	9	11	19
35–49	110	6.3	16	3	4	5	7	10	13	21
50–64	30	9.5	36	5	7	7	9	21	25	25
65+	30	10.0	31	3	6	9	15	17	19	21
GRAND TOTAL	434	6.1	20	3	3	5	7	10	15	27

94.1: PSYCH EVAL/CONSULT. Formerly included in operation group(s) 792.

Type of Patients	Observed Patients	Avg. Stay	Variance	Percentiles						
				10th	25th	50th	75th	90th	95th	99th
1. SINGLE DX										
0–19 Years	166	11.5	63	2	5	12	16	21	29	31
20–34	121	9.4	114	1	2	5	14	25	33	54
35–49	129	9.4	136	1	3	7	10	20	42	64
50–64	36	8.6	98	2	3	5	12	19	32	63
65+	12	13.8	102	6	6	11	19	26	44	44
2. MULTIPLE DX										
0–19 Years	553	12.6	109	2	6	10	16	26	34	50
20–34	563	6.4	41	1	2	4	9	16	19	30
35–49	636	7.6	70	1	2	5	10	17	22	41
50–64	235	8.8	72	2	3	7	11	18	26	39
65+	178	11.6	171	3	4	8	12	25	35	96
TOTAL SINGLE DX	464	10.5	94	1	3	8	14	21	29	54
MULTIPLE DX	2165	9.4	90	2	3	7	12	20	27	49
TOTAL										
0–19 Years	719	12.3	99	2	6	10	16	26	32	49
20–34	684	6.7	50	1	2	4	9	17	19	33
35–49	765	7.9	80	1	2	5	10	17	23	53
50–64	271	8.8	74	2	3	7	11	18	26	39
65+	190	11.7	168	3	4	8	13	25	35	96
GRAND TOTAL	2629	9.5	91	1	3	7	13	21	28	50

Length of Stay by Diagnosis and Operation, United States, 1997

United States, October 1995–September 1996 Data, by Operation

94.11: PSYCH MENTAL STATUS. Formerly included in operation group(s) 792.

Type of Patients	Observed Patients	Vari-ance	Avg. Stay	10th	25th	50th	75th	90th	95th	99th
1. SINGLE DX										
0–19 Years	62	24	5.9	1	2	4	8	12	15	23
20–34	72	86	8.3	1	2	4	10	25	31	41
35–49	92	112	8.4	1	2	5	8	20	40	54
50–64	27	112	9.2	2	3	6	12	19	32	63
65+	8	35	12.2	1	10	14	15	19	21	21
2. MULTIPLE DX										
0–19 Years	249	49	7.0	2	3	6	10	12	17	45
20–34	390	36	6.1	1	2	4	7	14	19	27
35–49	458	86	8.4	1	3	5	11	18	25	49
50–64	163	76	8.3	1	2	6	11	20	26	39
65+	129	194	14.2	4	5	8	18	32	40	64
TOTAL SINGLE DX	261	88	8.1	1	2	5	10	19	29	54
MULTIPLE DX	1389	77	8.0	1	3	5	10	18	25	45
TOTAL										
0–19 Years	311	46	6.9	2	3	6	9	12	16	45
20–34	462	42	6.4	1	2	4	8	15	20	31
35–49	550	90	8.4	1	3	5	11	18	26	53
50–64	190	80	8.4	1	3	6	11	19	26	39
65+	137	185	14.1	4	6	10	18	31	40	64
GRAND TOTAL	1650	78	8.0	1	3	5	10	18	25	45

94.2: PSYCH SOMATOTHERAPY. Formerly included in operation group(s) 792.

Type of Patients	Observed Patients	Vari-ance	Avg. Stay	10th	25th	50th	75th	90th	95th	99th
1. SINGLE DX										
0–19 Years	214	228	15.8	3	6	9	21	44	52	52
20–34	793	146	11.1	2	3	7	16	26	36	66
35–49	944	144	12.5	2	5	9	16	29	35	64
50–64	402	173	15.4	3	6	12	22	31	40	69
65+	397	139	19.1	5	13	16	26	33	37	62
2. MULTIPLE DX										
0–19 Years	1134	229	15.4	4	7	10	18	35	48	83
20–34	3513	143	12.3	2	4	9	16	27	36	65
35–49	4928	152	12.6	2	5	9	16	27	35	73
50–64	2167	181	16.0	4	7	12	22	34	45	91
65+	3720	185	20.0	6	10	17	27	39	48	>99
TOTAL SINGLE DX	2750	164	13.8	2	5	10	19	31	40	62
MULTIPLE DX	15462	179	15.1	3	6	11	20	33	44	80
TOTAL										
0–19 Years	1348	229	15.4	4	6	10	19	40	51	83
20–34	4306	143	12.0	2	4	8	16	27	36	65
35–49	5872	150	12.6	2	5	9	16	27	35	73
50–64	2569	180	15.9	4	7	12	22	34	44	85
65+	4117	181	20.0	6	10	17	27	39	47	94
GRAND TOTAL	18212	177	14.9	3	6	11	20	32	43	77

94.19: PSYCH INTERVIEW/EVAL NEC. Formerly included in operation group(s) 792.

Type of Patients	Observed Patients	Vari-ance	Avg. Stay	10th	25th	50th	75th	90th	95th	99th
1. SINGLE DX										
0–19 Years	98	62	12.9	2	7	13	16	23	29	31
20–34	46	86	9.3	1	3	4	14	19	33	43
35–49	29	41	6.6	1	1	5	10	15	21	21
50–64	9	25	5.5	2	2	3	8	15	15	15
65+	3	276	26.5	7	7	26	44	44	44	44
2. MULTIPLE DX										
0–19 Years	294	120	15.3	4	8	14	20	29	35	59
20–34	135	41	6.6	2	3	4	8	13	18	33
35–49	148	45	5.8	1	2	5	7	10	17	35
50–64	57	53	8.5	2	5	7	10	15	20	35
65+	38	39	10.0	4	7	10	11	12	19	48
TOTAL SINGLE DX	185	69	12.1	2	7	12	16	21	29	33
MULTIPLE DX	672	107	12.0	2	5	9	16	26	33	50
TOTAL										
0–19 Years	392	107	14.7	4	8	14	19	28	34	52
20–34	181	50	7.1	2	3	4	8	14	20	33
35–49	177	45	5.8	1	3	5	7	11	18	35
50–64	66	52	8.4	2	5	7	10	15	20	35
65+	41	52	10.5	4	7	11	11	15	20	48
GRAND TOTAL	857	100	12.0	2	5	10	16	25	32	49

94.22: LITHIUM THERAPY. Formerly included in operation group(s) 792.

Type of Patients	Observed Patients	Vari-ance	Avg. Stay	10th	25th	50th	75th	90th	95th	99th
1. SINGLE DX										
0–19 Years	14	95	8.0	2	2	6	7	18	25	51
20–34	45	216	16.4	5	7	11	21	50	50	>99
35–49	30	143	12.6	4	6	10	19	62	>99	>99
50–64	14	36	8.1	1	4	7	12	19	19	21
65+	2	39	13.5	9	9	14	18	18	18	18
2. MULTIPLE DX										
0–19 Years	75	112	14.9	6	9	11	23	27	35	60
20–34	150	112	10.5	2	4	8	14	21	29	56
35–49	185	89	10.9	3	6	9	13	22	28	50
50–64	71	142	14.8	6	10	14	14	21	27	99
65+	44	261	15.5	2	5	10	16	40	49	70
TOTAL SINGLE DX	105	166	13.0	3	6	9	18	33	51	>99
MULTIPLE DX	525	119	12.3	3	6	10	15	24	30	67
TOTAL										
0–19 Years	89	115	14.0	5	7	11	20	27	35	60
20–34	195	137	11.7	2	5	8	15	24	39	69
35–49	215	93	11.1	3	6	9	13	23	32	93
50–64	85	135	14.1	5	9	14	14	20	25	82
65+	46	256	15.4	2	5	10	17	40	49	70
GRAND TOTAL	630	125	12.4	3	6	10	15	25	33	77

Length of Stay by Diagnosis and Operation, United States, 1997

United States, October 1995–September 1996 Data, by Operation

94.23: NEUROLEPTIC THERAPY. Formerly included in operation group(s) 792.

Type of Patients	Observed Patients	Avg. Stay	Variance	Percentiles						
				10th	25th	50th	75th	90th	95th	99th
1. SINGLE DX										
0–19 Years	36	11.9	144	2	5	8	14	26	35	55
20–34	135	15.0	228	4	5	10	20	36	54	>99
35–49	136	17.7	304	2	5	12	28	39	50	83
50–64	33	15.3	230	3	7	10	19	35	59	>99
65+	13	25.3	671	1	5	18	36	59	85	85
2. MULTIPLE DX										
0–19 Years	129	17.5	389	4	6	10	18	50	74	>99
20–34	633	13.3	178	4	6	9	19	29	42	90
35–49	668	15.2	255	3	6	10	19	35	64	>99
50–64	226	14.3	220	4	6	8	17	45	52	>99
65+	146	15.2	115	7	9	13	18	24	50	78
TOTAL SINGLE DX	353	15.8	259	2	5	10	22	39	55	89
MULTIPLE DX	1802	14.7	217	3	6	10	18	33	50	>99
TOTAL										
0–19 Years	165	16.4	347	4	5	10	18	38	74	98
20–34	768	13.5	185	3	5	9	19	29	43	91
35–49	804	15.6	264	3	6	10	21	38	60	>99
50–64	259	14.4	221	4	6	9	17	45	59	>99
65+	159	15.5	131	7	9	13	18	25	50	78
GRAND TOTAL	2155	14.8	223	3	6	10	19	34	50	>99

94.25: PSYCH DRUG THERAPY NEC. Formerly included in operation group(s) 792.

Type of Patients	Observed Patients	Avg. Stay	Variance	Percentiles						
				10th	25th	50th	75th	90th	95th	99th
1. SINGLE DX										
0–19 Years	146	16.3	245	3	7	9	19	44	52	52
20–34	393	8.5	109	1	2	5	11	20	28	56
35–49	378	10.6	137	2	3	7	13	28	31	59
50–64	124	13.6	151	3	5	12	16	31	37	56
65+	53	18.0	257	4	10	14	19	31	66	88
2. MULTIPLE DX										
0–19 Years	898	15.0	213	4	7	10	18	35	44	83
20–34	1939	9.5	86	2	4	7	12	20	28	50
35–49	2478	9.4	94	2	4	7	11	20	27	56
50–64	849	11.9	132	2	5	8	14	24	34	64
65+	831	14.7	149	4	7	11	18	27	40	69
TOTAL SINGLE DX	1094	11.3	161	2	3	7	14	28	40	59
MULTIPLE DX	6995	11.2	126	2	4	8	14	23	33	66
TOTAL										
0–19 Years	1044	15.3	219	4	7	10	18	40	47	83
20–34	2332	9.3	91	2	3	7	11	20	28	52
35–49	2856	9.6	100	2	4	7	12	20	29	56
50–64	973	12.0	134	2	5	8	15	25	35	64
65+	884	14.8	155	4	7	11	19	28	40	70
GRAND TOTAL	8089	11.2	131	2	4	8	14	24	35	64

94.27: ELECTROSHOCK THERAPY NEC. Formerly included in operation group(s) 792.

Type of Patients	Observed Patients	Avg. Stay	Variance	Percentiles						
				10th	25th	50th	75th	90th	95th	99th
1. SINGLE DX										
0–19 Years	18	25.5	135	11	16	30	30	33	42	58
20–34	210	15.3	123	2	6	14	21	34	36	50
35–49	388	12.9	90	1	6	11	17	27	31	38
50–64	226	16.6	176	3	6	14	23	31	40	69
65+	327	19.2	109	5	14	17	26	33	37	46
2. MULTIPLE DX										
0–19 Years	29	16.5	153	3	9	12	22	33	47	50
20–34	772	18.7	201	5	9	16	25	36	42	84
35–49	1559	17.6	186	6	9	14	23	33	44	76
50–64	1005	20.2	186	6	10	18	28	39	46	>99
65+	2689	22.6	184	8	13	21	30	42	50	>99
TOTAL SINGLE DX	1169	16.2	125	3	8	15	23	31	35	54
MULTIPLE DX	6054	20.5	189	6	10	18	28	39	47	90
TOTAL										
0–19 Years	47	20.6	163	4	12	18	30	33	47	58
20–34	982	18.1	189	4	8	15	24	36	43	77
35–49	1947	16.8	163	5	8	14	22	32	40	73
50–64	1231	19.7	186	6	9	18	27	38	46	99
65+	3016	22.3	177	8	13	20	30	41	49	>99
GRAND TOTAL	7223	19.8	182	5	10	17	27	38	46	84

94.3: INDIVIDUAL PSYCHOTHERAPY. Formerly included in operation group(s) 792.

Type of Patients	Observed Patients	Avg. Stay	Variance	Percentiles						
				10th	25th	50th	75th	90th	95th	99th
1. SINGLE DX										
0–19 Years	334	7.8	50	1	3	6	10	15	20	27
20–34	453	7.3	51	2	3	5	9	15	19	41
35–49	435	8.8	78	3	4	7	11	16	20	43
50–64	153	9.2	66	2	3	6	14	19	25	35
65+	76	14.7	225	4	8	10	18	26	33	77
2. MULTIPLE DX										
0–19 Years	1897	8.1	52	2	4	6	10	16	22	37
20–34	2379	6.9	45	2	3	5	8	13	19	34
35–49	2379	7.5	45	2	3	6	9	14	19	39
50–64	830	11.1	118	2	5	7	13	27	42	45
65+	900	14.3	121	5	7	12	18	25	33	65
TOTAL SINGLE DX	1451	8.3	70	2	4	6	11	16	21	45
MULTIPLE DX	8385	8.4	65	2	4	6	10	17	23	42
TOTAL										
0–19 Years	2231	8.1	52	2	3	6	10	16	22	37
20–34	2832	6.9	46	2	3	5	8	14	19	35
35–49	2814	7.7	49	2	4	6	9	15	20	39
50–64	983	10.9	111	2	4	7	13	26	38	45
65+	976	14.3	127	5	7	12	18	25	33	71
GRAND TOTAL	9836	8.4	66	2	4	6	10	17	23	42

Length of Stay by Diagnosis and Operation, United States, 1997

94.31: PSYCHOANALYSIS. Formerly included in operation group(s) 792.

Type of Patients	Observed Patients	Avg. Stay	Vari-ance	Percentiles						
				10th	25th	50th	75th	90th	95th	99th
1. SINGLE DX										
0–19 Years	8	10.2	32	4	8	9	12	21	22	22
20–34	12	6.9	20	1	3	7	8	15	15	15
35–49	17	10.9	74	3	5	6	17	21	21	38
50–64	2	20.4	547	1	1	38	38	38	38	38
65+	1	1.0	0	1	1	1	1	1	1	1
2. MULTIPLE DX										
0–19 Years	72	13.2	132	2	4	11	19	32	40	>99
20–34	236	6.2	60	1	2	4	7	12	17	36
35–49	220	7.5	68	2	3	5	8	16	23	42
50–64	44	8.6	38	2	4	8	11	18	23	28
65+	30	11.7	57	5	6	11	14	21	28	42
TOTAL SINGLE DX	**40**	**9.7**	**68**	**1**	**5**	**8**	**13**	**21**	**22**	**38**
MULTIPLE DX	**602**	**8.3**	**75**	**2**	**3**	**6**	**11**	**18**	**27**	**55**
TOTAL										
0–19 Years	80	13.0	126	2	4	11	19	31	40	>99
20–34	248	6.3	58	1	2	4	7	12	17	36
35–49	237	7.7	69	2	3	5	9	18	21	42
50–64	46	8.8	45	2	4	8	11	18	23	30
65+	31	11.5	58	5	6	11	14	21	28	42
GRAND TOTAL	**642**	**8.3**	**75**	**2**	**3**	**6**	**11**	**18**	**27**	**54**

94.38: SUPP VERBAL PSYCHTX. Formerly included in operation group(s) 792.

Type of Patients	Observed Patients	Avg. Stay	Vari-ance	Percentiles						
				10th	25th	50th	75th	90th	95th	99th
1. SINGLE DX										
0–19 Years	15	7.4	28	3	3	6	10	13	21	24
20–34	59	15.4	252	3	5	9	20	56	56	>99
35–49	39	12.2	67	3	7	11	17	21	28	43
50–64	23	17.8	110	5	13	14	26	34	34	35
65+	9	36.5	942	8	8	23	77	77	77	77
2. MULTIPLE DX										
0–19 Years	147	8.1	46	2	4	6	9	16	27	30
20–34	198	11.6	235	2	4	6	13	28	34	94
35–49	244	9.3	99	2	3	6	11	23	31	45
50–64	101	14.0	106	4	7	12	19	25	32	61
65+	96	14.3	78	6	9	13	17	26	31	46
TOTAL SINGLE DX	**145**	**15.5**	**246**	**3**	**6**	**11**	**19**	**34**	**56**	**>99**
MULTIPLE DX	**786**	**11.4**	**122**	**2**	**4**	**8**	**15**	**23**	**30**	**54**
TOTAL										
0–19 Years	162	8.0	43	2	4	6	9	15	24	30
20–34	257	12.4	240	2	4	7	15	30	45	94
35–49	283	9.7	96	2	3	7	12	22	30	45
50–64	124	14.6	108	4	7	14	20	27	34	61
65+	105	15.3	139	6	9	13	17	28	40	77
GRAND TOTAL	**931**	**11.9**	**140**	**2**	**5**	**8**	**15**	**25**	**34**	**71**

94.39: INDIVIDUAL PSYCHTX NEC. Formerly included in operation group(s) 792.

Type of Patients	Observed Patients	Avg. Stay	Vari-ance	Percentiles						
				10th	25th	50th	75th	90th	95th	99th
1. SINGLE DX										
0–19 Years	308	7.6	50	1	3	6	10	15	20	27
20–34	365	6.9	37	2	3	5	9	13	19	29
35–49	358	8.7	80	3	4	7	10	15	19	45
50–64	122	8.0	49	2	3	6	11	16	21	31
65+	62	12.3	84	4	8	10	15	22	29	60
2. MULTIPLE DX										
0–19 Years	1616	7.8	45	2	3	6	10	16	21	34
20–34	1850	6.8	38	2	3	5	8	13	19	33
35–49	1846	7.4	40	2	4	6	9	14	18	38
50–64	660	11.1	125	2	4	7	12	27	42	45
65+	720	14.4	132	5	7	12	19	25	33	80
TOTAL SINGLE DX	**1215**	**7.9**	**57**	**2**	**4**	**6**	**10**	**15**	**19**	**38**
MULTIPLE DX	**6692**	**8.2**	**61**	**2**	**4**	**6**	**10**	**16**	**22**	**42**
TOTAL										
0–19 Years	1924	7.7	46	2	3	6	10	15	21	33
20–34	2215	6.8	38	2	3	5	8	13	19	33
35–49	2204	7.6	46	2	4	6	9	14	19	39
50–64	782	10.7	117	2	4	7	12	27	42	45
65+	782	14.3	129	5	7	12	19	25	33	71
GRAND TOTAL	**7907**	**8.1**	**60**	**2**	**4**	**6**	**10**	**16**	**22**	**42**

94.4: OTH PSYCHTX/COUNSELLING. Formerly included in operation group(s) 792.

Type of Patients	Observed Patients	Avg. Stay	Vari-ance	Percentiles						
				10th	25th	50th	75th	90th	95th	99th
1. SINGLE DX										
0–19 Years	65	10.5	66	3	4	9	15	21	22	40
20–34	104	9.4	169	2	3	5	10	23	31	78
35–49	90	10.3	128	2	5	7	10	26	26	63
50–64	33	12.9	108	4	6	10	16	34	34	47
65+	18	12.5	47	5	6	15	17	21	23	23
2. MULTIPLE DX										
0–19 Years	631	11.4	80	3	6	9	14	20	28	54
20–34	956	7.8	81	2	3	5	9	17	21	44
35–49	1001	7.1	34	2	3	6	8	14	18	26
50–64	399	9.9	88	3	4	6	13	21	32	60
65+	394	12.9	72	5	7	11	17	23	28	49
TOTAL SINGLE DX	**310**	**10.6**	**117**	**2**	**4**	**7**	**15**	**23**	**30**	**56**
MULTIPLE DX	**3381**	**8.9**	**69**	**2**	**4**	**7**	**11**	**18**	**23**	**45**
TOTAL										
0–19 Years	696	11.3	79	3	6	9	14	20	28	54
20–34	1060	7.9	87	2	3	5	9	17	25	49
35–49	1091	7.4	41	2	3	6	8	14	20	29
50–64	432	10.1	91	3	4	7	13	21	34	60
65+	412	12.9	71	5	7	11	17	23	28	49
GRAND TOTAL	**3691**	**9.0**	**73**	**2**	**4**	**7**	**11**	**18**	**24**	**46**

United States, October 1995–September 1996 Data, by Operation

94.44: OTHER GROUP THERAPY. Formerly included in operation group(s) 792.

Type of Patients	Observed Patients	Avg. Stay	Variance	Percentiles						
				10th	25th	50th	75th	90th	95th	99th
1. SINGLE DX										
0–19 Years	57	11.4	64	3	5	10	15	21	22	40
20–34	96	9.7	178	2	3	5	10	23	31	78
35–49	72	11.6	149	2	5	8	13	26	29	63
50–64	32	12.6	100	4	6	9	16	30	34	47
65+	14	11.9	45	5	6	11	17	19	23	23
2. MULTIPLE DX										
0–19 Years	562	12.0	84	4	6	10	15	21	29	54
20–34	897	7.8	69	2	3	6	9	17	19	44
35–49	912	7.2	33	2	4	6	8	14	18	27
50–64	373	10.1	86	3	4	7	13	21	33	>99
65+	352	12.3	66	5	7	10	15	22	28	43
TOTAL SINGLE DX	271	11.2	123	3	4	8	15	25	30	63
MULTIPLE DX	3096	9.0	66	3	4	7	11	18	22	45
TOTAL										
0–19 Years	619	11.9	82	4	6	10	15	21	28	54
20–34	993	7.9	76	2	3	6	8	17	20	50
35–49	984	7.5	42	2	4	6	8	15	19	30
50–64	405	10.3	88	3	5	7	13	22	34	60
65+	366	12.3	65	5	7	10	16	22	27	43
GRAND TOTAL	3367	9.2	70	3	4	7	11	18	23	47

94.6: ALCOHOL/DRUG REHAB/DETOX. Formerly included in operation group(s) 792.

Type of Patients	Observed Patients	Avg. Stay	Variance	Percentiles						
				10th	25th	50th	75th	90th	95th	99th
1. SINGLE DX										
0–19 Years	294	9.3	96	1	1	5	15	27	28	29
20–34	2903	4.6	23	1	2	5	5	9	14	26
35–49	3442	4.4	15	1	2	3	5	7	11	22
50–64	812	5.0	17	2	3	4	5	8	14	26
65+	157	6.8	28	2	4	4	10	13	18	25
2. MULTIPLE DX										
0–19 Years	2215	12.8	91	2	5	11	20	25	28	37
20–34	25335	6.5	37	2	3	4	7	14	21	28
35–49	37631	6.1	30	2	3	4	7	13	19	28
50–64	10320	6.4	31	2	3	5	8	13	18	28
65+	3831	8.8	54	2	4	6	11	18	26	34
TOTAL SINGLE DX	7608	4.8	23	1	2	4	5	9	14	27
MULTIPLE DX	79332	6.6	37	2	3	5	8	14	21	28
TOTAL										
0–19 Years	2509	12.4	93	2	4	11	19	25	28	36
20–34	28238	6.3	36	2	3	4	7	14	21	28
35–49	41073	6.0	29	2	3	4	7	13	18	28
50–64	11132	6.3	31	2	3	5	8	13	18	28
65+	3988	8.7	53	2	4	6	11	18	25	34
GRAND TOTAL	86940	6.4	36	2	3	4	7	14	21	28

94.5: REFFERAL PSYCH REHAB. Formerly included in operation group(s) 792.

Type of Patients	Observed Patients	Avg. Stay	Variance	Percentiles						
				10th	25th	50th	75th	90th	95th	99th
1. SINGLE DX										
0–19 Years	0									
20–34	2	1.7	<1	1	1	2	2	2	2	2
35–49	0									
50–64	0									
65+	0									
2. MULTIPLE DX										
0–19 Years	4	14.5	181	3	8	9	35	35	35	35
20–34	7	2.4	2	1	2	2	2	3	4	8
35–49	16	3.8	5	2	2	3	4	7	7	9
50–64	3	2.5	<1	2	3	3	4	3	3	3
65+	3	6.3	28	3	3	3	14	14	14	14
TOTAL SINGLE DX	2	1.7	<1	1	1	2	2	2	2	2
MULTIPLE DX	33	4.2	22	2	2	3	4	8	9	35
TOTAL										
0–19 Years	4	14.5	181	3	8	9	35	35	35	35
20–34	9	2.2	2	2	2	2	2	3	4	8
35–49	16	3.8	5	2	2	3	4	7	7	9
50–64	3	2.5	<1	2	3	3	4	3	3	3
65+	3	6.3	28	3	3	3	14	14	14	14
GRAND TOTAL	35	4.0	21	2	2	3	4	8	9	35

94.61: ALCOHOL REHABILITATION. Formerly included in operation group(s) 792.

Type of Patients	Observed Patients	Avg. Stay	Variance	Percentiles						
				10th	25th	50th	75th	90th	95th	99th
1. SINGLE DX										
0–19 Years	16	14.3	47	4	6	19	19	19	19	21
20–34	116	11.2	69	4	4	7	21	21	25	28
35–49	120	11.5	62	4	6	9	16	22	27	30
50–64	51	10.4	65	3	5	8	11	24	26	36
65+	19	11.5	64	2	7	8	15	25	25	25
2. MULTIPLE DX										
0–19 Years	88	16.0	106	1	8	17	24	25	33	42
20–34	591	14.8	64	4	8	15	21	24	28	30
35–49	806	13.9	69	4	8	14	19	25	28	32
50–64	288	13.6	66	4	9	12	20	23	28	48
65+	134	13.9	43	5	9	14	18	21	21	32
TOTAL SINGLE DX	322	11.5	65	3	4	9	19	21	25	28
MULTIPLE DX	1907	14.2	68	4	8	14	20	25	28	35
TOTAL										
0–19 Years	104	15.7	95	1	7	18	24	25	28	42
20–34	707	14.2	66	4	7	14	21	23	28	30
35–49	926	13.8	69	4	7	14	19	25	28	32
50–64	339	13.4	66	4	7	12	19	23	28	48
65+	153	13.7	45	5	9	14	18	21	24	32
GRAND TOTAL	2229	13.9	68	4	7	14	20	24	28	35

Length of Stay by Diagnosis and Operation, United States, 1997

United States, October 1995–September 1996 Data, by Operation

94.62: ALCOHOL DETOXIFICATION. Formerly included in operation group(s) 792.

Type of Patients	Observed Patients	Avg. Stay	Vari-ance	Percentiles 10th	25th	50th	75th	90th	95th	99th
1. SINGLE DX										
0–19 Years	79	1.2	<1	1	1	1	1	2	3	5
20–34	776	2.6	4	1	1	2	4	5	6	8
35–49	1302	3.0	3	1	1	3	4	5	6	8
50–64	437	3.9	4	2	3	4	5	5	6	12
65+	62	4.0	5	1	3	4	4	5	7	14
2. MULTIPLE DX										
0–19 Years	154	2.7	7	1	1	2	3	5	8	14
20–34	5513	3.9	13	1	2	3	5	7	10	23
35–49	13013	4.1	11	1	2	3	5	7	10	19
50–64	5797	4.6	14	2	3	4	5	8	11	21
65+	2296	7.2	36	2	3	5	8	14	19	28
TOTAL SINGLE DX	2656	3.0	4	1	1	3	4	5	6	8
MULTIPLE DX	26773	4.4	14	1	2	3	5	8	11	21
TOTAL										
0–19 Years	233	2.1	5	1	1	1	2	4	7	13
20–34	6289	3.8	12	1	2	3	5	7	9	21
35–49	14315	4.0	10	1	2	3	5	7	9	18
50–64	6234	4.6	14	2	3	4	5	8	11	20
65+	2358	7.1	35	2	3	5	8	14	18	28
GRAND TOTAL	29429	4.2	13	1	2	3	5	8	10	20

94.64: DRUG REHABILITATION. Formerly included in operation group(s) 792.

Type of Patients	Observed Patients	Avg. Stay	Vari-ance	Percentiles 10th	25th	50th	75th	90th	95th	99th
1. SINGLE DX										
0–19 Years	47	13.0	123	4	6	13	15	21	22	88
20–34	123	9.0	59	2	4	6	12	20	21	28
35–49	83	11.8	71	2	4	13	20	24	28	28
50–64	11	8.0	32	3	4	7	10	19	20	20
65+	1	17.0	0	17	17	17	17	17	17	17
2. MULTIPLE DX										
0–19 Years	257	13.9	61	5	8	14	19	22	25	33
20–34	478	13.5	66	3	7	13	21	27	28	28
35–49	346	12.7	66	3	6	13	17	25	28	32
50–64	37	15.6	178	4	5	11	29	29	29	81
65+	12	6.9	26	2	2	6	12	12	14	19
TOTAL SINGLE DX	265	11.1	88	3	5	9	15	21	24	35
MULTIPLE DX	1130	13.3	67	3	7	13	19	25	28	30
TOTAL										
0–19 Years	304	13.7	70	5	8	13	19	22	25	35
20–34	601	12.8	67	3	6	12	20	26	28	28
35–49	429	12.6	66	3	6	13	17	25	28	30
50–64	48	14.4	162	3	5	10	20	29	29	81
65+	13	7.5	30	2	2	6	12	17	17	19
GRAND TOTAL	1395	13.0	70	3	6	13	19	24	28	31

94.63: ALCOHOL REHAB/DETOX. Formerly included in operation group(s) 792.

Type of Patients	Observed Patients	Avg. Stay	Vari-ance	Percentiles 10th	25th	50th	75th	90th	95th	99th
1. SINGLE DX										
0–19 Years	21	14.2	81	3	10	12	22	28	28	28
20–34	323	5.6	31	1	2	4	7	13	19	28
35–49	558	6.0	24	3	3	4	7	11	18	28
50–64	195	6.8	36	2	3	5	8	16	20	28
65+	71	9.0	29	4	5	9	11	18	18	27
2. MULTIPLE DX										
0–19 Years	46	9.1	41	3	3	9	14	14	22	28
20–34	1718	8.6	44	2	3	6	12	20	24	27
35–49	4209	8.1	40	3	4	6	10	17	22	28
50–64	1951	9.2	44	3	4	7	13	19	22	31
65+	885	11.8	86	4	5	9	15	27	30	46
TOTAL SINGLE DX	1168	6.5	33	2	3	4	8	14	19	28
MULTIPLE DX	8809	8.7	46	3	4	6	12	19	23	30
TOTAL										
0–19 Years	67	11.0	62	3	3	12	14	27	28	28
20–34	2041	8.2	44	2	3	6	12	19	23	28
35–49	4767	7.9	39	3	4	6	10	17	21	28
50–64	2146	9.0	44	3	4	7	13	18	22	31
65+	956	11.6	82	4	5	9	14	24	30	46
GRAND TOTAL	9977	8.5	45	3	4	6	11	18	23	30

94.65: DRUG DETOXIFICATION. Formerly included in operation group(s) 792.

Type of Patients	Observed Patients	Avg. Stay	Vari-ance	Percentiles 10th	25th	50th	75th	90th	95th	99th
1. SINGLE DX										
0–19 Years	42	4.2	9	1	3	4	4	10	12	15
20–34	1105	3.9	6	1	2	4	5	6	8	13
35–49	976	4.3	4	3	3	4	5	6	8	12
50–64	83	4.3	6	3	3	3	5	8	10	13
65+	2	6.2	36	3	3	3	3	16	16	16
2. MULTIPLE DX										
0–19 Years	237	4.5	12	1	2	4	5	8	13	15
20–34	4684	4.7	10	2	3	4	5	8	10	15
35–49	5471	4.8	9	2	3	4	6	9	10	15
50–64	752	5.1	11	2	3	4	5	9	11	16
65+	233	8.7	64	3	3	6	9	15	34	34
TOTAL SINGLE DX	2208	4.1	5	2	3	4	5	6	8	13
MULTIPLE DX	11377	4.9	11	2	3	4	6	8	10	16
TOTAL										
0–19 Years	279	4.5	12	1	2	4	5	8	12	15
20–34	5789	4.6	9	2	3	4	5	8	10	14
35–49	6447	4.7	8	2	3	4	6	9	10	15
50–64	835	5.1	10	2	3	4	5	9	11	16
65+	235	8.7	64	3	3	6	9	15	34	34
GRAND TOTAL	13585	4.8	10	2	3	4	5	8	10	16

United States, October 1995–September 1996 Data, by Operation

94.66: DRUG REHAB/DETOX. Formerly included in operation group(s) 792.

Type of Patients	Observed Patients	Avg. Stay	Variance	10th	25th	50th	75th	90th	95th	99th
1. SINGLE DX										
0–19 Years	72	14.6	110	3	4	12	28	28	28	31
20–34	384	7.2	42	2	4	4	9	18	24	28
35–49	337	5.7	28	1	3	4	7	13	14	28
50–64	28	10.1	43	3	6	8	15	16	28	28
65+	1	7.0	0	7	7	7	7	7	7	7
2. MULTIPLE DX										
0–19 Years	161	10.3	102	3	4	7	12	28	28	51
20–34	1932	7.1	39	3	4	4	8	15	21	29
35–49	2103	7.4	30	3	4	6	9	14	19	28
50–64	307	11.1	104	3	5	8	12	27	43	43
65+	111	11.5	38	5	7	10	16	19	22	28
TOTAL SINGLE DX	822	7.1	47	1	3	4	9	17	26	28
MULTIPLE DX	4614	7.6	42	3	4	5	9	15	21	30
TOTAL										
0–19 Years	233	12.0	109	3	4	8	17	28	28	51
20–34	2316	7.1	40	2	4	4	8	16	22	28
35–49	2440	7.2	30	3	4	5	9	14	19	28
50–64	335	11.0	101	3	5	8	12	27	43	43
65+	112	11.5	38	5	7	10	16	19	22	28
GRAND TOTAL	5436	7.6	42	3	4	5	9	15	22	29

94.68: ALC/DRUG DETOXIFICATION. Formerly included in operation group(s) 792.

Type of Patients	Observed Patients	Avg. Stay	Variance	10th	25th	50th	75th	90th	95th	99th
1. SINGLE DX										
0–19 Years	3	4.0	8	1	1	4	7	7	7	7
20–34	28	4.3	9	2	2	4	5	10	12	12
35–49	28	4.5	5	1	3	4	6	7	7	14
50–64	4	4.5	2	3	4	4	4	7	7	7
65+	0									
2. MULTIPLE DX										
0–19 Years	202	4.9	24	1	2	4	5	9	15	31
20–34	5610	4.5	7	2	3	4	5	7	9	14
35–49	6726	4.7	8	2	3	4	6	8	10	15
50–64	699	5.5	8	3	4	5	7	8	9	15
65+	56	6.5	18	3	3	5	10	10	13	17
TOTAL SINGLE DX	63	4.4	7	1	3	4	6	7	10	12
MULTIPLE DX	13293	4.6	8	2	3	4	5	8	9	15
TOTAL										
0–19 Years	205	4.9	24	1	2	4	5	9	15	31
20–34	5638	4.4	7	2	3	4	5	7	9	14
35–49	6754	4.7	8	2	3	4	6	8	10	15
50–64	703	5.5	8	3	4	5	7	8	9	15
65+	56	6.5	18	3	3	5	10	10	13	17
GRAND TOTAL	13356	4.6	8	2	3	4	5	8	9	15

94.67: ALC/DRUG REHABILITATION. Formerly included in operation group(s) 792.

Type of Patients	Observed Patients	Avg. Stay	Variance	10th	25th	50th	75th	90th	95th	99th
1. SINGLE DX										
0–19 Years	7	16.4	52	9	11	15	15	29	29	29
20–34	9	13.9	77	5	5	10	25	25	28	28
35–49	1	1.0	0	1	1	1	1	1	1	1
50–64	0									
65+	0									
2. MULTIPLE DX										
0–19 Years	746	16.4	86	4	10	17	22	26	29	42
20–34	1367	15.3	82	4	8	14	22	28	28	33
35–49	1029	15.0	61	5	10	14	20	28	28	29
50–64	70	15.0	57	5	12	13	22	27	28	29
65+	14	14.4	36	6	12	14	16	27	28	28
TOTAL SINGLE DX	17	15.4	63	8	9	15	21	29	29	29
MULTIPLE DX	3226	15.6	77	4	9	14	22	28	28	35
TOTAL										
0–19 Years	753	16.4	86	4	10	17	22	26	29	42
20–34	1376	15.3	82	4	8	14	22	28	28	33
35–49	1030	15.1	61	5	10	14	20	28	28	29
50–64	70	15.0	57	5	12	13	22	27	28	29
65+	14	14.4	36	6	12	14	16	27	28	28
GRAND TOTAL	3243	15.6	77	4	9	14	22	28	28	35

94.69: ALC/DRUG REHAB/DETOX. Formerly included in operation group(s) 792.

Type of Patients	Observed Patients	Avg. Stay	Variance	10th	25th	50th	75th	90th	95th	99th
1. SINGLE DX										
0–19 Years	7	20.0	55	6	21	21	21	28	33	33
20–34	39	11.0	70	3	4	8	21	22	27	27
35–49	37	9.2	56	3	3	7	12	22	25	27
50–64	3	12.3	12	7	14	14	14	14	14	14
65+	1	5.0	0	5	5	5	5	5	5	5
2. MULTIPLE DX										
0–19 Years	324	12.7	81	3	6	10	21	25	28	37
20–34	3442	9.3	49	3	4	7	12	21	26	29
35–49	3928	9.1	46	3	4	7	11	19	26	29
50–64	419	9.6	36	4	6	8	12	19	22	28
65+	90	9.8	28	5	6	9	13	16	21	25
TOTAL SINGLE DX	87	10.9	68	3	4	7	20	22	27	28
MULTIPLE DX	8203	9.4	49	3	4	7	12	21	26	29
TOTAL										
0–19 Years	331	12.7	81	3	6	10	21	25	28	37
20–34	3481	9.3	49	3	4	7	12	21	26	29
35–49	3965	9.1	46	3	4	7	11	19	26	29
50–64	422	9.6	36	4	6	8	12	19	22	28
65+	91	9.7	28	3	6	8	13	16	20	25
GRAND TOTAL	8290	9.4	49	3	4	7	12	21	26	29

Length of Stay by Diagnosis and Operation

United States, 1997

United States, October 1995–September 1996 Data, by Operation

95.0: GEN/SUBJECTIVE EYE EXAM. Formerly included in operation group(s) 796.

Type of Patients	Observed Patients	Avg. Stay	Vari-ance	10th	25th	50th	75th	90th	95th	99th
1. SINGLE DX										
0–19 Years	19	1.5	1	1	1	1	2	2	2	8
20–34	0									
35–49	0									
50–64	0									
65+	0									
2. MULTIPLE DX										
0–19 Years	84	7.9	185	1	1	2	7	24	36	78
20–34	10	2.3	5	1	2	2	3	3	4	8
35–49	3	1.8	<1	1	2	2	2	2	2	2
50–64	6	5.0	3	2	3	6	6	6	6	6
65+	13	9.4	72	2	4	7	10	19	32	32
TOTAL SINGLE DX	19	1.5	1	1	1	1	2	2	2	8
MULTIPLE DX	116	7.2	148	1	1	2	6	24	36	58
TOTAL										
0–19 Years	103	6.4	149	1	1	1	4	24	36	58
20–34	10	2.3	1	1	2	2	2	3	4	8
35–49	3	1.8	<1	1	2	2	2	2	2	2
50–64	6	5.0	3	2	3	6	6	6	6	6
65+	13	9.4	72	2	4	7	10	19	32	32
GRAND TOTAL	135	6.1	125	1	1	2	5	24	36	58

95.1: FORM & STRUCT EYE EXAM. Formerly included in operation group(s) 796.

Type of Patients	Observed Patients	Avg. Stay	Vari-ance	10th	25th	50th	75th	90th	95th	99th
1. SINGLE DX										
0–19 Years	0									
20–34	3	2.9	1	2	2	2	4	4	4	4
35–49	1	1.0	0	1	1	1	1	1	1	1
50–64	0									
65+	0									
2. MULTIPLE DX										
0–19 Years	10	6.2	5	2	6	7	7	9	10	10
20–34	4	1.6	1	1	1	1	2	4	4	4
35–49	2	4.8	18	1	1	1	9	9	9	9
50–64	6	1.8	4	1	1	1	1	5	7	9
65+	9	4.8	20	3	3	3	4	8	11	28
TOTAL SINGLE DX	4	2.8	1	2	2	2	4	4	4	4
MULTIPLE DX	31	3.8	13	1	1	3	7	7	9	11
TOTAL										
0–19 Years	10	6.2	5	2	6	7	7	9	10	10
20–34	7	2.4	2	1	1	2	4	4	4	4
35–49	3	4.4	17	1	1	1	9	9	9	9
50–64	6	1.8	4	1	1	1	1	5	7	9
65+	9	4.8	20	3	3	3	4	8	11	28
GRAND TOTAL	35	3.8	12	1	1	3	6	7	9	11

95.2: OBJECTIVE FUNCT EYE TEST. Formerly included in operation group(s) 796.

Type of Patients	Observed Patients	Avg. Stay	Vari-ance	10th	25th	50th	75th	90th	95th	99th
1. SINGLE DX										
0–19 Years	0									
20–34	1	24.0	0	24	24	24	24	24	24	24
35–49	1	5.0	0	5	5	5	5	5	5	5
50–64	0									
65+	0									
2. MULTIPLE DX										
0–19 Years	0									
20–34	3	3.0	0	3	3	3	3	3	3	3
35–49	3	3.3	<1	3	3	3	4	4	4	4
50–64	2	2.2	2	1	1	3	3	3	3	3
65+	3	4.9	6	3	3	5	5	9	9	9
TOTAL SINGLE DX	2	11.1	115	5	5	5	24	24	24	24
MULTIPLE DX	11	3.8	4	3	3	3	4	5	9	9
TOTAL										
0–19 Years	0									
20–34	4	7.5	95	3	3	3	3	24	24	24
35–49	4	3.7	<1	3	3	3	4	5	5	5
50–64	2	2.2	2	1	1	3	3	3	3	3
65+	3	4.9	6	3	3	5	5	9	9	9
GRAND TOTAL	13	4.7	19	3	3	3	5	9	9	24

95.3: SPECIAL VISION SERVICES. Formerly included in operation group(s) 796.

Type of Patients	Observed Patients	Avg. Stay	Vari-ance	10th	25th	50th	75th	90th	95th	99th
1. SINGLE DX										
0–19 Years	0									
20–34	0									
35–49	0									
50–64	0									
65+	0									
2. MULTIPLE DX										
0–19 Years	0									
20–34	0									
35–49	0									
50–64	1	1.0	0	1	1	1	1	1	1	1
65+	1	3.0	0	3	3	3	3	3	3	3
TOTAL SINGLE DX	0									
MULTIPLE DX	2	2.1	1	1	1	3	3	3	3	3
TOTAL										
0–19 Years	0									
20–34	0									
35–49	0									
50–64	1	1.0	0	1	1	1	1	1	1	1
65+	1	3.0	0	3	3	3	3	3	3	3
GRAND TOTAL	2	2.1	1	1	1	3	3	3	3	3

Length of Stay by Diagnosis and Operation, United States, 1997

United States, October 1995–September 1996 Data, by Operation

95.4: NONOP HEARING PROCEDURE. Formerly included in operation group(s) 796.

Type of Patients	Observed Patients	Avg. Stay	Variance	10th	25th	50th	75th	90th	95th	99th
1. SINGLE DX										
0–19 Years	367	2.2	2	1	1	2	2	3	4	10
20–34	1	2.0	0	2	2	2	2	3	4	2
35–49	2	2.3	<1	2	2	2	3	3	3	3
50–64	1	1.0	0	1	1	1	1	1	1	1
65+	1	1.0	0	1	1	1	1	1	1	1
2. MULTIPLE DX										
0–19 Years	664	9.3	148	2	3	6	8	27	27	88
20–34	7	3.3	2	2	2	3	4	6	6	6
35–49	12	9.1	109	2	2	4	10	28	28	28
50–64	7	4.5	5	2	3	4	7	7	7	7
65+	28	8.2	32	4	7	8	8	10	15	43
TOTAL SINGLE DX	372	2.2	2	1	1	2	2	3	4	10
MULTIPLE DX	718	9.2	143	2	3	6	8	27	27	88
TOTAL										
0–19 Years	1031	8.4	136	2	3	5	7	27	27	88
20–34	8	3.0	2	2	2	2	4	4	6	6
35–49	14	7.6	93	2	2	3	6	28	28	28
50–64	8	4.2	6	1	3	4	7	7	7	7
65+	29	7.9	33	2	6	8	8	10	15	43
GRAND TOTAL	1090	8.4	131	2	3	5	7	27	27	88

95.41: AUDIOMETRY. Formerly included in operation group(s) 796.

Type of Patients	Observed Patients	Avg. Stay	Variance	10th	25th	50th	75th	90th	95th	99th
1. SINGLE DX										
0–19 Years	273	2.0	<1	1	1	2	2	3	4	6
20–34	1	2.0	0	2	2	2	2	2	2	2
35–49	2	2.0	0	2	2	2	2	2	2	2
50–64	0									
65+	0									
2. MULTIPLE DX										
0–19 Years	345	10.6	317	1	2	5	11	20	29	88
20–34	4	3.7	2	2	2	3	4	6	6	6
35–49	2	3.7	14	2	2	3	4	10	10	10
50–64	6	2.8	1	1	2	3	4	4	4	4
65+	13	8.5	38	2	6	9	10	10	17	33
TOTAL SINGLE DX	275	2.0	<1	1	1	2	2	3	4	6
MULTIPLE DX	370	10.5	306	1	2	5	11	20	28	88
TOTAL										
0–19 Years	618	8.4	249	2	2	3	8	20	21	88
20–34	5	3.1	2	2	2	2	4	6	6	6
35–49	6	2.8	6	2	2	2	4	4	10	10
50–64	6	2.8	1	1	2	3	4	4	4	4
65+	13	8.5	38	2	6	9	10	10	17	33
GRAND TOTAL	645	8.3	241	2	2	3	8	20	21	88

95.47: HEARING EXAMINATION NOS. Formerly included in operation group(s) 796.

Type of Patients	Observed Patients	Avg. Stay	Variance	10th	25th	50th	75th	90th	95th	99th
1. SINGLE DX										
0–19 Years	19	4.5	21	1	1	2	9	12	12	16
20–34	0									
35–49	0									
50–64	0									
65+	0									
2. MULTIPLE DX										
0–19 Years	201	9.1	76	3	3	7	7	27	27	27
20–34	0									
35–49	2	5.0	18	2	2	2	8	8	8	8
50–64	0									
65+	1	7.0	0	7	7	7	7	7	7	7
TOTAL SINGLE DX	19	4.5	21	1	1	2	9	12	12	16
MULTIPLE DX	204	9.0	75	3	3	7	7	27	27	27
TOTAL										
0–19 Years	220	9.0	76	3	3	7	7	27	27	27
20–34	0									
35–49	2	5.0	18	2	2	2	8	8	8	8
50–64	0									
65+	1	7.0	0	7	7	7	7	7	7	7
GRAND TOTAL	223	9.0	75	3	3	7	7	27	27	27

96.0: NONOP GI & RESP INTUB. Formerly included in operation group(s) 796.

Type of Patients	Observed Patients	Avg. Stay	Variance	10th	25th	50th	75th	90th	95th	99th
1. SINGLE DX										
0–19 Years	1688	2.4	21	1	1	2	2	3	6	33
20–34	143	2.7	5	1	1	2	4	7	7	7
35–49	151	3.0	6	1	1	3	3	6	7	14
50–64	120	3.3	13	2	2	2	3	6	8	24
65+	118	5.0	12	2	2	4	8	10	10	19
2. MULTIPLE DX										
0–19 Years	10628	12.0	347	1	2	4	12	44	64	>99
20–34	1880	5.1	46	1	2	3	6	11	17	37
35–49	2789	6.5	53	1	2	4	8	14	20	37
50–64	3457	8.5	65	2	3	6	11	18	24	38
65+	9403	9.0	62	2	4	7	11	18	23	40
TOTAL SINGLE DX	2220	2.6	18	1	1	2	3	5	7	20
MULTIPLE DX	28157	9.6	176	1	3	5	11	22	40	80
TOTAL										
0–19 Years	12316	10.3	303	1	2	3	9	38	58	>99
20–34	2023	4.9	43	1	1	3	5	10	17	37
35–49	2940	6.3	51	1	1	4	8	14	20	36
50–64	3577	8.2	63	2	3	6	10	18	24	37
65+	9521	9.0	62	2	4	7	11	18	23	39
GRAND TOTAL	30377	8.9	165	1	2	4	10	20	37	79

Length of Stay by Diagnosis and Operation, United States, 1997

United States, October 1995–September 1996 Data, by Operation

96.04: INSERT ENDOTRACHEAL TUBE. Formerly included in operation group(s) 796.

Type of Patients	Observed Patients	Avg. Stay	Vari- ance	10th	25th	50th	75th	90th	95th	99th
1. SINGLE DX										
0–19 Years	1305	2.4	20	1	1	2	2	3	6	22
20–34	42	2.6	4	1	1	2	4	6	6	8
35–49	38	5.2	19	1	3	4	5	14	18	18
50–64	20	7.4	108	1	2	3	9	17	39	46
65+	31	8.2	26	2	3	10	10	17	19	20
2. MULTIPLE DX										
0–19 Years	9462	12.8	369	1	2	4	13	45	67	>99
20–34	1172	6.3	65	1	2	4	7	15	22	37
35–49	1673	8.2	74	2	3	5	11	19	25	43
50–64	2208	11.2	82	3	5	9	14	22	28	46
65+	5827	11.4	80	4	6	9	14	21	26	51
TOTAL SINGLE DX	1436	2.5	21	1	1	2	2	4	6	22
MULTIPLE DX	20342	11.5	223	1	3	7	13	29	49	90
TOTAL										
0–19 Years	10767	11.0	325	1	2	3	10	42	61	>99
20–34	1214	6.2	63	1	2	3	7	14	22	37
35–49	1711	8.2	73	2	3	5	11	18	25	43
50–64	2228	11.2	82	3	5	9	14	22	28	46
65+	5858	11.4	79	4	6	9	14	21	26	50
GRAND TOTAL	21778	10.6	211	1	2	6	12	26	45	87

96.05: RESP TRACT INTUB NEC. Formerly included in operation group(s) 796.

Type of Patients	Observed Patients	Avg. Stay	Vari- ance	10th	25th	50th	75th	90th	95th	99th
1. SINGLE DX										
0–19 Years	120	4.3	79	1	1	2	3	11	33	>99
20–34	4	2.8	<1	2	2	3	3	4	4	4
35–49	2	1.0	0	1	1	1	1	1	1	1
50–64	1	3.0	0	3	3	3	3	3	3	3
65+	2	6.4	5	4	4	8	8	8	8	8
2. MULTIPLE DX										
0–19 Years	315	9.8	348	1	2	3	6	25	56	96
20–34	27	9.2	117	1	2	4	12	17	33	50
35–49	34	10.2	113	2	4	7	15	15	31	63
50–64	55	9.1	51	2	4	8	11	20	22	41
65+	128	11.2	37	4	7	11	13	18	22	34
TOTAL SINGLE DX	129	4.1	73	1	1	2	3	11	33	>99
MULTIPLE DX	559	10.1	208	1	2	5	12	20	39	82
TOTAL										
0–19 Years	435	8.1	272	1	1	2	4	23	55	98
20–34	31	8.8	112	1	2	4	12	17	33	50
35–49	36	8.7	106	1	2	7	12	15	31	63
50–64	56	9.1	51	2	4	8	11	20	22	41
65+	130	11.1	37	4	7	11	13	18	22	34
GRAND TOTAL	688	8.9	186	1	2	4	11	18	35	82

96.07: INSERT GASTRIC TUBE NEC. Formerly included in operation group(s) 796.

Type of Patients	Observed Patients	Avg. Stay	Vari- ance	10th	25th	50th	75th	90th	95th	99th
1. SINGLE DX										
0–19 Years	246	1.9	3	1	1	1	2	4	6	10
20–34	92	2.8	5	1	1	2	5	7	7	7
35–49	106	2.7	3	1	1	3	3	5	7	7
50–64	92	2.8	3	1	2	2	3	6	6	8
65+	82	3.7	4	2	2	4	4	6	8	9
2. MULTIPLE DX										
0–19 Years	756	6.1	122	1	1	3	5	12	21	58
20–34	655	3.2	12	1	1	2	4	6	9	20
35–49	1044	4.2	16	2	2	3	5	8	11	17
50–64	1106	4.5	15	2	2	3	5	10	11	18
65+	3201	5.5	18	2	3	4	7	10	13	21
TOTAL SINGLE DX	618	2.6	4	1	1	2	3	6	7	9
MULTIPLE DX	6762	4.9	33	1	2	3	6	10	13	29
TOTAL										
0–19 Years	1002	5.4	106	1	1	3	4	11	18	58
20–34	747	3.2	11	1	1	2	4	7	8	18
35–49	1150	4.0	15	1	2	3	5	8	10	16
50–64	1198	4.3	14	1	2	3	5	8	10	17
65+	3283	5.4	18	2	3	4	7	10	13	21
GRAND TOTAL	7380	4.7	31	1	2	3	6	9	12	26

96.1: OTHER NONOP INSERTION. Formerly included in operation group(s) 796.

Type of Patients	Observed Patients	Avg. Stay	Vari- ance	10th	25th	50th	75th	90th	95th	99th
1. SINGLE DX										
0–19 Years	2	1.4	<1	1	1	1	2	2	2	2
20–34	9	1.9	<1	1	1	2	2	3	3	3
35–49	10	1.6	<1	1	1	1	1	2	2	3
50–64	1	1.0	0	1	1	1	1	1	1	1
65+	1	1.0	0	1	1	1	1	1	1	1
2. MULTIPLE DX										
0–19 Years	13	2.0	4	1	1	1	1	6	6	8
20–34	23	2.4	4	1	1	2	3	4	7	9
35–49	18	2.6	2	2	2	3	3	4	5	7
50–64	13	4.7	63	1	1	3	5	7	28	28
65+	63	6.3	53	3	3	5	8	10	15	32
TOTAL SINGLE DX	23	1.6	<1	1	1	2	2	2	3	3
MULTIPLE DX	130	4.3	33	1	1	3	6	8	10	28
TOTAL										
0–19 Years	15	2.0	4	1	1	1	1	6	6	8
20–34	32	2.2	3	1	1	2	3	4	7	9
35–49	28	2.2	2	1	1	2	3	4	4	7
50–64	14	4.6	61	1	1	2	5	7	28	28
65+	64	6.3	52	1	3	4	8	10	15	32
GRAND TOTAL	153	3.9	30	1	1	2	5	8	10	28

Length of Stay by Diagnosis and Operation, United States, 1997

United States, October 1995–September 1996 Data, by Operation

96.2: NONOP DILATION & MANIP. Formerly included in operation group(s) 796.

Type of Patients	Observed Patients	Avg. Stay	Variance	Percentiles						
				10th	25th	50th	75th	90th	95th	99th
1. SINGLE DX										
0–19 Years	35	2.0	1	1	1	2	2	3	4	6
20–34	11	2.0	<1	2	1	2	2	2	3	4
35–49	13	2.3	<1	1	1	3	3	3	3	3
50–64	10	1.6	2	1	1	1	2	3	3	3
65+	25	1.9	<1	1	1	2	2	3	3	6
2. MULTIPLE DX										
0–19 Years	113	6.6	31	1	3	8	8	8	10	35
20–34	37	2.3	9	1	1	1	2	5	9	15
35–49	53	2.7	4	1	2	2	3	6	6	9
50–64	58	3.5	17	1	2	2	4	11	12	17
65+	238	5.0	31	1	2	3	6	10	17	25
TOTAL SINGLE DX	94	2.1	<1	1	1	2	3	3	3	6
MULTIPLE DX	499	4.9	27	1	1	3	8	8	12	35
TOTAL										
0–19 Years	148	5.9	30	1	2	6	8	8	8	35
20–34	48	2.3	7	1	1	2	2	4	5	15
35–49	66	2.5	2	1	1	2	3	4	4	9
50–64	68	3.4	16	1	2	2	3	10	12	17
65+	263	4.8	29	1	2	3	6	10	15	23
GRAND TOTAL	593	4.3	23	1	1	3	6	8	11	25

96.3: NONOP GI IRRIG/INSTILL. Formerly included in operation group(s) 796.

Type of Patients	Observed Patients	Avg. Stay	Variance	Percentiles						
				10th	25th	50th	75th	90th	95th	99th
1. SINGLE DX										
0–19 Years	700	1.7	2	1	1	1	2	3	4	8
20–34	66	1.3	<1	1	1	1	1	2	3	4
35–49	36	2.0	2	1	1	1	4	4	6	6
50–64	12	1.7	2	1	1	1	2	4	6	7
65+	13	2.5	2	1	2	3	4	4	4	4
2. MULTIPLE DX										
0–19 Years	1819	5.7	55	1	1	2	6	18	24	28
20–34	1530	2.4	11	1	1	1	2	5	7	21
35–49	1186	2.3	7	1	1	2	3	4	7	14
50–64	402	3.2	9	1	2	2	4	7	8	15
65+	709	6.0	42	2	2	4	7	13	18	32
TOTAL SINGLE DX	827	1.7	2	1	1	1	2	3	4	7
MULTIPLE DX	5646	4.1	32	1	1	2	4	10	18	28
TOTAL										
0–19 Years	2519	4.9	47	1	1	2	5	18	23	28
20–34	1596	2.4	11	1	1	1	3	4	7	21
35–49	1222	2.3	6	1	1	2	4	4	7	14
50–64	414	3.1	9	1	2	2	4	7	8	15
65+	722	5.9	42	1	2	4	7	13	18	32
GRAND TOTAL	6473	3.8	30	1	1	2	4	9	18	26

96.33: GASTRIC LAVAGE. Formerly included in operation group(s) 796.

Type of Patients	Observed Patients	Avg. Stay	Variance	Percentiles						
				10th	25th	50th	75th	90th	95th	99th
1. SINGLE DX										
0–19 Years	587	1.6	2	1	1	1	2	3	3	4
20–34	55	1.3	<1	1	1	1	1	3	3	4
35–49	26	1.3	<1	1	1	1	1	2	2	4
50–64	3	1.1	<1	1	1	1	1	1	1	7
65+	3	3.4	<1	2	2	4	4	4	4	4
2. MULTIPLE DX										
0–19 Years	1362	2.2	5	1	1	1	2	4	7	13
20–34	1435	2.4	11	1	1	1	2	5	7	21
35–49	1103	2.3	7	1	1	1	3	4	7	14
50–64	300	2.9	9	2	1	2	3	7	8	15
65+	216	6.2	41	1	2	4	8	12	23	30
TOTAL SINGLE DX	674	1.5	1	1	1	1	2	3	3	4
MULTIPLE DX	4416	2.5	10	1	1	1	3	5	8	17
TOTAL										
0–19 Years	1949	2.1	5	1	1	1	2	4	6	11
20–34	1490	2.4	11	1	1	1	2	4	7	21
35–49	1129	2.2	6	1	1	2	3	4	7	14
50–64	303	2.8	8	2	2	4	3	7	8	14
65+	219	6.1	41	1	2	4	8	12	23	30
GRAND TOTAL	5090	2.4	9	1	1	1	3	5	7	17

96.35: GASTRIC GAVAGE. Formerly included in operation group(s) 796.

Type of Patients	Observed Patients	Avg. Stay	Variance	Percentiles						
				10th	25th	50th	75th	90th	95th	99th
1. SINGLE DX										
0–19 Years	12	1.6	7	1	1	1	1	1	4	13
20–34	3	1.3	<1	1	1	1	1	3	3	3
35–49	1	3.0	0	3	3	3	3	3	3	3
50–64	0									
65+	0									
2. MULTIPLE DX										
0–19 Years	263	12.4	86	2	4	10	20	24	28	36
20–34	24	1.9	<1	1	1	1	2	3	3	4
35–49	25	3.0	7	1	1	2	5	6	10	10
50–64	12	8.4	35	2	4	8	12	14	15	26
65+	24	11.1	102	3	3	6	17	32	32	32
TOTAL SINGLE DX	16	1.6	7	1	1	1	1	2	4	13
MULTIPLE DX	348	11.8	87	2	3	9	20	24	28	36
TOTAL										
0–19 Years	275	11.5	88	1	3	8	19	24	28	36
20–34	27	1.9	<1	1	1	2	2	3	3	4
35–49	26	3.0	7	1	1	2	5	6	10	10
50–64	12	8.4	35	2	4	8	12	14	15	26
65+	24	11.1	102	3	3	6	17	32	32	32
GRAND TOTAL	364	11.0	88	1	2	7	18	24	28	35

Length of Stay by Diagnosis and Operation, United States, 1997

United States, October 1995–September 1996 Data, by Operation

96.38: IMPACTED FECES REMOVAL. Formerly included in operation group(s) 796.

Type of Patients	Observed Patients	Avg. Stay	Vari-ance	10th	25th	50th	75th	90th	95th	99th
1. SINGLE DX										
0–19 Years	46	2.3	2	1	1	2	3	4	5	7
20–34	7	1.2	<1	1	1	1	1	2	3	3
35–49	6	2.6	3	1	1	4	5	6	6	6
50–64	6	3.5	4	4	4	3	5	6	6	6
65+	8	2.0	2	1	1	1	4	4	4	4
2. MULTIPLE DX										
0–19 Years	118	3.4	10	1	2	3	5	6	10	10
20–34	24	3.4	8	1	2	2	5	5	8	18
35–49	24	3.3	6	1	1	3	4	8	8	10
50–64	59	3.9	6	2	2	3	6	7	8	11
65+	379	5.8	30	1	3	4	7	13	17	31
TOTAL SINGLE DX	73	2.4	2	1	1	2	4	4	5	7
MULTIPLE DX	604	4.8	22	1	2	4	6	10	15	20
TOTAL										
0–19 Years	164	3.0	8	1	1	2	4	5	7	10
20–34	31	3.0	7	1	1	2	4	5	5	18
35–49	30	2.8	4	1	1	3	4	4	6	10
50–64	65	3.9	6	2	2	3	6	7	8	11
65+	387	5.7	30	1	2	4	7	13	17	31
GRAND TOTAL	677	4.3	19	1	2	3	5	9	13	19

96.49: OTHER GU INSTILLATION. Formerly included in operation group(s) 796.

Type of Patients	Observed Patients	Avg. Stay	Vari-ance	10th	25th	50th	75th	90th	95th	99th
1. SINGLE DX										
0–19 Years	108	1.2	<1	1	1	1	1	2	3	3
20–34	605	1.2	<1	1	1	1	1	2	3	4
35–49	166	1.2	<1	1	1	1	1	2	2	4
50–64	2	3.0	0	3	3	3	3	3	3	3
65+	5	1.9	<1	1	2	2	2	3	3	3
2. MULTIPLE DX										
0–19 Years	176	1.7	1	1	1	1	2	3	4	6
20–34	1008	1.7	2	1	1	1	2	3	3	7
35–49	263	1.8	3	1	1	1	2	3	4	14
50–64	16	3.4	20	1	2	2	3	4	14	22
65+	77	4.5	50	1	1	2	4	8	24	46
TOTAL SINGLE DX	886	1.2	<1	1	1	1	1	2	2	3
MULTIPLE DX	1540	1.8	4	1	2	1	2	3	4	8
TOTAL										
0–19 Years	284	1.5	<1	1	1	1	2	3	3	5
20–34	1613	1.5	1	1	1	1	2	2	3	5
35–49	429	1.4	1	1	1	1	2	2	3	5
50–64	18	3.4	18	1	2	2	3	4	14	22
65+	82	4.4	49	1	2	2	4	8	11	46
GRAND TOTAL	2426	1.5	2	1	1	1	2	2	3	6

96.4: DIGEST/GU IRRIG/INSTILL. Formerly included in operation group(s) 796.

Type of Patients	Observed Patients	Avg. Stay	Vari-ance	10th	25th	50th	75th	90th	95th	99th
1. SINGLE DX										
0–19 Years	109	1.3	<1	1	1	1	1	2	3	3
20–34	612	1.2	<1	1	1	1	1	2	3	4
35–49	173	1.2	<1	1	1	1	1	2	2	4
50–64	4	3.9	<1	4	4	4	4	4	4	4
65+	11	2.5	3	1	1	2	3	3	7	7
2. MULTIPLE DX										
0–19 Years	188	1.9	2	1	1	1	2	3	6	7
20–34	1031	1.8	3	1	1	1	2	3	4	7
35–49	306	2.0	6	1	1	1	2	3	5	14
50–64	68	3.3	9	2	2	2	3	5	10	16
65+	246	4.8	29	1	2	3	6	11	15	28
TOTAL SINGLE DX	909	1.3	<1	1	1	1	1	2	3	4
MULTIPLE DX	1839	2.2	7	1	1	1	2	4	6	14
TOTAL										
0–19 Years	297	1.6	1	1	1	1	2	3	4	6
20–34	1643	1.5	2	1	1	1	2	3	3	6
35–49	479	1.6	3	1	1	1	2	3	5	10
50–64	72	3.4	7	2	2	3	4	4	8	16
65+	257	4.7	29	1	2	3	6	10	14	28
GRAND TOTAL	2748	1.7	4	1	1	1	2	3	4	10

96.5: OTHER NONOP IRRIG/CLEAN. Formerly included in operation group(s) 796.

Type of Patients	Observed Patients	Avg. Stay	Vari-ance	10th	25th	50th	75th	90th	95th	99th
1. SINGLE DX										
0–19 Years	71	2.5	8	1	1	2	3	5	7	11
20–34	50	3.2	46	1	1	2	2	4	5	38
35–49	30	2.7	4	1	1	2	4	6	7	9
50–64	10	3.1	6	1	1	2	5	8	8	8
65+	2	6.5	9	4	4	4	9	9	9	9
2. MULTIPLE DX										
0–19 Years	353	6.8	55	1	3	4	10	14	17	38
20–34	208	5.9	29	1	2	4	9	13	15	21
35–49	229	6.4	26	2	3	5	9	11	14	34
50–64	230	7.5	25	1	3	7	11	14	16	21
65+	528	9.3	39	3	5	7	12	17	20	34
TOTAL SINGLE DX	163	2.9	23	1	1	2	3	5	7	38
MULTIPLE DX	1548	7.4	39	1	3	6	10	14	19	28
TOTAL										
0–19 Years	424	6.2	51	1	2	4	9	12	17	35
20–34	258	5.3	34	1	1	3	7	13	15	27
35–49	259	6.1	26	2	3	4	8	11	14	34
50–64	240	7.4	25	1	3	7	11	14	16	21
65+	530	9.3	39	3	5	7	12	17	20	34
GRAND TOTAL	1711	7.0	39	1	3	5	10	14	18	29

Length of Stay by Diagnosis and Operation, United States, 1997

United States, October 1995–September 1996 Data, by Operation

96.56: BRONCH/TRACH LAVAGE NEC. Formerly included in operation group(s) 796.

Type of Patients	Observed Patients	Avg. Stay	Vari- ance	Percentiles						
				10th	25th	50th	75th	90th	95th	99th
1. SINGLE DX										
0–19 Years	19	2.3	4	1	1	1	2	7	7	7
20–34	10	1.6	2	1	1	1	2	2	4	8
35–49	6	4.2	10	1	1	4	6	9	9	9
50–64	3	2.9	4	1	1	3	5	5	5	5
65+	1	9.0	0	9	9	9	9	9	9	9
2. MULTIPLE DX										
0–19 Years	204	7.9	55	1	4	6	10	16	21	38
20–34	96	8.7	28	1	5	8	13	15	18	21
35–49	121	7.1	32	2	4	6	8	14	18	36
50–64	123	9.3	24	4	5	8	14	16	17	22
65+	261	10.5	38	4	6	9	14	19	21	32
TOTAL SINGLE DX	39	2.3	5	1	1	1	2	6	7	9
MULTIPLE DX	805	8.8	40	2	4	8	12	16	20	27
TOTAL										
0–19 Years	223	7.6	54	1	4	5	10	16	21	38
20–34	106	7.8	30	1	2	6	13	15	17	21
35–49	127	7.0	32	2	4	6	8	14	18	36
50–64	126	9.2	24	3	5	8	14	16	17	22
65+	262	10.5	38	4	6	9	14	19	21	32
GRAND TOTAL	844	8.5	40	2	4	7	12	16	20	27

96.6: ENTERAL NUTRITION. Formerly included in operation group(s) 796.

Type of Patients	Observed Patients	Avg. Stay	Vari- ance	Percentiles						
				10th	25th	50th	75th	90th	95th	99th
1. SINGLE DX										
0–19 Years	53	7.9	76	1	3	4	12	27	27	27
20–34	12	5.4	9	3	4	4	7	12	12	12
35–49	2	5.2	7	2	2	4	7	7	7	7
50–64	5	3.0	2	2	2	2	4	5	5	5
65+	8	3.9	8	1	2	3	7	7	10	10
2. MULTIPLE DX										
0–19 Years	1225	9.6	117	2	3	6	12	21	33	52
20–34	202	10.4	111	2	3	6	13	19	42	>99
35–49	262	11.4	185	3	4	8	28	>99	>99	>99
50–64	465	15.1	377	2	5	8	16	40	78	78
65+	2930	10.9	79	4	5	8	13	22	27	42
TOTAL SINGLE DX	80	7.2	64	1	2	4	10	17	27	27
MULTIPLE DX	5084	10.8	122	2	4	8	13	23	33	>99
TOTAL										
0–19 Years	1278	9.5	116	2	3	6	12	22	33	52
20–34	214	10.3	110	3	4	8	13	19	42	82
35–49	264	11.3	184	3	4	8	27	>99	>99	>99
50–64	470	15.0	375	2	5	8	16	39	78	78
65+	2938	10.9	79	4	5	8	13	22	27	42
GRAND TOTAL	5164	10.8	121	2	4	8	13	23	33	>99

96.59: WOUND IRRIGATION NEC. Formerly included in operation group(s) 796.

Type of Patients	Observed Patients	Avg. Stay	Vari- ance	Percentiles						
				10th	25th	50th	75th	90th	95th	99th
1. SINGLE DX										
0–19 Years	46	2.6	10	1	1	2	3	5	7	11
20–34	38	3.7	63	1	1	2	3	4	38	38
35–49	22	2.8	3	1	2	2	4	6	6	7
50–64	5	3.7	9	1	1	3	8	8	8	8
65+	0									
2. MULTIPLE DX										
0–19 Years	68	3.0	7	1	1	2	4	7	10	10
20–34	87	2.8	12	1	1	2	3	4	9	19
35–49	70	5.5	19	2	2	4	8	9	11	23
50–64	60	5.3	20	2	2	4	8	10	15	18
65+	79	8.4	43	3	4	6	10	17	20	29
TOTAL SINGLE DX	111	3.2	32	1	1	2	3	4	7	38
MULTIPLE DX	364	5.1	24	1	2	4	7	10	16	27
TOTAL										
0–19 Years	114	2.9	8	1	1	2	3	7	10	11
20–34	125	3.1	27	1	2	2	3	4	9	38
35–49	92	5.2	18	1	2	4	7	9	11	23
50–64	65	5.2	19	1	2	4	9	10	14	18
65+	79	8.4	43	3	4	6	10	17	20	29
GRAND TOTAL	475	4.7	26	1	2	3	6	9	14	29

96.7: CONT MECH VENT NEC. Formerly included in operation group(s) 790.

Type of Patients	Observed Patients	Avg. Stay	Vari- ance	Percentiles						
				10th	25th	50th	75th	90th	95th	99th
1. SINGLE DX										
0–19 Years	267	4.5	19	1	2	3	6	8	13	25
20–34	63	4.0	9	1	2	3	6	10	10	11
35–49	61	3.7	15	1	1	3	4	7	10	19
50–64	39	5.5	31	1	3	3	5	11	11	34
65+	57	15.1	372	1	3	9	17	64	90	>99
2. MULTIPLE DX										
0–19 Years	11565	20.1	475	2	5	11	28	61	80	>99
20–34	2797	7.5	76	2	3	4	10	17	23	48
35–49	4359	9.4	100	2	3	6	12	20	28	58
50–64	7390	11.3	83	3	5	9	15	22	28	46
65+	19366	12.3	83	4	6	10	16	23	29	50
TOTAL SINGLE DX	487	5.3	57	1	2	3	6	11	14	35
MULTIPLE DX	45477	13.7	209	3	5	9	17	29	48	92
TOTAL										
0–19 Years	11832	19.7	469	2	5	11	27	60	79	>99
20–34	2860	7.4	74	1	2	4	10	17	23	47
35–49	4420	9.3	99	2	3	6	12	20	28	58
50–64	7429	11.2	82	3	5	9	15	22	28	46
65+	19423	12.3	84	4	6	10	16	23	29	51
GRAND TOTAL	45964	13.6	208	3	5	9	17	29	47	92

United States, October 1995–September 1996 Data, by Operation

96.71: CONT MECH VENT-<96 HOURS. Formerly included in operation group(s) 790.

Type of Patients	Observed Patients	Avg. Stay	Vari-ance	Percentiles						
				10th	25th	50th	75th	90th	95th	99th
1. SINGLE DX										
0–19 Years	235	3.7	7	1	2	3	6	7	8	13
20–34	60	3.9	9	1	2	2	6	10	10	11
35–49	57	3.0	4	1	1	2	4	5	7	11
50–64	33	4.4	9	1	3	3	5	11	11	11
65+	34	7.1	42	1	1	7	10	14	17	35
2. MULTIPLE DX										
0–19 Years	7381	13.8	267	2	4	8	16	38	52	78
20–34	2150	5.0	24	1	2	6	6	10	15	26
35–49	3032	6.3	43	2	2	4	8	13	17	33
50–64	4810	8.2	37	3	4	6	10	16	20	29
65+	13333	9.8	48	4	6	8	12	17	22	36
TOTAL SINGLE DX	419	3.9	10	1	2	3	5	8	10	14
MULTIPLE DX	30706	9.8	108	2	4	7	11	19	28	60
TOTAL										
0–19 Years	7616	13.5	261	2	3	7	16	37	52	78
20–34	2210	5.0	24	1	2	3	6	10	15	26
35–49	3089	6.2	42	2	2	4	8	13	17	33
50–64	4843	8.2	37	3	4	6	10	16	20	29
65+	13367	9.8	48	4	5	8	12	17	22	36
GRAND TOTAL	31125	9.7	107	2	4	7	11	19	28	59

97.0: GI APPLIANCE REPLACEMENT. Formerly included in operation group(s) 796.

Type of Patients	Observed Patients	Avg. Stay	Vari-ance	Percentiles						
				10th	25th	50th	75th	90th	95th	99th
1. SINGLE DX										
0–19 Years	8	5.8	27	1	2	4	14	14	14	14
20–34	5	6.9	19	1	1	10	10	10	10	10
35–49	6	5.2	2	5	5	6	6	6	6	6
50–64	7	2.6	5	1	1	2	3	7	7	7
65+	10	3.4	11	1	1	2	5	10	10	10
2. MULTIPLE DX										
0–19 Years	385	7.3	46	2	2	6	12	12	15	34
20–34	114	9.0	129	1	2	6	10	19	35	>99
35–49	194	6.0	40	1	2	4	7	13	18	38
50–64	337	6.9	74	1	3	4	9	15	18	57
65+	1820	7.9	50	2	3	6	10	15	22	38
TOTAL SINGLE DX	36	5.0	14	1	2	5	6	10	14	14
MULTIPLE DX	2850	7.5	56	1	3	6	10	15	20	39
TOTAL										
0–19 Years	393	7.3	46	2	2	6	12	12	15	34
20–34	119	8.9	125	1	2	6	10	19	35	>99
35–49	200	5.9	38	1	2	5	7	13	17	38
50–64	344	6.8	74	1	2	4	9	15	18	50
65+	1830	7.8	50	2	3	6	10	15	22	38
GRAND TOTAL	2886	7.5	55	1	3	6	10	14	20	39

96.72: CONT MECH VENT->95 HOURS. Formerly included in operation group(s) 790.

Type of Patients	Observed Patients	Avg. Stay	Vari-ance	Percentiles						
				10th	25th	50th	75th	90th	95th	99th
1. SINGLE DX										
0–19 Years	27	12.5	50	7	7	11	14	25	28	31
20–34	3	5.9	5	5	5	5	5	10	10	10
35–49	3	14.2	54	8	8	8	19	28	28	28
50–64	6	18.7	135	4	6	18	26	34	34	34
65+	22	30.0	662	5	14	23	64	90	>99	>99
2. MULTIPLE DX										
0–19 Years	4083	32.2	649	8	13	24	56	86	>99	>99
20–34	625	17.9	158	6	10	15	22	31	48	>99
35–49	1294	18.5	155	8	11	16	22	34	44	93
50–64	2529	17.9	115	8	11	16	21	30	39	73
65+	5885	18.1	114	8	11	16	22	30	38	67
TOTAL SINGLE DX	61	17.5	278	6	7	13	23	34	66	>99
MULTIPLE DX	14416	22.4	326	8	12	17	26	54	78	>99
TOTAL										
0–19 Years	4110	32.0	647	8	13	24	56	85	>99	>99
20–34	628	17.8	158	6	10	15	22	31	48	>99
35–49	1297	18.4	155	8	11	16	22	34	44	93
50–64	2535	17.9	115	8	11	16	21	30	39	73
65+	5907	18.2	116	8	11	16	22	30	38	70
GRAND TOTAL	14477	22.4	326	8	12	17	26	54	78	>99

97.02: REPL GASTROSTOMY TUBE. Formerly included in operation group(s) 796.

Type of Patients	Observed Patients	Avg. Stay	Vari-ance	Percentiles						
				10th	25th	50th	75th	90th	95th	99th
1. SINGLE DX										
0–19 Years	5	7.8	30	1	4	4	14	14	14	14
20–34	0									
35–49	2	4.7	1	5	5	5	5	5	5	5
50–64	1	2.0	0	2	2	2	2	2	2	2
65+	7	4.2	13	1	1	3	5	10	10	10
2. MULTIPLE DX										
0–19 Years	343	7.1	68	1	2	4	9	15	19	45
20–34	78	10.9	164	2	2	8	16	22	35	72
35–49	101	6.6	35	1	3	5	9	14	18	26
50–64	199	10.1	113	3	4	7	13	18	30	75
65+	1505	8.4	50	2	4	7	10	16	23	35
TOTAL SINGLE DX	15	5.5	17	1	3	5	5	14	14	14
MULTIPLE DX	2226	8.4	65	2	4	6	10	17	23	43
TOTAL										
0–19 Years	348	7.1	67	1	2	4	9	15	19	45
20–34	78	10.9	164	2	2	8	16	22	35	72
35–49	103	6.6	33	1	3	5	8	14	18	26
50–64	200	10.1	113	3	4	7	13	18	30	75
65+	1512	8.4	50	2	4	6	10	16	23	35
GRAND TOTAL	2241	8.4	64	2	4	6	10	16	23	43

Length of Stay by Diagnosis and Operation, United States, 1997

United States, October 1995–September 1996 Data, by Operation

97.03: REPL SMALL INTEST TUBE. Formerly included in operation group(s) 796.

Type of Patients	Observed Patients	Avg. Stay	Variance	10th	25th	50th	75th	90th	95th	99th
1. SINGLE DX										
0–19 Years	2	2.3	<1	2	2	2	3	3	3	3
20–34	0									
35–49	1	6.0	0	6	6	6	6	6	6	6
50–64	0									
65+	0									
2. MULTIPLE DX										
0–19 Years	22	7.8	22	2	2	10	12	12	12	15
20–34	15	6.0	29	2	3	4	7	11	11	23
35–49	19	6.4	65	1	1	3	8	19	29	33
50–64	26	6.3	42	1	4	4	5	13	26	26
65+	98	9.0	80	2	3	7	10	19	39	39
TOTAL SINGLE DX	3	3.5	3	2	2	3	6	6	6	6
MULTIPLE DX	180	7.8	41	2	2	8	12	12	14	39
TOTAL										
0–19 Years	24	7.7	22	2	2	10	12	12	12	15
20–34	15	6.0	29	2	3	4	7	11	23	23
35–49	20	6.4	62	1	1	4	8	13	29	33
50–64	26	6.3	42	1	4	4	5	13	26	26
65+	98	9.0	80	2	3	7	10	19	39	39
GRAND TOTAL	183	7.8	41	2	2	8	12	12	14	39

97.05: REPL PANC/BILIARY STENT. Formerly included in operation group(s) 796.

Type of Patients	Observed Patients	Avg. Stay	Variance	10th	25th	50th	75th	90th	95th	99th
1. SINGLE DX										
0–19 Years	0									
20–34	5	6.9	19	1	6	10	10	10	10	10
35–49	3	5.4	3	6	6	6	6	7	7	7
50–64	6	2.7	6	1	1	1	5	6	7	7
65+	3	1.3	<1	1	1	1	2	2	2	2
2. MULTIPLE DX										
0–19 Years	15	5.5	16	1	2	3	10	10	10	10
20–34	18	3.7	9	1	1	1	6	8	8	8
35–49	68	3.8	9	1	1	3	5	7	8	14
50–64	109	3.2	12	1	1	2	4	6	12	15
65+	200	3.9	14	1	1	3	5	9	11	18
TOTAL SINGLE DX	17	5.0	12	1	1	6	7	10	10	10
MULTIPLE DX	410	3.7	13	1	1	2	5	9	11	18
TOTAL										
0–19 Years	15	5.5	16	1	2	3	10	10	10	10
20–34	23	4.2	12	1	1	2	6	7	10	10
35–49	71	3.9	9	1	1	3	6	7	10	14
50–64	115	3.2	12	1	1	2	4	6	12	15
65+	203	3.9	14	1	1	3	5	9	11	18
GRAND TOTAL	427	3.8	13	1	1	3	5	9	11	18

97.1: REPL MS APPLIANCE. Formerly included in operation group(s) 796.

Type of Patients	Observed Patients	Avg. Stay	Variance	10th	25th	50th	75th	90th	95th	99th
1. SINGLE DX										
0–19 Years	21	3.6	36	1	1	1	2	11	24	24
20–34	8	2.4	4	1	1	2	3	7	7	7
35–49	2	2.0	0	1	1	1	1	2	2	2
50–64	3	1.0	0	2	1	1	1	1	1	1
65+	1	1.0	0	1	1	1	1	1	1	1
2. MULTIPLE DX										
0–19 Years	60	3.6	14	1	1	2	4	7	12	17
20–34	12	4.6	14	1	3	4	5	7	8	24
35–49	13	7.3	121	2	2	4	7	13	49	49
50–64	8	4.2	4	2	2	4	5	8	8	8
65+	42	7.9	38	3	5	6	8	16	24	31
TOTAL SINGLE DX	34	2.7	16	1	1	2	2	7	11	24
MULTIPLE DX	135	5.6	37	1	2	4	6	11	17	31
TOTAL										
0–19 Years	81	3.6	17	1	1	2	4	8	12	23
20–34	20	4.0	12	1	2	4	4	7	24	24
35–49	14	6.0	97	2	2	4	6	10	24	49
50–64	11	3.3	5	2	2	4	5	6	8	8
65+	43	7.8	38	3	5	6	8	16	24	31
GRAND TOTAL	169	5.2	35	1	2	4	6	11	16	31

97.2: OTHER NONOP REPLACEMENT. Formerly included in operation group(s) 796.

Type of Patients	Observed Patients	Avg. Stay	Variance	10th	25th	50th	75th	90th	95th	99th
1. SINGLE DX										
0–19 Years	0									
20–34	2	1.0	0	1	1	1	1	1	1	1
35–49	3	2.3	2	1	1	2	4	4	4	4
50–64	1	4.0	0	4	4	4	4	4	4	4
65+	2	3.3	5	1	1	5	5	5	5	5
2. MULTIPLE DX										
0–19 Years	104	4.5	33	1	1	3	5	9	13	27
20–34	34	10.7	233	2	4	7	13	80	>99	>99
35–49	54	10.3	119	2	3	7	16	18	35	>99
50–64	96	8.8	58	1	4	6	13	15	28	>99
65+	165	9.0	92	1	6	9	14	23	28	54
TOTAL SINGLE DX	8	2.5	3	1	1	2	4	5	5	5
MULTIPLE DX	453	8.1	83	1	2	5	11	23	28	>99
TOTAL										
0–19 Years	104	4.5	33	1	1	3	5	9	13	27
20–34	36	10.5	229	2	4	7	13	80	>99	>99
35–49	57	10.0	117	2	3	7	16	18	35	>99
50–64	97	8.7	58	1	4	5	13	15	28	>99
65+	167	9.0	91	1	5	6	14	23	28	52
GRAND TOTAL	461	8.0	83	1	2	5	10	23	28	>99

Length of Stay by Diagnosis and Operation, United States, 1997

United States, October 1995–September 1996 Data, by Operation

97.23: REPL TRACH TUBE. Formerly included in operation group(s) 796.

Type of Patients	Observed Patients	Avg. Stay	Vari-ance	Percentiles						
				10th	25th	50th	75th	90th	95th	99th
1. SINGLE DX										
0–19 Years	0									
20–34	2	1.0	0	1	1	1	1	1	1	1
35–49	2	1.3	<1	1	1	1	2	2	2	2
50–64	1	4.0	0	4	4	4	4	4	4	4
65+	2	3.3	5	1	1	5	5	5	5	5
2. MULTIPLE DX										
0–19 Years	100	4.5	35	1	1	3	5	10	14	27
20–34	30	12.0	264	3	6	9	13	80	>99	>99
35–49	46	10.1	134	2	3	7	13	18	35	>99
50–64	86	9.0	64	1	4	7	14	15	28	>99
65+	137	9.3	96	1	1	6	15	23	28	54
TOTAL SINGLE DX	7	2.2	3	1	1	1	4	5	5	5
MULTIPLE DX	399	8.3	89	1	2	5	11	23	28	>99
TOTAL										
0–19 Years	100	4.5	35	1	1	3	5	10	14	27
20–34	32	11.6	259	2	5	9	13	80	>99	>99
35–49	48	9.8	132	2	3	7	12	18	35	>99
50–64	87	9.0	64	1	4	7	14	15	28	>99
65+	139	9.3	96	1	1	6	15	23	28	54
GRAND TOTAL	406	8.2	88	1	2	5	11	23	28	>99

97.4: RMVL THOR THER DEVICE. Formerly included in operation group(s) 796.

Type of Patients	Observed Patients	Avg. Stay	Vari-ance	Percentiles						
				10th	25th	50th	75th	90th	95th	99th
1. SINGLE DX										
0–19 Years	4	1.7	2	1	1	1	1	4	4	4
20–34	5	4.9	37	1	1	4	5	19	19	19
35–49	1	3.0	0	3	3	3	3	3	3	3
50–64	2	1.5	<1	1	1	1	2	2	2	2
65+	0									
2. MULTIPLE DX										
0–19 Years	51	7.5	45	2	3	4	12	16	17	34
20–34	74	8.4	51	2	3	6	12	22	23	30
35–49	97	7.4	64	2	3	6	8	17	19	46
50–64	119	7.3	54	2	3	4	8	19	25	34
65+	112	6.9	37	2	3	4	9	17	20	28
TOTAL SINGLE DX	12	3.3	20	1	1	1	4	5	19	19
MULTIPLE DX	453	7.5	50	2	3	5	9	18	23	34
TOTAL										
0–19 Years	55	7.1	44	1	3	4	11	16	17	34
20–34	79	8.3	51	2	3	6	11	20	23	30
35–49	98	7.4	63	2	3	6	8	17	19	46
50–64	121	7.3	53	2	3	4	8	19	25	34
65+	112	6.9	37	2	3	4	9	17	20	28
GRAND TOTAL	465	7.4	50	2	3	5	9	18	23	31

97.3: RMVL THER DEV-HEAD/NK. Formerly included in operation group(s) 796.

Type of Patients	Observed Patients	Avg. Stay	Vari-ance	Percentiles						
				10th	25th	50th	75th	90th	95th	99th
1. SINGLE DX										
0–19 Years	26	1.4	<1	1	1	1	1	2	3	4
20–34	4	4.1	3	3	3	3	4	7	7	7
35–49	7	1.8	7	1	1	1	2	2	2	14
50–64	3	6.3	20	4	4	10	10	10	10	10
65+	1	6.0	0	6	6	6	6	6	6	6
2. MULTIPLE DX										
0–19 Years	129	3.6	46	1	2	2	3	7	10	78
20–34	29	9.3	118	2	4	5	6	27	33	45
35–49	44	11.4	341	1	1	4	7	56	56	58
50–64	49	3.4	6	1	1	3	5	7	7	13
65+	118	10.3	53	2	3	8	18	18	18	32
TOTAL SINGLE DX	41	1.9	5	1	1	1	2	3	6	10
MULTIPLE DX	369	7.0	88	1	2	3	8	18	18	56
TOTAL										
0–19 Years	155	3.3	40	1	1	2	3	6	10	50
20–34	33	8.9	111	2	4	5	6	26	33	45
35–49	51	9.7	294	1	1	3	7	56	56	56
50–64	52	3.5	7	1	1	3	5	7	7	13
65+	119	10.2	53	2	3	8	18	18	18	32
GRAND TOTAL	410	6.5	83	1	2	3	7	18	18	56

97.49: RMVL OTH DEV FROM THORAX. Formerly included in operation group(s) 796.

Type of Patients	Observed Patients	Avg. Stay	Vari-ance	Percentiles						
				10th	25th	50th	75th	90th	95th	99th
1. SINGLE DX										
0–19 Years	4	1.7	2	1	1	1	1	4	4	4
20–34	4	5.0	42	1	1	1	5	19	19	19
35–49	0									
50–64	1	2.0	0	2	2	2	2	2	2	2
65+	0									
2. MULTIPLE DX										
0–19 Years	46	7.9	47	2	3	6	12	16	17	34
20–34	69	8.6	52	2	3	6	12	23	23	30
35–49	87	7.6	69	2	3	6	8	18	20	46
50–64	104	7.4	57	2	3	4	8	19	25	34
65+	94	6.6	38	2	3	4	9	14	21	28
TOTAL SINGLE DX	9	3.4	24	1	1	1	4	5	19	19
MULTIPLE DX	400	7.6	53	2	3	5	9	19	23	34
TOTAL										
0–19 Years	50	7.4	46	1	3	4	12	16	17	34
20–34	73	8.4	52	2	3	6	12	22	23	30
35–49	87	7.6	69	2	3	6	8	18	20	46
50–64	105	7.4	56	2	3	4	8	19	25	34
65+	94	6.6	38	2	3	4	9	14	21	28
GRAND TOTAL	409	7.5	53	2	3	5	9	19	23	34

Length of Stay by Diagnosis and Operation, United States, 1997

United States, October 1995–September 1996 Data, by Operation

97.5: NONOP RMVL GI THER DEV. Formerly included in operation group(s) 796.

Type of Patients	Observed Patients	Avg. Stay	Vari-ance	10th	25th	50th	75th	90th	95th	99th
1. SINGLE DX										
0–19 Years	2	4.0	21	1	1	1	8	8	8	8
20–34	1	4.0	0	4	4	4	4	4	4	4
35–49	3	2.3	<1	2	2	2	2	4	4	4
50–64	2	1.0	0	1	1	1	1	1	1	1
65+	2	2.5	<1	2	2	2	3	3	3	3
2. MULTIPLE DX										
0–19 Years	43	10.6	313	1	3	4	8	32	64	79
20–34	25	10.1	256	1	2	2	12	22	47	75
35–49	54	15.0	419	1	3	7	22	30	59	94
50–64	70	13.6	205	2	3	7	25	44	44	44
65+	229	9.6	87	2	4	7	13	20	28	56
TOTAL SINGLE DX	10	2.7	3	1	2	2	4	4	4	8
MULTIPLE DX	421	11.1	186	1	3	7	13	28	44	75
TOTAL										
0–19 Years	45	10.5	309	1	3	4	8	32	64	79
20–34	26	9.8	246	1	2	2	12	22	47	75
35–49	57	14.0	398	1	3	6	20	30	47	94
50–64	72	13.5	205	2	3	7	25	44	44	44
65+	231	9.5	87	2	4	7	13	20	27	56
GRAND TOTAL	431	10.9	184	1	3	6	13	28	44	75

97.62: RMVL URETERAL DRAIN. Formerly included in operation group(s) 796.

Type of Patients	Observed Patients	Avg. Stay	Vari-ance	10th	25th	50th	75th	90th	95th	99th
1. SINGLE DX										
0–19 Years	5	1.6	<1	1	1	1	2	3	3	3
20–34	16	1.4	<1	1	1	1	3	3	5	5
35–49	25	2.1	1	1	1	2	3	3	4	5
50–64	9	2.0	<1	2	2	2	2	2	2	5
65+	7	5.3	58	1	1	2	2	20	20	20
2. MULTIPLE DX										
0–19 Years	37	15.0	499	1	2	3	27	27	99	99
20–34	67	3.0	13	1	2	3	3	3	9	17
35–49	115	3.4	6	2	2	3	5	6	7	14
50–64	78	5.5	33	1	2	4	7	11	15	34
65+	154	6.9	43	2	4	6	9	12	15	29
TOTAL SINGLE DX	62	2.3	8	1	1	2	2	3	5	20
MULTIPLE DX	451	5.4	64	1	2	3	6	10	15	29
TOTAL										
0–19 Years	42	13.6	466	1	1	3	27	27	33	99
20–34	83	2.7	11	1	1	2	3	4	5	17
35–49	140	3.1	5	1	2	2	4	6	7	14
50–64	87	4.6	26	1	2	4	6	10	14	34
65+	161	6.8	44	2	3	6	9	12	18	29
GRAND TOTAL	513	4.8	56	1	2	3	5	10	14	27

97.6: NONOP RMVL URIN THER DEV. Formerly included in operation group(s) 796.

Type of Patients	Observed Patients	Avg. Stay	Vari-ance	10th	25th	50th	75th	90th	95th	99th
1. SINGLE DX										
0–19 Years	7	1.4	<1	1	1	1	2	2	3	3
20–34	18	1.3	<1	1	1	1	1	2	3	5
35–49	28	2.1	<1	1	1	2	3	3	4	5
50–64	10	1.4	<1	1	1	1	2	3	4	5
65+	8	5.0	55	1	1	1	2	20	20	20
2. MULTIPLE DX										
0–19 Years	56	13.9	451	1	1	3	27	27	53	99
20–34	80	3.1	15	1	2	2	3	4	9	27
35–49	140	3.6	8	1	2	2	5	6	6	15
50–64	98	5.4	29	2	2	4	5	11	15	34
65+	215	6.6	36	3	3	5	9	12	16	22
TOTAL SINGLE DX	71	2.0	7	1	1	2	2	3	4	20
MULTIPLE DX	589	5.6	66	1	2	3	6	10	16	35
TOTAL										
0–19 Years	63	12.7	420	1	1	3	20	27	53	99
20–34	98	2.9	13	1	2	2	3	4	7	27
35–49	168	3.3	7	1	2	2	5	6	8	15
50–64	108	3.9	22	1	1	2	5	9	13	20
65+	223	6.5	37	1	3	5	9	12	16	22
GRAND TOTAL	660	4.9	57	1	2	3	5	10	15	34

97.7: RMVL THER DEV GENIT SYST. Formerly included in operation group(s) 796.

Type of Patients	Observed Patients	Avg. Stay	Vari-ance	10th	25th	50th	75th	90th	95th	99th
1. SINGLE DX										
0–19 Years	1	3.0	0	3	3	3	3	3	3	3
20–34	17	1.9	<1	1	1	2	2	3	3	3
35–49	8	1.6	1	1	1	1	2	3	5	5
50–64	1	4.0	0	4	4	4	4	4	4	4
65+	0									
2. MULTIPLE DX										
0–19 Years	1	5.0	0	5	5	5	5	5	5	5
20–34	29	4.2	22	1	2	3	6	7	7	25
35–49	61	4.1	11	2	2	4	4	8	9	16
50–64	23	5.7	29	1	3	4	10	13	25	25
65+	34	7.3	36	3	4	5	8	13	22	28
TOTAL SINGLE DX	27	1.9	<1	1	1	2	3	3	3	5
MULTIPLE DX	148	4.9	21	2	2	4	5	8	13	28
TOTAL										
0–19 Years	2	4.1	2	3	3	5	5	5	5	5
20–34	46	3.5	17	1	2	2	3	6	7	27
35–49	69	3.9	11	2	2	4	4	8	9	16
50–64	24	5.6	29	1	3	4	6	8	25	25
65+	34	7.3	36	3	4	5	8	13	22	28
GRAND TOTAL	175	4.5	20	1	2	4	5	8	12	28

Length of Stay by Diagnosis and Operation, United States, 1997

418

United States, October 1995–September 1996 Data, by Operation

97.8: OTH NONOP RMVL THER DEV. Formerly included in operation group(s) 796.

Type of Patients	Observed Patients	Avg. Stay	Variance	10th	25th	50th	75th	90th	95th	99th
1. SINGLE DX										
0–19 Years	38	7.2	63	1	2	3	11	16	24	28
20–34	11	2.6	4	1	1	2	3	6	9	9
35–49	11	4.5	8	1	1	7	7	7	8	8
50–64	8	2.0	2	1	1	1	2	5	5	5
65+	6	2.7	5	1	1	2	4	7	7	7
2. MULTIPLE DX										
0–19 Years	282	6.2	43	1	2	3	9	13	18	31
20–34	143	6.6	44	1	3	5	8	15	23	24
35–49	223	8.1	69	2	3	7	11	15	19	34
50–64	194	7.8	50	2	3	5	10	20	20	36
65+	310	7.4	56	1	3	5	9	17	22	31
TOTAL SINGLE DX	74	5.5	43	1	1	2	7	16	21	28
MULTIPLE DX	1152	7.2	53	1	3	5	9	15	22	31
TOTAL										
0–19 Years	320	6.3	46	1	2	3	10	13	21	31
20–34	154	6.4	43	1	3	5	8	12	23	24
35–49	234	7.9	67	2	3	7	11	14	19	28
50–64	202	7.7	50	2	3	5	9	20	20	36
65+	316	7.3	55	1	3	5	9	16	22	30
GRAND TOTAL	1226	7.1	53	1	2	5	9	16	22	30

98.0: RMVL INTRALUM GI FB. Formerly included in operation group(s) 793.

Type of Patients	Observed Patients	Avg. Stay	Variance	10th	25th	50th	75th	90th	95th	99th
1. SINGLE DX										
0–19 Years	243	1.1	<1	1	1	1	1	1	2	2
20–34	24	1.2	<1	1	1	1	1	2	2	4
35–49	22	1.0	<1	1	1	1	1	1	1	2
50–64	12	1.2	<1	1	1	1	1	2	2	2
65+	5	1.1	<1	1	1	1	1	2	2	2
2. MULTIPLE DX										
0–19 Years	117	2.4	7	1	1	1	3	4	8	18
20–34	24	7.3	31	1	2	5	13	13	13	13
35–49	42	1.9	2	1	1	1	3	3	4	8
50–64	45	3.1	39	1	1	2	2	4	15	37
65+	141	3.3	7	1	1	3	4	6	8	12
TOTAL SINGLE DX	306	1.1	<1	1	1	1	1	1	2	2
MULTIPLE DX	369	3.3	16	1	1	2	4	7	13	16
TOTAL										
0–19 Years	360	1.5	3	1	1	1	1	3	4	8
20–34	48	5.1	28	1	1	2	13	13	13	13
35–49	64	1.5	1	1	1	1	1	3	3	8
50–64	57	3.0	36	1	1	3	2	4	15	37
65+	146	3.3	7	1	1	3	4	6	8	12
GRAND TOTAL	675	2.3	10	1	1	1	2	4	8	13

97.89: RMVL OTH THER DEV. Formerly included in operation group(s) 796.

Type of Patients	Observed Patients	Avg. Stay	Variance	10th	25th	50th	75th	90th	95th	99th
1. SINGLE DX										
0–19 Years	10	1.9	2	1	1	2	2	2	2	7
20–34	3	6.3	9	2	6	6	9	9	9	9
35–49	3	5.9	9	1	7	7	8	8	8	8
50–64	2	3.5	<1	3	3	3	4	4	5	8
65+	1	1.0	0	1	1	1	1	1	1	1
2. MULTIPLE DX										
0–19 Years	150	7.3	49	2	2	5	10	13	22	42
20–34	88	5.9	25	2	3	4	8	10	14	24
35–49	134	8.3	84	2	3	7	11	16	20	51
50–64	98	5.8	25	1	3	5	7	12	14	25
65+	173	6.8	40	1	3	5	9	13	18	30
TOTAL SINGLE DX	19	2.8	6	1	1	2	2	7	8	9
MULTIPLE DX	643	7.0	48	2	3	5	9	13	18	34
TOTAL										
0–19 Years	160	6.9	48	2	2	4	10	13	19	42
20–34	91	5.9	25	2	3	5	8	10	12	24
35–49	137	8.3	83	2	3	7	11	16	20	51
50–64	100	5.8	25	1	3	5	7	12	14	25
65+	174	6.8	40	1	3	5	9	13	18	30
GRAND TOTAL	662	6.9	47	2	3	5	9	13	18	31

98.02: RMVL INTRALUM ESOPH FB. Formerly included in operation group(s) 793.

Type of Patients	Observed Patients	Avg. Stay	Variance	10th	25th	50th	75th	90th	95th	99th
1. SINGLE DX										
0–19 Years	231	1.1	<1	1	1	1	1	1	2	2
20–34	10	1.2	<1	1	1	1	1	2	2	2
35–49	6	1.5	<1	1	1	1	2	3	3	3
50–64	9	1.1	<1	1	1	1	1	1	2	2
65+	5	1.1	<1	1	1	1	1	2	2	2
2. MULTIPLE DX										
0–19 Years	105	2.1	6	1	1	1	2	4	6	18
20–34	12	2.2	6	1	1	2	2	3	4	16
35–49	19	1.5	<1	1	1	1	2	2	3	3
50–64	34	2.4	7	1	1	2	2	4	6	15
65+	122	3.2	7	1	1	3	4	5	7	12
TOTAL SINGLE DX	261	1.1	<1	1	1	1	1	1	2	2
MULTIPLE DX	292	2.6	7	1	1	2	4	5	7	15
TOTAL										
0–19 Years	336	1.4	2	1	1	1	2	3	3	8
20–34	22	1.7	3	1	1	2	2	3	3	16
35–49	25	1.5	<1	1	1	1	2	3	3	3
50–64	43	2.3	7	1	1	2	2	4	6	15
65+	127	3.2	7	1	1	3	4	5	7	12
GRAND TOTAL	553	1.9	4	1	1	1	2	4	5	11

Length of Stay by Diagnosis and Operation, United States, 1997

United States, October 1995–September 1996 Data, by Operation

98.1: RMVL INTRALUM FB NEC. Formerly included in operation group(s) 793.

Type of Patients	Observed Patients	Avg. Stay	Vari-ance	10th	25th	50th	75th	90th	95th	99th
1. SINGLE DX										
0–19 Years	151	1.2	<1	1	1	1	1	1	2	5
20–34	24	1.0	0	1	1	1	1	1	1	1
35–49	6	1.3	<1	1	1	1	1	2	3	3
50–64	2	1.0	0	1	1	1	1	1	1	1
65+	4	1.0	<1	1	1	1	1	1	1	2
2. MULTIPLE DX										
0–19 Years	129	4.3	30	1	1	2	4	18	19	19
20–34	24	3.6	19	1	2	2	3	10	14	23
35–49	27	3.4	12	1	1	2	5	7	11	16
50–64	21	3.1	13	1	1	2	5	9	9	16
65+	69	5.9	37	1	2	3	10	15	17	28
TOTAL SINGLE DX	165	1.2	<1	1	1	1	1	1	2	5
MULTIPLE DX	270	4.6	29	1	1	2	5	11	18	20
TOTAL										
0–19 Years	280	2.3	13	1	1	1	2	4	8	19
20–34	26	3.5	18	1	2	2	3	7	14	23
35–49	33	3.2	11	1	1	2	5	7	11	16
50–64	23	3.0	13	1	1	1	3	9	10	16
65+	73	5.2	35	1	2	3	8	12	17	28
GRAND TOTAL	435	3.0	19	1	1	1	3	8	14	19

98.2: RMVL OTH FB W/O INC. Formerly included in operation group(s) 793.

Type of Patients	Observed Patients	Avg. Stay	Vari-ance	10th	25th	50th	75th	90th	95th	99th
1. SINGLE DX										
0–19 Years	33	1.5	2	1	1	1	2	3	3	8
20–34	25	1.4	<1	1	1	1	1	2	3	4
35–49	14	2.7	3	1	2	3	3	8	8	8
50–64	2	2.0	0	2	2	3	3	2	2	2
65+	3	1.6	<1	1	1	2	2	2	2	2
2. MULTIPLE DX										
0–19 Years	76	3.9	34	1	1	2	5	6	15	38
20–34	66	3.0	25	1	1	1	3	6	8	23
35–49	63	4.7	40	2	2	3	7	7	8	40
50–64	28	5.4	64	2	2	2	7	10	18	29
65+	41	8.7	64	3	4	5	10	27	27	27
TOTAL SINGLE DX	77	1.7	2	1	1	1	2	3	3	8
MULTIPLE DX	274	4.5	39	1	1	3	5	8	15	31
TOTAL										
0–19 Years	109	3.2	26	1	1	2	4	5	9	26
20–34	91	2.6	19	1	1	1	3	6	8	23
35–49	77	4.3	33	1	2	3	6	7	8	40
50–64	30	5.2	33	2	2	4	7	10	18	29
65+	44	8.3	63	2	4	4	10	27	27	27
GRAND TOTAL	351	3.9	32	1	1	2	4	7	11	27

98.5: ESWL. Formerly included in operation group(s) 629, 662, 793.

Type of Patients	Observed Patients	Avg. Stay	Vari-ance	10th	25th	50th	75th	90th	95th	99th
1. SINGLE DX										
0–19 Years	18	2.0	2	1	1	1	3	5	5	5
20–34	136	1.8	2	1	1	1	3	5	4	7
35–49	202	2.0	1	1	1	2	2	3	4	7
50–64	107	2.0	1	1	1	2	2	3	4	7
65+	60	1.8	1	1	1	1	2	4	5	5
2. MULTIPLE DX										
0–19 Years	33	3.6	7	1	2	3	4	7	11	11
20–34	169	3.5	14	1	2	3	4	7	11	15
35–49	339	2.6	5	1	1	2	3	5	6	13
50–64	348	4.1	33	1	1	2	4	8	16	31
65+	435	4.0	14	1	1	3	5	9	10	17
TOTAL SINGLE DX	523	1.9	2	1	1	2	2	3	4	7
MULTIPLE DX	1324	3.5	17	1	1	2	4	7	10	28
TOTAL										
0–19 Years	51	3.2	6	1	1	3	4	5	11	11
20–34	305	2.7	9	1	1	2	3	6	8	14
35–49	541	2.4	4	1	1	2	3	5	6	12
50–64	455	3.7	27	1	1	2	4	7	13	28
65+	495	3.7	13	1	1	2	5	8	10	17
GRAND TOTAL	1847	3.0	13	1	1	2	3	6	9	19

98.51: RENAL/URETER/BLAD ESWL. Formerly included in operation group(s) 662.

Type of Patients	Observed Patients	Avg. Stay	Vari-ance	10th	25th	50th	75th	90th	95th	99th
1. SINGLE DX										
0–19 Years	18	2.0	2	1	1	1	3	5	5	5
20–34	136	1.8	2	1	1	1	3	5	4	7
35–49	201	2.0	1	1	1	2	2	3	4	7
50–64	106	1.9	<1	1	1	2	2	3	4	4
65+	59	1.7	1	1	1	1	2	3	5	5
2. MULTIPLE DX										
0–19 Years	33	3.6	7	1	2	3	4	7	11	11
20–34	169	3.5	14	1	2	3	4	7	10	15
35–49	335	2.6	5	1	1	2	3	5	6	13
50–64	344	4.2	34	1	1	2	4	8	17	31
65+	433	4.0	14	1	1	3	5	9	10	17
TOTAL SINGLE DX	520	1.9	1	1	1	2	2	3	4	7
MULTIPLE DX	1314	3.5	17	1	1	2	4	7	10	28
TOTAL										
0–19 Years	51	3.2	6	1	1	3	4	5	11	11
20–34	305	2.7	9	1	1	2	3	6	8	14
35–49	536	2.4	4	1	1	2	3	5	6	12
50–64	450	3.7	28	1	1	2	3	7	13	28
65+	492	3.7	13	1	1	2	5	8	10	17
GRAND TOTAL	1834	3.0	13	1	1	2	3	6	9	19

Length of Stay by Diagnosis and Operation, United States, 1997

United States, October 1995–September 1996 Data, by Operation

99.0: BLOOD TRANSFUSION. Formerly included in operation group(s) 794.

Type of Patients	Observed Patients	Avg. Stay	Vari-ance	10th	25th	50th	75th	90th	95th	99th
1. SINGLE DX										
0–19 Years	574	2.9	7	1	1	2	3	6	8	12
20–34	360	4.4	13	1	2	3	6	9	12	15
35–49	208	3.8	27	1	2	3	4	7	9	17
50–64	117	2.8	4	1	1	3	4	5	8	10
65+	244	3.1	16	1	1	1	3	10	13	13
2. MULTIPLE DX										
0–19 Years	4238	5.9	59	1	2	4	7	11	16	45
20–34	3316	5.4	30	1	2	4	7	11	15	26
35–49	5561	5.3	24	1	2	4	7	11	14	24
50–64	6835	5.7	26	1	2	4	7	11	15	28
65+	26516	6.3	30	2	3	5	8	12	16	27
TOTAL SINGLE DX	1503	3.4	13	1	1	2	4	7	9	15
MULTIPLE DX	46466	6.0	31	1	3	4	8	12	16	28
TOTAL										
0–19 Years	4812	5.5	54	1	2	4	6	11	15	44
20–34	3676	5.3	28	1	2	4	7	11	14	26
35–49	5769	5.3	25	1	2	4	7	11	14	24
50–64	6952	5.6	25	1	2	4	7	11	15	28
65+	26760	6.3	30	2	3	5	8	12	16	27
GRAND TOTAL	47969	5.9	31	1	3	4	7	12	15	28

99.01: EXCHANGE TRANSFUSION. Formerly included in operation group(s) 794.

Type of Patients	Observed Patients	Avg. Stay	Vari-ance	10th	25th	50th	75th	90th	95th	99th
1. SINGLE DX										
0–19 Years	26	4.5	20	1	2	3	5	7	20	20
20–34	9	8.9	39	1	2	10	15	15	15	15
35–49	5	7.0	22	4	4	7	7	17	17	17
50–64	0									
65+	1	25.0	0	25	25	25	25	25	25	25
2. MULTIPLE DX										
0–19 Years	284	6.8	47	2	3	5	8	12	15	38
20–34	50	6.6	53	1	3	5	8	10	14	46
35–49	21	7.4	72	1	3	5	9	22	24	41
50–64	9	6.9	21	2	5	6	10	10	20	20
65+	11	7.1	24	2	3	6	8	17	17	17
TOTAL SINGLE DX	41	6.2	33	1	2	4	7	15	20	25
MULTIPLE DX	375	6.8	47	2	3	5	8	12	17	39
TOTAL										
0–19 Years	310	6.6	46	2	3	5	8	12	16	38
20–34	59	7.1	51	1	3	5	9	15	15	39
35–49	26	7.3	58	1	3	5	7	17	24	41
50–64	9	6.9	21	2	5	6	10	10	20	20
65+	12	8.0	38	2	3	6	8	17	20	25
GRAND TOTAL	416	6.8	46	2	3	5	8	12	17	39

99.03: WHOLE BLOOD TRANSFUS NEC. Formerly included in operation group(s) 794.

Type of Patients	Observed Patients	Avg. Stay	Vari-ance	10th	25th	50th	75th	90th	95th	99th
1. SINGLE DX										
0–19 Years	11	1.6	<1	1	1	1	2	3	3	4
20–34	4	4.8	17	2	2	2	10	10	10	10
35–49	4	2.9	2	3	2	3	4	4	4	4
50–64	2	1.4	1	1	1	1	1	4	4	4
65+	1	1.0	0	1	1	1	1	1	1	1
2. MULTIPLE DX										
0–19 Years	50	9.9	233	2	2	5	9	21	44	73
20–34	39	5.7	27	2	3	4	6	14	16	24
35–49	64	3.7	7	2	2	3	4	8	8	12
50–64	73	5.0	13	1	3	4	6	9	11	17
65+	279	5.6	24	1	2	4	7	12	15	24
TOTAL SINGLE DX	22	2.2	4	1	1	1	2	4	4	10
MULTIPLE DX	505	5.6	35	1	2	4	7	11	15	24
TOTAL										
0–19 Years	61	8.4	201	1	2	4	7	14	40	73
20–34	43	5.6	26	2	3	4	6	14	16	24
35–49	68	3.7	7	2	2	3	4	8	8	12
50–64	75	4.9	13	1	3	4	6	9	11	17
65+	280	5.6	24	1	2	4	7	12	15	24
GRAND TOTAL	527	5.5	34	1	2	4	7	11	15	24

99.04: PACKED CELL TRANSFUSION. Formerly included in operation group(s) 794.

Type of Patients	Observed Patients	Avg. Stay	Vari-ance	10th	25th	50th	75th	90th	95th	99th
1. SINGLE DX										
0–19 Years	443	2.8	6	1	1	2	4	7	9	10
20–34	322	4.3	12	1	2	3	6	9	11	15
35–49	179	4.1	31	1	2	3	6	7	10	25
50–64	103	2.9	4	1	1	2	4	5	8	10
65+	226	3.1	15	1	1	1	3	11	13	13
2. MULTIPLE DX										
0–19 Years	2997	5.8	55	1	2	4	6	11	16	42
20–34	2923	5.5	30	1	2	4	7	11	15	26
35–49	4904	5.3	25	1	2	4	7	11	14	25
50–64	6022	5.5	24	1	2	4	7	11	14	28
65+	24653	6.3	30	2	3	5	8	12	16	27
TOTAL SINGLE DX	1273	3.4	13	1	1	2	4	7	10	14
MULTIPLE DX	41499	6.0	31	1	3	4	8	12	15	28
TOTAL										
0–19 Years	3440	5.5	50	1	2	4	6	10	15	41
20–34	3245	5.4	29	1	2	4	7	11	14	26
35–49	5083	5.3	26	1	2	4	7	11	15	25
50–64	6125	5.5	24	1	2	4	7	11	14	28
65+	24879	6.3	30	2	3	5	8	12	16	27
GRAND TOTAL	42772	5.9	30	1	3	4	7	12	15	28

Length of Stay by Diagnosis and Operation, United States, 1997

United States, October 1995–September 1996 Data, by Operation

99.05: PLATELET TRANSFUSION. Formerly included in operation group(s) 794.

Type of Patients	Observed Patients	Avg. Stay	Variance	10th	25th	50th	75th	90th	95th	99th
1. SINGLE DX										
0–19 Years	26	3.8	10	1	3	3	5	5	9	18
20–34	10	5.0	5	2	5	5	5	6	11	16
35–49	7	1.6	<1	1	1	2	2	2	2	4
50–64	7	1.6	<1	1	1	1	3	3	3	3
65+	12	1.5	<1	1	1	1	2	2	4	4
2. MULTIPLE DX										
0–19 Years	665	5.1	27	1	2	4	6	11	15	29
20–34	171	6.1	30	1	2	4	9	13	16	29
35–49	323	6.0	21	1	2	5	9	12	14	20
50–64	400	7.6	45	1	3	6	10	19	19	26
65+	714	6.3	22	1	3	5	9	11	14	22
TOTAL SINGLE DX	62	3.1	7	1	1	3	5	5	5	18
MULTIPLE DX	2273	6.2	30	1	2	5	9	12	16	24
TOTAL										
0–19 Years	691	5.0	26	1	2	4	6	10	15	29
20–34	181	6.0	27	1	2	5	8	12	16	29
35–49	330	5.7	21	1	2	4	9	12	14	19
50–64	407	7.6	45	1	3	6	10	19	19	26
65+	726	6.3	22	1	3	5	9	11	14	22
GRAND TOTAL	2335	6.1	29	1	2	5	8	12	16	24

99.07: SERUM TRANSFUSION NEC. Formerly included in operation group(s) 794.

Type of Patients	Observed Patients	Avg. Stay	Variance	10th	25th	50th	75th	90th	95th	99th
1. SINGLE DX										
0–19 Years	22	1.0	<1	1	1	1	1	1	1	2
20–34	5	6.3	14	1	1	8	9	10	10	10
35–49	2	3.0	2	1	3	3	4	4	4	4
50–64	4	3.1	<1	3	3	3	4	4	4	4
65+	3	1.9	<1	1	1	2	3	3	3	3
2. MULTIPLE DX										
0–19 Years	60	12.0	389	1	3	5	7	65	65	65
20–34	52	5.4	12	2	3	4	7	10	11	18
35–49	181	5.2	15	2	3	4	6	10	12	22
50–64	262	5.2	20	2	3	4	7	10	11	23
65+	730	6.5	26	2	3	5	9	13	17	24
TOTAL SINGLE DX	36	2.0	3	1	1	1	3	4	4	9
MULTIPLE DX	1285	6.1	38	2	2	4	8	11	15	26
TOTAL										
0–19 Years	82	9.0	306	1	1	3	6	15	65	65
20–34	57	5.5	12	2	3	4	7	10	11	18
35–49	183	5.2	15	2	3	4	6	10	12	22
50–64	266	5.2	20	1	2	4	7	10	11	23
65+	733	6.5	26	2	3	5	9	13	17	24
GRAND TOTAL	1321	6.0	38	1	2	4	8	11	15	26

99.1: INJECT/INFUSE THER SUBST. Formerly included in operation group(s) 794.

Type of Patients	Observed Patients	Avg. Stay	Variance	10th	25th	50th	75th	90th	95th	99th
1. SINGLE DX										
0–19 Years	779	2.6	4	1	1	2	3	5	6	11
20–34	489	3.5	8	1	2	2	3	5	8	13
35–49	254	3.9	12	1	2	3	5	7	10	14
50–64	168	4.0	6	1	2	4	5	7	8	12
65+	113	4.6	16	1	2	4	6	9	12	14
2. MULTIPLE DX										
0–19 Years	3352	7.9	100	1	2	4	9	18	28	53
20–34	1744	6.0	55	1	2	4	7	13	19	36
35–49	2154	6.8	46	2	3	5	8	14	19	34
50–64	2496	6.8	53	2	3	5	8	13	20	36
65+	4642	7.5	43	2	4	6	9	15	21	33
TOTAL SINGLE DX	1803	3.3	7	1	1	2	4	7	8	13
MULTIPLE DX	14388	7.2	61	2	3	5	8	15	21	40
TOTAL										
0–19 Years	4131	6.9	88	1	2	4	8	16	25	50
20–34	2233	5.5	46	1	2	3	7	12	18	34
35–49	2408	6.5	44	1	3	5	8	13	18	33
50–64	2664	6.6	51	2	3	5	8	12	19	36
65+	4755	7.5	42	2	4	6	9	15	21	32
GRAND TOTAL	16191	6.8	56	1	3	5	8	14	20	38

99.11: INJECT RH IMMUNE GLOB. Formerly included in operation group(s) 794.

Type of Patients	Observed Patients	Avg. Stay	Variance	10th	25th	50th	75th	90th	95th	99th
1. SINGLE DX										
0–19 Years	27	1.5	<1	1	1	1	2	2	4	4
20–34	107	1.5	<1	1	1	1	2	2	3	4
35–49	6	1.2	<1	1	1	1	1	2	2	3
50–64	1	4.0	0	4	4	4	4	4	4	4
65+	1	4.0	0	4	4	4	4	4	4	4
2. MULTIPLE DX										
0–19 Years	61	3.0	6	2	2	2	4	6	10	10
20–34	238	2.1	13	1	2	2	2	3	4	13
35–49	46	3.0	5	1	3	5	5	8	8	12
50–64	3	3.0	6	1	1	1	5	5	5	5
65+	6	7.5	100	1	1	5	12	27	27	27
TOTAL SINGLE DX	142	1.5	<1	1	1	1	2	2	3	4
MULTIPLE DX	353	2.3	12	1	1	2	2	4	6	13
TOTAL										
0–19 Years	88	2.5	5	1	1	2	3	4	7	10
20–34	345	2.0	10	1	1	1	2	3	4	13
35–49	52	2.7	5	1	1	1	5	5	5	12
50–64	3	3.3	4	1	1	4	5	5	5	5
65+	7	7.1	88	1	3	3	12	27	27	27
GRAND TOTAL	495	2.1	10	1	1	2	2	4	5	12

Length of Stay by Diagnosis and Operation, United States, 1997

United States, October 1995–September 1996 Data, by Operation

99.14: INJECT GAMMA GLOBULIN. Formerly included in operation group(s) 794.

Type of Patients	Observed Patients	Avg. Stay	Vari-ance	Percentiles						
				10th	25th	50th	75th	90th	95th	99th
1. SINGLE DX										
0–19 Years	442	2.1	1	1	1	2	2	3	4	7
20–34	34	2.1	1	1	2	2	2	3	3	8
35–49	36	2.2	<1	1	2	2	3	3	4	4
50–64	26	2.8	6	1	1	2	3	5	5	17
65+	22	2.8	1	2	2	2	4	5	5	5
2. MULTIPLE DX										
0–19 Years	442	3.4	18	1	1	3	4	5	10	15
20–34	50	4.3	15	1	1	3	6	9	14	14
35–49	107	4.1	11	1	2	4	5	7	9	21
50–64	143	3.6	5	1	2	4	4	5	7	12
65+	176	4.8	20	1	1	4	7	10	12	21
TOTAL SINGLE DX	560	2.1	2	1	1	2	2	3	4	7
MULTIPLE DX	918	3.8	16	1	2	3	4	7	10	16
TOTAL										
0–19 Years	884	2.7	10	1	1	2	3	5	6	13
20–34	84	3.1	9	1	2	2	3	6	9	14
35–49	143	3.6	9	1	2	3	5	7	7	18
50–64	169	3.5	5	1	2	4	4	5	7	12
65+	198	4.6	19	1	1	3	6	10	10	21
GRAND TOTAL	1478	3.2	11	1	1	2	4	5	9	14

99.15: PARENTERAL NUTRITION. Formerly included in operation group(s) 794.

Type of Patients	Observed Patients	Avg. Stay	Vari-ance	Percentiles						
				10th	25th	50th	75th	90th	95th	99th
1. SINGLE DX										
0–19 Years	39	5.7	10	2	4	5	7	9	13	15
20–34	46	5.1	13	1	2	4	7	12	12	18
35–49	26	8.3	31	3	5	6	11	14	15	28
50–64	10	6.6	5	3	4	8	8	8	8	10
65+	9	13.2	95	6	7	8	13	31	33	33
2. MULTIPLE DX										
0–19 Years	1482	11.9	142	2	4	8	14	26	37	57
20–34	548	10.6	98	3	4	8	13	19	30	60
35–49	801	10.6	80	3	5	8	13	20	25	47
50–64	718	10.3	106	3	4	7	12	21	27	59
65+	1285	11.7	68	4	6	10	15	23	28	42
TOTAL SINGLE DX	130	6.4	21	2	3	6	8	12	14	28
MULTIPLE DX	4834	11.2	105	3	5	8	14	23	31	54
TOTAL										
0–19 Years	1521	11.8	140	2	4	8	14	26	37	56
20–34	594	10.2	94	3	5	7	12	19	27	60
35–49	827	10.5	78	3	5	8	13	20	25	43
50–64	728	10.2	105	3	4	7	12	21	27	59
65+	1294	11.7	68	4	6	10	15	23	28	42
GRAND TOTAL	4964	11.1	104	3	5	8	14	22	31	53

99.17: INJECT INSULIN. Formerly included in operation group(s) 794.

Type of Patients	Observed Patients	Avg. Stay	Vari-ance	Percentiles						
				10th	25th	50th	75th	90th	95th	99th
1. SINGLE DX										
0–19 Years	117	3.1	3	1	2	3	4	5	7	9
20–34	146	3.1	4	1	2	3	4	5	6	10
35–49	70	3.0	6	1	1	2	4	6	8	10
50–64	27	4.3	2	2	3	5	5	5	5	6
65+	13	5.4	10	2	4	4	6	10	13	13
2. MULTIPLE DX										
0–19 Years	240	4.5	18	1	2	4	6	6	10	34
20–34	378	3.6	7	1	2	3	4	7	8	14
35–49	432	4.2	14	2	2	3	5	8	11	20
50–64	504	5.3	21	1	3	4	7	10	12	16
65+	565	6.2	50	2	3	4	8	12	16	27
TOTAL SINGLE DX	373	3.3	4	1	2	3	4	5	7	10
MULTIPLE DX	2119	4.8	24	1	2	4	6	9	12	22
TOTAL										
0–19 Years	357	4.2	15	1	2	3	5	6	8	21
20–34	524	3.5	6	1	2	3	4	7	8	14
35–49	502	4.0	13	1	2	3	5	8	10	19
50–64	531	5.2	19	1	3	4	7	10	12	15
65+	578	6.2	49	2	3	4	8	12	16	27
GRAND TOTAL	2492	4.6	21	1	2	3	6	8	12	20

99.18: INJECT ELECTROLYTES. Formerly included in operation group(s) 794.

Type of Patients	Observed Patients	Avg. Stay	Vari-ance	Percentiles						
				10th	25th	50th	75th	90th	95th	99th
1. SINGLE DX										
0–19 Years	101	2.8	8	1	1	2	3	6	9	21
20–34	88	2.7	5	1	1	2	3	4	5	14
35–49	29	2.1	3	1	1	2	2	5	6	7
50–64	8	1.5	2	1	1	1	1	2	7	7
65+	6	1.9	4	1	1	1	1	3	8	8
2. MULTIPLE DX										
0–19 Years	1003	2.6	5	1	1	2	3	4	6	10
20–34	256	3.7	25	1	2	2	4	7	10	30
35–49	234	4.1	11	1	2	3	5	8	11	16
50–64	179	4.6	42	2	2	3	5	8	11	40
65+	466	5.9	39	1	2	4	7	12	17	34
TOTAL SINGLE DX	232	2.5	6	1	1	2	3	5	6	13
MULTIPLE DX	2138	3.8	21	1	2	3	4	8	10	23
TOTAL										
0–19 Years	1104	2.6	5	1	1	2	3	4	6	11
20–34	344	3.4	20	1	2	2	4	6	10	30
35–49	263	3.8	10	1	2	3	5	8	11	16
50–64	187	4.3	38	1	2	3	5	8	10	40
65+	472	5.9	39	1	2	4	7	12	17	34
GRAND TOTAL	2370	3.6	19	1	2	2	4	7	10	22

Length of Stay by Diagnosis and Operation, United States, 1997

United States, October 1995–September 1996 Data, by Operation

99.21: INJECT ANTIBIOTIC. Formerly included in operation group(s) 794.

Type of Patients	Observed Patients	Avg. Stay	Variance	10th	25th	50th	75th	90th	95th	99th
1. SINGLE DX										
0–19 Years	2259	3.4	8	1	2	3	4	6	7	14
20–34	968	3.2	6	1	2	3	4	6	7	13
35–49	539	3.7	12	2	2	3	4	7	10	14
50–64	245	4.7	14	2	3	3	6	11	14	17
65+	151	4.5	15	2	3	4	5	7	8	22
2. MULTIPLE DX										
0–19 Years	9031	4.6	22	1	2	3	5	8	11	23
20–34	3888	4.5	18	2	2	3	6	8	11	23
35–49	4452	5.6	27	2	3	4	7	11	15	28
50–64	3774	5.8	31	2	3	4	7	10	15	27
65+	8808	7.1	38	2	4	6	9	14	18	33
TOTAL SINGLE DX	4162	3.5	9	1	2	3	4	6	8	14
MULTIPLE DX	29953	5.7	29	2	3	4	7	11	15	28
TOTAL										
0–19 Years	11290	4.3	19	2	2	3	5	8	11	22
20–34	4856	4.2	16	2	3	3	5	7	10	21
35–49	4991	5.4	25	2	3	4	6	10	14	27
50–64	4019	5.7	30	2	3	4	7	10	14	26
65+	8959	7.1	38	2	4	6	8	14	17	33
GRAND TOTAL	34115	5.4	27	2	3	4	6	10	14	27

99.23: INJECT STEROID. Formerly included in operation group(s) 794.

Type of Patients	Observed Patients	Avg. Stay	Variance	10th	25th	50th	75th	90th	95th	99th
1. SINGLE DX										
0–19 Years	535	2.6	2	1	2	2	3	4	5	8
20–34	171	3.2	4	1	2	3	4	6	7	9
35–49	188	3.2	4	2	2	3	4	5	7	13
50–64	58	3.4	5	1	2	3	4	5	7	13
65+	51	3.9	8	1	3	3	5	7	10	14
2. MULTIPLE DX										
0–19 Years	648	3.5	7	1	2	3	4	6	8	14
20–34	466	4.3	9	1	2	3	6	7	10	15
35–49	619	5.2	12	2	3	5	6	8	11	19
50–64	583	5.2	12	2	3	5	6	9	12	18
65+	932	6.4	23	2	3	5	8	12	15	24
TOTAL SINGLE DX	1003	3.0	4	1	2	3	4	5	7	9
MULTIPLE DX	3248	5.1	15	2	3	4	6	9	12	20
TOTAL										
0–19 Years	1183	3.2	5	1	2	3	4	6	7	12
20–34	637	4.0	8	1	2	3	6	7	9	15
35–49	807	4.8	11	2	3	4	6	8	10	18
50–64	641	5.0	12	2	3	5	6	9	11	17
65+	983	6.3	23	2	3	5	8	11	15	24
GRAND TOTAL	4251	4.6	13	1	2	4	6	8	11	18

99.19: INJECT ANTICOAGULANT. Formerly included in operation group(s) 794.

Type of Patients	Observed Patients	Avg. Stay	Variance	10th	25th	50th	75th	90th	95th	99th
1. SINGLE DX										
0–19 Years	12	6.0	4	4	5	7	7	8	8	8
20–34	66	6.0	7	3	5	6	8	8	10	20
35–49	85	5.1	5	2	4	5	7	8	9	10
50–64	95	4.4	5	2	3	4	5	7	8	14
65+	62	4.8	9	1	2	4	6	9	12	14
2. MULTIPLE DX										
0–19 Years	58	5.4	29	1	3	4	7	10	15	44
20–34	245	4.8	13	2	2	4	7	8	10	16
35–49	520	5.1	16	1	3	5	6	10	12	16
50–64	942	5.4	19	1	3	5	6	8	12	26
65+	2141	6.0	19	2	4	5	7	10	14	22
TOTAL SINGLE DX	320	5.2	7	2	3	5	7	8	9	13
MULTIPLE DX	3906	5.6	18	2	3	5	7	10	13	24
TOTAL										
0–19 Years	70	5.5	26	1	3	4	7	10	13	20
20–34	311	5.1	12	2	3	5	7	8	10	16
35–49	605	5.1	15	1	3	5	6	8	12	16
50–64	1037	5.3	18	1	3	5	6	8	12	26
65+	2203	6.0	18	2	4	5	7	10	14	22
GRAND TOTAL	4226	5.6	17	2	3	5	7	10	12	22

99.2: OTH INJECT THER SUBST. Formerly included in operation group(s) 794.

Type of Patients	Observed Patients	Avg. Stay	Variance	10th	25th	50th	75th	90th	95th	99th
1. SINGLE DX										
0–19 Years	3999	3.2	7	1	2	3	4	5	7	13
20–34	2537	3.0	7	1	1	2	4	5	7	12
35–49	1238	3.5	13	1	1	3	4	6	7	16
50–64	676	3.9	12	1	2	3	5	6	10	17
65+	411	3.8	9	1	2	3	5	7	8	13
2. MULTIPLE DX										
0–19 Years	29466	3.9	16	1	2	3	5	6	9	21
20–34	11073	4.6	25	1	2	4	5	8	12	29
35–49	18787	4.7	24	2	2	4	5	8	12	28
50–64	28613	4.6	28	1	2	4	5	8	12	29
65+	37725	5.3	32	1	2	4	6	10	14	30
TOTAL SINGLE DX	8861	3.2	9	1	2	3	4	6	7	14
MULTIPLE DX	125664	4.6	25	1	2	4	5	8	12	28
TOTAL										
0–19 Years	33465	3.8	15	1	2	3	4	6	9	21
20–34	13610	4.2	22	1	2	4	5	7	10	26
35–49	20025	4.6	24	1	2	4	5	8	12	28
50–64	29289	4.5	28	1	2	4	5	8	12	29
65+	38136	5.3	32	1	2	4	6	10	14	30
GRAND TOTAL	134525	4.5	24	1	2	3	5	8	12	27

Length of Stay by Diagnosis and Operation, United States, 1997

United States, October 1995–September 1996 Data, by Operation

99.24: INJECT HORMONE NEC. Formerly included in operation group(s) 794.

Type of Patients	Observed Patients	Avg. Stay	Vari-ance	10th	25th	50th	75th	90th	95th	99th
1. SINGLE DX										
0–19 Years	18	1.7	<1	1	1	2	2	3	3	3
20–34	34	2.7	7	1	1	2	2	10	10	10
35–49	37	4.1	6	1	2	4	5	6	10	13
50–64	6	6.1	7	2	5	5	9	9	9	9
65+	2	2.9	6	1	1	1	5	5	5	5
2. MULTIPLE DX										
0–19 Years	35	2.7	3	2	2	2	3	5	5	10
20–34	74	2.3	3	1	1	2	3	4	5	7
35–49	46	3.9	21	1	1	2	5	9	16	19
50–64	17	7.6	34	4	4	5	9	11	14	30
65+	12	10.0	214	2	4	5	8	52	52	52
TOTAL SINGLE DX	97	2.8	6	1	1	2	3	5	10	10
MULTIPLE DX	184	3.2	19	1	1	2	3	5	9	19
TOTAL										
0–19 Years	53	2.4	2	1	2	2	3	4	5	10
20–34	108	2.4	4	1	1	2	3	4	6	10
35–49	83	3.9	18	1	1	2	5	9	15	19
50–64	23	7.2	28	4	5	5	9	11	14	30
65+	14	9.3	197	2	4	5	8	52	52	52
GRAND TOTAL	281	3.1	16	1	1	2	3	5	9	19

99.25: INJECT CA CHEMO AGENT. Formerly included in operation group(s) 794.

Type of Patients	Observed Patients	Avg. Stay	Vari-ance	10th	25th	50th	75th	90th	95th	99th
1. SINGLE DX										
0–19 Years	300	3.5	8	1	1	3	5	7	8	11
20–34	96	4.9	46	1	2	4	6	8	11	55
35–49	107	4.5	52	1	1	3	5	7	9	64
50–64	190	3.9	14	1	2	4	5	6	9	17
65+	89	2.8	6	1	1	2	4	6	8	12
2. MULTIPLE DX										
0–19 Years	17557	3.8	14	1	2	3	4	6	8	21
20–34	4465	5.0	36	1	3	4	5	7	15	35
35–49	11347	4.3	26	1	2	3	5	7	11	31
50–64	21333	4.2	31	1	2	3	5	7	11	32
65+	22740	4.4	31	1	2	3	5	8	12	30
TOTAL SINGLE DX	782	3.8	19	1	1	3	5	7	9	17
MULTIPLE DX	77442	4.2	26	1	2	3	5	7	10	29
TOTAL										
0–19 Years	17857	3.8	14	1	1	3	4	6	8	21
20–34	4561	5.0	37	1	3	4	5	7	15	35
35–49	11454	4.3	26	1	2	3	5	7	11	31
50–64	21523	4.2	30	1	2	3	5	7	11	31
65+	22829	4.4	31	1	2	3	5	8	12	30
GRAND TOTAL	78224	4.2	26	1	2	3	5	7	10	29

99.28: INJECT BRM/ANTINEO AGENT. Formerly included in operation group(s) 794.

Type of Patients	Observed Patients	Avg. Stay	Vari-ance	10th	25th	50th	75th	90th	95th	99th
1. SINGLE DX										
0–19 Years	5	1.3	<1	1	1	1	1	2	3	3
20–34	5	4.7	21	1	1	4	11	12	12	12
35–49	16	6.1	19	1	2	5	10	11	11	11
50–64	10	4.4	10	1	2	4	7	9	11	11
65+	1	1.0	0	1	1	1	1	1	1	1
2. MULTIPLE DX										
0–19 Years	33	5.2	5	2	4	5	6	7	11	12
20–34	35	6.3	21	3	4	5	7	8	11	25
35–49	139	6.2	20	2	4	5	7	12	17	25
50–64	194	5.9	17	2	4	5	7	10	11	23
65+	109	7.0	77	3	4	5	7	9	16	58
TOTAL SINGLE DX	37	4.5	16	1	1	2	10	11	11	12
MULTIPLE DX	510	6.2	31	3	4	5	7	9	14	25
TOTAL										
0–19 Years	38	4.8	6	2	3	5	6	7	9	12
20–34	40	6.1	21	3	4	5	7	10	18	25
35–49	155	6.1	20	2	4	5	7	11	17	25
50–64	204	5.8	16	2	4	5	7	10	11	23
65+	110	7.0	76	3	4	5	7	9	16	58
GRAND TOTAL	547	6.0	30	2	4	5	7	10	14	25

99.29: INJECT/INFUSE NEC. Formerly included in operation group(s) 794.

Type of Patients	Observed Patients	Avg. Stay	Vari-ance	10th	25th	50th	75th	90th	95th	99th
1. SINGLE DX										
0–19 Years	868	2.8	8	1	1	2	3	5	6	18
20–34	1258	2.7	6	1	1	2	3	5	6	12
35–49	349	3.1	10	1	1	2	4	6	7	16
50–64	166	3.3	8	1	2	3	4	6	7	15
65+	117	3.8	4	1	2	4	5	6	7	8
2. MULTIPLE DX										
0–19 Years	2137	3.2	12	1	1	2	4	6	8	18
20–34	2110	4.1	20	1	2	3	5	8	11	22
35–49	2122	4.7	17	1	2	4	6	8	11	21
50–64	2688	5.0	12	2	3	5	6	8	11	17
65+	5105	5.8	20	2	3	5	7	10	13	22
TOTAL SINGLE DX	2758	2.8	7	1	1	2	3	5	7	16
MULTIPLE DX	14162	4.8	18	1	2	4	6	9	11	21
TOTAL										
0–19 Years	3005	3.1	11	1	1	2	4	6	8	18
20–34	3368	3.6	15	1	1	3	4	7	10	20
35–49	2471	4.5	16	1	2	4	6	8	11	21
50–64	2854	4.9	12	1	3	4	6	8	11	17
65+	5222	5.8	20	2	3	5	7	10	13	22
GRAND TOTAL	16920	4.5	16	1	2	4	6	8	11	20

United States, October 1995–September 1996 Data, by Operation

99.3: PROPHYL VACC-BACT DIS. Formerly included in operation group(s) 794.

Type of Patients	Observed Patients	Avg. Stay	Vari-ance	10th	25th	50th	75th	90th	95th	99th
1. SINGLE DX										
0–19 Years	6	1.2	<1	1	1	1	1	2	2	2
20–34	4	3.6	<1	3	3	3	5	5	5	5
35–49	4	1.8	<1	1	1	2	2	3	3	3
50–64	1	2.0	0	2	2	2	2	2	2	2
65+	1	1.0	0	1	1	1	1	1	1	1
2. MULTIPLE DX										
0–19 Years	29	3.7	14	1	1	3	4	8	12	17
20–34	24	2.6	3	1	1	2	4	5	7	7
35–49	27	3.8	6	1	2	3	6	6	6	13
50–64	17	4.5	42	1	2	4	6	10	17	35
65+	57	5.0	20	1	3	3	5	13	18	20
TOTAL SINGLE DX	16	2.1	2	1	1	2	3	5	5	5
MULTIPLE DX	154	3.9	14	1	1	3	5	7	11	18
TOTAL										
0–19 Years	35	3.5	14	1	1	2	4	8	11	17
20–34	28	2.7	3	1	2	3	4	5	7	7
35–49	31	3.7	6	1	2	3	6	6	6	13
50–64	18	4.4	41	1	1	2	4	10	17	35
65+	58	5.0	20	1	3	3	5	11	15	20
GRAND TOTAL	170	3.8	13	1	1	3	5	7	11	18

99.5: OTHER IMMUNIZATION. Formerly included in operation group(s) 794.

Type of Patients	Observed Patients	Avg. Stay	Vari-ance	10th	25th	50th	75th	90th	95th	99th
1. SINGLE DX										
0–19 Years	15422	1.7	<1	1	1	2	2	3	3	4
20–34	7	1.6	<1	1	1	2	2	3	3	3
35–49	1	1.0	0	1	1	1	1	1	1	1
50–64	2	10.3	23	8	8	8	8	18	18	18
65+	3	6.7	32	4	4	4	4	16	16	16
2. MULTIPLE DX										
0–19 Years	79808	2.0	4	1	1	2	2	3	4	9
20–34	23	5.9	6	3	4	7	7	9	10	11
35–49	24	3.4	6	1	1	3	4	7	8	13
50–64	33	5.0	7	2	3	5	7	7	10	15
65+	102	5.3	51	1	2	4	7	9	14	66
TOTAL SINGLE DX	15435	1.7	<1	1	1	2	2	3	3	4
MULTIPLE DX	79990	2.0	4	1	1	2	2	3	4	9
TOTAL										
0–19 Years	95230	2.0	4	1	1	2	2	3	4	9
20–34	30	5.4	7	1	3	7	7	8	10	11
35–49	25	3.1	6	1	1	3	4	7	7	13
50–64	35	5.3	8	2	3	5	7	8	10	18
65+	105	5.3	50	2	2	4	7	9	14	23
GRAND TOTAL	95425	2.0	4	1	1	2	2	3	4	9

99.4: VIRAL IMMUNIZATION. Formerly included in operation group(s) 794.

Type of Patients	Observed Patients	Avg. Stay	Vari-ance	10th	25th	50th	75th	90th	95th	99th
1. SINGLE DX										
0–19 Years	8	1.2	<1	1	1	1	1	2	2	3
20–34	10	1.9	<1	1	2	2	2	2	2	4
35–49	1	1.0	0	1	1	1	1	1	1	1
50–64	0									
65+	0									
2. MULTIPLE DX										
0–19 Years	22	1.6	1	1	1	1	2	3	3	8
20–34	30	2.5	4	1	2	2	3	3	8	8
35–49	3	1.8	<1	1	2	2	2	2	2	2
50–64	1	12.0	0	12	12	12	12	12	12	12
65+	2	4.6	11	2	2	2	8	8	12	12
TOTAL SINGLE DX	19	1.3	<1	1	1	1	1	2	3	3
MULTIPLE DX	58	2.3	5	1	1	2	2	3	8	12
TOTAL										
0–19 Years	30	1.4	1	1	1	1	1	3	3	8
20–34	40	2.4	4	1	2	2	3	3	8	8
35–49	4	1.7	<1	1	1	2	3	3	2	2
50–64	1	12.0	0	12	12	12	12	12	12	12
65+	2	4.6	11	2	2	2	8	8	12	12
GRAND TOTAL	77	2.0	4	1	1	1	2	3	5	12

99.55: VACCINATION NEC. Formerly included in operation group(s) 794.

Type of Patients	Observed Patients	Avg. Stay	Vari-ance	10th	25th	50th	75th	90th	95th	99th
1. SINGLE DX										
0–19 Years	13192	1.7	<1	1	1	1	2	3	3	4
20–34	6	1.4	<1	1	1	1	2	3	3	3
35–49	1	1.0	0	1	1	1	1	1	1	1
50–64	0									
65+	0									
2. MULTIPLE DX										
0–19 Years	77106	2.0	4	1	1	2	2	3	4	9
20–34	7	5.5	12	3	3	4	6	11	13	13
35–49	14	3.1	6	1	1	2	5	7	8	8
50–64	18	4.4	8	2	2	4	5	10	10	10
65+	13	2.0	1	1	1	2	2	2	5	6
TOTAL SINGLE DX	13199	1.7	<1	1	1	1	2	3	3	4
MULTIPLE DX	77158	2.0	4	1	1	2	2	3	4	9
TOTAL										
0–19 Years	90298	2.0	4	1	1	2	2	3	4	9
20–34	13	3.8	11	1	1	3	4	11	11	13
35–49	15	2.7	5	1	1	2	4	7	7	8
50–64	18	4.4	8	2	2	4	5	10	10	10
65+	13	2.0	1	1	1	2	2	2	5	6
GRAND TOTAL	90357	2.0	4	1	1	2	2	3	4	9

Length of Stay by Diagnosis and Operation, United States, 1997

United States, October 1995–September 1996 Data, by Operation

99.59: VACC/INOCULATION NEC. Formerly included in operation group(s) 794.

Type of Patients	Observed Patients	Avg. Stay	Vari-ance	10th	25th	50th	75th	90th	95th	99th
1. SINGLE DX										
0–19 Years	2200	2.0	<1	1	1	2	2	3	3	6
20–34	1	2.0	0	2	2	2	2	3	2	2
35–49	0									
50–64	1	8.0	0	8	8	8	8	8	8	8
65+	0									
2. MULTIPLE DX										
0–19 Years	2614	2.0	2	1	1	2	2	3	4	7
20–34	4	6.5	2	7	7	7	7	7	7	7
35–49	3	3.2	7	1	1	3	3	7	7	7
50–64	4	5.8	3	5	5	5	7	8	8	11
65+	6	4.1	14	2	3	3	3	4	14	17
TOTAL SINGLE DX	2202	2.0	1	1	1	2	2	3	4	6
MULTIPLE DX	2631	2.0	3	1	1	2	2	3	4	7
TOTAL										
0–19 Years	4814	2.0	2	1	1	2	2	3	4	7
20–34	5	6.4	3	4	7	7	7	7	7	7
35–49	3	3.2	7	1	1	3	3	7	7	7
50–64	5	6.0	3	5	5	7	7	8	8	11
65+	6	4.1	14	2	3	3	3	4	14	17
GRAND TOTAL	4833	2.0	2	1	1	2	2	3	4	7

99.60: CPR NOS. Formerly included in operation group(s) 794.

Type of Patients	Observed Patients	Avg. Stay	Vari-ance	10th	25th	50th	75th	90th	95th	99th
1. SINGLE DX										
0–19 Years	8	1.5	<1	1	1	1	2	2	3	3
20–34	2	15.5	156	1	1	25	25	25	25	25
35–49	0									
50–64	0									
65+	2	6.2	62	1	1	1	14	14	14	14
2. MULTIPLE DX										
0–19 Years	87	8.0	83	1	3	6	10	24	53	>99
20–34	21	5.4	29	1	2	3	5	16	16	19
35–49	30	8.8	147	1	2	7	9	15	20	93
50–64	80	8.2	44	1	4	6	10	17	24	29
65+	274	9.8	61	3	5	9	11	18	23	40
TOTAL SINGLE DX	12	2.5	22	1	1	1	2	3	3	25
MULTIPLE DX	492	8.8	71	2	4	8	11	17	27	>99
TOTAL										
0–19 Years	95	6.8	74	1	2	4	10	13	33	>99
20–34	23	6.9	59	1	2	3	11	19	25	25
35–49	30	8.8	147	1	2	7	9	15	20	93
50–64	80	8.2	44	1	4	6	10	17	24	29
65+	276	9.7	61	3	5	9	11	18	23	40
GRAND TOTAL	504	8.3	70	1	3	7	10	17	25	>99

99.6: CARD RHYTHM CONVERSION. Formerly included in operation group(s) 794.

Type of Patients	Observed Patients	Avg. Stay	Vari-ance	10th	25th	50th	75th	90th	95th	99th
1. SINGLE DX										
0–19 Years	36	1.6	<1	1	1	1	2	2	3	4
20–34	43	3.3	33	1	1	2	2	5	25	25
35–49	138	1.6	<1	1	1	1	2	3	3	5
50–64	290	1.8	1	1	1	1	3	3	3	6
65+	309	1.8	1	1	1	1	2	3	3	6
2. MULTIPLE DX										
0–19 Years	271	7.5	106	1	2	5	10	14	32	>99
20–34	299	3.2	7	1	1	2	5	6	8	16
35–49	963	3.8	17	1	2	3	5	8	9	16
50–64	3308	3.9	14	1	2	3	5	8	10	16
65+	9773	5.1	22	1	2	4	7	11	14	23
TOTAL SINGLE DX	816	1.8	2	1	1	1	2	3	4	6
MULTIPLE DX	14614	4.8	22	1	2	3	6	10	13	23
TOTAL										
0–19 Years	307	6.7	96	1	2	4	8	14	31	>99
20–34	342	3.2	10	1	1	2	5	6	8	19
35–49	1101	3.6	15	1	1	2	5	7	9	16
50–64	3598	3.7	13	1	2	3	5	8	10	16
65+	10082	5.0	21	1	2	4	6	10	13	23
GRAND TOTAL	15430	4.6	21	1	2	3	6	10	12	23

99.61: ATRIAL CARDIOVERSION. Formerly included in operation group(s) 794.

Type of Patients	Observed Patients	Avg. Stay	Vari-ance	10th	25th	50th	75th	90th	95th	99th
1. SINGLE DX										
0–19 Years	11	1.7	<1	1	1	2	2	2	3	3
20–34	14	1.7	2	1	1	1	2	5	5	5
35–49	68	1.7	1	1	1	1	2	3	4	5
50–64	159	1.8	1	1	1	2	2	3	5	6
65+	157	1.8	1	1	1	2	2	3	3	6
2. MULTIPLE DX										
0–19 Years	67	4.6	14	1	1	4	7	8	12	14
20–34	126	3.4	4	1	2	3	5	5	6	8
35–49	396	3.2	6	1	1	3	4	6	7	13
50–64	1502	3.6	10	1	2	3	6	7	10	15
65+	4136	4.9	19	1	2	3	6	10	14	21
TOTAL SINGLE DX	409	1.8	1	1	1	2	2	3	4	6
MULTIPLE DX	6227	4.5	16	1	2	3	6	9	12	18
TOTAL										
0–19 Years	78	4.3	14	1	1	3	7	8	12	14
20–34	140	3.3	4	1	1	3	5	5	6	8
35–49	464	3.0	6	1	1	2	4	6	7	12
50–64	1661	3.4	10	1	2	3	4	7	9	14
65+	4293	4.7	18	2	2	3	6	10	13	20
GRAND TOTAL	6636	4.3	16	1	2	3	5	9	12	18

Length of Stay by Diagnosis and Operation, United States, 1997

United States, October 1995–September 1996 Data, by Operation

99.62: HEART COUNTERSHOCK NEC. Formerly included in operation group(s) 794.

Type of Patients	Observed Patients	Avg. Stay	Vari-ance	Percentiles						
				10th	25th	50th	75th	90th	95th	99th
1. SINGLE DX										
0–19 Years	8	2.0	8	1	1	1	2	2	11	11
20–34	26	2.0	2	1	1	2	2	4	4	8
35–49	61	1.5	<1	1	1	1	2	2	3	5
50–64	121	1.8	1	1	1	1	3	3	3	5
65+	142	1.7	1	1	1	1	3	3	4	6
2. MULTIPLE DX										
0–19 Years	68	4.8	35	1	1	3	5	14	19	28
20–34	134	2.7	9	1	1	1	3	6	8	19
35–49	480	4.1	17	1	2	3	6	9	9	18
50–64	1624	4.0	16	1	2	3	5	8	11	16
65+	4925	5.1	21	1	2	4	7	10	13	23
TOTAL SINGLE DX	358	1.7	1	1	1	1	3	3	3	5
MULTIPLE DX	7231	4.7	20	1	2	3	6	10	12	22
TOTAL										
0–19 Years	76	4.7	34	1	1	3	5	14	19	28
20–34	160	2.6	8	1	1	1	3	6	8	19
35–49	541	3.9	16	1	2	2	5	8	9	16
50–64	1745	3.8	15	1	2	3	5	8	11	15
65+	5067	4.9	21	1	2	4	6	10	13	23
GRAND TOTAL	7589	4.5	19	1	2	3	6	9	12	22

99.7: THERAPEUTIC APHERESIS. Formerly included in operation group(s) 794.

Type of Patients	Observed Patients	Avg. Stay	Vari-ance	Percentiles						
				10th	25th	50th	75th	90th	95th	99th
1. SINGLE DX										
0–19 Years	32	3.2	7	1	1	2	4	7	9	15
20–34	30	8.3	4	5	9	9	9	9	9	11
35–49	37	6.9	13	3	5	8	9	11	11	17
50–64	23	4.8	14	1	3	5	5	6	15	21
65+	32	3.6	5	1	1	3	5	6	8	9
2. MULTIPLE DX										
0–19 Years	147	7.7	67	1	3	5	11	19	24	47
20–34	122	10.3	47	3	6	9	14	19	23	36
35–49	257	8.7	57	3	5	7	10	21	24	34
50–64	242	10.6	68	2	5	9	15	20	30	37
65+	276	7.7	69	2	3	5	9	17	20	49
TOTAL SINGLE DX	154	6.1	12	1	3	6	9	9	10	17
MULTIPLE DX	1044	8.8	65	2	4	6	11	19	24	40
TOTAL										
0–19 Years	179	6.9	59	1	2	4	9	15	24	35
20–34	152	9.5	31	3	7	9	10	15	20	26
35–49	294	8.3	48	3	5	7	10	18	21	34
50–64	265	9.9	65	2	5	7	15	18	30	37
65+	308	7.5	66	2	3	5	8	16	20	49
GRAND TOTAL	1198	8.3	57	2	4	6	10	17	22	37

99.69: CARDIAC RHYTHM CONV NEC. Formerly included in operation group(s) 794.

Type of Patients	Observed Patients	Avg. Stay	Vari-ance	Percentiles						
				10th	25th	50th	75th	90th	95th	99th
1. SINGLE DX										
0–19 Years	6	1.8	<1	1	1	2	2	2	4	4
20–34	1	2.0	0	2	2	2	2	2	2	2
35–49	8	1.7	<1	1	1	1	1	2	2	3
50–64	10	1.2	<1	1	1	1	1	1	3	3
65+	8	2.2	3	1	1	2	2	7	7	7
2. MULTIPLE DX										
0–19 Years	24	6.7	126	2	3	4	6	15	15	80
20–34	14	2.0	1	1	1	2	3	3	4	4
35–49	51	3.1	6	1	2	3	4	6	8	12
50–64	96	3.2	4	1	2	3	4	6	7	10
65+	400	5.3	24	1	2	4	6	9	16	24
TOTAL SINGLE DX	33	1.7	<1	1	1	2	2	2	3	7
MULTIPLE DX	585	4.9	26	1	2	3	6	9	15	24
TOTAL										
0–19 Years	30	5.9	108	1	2	3	6	15	15	80
20–34	15	2.0	<1	1	1	2	3	3	4	4
35–49	59	2.8	5	1	1	2	3	6	8	12
50–64	106	3.1	4	1	1	3	4	5	7	10
65+	408	5.3	24	1	2	4	6	9	16	24
GRAND TOTAL	618	4.8	25	1	2	3	6	9	15	24

99.71: THER PLASMAPHERESIS. Formerly included in operation group(s) 794.

Type of Patients	Observed Patients	Avg. Stay	Vari-ance	Percentiles						
				10th	25th	50th	75th	90th	95th	99th
1. SINGLE DX										
0–19 Years	20	3.7	9	1	1	2	7	7	9	15
20–34	23	8.6	2	8	9	9	9	9	9	11
35–49	30	7.3	12	3	5	8	9	11	17	17
50–64	22	4.9	14	1	3	5	5	6	15	21
65+	29	3.6	5	1	1	4	5	6	8	8
2. MULTIPLE DX										
0–19 Years	55	8.8	39	2	3	7	13	16	21	35
20–34	92	10.0	47	4	6	9	13	19	23	26
35–49	194	8.3	55	2	4	7	10	16	26	40
50–64	151	11.4	64	3	6	9	15	19	30	34
65+	221	8.5	85	1	3	7	11	19	20	49
TOTAL SINGLE DX	124	6.5	12	1	4	7	9	9	10	17
MULTIPLE DX	713	9.3	68	2	4	7	12	19	24	40
TOTAL										
0–19 Years	75	7.4	36	1	3	6	12	15	20	27
20–34	115	9.3	26	4	7	9	9	14	20	26
35–49	224	8.1	44	3	5	7	10	14	20	39
50–64	173	10.4	62	2	5	9	15	18	30	34
65+	250	8.1	81	2	3	6	10	19	20	49
GRAND TOTAL	837	8.7	57	2	4	7	11	16	21	39

Length of Stay by Diagnosis and Operation, United States, 1997

United States, October 1995–September 1996 Data, by Operation

99.8: MISC PHYSICAL PROCEDURES. Formerly included in operation group(s) 794.

Type of Patients	Observed Patients	Avg. Stay	Variance	10th	25th	50th	75th	90th	95th	99th
1. SINGLE DX										
0–19 Years	4154	2.1	4	1	1	2	2	3	3	6
20–34	46	9.9	118	1	4	7	14	17	21	84
35–49	45	7.5	28	1	2	8	11	14	15	17
50–64	28	8.1	56	1	3	7	9	17	24	32
65+	15	4.0	10	2	2	2	7	8	8	12
2. MULTIPLE DX										
0–19 Years	12688	7.4	83	2	3	4	7	16	24	48
20–34	211	6.7	70	1	1	4	8	15	19	32
35–49	362	6.0	42	1	1	4	9	14	17	35
50–64	273	9.1	56	2	3	9	13	15	24	30
65+	597	7.2	28	2	2	7	10	13	15	26
TOTAL SINGLE DX	4288	2.1	5	1	1	2	2	3	4	10
MULTIPLE DX	14131	7.4	80	2	3	5	8	16	23	48
TOTAL										
0–19 Years	16842	5.9	67	1	2	3	6	13	21	43
20–34	257	7.0	75	1	2	4	9	16	21	32
35–49	407	6.1	42	1	1	4	9	14	17	35
50–64	301	9.0	56	2	3	8	13	15	24	30
65+	612	7.1	28	2	2	7	10	13	15	26
GRAND TOTAL	18419	6.0	65	1	2	3	6	13	21	43

99.83: OTHER PHOTOTHERAPY. Formerly included in operation group(s) 794.

Type of Patients	Observed Patients	Avg. Stay	Variance	10th	25th	50th	75th	90th	95th	99th
1. SINGLE DX										
0–19 Years	3843	2.0	2	1	1	2	2	3	3	5
20–34	46	8.0	0	8	8	8	8	8	8	8
35–49	1	15.0	0	15	15	15	15	15	15	15
50–64	3	5.6	5	2	6	6	7	7	7	7
65+	2	2.0	0	2	2	2	2	2	2	2
2. MULTIPLE DX										
0–19 Years	12013	7.5	86	2	3	5	7	17	25	48
20–34	0									
35–49	3	8.2	68	2	2	3	18	18	18	18
50–64	6	17.0	116	2	7	12	27	27	27	27
65+	6	3.4	5	1	2	3	5	7	7	7
TOTAL SINGLE DX	3850	2.0	2	1	1	2	2	3	3	5
MULTIPLE DX	12028	7.5	86	2	3	5	7	17	25	48
TOTAL										
0–19 Years	15856	6.0	69	1	2	3	6	13	21	44
20–34	1	8.0	0	8	8	8	8	8	8	8
35–49	4	9.3	62	2	3	3	18	18	18	18
50–64	9	13.7	109	2	6	7	27	27	27	27
65+	8	3.1	4	1	2	2	5	7	7	7
GRAND TOTAL	15878	6.0	69	1	2	3	6	13	21	44

99.82: UV LIGHT THERAPY. Formerly included in operation group(s) 794.

Type of Patients	Observed Patients	Avg. Stay	Variance	10th	25th	50th	75th	90th	95th	99th
1. SINGLE DX										
0–19 Years	299	2.8	21	1	1	2	2	3	3	6
20–34	10	11.4	27	5	5	14	14	14	21	21
35–49	18	10.2	5	8	8	10	12	13	14	14
50–64	8	12.8	78	5	9	11	11	32	32	32
65+	2	9.7	11	6	6	12	12	12	12	12
2. MULTIPLE DX										
0–19 Years	587	6.4	48	2	3	4	7	14	21	37
20–34	42	9.4	8	6	7	9	12	14	14	15
35–49	135	9.2	16	4	7	9	12	14	17	18
50–64	154	11.1	12	7	9	10	14	15	15	22
65+	150	9.5	8	6	7	10	11	13	14	16
TOTAL SINGLE DX	337	3.2	25	1	1	2	2	6	12	31
MULTIPLE DX	1068	7.6	37	2	3	6	10	14	18	31
TOTAL										
0–19 Years	886	5.2	42	1	2	3	5	12	19	34
20–34	52	9.7	11	6	7	9	13	14	15	21
35–49	153	9.4	14	5	7	9	12	14	17	18
50–64	162	11.2	15	7	9	10	14	15	16	24
65+	152	9.5	8	6	7	10	11	13	14	16
GRAND TOTAL	1405	6.5	38	1	2	4	9	14	17	31

99.84: ISOLATION. Formerly included in operation group(s) 794.

Type of Patients	Observed Patients	Avg. Stay	Variance	10th	25th	50th	75th	90th	95th	99th
1. SINGLE DX										
0–19 Years	8	4.5	18	1	1	1	10	10	10	12
20–34	31	10.2	158	1	4	7	15	20	32	84
35–49	14	7.2	40	2	3	3	12	17	17	29
50–64	7	8.9	46	3	5	7	9	24	24	24
65+	6	4.0	8	2	2	2	8	8	8	8
2. MULTIPLE DX										
0–19 Years	80	6.0	40	1	2	3	10	14	17	32
20–34	162	6.5	79	1	1	3	7	17	31	32
35–49	205	5.1	48	1	1	5	7	12	17	35
50–64	71	8.5	104	3	3	5	12	21	25	85
65+	253	8.9	38	3	5	7	11	19	22	35
TOTAL SINGLE DX	66	7.2	72	1	2	5	9	16	17	33
MULTIPLE DX	771	6.7	58	1	2	4	9	15	21	35
TOTAL										
0–19 Years	88	5.9	39	1	1	3	10	14	15	32
20–34	193	6.8	86	1	1	4	8	17	31	38
35–49	219	5.2	47	1	2	2	7	13	17	35
50–64	78	8.5	100	3	3	5	11	24	25	85
65+	259	8.7	38	3	4	7	11	18	22	35
GRAND TOTAL	837	6.7	59	1	2	4	9	15	21	35

Length of Stay by Diagnosis and Operation, United States, 1997

United States, October 1995–September 1996 Data, by Operation

99.9: OTHER MISC PROCEDURES. Formerly included in operation group(s) 794.

Type of Patients	Observed Patients	Avg. Stay	Vari-ance	Percentiles						
				10th	25th	50th	75th	90th	95th	99th
1. SINGLE DX										
0–19 Years	8	1.2	<1	1	1	1	1	2	2	2
20–34	47	3.6	12	1	1	2	4	8	11	14
35–49	88	5.3	29	1	2	4	6	13	16	31
50–64	29	3.4	4	1	2	3	5	6	8	9
65+	5	4.4	9	1	2	3	7	8	8	8
2. MULTIPLE DX										
0–19 Years	22	4.1	43	1	1	2	4	9	9	44
20–34	66	4.1	20	1	2	2	4	10	16	21
35–49	85	6.9	32	1	2	5	14	14	16	17
50–64	54	9.5	39	2	5	7	13	19	20	26
65+	191	8.4	44	3	4	6	11	17	23	29
TOTAL SINGLE DX	177	4.4	19	1	2	3	6	10	13	22
MULTIPLE DX	418	7.8	42	2	3	6	11	16	21	29
TOTAL										
0–19 Years	30	3.3	33	1	1	2	3	9	9	44
20–34	113	3.9	16	1	1	2	4	9	14	18
35–49	173	6.1	31	1	2	4	9	14	16	27
50–64	83	7.3	35	2	3	5	11	15	20	26
65+	196	8.4	44	3	4	6	11	17	23	29
GRAND TOTAL	595	6.9	38	1	3	5	9	16	20	29

99.99: MISC PROCEDURES NEC. Formerly included in operation group(s) 794.

Type of Patients	Observed Patients	Avg. Stay	Vari-ance	Percentiles						
				10th	25th	50th	75th	90th	95th	99th
1. SINGLE DX										
0–19 Years	6	1.2	<1	1	1	1	1	2	2	2
20–34	46	3.6	12	1	1	2	4	8	11	14
35–49	87	5.2	29	1	2	3	6	13	14	31
50–64	29	3.4	4	1	2	3	5	6	8	9
65+	4	4.6	10	1	2	7	8	8	8	8
2. MULTIPLE DX										
0–19 Years	9	6.9	103	1	1	4	9	9	26	44
20–34	62	4.1	20	1	2	2	4	10	16	21
35–49	79	7.1	33	1	2	5	14	14	16	17
50–64	47	9.9	42	2	5	10	13	19	20	26
65+	177	8.5	45	3	4	6	11	17	23	29
TOTAL SINGLE DX	172	4.3	19	1	2	3	6	9	13	22
MULTIPLE DX	374	8.0	43	2	3	6	12	16	23	29
TOTAL										
0–19 Years	15	4.2	62	1	1	1	4	9	9	44
20–34	108	3.9	16	1	1	2	4	9	14	18
35–49	166	6.1	31	1	2	4	9	14	16	27
50–64	76	7.4	37	1	3	5	13	17	20	26
65+	181	8.4	45	3	4	6	11	17	23	29
GRAND TOTAL	546	7.0	40	1	3	5	9	16	21	29

Length of Stay by Diagnosis and Operation, United States, 1997

APPENDIX A
Hospital Characteristics
Short-Term, General, Nonfederal Hospitals[1]

HOSPITAL CATEGORY	U.S. TOTAL
Bed Size	
6–24	311
25–49	1,049
50–99	1,579
100–199	1,467
200–299	793
300–399	433
400–499	224
500+	263
Unknown	12
Total	**6,131**
Region and Census Division	
Northeast	**927**
New England	279
Middle Atlantic	648
North Central	**1,651**
East North Central	950
West North Central	701
South	**2,396**
South Atlantic	978
East South Central	517
West South Central	901
West	**1,157**
Mountain	398
Pacific	759
Location	
Urban	3,685
Rural	2,446
Teaching Intensity	
High/Medium	1,048
Low	5,083

---

[1] For a definition of short-term, general, and nonfederal hospitals, see page viii.

APPENDIX B
States Included in Each Region

Northeast	North Central	South	West
Connecticut	Illinois	Alabama	Alaska
Maine	Indiana	Arkansas	Arizona
Massachusetts	Iowa	Delaware	California
New Hampshire	Kansas	District of Columbia	Colorado
New Jersey	Michigan	Florida	Hawaii
New York	Minnesota	Georgia	Idaho
Pennsylvania	Missouri	Kentucky	Montana
Rhode Island	Nebraska	Louisiana	Nevada
Vermont	North Dakota	Maryland	New Mexico
	Ohio	Mississippi	Oregon
	South Dakota	North Carolina	Utah
	Wisconsin	Oklahoma	Washington
		South Carolina	Wyoming
		Tennessee	
		Texas	
		Virginia	
		West Virginia	

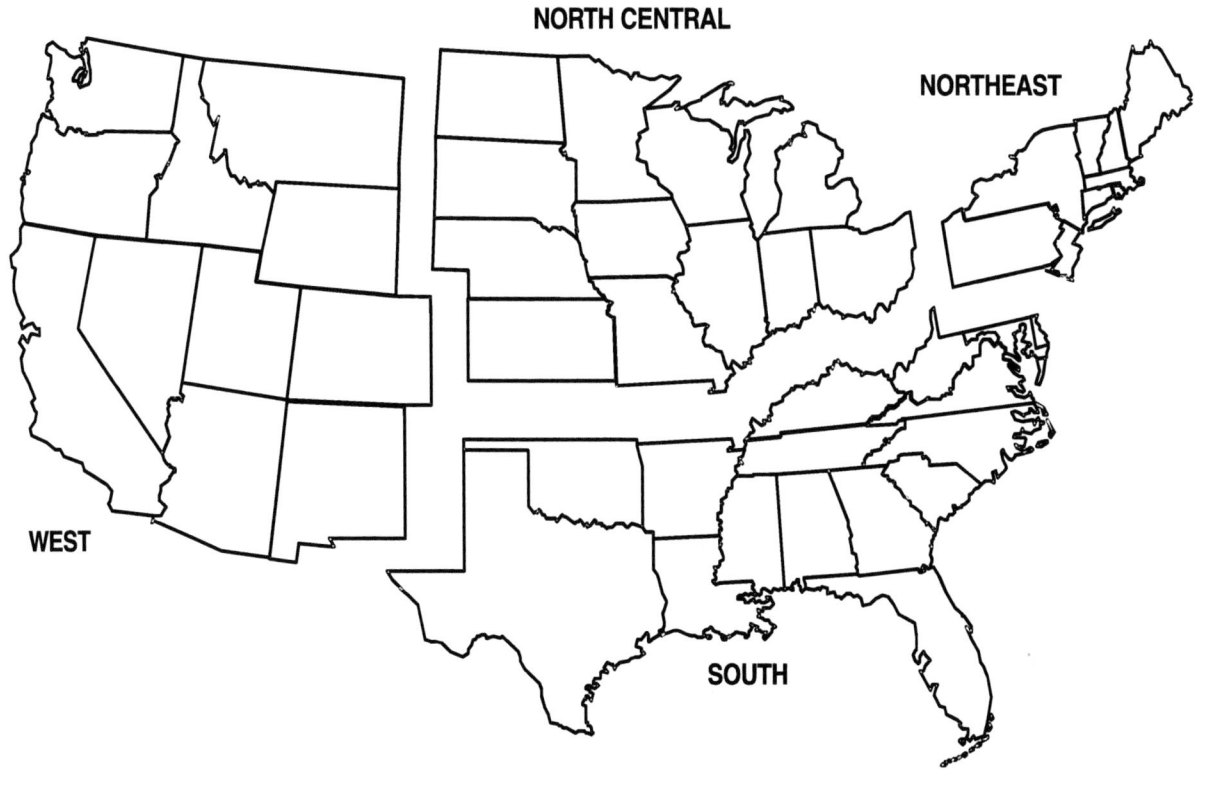

APPENDIX C
Operative Status of Procedure Codes

The following table lists every ICD-9-CM procedure code included in this book, its description, and its HCFA-defined operative status (*i.e.,* operative or non-operative). Operative procedures are those classified by HCFA as "operating room" procedures. HCFA physician panels classify every ICD-9-CM procedure code according to whether the procedure would, in most hospitals, be performed in the operating room. For summary (3-digit) codes that contain both operative and non-operative detail (four-digit) codes, the notation "Mixed," followed by the number of each type, will appear in the "Operative Status" column. For example, a summary code containing three operative and two non-operative detail codes will be identified as "Mixed (3, 2)."

Code	Description	Operative Status	Code	Description	Operative Status
01.0	Cranial puncture	Non-Operative	03.7	Spinal thecal shunt	Operative
01.02	Ventriculopunct via cath	Non-Operative	03.71	Subarach-periton shunt	Operative
01.09	Cranial puncture NEC	Non-Operative	03.8	Destr inject-spine canal	Non-Operative
01.1	Dxtic px on skull/brain	Mixed (5, 2)	03.9	Spinal cord ops NEC	Mixed (5, 5)
01.13	Clsd (PERC) brain Bx	Non-Operative	03.90	Insert spinal canal cath	Non-Operative
01.14	Open biopsy of brain	Operative	03.91	Inject anes-spinal canal	Non-Operative
01.18	Dxtic px brain/cereb NEC	Operative	03.92	Inject spinal canal NEC	Non-Operative
01.2	Craniotomy & craniectomy	Operative	03.93	Insert spinal neurostim	Operative
01.24	Other craniotomy	Operative	03.95	Spinal blood patch	Non-Operative
01.25	Other craniectomy	Operative	04.0	Periph nerve inc/div/exc	Operative
01.3	Inc brain/cereb meninges	Operative	04.01	Exc acoustic neuroma	Operative
01.31	Inc cerebral meninges	Operative	04.07	Periph/cran nerv exc NEC	Operative
01.39	Other brain incision	Operative	04.1	Dxtic px periph nerv	Mixed (2, 1)
01.4	Thalamus/globus pall ops	Operative	04.2	Destr periph/cran nerves	Non-Operative
01.42	Globus pallidus ops	Operative	04.3	Cran/periph nerve suture	Operative
01.5	Exc/destr brain/meninges	Operative	04.4	Periph nerv adhesiolysis	Operative
01.51	Exc cereb meningeal les	Operative	04.41	Decomp trigeminal root	Operative
01.53	Brain lobectomy	Operative	04.43	Carpal tunnel release	Operative
01.59	Exc/destr brain les NEC	Operative	04.49	Periph nerv ADHESIO NEC	Operative
01.6	Excision of skull lesion	Operative	04.5	Cran or periph nerv grft	Operative
02.0	Cranioplasty	Operative	04.6	Periph nerves transpos	Operative
02.01	Opening cranial suture	Operative	04.7	Other periph neuroplasty	Operative
02.02	Elevation skull fx frag	Operative	04.8	Peripheral nerve inject	Non-Operative
02.06	Cranial osteoplasty NEC	Operative	04.81	Anes inject periph nerve	Non-Operative
02.1	Cerebral meninges repair	Operative	04.9	Oth periph nerve ops	Operative
02.12	REP cerebral mening NEC	Operative	05.0	Sympath nerve division	Operative
02.2	Ventriculostomy	Operative	05.1	Sympath nerve dxtic px	Operative
02.3	Extracranial vent shunt	Operative	05.2	Sympathectomy	Operative
02.34	Vent shunt to abd cavity	Operative	05.23	Lumbar sympathectomy	Operative
02.4	Vent shunt rev/rmvl	Mixed (2, 1)	05.3	Sympath nerve injection	Non-Operative
02.42	Repl ventriclular shunt	Operative	05.31	Anes inject sympath nerv	Non-Operative
02.43	Rmvl ventriclular shunt	Operative	05.8	Oth sympath nerve ops	Operative
02.9	Skull & brain ops NEC	Mixed (5, 2)	05.9	Other nervous system ops	Operative
02.94	Insert/repl skull tongs	Operative	06.0	Thyroid field incision	Mixed (2, 1)
02.96	Insert sphenoid electrod	Non-Operative	06.09	Inc thyroid field NEC	Operative
03.0	Spinal canal exploration	Operative	06.1	Thyroid/parathy dxtic px	Mixed (3, 1)
03.02	Reopen laminectomy site	Operative	06.2	Unilat thyroid lobectomy	Operative
03.09	Spinal canal explor NEC	Operative	06.3	Other part thyroidectomy	Operative
03.1	Intraspin nerve root div	Operative	06.31	Excision thyroid lesion	Operative
03.2	Chordotomy	Operative	06.39	Part thyroidectomy NEC	Operative
03.3	Dxtic px on spinal canal	Mixed (2, 1)	06.4	Complete thyroidectomy	Operative
03.31	Spinal tap	Non-Operative	06.5	Substernal thyroidectomy	Operative
03.4	Exc spinal cord lesion	Operative	06.51	Part substern thyroidect	Operative
03.5	Spinal cord plastic ops	Operative	06.6	Lingual thyroid excision	Operative
03.53	Vertebral fx repair	Operative	06.7	Thyroglossal duct exc	Operative
03.59	Spinal struct repair NEC	Operative	06.8	Parathyroidectomy	Operative
03.6	Spinal cord adhesiolysis	Operative	06.81	Total parathyroidectomy	Operative

Code	Description	Operative Status	Code	Description	Operative Status
06.89	Other parathyroidectomy	Operative	12.4	Destr iris/cil body les	Operative
06.9	Thyroid/parathy ops NEC	Operative	12.5	InOc circulat facilitat	Operative
07.0	Adrenal field explor	Operative	12.6	Scleral fistulization	Operative
07.1	Oth endocrine dxtic px	Mixed (7, 1)	12.64	Trabeculect ab externo	Operative
07.2	Partial adrenalectomy	Operative	12.7	Elevat inOc press relief	Operative
07.22	Unilateral adrenalectomy	Operative	12.8	Operations on sclera	Operative
07.3	Bilateral adrenalectomy	Operative	12.9	Oth anterior segment ops	Operative
07.4	Other adrenal operations	Operative	13.0	Removal FB from lens	Operative
07.5	Pineal gland operations	Operative	13.1	Intracap lens extraction	Operative
07.6	Hypophysectomy	Operative	13.2	Lin extracaps lens extr	Operative
07.62	Exc pit les-transsphen	Operative	13.3	Simp asp lens extraction	Operative
07.65	Tot exc pit-transsphen	Operative	13.4	Frag-asp extracaps lens	Operative
07.7	Other hypophysis ops	Operative	13.41	Cataract PHACO & asp	Operative
07.8	Thymectomy	Operative	13.5	Oth extracaps lens extr	Operative
07.82	Total excision of thymus	Operative	13.59	Extracaps lens extr NEC	Operative
07.9	Other thymus operations	Operative	13.6	Oth cataract extraction	Operative
08.0	Eyelid incision	Non-Operative	13.7	Insert prosthetic lens	Operative
08.1	Dxtic px on eyelid	Mixed (1, 1)	13.8	Implanted lens removal	Operative
08.2	Exc/destr eyelid lesion	Operative	13.9	Other operations on lens	Operative
08.3	Ptosis/lid retract REP	Operative	14.0	Rmvl of post segment FB	Operative
08.4	Entropion/ectropion REP	Operative	14.1	Dxtic px posterior SEG	Operative
08.5	Oth adjust lid position	Operative	14.2	Retina-choroid les destr	Mixed (5, 3)
08.6	Eyelid reconst w graft	Operative	14.27	Chorioret radiat implant	Operative
08.7	Other eyelid reconst	Operative	14.3	Repair of retinal tear	Mixed (3, 3)
08.70	Lid reconstruction NOS	Operative	14.4	REP retina detach/buckle	Operative
08.8	Other repair of eyelid	Operative	14.41	Scleral buckling w impl	Operative
08.81	Linear REP eyelid lac	Operative	14.49	Scleral buckling NEC	Operative
08.9	Other eyelid operations	Operative	14.5	Oth repair retina detach	Operative
09.0	Lacrimal gland incision	Operative	14.54	Detach retina laser coag	Operative
09.1	Lacrimal system dxtic px	Operative	14.6	Rmvl prosth mat post SEG	Operative
09.2	Lacrimal gland les exc	Operative	14.7	Operations on vitreous	Operative
09.3	Other lacrimal gland ops	Operative	14.72	Vitreous removal NEC	Operative
09.4	Lacrimal passage manip	Operative	14.74	Mech vitrectomy NEC	Operative
09.5	Inc lacrimal sac/passg	Operative	14.9	Other post segment ops	Operative
09.6	Lacrimal sac/passage exc	Operative	15.0	ExOc musc-tend dxtic px	Operative
09.7	Canaliculus/punctum REP	Operative	15.1	1 ExOc musc ops w detach	Operative
09.8	NL fistulization	Operative	15.2	Oth ops on 1 ExOc muscle	Operative
09.9	Oth lacrimal syst ops	Operative	15.3	Temp detach >1 ExOc musc	Operative
10.0	Inc/rmvl FB-conjunctiva	Operative	15.4	Oth ops on >1 ExOc musc	Operative
10.1	Conjunctiva incision NEC	Operative	15.5	ExOc musc transposition	Operative
10.2	Conjunctiva dxtic px	Operative	15.6	Rev ExOc muscle surgery	Operative
10.3	Exc/destr conjunct les	Operative	15.7	ExOc muscle injury REP	Operative
10.4	Conjunctivoplasty	Operative	15.9	Oth ExOc musc-tend ops	Operative
10.5	Conjunct/lid ADHESIO	Operative	16.0	Orbitotomy	Operative
10.6	Repair conjunct lac	Operative	16.09	Orbitotomy NEC	Operative
10.9	Other conjunctival ops	Operative	16.1	Rmvl penetr FB eye NOS	Operative
11.0	Magnet removal cornea FB	Operative	16.2	Orbit & eyeball dxtic px	Mixed (3, 1)
11.1	Corneal incision	Operative	16.3	Evisceration of eyeball	Operative
11.2	Dxtic px on cornea	Operative	16.4	Enucleation of eyeball	Operative
11.3	Excision of pterygium	Operative	16.5	Exenteration of orbit	Operative
11.4	Exc/destr corneal lesion	Operative	16.6	2nd px post rmvl eyeball	Operative
11.5	Corneal repair	Operative	16.7	Ocular/orbital impl rmvl	Operative
11.51	Suture of corneal lac	Operative	16.8	Eyeball/orbit inj repair	Operative
11.6	Corneal transplant	Operative	16.82	Repair eyeball rupture	Operative
11.64	Penetr keratoplasty NEC	Operative	16.89	Eye/orbit inj repair NEC	Operative
11.7	Other cornea reconst	Operative	16.9	Other eye & orbit ops	Mixed (4, 1)
11.9	Other corneal operations	Operative	18.0	External ear incision	Non-Operative
12.0	Rmvl inOc FB ant segment	Operative	18.09	External ear inc NEC	Non-Operative
12.1	Iridotomy/smp iridectomy	Operative	18.1	External ear dxtic px	Non-Operative
12.2	Anterior SEG dxtic px	Operative	18.2	Exc/destr ext ear lesion	Mixed (1, 1)
12.3	Iridoplasty/coreoplasty	Operative	18.29	Destr ext ear les NEC	Non-Operative

Code	Description	Operative Status	Code	Description	Operative Status
18.3	Other external ear exc	Operative	23.0	Forceps tooth extraction	Non-Operative
18.4	Suture ext ear lac	Non-Operative	23.09	Tooth extraction NEC	Non-Operative
18.5	Correction prominent ear	Operative	23.1	Surg removal of tooth	Non-Operative
18.6	Ext audit canal reconst	Operative	23.19	Surg tooth extract NEC	Non-Operative
18.7	Oth plastic REP ext ear	Operative	23.2	Tooth restor by filling	Non-Operative
18.71	Construction ear auricle	Operative	23.3	Tooth restor by inlay	Non-Operative
18.79	Plastic REP ext ear NEC	Operative	23.4	Other dental restoration	Non-Operative
18.9	Other ext ear operations	Operative	23.5	Tooth implantation	Non-Operative
19.0	Stapes mobilization	Operative	23.6	Prosthetic dental impl	Non-Operative
19.1	Stapedectomy	Operative	23.7	Root canal Tx & apicoect	Non-Operative
19.19	Stapedectomy NEC	Operative	24.0	Gum or alveolar incision	Non-Operative
19.2	Stapedectomy revision	Operative	24.1	Tooth & gum dxtic px	Non-Operative
19.3	Ossicular chain ops NEC	Operative	24.2	Gingivoplasty	Operative
19.4	Myringoplasty	Operative	24.3	Other operations on gums	Non-Operative
19.5	Other tympanoplasty	Operative	24.4	Exc of dental les of jaw	Operative
19.6	Tympanoplasty revision	Operative	24.5	Alveoloplasty	Operative
19.9	Middle ear repair NEC	Operative	24.6	Exposure of tooth	Non-Operative
20.0	Myringotomy	Mixed (1, 1)	24.7	Appl orthodont appliance	Non-Operative
20.01	Myringotomy w intubation	Operative	24.8	Other orthodontic op	Non-Operative
20.1	Tympanostomy tube rmvl	Non-Operative	24.9	Other dental operation	Non-Operative
20.2	Mastoid & mid ear inc	Operative	25.0	Dxtic px on tongue	Mixed (1, 2)
20.3	Mid & inner ear dxtic px	Mixed (2, 1)	25.1	Exc/destr tongue les	Operative
20.4	Mastoidectomy	Operative	25.2	Partial glossectomy	Operative
20.42	Radical mastoidectomy	Operative	25.3	Complete glossectomy	Operative
20.49	Mastoidectomy NEC	Operative	25.4	Radical glossectomy	Operative
20.5	Oth middle ear excision	Operative	25.5	Repair of tongue	Mixed (1, 1)
20.6	Fenestration inner ear	Operative	25.9	Other tongue operations	Mixed (2, 3)
20.7	Inc/exc/destr inner ear	Operative	26.0	Inc salivary gland/duct	Non-Operative
20.8	Eustachian tube ops	Non-Operative	26.1	Salivary gland dxtic px	Mixed (1, 2)
20.9	Other ME & IE ops	Mixed (8, 1)	26.2	Exc of SG lesion	Operative
21.0	Control of epistaxis	Mixed (5, 4)	26.29	Salivary les exc NEC	Operative
21.01	Ant NAS pack for epistx	Non-Operative	26.3	Sialoadenectomy	Operative
21.02	Post NAS pack for epistx	Non-Operative	26.30	Sialoadenectomy NOS	Operative
21.03	Caut to cntrl epistaxis	Non-Operative	26.31	Partial sialoadenectomy	Operative
21.1	Incision of nose	Non-Operative	26.32	Complete sialoadenectomy	Operative
21.2	Nasal diagnostic px	Non-Operative	26.4	SG & duct repair	Operative
21.3	Nasal lesion destr/exc	Non-Operative	26.9	Oth salivary operations	Mixed (1, 1)
21.4	Resection of nose	Operative	27.0	Drain face & mouth floor	Operative
21.5	Submuc NAS septum resect	Operative	27.1	Incision of palate	Operative
21.6	Turbinectomy	Operative	27.2	Oral cavity dxtic px	Mixed (2, 3)
21.69	Turbinectomy NEC	Operative	27.3	Exc bony palate les/tiss	Operative
21.7	Nasal fracture reduction	Mixed (1, 1)	27.4	Other excision of mouth	Mixed (3, 1)
21.71	Clsd reduction nasal fx	Non-Operative	27.49	Excision of mouth NEC	Operative
21.72	Open reduction nasal fx	Operative	27.5	Plastic repair of mouth	Mixed (6, 2)
21.8	Nasal REP & plastic ops	Mixed (8, 1)	27.51	Suture of lip laceration	Non-Operative
21.81	Nasal laceration suture	Non-Operative	27.54	Repair of cleft lip	Operative
21.88	Septoplasty NEC	Operative	27.59	Mouth repair NEC	Operative
21.9	Other nasal operations	Mixed (1, 1)	27.6	Palatoplasty	Operative
22.0	Nasal sinus asp & lavage	Non-Operative	27.62	Cleft palate correction	Operative
22.1	Nasal sinus dxtic px	Mixed (1, 2)	27.63	Rev cleft palate repair	Operative
22.2	Intranasal antrotomy	Non-Operative	27.69	Other plastic REP palate	Operative
22.3	Ext maxillary antrotomy	Operative	27.7	Operations on uvula	Operative
22.39	Ext max antrotomy NEC	Operative	27.9	Oth ops on mouth & face	Mixed (2, 1)
22.4	Front sinusot & sinusect	Operative	28.0	Tonsil/peritonsillar I&D	Operative
22.42	Frontal sinusectomy	Operative	28.1	Tonsil adenoid dxtic px	Operative
22.5	Other nasal sinusotomy	Operative	28.2	Tonsillectomy	Operative
22.6	Other nasal sinusectomy	Operative	28.3	T&A	Operative
22.62	Exc max sinus lesion NEC	Operative	28.4	Excision of tonsil tag	Operative
22.63	Ethmoidectomy	Operative	28.5	Excision lingual tonsil	Operative
22.7	Nasal sinus repair	Operative	28.6	Adenoidectomy	Operative
22.9	Other nasal sinus ops	Operative	28.7	Hemor control post T&A	Operative

Code	Description	Operative Status	Code	Description	Operative Status
28.9	Other tonsil/adenoid ops	Operative	34.1	Incision of mediastinum	Operative
29.0	Pharyngotomy	Operative	34.2	Thorax dxtic procedures	Mixed (6, 3)
29.1	Pharyngeal dxtic px	Non-Operative	34.21	Transpleura thoracoscopy	Operative
29.11	Pharyngoscopy	Non-Operative	34.22	Mediastinoscopy	Operative
29.2	Exc branchial cleft cyst	Operative	34.24	Pleural biopsy	Non-Operative
29.3	Exc/destr pharyngeal les	Operative	34.26	Open mediastinal biopsy	Operative
29.4	Plastic op on pharynx	Operative	34.3	Destr mediastinum les	Operative
29.5	Other pharyngeal repair	Operative	34.4	Exc/destr chest wall les	Operative
29.9	Other pharyngeal ops	Mixed (2, 1)	34.5	Pleurectomy	Operative
30.0	Exc/destr les larynx	Operative	34.51	Decortication of lung	Operative
30.09	Exc/destr larynx les NEC	Operative	34.59	Other pleural excision	Operative
30.1	Hemilaryngectomy	Operative	34.6	Scarification of pleura	Operative
30.2	Partial laryngectomy NEC	Operative	34.7	Repair of chest wall	Mixed (3, 2)
30.3	Complete laryngectomy	Operative	34.74	Pectus deformity repair	Operative
30.4	Radical laryngectomy	Operative	34.8	Operations on diaphragm	Operative
31.0	Injection of larynx	Non-Operative	34.9	Other ops on thorax	Mixed (2, 2)
31.1	Temporary tracheostomy	Non-Operative	34.91	Thoracentesis	Non-Operative
31.2	Permanent tracheostomy	Operative	34.92	Inject into thor cavit	Non-Operative
31.29	Other perm tracheostomy	Operative	35.0	Closed heart valvotomy	Operative
31.3	Inc larynx/trachea NEC	Operative	35.1	Open heart valvuloplasty	Operative
31.4	Larynx/trachea dxtic px	Mixed (1, 6)	35.11	Opn aortic valvuloplasty	Operative
31.42	Laryngoscopy/tracheoscop	Non-Operative	35.12	Opn mitral valvuloplasty	Operative
31.43	Clsd (endo) Bx larynx	Non-Operative	35.2	Heart valve replacement	Operative
31.5	Loc exc/destr larynx les	Operative	35.21	Repl aortic valve-tissue	Operative
31.6	Repair of larynx	Operative	35.22	Repl aortic valve NEC	Operative
31.69	Other laryngeal repair	Operative	35.23	Repl mitral valve w tiss	Operative
31.7	Repair of trachea	Operative	35.24	Repl mitral valve NEC	Operative
31.73	Trach fistula close NEC	Operative	35.3	Tiss adj to hrt valv ops	Operative
31.74	Revision of tracheostomy	Operative	35.33	Annuloplasty	Operative
31.9	Other larynx/trachea ops	Mixed (4, 3)	35.4	Septal defect production	Mixed (1, 1)
32.0	Loc exc/destr bronch les	Mixed (1, 1)	35.5	Prosth REP heart septa	Operative
32.1	Other bronchial excision	Operative	35.53	Prosth REP VSD	Operative
32.2	Loc exc/destr lung les	Mixed (3, 1)	35.6	Tiss grft REP hrt septa	Operative
32.21	Emphysem bleb plication	Operative	35.61	Repair ASD w tiss graft	Operative
32.22	Lung volume red surgery	Operative	35.7	Heart septa REP NEC/NOS	Operative
32.28	Endo exc/destr lung les	Non-Operative	35.71	Repair ASD NEC	Operative
32.29	Loc exc lung les NEC	Operative	35.72	Repair VSD NEC	Operative
32.3	Segmental lung resection	Operative	35.8	Tot REP cong card anom	Operative
32.4	Lobectomy of lung	Operative	35.81	Tot REP tetralogy fallot	Operative
32.5	Complete pneumonectomy	Operative	35.9	Valves & septa ops NEC	Operative
32.6	RAD dissect thor struct	Operative	35.94	Creat conduit atrium-PA	Operative
32.9	Other excision of lung	Operative	35.96	PERC valvuloplasty	Operative
33.0	Incision of bronchus	Operative	36.0	Rmvl coronary art obstr	Mixed (5, 2)
33.1	Incision of lung	Operative	36.01	1 PTCA/atherect w/o TL	Operative
33.2	Bronchial/lung dxtic px	Mixed (4, 5)	36.02	1 PTCA/atherect w TL	Operative
33.22	Fiber-optic bronchoscopy	Non-Operative	36.05	PTCA/atherect->1 vessel	Operative
33.23	Other bronchoscopy	Non-Operative	36.06	Insert coronary stent	Non-Operative
33.24	Clsd (endo) bronchus Bx	Non-Operative	36.1	Hrt revasc bypass anast	Operative
33.26	Closed lung biopsy	Non-Operative	36.11	Ao-cor bypass-1 cor art	Operative
33.27	Endo lung Bx (closed)	Operative	36.12	Ao-cor bypass-2 cor art	Operative
33.28	Open biopsy of lung	Operative	36.13	Ao-cor bypass-3 cor art	Operative
33.3	Surg collapse of lung	Mixed (2, 3)	36.14	Ao-cor bypass-4+ cor art	Operative
33.4	Lung and bronchus repair	Operative	36.15	1 int mam-cor art bypass	Operative
33.5	Lung transplantion	Operative	36.16	2 int mam-cor art bypass	Operative
33.6	Heart-lung transplant	Operative	36.2	Arterial implant revasc	Operative
33.9	Other bronchial lung ops	Mixed (4, 1)	36.3	Heart revasc NEC	Operative
34.0	Inc chest wall & pleura	Mixed (2, 4)	36.9	Other heart vessel ops	Operative
34.01	Incision of chest wall	Non-Operative	37.0	Pericardiocentesis	Non-Operative
34.02	Exploratory thoracotomy	Operative	37.1	Cardiotomy & pericardiot	Operative
34.04	Insert intercostal cath	Non-Operative	37.12	Pericardiotomy	Operative
34.09	Other pleural incision	Non-Operative	37.2	Dxtic px hrt/pericardium	Mixed (1, 7)

Code	Description	Operative Status	Code	Description	Operative Status
37.21	Rt heart cardiac cath	Non-Operative	38.95	Venous cath for RD	Non-Operative
37.22	Left heart cardiac cath	Non-Operative	38.98	Arterial puncture NEC	Non-Operative
37.23	Rt/left heart card cath	Non-Operative	38.99	Venous puncture NEC	Non-Operative
37.25	Cardiac biopsy	Non-Operative	39.0	Systemic to PA shunt	Operative
37.26	Card EPS/record studies	Non-Operative	39.1	Intra-abd venous shunt	Operative
37.3	Pericardiect/exc hrt les	Operative	39.2	Other shunt/vasc bypass	Operative
37.31	Pericardiectomy	Operative	39.21	Caval-PA anastomosis	Operative
37.33	Heart les exc/destr NEC	Operative	39.22	Aorta-scl-carotid bypass	Operative
37.34	Cath ablation heart les	Operative	39.25	Aorta-iliac-femoral byp	Operative
37.4	REP heart & pericardium	Operative	39.27	Arteriovenostomy for RD	Operative
37.5	Heart transplantation	Operative	39.29	Vasc shunt & bypass NEC	Operative
37.6	Impl heart assist syst	Operative	39.3	Suture of vessel	Operative
37.61	Pulsation balloon impl	Operative	39.31	Suture of artery	Operative
37.7	Cardiac pacer lead op	Mixed (5, 5)	39.4	Vascular px revision	Operative
37.71	Insert TV lead-ventricle	Non-Operative	39.42	Rev AV shunt for RD	Operative
37.72	Insert TV lead-ATR&vent	Non-Operative	39.43	Rmvl AV shunt for RD	Operative
37.75	Revision pacemaker lead	Operative	39.49	Vascular px revision NEC	Operative
37.76	Replace transvenous lead	Operative	39.5	Other vessel repair	Operative
37.78	Insert temp TV pacer	Non-Operative	39.50	PTA/atherectomy oth vsl	Operative
37.8	Cardiac pacemaker dev op	Mixed (5, 3)	39.51	Clipping of aneurysm	Operative
37.80	Insert pacemaker dev NOS	Operative	39.52	Aneurysm repair NEC	Operative
37.81	Insert single chamb dev	Non-Operative	39.53	AV fistula repair	Operative
37.82	Insert rate-respon dev	Non-Operative	39.56	REP vess w tiss patch	Operative
37.83	Insert dual-chamber dev	Non-Operative	39.57	REP vess w synth patch	Operative
37.85	Repl w 1-chamber device	Operative	39.59	Repair of vessel NEC	Operative
37.86	Repl w rate-respon dev	Operative	39.6	Open heart auxiliary px	Non-Operative
37.87	Repl w dual-chamb device	Operative	39.8	Vascular body operations	Operative
37.9	Hrt/pericardium ops NEC	Mixed (7, 2)	39.9	Other vessel operations	Mixed (6, 3)
37.94	Impl/repl AICD tot syst	Operative	39.93	Insert vess-vess cannula	Operative
37.98	Repl AICD generator only	Operative	39.95	Hemodialysis	Non-Operative
38.0	Incision of vessel	Operative	39.97	Other perfusion	Non-Operative
38.03	Upper limb vessel inc	Operative	39.98	Hemorrhage control NOS	Operative
38.08	Lower limb artery inc	Operative	40.0	Inc lymphatic structure	Operative
38.1	Endarterectomy	Operative	40.1	Lymphatic dxtic px	Operative
38.12	Head/nk endarterect NEC	Operative	40.11	Lymphatic struct biopsy	Operative
38.16	Abdominal endarterectomy	Operative	40.2	Smp exc lymphatic struct	Operative
38.18	Lower limb endarterect	Operative	40.21	Exc deep cervical node	Operative
38.2	Dxtic px on blood vessel	Mixed (2, 1)	40.23	Exc axillary lymph node	Operative
38.21	Blood vessel biopsy	Operative	40.24	Exc inguinal lymph node	Operative
38.3	Vessel resect w anast	Operative	40.29	Smp exc lymphatic NEC	Operative
38.34	Aorta resection & anast	Operative	40.3	Regional lymph node exc	Operative
38.4	Vessel resect w repl	Operative	40.4	RAD exc cerv lymph node	Operative
38.44	Abd aorta resect w repl	Operative	40.41	Unilat RAD neck dissect	Operative
38.45	Thor vess resect w repl	Operative	40.5	Oth RAD node dissection	Operative
38.46	Abd artery resect w repl	Operative	40.6	Thoracic duct operations	Operative
38.48	Leg artery resect w repl	Operative	40.9	Lymphatic struct ops NEC	Operative
38.5	Lig&strip varicose veins	Operative	41.0	Bone marrow transplant	Mixed (4, 1)
38.59	Lower limb VV lig&strip	Operative	41.01	Autolog marrow transpl	Operative
38.6	Other vessel excision	Operative	41.03	Allo marrow transpl NEC	Operative
38.64	Excision of aorta	Operative	41.04	Stem cell transplant	Non-Operative
38.68	Lower limb artery exc	Operative	41.1	Puncture of spleen	Non-Operative
38.7	Interruption vena cava	Operative	41.2	Splenotomy	Operative
38.8	Other surg vessel occl	Operative	41.3	Marrow & spleen dxtic px	Mixed (1, 4)
38.82	Occl head/neck vess NEC	Operative	41.31	Bone marrow biopsy	Non-Operative
38.85	Occl thoracic vess NEC	Operative	41.4	Exc/destr splenic tissue	Operative
38.86	Surg occl abd artery NEC	Operative	41.5	Total splenectomy	Operative
38.9	Puncture of vessel	Non-Operative	41.9	Oth spleen & marrow ops	Mixed (4, 3)
38.91	Arterial catheterization	Non-Operative	41.91	Donor marrow aspiration	Non-Operative
38.92	Umbilical vein cath	Non-Operative	42.0	Esophagotomy	Operative
38.93	Venous catheter NEC	Non-Operative	42.1	Esophagostomy	Operative
38.94	Venous cutdown	Non-Operative	42.2	Esophageal dxtic px	Mixed (2, 4)

Code	Description	Operative Status	Code	Description	Operative Status
42.23	Esophagoscopy NEC	Non-Operative	45.33	Loc exc sm bowel les NEC	Operative
42.29	Esophageal dxtic px NEC	Non-Operative	45.4	Loc destr lg bowel les	Mixed (2, 2)
42.3	Exc/destr esoph les/tiss	Mixed (3, 1)	45.41	Loc exc lg bowel les	Operative
42.31	Exc esoph diverticulum	Operative	45.42	Endo colon polypectomy	Non-Operative
42.33	Endo exc/destr esoph les	Non-Operative	45.43	Endo destr colon les NEC	Non-Operative
42.4	Excision of esophagus	Operative	45.5	Intestinal SEG isolation	Operative
42.41	Partial esophagectomy	Operative	45.6	Other sm bowel excision	Operative
42.42	Total esophagectomy	Operative	45.61	Mult SEG sm bowel resect	Operative
42.5	Intrathor esoph anast	Operative	45.62	Part sm bowel resect NEC	Operative
42.6	Antesternal esoph anast	Operative	45.7	Part lg bowel excision	Operative
42.7	Esophagomyotomy	Operative	45.71	Mult SEG lg bowel resect	Operative
42.8	Other esophageal repair	Mixed (7, 1)	45.72	Cecectomy	Operative
42.9	Other esophageal ops	Mixed (1, 2)	45.73	Right hemicolectomy	Operative
42.92	Esophageal dilation	Non-Operative	45.74	Transverse colon resect	Operative
43.0	Gastrotomy	Operative	45.75	Left hemicolectomy	Operative
43.1	Gastrostomy	Non-Operative	45.76	Sigmoidectomy	Operative
43.11	PERC (endo) gastrostomy	Non-Operative	45.79	Part lg bowel exc NEC	Operative
43.19	Gastrostomy NEC	Non-Operative	45.8	Tot intra-abd colectomy	Operative
43.3	Pyloromyotomy	Operative	45.9	Intestinal anastomosis	Operative
43.4	Loc exc gastric les	Mixed (2, 1)	45.91	Sm-to-sm bowel anast	Operative
43.41	Endo exc gastric les	Non-Operative	45.93	Small-to-large bowel NEC	Operative
43.42	Loc gastric les exc NEC	Operative	45.94	Lg-to-lg bowel anast	Operative
43.5	Proximal gastrectomy	Operative	46.0	Exteriorization of bowel	Operative
43.6	Distal gastrectomy	Operative	46.01	Sm bowel exteriorization	Operative
43.7	Part gastrectomy w anast	Operative	46.03	Lg bowel exteriorization	Operative
43.8	Oth partial gastrectomy	Operative	46.1	Colostomy	Mixed (3, 1)
43.89	Partial gastrectomy NEC	Operative	46.10	Colostomy NOS	Operative
43.9	Total gastrectomy	Operative	46.11	Temporary colostomy	Operative
43.99	Total gastrectomy NEC	Operative	46.13	Permanent colostomy	Operative
44.0	Vagotomy	Operative	46.2	Ileostomy	Mixed (4, 1)
44.01	Truncal vagotomy	Operative	46.3	Other enterostomy	Non-Operative
44.1	Gastric dxtic px	Mixed (2, 4)	46.32	PERC (endo) jejunostomy	Non-Operative
44.13	Gastroscopy NEC	Non-Operative	46.39	Enterostomy NEC	Non-Operative
44.14	Clsd (endo) gastric Bx	Non-Operative	46.4	Intestinal stoma rev	Operative
44.2	Pyloroplasty	Mixed (2, 1)	46.41	Sm bowel stoma revision	Operative
44.29	Other pyloroplasty	Operative	46.42	Pericolostomy hernia REP	Operative
44.3	Gastroenterostomy	Operative	46.43	Lg bowel stoma rev NEC	Operative
44.31	High gastric bypass	Operative	46.5	Closure intestinal stoma	Operative
44.39	Gastroenterostomy NEC	Operative	46.51	Sm bowel stoma closure	Operative
44.4	Cntrl peptic ulcer hemor	Mixed (3, 3)	46.52	Lg bowel stoma closure	Operative
44.41	Sut gastric ulcer site	Operative	46.6	Fixation of intestine	Operative
44.42	Sut duodenal ulcer site	Operative	46.7	Other intestinal repair	Operative
44.43	Endo cntrl gastric bleed	Non-Operative	46.73	Small bowel suture NEC	Operative
44.5	Revision gastric anast	Operative	46.74	Closure SmB fistula NEC	Operative
44.6	Other gastric repair	Mixed (6, 1)	46.75	Suture lg bowel lac	Operative
44.63	Close stom fistula NEC	Operative	46.79	Repair of intestine NEC	Operative
44.66	Creat EG sphinct compet	Operative	46.8	Bowel dilation & manip	Mixed (3, 1)
44.69	Gastric repair NEC	Operative	46.81	Intra-abd sm bowel manip	Operative
44.9	Other stomach operations	Mixed (3, 2)	46.82	Intra-abd lg bowel manip	Operative
45.0	Enterotomy	Operative	46.85	Dilation of intestine	Non-Operative
45.1	Small bowel dxtic px	Mixed (2, 5)	46.9	Other intestinal ops	Mixed (5, 2)
45.13	Sm bowel endoscopy NEC	Non-Operative	47.0	Appendectomy	Operative
45.14	Clsd (endo) sm intest Bx	Non-Operative	47.1	Incidental appendectomy	Operative
45.16	EGD with closed biopsy	Non-Operative	47.2	Drain appendiceal absc	Operative
45.2	Lg intestine dxtic px	Mixed (2, 7)	47.9	Other appendiceal ops	Operative
45.22	Endo lg bowel thru stoma	Non-Operative	48.0	Proctotomy	Operative
45.23	Colonoscopy	Non-Operative	48.1	Proctostomy	Operative
45.24	Flexible sigmoidoscopy	Non-Operative	48.2	Rectal/perirect dxtic px	Mixed (2, 5)
45.25	Clsd (endo) lg intest Bx	Non-Operative	48.23	Rigid proctsigmoidoscopy	Non-Operative
45.3	Loc exc/destr SmB les	Mixed (4, 1)	48.24	Clsd (endo) rectal Bx	Non-Operative
45.30	Endo exc/destr duod les	Non-Operative	48.3	Loc destr rectal lesion	Mixed (1, 5)

Code	Description	Operative Status	Code	Description	Operative Status
48.35	Loc exc rectal les/tiss	Operative	51.85	Endo sphinctot/papillot	Non-Operative
48.36	Endo rectal polypectomy	Non-Operative	51.87	Endo insert BD stent	Non-Operative
48.4	Pull-thru rect resection	Operative	51.88	Endo rmvl biliary stone	Non-Operative
48.5	Abd-perineal rect resect	Operative	51.9	Other biliary tract ops	Mixed (6, 2)
48.6	Other rectal resection	Operative	51.98	PERC op on bil tract NEC	Non-Operative
48.62	Ant rect resect w colost	Operative	52.0	Pancreatotomy	Operative
48.63	Anterior rect resect NEC	Operative	52.1	Pancreatic dxtic px	Mixed (2, 3)
48.69	Rectal resection NEC	Operative	52.11	Panc asp (needle) Bx	Non-Operative
48.7	Repair of rectum	Operative	52.2	Panc/panc duct les destr	Mixed (1, 1)
48.76	Proctopexy NEC	Operative	52.3	Pancreatic cyst marsup	Operative
48.8	Perirect tiss inc/exc	Operative	52.4	Int drain panc cyst	Operative
48.81	Perirectal incision	Operative	52.5	Partial pancreatectomy	Operative
48.9	Oth rectal/perirect op	Operative	52.52	Distal pancreatectomy	Operative
49.0	Perianal tiss inc/exc	Mixed (3, 1)	52.6	Total pancreatectomy	Operative
49.01	Inc perianal abscess	Operative	52.7	RAD panc/duodenectomy	Operative
49.1	Inc/exc of anal fistula	Operative	52.8	Transplant of pancreas	Operative
49.11	Anal fistulotomy	Operative	52.9	Other ops on pancreas	Mixed (4, 4)
49.12	Anal fistulectomy	Operative	52.93	Endo insert panc stent	Non-Operative
49.2	Anal & perianal dxtic px	Non-Operative	52.96	Pancreatic anastomosis	Operative
49.21	Anoscopy	Non-Operative	53.0	Unilat IH repair	Operative
49.3	Loc destr anal les NEC	Mixed (1, 1)	53.00	Unilat IH repair NOS	Operative
49.39	Oth loc destr anal les	Operative	53.01	Unilat REP direct IH	Operative
49.4	Hemorrhoid procedures	Mixed (4, 4)	53.02	Unilat REP indirect IH	Operative
49.46	Exc of hemorrhoids	Operative	53.03	Unilat REP DIR IH/graft	Operative
49.5	Anal sphincter division	Operative	53.04	Unilat indirect IH/graft	Operative
49.6	Excision of anus	Operative	53.05	Unilat REP IH/graft NOS	Operative
49.7	Repair of anus	Operative	53.1	Bilat IH repair	Operative
49.79	Anal sphincter REP NEC	Operative	53.10	Bilat IH repair NOS	Operative
49.9	Oth operations on anus	Operative	53.12	Bilat indirect IH repair	Operative
50.0	Hepatotomy	Operative	53.14	Bilat direct IH REP-grft	Operative
50.1	Hepatic dxtic px	Mixed (2, 1)	53.17	Bilat IH REP-graft NOS	Operative
50.11	Clsd (PERC) liver biopsy	Non-Operative	53.2	Unilat FH repair	Operative
50.12	Open biopsy of liver	Operative	53.21	Unilat FH REP w graft	Operative
50.2	Loc exc/destr liver les	Operative	53.29	Unilat FH REP NEC	Operative
50.22	Partial hepatectomy	Operative	53.3	Bilat FH repair	Operative
50.29	Destr hepatic lesion NEC	Operative	53.4	Umbilical hernia repair	Operative
50.3	Hepatic lobectomy	Operative	53.41	Umb hernia repair-graft	Operative
50.4	Total hepatectomy	Operative	53.49	Umb hernia repair NEC	Operative
50.5	Liver transplant	Operative	53.5	REP oth abd wall hernia	Operative
50.59	Liver transplant NEC	Operative	53.51	Incisional hernia repair	Operative
50.6	Repair of liver	Operative	53.59	Abd wall hernia REP NEC	Operative
50.61	Closure of liver lac	Operative	53.6	REP oth abd hernia-graft	Operative
50.9	Other liver operations	Non-Operative	53.61	Inc hernia repair-graft	Operative
50.91	PERC liver aspiration	Non-Operative	53.69	Abd hernia REP-grft NEC	Operative
51.0	GB inc & cholecystostomy	Mixed (3, 1)	53.7	Abd REP-diaph hernia	Operative
51.1	Biliary tract dxtic px	Mixed (2, 5)	53.8	Repair DH, thor appr	Operative
51.10	ERCP	Non-Operative	53.9	Other hernia repair	Operative
51.14	Clsd BD/sphinct Oddi Bx	Non-Operative	54.0	Abdominal wall incision	Operative
51.2	Cholecystectomy	Operative	54.1	Laparotomy	Operative
51.22	Cholecystectomy NOS	Operative	54.11	Exploratory laparotomy	Operative
51.23	Lapscp cholecystectomy	Operative	54.12	Reopen recent LAP site	Operative
51.3	Biliary tract anast	Operative	54.19	Laparotomy NEC	Operative
51.32	GB-to-intestine anast	Operative	54.2	Abd region dxtic px	Mixed (4, 2)
51.36	Choledochoenterostomy	Operative	54.21	Laparoscopy	Operative
51.4	Inc bile duct obstr	Operative	54.23	Peritoneal biopsy	Operative
51.43	Insert CBD-hep tube	Operative	54.24	Clsd Bx intra-abd mass	Non-Operative
51.5	Other bile duct incision	Operative	54.25	Peritoneal lavage	Non-Operative
51.6	Loc exc BD & S of O les	Mixed (4, 1)	54.3	Exc/destr abd wall les	Operative
51.7	Repair of bile ducts	Operative	54.4	Exc/destr periton tiss	Operative
51.8	Sphincter of Oddi op NEC	Mixed (4, 5)	54.5	Peritoneal adhesiolysis	Operative
51.84	Endo ampulla & BD dilat	Non-Operative	54.6	Abd wall/periton suture	Operative

Code	Description	Operative Status	Code	Description	Operative Status
54.61	Reclose postop disrupt	Operative	57.71	Radical cystectomy	Operative
54.7	Oth abd wall periton REP	Operative	57.8	Oth urin bladder repair	Operative
54.9	Other abd region ops	Mixed (4, 5)	57.84	REP oth fistula bladder	Operative
54.91	PERC abd drainage	Non-Operative	57.87	Urinary bladder reconst	Operative
54.92	Rmvl FB periton cavity	Operative	57.89	Bladder repair NEC	Operative
54.93	Create cutaneoperit fist	Operative	57.9	Other bladder operations	Mixed (6, 3)
54.94	Creat peritoneovas shunt	Operative	57.91	Bladder sphincterotomy	Operative
54.95	Peritoneal incision	Operative	57.93	Control bladder hemor	Operative
54.98	Peritoneal dialysis	Non-Operative	57.94	Insert indwell urin cath	Non-Operative
55.0	Nephrotomy & nephrostomy	Operative	58.0	Urethrotomy	Operative
55.01	Nephrotomy	Operative	58.1	Urethral meatotomy	Operative
55.02	Nephrostomy	Operative	58.2	Urethral diagnostic px	Non-Operative
55.03	PERC nephrostomy-no frag	Operative	58.3	Exc/destr urethral les	Non-Operative
55.04	PERC nephrostomy w frag	Operative	58.31	Endo urethral les destr	Non-Operative
55.1	Pyelotomy & pyelostomy	Operative	58.39	Urethra les destr NEC	Non-Operative
55.11	Pyelotomy	Operative	58.4	Repair of urethra	Operative
55.2	Renal diagnostic px	Mixed (2, 3)	58.45	Hypospad/epispadias REP	Operative
55.23	Clsd (PERC) renal biopsy	Non-Operative	58.49	Urethral repair NEC	Operative
55.24	Open biopsy of kidney	Operative	58.5	Urethral stricture rel	Operative
55.3	Loc exc/destr renal les	Operative	58.6	Urethral dilation	Non-Operative
55.39	Loc destr renal les NEC	Operative	58.9	Other urethral ops	Operative
55.4	Partial nephrectomy	Operative	58.93	Implantation of AUS	Operative
55.5	Complete nephrectomy	Operative	59.0	Retroperiton dissection	Operative
55.51	Nephroureterectomy	Operative	59.1	Perivesical incision	Operative
55.53	Rejected kid nephrectomy	Operative	59.2	Perirenal dxtic px	Operative
55.6	Kidney transplant	Operative	59.3	Urethroves junct plicat	Operative
55.69	Kidney transplant NEC	Operative	59.4	Suprapubic sling op	Operative
55.7	Nephropexy	Operative	59.5	Retropubic urethral susp	Operative
55.8	Other kidney repair	Operative	59.6	Paraurethral suspension	Operative
55.87	Correction of UPJ	Operative	59.7	Oth urinary incont REP	Mixed (2, 1)
55.9	Other renal operations	Mixed (4, 5)	59.71	Levator musc suspension	Operative
55.93	Repl nephrostomy tube	Non-Operative	59.79	Urin incont repair NEC	Operative
56.0	TU rmvl ureteral obstr	Operative	59.8	Ureteral catheterization	Non-Operative
56.1	Ureteral meatotomy	Operative	59.9	Other urinary system ops	Mixed (2, 4)
56.2	Ureterotomy	Operative	60.0	Incision of prostate	Operative
56.3	Ureteral diagnostic px	Mixed (2, 4)	60.1	Pros/sem vesicl dxtic px	Mixed (5, 2)
56.31	Ureteroscopy	Non-Operative	60.11	Clsd (PERC) prostatic Bx	Non-Operative
56.4	Ureterectomy	Operative	60.2	TU prostatectomy	Operative
56.41	Partial ureterectomy	Operative	60.21	TULIP procedure	Operative
56.5	Cutan uretero-ileostomy	Operative	60.29	TU prostatectomy NEC	Operative
56.51	Form cutan ileoureterost	Operative	60.3	Suprapubic prostatectomy	Operative
56.6	Ext urin diversion NEC	Operative	60.4	Retropubic prostatectomy	Operative
56.7	Other ureteral anast	Operative	60.5	Radical prostatectomy	Operative
56.74	Ureteroneocystostomy	Operative	60.6	Other prostatectomy	Operative
56.8	Repair of ureter	Operative	60.7	Seminal vesicle ops	Mixed (3, 1)
56.9	Other ureteral operation	Mixed (5, 1)	60.8	Periprostatic inc or exc	Operative
57.0	TU bladder clearance	Non-Operative	60.9	Other prostatic ops	Mixed (4, 2)
57.1	Cystotomy & cystostomy	Mixed (3, 2)	60.94	Cntrl postop pros hemor	Operative
57.17	Percutaneous cystostomy	Non-Operative	61.0	Scrotum & tunica vag I&D	Non-Operative
57.18	S/P cystostomy NEC	Operative	61.1	Scrotum/tunica dxtic px	Non-Operative
57.19	Cystotomy NEC	Operative	61.2	Excision of hydrocele	Operative
57.2	Vesicostomy	Operative	61.3	Scrotal les exc/destr	Non-Operative
57.3	Bladder diagnostic px	Mixed (3, 2)	61.4	Scrotum & tunica vag REP	Mixed (2, 1)
57.32	Cystoscopy NEC	Non-Operative	61.9	Oth scrot/tunica vag ops	Mixed (2, 1)
57.33	Clsd (TU) bladder biopsy	Operative	62.0	Incision of testis	Operative
57.4	TU exc/destr bladder les	Operative	62.1	Testes dxtic px	Mixed (2, 1)
57.49	TU destr bladder les NEC	Operative	62.2	Testicular les destr/exc	Operative
57.5	Bladder les destr NEC	Operative	62.3	Unilateral orchiectomy	Operative
57.59	Oth bladder lesion destr	Operative	62.4	Bilateral orchiectomy	Operative
57.6	Partial cystectomy	Operative	62.41	Rmvl both testes	Operative
57.7	Total cystectomy	Operative	62.5	Orchiopexy	Operative

Code	Description	Operative Status	Code	Description	Operative Status
62.6	Repair of testes	Operative	67.1	Cervical diagnostic px	Operative
62.7	Insert testicular prosth	Operative	67.12	Cervical biopsy NEC	Operative
62.9	Other testicular ops	Mixed (1, 2)	67.2	Conization of cervix	Operative
63.0	Spermatic cord dxtic px	Mixed (1, 1)	67.3	Exc/destr cerv les NEC	Operative
63.1	Exc spermatic varicocele	Operative	67.39	Cerv les exc/destr NEC	Operative
63.2	Exc epididymis cyst	Operative	67.4	Amputation of cervix	Operative
63.3	Exc sperm cord les NEC	Operative	67.5	Int cervical os repair	Operative
63.4	Epididymectomy	Operative	67.6	Other repair of cervix	Operative
63.5	Sperm cord/epid repair	Mixed (3, 1)	68.0	Hysterotomy	Operative
63.6	Vasotomy	Non-Operative	68.1	Uter/adnexa dxtic px	Mixed (5, 2)
63.7	Vasectomy & vas def lig	Non-Operative	68.16	Clsd uterine Bx	Operative
63.8	Vas def & epid repair	Mixed (5, 1)	68.2	Uterine les exc/destr	Operative
63.9	Oth sperm cord/epid ops	Mixed (5, 1)	68.29	Uter les exc/destr NEC	Operative
64.0	Circumcision	Operative	68.3	Subtot abd hysterectomy	Operative
64.1	Penile diagnostic px	Mixed (1, 1)	68.4	Total abd hysterectomy	Operative
64.2	Loc exc/destr penile les	Operative	68.5	Vaginal hysterectomy	Operative
64.3	Amputation of penis	Operative	68.6	Radical abd hysterectomy	Operative
64.4	Penile REP/plastic ops	Operative	68.7	Radical vag hysterectomy	Operative
64.5	Sex transformation NEC	Operative	68.8	Pelvic evisceration	Operative
64.9	Other male genital ops	Mixed (7, 2)	68.9	Hysterectomy NEC & NOS	Operative
64.95	Insert/repl non-IPP NOS	Operative	69.0	Uterine D&C	Operative
64.96	Rmvl int penile prosth	Operative	69.01	D&C for term of preg	Operative
64.97	Insert or repl IPP	Operative	69.02	D&C post del or AB	Operative
65.0	Oophorotomy	Operative	69.09	D&C NEC	Operative
65.1	Dxtic px on ovaries	Operative	69.1	Exc/destr uter/supp les	Operative
65.2	Loc exc/destr ovary les	Operative	69.19	Exc uter/supp struct NEC	Operative
65.22	Ovarian wedge resection	Operative	69.2	Uterine supp struct REP	Operative
65.29	Loc exc/destr ov les NEC	Operative	69.3	Paracerv uterine denerv	Operative
65.3	Unilateral oophorectomy	Operative	69.4	Uterine repair	Operative
65.4	Unilateral S-O	Operative	69.5	Asp curettage uterus	Mixed (2, 1)
65.5	Bilateral oophorectomy	Operative	69.51	Asp curettage-preg term	Operative
65.51	Rmvl both ov-same op	Operative	69.52	Asp curette post del/AB	Operative
65.52	Rmvl remaining ovary	Operative	69.59	Asp curettage uterus NEC	Non-Operative
65.6	Bilat salpingo-oophorect	Operative	69.6	Menstrual extraction	Non-Operative
65.61	Rmvl both ov & FALL-1 op	Operative	69.7	Insertion of IUD	Non-Operative
65.62	Rmvl rem ovary & tube	Operative	69.9	Other ops uterus/adnexa	Mixed (4, 5)
65.7	Repair of ovary	Operative	69.93	Insertion of laminaria	Non-Operative
65.8	Tubo-ovarian ADHESIO	Operative	69.96	Rmvl cervical cerclage	Non-Operative
65.9	Other ovarian operations	Operative	70.0	Culdocentesis	Non-Operative
65.91	Aspiration of ovary	Operative	70.1	Inc vagina & cul-de-sac	Mixed (3, 1)
66.0	Salpingostomy/salpingot	Operative	70.12	Culdotomy	Operative
66.01	Salpingotomy	Operative	70.2	Vag/cul-de-sac dxtic px	Mixed (3, 2)
66.02	Salpingostomy	Operative	70.3	Loc exc/destr vag/cul	Operative
66.1	Fallopian tube dxtic px	Operative	70.33	Exc/destr vag lesion	Operative
66.2	Bilat endo occl FALL	Operative	70.4	Vaginal obliteration	Operative
66.22	Bilat endo lig/div FALL	Operative	70.5	Cystocele/rectocele REP	Operative
66.29	Bilat endo occl FALL NEC	Operative	70.50	REP cystocele/rectocele	Operative
66.3	Oth bilat FALL destr/exc	Operative	70.51	Cystocele repair	Operative
66.32	Bilat FALL lig & div NEC	Operative	70.52	Rectocele repair	Operative
66.39	Bilat FALL destr NEC	Operative	70.6	Vaginal constr/reconst	Operative
66.4	Tot unilat salpingectomy	Operative	70.7	Other vaginal repair	Operative
66.5	Tot bilat salpingectomy	Operative	70.71	Suture vagina laceration	Operative
66.6	Other salpingectomy	Operative	70.73	REP rectovaginal fistula	Operative
66.61	Exc/destr FALL les	Operative	70.77	Vaginal susp & fixation	Operative
66.62	Rmvl FALL & tubal preg	Operative	70.79	Vaginal repair NEC	Operative
66.69	Partial FALL rmvl NEC	Operative	70.8	Vaginal vault oblit	Operative
66.7	Repair of fallopian tube	Operative	70.9	Oth vag & cul-de-sac ops	Operative
66.79	FALL tube repair NEC	Operative	70.92	Cul-de-sac operation NEC	Operative
66.8	FALL tube insufflation	Non-Operative	71.0	Inc vulva & perineum	Operative
66.9	Other fallopian tube ops	Mixed (7, 1)	71.09	Inc vulva/perineum NEC	Operative
67.0	Cervical canal dilation	Non-Operative	71.1	Vulvar diagnostic px	Operative

Code	Description	Operative Status	Code	Description	Operative Status
71.2	Bartholin's gland ops	Mixed (4, 1)	75.7	PP manual explor uterus	Non-Operative
71.3	Loc vulvar/peri exc NEC	Operative	75.8	OB tamponade uterus/vag	Non-Operative
71.4	Operations on clitoris	Operative	75.9	Other obstetrical ops	Mixed (2, 3)
71.5	Radical vulvectomy	Operative	76.0	Facial bone incision	Operative
71.6	Other vulvectomy	Operative	76.1	Dxtic px facial bone/jt	Operative
71.61	Unilateral vulvectomy	Operative	76.2	Destr facial bone les	Operative
71.7	Vulvar & perineal repair	Operative	76.3	Partial facial ostectomy	Operative
71.71	Suture vulvar/peri lac	Operative	76.31	Partial mandibulectomy	Operative
71.79	Vulvar/perineum REP NEC	Operative	76.4	Facial bone exc/reconst	Operative
71.8	Other vulvar operations	Operative	76.5	TMJ arthroplasty	Operative
71.9	Other female genital ops	Operative	76.6	Other facial bone repair	Operative
72.0	Low forceps operation	Non-Operative	76.62	Opn osty mand ramus	Operative
72.1	Low forceps w episiotomy	Non-Operative	76.64	Mand orthognathic op NEC	Operative
72.2	Mid forceps operation	Non-Operative	76.65	SEG osteoplasty maxilla	Operative
72.21	Mid forceps w episiotomy	Non-Operative	76.66	Tot osteoplasty maxilla	Operative
72.3	High forceps operation	Non-Operative	76.7	Reduction of facial fx	Mixed (6, 4)
72.4	Forceps ROT fetal head	Non-Operative	76.72	Open red malar/ZMC fx	Operative
72.5	Breech extraction	Non-Operative	76.74	Open red maxillary fx	Operative
72.52	Part breech extract NEC	Non-Operative	76.75	Clsd red mandibular fx	Non-Operative
72.54	Tot breech extract NEC	Non-Operative	76.76	Open red mandibular fx	Operative
72.6	Forceps-aftercoming head	Non-Operative	76.79	Open red facial fx NEC	Operative
72.7	Vacuum extraction del	Non-Operative	76.9	Oth ops facial bone/jt	Mixed (5, 3)
72.71	VED w episiotomy	Non-Operative	77.0	Sequestrectomy	Operative
72.79	Vacuum extract del NEC	Non-Operative	77.1	Other bone inc w/o div	Operative
72.8	Instrumental del NEC	Non-Operative	77.2	Wedge osteotomy	Operative
72.9	Instrumental del NOS	Non-Operative	77.25	Femoral wedge osteotomy	Operative
73.0	Artificial rupt membrane	Non-Operative	77.27	Tib & fib wedge osty	Operative
73.01	Induction labor by AROM	Non-Operative	77.3	Other division of bone	Operative
73.09	Artif rupt membranes NEC	Non-Operative	77.35	Femoral division NEC	Operative
73.1	Surg induction labor NEC	Non-Operative	77.37	Tibia/fibula div NEC	Operative
73.2	Int/comb version/extract	Non-Operative	77.39	Bone division NEC	Operative
73.3	Failed forceps	Non-Operative	77.4	Biopsy of bone	Operative
73.4	Medical induction labor	Non-Operative	77.45	Femoral biopsy	Operative
73.5	Manually assisted del	Non-Operative	77.47	Tibia & fibula biopsy	Operative
73.51	Manual ROT fetal head	Non-Operative	77.49	Bone biopsy NEC	Operative
73.59	Manual assisted del NEC	Non-Operative	77.5	Toe deformity exc/REP	Operative
73.6	Episiotomy	Non-Operative	77.51	Bunionect/STC/osty	Operative
73.8	Fetal ops-facilitate del	Non-Operative	77.6	Loc exc bone lesion	Operative
73.9	Oth ops assisting del	Mixed (2, 3)	77.61	Exc chest cage bone les	Operative
73.91	Ext version-assist del	Non-Operative	77.62	Loc exc bone les humerus	Operative
74.0	Classical CD	Operative	77.65	Loc exc bone les femur	Operative
74.1	Low cervical CD	Operative	77.67	Loc exc les tibia/fibula	Operative
74.2	Extraperitoneal CD	Operative	77.68	Loc exc les MT/tarsal	Operative
74.3	Rmvl extratubal preg	Operative	77.69	Loc exc bone lesion NEC	Operative
74.4	Cesarean section NEC	Operative	77.7	Exc bone for graft	Operative
74.9	Cesarean section NOS	Operative	77.79	Exc bone for graft NEC	Operative
74.99	Other CD type NOS	Operative	77.8	Other partial ostectomy	Operative
75.0	Intra-amnio inject-AB	Non-Operative	77.81	Oth chest cage ostectomy	Operative
75.1	Diagnostic amniocentesis	Non-Operative	77.83	Part ostectomy rad/ulna	Operative
75.2	Intrauterine transfusion	Non-Operative	77.85	Part ostectomy-femur	Operative
75.3	IU ops fetus & amnio NEC	Mixed (1, 5)	77.86	Partial patellectomy	Operative
75.32	Fetal EKG (scalp)	Non-Operative	77.87	Part ostectomy tib/fib	Operative
75.34	Fetal monitoring NOS	Non-Operative	77.88	Part ostectomy-MT/tarsal	Operative
75.35	Dxtic px fetus/amnio NEC	Non-Operative	77.89	Partial ostectomy NEC	Operative
75.4	Man rmvl of ret placenta	Non-Operative	77.9	Total ostectomy	Operative
75.5	REP current OB lac uter	Operative	77.91	Tot chest cage ostectomy	Operative
75.51	REP current OB lac cerv	Operative	77.96	Total patellectomy	Operative
75.6	REP oth current OB lac	Mixed (1, 2)	78.0	Bone graft	Operative
75.61	REP OB lac blad/urethra	Operative	78.05	Bone graft to femur	Operative
75.62	REP OB lac rectum/anus	Non-Operative	78.07	Bone graft tibia/fibula	Operative
75.69	REP current OB lac NEC	Non-Operative	78.1	Appl ext fixation device	Operative

Code	Description	Operative Status	Code	Description	Operative Status
78.13	Appl ext fix rad/ulna	Operative	80.1	Other arthrotomy	Operative
78.15	Appl ext fix dev femur	Operative	80.11	Oth arthrotomy shoulder	Operative
78.17	Appl ext fix dev tib/fib	Operative	80.12	Oth arthrotomy elbow	Operative
78.2	Limb shortening px	Operative	80.14	Oth arthrotomy hand	Operative
78.25	Limb short px femur	Operative	80.15	Oth arthrotomy hip	Operative
78.3	Limb lengthening px	Operative	80.16	Oth arthrotomy knee	Operative
78.4	Other bone repair	Operative	80.17	Oth arthrotomy ankle	Operative
78.5	Int fix w/o fx reduction	Operative	80.2	Arthroscopy	Operative
78.52	Int fix w/o red humerus	Operative	80.21	Shoulder arthroscopy	Operative
78.55	Int fix w/o red femur	Operative	80.26	Knee arthroscopy	Operative
78.57	Int fix w/o red tib/fib	Operative	80.3	Biopsy joint structure	Non-Operative
78.59	Int fix w/o fx red NEC	Operative	80.4	Jt capsule/LIG/cart div	Operative
78.6	Rmvl impl dev from bone	Operative	80.46	Knee structure division	Operative
78.63	Rmvl impl dev rad/ulna	Operative	80.48	Foot joint struct div	Operative
78.65	Rmvl impl dev femur	Operative	80.5	IV disc exc/destruction	Mixed (3, 1)
78.67	Rmvl impl dev tib & fib	Operative	80.51	IV disc excision	Operative
78.69	Rmvl impl dev site NEC	Operative	80.59	IV disc destruction NEC	Operative
78.7	Osteoclasis	Operative	80.6	Exc knee semilunar cart	Operative
78.8	Other bone diagnostic px	Operative	80.7	Synovectomy	Operative
78.9	Insert bone growth stim	Operative	80.76	Knee synovectomy	Operative
79.0	Clsd fx red w/o int fix	Non-Operative	80.8	Oth exc/destr joint les	Operative
79.01	Clsd fx red humerus	Non-Operative	80.81	Destr shoulder les NEC	Operative
79.02	Clsd red fx radius/ulna	Non-Operative	80.85	Destr hip lesion NEC	Operative
79.05	Clsd fx red femur	Non-Operative	80.86	Destr knee lesion NEC	Operative
79.06	Clsd fx red tibia/fibula	Non-Operative	80.9	Other joint excision	Operative
79.07	Clsd fx red MT/tarsal	Non-Operative	81.0	Spinal fusion	Operative
79.1	Clsd fx red w int fix	Operative	81.01	Atlas-axis sp fusion	Operative
79.11	CRIF humerus	Operative	81.02	Anterior cerv fusion NEC	Operative
79.12	CRIF radius/ulna	Operative	81.03	Post cervical fusion NEC	Operative
79.15	CRIF femur	Operative	81.04	Anterior dorsal fusion	Operative
79.16	CRIF tibia & fibula	Operative	81.05	Posterior dorsal fusion	Operative
79.17	CRIF metatarsal/tarsal	Operative	81.06	Anterior lumbar fusion	Operative
79.2	Open fracture reduction	Operative	81.07	Lat trans lumbar fusion	Operative
79.22	Open red radius/ulna fx	Operative	81.08	Posterior lumbar fusion	Operative
79.26	Open red tibia/fib fx	Operative	81.09	Refusion of spine	Operative
79.3	Open fx reduct w int fix	Operative	81.1	Foot & ankle arthrodesis	Operative
79.31	ORIF humerus	Operative	81.11	Ankle fusion	Operative
79.32	ORIF radius/ulna	Operative	81.12	Triple arthrodesis	Operative
79.33	ORIF carpals/metacarpals	Operative	81.13	Subtalar fusion	Operative
79.34	ORIF finger	Operative	81.2	Arthrodesis of oth joint	Operative
79.35	ORIF femur	Operative	81.26	Metacarpocarpal fusion	Operative
79.36	ORIF tibia & fibula	Operative	81.4	Low limb joint REP NEC	Operative
79.37	ORIF metatarsal/tarsal	Operative	81.40	Repair of hip NEC	Operative
79.39	ORIF bone NEC X facial	Operative	81.44	Patellar stabilization	Operative
79.4	CR sep epiphysis	Operative	81.45	Cruciate LIG repair NEC	Operative
79.45	CR sep epiph femur	Operative	81.46	Collateral LIG REP NEC	Operative
79.5	Open red sep epiphysis	Operative	81.47	Other repair of knee	Operative
79.6	Open fx site debridement	Operative	81.49	Other repair of ankle	Operative
79.62	Debride open fx rad/ulna	Operative	81.5	Joint repl lower EXT	Operative
79.64	Debride open fx finger	Operative	81.51	Total hip replacement	Operative
79.65	Debride open fx femur	Operative	81.52	Partial hip replacement	Operative
79.66	Debride opn fx tibia/fib	Operative	81.53	Hip replacement revision	Operative
79.7	Closed red dislocation	Non-Operative	81.54	Total knee replacement	Operative
79.71	Clsd red disloc shoulder	Non-Operative	81.55	Knee replacement rev	Operative
79.75	Clsd red disloc hip	Non-Operative	81.7	Hand/finger arthroplasty	Operative
79.8	Open red dislocation	Operative	81.75	Carpal/CMC arthroplasty	Operative
79.85	Open red disloc hip	Operative	81.8	Should/elb arthroplasty	Operative
79.9	Bone injury op NOS	Operative	81.80	Total shoulder repl	Operative
80.0	Arthrotomy rmvl prosth	Operative	81.81	Partial shoulder repl	Operative
80.05	Rmvl prosth hip inc	Operative	81.82	REP recur should disloc	Operative
80.06	Rmvl prosth knee inc	Operative	81.83	Should arthroplasty NEC	Operative

Code	Description	Operative Status	Code	Description	Operative Status
81.84	Total elbow replacement	Operative	85.1	Breast diagnostic px	Mixed (1, 2)
81.9	Other joint structure op	Mixed (7, 2)	85.11	PERC breast biopsy	Non-Operative
81.91	Arthrocentesis	Non-Operative	85.12	Open biopsy of breast	Operative
81.92	Injection into joint	Non-Operative	85.2	Exc/destr breast tiss	Operative
82.0	Inc hand soft tissue	Mixed (4, 1)	85.21	Local exc breast lesion	Operative
82.01	Explor tend sheath hand	Operative	85.22	Quadrant resect breast	Operative
82.09	Inc soft tissue hand NEC	Operative	85.23	Subtotal mastectomy	Operative
82.1	Div hand musc/tend/fasc	Operative	85.3	Red mammoplasty/ectomy	Operative
82.2	Exc les hand soft tissue	Operative	85.32	Bilat red mammoplasty	Operative
82.3	Oth exc hand soft tiss	Operative	85.4	Mastectomy	Operative
82.4	Suture hand soft tissue	Operative	85.41	Unilat simple mastectomy	Operative
82.44	Sut flexor tend hand NEC	Operative	85.42	Bilat simple mastectomy	Operative
82.45	Suture hand tendon NEC	Operative	85.43	Unilat exten smp MAST	Operative
82.5	Hand musc/tend transpl	Operative	85.44	Bilat exten smp MAST	Operative
82.6	Reconstruction of thumb	Operative	85.45	Unilat RAD mastectomy	Operative
82.7	Plastic op hnd grft/impl	Operative	85.5	Augmentation mammoplasty	Mixed (3, 2)
82.8	Other plastic ops hand	Operative	85.6	Mastopexy	Operative
82.9	Oth hand soft tissue ops	Mixed (2, 5)	85.7	Total breast reconst	Operative
83.0	Inc musc/tend/fasc/bursa	Operative	85.8	Other breast repair	Mixed (7, 1)
83.02	Myotomy	Operative	85.85	Breast muscle flap graft	Operative
83.03	Bursotomy	Operative	85.9	Other breast operations	Mixed (5, 2)
83.09	Soft tissue incision NEC	Operative	85.94	Breast implant removal	Operative
83.1	Musc/tend/fasc division	Operative	86.0	Incision skin & subcu	Mixed (1, 7)
83.12	Adductor tenotomy of hip	Operative	86.01	Aspiration skin & subcu	Non-Operative
83.13	Other tenotomy	Operative	86.03	Incision pilonidal sinus	Non-Operative
83.14	Fasciotomy	Operative	86.04	Other skin & subcu I&D	Non-Operative
83.19	Soft tissue division NEC	Operative	86.05	Inc w rmvl FB skin/subcu	Non-Operative
83.2	Soft tissue dxtic px	Operative	86.06	Insertion infusion pump	Operative
83.21	Soft tissue biopsy	Operative	86.07	VAD insertion	Non-Operative
83.3	Exc les soft tissue	Operative	86.09	Skin/subcu incision NEC	Non-Operative
83.32	Exc lesion of muscle	Operative	86.1	Skin & subcu dxtic px	Non-Operative
83.39	Exc les soft tissue NEC	Operative	86.11	Skin & subcu biopsy	Non-Operative
83.4	Other exc musc/tend/fasc	Operative	86.2	Exc/destr skin lesion	Mixed (3, 5)
83.45	Other myectomy	Operative	86.21	Excision of pilonid cyst	Operative
83.5	Bursectomy	Operative	86.22	Exc debride WND/infect	Operative
83.6	Suture musc/tendon/fasc	Operative	86.23	Nail removal	Non-Operative
83.63	Rotator cuff repair	Operative	86.26	Lig dermal appendage	Non-Operative
83.64	Other suture of tendon	Operative	86.27	Debridement of nail	Non-Operative
83.65	Other muscle/fasc suture	Operative	86.28	Nonexc debridement wound	Non-Operative
83.7	Muscle/tendon reconst	Operative	86.3	Oth loc exc/destr skin	Non-Operative
83.75	Tendon transf/transpl	Operative	86.4	RAD excision skin lesion	Operative
83.8	Musc/tend/fasc op NEC	Operative	86.5	Skin & subcu suture	Non-Operative
83.84	Clubfoot release NEC	Operative	86.59	Skin suture NEC	Non-Operative
83.85	Change in m/t length NEC	Operative	86.6	Free skin graft	Mixed (7, 1)
83.86	Quadricepsplasty	Operative	86.62	Hand skin graft NEC	Operative
83.88	Other plastic ops tendon	Operative	86.63	Fthick skin graft NEC	Operative
83.9	Other conn tissue ops	Mixed (4, 5)	86.69	Free skin graft NEC	Operative
83.94	Aspiration of bursa	Non-Operative	86.7	Pedicle grafts or flaps	Operative
83.95	Soft tissue asp NEC	Non-Operative	86.72	Pedicle graft adv	Operative
84.0	Amputation of upper limb	Operative	86.74	Attach pedicle graft NEC	Operative
84.01	Finger amputation	Operative	86.75	Rev pedicle/flap graft	Operative
84.1	Amputation of lower limb	Operative	86.8	Other skin & subcu REP	Operative
84.11	Toe amputation	Operative	86.82	Facial rhytidectomy	Operative
84.12	Amputation through foot	Operative	86.83	Size red plastic op	Operative
84.15	BK amputation NEC	Operative	86.89	Skin REP & reconst NEC	Operative
84.17	Above knee amputation	Operative	86.9	Other skin & subcu ops	Mixed (2, 2)
84.2	Extremity reattachment	Operative	87.0	Head/neck sft tiss x-ray	Non-Operative
84.3	Amputation stump rev	Operative	87.03	CAT scan head	Non-Operative
84.4	Impl or fit prosth limb	Mixed (3, 6)	87.1	Other head/neck x-ray	Non-Operative
84.9	Other musculoskeletal op	Operative	87.2	X-ray of spine	Non-Operative
85.0	Mastotomy	Non-Operative	87.21	Contrast myelogram	Non-Operative

Code	Description	Operative Status	Code	Description	Operative Status
87.3	Thorax soft tissue x-ray	Non-Operative	89.17	Polysomnogram	Non-Operative
87.4	Other x-ray of thorax	Non-Operative	89.19	Video/telemetric EEG MON	Non-Operative
87.41	CAT scan thorax	Non-Operative	89.2	GU system-examination	Non-Operative
87.44	Routine chest x-ray	Non-Operative	89.22	Cystometrogram	Non-Operative
87.49	Chest x-ray NEC	Non-Operative	89.3	Other examinations	Non-Operative
87.5	Biliary tract x-ray	Mixed (1, 4)	89.37	Vital capacity	Non-Operative
87.51	PERC hepat cholangiogram	Non-Operative	89.38	Respiratory measure NEC	Non-Operative
87.6	Oth digestive syst x-ray	Non-Operative	89.39	Nonoperative exams NEC	Non-Operative
87.61	Barium swallow	Non-Operative	89.4	Pacer/card stress test	Non-Operative
87.62	Upper GI series	Non-Operative	89.41	Treadmill stress test	Non-Operative
87.63	Small bowel series	Non-Operative	89.44	CV stress test NEC	Non-Operative
87.64	Lower GI series	Non-Operative	89.5	Other cardiac funct test	Non-Operative
87.7	X-ray of urinary system	Non-Operative	89.50	Ambulatory card monitor	Non-Operative
87.73	IV pyelogram	Non-Operative	89.51	Rhythm electrocardiogram	Non-Operative
87.74	Retrograde pyelogram	Non-Operative	89.52	Electrocardiogram	Non-Operative
87.76	Retro cystourethrogram	Non-Operative	89.54	ECG monitoring	Non-Operative
87.77	Cystogram NEC	Non-Operative	89.59	Nonop card/vasc exam NEC	Non-Operative
87.79	Urinary system x-ray NEC	Non-Operative	89.6	Circulatory monitoring	Non-Operative
87.8	Female genital x-ray	Non-Operative	89.62	CVP monitoring	Non-Operative
87.9	Male genital x-ray	Non-Operative	89.64	PA wedge monitoring	Non-Operative
88.0	Soft tissue x-ray abd	Non-Operative	89.65	Arterial bld gas measure	Non-Operative
88.01	CAT scan of abdomen	Non-Operative	89.66	Mix venous bld gas meas	Non-Operative
88.1	Other x-ray of abdomen	Non-Operative	89.68	Cardiac output monit NEC	Non-Operative
88.19	Abdominal x-ray NEC	Non-Operative	89.7	General physical exam	Non-Operative
88.2	Skel x-ray-EXT & pelvis	Non-Operative	89.8	Autopsy	Non-Operative
88.3	Other x-ray	Non-Operative	90.0	Micro exam-nervous syst	Non-Operative
88.38	Other C.A.T. scan	Non-Operative	90.1	Micro exam-endocrine NEC	Non-Operative
88.4	Contrast arteriography	Non-Operative	90.2	Micro exam-eye	Non-Operative
88.41	Cerebral arteriogram	Non-Operative	90.3	Micro exam-ENT/larynx	Non-Operative
88.42	Contrast aortogram	Non-Operative	90.4	Micro exam-lower resp	Non-Operative
88.43	Pulmonary arteriogram	Non-Operative	90.5	Micro exam-blood	Non-Operative
88.45	Renal arteriogram	Non-Operative	90.52	Culture-blood	Non-Operative
88.47	Abd arteriogram NEC	Non-Operative	90.6	Micro exam-spleen/marrow	Non-Operative
88.48	Contrast arteriogram-leg	Non-Operative	90.7	Micro exam-lymph system	Non-Operative
88.49	Contrast arteriogram NEC	Non-Operative	90.8	Micro exam-upper GI	Non-Operative
88.5	Contrast angiocardiogram	Non-Operative	90.9	Micro exam-lower GI	Non-Operative
88.53	Lt heart angiocardiogram	Non-Operative	91.0	Micro exam-bil/pancreas	Non-Operative
88.56	Cor arteriogram-2 cath	Non-Operative	91.1	Micro exam-peritoneum	Non-Operative
88.57	Coronary arteriogram NEC	Non-Operative	91.2	Micro exam-upper urinary	Non-Operative
88.6	Phlebography	Non-Operative	91.3	Micro exam-lower urinary	Non-Operative
88.66	Contrast phlebogram-leg	Non-Operative	91.32	Culture-lower urinary	Non-Operative
88.67	Contrast phlebogram NEC	Non-Operative	91.33	C&S-lower urinary	Non-Operative
88.7	Diagnostic ultrasound	Non-Operative	91.4	Micro exam-female genit	Non-Operative
88.71	Dxtic US-head/neck	Non-Operative	91.5	Micro exam-MS/jt fluid	Non-Operative
88.72	Dxtic ultrasound-heart	Non-Operative	91.6	Micro exam-integument	Non-Operative
88.73	Dxtic US-thorax NEC	Non-Operative	91.7	Micro exam-op wound	Non-Operative
88.74	Dxtic ultrasound-digest	Non-Operative	91.8	Micro exam NEC	Non-Operative
88.75	Dxtic ultrasound-urinary	Non-Operative	91.9	Micro exam NOS	Non-Operative
88.76	Dxtic ultrasound-abd	Non-Operative	92.0	Isotope scan & function	Non-Operative
88.77	Dxtic ultrasound-vasc	Non-Operative	92.02	Liver scan/isotope funct	Non-Operative
88.78	Dxtic US-gravid uterus	Non-Operative	92.03	Renal scan/isotope study	Non-Operative
88.79	Dxtic ultrasound NEC	Non-Operative	92.04	GI scan & isotope study	Non-Operative
88.8	Thermography	Non-Operative	92.05	CV scan/isotope study	Non-Operative
88.9	Other diagnostic imaging	Non-Operative	92.1	Other radioisotope scan	Non-Operative
88.91	MRI-brain & brain stem	Non-Operative	92.14	Bone scan	Non-Operative
88.93	MRI-spinal canal	Non-Operative	92.15	Pulmonary scan	Non-Operative
88.94	MRI-musculoskeletal	Non-Operative	92.18	Total body scan	Non-Operative
88.97	MRI site NEC&NOS	Non-Operative	92.19	Scan of other sites	Non-Operative
89.0	Dx interview/consul/exam	Non-Operative	92.2	Ther radiology & nu med	Mixed (1, 8)
89.1	Nervous system exams	Non-Operative	92.23	Isotope teleradiotherapy	Non-Operative
89.14	Electroencephalogram	Non-Operative	92.24	Photon teleradiotherapy	Non-Operative

Code	Description	Operative Status	Code	Description	Operative Status
92.27	Radioactive element impl	Operative	94.65	Drug detoxification	Non-Operative
92.28	Isotope inject/instill	Non-Operative	94.66	Drug rehab/detox	Non-Operative
92.29	Radiotherapeutic px NEC	Non-Operative	94.67	ALC/drug rehabilitation	Non-Operative
92.3	Stereotactic radiosurg	Non-Operative	94.68	ALC/drug detoxification	Non-Operative
93.0	Dxtic physical Tx	Non-Operative	94.69	ALC/drug rehab/detox	Non-Operative
93.01	Functional PT evaluation	Non-Operative	95.0	Gen/subjective eye exam	Mixed (1, 7)
93.08	Electromyography	Non-Operative	95.1	Form & struct eye exam	Non-Operative
93.1	PT exercises	Non-Operative	95.2	Objective funct eye test	Non-Operative
93.2	Oth PT MS manipulation	Non-Operative	95.3	Special vision services	Non-Operative
93.22	Amb & gait training	Non-Operative	95.4	Nonop hearing procedure	Non-Operative
93.26	Manual rupt joint adhes	Non-Operative	95.41	Audiometry	Non-Operative
93.3	Other PT therapeutic px	Non-Operative	95.47	Hearing examination NOS	Non-Operative
93.32	Whirlpool treatment	Non-Operative	96.0	Nonop GI & resp intub	Non-Operative
93.38	Combined PT NOS	Non-Operative	96.04	Insert endotracheal tube	Non-Operative
93.39	Physical therapy NEC	Non-Operative	96.05	Resp tract intub NEC	Non-Operative
93.4	Skeletal & oth traction	Non-Operative	96.07	Insert gastric tube NEC	Non-Operative
93.44	Other skeletal traction	Non-Operative	96.1	Other nonop insertion	Non-Operative
93.46	Limb skin traction NEC	Non-Operative	96.2	Nonop dilation & manip	Non-Operative
93.5	Oth immob/press/WND attn	Non-Operative	96.3	Nonop GI irrig/instill	Non-Operative
93.51	Plaster jacket appl	Non-Operative	96.33	Gastric lavage	Non-Operative
93.53	Other cast application	Non-Operative	96.35	Gastric gavage	Non-Operative
93.54	Application of splint	Non-Operative	96.38	Impacted feces removal	Non-Operative
93.57	Appl oth WND dressing	Non-Operative	96.4	Digest/GU irrig/instill	Non-Operative
93.59	Immob/press/WND attn NEC	Non-Operative	96.49	Other GU instillation	Non-Operative
93.6	Osteopathic manipulation	Non-Operative	96.5	Other nonop irrig/clean	Non-Operative
93.61	OMT for gen mobil	Non-Operative	96.56	Bronch/trach lavage NEC	Non-Operative
93.7	Speech/read/blind rehab	Non-Operative	96.59	Wound irrigation NEC	Non-Operative
93.75	Other speech therapy	Non-Operative	96.6	Enteral nutrition	Non-Operative
93.8	Other rehab therapy	Non-Operative	96.7	Cont mech vent NEC	Non-Operative
93.81	Recreational therapy	Non-Operative	96.71	Cont mech vent-<96 hours	Non-Operative
93.83	Occupational therapy	Non-Operative	96.72	Cont mech vent->95 hours	Non-Operative
93.89	Rehabilitation NEC	Non-Operative	97.0	GI appliance replacement	Non-Operative
93.9	Respiratory therapy	Non-Operative	97.02	Repl gastrostomy tube	Non-Operative
93.90	CPAP	Non-Operative	97.03	Repl small intest tube	Non-Operative
93.93	Nonmech resuscitation	Non-Operative	97.05	Repl panc/biliary stent	Non-Operative
93.94	Nebulizer therapy	Non-Operative	97.1	Repl MS appliance	Non-Operative
93.95	Hyperbaric oxygenation	Non-Operative	97.2	Other nonop replacement	Non-Operative
93.96	Oxygen enrichment NEC	Non-Operative	97.23	Repl TRACH tube	Non-Operative
93.99	Other resp procedures	Non-Operative	97.3	Rmvl ther dev-head/nk	Non-Operative
94.0	Psych eval & testing	Non-Operative	97.4	Rmvl thor ther device	Non-Operative
94.08	Psych eval & test NEC	Non-Operative	97.49	Rmvl oth dev from thorax	Non-Operative
94.1	Psych eval/consult	Non-Operative	97.5	Nonop rmvl GI ther dev	Non-Operative
94.11	Psych mental status	Non-Operative	97.6	Nonop rmvl urin ther dev	Non-Operative
94.19	Psych interview/eval NEC	Non-Operative	97.62	Rmvl ureteral drain	Non-Operative
94.2	Psych somatotherapy	Non-Operative	97.7	Rmvl ther dev genit syst	Non-Operative
94.22	Lithium therapy	Non-Operative	97.8	Oth nonop rmvl ther dev	Non-Operative
94.23	Neuroleptic therapy	Non-Operative	97.89	Rmvl oth ther dev	Non-Operative
94.25	Psych drug therapy NEC	Non-Operative	98.0	Rmvl intralum GI FB	Non-Operative
94.27	Electroshock therapy NEC	Non-Operative	98.02	Rmvl intralum esoph FB	Non-Operative
94.3	Individual psychotherapy	Non-Operative	98.1	Rmvl intralum FB NEC	Non-Operative
94.31	Psychoanalysis	Non-Operative	98.2	Rmvl oth FB w/o inc	Non-Operative
94.38	Supp verbal psychTx	Non-Operative	98.5	ESWL	Non-Operative
94.39	Individual psychTx NEC	Non-Operative	98.51	Renal/ureter/blad ESWL	Non-Operative
94.4	Oth psychTx/counselling	Non-Operative	99.0	Blood transfusion	Non-Operative
94.44	Other group therapy	Non-Operative	99.01	Exchange transfusion	Non-Operative
94.5	Refferal psych rehab	Non-Operative	99.03	Whole blood transfus NEC	Non-Operative
94.6	Alcohol/drug rehab/detox	Non-Operative	99.04	Packed cell transfusion	Non-Operative
94.61	Alcohol rehabilitation	Non-Operative	99.05	Platelet transfusion	Non-Operative
94.62	Alcohol detoxification	Non-Operative	99.07	Serum transfusion NEC	Non-Operative
94.63	Alcohol rehab/detox	Non-Operative	99.1	Inject/infuse ther subst	Non-Operative
94.64	Drug rehabilitation	Non-Operative	99.11	Inject Rh immune glob	Non-Operative

Code	Description	Operative Status	Code	Description	Operative Status
99.14	Inject gamma globulin	Non-Operative	99.55	Vaccination NEC	Non-Operative
99.15	Parenteral nutrition	Non-Operative	99.59	Vacc/inoculation NEC	Non-Operative
99.17	Inject insulin	Non-Operative	99.6	Card rhythm conversion	Non-Operative
99.18	Inject electrolytes	Non-Operative	99.60	CPR NOS	Non-Operative
99.19	Inject anticoagulant	Non-Operative	99.61	Atrial cardioversion	Non-Operative
99.2	Oth inject ther subst	Non-Operative	99.62	Heart countershock NEC	Non-Operative
99.21	Inject antibiotic	Non-Operative	99.69	Cardiac rhythm conv NEC	Non-Operative
99.23	Inject steroid	Non-Operative	99.7	Therapeutic apheresis	Non-Operative
99.24	Inject hormone NEC	Non-Operative	99.71	Ther plasmapheresis	Non-Operative
99.25	Inject CA chemo agent	Non-Operative	99.8	Misc physical procedures	Non-Operative
99.28	Inject BRM/antineo agent	Non-Operative	99.82	UV light therapy	Non-Operative
99.29	Inject/infuse NEC	Non-Operative	99.83	Other phototherapy	Non-Operative
99.3	Prophyl vacc-bact dis	Non-Operative	99.84	Isolation	Non-Operative
99.4	Viral immunization	Non-Operative	99.9	Other misc procedures	Non-Operative
99.5	Other immunization	Non-Operative	99.99	Misc procedures NEC	Non-Operative

GLOSSARY

Average Length of Stay: Calculated from the admission and discharge dates by counting the day of admission as the first day; the day of discharge is not included. The average is figured by adding the lengths of stay for each patient and then dividing by the total number of patients. Patients discharged on the day of admission are counted as staying one day in the calculation of average length of stay. Patients with stays over 99 days (>99) are excluded from this calculation.

Distribution Percentiles: A length of stay percentile for a stratified group of patients is determined by arranging the individual patient stays from low to high. Counting up from the lowest stay to the point where one-half of the patients have been counted yields the value of the 50th percentile. Counting one-tenth of the total patients gives the 10th percentile, and so on. The 10th, 25th, 50th, 75th, 90th, 95th, and 99th percentiles of stay are displayed in days. If, for example, the 10th percentile for a group of patients is four, then 10 percent of the patients stayed four days or less. The 50th percentile is the median. Any percentile with a value of 100 days or more is listed as >99. Patients who were hospitalized more than 99 days (>99) are not included in the total patients, average stay, and variance categories. The percentiles, however, do include these patients.

Multiple Diagnoses Patients: Patients are classified in the multiple diagnoses category if they had at least one valid secondary diagnosis in addition to the principal one. The following codes are not considered valid secondary diagnoses for purposes of this classification:

1. Manifestation codes (conditions that evolved from underlying diseases [etiology] and are in italics in ICD-9-CM, Volume 1)

2. Codes V27.0-V27.9 (outcome of delivery)

3. E Codes (external causes of injury and poisoning)

Observed Patients: The number of observed patients in the stratified group. Patients with stays longer than 99 days (>99) are not included. This data element does not use the projection factor.

Operated Patients: In the diagnosis tables, operated patients are those who had at least one procedure that is classified by HCFA as an operating room procedure. HCFA physician panels classify every ICD-9-CM procedure code according to whether the procedure would in most hospitals be performed in the operating room. This classification system differs slightly from that used in Length of Stay publications published previous to 1995, in which patients were categorized as operated if any of their procedures were labeled as Uniform Hospital Discharge Data Set (UHDDS) Class 1. Appendix C contains a list of procedure codes included in this book and their HCFA-defined operative status.

Variance: A measure of the spread of the data around the average. The smallest variance is zero, indicating that all lengths of stay are equal. In tables in which there is a large variance and the patient group size is relatively small, the average stay may appear high. This sometimes occurs when one or two patients with long hospitalizations fall into the group.

ALPHABETIC INDEX

This index provides an alphabetical listing by descriptive title for all ICD-9-CM diagnoses and procedures codes included in the book. For ease of use, titles are grouped into major classification categories (i.e., *Diseases of the Circulatory System*). These classification categories are listed for your reference below.

ICD-9-CM Classification Categories

Diagnosis Categories

Infectious and Parasitic Diseases	Codes 001–139
Neoplasms	Codes 140–239
Endocrine, Nutritional and Metabolic Diseases, and Immunity Disorders	Codes 240–279
Diseases of the Blood and Blood-Forming Organs	Codes 280–289
Mental Disorders	Codes 290–319
Diseases of the Nervous System and Sense Organs	Codes 320–389
Diseases of the Circulatory System	Codes 390–459
Diseases of the Respiratory System	Codes 460–519
Diseases of the Digestive System	Codes 520–579
Diseases of the Genitourinary System	Codes 580–629
Complications of Pregnancy, Childbirth, and the Puerperium	Codes 630–676
Diseases of the Skin and Subcutaneous Tissue	Codes 680–709
Diseases of the Musculoskeletal System and Connective Tissue	Codes 710–739
Congenital Anomalies	Codes 740–759
Certain Conditions Originating in the Perinatal Period	Codes 760–779
Symptoms, Signs, and Ill-Defined Conditions	Codes 780–799
Injury and Poisoning	Codes 800–999
Supplementary Classification of Factors Influencing Health Status and Contact with Health Services	Codes V01–V82

Procedure Categories

Operations on the Nervous System	Codes 01–05
Operations on the Endocrine System	Codes 06–07
Operations on the Eye	Codes 08–16
Operations on the Ear	Codes 18–20
Operations on the Nose, Mouth, and Pharynx	Codes 21–29
Operations on the Respiratory System	Codes 30–34
Operations on the Cardiovascular System	Codes 35–39
Operations on the Hemic and Lymphatic System	Codes 40–41
Operations on the Digestive System	Codes 42–54
Operations on the Urinary System	Codes 55–59
Operations on the Male Genital Organs	Codes 60–64
Operations on the Female Genital Organs	Codes 65–71
Obstetrical Procedures	Codes 72–75
Operations on the Musculoskeletal System	Codes 76–84
Operations on the Integumentary System	Codes 85–86
Miscellaneous Diagnostic and Therapeutic Procedures	Codes 87–99

Diagnosis Codes

Diagnosis Codes

Diagnosis Codes

Diagnosis Codes

Diagnosis Codes

Code	Description	Page	Code	Description	Page
575	Oth gallbladder disorder	376	589	Small kidney	386
537	Oth gastroduod disorder	342	598	Urethral stricture	393
569	Oth intestinal disorders	365	597	Urethritis/urethral synd	393
573	Oth liver disorders	371	615	Uterine inflammatory dis	404
558	Oth noninf gastroenterit	356			
568	Oth peritoneal disorders	364			

Code	Description	Page	Code	Description	Page
553	Other abdominal hernia	350		**COMPLICATIONS OF PREGNANCY, CHILDBIRTH, AND**	
542	Other appendicitis	344		**THE PUERPERIUM (630-676)**	
525	Other dental disorder	323	641	AP hemor & plac prev	425
533	Peptic ulcer, site NOS	334	654	Abn pelvic organ in preg	447
567	Peritonitis	363	661	Abnormal forces of labor	460
522	Pulp & periapical dis	321	668	Comp anes in delivery	472
555	Regional enteritis	351	639	Comp following abortion	424
527	Salivary gland diseases	324	653	Disproportion	446
572	Sequela of chr liver dis	370	644	Early/threatened labor	432
536	Stomach function disord	340	633	Ectopic pregnancy	420
529	Tongue disorders	326	643	Excess vomiting in preg	431
520	Tooth develop/erupt pbx	320	638	Failed attempted AB	423
556	Ulcerative colitis	353	655	Fetal abn affect mother	449
557	Vasc insuff intestine	354	640	Hemorrhage in early preg	424
			630	Hydatidiform mole	419
	DISEASES OF THE GENITOURINARY SYSTEM (580-629)		642	Hypertension compl preg	427
			636	Illegal induced abortion	422
580	Acute nephritis	382	675	Infect breast in preg	476
584	Acute renal failure	383	647	Infective dis in preg	436
610	Benign mammary dysplasia	400	635	Legally induced abortion	422
582	Chronic nephritis	383	662	Long labor	463
585	Chronic renal failure	384	670	Major puerperal infect	474
595	Cystitis	391	652	Malposition of fetus	444
593	Disord kidney/ureter NEC	388	632	Missed abortion	419
626	Disorder of menstruation	416	651	Multiple gestation	443
607	Disorders of penis	399	650	Normal delivery	443
621	Disorders of uterus NEC	413	673	OB pulmonary embolism	475
617	Endometriosis	405	660	Obstructed labor	458
619	Female genital fistula	410	658	Oth amniotic cavity prob	453
625	Female genital symptoms	415	676	Oth breast/lact dis preg	476
628	Female infertility	418	669	Oth comp labor/delivery	473
614	Female pelvic inflam dis	402	648	Oth current cond in preg	438
618	Genital prolapse	407	656	Oth fetal pbx aff moth	450
603	Hydrocele	397	659	Oth indication care-del	455
591	Hydronephrosis	387	631	Other abnmal POC	419
600	Hyperplasia of prostate	395	646	Other comp of pregnancy	434
588	Impaired renal function	385	665	Other obstetrical trauma	469
590	Kidney infection	386	664	Perineal trauma w del	466
594	Lower urinary calculus	390	657	Polyhydramnios	453
606	Male infertility	398	666	Postpartum hemorrhage	470
627	Menopausal disorders	417	645	Prolonged pregnancy	433
583	Nephritis NOS	383	674	Puerperal comp NEC/NOS	475
581	Nephrotic syndrome	382	672	Puerperal pyrexia NOS	475
620	Noninfl disord a.uterine	411	667	Ret placenta w/o hemor	472
622	Noninfl disord cervix	414	634	Spontaneous abortion	420
624	Noninfl disord vulva	415	663	Umbilical cord comp	464
623	Noninflam disord vagina	414	637	Unspecified abortion	423
604	Orchitis & epididymitis	397	671	Venous comp in preg & PP	474
608	Oth disordr male genital	399			
616	Oth female genit inflam	405		**DISEASES OF THE SKIN AND SUBCUTANEOUS TISSUE**	
629	Oth female genital dis	418		**(680-709)**	
602	Oth prostatic disorders	396	683	Acute lymphadenitis	482
599	Oth urinary tract disord	394	691	Atopic dermatitis	483
596	Other bladder disorders	392	694	Bullous dermatoses	485
611	Other breast disorders	401	680	Carbuncle and furuncle	477
601	Prostatic inflammation	396	681	Cellulitis, finger/toe	477
605	Redun prepuce & phimosis	398	707	Chronic ulcer of skin	490
586	Renal failure NOS	385	692	Contact dermatitis	484
587	Renal sclerosis NOS	385	700	Corns and callosities	487
592	Renal/ureteral calculus	387	693	Derm D/T internal agent	484

Diagnosis Codes

Diagnosis Codes

Code	Description	Page	Code	Description	Page
946	Burn of multiple site	656	869	Internal injury NOS	625
942	Burn of trunk	655	862	Intrathoracic injury NEC	622
949	Burn unspecified	657	830	Jaw dislocation	604
814	Carpal fracture	588	866	Kidney injury	623
851	Cerebral lac/contusion	615	909	Late eff ext cause NEC	641
995	Certain adverse eff NEC	681	908	Late eff injury NEC/NOS	641
810	Clavicle fracture	582	907	Late eff nerv system inj	641
999	Comp medical care NEC	697	906	Late eff skin/subcut inj	640
850	Concussion	614	905	Late effect MS injury	640
921	Contusion eye & adnexa	645	864	Liver injury	622
920	Contusion face/scalp/nck	645	827	Lower limb fracture NEC	603
924	Contusion leg & oth site	648	852	Meningeal hemor post inj	616
922	Contusion of trunk	646	815	Metacarpal fracture	588
923	Contusion of upper limb	647	804	Mult fx skull w oth bone	576
951	Cranial nerve injury NEC	658	817	Multiple hand fractures	590
925	Crush inj face/scalp/nck	649	870	Ocular adnexa open wound	625
929	Crush inj mult/site NOS	650	891	Open wnd knee/leg/ankle	635
927	Crushing inj upper limb	649	884	Open wound arm mult/NOS	633
928	Crushing injury of leg	650	878	Open wound genital organ	629
926	Crushing injury of trunk	649	876	Open wound of back	629
839	Dislocation NEC	608	877	Open wound of buttock	629
837	Dislocation of ankle	607	875	Open wound of chest	628
834	Dislocation of finger	606	872	Open wound of ear	626
838	Dislocation of foot	608	883	Open wound of finger	632
835	Dislocation of hip	606	892	Open wound of foot	636
836	Dislocation of knee	606	882	Open wound of hand	631
958	Early comp of trauma	660	890	Open wound of hip/thigh	634
991	Eff reduced temperature	679	894	Open wound of leg NEC	637
994	Effect ext cause NEC	680	881	Open wound of lower arm	631
992	Effect of heat/light	679	874	Open wound of neck	627
993	Effects of air pressure	680	893	Open wound of toe	637
990	Effects radiation NOS	679	879	Open wound site NEC	630
832	Elbow dislocation	605	880	Opn WND should/upper arm	630
871	Eyeball open wound	625	868	Oth intra-abdominal inj	624
930	FB external eye	650	998	Oth surgical comp NEC	694
936	FB in intestine & colon	653	854	Other brain injury	618
935	FB mouth/esoph/stomach	652	821	Other femoral fracture	594
933	FB pharynx & larynx	651	873	Other open wound of head	626
934	FB trachea/bronchus/lung	652	803	Other skull fracture	575
938	Foreign body GI NOS	653	822	Patella fracture	596
939	Foreign body GU tract	654	808	Pelvic fracture	580
937	Foreign body anus/rectum	653	867	Pelvic organ injury	624
931	Foreign body in ear	651	964	Pois-agent aff blood	664
932	Foreign body in nose	651	965	Pois-analgesic/antipyr	664
829	Fracture NOS	604	977	Pois-medicinal NEC/NOS	673
818	Fracture arm mult/NOS	590	979	Pois-oth vacc/biological	674
820	Fracture neck of femur	591	969	Pois-psychotropic agent	669
802	Fracture of face bones	573	976	Pois-skin/EENT agent	673
809	Fracture of trunk bones	581	974	Pois-water metab agent	672
826	Fracture phalanges, foot	603	972	Poison-CV agent	671
816	Fracture phalanges, hand	589	961	Poison-anti-infect NEC	662
819	Fx arms w rib/sternum	590	966	Poison-anticonvulsants	666
828	Fx legs w arm/rib	604	971	Poison-autonomic agent	670
825	Fx of tarsal/metatarsal	602	967	Poison-sedative/hypnotic	667
807	Fx rib/stern/lar/trach	578	960	Poisoning by antibiotics	662
863	GI tract injury	622	962	Poisoning by hormones	662
900	Head/neck vessel injury	638	968	Poisoning-CNS depressant	668
861	Heart & lung injury	621	970	Poisoning-CNS stimulants	670
812	Humerus fracture	582	973	Poisoning-GI agents	672
955	Inj PNS should/arm	659	978	Poisoning-bact vaccines	674
953	Inj nerve root/sp plexus	658	975	Poisoning-muscle agent	672
950	Inj optic nerv/pathways	657	963	Poisoning-systemic agent	663
956	Inj periph nerv pelv/leg	659	813	Radius & ulna fracture	585
959	Injury NEC/NOS	661	996	Replacement & graft comp	682
954	Injury oth trunk nerve	659	811	Scapula fracture	582
957	Injury to nerve NEC/NOS	660	831	Shoulder dislocation	605

Diagnosis Codes

Code	Description	Page	Code	Description	Page
801	Skull base fracture	572	V19	Fam hx-other conditions	703
800	Skull vault fracture	572	V16	Family hx-malignancy	702
952	Spinal cord inj w/o fx	658	V52	Fitting of prosthesis	718
865	Spleen injury	623	V67	Follow-up examination	727
848	Sprain & strain NEC	613	V70	General medical exam	728
841	Sprain elbow & forearm	609	V48	Head/neck/trunk problems	716
845	Sprain of ankle & foot	611	V20	Health supervision child	704
847	Sprain of back NEC/NOS	612	V60	Household circumstances	725
843	Sprain of hip & thigh	610	V12	Hx of disease NEC	701
844	Sprain of knee & leg	610	V14	Hx of drug allergy	702
846	Sprain sacroiliac region	612	V10	Hx of malignant neoplasm	700
840	Sprain shoulder & arm	608	V11	Hx of mental disorder	701
842	Sprain wrist & hand	609	V13	Hx of other diseases	701
918	Superf inj eye/adnexa	644	V09	Inf w drug-resistent org	700
912	Superf inj should/arm	642	V02	Infectious dis carrier	698
915	Superficial inj finger	643	V69	Lifestyle problems	728
917	Superficial inj foot/toe	644	V49	Limb problem/problem NEC	717
913	Superficial inj forearm	643	V39	Liveborn NOS	713
916	Superficial inj hip/leg	644	V40	Mental/behavioral pbx	714
914	Superficial inj of hand	643	V37	Mult birth NEC&NOS	713
919	Superficial inj oth site	645	V63	No med facility for care	726
910	Superficial injury head	642	V22	Normal pregnancy	704
911	Superficial injury trunk	642	V29	Obs-infnt suspected cond	707
997	Surg comp-body syst NEC	691	V71	Observation-suspect cond	729
901	Thor blood vessel inj	639	V43	Organ replacement NEC	715
823	Tibia & fibula fracture	596	V42	Organ transplant status	714
986	Tox eff carbon monoxide	677	V61	Oth family circumstances	725
989	Tox eff oth nonmed subst	678	V15	Oth hx of health hazards	702
987	Toxic eff gas/vapor NEC	677	V34	Oth mult birth, all LB	712
984	Toxic eff lead/compound	676	V36	Oth mult, LB&SB	713
988	Toxic eff noxious food	678	V35	Oth mult-mates stillborn	712
981	Toxic eff petroleum prod	675	V54	Oth orthopedic aftercare	719
983	Toxic effect caustics	676	V45	Oth postsurgical states	715
985	Toxic effect oth metals	677	V47	Oth probl w internal org	716
982	Toxic effect solvent NEC	676	V62	Oth psychosocial circum	725
853	Traum ICH NEC & NOS	617	V05	Oth vacc for singl dis	699
886	Traum amputation finger	633	V50	Other elective surgery	717
885	Traum amputation thumb	633	V46	Other machine dependence	716
860	Traum pneumohemothorax	619	V65	Other reason for consult	726
887	Traumatic amp arm/hand	634	V27	Outcome of delivery	707
896	Traumatic amp foot	638	V41	Pbx w special functions	714
897	Traumatic amputation leg	638	V24	Postpartum care/exam	705
895	Traumatic amputation toe	637	V64	Procedures not done	726
806	Vertebral fx w cord inj	577	V26	Procreative management	706
805	Vertebrl fx w/o cord inj	576	V07	Prophylactic measures	699
833	Wrist dislocation	605	V57	Rehabilitation procedure	721
			V77	Screen-endocr/nutr/metab	731
SUPPLEMENTARY CLASSIFICATION OF FACTORS			V81	Screen-heart/resp/GU dis	733
INFLUENCING HEALTH STATUS (V01-V82)			V80	Screen-neuro/eye/ear dis	732
			V75	Screen-oth infective dis	731
V53	Adjustment of oth device	718	V82	Screen-other conditions	733
V68	Administrative encounter	727	V78	Screening for blood dis	732
V51	Aftercare w plastic surg	717	V76	Screening mal neoplasm	731
V28	Antenatal screening	707	V73	Screening viral/chlamyd	730
V44	Artif opening status	715	V74	Screening-bacterial dis	730
V08	Asymptomatic HIV status	700	V79	Screening-mental disord	732
V55	Atten to artif opning	719	V30	Single liveborn	709
V01	Communicable dis contact	697	V72	Special examinations	730
V21	Constitut state in devel	704	V23	Supervis high-risk preg	705
V25	Contraceptive management	706	V33	Twin NOS	711
V66	Convalescence	727	V31	Twin, mate liveborn	710
V56	Dialysis encounter	721	V32	Twin, mate stillborn	711
V59	Donor	724	V06	Vac for dis combination	699
V58	Encounter px/aftrcr NEC	722	V03	Vacc for bacterial dis	698
V17	Fam hx-chr disabling dis	703	V04	Vacc for viral disease	698
V18	Fam hx-oth specific cond	703			

Procedure Codes

Procedure Codes

Procedure Codes

OPERATIONS ON THE HEMIC AND LYMPHATIC SYSTEM (40-41)

OPERATIONS ON THE DIGESTIVE SYSTEM (42-54)

Procedure Codes

Procedure Codes

Procedure Codes

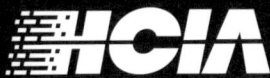
HCIA Inc.
300 East Lombard Street
Baltimore, MD 21202

The Comparative Performance of U.S. Hospitals: The Sourcebook

The Sourcebook features comprehensive information on the performance of the U.S. hospital industry for the latest five-year period. Included in the book are 52 key measures of hospital performance, with median and quartile values presented for more than 160 hospital comparison groups. Published with Deloitte & Touche every fall. $399*

The DRG Handbook: Comparative Clinical and Financial Standards

The Handbook focuses on key clinical and financial measures for the 50 highest volume Diagnosis-Related Groups (DRGs). For each DRG, *The Handbook* identifies the top 20 hospitals (based on volume of cases) and provides average charge and length of stay information for more than 90 hospital comparison groups. Includes all-payor data. Published with Ernst & Young every winter. $399*

The Guide to the Nursing Home Industry

The Guide presents aggregate financial operating performance data for more than 10,000 nursing homes. It provides an overview of each state's Medicaid and certificate of need programs, with median values presented for 19 key financial and operating indicators. Published with Arthur Andersen every summer. $249*

Profiles of U.S. Hospitals

This publication presents more than 30 key measures of financial, clinical, and operating performance for every U.S. hospital. Decile rankings for financial indicators such as profitability, leverage, and liquidity are also included. In addition, *Profiles of U.S. Hospitals* lists the number of cases, average charge, and average length of stay for each of the hospital's top five DRGs. Published every fall. $299*

Length of Stay Publications

Organized by individual ICD-9-CM codes or by DRGs, and broken down by diagnosis, operation, and payment source, *LOS* publications serve as a comprehensive guide to one of the most important issues in hospital care. The publications contain detailed patient and clinical data, including breakouts by age groups, single versus multiple diagnoses, and operated versus non-operated populations. Published every summer. Please call for prices.*

The Guide to the Managed Care Industry

A comprehensive listing of the nation's HMOs and PPOs, *The Guide* features enrollment information, names of key industry contacts, and an analysis of major industry trends. Published every fall. $245*

* Also available on magnetic tape and diskette. Please call for prices.

(continued on other side)

3 WAYS TO ORDER

❶ Call (800) 324-1746

❷ Fax Your Order to (410) 865-4321

❸ Return the Attached Order Cards

Essential Information for the Health Care Industry

Item	Qty.	Price	Total
❏ The Comparative Performance of U.S. Hospitals: The Sourcebook		$ 399	
❏ The DRG Handbook: Comparative Clinical and Financial Standards		399	
❏ The Guide to the Nursing Home Industry		249	
❏ Profiles of U.S. Hospitals		299	
❏ Length of Stay Publications		*call*	
❏ The Guide to the Managed Care Industry		245	
❏ 50 Top Outpatient Procedures: Benchmarks, Standards & Trends		245	
❏ The APG Handbook		295	
❏ Market Profiles for Medicare Risk Contracting: A Provider Perspective		310	

Subtotal _____

(AL, CA, CT, FL, GA, IL, KY, MA, MD, MI, NC, OH, RI, SC, TN, TX, UT, WA) Sales Tax _____

Shipping and Handling ___$7.95___

Total _____

❏ Enclosed is a check made payable to HCIA Inc. for $_____

❏ Please bill my: ❏ VISA ❏ MasterCard ❏ American Express

Account #_____ Expiration Date_____

Purchase Order #_____ Signature *(required)*_____

Name and Title_____

Company_____

Address_____
(cannot be delivered to a P.O. box)

City_____ State_____ Zip_____

Telephone_____ Fax_____

Target Selected Markets — With HCIA's Specialized Directories

Item	Qty.	Price	Total
❏ The Directory of Nursing Homes		$ 249	
❏ The Directory of Retirement Facilities		249	
❏ The Directory of Health Care Professionals		299	

Subtotal _____

(AL, CA, CT, FL, GA, IL, KY, MA, MD, MI, NC, OH, RI, SC, TN, TX, UT, WA) Sales Tax _____

Shipping and Handling ___$7.95___

Total _____

❏ Enclosed is a check made payable to HCIA Inc. for $_____

❏ Please bill my: ❏ VISA ❏ MasterCard ❏ American Express

Account #_____ Expiration Date_____

Purchase Order #_____ Signature *(required)*_____

Name and Title_____

Company_____

Address_____
(cannot be delivered to a P.O. box)

City_____ State_____ Zip_____

Telephone_____ Fax_____

HCIA Inc.
300 East Lombard Street
Baltimore, MD 21202

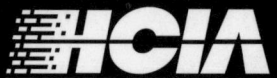

HCIA

Your Complete Resource For Health Care Information

3 WAYS TO ORDER

❶ Call (800) 324-1746

❷ Fax Your Order to (410) 865-4321

❸ Return the Attached Order Cards

NO POSTAGE
NECESSARY
IF MAILED
IN THE
UNITED STATES

BUSINESS REPLY MAIL

FIRST CLASS MAIL   PERMIT NO. 302   BALTIMORE, MD

POSTAGE WILL BE PAID BY ADDRESSEE

ATTN PUBLICATION SALES
HCIA INC
300 EAST LOMBARD ST
BALTIMORE MD 21298-6213

NO POSTAGE
NECESSARY
IF MAILED
IN THE
UNITED STATES

BUSINESS REPLY MAIL

FIRST CLASS MAIL   PERMIT NO. 302   BALTIMORE, MD

POSTAGE WILL BE PAID BY ADDRESSEE

ATTN PUBLICATION SALES
HCIA INC
300 EAST LOMBARD ST
BALTIMORE MD 21298-6213

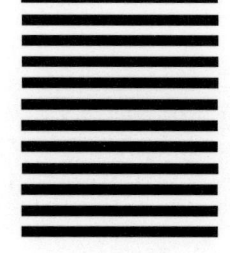

The APG Handbook

The APG Handbook is the complete guide to both the implementation and use of an APG system. Beginning with a detailed overview of the history and implementation requirements of APGs, *The Handbook* provides detailed information on APG Initial Classification Variable, Significant Surgical Procedures, and Medical and Ancillary APGs. $295*

Market Profiles for Medicare Risk Contracting: A Provider Perspective

Market Profiles presents charge, reimbursement, and utilization figures on the county level. Use it to investigate regional markets prior to negotiating a risk contract. Available in regional editions. $310*

50 Top Outpatient Procedures: Benchmarks, Standards & Trends

50 Top Outpatient Procedures provides a broad range of information on 50 of the most significant outpatient procedures. Reflective of the heavy growth in outpatient services, it is an excellent tool for analyzing ongoing shifts in use rates, charges, and reimbursement — by setting, patient demographics, or region. For each studied procedure, detailed information is broken down across hospital-based outpatient, physician office, ambulatory surgery center, and inpatient settings. $245*

HCIA DIRECTORIES

The Directory of Nursing Homes

This publication lists more than 16,000 licensed nursing homes across the U.S., alphabetically arranged by state and city. *The Directory* features addresses, contact names, service offerings, and ownership/management information. Published every winter. $249*

The Directory of Retirement Facilities

Profiles of more than 18,000 assisted living, congregate care, independent living, and continuing care facilities in the U.S. are featured. Conveniently catalogued by state and city, facilities are listed with addresses, contact names, number of residents, average monthly fees, social/recreational service offerings, ownership, and affiliation. Published every fall. $249*

The Directory of Health Care Professionals

The Directory is a comprehensive source of contact names arranged by hospital, system headquarters, and primary job function. More than 175,000 hospital professionals and 7,000 hospitals are listed in an easy-to-use format. Published every fall. $299*

* Also available on magnetic tape and diskette. Please call for prices.

Prices are subject to change without notice.

HCIA GUARANTEE

Books may be returned for a full refund if they are returned in good condition within 10 business days of receipt. Books damaged in shipping should be returned to HCIA within 5 business days for replacement. If you need to return a book, please contact HCIA Customer Service at (800) 568-3282 for return authorization. Diskettes and magnetic tapes are not returnable.